W9-DHY-439

Health & Wellness

TENTH EDITION

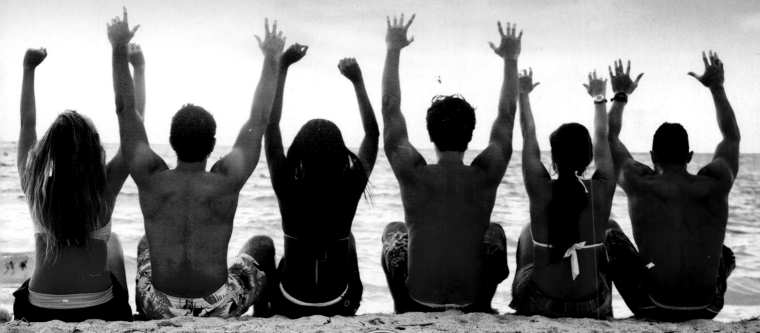

Gordon Edlin
John A. Burns School of Medicine
University of Hawaii at Manoa
Honolulu, Hawaii

Eric Golanty
Las Positas College
Livermore, California

JONES AND BARTLETT PUBLISHERS
Sudbury, Massachusetts
BOSTON   TORONTO   LONDON   SINGAPORE

World Headquarters

Jones and Bartlett Publishers
40 Tall Pine Drive
Sudbury, MA 01776
978-443-5000
info@jbpub.com
www.jbpub.com

Jones and Bartlett Publishers
 Canada
6339 Ormindale Way
Mississauga, ON L5V IJ2
Canada

Jones and Bartlett Publishers
 International
Barb House, Barb Mews
London W6 7PA
United Kingdom

Jones and Bartlett's books and products are available through most bookstores and online booksellers. To contact Jones and Bartlett Publishers directly, call 800-832-0034, fax 978-443-8000, or visit our website, www.jbpub.com.

Substantial discounts on bulk quantities of Jones and Bartlett's publications are available to corporations, professional associations, and other qualified organizations. For details and specific discount information, contact the special sales department at Jones and Bartlett via the above contact information or send an email to specialsales@jbpub.com.

Copyright © 2010 by Jones and Bartlett Publishers, LLC

All rights reserved. No part of the material protected by this copyright may be reproduced or utilized in any form, electronic or mechanical, including photocopying, recording, or by any information storage and retrieval system, without written permission from the copyright owner.

Production Credits
Chief Executive Officer: Clayton Jones
Chief Operating Officer: Don W. Jones, Jr.
President, Higher Education and Professional Publishing: Robert W. Holland, Jr.
V.P., Sales: William J. Kane
V.P., Design and Production: Anne Spencer
V.P., Manufacturing and Inventory Control: Therese Connell
Publisher, Higher Education: Cathleen Sether
Acquisitions Editor: Shoshanna Goldberg
Senior Associate Editor: Amy L. Bloom
Editorial Assistant: Kyle Hoover
Production Manager: Julie Champagne Bolduc
Production Assistant: Jessica Steele Newfell
Associate Marketing Manager: Jody Sullivan
Composition: Publishers' Design and Production Services, Inc.
Cover Design: Kristin E. Parker
Photo Research and Permissions Manager: Kimberly Potvin
Senior Photo Researcher and Photographer: Christine McKeen
Cover Image: © Andresr/ShutterStock, Inc. (main) and © Shanaka Wijesooriya/Dreamstime.com (top right)
Printing and Binding: Courier Kendallville
Cover Printing: Courier Kendallville

Library of Congress Cataloging-in-Publication Data
Edlin, Gordon, 1932–
    Health and wellness / Gordon Edlin, Eric Golanty—10th ed.
       p. ; cm.
    Includes bibliographical references and index.
    ISBN 978-0-7637-6593-4 (pbk. : alk. paper)
    1. Health.   2. Holistic medicine.   I. Golanty, Eric.   II. Title.
    [DNLM: 1. Holistic Health.   2. Health Behavior.   3. Life Style.   4. Mind-Body Relations (Metaphysics)
W 61 E23h 2010]
    RA776.E24   2010
    613—dc22

6048   2009020229

Printed in the United States of America
14 13 12 11 10   10 9 8 7 6 5 4 3 2

Brief Contents

Contents

Part 5 Explaining Drug Use and Abuse 361

Features

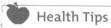 Health Tips

🧘 Managing Stress

☯ Wellness Guide

🌐 Global Wellness

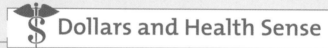

$ Dollars and Health Sense

Preface

Our goal in writing this textbook has always been to provide you with information to understand and implement the basic principles of physical, mental, and spiritual wellness. For the 10th edition, we have provided up-to-date tools, information, exercises, and humor to motivate you toward making healthy changes in your life and developing a lifestyle that will promote lifelong wellness. We believe that the major factors to living healthfully are the following:

- Being responsible for one's behaviors; for example, not smoking cigarettes or overusing alcohol and other drugs, maintaining healthy body weight, getting sufficient exercise, consuming nutritious foods rather than fast and junk foods, managing stress, and living in harmony within oneself.
- Contributing to the health of one's social and physical environments; for example, supporting laws that enhance the health and safety of children, ensuring safe food and medicines, and making the air, water, and land healthy and safe for everyone.
- Realizing that health and wellness encompass one's entire being—body, mind, spirit, and relationships with the environment—rather than the medical management of illness and the repair of diseased and broken body parts.

What does it mean to be healthy and well? Often, the answers students give to that question are eating right, not being sick, and being physically fit. But a holistic view of health encompasses many more of our behaviors. Answer the following questions and see if your opinion about your health changes:

- Are you able to cope with stress without getting angry, anxious, or depressed?
- Do you get enough sleep (at least eight hours a night)?
- Does your diet consist of several daily servings of fruit, vegetables, and whole grains or fast food, pizza, and ice cream?

- Do you exercise regularly?
- Do you take time to enjoy nature?
- If you drink, do you drink responsibly (e.g., you do not get drunk or drink and then drive)?
- If you are sexually active, do you use fertility control and practice safer sex?
- Are your interpersonal relationships satisfying?
- Are you involved in your community?
- Do you not smoke cigarettes?

We all engage in unhealthy behaviors from time to time, but you should know that these behaviors can be changed. Wellness is a process, not a place. We hope that this textbook will help you become aware of your unhealthy behaviors, and we hope that it can motivate you to change and give you some strategies for making changes. We want you to be healthy and well now and for the rest of your life.

We have developed a number of features to help you learn about health and wellness in this book.

Each chapter begins with a list of **Learning Objectives** to help you focus on the most important concepts in that chapter and a list of **Self-Assessment Activities** offered in the back of the book.

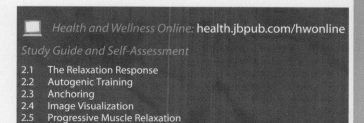

Health and Wellness Online: **health.jbpub.com/hwonline**

Study Guide and Self-Assessment

2.1	The Relaxation Response
2.2	Autogenic Training
2.3	Anchoring
2.4	Image Visualization
2.5	Progressive Muscle Relaxation
2.6	Quiet Time Exploration
2.7	The Power Write
2.8	Massage
2.9	Leaving It at the River

Key Terms are defined on or near the page on which they are introduced as well as in the glossary at the end of the book. For review, terms are available on the text's Web site (health.jbpub.com/hwonline) in the form of flashcards, crossword puzzles, and an interactive glossary.

Epigrams enliven each chapter with thought-provoking (and often humorous) quotations about health.

Health Tips in every chapter enable students to make immediate changes in their behavior.

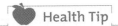

TERMS

communicable disease: an infectious disease that is usually transmitted from person to person

etiology: specific cause of disease

malaria: a disease of red blood cells that produces fever, anemia, and death

pathogen: a disease-causing organism

probiotic therapy: ingesting beneficial bacteria to help treat digestive disorders or other problems

vector: the carrier of infectious organisms from animals to people or from person to person

One of the major arguments for keeping marijuana illegal is that early use of marijuana leads to the use of other illegal drugs, the so-called gateway hypothesis. A number of scientific studies have addressed this question, but the results are conflicting and it still cannot be concluded that use of marijuana, especially by adolescents, inevitably leads to the use of other, more dangerous drugs (Maccoun, 2006).

> Insanity is doing the same thing over and over again and expecting a different outcome.
>
> *Albert Einstein*

Despite the confusions and caveats over the use of marijuana, as of 2008 12 states had legalized medical marijuana use: Alaska, California, Colorado, Hawaii, Maine, Montana, Nevada, New Mexico, Oregon, Rhode

🍎 Health Tip

Laughter Helps Heart Stay Healthier

In 1979, a well-known magazine editor, Norman Cousins, published a memoir called *Anatomy of an Illness*. In this book he described how he cured himself of a rare, untreatable disease called ankylosing spondylitis by watching humorous movies over an extended period of time. He became famous for advocating laughter as a cure for most serious diseases, including cancer and heart disease. Since his original account, scientists have been pursuing evidence that laughter heals. One of the best demonstrations that laughter is good for the heart comes from experiments in which volunteers were asked to watch "happy" or "sad" movies (Miller et al., 2006). After watching a happy, humorous movie, blood flow to the heart increased in 19 of 20 subjects. Conversely, after watching a sad, depressing move, blood flow to the heart decreased in 14 of the 20 subjects. Overall, blood flow levels to the heart changed by as much as 50 percent. Anyone at risk for heart disease should probably watch more comedies than war movies.

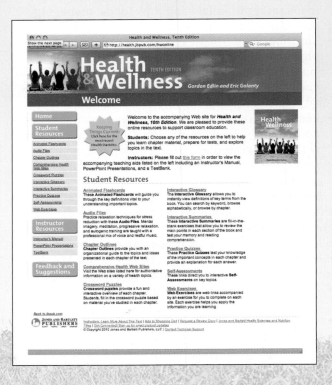

Current topics are highlighted in boxes to give a complete perspective in your study of health and wellness.

- **Global Wellness** boxes explore health and wellness topics as they affect different countries and cultures.
- **Wellness Guides** offer tips, techniques, and steps toward a healthy lifestyle and self-responsibility.
- **Managing Stress** boxes give you practical strategies for coping with stress.

- **Dollars and Health Sense** boxes focus on the influence of economic forces on individual and community health; for example, the marketing of worthless and sometimes dangerous supplements and devices for weight management, fitness, and stress relief, direct-to-consumer advertising in the marketing of minimally effective and sometimes dangerous pharmaceuticals, and cigarette advertising to encourage youth to start smoking.

 Global Wellness

Lactose Intolerance: A Mutation That Influenced Human Evolution

The sugar *lactose* is present in mother's milk and is the primary source of energy for all babies when breastfed. Digestion of the sugar lactose is accomplished by an enzyme—called *lactase*—that is present in the digestive system of all newborns. The gene for producing the enzyme that digests lactose is situated on chromosome 2, and almost all babies are born with this gene activated so that they can diges[t] milk. Very infrequently, a baby is bor[n] that causes a condition known as *ala[...]* cannot digest lactose in breast milk o[...] they are breast fed or given cow's mi[lk...] watery diarrhea, which can be life-thr[...]

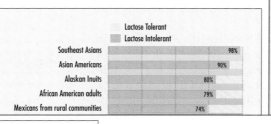

Lactose Tolerant
Lactose Intolerant

Southeast Asians	98%
Asian Americans	90%
Alaskan Inuits	80%
African American adults	79%
Mexicans from rural communities	74%

 Wellness Guide

Home Blood Pressure Monitors and Internet Consultations to Help Patients Reduce Hypertension

High blood pressure is the leading reversible risk factor for heart attacks and brain attacks. For people with high blood pressure, a 10-mm reduction in systolic blood pressure means a 30% to 40% reduced risk of dying from a heart attack or brain attack (Jones & Peterson, 2008). Despite effective therapies for reducing high blood pressure, efforts to do so are largely unsuccessful. Physicians who diagnose high blood pressure in patients usually recommend lifestyle changes if people smoke, are overweight, or do not exercise. Medications are also [...] effective in lowering blood pressure to

more acceptable levels. Yet, fewer than a third of patients with high blood pressure achieve goals for lower blood pressure. A new strategy is to supply patients with a home blood pressure monitor with which to take frequent measurements. They also are supplied with an Internet site where their progress is monitored and questions answered by a health professional. It is hoped that increased patient involvement with controlling their high blood pressure will increase the number of patients who successfully lower their blood pressure and thus their risk of cardiovascular disease.

 Managing Stress

Breaking Addictive Behaviors

It's a little known fact, but it was psychologist Carl Jung who inspired the Alcoholics Anonymous program. Frustrated with a client unable to change his alcoholism, Jung suggested that his only hope for recovery was to purposefully have a spiritual experience to rid himself of this addictive habit. So, Roland H. did just that. After conquering his addiction, he went on to share this experience with Edwin T., then Bill W., who then went on to co-found Alcoholics Anonymous.

In response to a letter from Bill W[...] craving for alcohol was the equivalen[t...] spiritual thirst of our being for whole[...] medieval language: the union with G[...] Latin is *spiritus*, and we use the same[...] religious experience as well as for the[...] poison. The helpful formula therefor[e...] *spiritum.*" (Spiritual crises require spir[...]

 Dollars and Health Sense

Junk Food Marketing and the Childhood Obesity Epidemic

Approximately 18% of American children between the ages of 6 and 19 are overweight, a tripling in prevalence since 1980 (see accompanying figure). Although a variety of social factors have been offered to explain it, a report from the United States Institute of Medicine (IOM), a division of the U.S. National Academy of Sciences, concludes that the marketing of high-calorie, low-nutrient "junk" food to kids is a major contributor to this disturbing trend (McGinnis et al., 2006).

The IOM report shows that 30% of the calories in an average child's diet come from sweets, salty snacks, fast food, and sodas, which together account for 10% of the average daily calories ingested. Beverage companies spend millions of dollars per year to market their products to youth via TV (American children see between 10 and 20 food-related TV

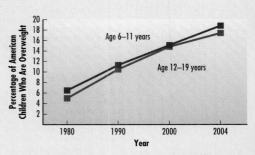

Prevalence of Overweight Among American Children, 1980–2004
Source: U.S. National Center for Health Statistics.

Chapters conclude with **Critical Thinking About Health**—a set of questions that present controversial or thought-provoking situations and ask you to examine your opinions and explore your biases.

End-of-chapter material includes **Health in Review**, a brief review of the chapter, **Health and Wellness Online**, a glimpse at the resources available on the Web, **References**, **Suggested Readings**, and **Recommended Web Sites** where you can find additional health information.

The text also includes appendixes on relaxation exercises and stress management techniques (including guides for yoga and t'ai chi).

A workbook has been included at the end of the text to provide you with self-assessments and activities to explore your own health.

We are pleased to provide the Health Statistics Web site as a new resource to accompany the *Tenth Edition* of *Health and Wellness*. The Web site was created to help instructors and students obtain statistical data on a variety of health issues including the morbidity, mortality, incidence, and prevalence of a particular health concern. The Web site is updated frequently.

Below are some examples of topics that are new to this edition or have been expanded upon from prior editions:

- Chapter 2 has been updated to include new information on the power of prayer; relaxation; and managing stress with music
- Chapter 4 includes new information on the biological roots of some mental illnesses
- Chapter 5 provides new information on vitamin D deficiency and food additives
- Chapter 6 contains a new "Dollars and Sense" health box on overweight children and new coverage of body dysmorphic disorder
- Chapter 7 includes an expanded discussion of the role of sedentary lifestyle and feasible ways to include physical activity in one's life, what constitutes physical activity, components of physical activity, flexibility, body composition, and physical activity and college students
- Chapter 12 has the latest information on bacteria and health; new vaccines including the HPV vaccine to prevent cervical cancer, the vaccines against herpes zoster and hepatitis E; updated information on preventing and treating asthma; and discussion of the 2009 "swine flu" pandemic
- Chapter 13 includes new information on lung cancer and curing childhood cancer

Critical Thinking About Health

1. Dr. Razmataz's book, *30 Days to Exceptional Mental Health*, had been on the best-seller charts for 10 weeks, but after his appearance on TV's *Inside This Week*, sales went through the roof. Entertainers, business executives, professional athletes, and political leaders extolled the value of his program to lessen needless worry, improve sleep, and enhance mood, self-esteem, memory, and mental acuity.

   Dr. Razmataz based his program on 10 years of research he conducted as director of the Ersatz Mental Health Clinic. In his book and his media appearances, Dr. Razmataz explained that the type and severity of a particular mental illness were caused by either the over- or underactivity of the genes that controlled the production of the six basic neurotransmitter chemicals in the brain. The key to his method was determining a patient's genetic profile and matching it to one of six specific organic food diets.

   Questions:
   a. What factors are mentioned in the description above that might suggest to someone that Dr. Razmataz's method is credible and efficacious?
   b. Which of these factors do you find influence you when you are making a health decision?
   c. What additional information, if any, would you want before trying Dr. Razmataz's method yourself or recommending it to someone else? How would you find such information?

2. List five characteristics of a mentally healthy person. If you were a parent, how would you ensure that your child(ren) grow(s) up to manifest the five characteristics on your list? Also discuss how individuals can contribute to the mental health of people in their community.

3. John hasn't liked being Margie's supervisor since her first day of work. She just doesn't get it. And because she's the boss's niece, there is little he can do. In the past six months, whenever Margie is on John's shift-team, his finds himself so distressed that he doesn't want to go to work.
   a. The chapter describes several ways to cope with emotional distress, including (1) changing the situation that is causing the distress, (2) altering the significance one places on the distressing situation, and (3) lessening the distressing emotions. Discuss how John could employ each of these coping strategies to lessen his emotional distress. Also, describe the consequences for John of implementing each coping strategy.
   b. When you experience emotional distress, which of the three coping strategies do you employ most often? Do you notice situations in which one coping strategy works better than others?

4. Many people equate mental and emotional well-being with happiness. If they feel happy, they identify themselves as emotionally well. In your opinion, what is the relationship of emotional well-being and happiness? How do unpleasant emotions, such as sadness, grief, shame, guilt, and anger, affect one's sense of emotional well-being? Would you argue that the path to mental and emotional well-being is the pursuit of happiness? If not, in your view, what constitutes the path to mental and emotional well-being?

Health in Review

- Mental health is when your mental functions produce a sense of optimism, vitality, and well-being, and when your intentional behaviors lead to productive activities (including healthy behaviors), fulfilling relationships with others, and the ability to adapt to change and to cope with adversity.
- Mental illness refers to alterations in thinking, emotions, and/or intentional behaviors that produce psychological distress and/or impaired functioning.
- Mental and emotional health depend on how well

- Emotional distress occurs when needs are not met. People cope with emotional distress by changing their modes of interaction with the environment, changing the importance of their unmet needs, or changing the distressing feelings.
- Positive thoughts and emotions, including beliefs in one's worth (self-esteem) and abilities (self-efficacy and agency), motivate people to engage in healthy behaviors and to avoid unhealthy ones.
- Optimism is associated with perceiving negative

- Chapter 14 provides new information on arterial fibrillation, the connection between laughter and heart health, and the connection between caffeine and hypertension
- Chapter 15 has added information on lactose intolerance and biomarkers for disease susceptibility
- Chapter 16 now explores pharmacogenetics and the legalization of marijuana use in some states
- Chapter 17 discusses the contribution of cigarette smoking to the global burden of disease and provides information on the Family Smoking Prevention and Tobacco Act
- Chapter 19 explores the growing popularity of having medical procedures done overseas and the medicalization of human traits and behaviors
- Chapter 22 discusses new herbal supplements being used to treat Alzheimer's; how exercise can slow aging; and anti-aging hormones
- Chapter 24 provides information on how air pollution in Beijing affected the summer Olympic Games; how to reduce one's carbon footprint; and health risks associated with different plastics used in the manufacture of water bottles

A Note of Thanks

Throughout all of the editions of *Health and Wellness*, many people have contributed support and guidance. This book has benefited greatly from their comments, opinions, thoughtful critiques, expert knowledge, and constructive suggestions. We are most appreciative for their participation in this project. We also want to thank our editors (past and present) and all of the people at Jones and Bartlett Publishers for their unflagging support of this textbook over the years.

Reviewers

Pat Alsader, Planned Parenthood of West Central Illinois
David Anspaugh, Memphis State University
Catherine G. Ansuini, Buffalo State College
Jennifer Austin, PhD, ATC, N.H. LAT, Colby-Sawyer College
Judy B. Baker, East Carolina University
N. K. Bhagavan, University of Hawaii Medical School
Barbara Brehm-Curtis, Smith College
Nancy J. Binkin, Centers for Disease Control and Prevention, Atlanta
David Birch, Indiana University
Donald Calitri, Eastern Kentucky University
Barbara Coombs, San Francisco City College
Linda Chaput, W. H. Freeman, New York
Dorothy Coltrin, De Anza College
Geoffrey Cooper, Harvard Medical School
Judy Drolet, Southern Illinois University at Carbondale
Philip Duryea, University of New Mexico

Seymour Eiseman, California State University–Northridge
Carol Ellison, Berkeley, California
Marianne Frauenknecht, Western Michigan University
Laura Fox Fudacz, Ivy Tech Community College of Indiana
Nicole Gegel, Illinois State University
Mai Goldsmith, Southern Illinois University at Edwardsville
Allan C. Henderson, California State University–Long Beach
Catherine M. Headley, Judson College
Sherry Hineman, University of California–San Diego
Leo Hollister, Stanford Medical Center
Stanley Inkelis, Harbor General Hospital
William Kane, University of New Mexico
Mark Kittleson, Southern Illinois University at Carbondale
Tim Knickelbein, Normandale Community College
Dawn Larsen, Mankato State University
Will Lotter, University of California, Davis
Beverly Saxton Mahoney, The Pennsylvania State University
Mary Martin, University of California–San Francisco
Sharon Mathis, Benedictine College
Patricia L. McDiarmid, EdD, Springfield College
Marion Micke, Illinois State University
Peter J. Morano, Central Connecticut State University
Richard P. Morris, Rollins College
Linda J. Mukina Felker, PhD, Edinboro University of Pennsylvania
Debra J. C. Murray, University of North Carolina at Chapel Hill
Anne Nadakavukaren, Illinois State University
Ann Neilson, PhD, College of Saint Rose
Marion Nestle, New York University
Roberta Ogletree, Southern Illinois University at Carbondale
Larry Olsen, The Pennsylvania State University
Elizabeth O'Neill, Central Connecticut State University
David Phelps, Oregon State University
Richard Plant, South Middlesex Community College
Bruce Ragon, Indiana University
Kerry J. Redican, Virginia Technical University
Dwayne Reed, Buck Center for Research in Aging
Janet Reis, University of Illinois at Urbana-Champaign
Russell E. Robinson, PhD, Shippensburg University
Brian Luke Seaward, University of Northern Colorado–Greeley
Sam Singer, University of California–Santa Cruz
Susan Spreecher, Illinois State University
Chris Stratford, RN, BS, EMT, University of Utah
David Stronk, California State University–Hayward
John Struthers, Planned Parenthood of Sacramento County
Michael Teague, University of Iowa
Amy Thompson, Mississippi State University

Eric Triffin, MPH, Southern Connecticut State University

Aleida Whittaker-Gordon, RD, MPH, MBA, California Polytechnic University–Pomona

Bryan Williams, University of Arkansas

Malinda Williams, MS, ACSM-HFI, NSCA-CPT*D, University of Oklahoma

Carol Wilson, University of Nevada at Las Vegas

Richard Wilson, Western Kentucky University

Acknowledgments

This book could not have been published without the efforts of the staff at Jones and Bartlett Publishers and the Health and Wellness team: Shoshanna Goldberg, Amy Bloom, Kyle Hoover, Julie Bolduc, Jess Newfell, and Christine McKeen. We would also like to thank Brian Luke Seaward, PhD, University of Northern Colorado–Greeley; James Walsh; Esther M. Weekes; Martin Schulz; Shae Bearden; Rocky Young; Bharti Temkin; Laura Jones-Swann, MEd, LCDC, Texas Tech University; and Scott O. Roberts, PhD, FAACVPR, Texas Tech University. To all we express our appreciation. A special thanks goes to Paul Wermager, Head, Science and Technology Reference Department, Hamilton Library, University of Hawaii at Manoa, for valuable research on health statistics.

Part One

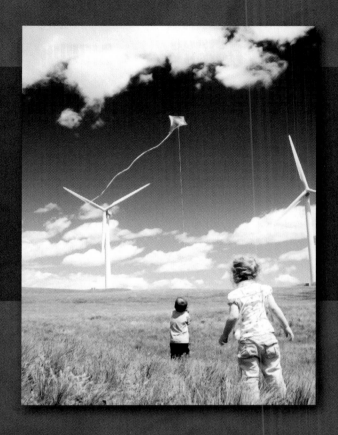

Achieving Wellness

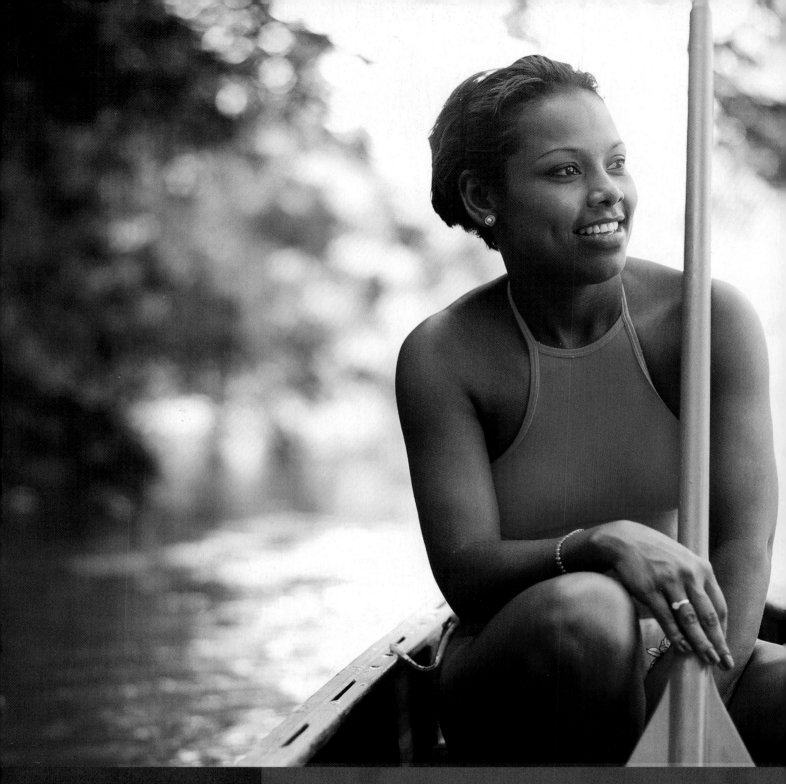

Chapter One

Achieving Personal Health

Learning Objectives

1. List the key points of the World Health Organization definition of health.

2. Describe the medical, environmental, and holistic models of health.

3. List and describe the six dimensions of wellness.

4. List the three health behaviors responsible for most of the actual causes of death.

5. Define lifestyle disease.

6. Identify the goals of Healthy People 2010.

7. List and describe the major health issues of college students.

8. Describe the Health Belief Model, Transtheoretical Model, and Theory of Reasoned Action/Theory of Planned Behavior.

Ask people what they mean by "being healthy" or "feeling well" and you probably will get a variety of answers. Most people usually think of health as the absence of disease. But what about someone who has a relatively harmless genetic disorder, such as an extra toe? Is this individual less healthy than a person with the usual number of toes? Different perhaps, but not necessarily less healthy. Are you less well when you are struggling with a personal problem than when you are out having fun? Finding an acceptable, generally useful definition of health or wellness is not a simple task.

> The health of a people is really the foundation upon which all their happiness and all their powers as a state depend.
>
> *Benjamin Disraeli*

It is true that not feeling sick is one important aspect of health. Just as important, however, is the idea that health is a sense of optimum well-being—a state of physical, mental, emotional, social, and spiritual wellness. Contained in this view is the idea that health can be obtained by living in harmony with yourself, with other people, and with your social and physical environments. You foster your own health and well-being when you take responsibility for avoiding harmful behaviors (e.g., not smoking cigarettes) and limiting your exposure to health risks (e.g., not drinking alcohol and driving; limiting the consumption of junk food), and by undertaking healthy behaviors and practices such as consuming nutritious food, exercising regularly, attending to your mental well-being, and supporting actions that contribute to the health and well-being of your community (e.g., replacing junk food with nutritious foods in schools).

Throughout this book, we show you ways to maximize your health by understanding how your mind and body function, how to limit exposure to pollution and toxic substances, how to make informed decisions about health and health care, how to be responsible for your actions and behaviors, and how social, economic, and political forces affect your ability to lead a healthy life. Learning to be responsible for the degree of health and vitality you want while you are young helps to ensure lifelong wellness and the capacity to cope with sickness when it does occur.

The Definition of Health

Health, like love or happiness, is a quality of life that is difficult to define and virtually impossible to measure. The World Health Organization (WHO) defines **health** as "a state of complete physical, mental, and social well-being and not merely the absence of disease and infirmity." This definition is so broad and covers so much that some people find it meaningless. Its universality, however, is exactly right. People's lives, and therefore their health, are affected by every aspect of life: environmental influences such as climate; the availability of nutritious food, comfortable shelter, clean air to breathe, and pure water to drink; and other people, including family, lovers, employers, coworkers, friends, and associates of various kinds.

The WHO definition of health takes into account not only the condition of your body but also the state of your mind. Your mental processes are perhaps the most important influences on your health, because they determine how you deal with your physical and social surroundings, what attitudes about life you have, and how you interact with others.

Health as the totality of a person's existence recognizes the interrelatedness of the physical, psychological, emotional, social, spiritual, and environmental factors that contribute to the overall quality of a person's life. All parts of the mind, body, and environment are interdependent.

Health is not static; it is a dynamic process that takes into account all the decisions we make daily, such as which foods we eat, the amount of exercise we get, whether we drink alcohol before driving, wear seat belts, or smoke cigarettes. Every choice we make potentially affects health and wellness. Sometimes the social and physical environments present obstacles to making healthful choices. For example, a person may know not to eat fatty, fast food every day, but this kind of food may be easier to obtain than healthier alternatives. Wellness includes recognizing that some social influences are not healthy and finding healthier alternatives. It also includes taking actions to make the social and physical environments healthier for all.

Health is not something suddenly achieved at a specific time, like getting a college degree. Rather, health is a *process*—indeed, a way of life—through which you develop and encourage every aspect of your body, mind, and spirit to interrelate harmoniously as much of the time as possible. Health means (1) being free from symptoms of disease and pain as much as possible; (2) being active, able to do what you want and what you must at the appropriate time; and (3) being in good spirits and feeling emotionally healthy most of the time.

Jesse Williams (1939), one of the founders of modern health education, described health as

> that condition of the individual that makes possible the highest enjoyment of life, the greatest constructive work, and that shows itself in the best service to the world. . . . Health as freedom from disease is a standard of mediocrity; health as a quality of life is a standard of inspiration and increasing achievement.

This is a goal we believe in, and the content of this book reflects this view.

Homeostasis and Health

Many of the vital functions in the body, such as breathing, heartbeat, blood circulation, digestion, and elimination, require no conscious effort. Rarely do you think about how often to breathe, or whether your heart needs to beat faster or slower. Your body has mechanisms for controlling and integrating its functions without conscious control, so that it maintains a relatively constant internal physiological environment. The tendency for body systems to interact and to maintain a constant physiological state is called **homeostasis.**

When you are well and healthy, your body systems function harmoniously. It is similar to the members of a team playing together in a coordinated way to accomplish the goals of the game. If one of your organs is not functioning properly, however, the other organs may not be able to function correctly either, and you may become ill. Thus, in Western medicine disease may be regarded as the disruption of homeostasis.

Many Asian philosophies embody an idea of mind–body harmony that is similar to the concept of homeostasis. This idea is based on a universal energy called **chi** *(qi),* which must be distributed harmoniously throughout the mind–body to attain and maintain health. Harmony is expressed as a balance of forces called *yin* and *yang* (**Figure 1.1**). Yin and yang represent the opposing and complementary aspects of the universal *chi* that is present in everything, including our bodies. Yang forces are characterized as light, positive, creative, full of movement, and having the nature of heaven. Yin forces are characterized as dark, negative, quiet, receptive, and having the nature of earth.

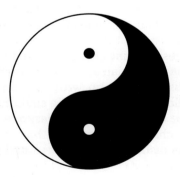

■ **Figure 1.1**

The Yin–Yang Symbol

This symbol represents the harmonious balance of forces in nature and in people. The white and dark dots show that there is always some yin in a person's yang component and vice versa. The goal in life and nature, according to the traditional Asian view, is to maintain a harmonious balance between yin and yang forces.

Traditional Asian medicine classifies the organs of the body as predominantly yin or yang. Hollow organs, such as the stomach, intestines, and bladder, are yang; solid organs, such as the heart, spleen, liver, and lungs, are yin. Food and herbs also are classified as having mostly yin or yang properties. When yin and yang forces are in balance in an individual, a state of harmony exists and the person experiences health and wellness. However, if either yin or yang forces come to predominate in a person, a state of disharmony is produced and disease may result.

In Asian philosophies and medicine, body and mind are regarded as inseparable. Yin and yang apply to both mental and physical processes. Treatment of disease involves the whole person and is designed to reestablish harmony of the mind and body. The balance of yin and yang forces must be restored so that health returns.

T'ai chi ch'uan and *qigong* (pronounced jê-kung) are two Chinese mind–body exercise techniques that are being practiced by more and more North Americans to help maintain health and harmony. These exercises are especially useful for older persons whose bodies can no longer tolerate vigorous exercise. People who practice *qigong* experience lower blood pressure, improved circulation, and enhanced immune system functions.

Models of Health

Scientists and health educators have developed three main ways to define health: (1) the medical model, (2) the environmental model, and (3) the wellness, or holistic, model. In this book, we discuss aspects of the major models of health wherever appropriate. The models themselves are abstractions of ideas, but in real life one needs to use whatever is practical to optimize health and well-being.

The Medical Model

The **medical model's** main tenet is that health is the absence of one or more of the "five Ds"—death, disease, discomfort, disability, and dissatisfaction. In other words,

---

TERMS

chi: a Chinese term referring to the balance of energy in the body

health: state of sound physical, mental, and social well-being

homeostasis: the tendency for body systems to interact in ways that maintain a constant physiological state

medical model: interprets health in terms of the absence of disease and disability if you are not sick, disabled, or clinically depressed, you are defined as healthy. The medical model relies almost exclusively on biological explanations of disease and illness and is interpreted in terms of malfunction of organs, cells, and other biological systems (e.g., liver disease, heart disease, or osteoporosis).

Within the medical model, the health of a population is measured in terms of **vital statistics,** which are data on the degree of illness (**morbidity**) and the numbers of deaths (**mortality**) in a given population. Vital statistics include the following:

> **Incidence:** the number of new cases of disease or illness during a particular time period, generally expressed per 100,000 population. Example: The annual incidence of chlamydia infection among U.S. college students is about 1,000/100,000.
>
> **Prevalence:** the total number of people in a community, country, or other group with a particular health status. Example: The prevalence of high blood pressure among U.S. adults is about 50 million.

These statistical measurements allow comparisons between populations and also within the same population over time.

The medical model tends not to deal with social problems that affect health and only with difficulty integrates mental and behavioral issues that do not derive from diseased organs. In the medical model, health is restored by curing a disease or by restoring function to a damaged body part. Because it rarely considers psychological and social factors in the cause, diagnosis, treatment, and prevention of illness and disease, the medical model is limited.

The reliance on biological interpretations of illness has contributed greatly to the success of the medical model. Anyone who has been cured of a serious infec-

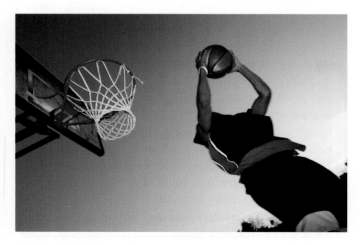

A healthy lifestyle depends on exercise.

tion by taking antibiotics or undergone a lifesaving surgical procedure can attest to that. On the other hand, that same reliance on biological thinking has not furthered understanding of health and illness in terms of psychological and social factors, nor has it been very successful in encouraging healthy lifestyles and reducing unhealthy behaviors.

For example, type 2 diabetes, which is now a worldwide pandemic, is caused by the excess consumption of high-fat, low-nutrient food and by modern lifestyles that lack most forms of physical activity. Walter Willett of the Harvard School of Public Health estimates that 92% of all type 2 diabetes cases could be avoided by changes in diet and lifestyle (Liebman, 2008). Rather than addressing personal living habits and social conditions, the response of the medical model to type 2 diabetes is to treat patients with drugs, surgery, or both to alter the biological aspects of the disease. In fact, surgically tying off most of the stomach in obese individuals is the fastest-growing surgical procedure in the United States. This surgery can lessen the symptoms of type 2 diabetes within days but does not resolve other dietary, lifestyle, and medical problems that persist.

The Environmental Model

The **environmental model** of health emerged with modern analyses of ecosystems and environmental risks to human health. In this model, health is defined in terms of the quality of a person's adaptation to the environment as conditions change. This model (**Figure 1.2**) includes the effects on personal health of socioeconomic status, education, and multiple environmental factors.

Unlike the medical model, which focuses on diseased organs and biological abnormalities, the environmental model focuses on conditions outside the individual that affect his or her health. These conditions include the quality of air and water, living conditions, access to nutritious food, exposure to harmful substances, socioeconomic conditions, social relationships, and the health care system.

In many respects the environmental model of health is similar to ancient Asian and Native American philosophies that associate health with harmonious interactions with fellow creatures and the environment. In particular, as the environment changes, one's interaction with it must change to remain in harmony. Illness is interpreted as disharmony of human and environmental interactions.

The Holistic Model

The holistic, or wellness, model defines health in terms of the whole person, not just in terms of diseased parts of the body or environmental condition. The **holistic model** encompasses the physiological, mental, emotional, social, spiritual, and environmental aspects of individuals and communities. It focuses on optimal

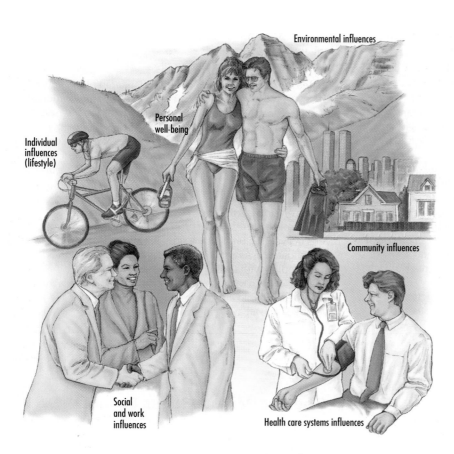

Environmental influences

Personal well-being

Individual influences (lifestyle)

Community influences

Social and work influences

Health care systems influences

■ **Figure 1.2**

Environmental Health Model
This model takes into account all environmental factors that interact with one another to affect health.

health, prevention of disease, and positive mental and emotional states.

The holistic model incorporates the idea of spiritual health, which is not considered in the medical model.

> You can observe a lot just by watching.
>
> *Yogi Berra*

Unlike the medical model, which assumes that a person who is not sick or not suffering from a disease is as healthy as possible, the holistic model proposes that health is a state of optimum or positive wellness.

The holistic model emphasizes the unity of the mind, spirit, and body. Therefore, symptoms of illness and disease may be viewed as an imbalance in a person's total state of being and not simply as the malfunction of a particular part of the body. Consider, for example, a common minor illness: the headache. About 80% to 90% of American adults experience at least one headache each year. Although a headache can be the result of brain injury or the symptom of another illness, more often it is caused by emotional stress that produces a tightening of the muscles in the head and neck. These contracting muscles increase the blood pressure in the head, thereby causing the pain of headache.

Most people try to relieve a headache by taking aspirin or some other analgesic drug that can alter the physiological mechanisms that produce the pain. In contrast, someone using the holistic approach would first try

to determine the *source* of the tensions—worry, anger, or frustration—and then work to reduce or eliminate the tensions. Similarly, an upset stomach cannot be regarded as simply the result of excessive secretion of stomach

TERMS

environmental model: modern analyses of ecosystems and environmental risks to health, such as socioeconomic status, education, and various environmental factors

holistic model: encompasses the physiological, mental, emotional, social, spiritual, and environmental aspects of health

incidence: the number of new cases of a particular disease

morbidity: the number of persons in a population who are ill

mortality: death rate; number of deaths per unit of population (e.g., per 100, 10,000, or 1,000,000) in a specific region, age range, or other group

prevalence: the number of people within a population with a particular disease

vital statistics: numerical data relating to birth, death, disease, marriage, and health

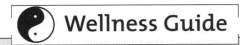

Wellness Guide

Oh, My Aching Head!

Headaches are one of the most common causes of human discomfort. Although headaches can be a symptom of a brain disease or injury, the vast majority of headaches are caused by anxiety, tension, and emotional distress.

Tension headache is the most common type of headache. It is caused by persistent contractions of the muscles in the neck and scalp, brought on by anxiety, stress, or allergic reactions to drugs and foods. Tension headaches may last for hours, may occur frequently, and may be a problem over the course of several years. The pain of a tension headache often can be relieved by experiencing a few minutes of deep mental relaxation or by massaging the tense muscles in the neck and scalp.

Migraine headache, or vascular headache, is characterized by throbbing pain that can last for hours and even days.

Migraine headaches are accompanied by altered blood flow to the brain's blood vessels. They are treatable with medications. Also, massaging the neck and scalp can help relieve the pain, as can mental relaxation and visualizing normal blood flow to the head. Autosuggestion and visualizing the hands becoming warmer may also help relieve pain, because some blood flow is diverted from the brain to the hands, thereby reducing blood pressure in the brain.

Identifying and eliminating the sources of tension and anxiety in your life is the surest way to prevent headaches. Some people have learned to use "having a headache" as a means of avoiding unpleasant situations, such as school or work obligations. As children they may have observed their parents coping with tension and stress by "getting a headache," and so they too learned that "having a headache" can be used to avoid anxiety-provoking experiences. Have you developed such an avoidance mechanism?

---

acid, requiring an antacid to bring relief. In many cases, the upset results from unexpressed hostility or fear. You are probably aware that such common events as taking an examination or having a dispute with someone can cause uncomfortable feelings in the stomach.

The holistic approach emphasizes self-healing, the maintenance of health, and the prevention of illness, rather than solely the treatment of symptoms and disease. A holistic approach integrates medical technology into a broader treatment that looks not only at a person's symptoms, but also at the sources of disharmony. From the holistic point of view, illness is the result of some imbalance in the harmonious interaction of the body, mind, and environment. Thus, to the extent that we can follow a program of positive wellness and create a healthy environment, we can be free of disease.

Some of the great advances in medicine have resulted from considering illness solely in terms of the affected body organ. Indeed, devoting medical attention to one specific ailing part of the body is sometimes the most efficient way to treat a medical problem, which is why we have specialists who are experts in treating diseases of different body parts, such as heart specialists, gastrointestinal specialists, gynecologists, and so on.

Some health professionals have criticized those who advocate holistic health practices and holistic medicine, arguing that the concepts and methods are antiscientific and hence harmful. Holistic medicine is not antiscientific. By encouraging individuals to take personal command of their health, including how they use medical services, holistic health practices are likely to be less harmful than some modern medical practices, such as unnecessary surgery (see Chapter 19).

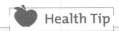 Health Tip

The Two-Minute Stress Reducer

Stressed out?
Be still.
          And take a
                D
                 E
                  E
                   P
                     Breath.

Center Yourself
Focus your attention inward. Allow thoughts, ideas, and sensations to pass through your mind without reacting to any of them. You will notice them pass out of your mind, only to be replaced by new thoughts and sensations. Continue to breathe deeply and slowly and watch the passing of the thoughts that stress you.

Empty Your Mind
Acknowledge that you have preconceived ideas and ingrained habits of perceiving. Know that you can empty your mind of distressing thoughts and replace them with ones that create inner harmony.

Ground Yourself
Feel the sensation of your body touching the earth. Place your feet (or your bottom if you are sitting, or your entire body if you are lying down) firmly on the earth. Let your awareness come to your point of contact with the earth, and feel gravity connecting you to Mother Earth and stabilizing you.

Connect
Allow yourself to feel your physical and spiritual connection with all living things. Remind yourself that with every breath you are reestablishing your connection with all of nature.

🧘 Managing Stress

Harmony and Peace

Many Native American cultures and tribes incorporate the idea of harmonious interactions with nature, animals, and other people in their religions.

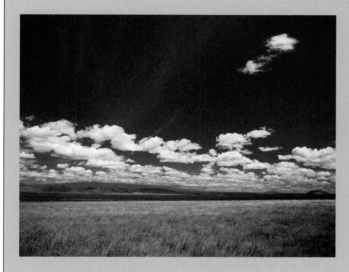

The first peace,
which is the most important,
is that which comes from
within the souls of men when they
realize their relationship,
their oneness, with the universe
and all its powers,
and when they realize that
at the center of the universe dwells
Wakan-Tanka, and that
this center is really everywhere,
it is within each of us.
This is the real peace, and the others are
but reflections of this.
The second peace is that which is
made between two individuals,
and the third is that
which is made between two nations.
But above all you should
understand that there can never be peace
between nations until there is
first known that true peace which . . .
is within the souls of men.

Black Elk
The Sacred Pipe

Source: From *The Sacred Pipe: Black Elk's Account of the Seven Rites of the Oglala Sioux,* by Joseph Epes Brown. Copyright © 1953, 1989 by the University of Oklahoma Press.

Holistic health is not incompatible with the practice of conventional medicine. Rather, it emphasizes a view that has gained wide acceptance among members of the medical community—that each person has the capacity and the responsibility for optimizing his or her sense of well-being, for self-healing, and for the creation of conditions and feelings that help prevent disease. Holistic health is hardly a revolutionary idea; the Old English root of our word *health* (*hal,* meaning sound or whole) implies that there is more to health than freedom from sickness.

Dimensions of Health and Wellness

Because wellness is dynamic and continuous, no dimension of wellness functions in isolation. When you have a high level of wellness or optimal health, all dimensions are integrated and functioning together. The person's environment (including work, school, family, community) and his or her physical, emotional, intellectual, occupational, spiritual, and social dimensions of wellness are in tune with one another to produce harmony.

However, health is more than a matter of individual choices. Family and other social relationships also influence a person's health. If a spouse has a serious illness, the chances that the marital partner will acquire a serious illness doubles (Strobe et al., 2007). If a couple has a child with a serious illness, the strain on the family can be enormous. Marital partners may ignore the well-being of other children, fight, and even divorce. Research suggests that as much as 25% of a person's health is a direct consequence of family interactions.

Health educators commonly refer to six dimensions of health and wellness: emotional, intellectual, spiritual, occupational, social, and physical:

- **Emotional wellness** requires understanding emotions and coping with problems that arise in everyday life.
- **Intellectual wellness** involves having a mind open to new ideas and concepts. If you are intellectually healthy, you seek new experiences and challenges.

TERMS

emotional wellness: understanding emotions and knowing how to cope with problems that arise in everyday life, and how to manage stress

intellectual wellness: having a mind open to new ideas and concepts

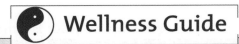

Wellness Guide

Whole-Person Wellness

A person with emotional wellness is able to
- Maintain a sense of humor
- Recognize feelings and appropriately express them
- Strive to meet emotional needs
- Take responsibility for his or her behavior

A person with intellectual wellness is able to
- Communicate effectively in speaking and in writing
- See more than one side of an issue
- Keep abreast of global issues
- Exhibit good time-management skills

A person with spiritual wellness is able to
- Examine personal values and beliefs
- Search for meanings that help explain the purpose of life
- Have a clear understanding of right and wrong
- Appreciate natural forces in the universe

A person with occupational wellness is able to
- Feel a sense of accomplishment in his or her work
- Balance work and other aspects of life
- Find satisfaction in being creative and innovative
- Seek challenges at work

A person with social wellness is able to
- Develop positive relationships with loved ones
- Develop relationships with friends
- Enjoy being with others
- Effectively communicate with others who may be different

A person with physical wellness is able to
- Exercise regularly and select a well-balanced diet
- Participate in safe, responsible sexual behavior
- Make informed choices about medicinal use and medical care
- Maintain a positive, health-promoting lifestyle

- **Spiritual wellness** is the state of harmony with yourself and others. It is the ability to balance inner needs with the demands of the rest of the world.
- **Occupational wellness** is being able to enjoy what you are doing to earn a living and contribute to society, whether it be going to college or working as a secretary, doctor, construction manager, or accountant. In a job, it means having skills such as critical thinking, problem solving, and communicating well.
- **Social wellness** refers to the ability to perform social roles effectively, comfortably, and without harming others.
- **Physical wellness** is a healthy body maintained by eating right, exercising regularly, avoiding harmful habits, making informed and responsible decisions about health, seeking medical care when needed, and participating in activities that help prevent illness.

Taking Responsibility for Your Health

Not so many years ago, people were subject to a variety of diseases over which they had little or no control. In the early part of the twentieth century, infectious diseases caused by organisms were the leading causes of death in the United States. Modern public health methods and modern drugs, such as antibiotics, were not available. In 1918, millions of people around the world died from influenza, the cause of which was unknown at that time, but is now known to be caused by a virus.

Today, the leading causes of illness and death in the United States and much of the industrialized world are not due to infections, but to "lifestyle diseases" (**Table 1.1**). These diseases, such as heart disease and cancer, mostly result from people's behaviors and the ways in which they live. The idea that lifestyle is a major cause of disease and death in modern societies is not new. A generation ago, Lewis Thomas (1978), an eminent physician and author, observed that our lifestyles were killing us.

> The new theory is that most of today's human illnesses, the infectious ones aside, are multifactoral in nature, caused by two great arrays of causative mechanisms: the influence of things in the environment; and one's personal lifestyle. For medicine to become effective in dealing with such disease, it has become common belief that the environment will have to be changed, and personal ways of living also have to be transformed, and radically.

Unfortunately, in the years since Dr. Thomas's pronouncement, the radical transformation he envisioned has yet to occur as pollution and unhealthy lifestyles continue to cause health problems. Continued massive burning of fossil fuels has ushered in global warming (see Chapter 24), heart disease is still the top cause of death, cigarette smoking is still increasing worldwide, and the prevalence of overweight and type 2 diabetes is increasing rapidly (see Chapter 6).

Heart disease results primarily from today's lifestyles, which include overweight (see Chapter 6), cigarette smoking (see Chapter 17), lack of exercise (see Chapter 7), high levels of stress (see Chapter 3), and high blood pressure and high levels of blood cholesterol (see Chapter 14). Cancer is associated with both nutritional (see Chapter 5) and environmental factors (see Chapter 13). Poor nutrition, smoking cigarettes, and exposure to haz-

Table 1.1

Ten Leading Causes of Death for All Ages, All Races, and Both Sexes, 1900, 1987, and 2002

1900	1987	2005
1. Tuberculosis	Heart disease	Heart disease
2. Pneumonia	Cancer	Cancer
3. Diarrhea and enteritis	Stroke	Stroke
4. Heart disease	Injuries	Chronic lower respiratory disease
5. Liver disease	Bronchitis and emphysema	Accidents
6. Injuries	Pneumonia and influenza	Diabetes
7. Stroke	Diabetes	Alzheimer's disease
8. Cancer	Suicide	Pneumonia and influenza
9. Bronchitis	Chronic liver disease	Kidney diseases
10. Diphtheria	Arteriosclerosis	Septicemia

Source: National Center for Health Statistics.

ardous substances in the environment initiate biological changes that can result in cancer. An unhealthy lifestyle is also at the root of some instances of suicide and homicide (alcohol, drugs, and stress), accidents (alcohol use and stress), and cirrhosis of the liver (alcohol abuse).

A major characteristic of many lifestyle diseases is that they are **chronic diseases** that persist for years or life. Chronic diseases lower the quality of life of the affected person and usually shorten the life span. A chronic disease also tend's to affect a patient's family and is costly to the health care system (DeVol & Bedroussian, 2007; U.S. Centers for Disease Control and Prevention, 2008).

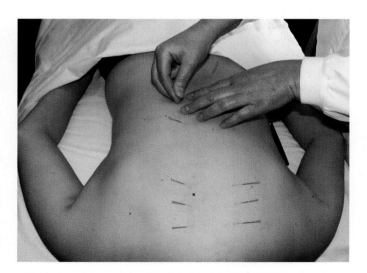

Many alternative medical practices, such as chiropractic, massage, and acupuncture, are now considered legitimate medical treatments and are often covered by insurance.

Lifestyle and Health

When a person dies, the cause of death is generally identified in terms of the organ system(s) that failed and resulted in the person's death, for example, heart disease, cirrhosis of the liver, cancer of the lung. This may not, however, identify the root causes of that death. For example, saying someone died of lung cancer does not tell us that the *actual* cause of death was smoking. When deaths are examined for their actual causes and not simply what is reported on death certificates, the results show that approximately *half* of the 2.4 million deaths in the United States each year are due to lifestyle factors (**Figure 1.3**) and, by extension, that many, many deaths could be prevented if people lived more healthfully.

Leading the list of life-shortening behaviors is tobacco use, which is responsible for more than 435,000 American deaths per year. Smoking cigarettes and

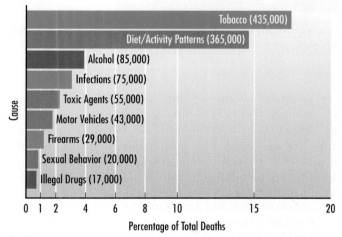

■ **Figure 1.3**

Number of Preventable Deaths in the United States in 2000
Estimates are from data including actual numbers (firearm deaths) and calculated risks (tobacco deaths). More than 1 million deaths are caused by lifestyles and behaviors—all preventable deaths.

Source: Data from A. H. Mokdad, et al. (2004). Actual causes of death in the United States, 2000. *Journal of the American Medical Association, 291*, 1238–1243.

TERMS

chronic disease: a disease that persists for years or even a lifetime

occupational wellness: enjoyment of what you are doing to earn a living and contribute to society

physical wellness: maintenance of your body in good condition by eating right, exercising regularly, avoiding harmful habits, and making informed, responsible decisions about your health

social wellness: ability to perform social roles effectively, comfortably, and without harming others

spiritual wellness: state of balance and harmony with yourself and others

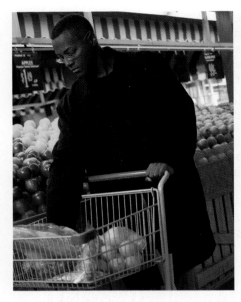
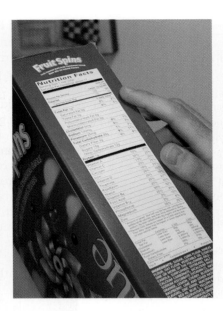
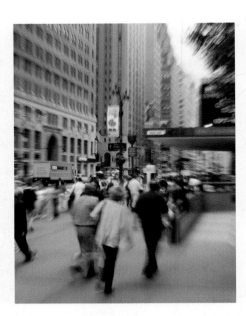

Simple behaviors in our everyday lives can positively affect health: Eat five servings of fruits and vegetables every day, read food labels to make wise choices, and walk instead of drive whenever possible.

cigars, chewing tobacco, and being exposed to second-hand smoke contribute substantially to deaths caused by cancer of all kinds, heart disease, high blood pressure, stroke, bronchitis, chronic obstructive pulmonary disease (COPD), pneumonia, low birth weight, and burns from fires. The enormous toll on life and health exacted by tobacco use is the reason that health agencies, doctors, and governments overwhelmingly recommend limiting tobacco use (see Chapter 17).

Next to tobacco use, unhealthy diet and activity patterns contribute the most to death in the United States. Consumption of high levels of cholesterol and saturated fat in foods is associated with heart disease, several types of cancer, and stroke. High-calorie consumption coupled with low levels of physical activity predisposes people to overweight, diabetes, and high blood pressure. A sedentary lifestyle is responsible for 23% of deaths from the leading chronic diseases (heart disease, high blood pressure, stroke, and diabetes).

Alcohol abuse accounts for nearly 85,000 deaths each year from alcohol toxicity, motor vehicle and other types of accidents, and homicides. In contrast, only 20,000 deaths annually are attributable to the use of illegal drugs. Unsafe sex and injection drug use contribute to thousands of new cases of AIDS each year. Transmission of hepatitis B and C viruses results in thousands of cases of liver disease. Overuse of antibiotics has produced bacterial strains that are resistant to antibiotics, resulting in infections that are difficult to treat.

Environmental factors also cause fatalities. For example, exposure to toxic agents in the workplace and elsewhere accounts for more than 50,000 deaths per year. Firearms used in homicides, suicides, and accidental shootings are responsible for 29,000 deaths. Motor vehicle accidents cause nearly 43,000 deaths. Lack of access to medical care—which affects the 47 million American families who have no health insurance—contributes to thousands of deaths each year as well.

Type 2 Diabetes as a Lifestyle Disease

Diabetes is a disease in which the amount of sugar in the blood increases to unhealthy levels as a result of malfunctions in the body's sugar-regulating system. Diabetes can cause blindness, blood vessel problems, kidney failure, heart damage, and death. There are two forms of diabetes:

Type 1 (insulin-dependent). The pancreas (a digestive organ) is diseased and is unable to manufacture the hormone insulin, which regulates the level of sugar in the blood. Medical treatment involves frequent injections of insulin.

Type 2 (non-insulin-dependent). Too much fat in the blood (generally from being overweight) causes body cells to resist the actions of insulin (*insulin resistance*). This causes blood levels of sugar to rise. Over time, insulin-producing cells in the pancreas become damaged and produce less insulin. Treatment includes increasing exercise, decreasing the consumption of calories to produce weight (fat) loss, and possibly injections of insulin or drugs that decrease insulin resistance.

Evidence that type 2 diabetes is a disease of lifestyle comes from studies of populations that have dramatically altered their lifestyle over a brief time span. For

$ Dollars and Health Sense

Large Corporations Profit from Products That Make People Sick

Heart disease, stroke, lung cancer, colon cancer, type 2 diabetes, and chronic obstructive pulmonary disease account for nearly half of all deaths in the United States. These diseases are caused in large part by unhealthy lifestyle choices: eating poorly, smoking cigarettes, being overweight, and not exercising. Unfortunately, many large corporations profit from individuals' unhealthy lifestyles—indeed, some encourage unhealthy behavior as the basis of their business.

The tobacco industry is the prime example of companies profiting financially from harming others. No other industry makes a product that, when used as directed, causes disease and death. In the late 1990s, the major tobacco companies were sued by the federal government, state governments, and individuals for lying to the public for nearly 50 years about the addictive properties of their products and the harm that tobacco use causes. Knowing that long-term smokers (i.e., their best customers) tend to begin smoking as teens, the tobacco industry uses sophisticated marketing methods to lure young people to smoke and to get them hooked. The tobacco industry is a friend to no one.

Whereas it is not as obvious as with tobacco, some food companies—particularly fast-food companies—also profit from harming their customers. A typical serving of fast food (e.g., burger, fries, and a soft drink or shake) contains around 1,000 calories. Approximately one-third to one-half of those calories are from fat, a prime contributor to heart and blood vessel disease. Fast food also contains large amounts of cholesterol and salt, which also contribute to heart and blood vessel disease. Studies show that the blood vessels of young people who consume typical fast foods show the beginning stages of blood vessel disease, with the degree of damage proportional to the amount of fast food consumed. Moreover, the calories in a typical serving of fast food provide about half or more of most individuals' energy requirement for one day. This is why a steady diet of fast food can lead to weight problems and associated illnesses like type 2 diabetes.

Some fast-food companies have been legally challenged for causing disease. But you need not wait for legal challenges to be a healthy person. You can become aware that in some instances the quest for corporate profits is based on encouraging people to adopt unhealthy living habits, and you can choose a healthier way to live.

---

example, Yemenite Jews who emigrated to Israel in 1949 had one of the lowest rates of type 2 diabetes in the world—less than 1 case per 1,000 individuals. Thirty years later, the same population, now adapted to a Western lifestyle in Israel, had a rate of almost 12 cases of type 2 diabetes per 1,000 individuals.

Another example is the prevalence of type 2 diabetes among the Pima Indians of the southwestern United States. Traditionally, these Native Americans lived mostly on maize, beans, wild game, and vegetables. They were active, lean, and strong. Today many Pima Indians are sedentary, obese, and have the highest rate of diabetes in the world. As a result of their changed lifestyle, nearly 40% of Pima Indians suffer from diabetes. That the prevalence of type 2 diabetes among Pima Indians living in Mexico is approximately 6% indicates that the disease is determined mostly by environmental circumstances and not by genetics (Schulz et al., 2006).

Type 2 diabetes is an increasingly prevalent lifestyle disease. Currently, about 23.6 million Americans are affected and millions more have prediabetes, a risk factor for developing diabetes in 10 years. Diabetes is strongly associated with being overweight: For every 20% increase in weight gain, the chance of diabetes doubles. As a consequence of the epidemic of overweight and obesity in the United States, diabetes has become a

major health problem. For Americans born in 2000, the average lifetime risk of developing diabetes is 32.8% for men and 38.5% for women (Narayan et al., 2003). Hispanics have the highest risk (men, 45%; women, 52%). The consequences of developing diabetes in midlife are substantial. For example, if diagnosed with diabetes at age 40, men will die 11.6 years prematurely and women will die 14.3 years prematurely.

Diabetes is a problem not only in the United States but also around the world. In 2000, the global number of people with diabetes was about 171 million (2.5% of the world's population). In 2007, it was estimated that 246 million people worldwide had diabetes (about 7.3% of the world's population). In the years to come, as less developed countries develop economically and their populations adopt the dietary and physical activity patterns of the most developed countries, by the year 2025 the number of people with diabetes is expected to increase to 366 million (World Health Organization, 2008).

Research has conclusively shown that eating healthfully and regularly engaging in a moderate physical activity can reverse and prevent type 2 diabetes (Schwarz et al., 2008). The 2005 revision of its Food Guide Pyramid reflects the U.S. government's efforts to help people alter their lifestyles to reduce overweight and the risk of type 2 diabetes (see Chapter 5). Everyone is encouraged to learn more about healthy eating and the value of moderate physical activity.

Whereas each individual is responsible for her or his lifestyle decisions, scientists and health professionals know that many lifestyle diseases, including type 2 diabetes, require community-wide efforts to help individuals make healthy choices (Vinicor, 2005). For example, institutions can insist that vending machines contain healthy foods instead of junk food. Stairwells can be made visually attractive and have music or video to encourage walking instead of riding elevators. Municipalities can ensure that subdivisions have sidewalks and many parks. Rather than being at a centralized location, food service can be located at the periphery of large institutions to encourage walking.

Many health insurers and employers have begun to offer financial incentives to employees to make healthy changes in their lifestyles. Some companies give employees time off to exercise during work hours and financial rewards for losing weight. Some companies also penalize and even fire employees who violate no-smoking rules. In a 2008 poll, 91% of American employers believed that they could reduce their health care costs by getting employees to adopt healthier lifestyles (Mello & Rosenthal, 2008).

Nearsightedness

Another dramatic example of how modern lifestyles affect health concerns vision. Many children and a majority of adults in modern societies wear glasses or contact lenses to correct for nearsightedness (myopia). When our ancestors had to forage and hunt for food, acute vision was probably essential to survival and, of course, corrective lenses were unknown. During early development, a child's eye adapts to the visual information the eyes receive from the environment. Looking at distant objects tends to produce normal vision or eyes that are slightly farsighted. Today, almost all children watch TV and computer screens for many hours a day and also read books, magazines, and newspapers—all of which require close-up vision. These activities tend to cause myopia in many children.

The influence of modern lifestyles on vision was documented by measuring the vision of young people in rural China compared with the vision of Chinese students in Hong Kong (Wallman, 1994). Most of the young people in the rural environment had normal vision or were slightly farsighted (**Figure 1.4**). In contrast, most of the Chinese students in Hong Kong were nearsighted, many to a considerable degree. Thus, if one considers 20/20 vision desirable, our modern lifestyle, which involves much close-up vision, is likely to affect eye development and may produce myopia. Until we understand more about the environmental and genetic cues that affect visual development, children should be encouraged to spend time outdoors, where their eyes are more likely to focus on distant objects.

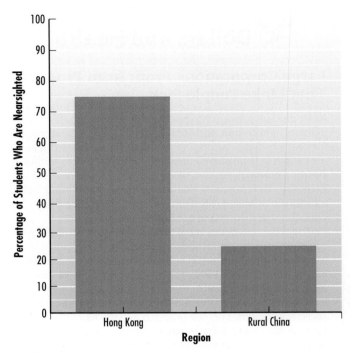

■ **Figure 1.4**

Comparison of visual acuity of 18- to 28-year-old students in Hong Kong with youths in rural areas of China. Most of the rural youths have normal vision, whereas most of the Hong Kong students are myopic.

Source: Data from J. Wallman (1994). Nature and nurture of myopia. *Nature, 371,* 201–202.

Healthy People 2010

Periodically, the U.S. government issues health objectives for the nation, the latest of which is Healthy People 2010 (Office of Disease Prevention and Health Promotion, 2000). The main goals of Healthy People 2010 are (1) to help individuals of all ages live longer and improve their quality of life, and (2) to eliminate health disparities among segments of the U.S. population, including differences by gender, race or ethnicity, education or income, disability, geographic location, or sexual orientation.

To foster the health of the diverse American population, Healthy People 2010 recognizes that families, schools, worksites, communities, states, and national organizations must help individuals live healthfully. This means that not only are individuals asked to make healthy lifestyle choices based on sound health knowledge, but also that communities strive to provide quality education, housing, and transportation; health-promoting social and physical environments; and access to quality medical care. For example, informing

> The only way to keep your health is to eat what you don't want, drink what you don't like, and do what you'd rather not.
>
> *Mark Twain*

1. Access to Quality Health Service
2. Arthritis, Osteoporosis, and Chronic Back Conditions
3. Cancer
4. Chronic Kidney Disease
5. Diabetes
6. Disability and Secondary Conditions
7. Educational and Community-Based Programs
8. Environmental Health
9. Family Planning and Sexual Health
10. Food Safety
11. Health Communication
12. Heart Disease and Stroke
13. HIV
14. Immunizations and Infectious Diseases
15. Injury and Violence Prevention
16. Maternal, Infant, and Child Health
17. Medical Product Safety
18. Mental Health and Mental Disorders
19. Nutrition
20. Occupational Safety and Health
21. Oral Health
22. Physical Activity and Fitness
23. Public Health Infrastructure
24. Respiratory Diseases
25. Sexually Transmitted Diseases
26. Substance Abuse
27. Tobacco Use
28. Vision and Hearing

■ **Figure 1.5**

Focus Areas for Healthy People 2010

1. **Healthy Weight.** Percentage of the population with a body mass index that is no more than 20% lower and no more than 20% higher than that recommended for age and gender
2. **Physical Activity.** Percentage of the population regularly participating in exercise that offers significant cardiovascular benefits.
3. **Immunization.** Percentage of the adult, teenage, and childhood population that is up-to-date for the currently recommended immunization schedule.
4. **Teen Smoking.** Prevalence of any use of tobacco products among youth up to age 17.
5. **Substance Abuse.** Percentage of youth aged 12–17 that used alcohol or illicit drugs during the previous 12 months.
6. **Mental Health.** Percentage of the population with diagnosed clinical depression or severe depressive symptoms.
7. **Preventable Injury Deaths.** Percentage of preventable deaths attributed to injuries.
8. **Clean Air and Water.** Percentage of the population living in areas where air and water quality meet or exceed federal standards.
9. **Access to Health Care.** Percentage of the population with health insurance and/or a regular source of medical care.
10. **Social Environment.** Percentage of the population with household incomes less than 100% of the federal poverty limit or percentage of the population aged 18–24 that has completed high school.

■ **Figure 1.6**

Healthy People 2010 Leading Health Indicators

people that it is healthy to consume five servings of fresh fruits and vegetables each day is insufficient if their community does not have stores or other sources of healthy food. Also, advising people to walk more is insufficient if their communities are not safe or lack parks or sidewalks.

Healthy People 2010 consists of 467 specific health objectives grouped into 28 focus areas (**Figure 1.5**) each with a specific goal. Examples of specific goals are the following:

- *Cancer:* reduce the number of new cancer cases as well as the illness, disability, and death caused by cancer.
- *Disability and Secondary Conditions:* promote the health of people with disabilities, prevent secondary conditions, and eliminate disparities between people with and without disabilities in the U.S. population.
- *Food Safety:* reduce foodborne illnesses.

Several of the goals in Healthy People 2010 are grouped into 10 categories, called **Leading Health Indicators,** which reflect the major health concerns in the United States (**Figure 1.6**). The Leading Health Indicators are intended to help everyone more easily understand the overall health of the U.S. population and the most important changes required to improve individual health and the health of families and communities. Each of the indicators depends to some extent on the following factors:

- The information people have about their health and how to make improvements
- Choices people make (behavioral factors)

▌TERMS▐

Leading Health Indicators: ten categories of health goals that represent the major public health concerns in the United States

Table 1.2

Some Health Goals with Prevalence in Year 2000 and Goals for 2010 in Healthy Campus 2010

Health goal	Year 2000 data	Year 2010 goal
Increase the proportion of college students with health insurance.	83.3%	100%
Increase the proportion of college students receiving information from their institution on each of 11 priority health risk behavior areas.*	3.1%	17.4%
Increase the proportion of females at risk of unintended pregnancy (and their partners) who use contraception.	95.1%	100%
Reduce unintentional pregnancies among college women.	25.3%	17.5%
Increase the proportion of sexually active women/men who used condoms at last intercourse.	40/46.8%	60/60%
Increase use of safety belts.	69.5%	94%
Decrease the proportion of college students who have been in an emotionally abusive relationship (per 1,000).	124	93.9
Reduce the annual rate of rape or attempted rape (per 1,000).	34.6	23.3
Reduce sexual assault/unwanted sexual touching other than rape (per 1,000).	96	56.4
Reduce physical assaults (per 1,000).	37	21.3
Reduce the proportion of college students who report that they drove after drinking any alcohol at all during the previous 30 days.	30.9%	15.3%
Reduce the proportion of college students engaging in high-risk (binge) drinking of alcoholic beverages during the past two weeks.	39%	20%
Reduce tobacco use by college students.	25.1%	10.5%
Reduce the rate of suicide attempts by adolescents and college students (12-month average rate).	1.5%	0.53%
Increase the proportion of adults and college students who are at a healthy weight. Healthy weight is defined as a body mass index [BMI] equal to or greater than 18.5 and less than 25.	66.8%	75%
Increase the proportion of college students who consume at least five daily servings of fruit and vegetables.	7.4%	25.5%
Increase the proportion of adults and college students who use the oral health care system each year.	77%	92%
Increase the proportion of college students who engage in physical activity at least three days per week that includes moderate physical activity for at least 30 minutes, or vigorous physical activity for 20 or more minutes per occasion.	40.3%	55%

*Eleven priority health risk behaviors: tobacco use, alcohol use, sexual assault/relationship violence, violence prevention, injury prevention and safety, suicide prevention, pregnancy prevention, HIV/AIDS prevention, STD prevention, dietary behaviors and nutrition, physical activity and fitness.

Source: Modified from American College Health Association. (2002). *Healthy Campus 2010*. Baltimore, MD: American College Health Association.

- Where and how people live (environmental, economic, and social conditions)
- The type, amount, and quality of health care people receive (access to health care and characteristics of the health care system)

The Leading Health Indicators illuminate what each person can do individually and within the home, communities, school, and worksite to promote the health of everyone.

Applying the goals and strategies of Healthy People 2010 to American colleges and universities has resulted in identifying 167 health goals, some of which are listed in Table 1.2.

Health Issues of College Students

About 16 million people attend U.S. colleges and universities. About half are "traditional" students, those who enrolled in college directly from high school; others are "nontraditional students," those who enrolled in college after having devoted months or years to working, military service, traveling, and/or raising a family. Some health issues, such as time pressures and academic and financial stress, can affect students of any age (Table 1.3). Other health issues, such as the risk of acquiring a sexually transmitted disease (STD), may be more pertinent to students within a certain age group. Some typical health issues for college students include the following:

Mental health. Students are exposed to a variety of stressors and pressures that can impair their mental health. Academic overload, tests, and competition can create feelings of insecurity, anxiety, inferiority, and depression. Traditional students may be lonely and have difficulty adjusting to early adulthood. Nontraditional students may feel isolated and without social support. Stress can impair sleep and lead to depression.

Table 1.3

Health Impediments to Academic Performance Reported by American College Students

Health issue	Percentage reporting
Stress	33
Cold/flu/sore throat	25
Sleep difficulties	26
Concern about family/friend	18
Relationship difficulties	16
Depression/anxiety	16
Internet use/games	15
Sinus infection	9
Death of friend/family member	10
Alcohol use	6

Source: Modified from American College Health Association—National College Health Assessment. (2007). Nearly 20,000 students were asked "Within the last school year, have any of the following affected your academic performance?" Available: http://www.acha.org/projects_programs/assessment.cfm.

Food and weight. Time pressures and the easy availability of junk food cause many to consume lots of sugar (candy, sodas) and fat (fast food) and insufficient amounts of fruits and vegetables. Students may use food as a way to cope with stress and uncomfortable emotions. Many students are overly concerned about their body size and shape to meet social expectations of attractiveness, causing some to develop eating disorders. Because more than half of North American adults are overweight, weight control is an issue for many students.

Health care. A large proportion of U.S. college students has limited access to health care because their colleges do not have comprehensive services and they are without health insurance.

Substance use and abuse. Many students use tobacco, alcohol, and other drugs to cope with stress and unpleasant feelings or to fit in socially. Alcohol abuse is related to sexual assault and date rape, unintended pregnancies (from not using contraceptives properly or at all), and acquiring an STD (from not practicing safer sex).

Sexual and relationship health. Sexually active students of any age are at risk for acquiring an STD, becoming unintentionally pregnant, or becoming involved in sexual assault, especially acquaintance or date rape. Sexual activity to relieve academic stress, increase self-esteem, gain peer acceptance, or relieve loneliness can be mentally and spiritually damaging. Married students may find that the time and energy demands of college work create stress in their marital relationships.

Accidents and injuries. Many students commute to school, often rushing to and from work and home, and hence are at risk for automobile accidents.

Alcohol-using students are at risk for auto and other kinds of accidents. Athletically active students are at risk for sports injuries.

Also, a variety of environmental and social forces present barriers to healthful living. For example, someone may want to become more physically active to manage weight and reduce the risks of heart disease and cancer. However, that person may live in a car-dependent community where work, school, and services are located miles away and where there are no sidewalks, bike lanes, or nearby parks.

Making Healthy Changes

A major assumption of health education is that nearly everyone has a basic desire to be healthy and well, but that many people acquire habits of thought and behavior that may make them less well rather than more. One goal of health education, therefore, is to provide knowledge and information to people so they can develop healthful attitudes and skills. With healthful attitudes and skills, it is reasoned, people will adopt healthy behaviors because they naturally want to do what is best for themselves.

> If you find yourself in a hole, stop digging.
> *Will Rogers*

It is said that knowledge is power, but with regard to living healthfully, that isn't always the case. Almost everyone knows that smoking cigarettes, driving after drinking alcohol, and eating junk food are unhealthy, but many people do those things anyway. Simply knowing what to do is no guarantee that a person will do it. One reason for this is that an unhealthy attitude or behavior is rewarding in some way, even if it is harmful in some other way (for example, smoking cigarettes to relieve stress). To change a health behavior, a person must believe that the benefits of change outweigh the costs and that she or he is capable of making the desired change. Rituals such as New Year's resolutions and slogans such as "just do it" offer unrealistic models of how habits are changed. Desire and willpower alone are insufficient; research, planning, and enlisting social support are required as well. Following are three models that describe the process of health behavior change.

The Health Belief Model

The Health Belief Model (HBM) was originally developed as a systematic method to explain and predict preventive health behavior, but it has been revised to include general health motivation for the purpose of distinguishing illness and sick-role behavior from healthy behavior. Key aspects of the model are described as follows:

- **Perceived susceptibility.** Each individual has his or her own perception of the likelihood of experiencing

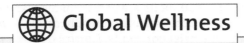

Global Wellness

Chronic Diseases in Rich and Poor Countries—the Causes Differ

Chronic diseases are the leading causes of death throughout the world. Besides causing death, chronic diseases reduce the quality of life of affected individuals, often for many years. In 2005, four chronic diseases—heart disease, cancer, respiratory disease, and type 2 diabetes—accounted for 35 million deaths worldwide (World Health Organization, 2005). By 2025, the number of deaths worldwide from those four chronic diseases is expected to increase to nearly 50 million annually.

In economically developed countries, such as Japan, the United States, Australia, and most of Europe, nearly 50% of the chronic disease burden is associated with five risk factors: tobacco use, high blood pressure, alcohol use, high cholesterol, and overweight (Table 1.4). On the other hand, in the least economically developed countries, deaths from chronic disease result from different risk factors: underweight, unsafe sex (causing HIV/AIDS), unsafe water and sanitation, and indoor smoke from cooking. As poor countries develop economically, the risk factors for chronic disease resemble those of developed countries.

Recognizing that heart disease, cancer, respiratory disease, and type 2 diabetes are largely preventable, international health organizations are searching for ways to stem the rising tide of chronic disease in developing countries. Not only is there a desire to offer people an improved quality of life, but

also there is the recognition that economic development is slowed or stalled when a country carries a large burden of disease. The more a poor country's meager financial resources are used to deal with an increasing number of people with chronic diseases, the less money there is to build schools, roads, electricity generating plants, and other infrastructure. To the degree that disease retards economic advancement, it contributes to poverty and its discontents, including terrorism born of frustration.

To reduce the burden of chronic disease in developing countries, individuals must be encouraged and taught how to live more healthfully. Moreover, governments will need to regulate transnational economic activities that can negatively affect the public health. For example, to limit the damage caused by tobacco smoking, in 2003, the World Health Organization sponsored the Framework Treaty on Tobacco Control, agreed to by 168 countries, which includes a comprehensive ban on all tobacco advertising, promotion, and sponsorship, elimination of illicit trade in tobacco products, banning of tobacco sales to and by minors, agricultural diversification and the promotion of alternative livelihoods, and an increase in taxes on tobacco products to discourage consumption. Similar efforts will be required to limit consumption of sugar, fat, and cholesterol and thereby reduce the burdens of heart disease, high blood pressure, type 2 diabetes, and overweight (Yach et al., 2004).

Table 1.4

Percentage of Deaths from Chronic Disease Risk Factors in Developed and Developing Countries

Risk factor	Developed countries (1.4 billion people)	Developing countries (2.4 billion people)	Least developed countries (2.3 billion people)
Tobacco use	12.2	4.0	2.0
High blood pressure	10.9	5.0	2.5
Alcohol use	9.2	6.2	***
High cholesterol	7.6	2.1	1.9
Overweight	7.4	2.7	***
Low fruit and vegetable consumption	3.9	1.9	***
Physical inactivity	3.3	***	***
Underweight	***	3.1	14.9
Unsafe water, sanitation, hygiene	***	1.7	5.5
Unsafe sex	10.2	***	0.8
Indoor smoke	***	1.9	3.9

Developed countries include the United States, Japan, and Australia.

Developing countries include China, Brazil, and Thailand.

Least developed countries include India, Mali, and Nigeria.

***Indicates a low percentage of deaths.

Source: Adapted from D. Yach et al. (2004). The global burden of chronic diseases. *Journal of the American Medical Association, 291,* 2616–2622.

a condition that would adversely affect his or her health. Individuals vary widely in their perception of susceptibility to a disease or condition. Those at one end deny the possibility of contracting an adverse condition. Individuals in the middle admit to a statistical possibility of disease susceptibility. Individuals at the high end of susceptibility feel there is real danger that they will experience an adverse condition or contract a given disease.

- **Perceived seriousness.** Perceived seriousness refers to the beliefs a person holds concerning the effects of a given disease or condition on his or her state of affairs. These effects can be considered from the point of view of the differences that a disease would create—for instance, pain and discomfort, loss of work time, financial burdens, difficulties with family, problems with relationships, and susceptibility to future conditions. It is important to include these emotional and financial burdens when considering the seriousness of a disease or condition.
- **Perceived benefits of taking action.** Taking action toward the prevention of disease or toward dealing with an illness is the next step after an individual has accepted the susceptibility to a disease and recognized its seriousness. The action a person chooses will be influenced by his or her beliefs regarding the benefits of the action.
- **Barriers to taking action.** Action may not take place even though an individual may believe that the benefits to taking action are significant. This may be because of barriers, which can include inconvenience, cost, unpleasantness, pain, or upset. These characteristics may lead a person away from taking the desired action.
- **Cues to action.** An individual's perception of the levels of susceptibility and seriousness provides the force to act. Benefits, minus barriers, provide the path of action. However, "cues to action" may be required for the desired behavior to occur. These cues to action may be internal or external.

The Transtheoretical Model

One of the most influential models of health behavior change is the Transtheoretical Model, or Process of Change Model (Prochaska, DiClemente, & Norcross, 1992). This model recognizes that change occurs through the following stages:

- **Precontemplation.** The person is not considering changing a particular behavior any time in the foreseeable future. Many individuals in this stage are unaware or underaware of their problems. Information is important during this stage.
- **Contemplation.** The person becomes aware that change is desirable but has not committed to act. The person often focuses on why it would be difficult to change. Information on options on how to change the behavior can be helpful during this stage.
- **Preparation.** The person desires change and commits to making that change in the near future, usually within the next 30 days. Instead of thinking why he or she can't take action, the focus is on what can be done to begin. The person creates a realistic plan for making a change, including overcoming obstacles. This stage may include announcing the change to friends and family, researching how to make the change, making a calendar, or setting up a diary or journal to record progress and obstacles to progress.
- **Action.** The person implements the plan. The old behavior and the environmental situations that reinforced that behavior are stopped and new behaviors and environmental supports are adopted. Obstacles are expected and noted, and strategies for overcoming them are implemented. Progress through this stage may take six months or more.
- **Maintenance.** The person strengthens the change, recognizing that lapses and even temptations to give up will occur. "Ebb and flow" are to be expected and are not to be seen as failures. The person can remind himself or herself of the many benefits of and gains from the behavior change to help combat relapse.
- **Termination.** The person is not tempted to return to the previous behavior.

The Theory of Reasoned Action/Theory of Planned Behavior

The Theory of Reasoned Action/Theory of Planned Behavior posits that changing a health behavior begins with an intention to adopt a new behavior (e.g., stop smoking). The intention is a combination of a positive attitude about performing the behavior (e.g., "not smoking is good") and the person's thoughts about how others will respond to the behavior (e.g., "my girlfriend will be happy if I stop"). Furthermore, change is affected by the person's perceptions of how much control the person has over successfully bringing about the desired change (e.g., "I can do this if I get some support").

It Starts with You

Being healthy and well starts with you. The medical care system—doctors and other medical providers, pharmaceutical companies, hospitals, clinics, insurance companies, and to some degree the government—can help you when you are sick. However, only you can make life goals to be healthy and well; to take responsibility for the ways that your thoughts, feelings, and behaviors affect your life; to care for rather than harm yourself; and to choose to learn and adopt health-promoting behaviors, and contribute to the development and maintenance of a health-promoting culture.

Scientists at the University of California at Berkeley undertook a multiyear study to determine, among other things, behaviors that contribute to health and longevity. Their findings include the following:

- No smoking
- Getting seven to eight hours of sleep per night
- Maintaining body weight not less than 10% and not more than 30% of recommended for height and body frame
- Regular exercise
- Little or no alcohol consumption
- Eating breakfast regularly
- Little between-meal snacking

Much research shows that people could do more to maintain and improve their health. For example, data from the U.S. Centers for Disease Control and Prevention Behavioral Risk Surveillance System show that less than 50% of American adults practice one of four basic health behaviors—not smoking, maintaining a healthy body weight, eating five servings of fruits and vegetables per day, and getting regular exercise—and only 3% practice all four (**Table 1.5**) (Reeves & Rafferty, 2005). The coronary arteries of young adults with one or more of these risk factors—smoking, high cholesterol, high blood pressure, and overweight—show damage in blood vessels consistent with developing heart disease (McMahan et al., 2006).

It is clear from many kinds of health research that each one of us needs to do more to maintain and improve our health. When one is young, thinking about health is the last thing one is interested in doing. We (the authors) certainly did not worry about our health when we were teenagers or even in college. Moreover, 50 years ago, eating as much meat as you could afford, smoking cigarettes, and getting drunk were generally accepted behaviors. When you are 20 years old, thinking about being 60 or 70 years old is unimaginable. Unlike 50 years ago, we now know that protecting health is something that has to begin while you are young. Making

Table 1.5

Prevalence of Health Lifestyle Characteristics, by Age

Age (years)	Nonsmoking	Healthy weight	Fruits and vegetables	Regular physical activity
18–24	69.9%	57.5%	22.0%	26.8%
25–34	74.2%	44.2%	19.8%	21.5%
35–44	73.7%	38.5%	21.5%	20.1%
45–54	80.5%	32.0%	26.5%	22.6%

Source: Modified from M. J. Reeves & A. P. Rafferty. (2005). Healthy lifestyle characteristics among adults in the United States, 2000. *Archives of Internal Medicine, 165,* 854–857.

lifestyle changes when you already are old (and presumably wiser) is mostly too late.

Health is similar to retirement: It is something you have to plan for and pay attention to while you are young. For example, putting away just a few dollars every month adds up to an enormous sum in 50 years, but most of us never think about doing it. The same holds true for health. Making small, positive changes in your health and lifestyle now will pay enormous dividends in the future.

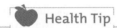 Health Tip

Reduce Stress When Sitting in Front of a Computer

If you sit at a computer for more than 30 minutes at a time, remember to stand up and stretch the muscles of your neck, shoulders, and back. Do stretches for at least 5 minutes to avoid headaches, fatigue, and muscle cramps. Studies show that virtually everyone raises and hunches their shoulders as soon as they sit down at a computer. About one-third start breathing shallowly. The American Institute of Stress recommends practicing slow, deep breathing while using a computer.

Critical Thinking About Health

1. As pointed out in this chapter, the major health issues of college students are sexual health, mental health, substance abuse, weight, accidents and injuries, and health care. Discuss which of these issues is of most concern to you personally. Explain your reasons and worries. How can you deal with your concerns in a way that will improve your health?

2. Describe one lifestyle behavior you routinely engage in that you regard as harmful to your health (smoking, for example). Discuss your reasons for continuing to engage in this unhealthy behavior. Consider what you might do to change this behavior and list the steps you would take to accomplish the healthy change. Do you believe that you can make the healthy change?

3. What is the significance to American society of the data in Figure 1.3?

4. Imagine that you are the Surgeon General of the United States, who formulates national health policy. (A former surgeon general, C. Everett Koop, formulated the crusade against tobacco smoking a generation ago.) Describe what you believe is the primary health problem in the United States today. Justify your choice with as many facts as you can find. Describe the steps you believe should be taken by government, private companies, organizations, and individuals to eradicate this health problem.

Health in Review

- Health is not only the absence of disease but also is living in harmony with oneself, friends and relatives, and the social and physical environments.
- Health means being responsible for preventing personal illness and injuries as well as knowing when to seek medical help.
- Three models used to describe health are medical, environmental, and holistic, or wellness.
- A holistic approach to health emphasizes prevention of disease and injury and self-responsibility for nutrition, exercise, and other aspects of lifestyle that promote wellness.
- The dimensions of wellness are emotional, intellectual, spiritual, occupational, social, and physical.
- Many illnesses (e.g., diabetes, heart disease, cancer) are "lifestyle diseases," that is, primarily attributable to unhealthy living habits. Taking responsibility for your health while you are young is the best way to reduce the risk of chronic disease later in life.
- Unhealthy lifestyles and behaviors are responsible for half of all deaths in the United States each year.
- Healthy People 2010 is a set of national health objectives characterized by enhancing the quality of life, reducing the incidence of preventable diseases and premature deaths, and reducing disparity in health status among different demographic groups.
- Changing health behaviors requires knowledge, planning, and social support.

Health and Wellness Online

The Web contains a wealth of information about health and wellness. By accessing the Internet using Web browser software, you can gain a new perspective on many topics presented in *Health and Wellness*, Tenth Edition. Access the Jones and Bartlett Publishers Web site at **health.jbpub.com/hwonline.**

References

DeVol, R., & Bedroussian, A. (2007). An unhealthy America: The economic burden of chronic disease. Milken Institute. Retrieved May 5, 2008, from http://www.milkeninstitute.org/publications/publications.taf?function=detail&ID=38801018&cat=ResRep

Liebman, B. (2008, September). Diabetes. *Nutrition Action Health Letter*, 1–7.

McMahan, C. A., et al. (2006). Pathobiological determinants of atherosclerosis in youth risk scores are associated with early and advanced atherosclerosis. *Pediatrics, 118*, 1447–1455.

Mello, M. M., & Rosenthal, M. B. (2008). Wellness programs and lifestyle discrimination: The legal limits. *New England Journal of Medicine, 359*, 192–199.

Mokdad, A. H., et al. (2004). Actual causes of death in the United States. *Journal of the American Medical Association, 291*, 1238–1245.

Narayan, K. M. V., et al. (2003). Lifetime risk for diabetes mellitus in the United States. *Journal of the American Medical Association, 290*, 1884–1890.

Office of Disease Prevention and Health Promotion, U.S. Department of Health and Human Services. (2000). Healthy People 2010. Retrieved February 8, 2006, from www.healthypeople.gov

Prochaska, J. O., DiClemente, C. C., & Norcross, J. C. (1992). In search of how people change. *American Psychologist, 47*, 1102–1104.

Reeves, M. J., & Rafferty, A. P. (2005). Healthy lifestyle characteristics among adults in the United States, 2000. *Archives of Internal Medicine, 165*, 854–857.

Schulz, L. O., et al. (2006). Effects of traditional and Western environments on prevalence of type 2 diabetes in Pima Indians in Mexico and the U.S. *Diabetes Care, 29*, 1866–1871.

Schwarz, P. E., et al. (2008). The European perspective on type 2 diabetes prevention. *Experimental and Clinical Endocrinology and Diabetes, 116*, 167–172.

Strobe, M., et al. (2007). Health outcomes of bereavement. *Lancet, 370*, 1960–1973.

Thomas, L. (1978). On magic and medicine. *New England Journal of Medicine, 299*, 461–463.

U.S. Centers for Disease Control and Prevention. (2008). Costs of chronic disease. Retrieved May 5, 2008, from http://www.cdc.gov/nccdphp/overview.htm#2

Vinicor, F. (2005). Primary prevention of type 2 diabetes: Are we there yet? *Johns Hopkins Advanced Studies in Medicine, 5*, 260–261.

Wallman, J. (1994). Nature and nurture of myopia. *Nature, 371*, 201–202.

Williams, J. F. (1939). *Personal hygiene applied.* Philadelphia: W. B. Saunders.

World Health Organization. (2005). *Preventing chronic diseases.* Retrieved May 2, 2008, from http://www.who.int/chp/chronic_disease_report/contents/en/index.html

World Health Organization. (2008). Prevalence of diabetes worldwide. Retrieved May 2, 2008, from http://www.who.int/diabetes/facts/world_figures/en/

Yach, D., et al. (2004). The global burden of chronic diseases. *Journal of the American Medical Association, 291*, 2616–2622.

Suggested Readings

Barondess, J. A. (2005). On the preservation of health. *Journal of the American Medical Association, 294,* 3024–3026. Presents the idea that health is best maintained by adopting healthy living habits early in life and practicing them consistently as one grows older.

Breslow, L. (1999). From disease prevention to health promotion. *Journal of the American Medical Association, 281,* 1030–1033. Discusses why health promotion is more important than disease prevention.

Cohen, J. T., et al. (2008). Does preventive care save money? *New England Journal of Medicine, 358,* 661–663. Quantifies the costs savings of many preventive health measures (e.g., smoking relapse, screening all 65-year-olds for diabetes).

Fraser, G. F., & Shavlik, D. J. (2001). Ten years of life. *Archives of Internal Medicine, 161,* 1645–1652. An investigative study of Seventh-Day Adventists concludes that making lifestyle changes regarding exercise, diet, and weight does result in extension of life expectancy.

King, D. E., et al. (2007). Turning back the clock: Adopting a healthy lifestyle in middle age. *American Journal of Medicine, 120,* 598–603. Shows that middle aged Americans who newly adopt four healthy behaviors (consuming five or more servings of fruits and vegetables per day, exercising regularly, maintaining a normal body weight, and not smoking cigarettes) are healthier and live longer than those who do not.

Mokdad, A. H., et al. (2004). Actual causes of death in the United States. *Journal of the American Medical Association, 291,* 1238–1245. Demonstrates how lifestyle contributes to nearly 50% of illness in the United States.

Recommended Web Sites

Please visit **health.jbpub.com/hwonline** for links to these Web sites.

American Holistic Health Association

Information on healthy lifestyle choices and enhancing your level of wellness.

Healthy People 2010 Goals

The U.S. government's national health objectives, which are designed to identify the most significant preventable threats to health and to establish national goals to reduce these health risks.

The Mayo Clinic

This site carries authoritative information on a variety of health topics.

MedlinePlus

The U.S. National Library of Medicine offers information and education on more than 600 health topics.

National Center for Health Statistics

Data on all aspects of health and disease in the United States, from the Centers for Disease Control and Prevention.

The Partnership to Fight Chronic Disease

A national coalition of patients, health care providers, community organizations, business and labor groups, and health policy experts committed to raising awareness of the number one cause of death, disability, and rising health care costs in the United States: rising rates of preventable and treatable chronic diseases.

World Health Organization Global Health Atlas

Standardized data and statistics for infectious diseases at country, regional, and global levels supported through information on demography, socioeconomic conditions, and environmental factors. Data can be accessed in the form of reports, charts, and interactive maps.

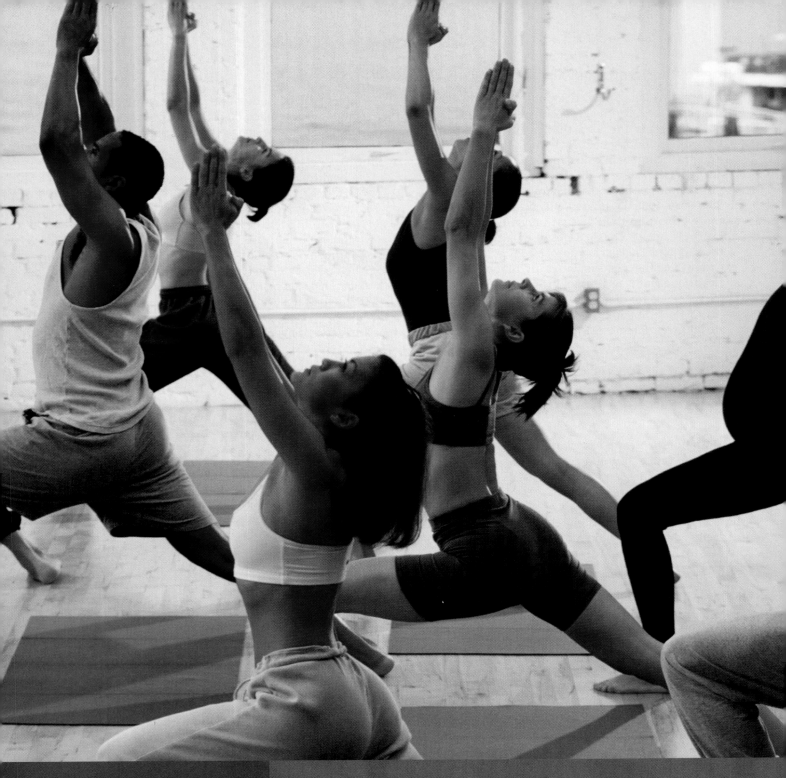

Chapter Two

Mind–Body Communications Maintain Wellness

Learning Objectives

1. Describe three ways the mind and body communicate biologically.
2. Define psychosomatic illness.
3. Describe and give examples of the placebo effect.
4. Describe how faith, religion, and spirituality affect health.
5. Explain hypnotherapy.
6. Describe meditation and image visualization.

Many people believe that good health is related primarily to proper nutrition and physical fitness. Whereas both are vital to health, another important factor that determines your state of health is your mind. Positive thoughts about yourself and others and positive emotions such as happiness and love contribute to vitality, optimism, and joy, which can motivate living healthfully, aid healing and recovery from illness and injury, and increase longevity (Steptoe, Wardle, & Marmot, 2005). Negative thoughts and emotions contribute to depression, pessimism, and decreased health and longevity (Astin et al., 2003).

> Life is not measured by the number of breaths we take, but by the moments that take our breaths away.
>
> *George Carlin*

In Western culture, we are accustomed to thinking of health and healing in terms of drugs, medical treatments, and surgery. In other cultures, past and present, health and healing are accomplished by mental processes such as faith, magic, and spiritual practices. Even in our culture we recognize that attitudes play an important role in promoting health and recovering from illness. Most physicians are aware that a person's attitude greatly affects the probability of recovery from illness. We've all heard of the patient's "will to live."

The mind affects health and well-being because the mind and body make up a single, unified organism. No body exists without a mind; no mind exists without a body. The mind and body communicate with each other by means of the nervous, endocrine (hormone), and immune systems, allowing thoughts, beliefs, and feelings to change body chemistry and physiology.

There are ways to focus the mind to promote health, prevent disease, and foster healing in times of illness. Among them are biofeedback, relaxation, hypnosis, guided imagery, autogenic training, and meditation (**Table 2.1**). Recognizing their effectiveness, mainstream medicine has begun to utilize mind–body techniques, and researchers are elucidating the biological mechanisms that underlie mind–body communications and their effects on health and wellness. In this chapter we discuss mind–body interactions and their contributions to health and well-being.

Mind–Body Communication

Advances in identifying the biological mechanisms of mind–body communication confirm that the mind can affect health in powerful ways. Joy, creativity, and contentment lead to a state of mind–body harmony, which we experience as bodily health and subjective well-being. Fear, anxiety, stress, and depression contribute to mind–body disharmony, which increases risks for a

Table 2.1

Mind–Body Methods for Promoting Health and Preventing and Recovering from Illness

Method	Description
Autogenic training	Silent repetition of one of six autogenic phrases to produce a state of deep relaxation
Biofeedback	Using an electronic device to "feed back" information about the activity of a particular region of the body to alter that activity
Guided imagery	Using mental images suggested by a "guide" to produce relaxation and/or develop a skill
Hypnosis	Focusing attention and lessening awareness of surroundings to produce a relaxed state that is open to suggestion
Image visualization	Using self-generated mental images to produce relaxation and/or develop a skill
Meditation	Focusing awareness on a self-produced inner sound ("mantra") or an external sound, or image, or one's breathing to lessen attentiveness to external stimuli
Progressive muscle relaxation	Progressive tensing and relaxing of muscles in the body to produce relaxation

variety of illnesses, impedes healing, and fosters a sense that life is difficult and unpleasant.

Nerve cells in the brain's thought and feeling centers connect to other nerve cells in the brain and body, hormone-producing tissues and organs, and immune cells throughout the body. In this way, mental activity is able to influence many of the body's physiological processes and maintain homeostasis.

A classic method for using the mind to alter bodily functions is **biofeedback.** This method employs a recording device to facilitate learned self-control of physiological activities (see the Managing Stress feature "Biofeedback"). The recording device is connected to a region of the body (e.g., forehead, arm), and information about biological activity in that region is "fed back" on a screen or by means of a sound to the person in whose body the activity is taking place. Using this visual or auditory information about the activity, the person can learn to control the activity in a desired way. Biofeedback has been used successfully to treat more than 150 medical conditions, including high blood pressure, back pain, panic attacks, asthma, and headaches (Mayo Clinic, 2008). Biofeedback also can be used to produce changes in the brain's electrical activity (*alpha waves*) to bring about a state of relaxation.

The Autonomic Nervous System

A major way by which the mind and body communicate is through the **autonomic nervous system** (ANS), a group

‎🧘 Managing Stress

Biofeedback

Dan was a first-year graduate student who experienced frequent headaches, for which he sought help from the Student Health Center. Medical tests showed no brain pathology, such as a tumor, or brain infection or injury. Diagnosis: Dan's headaches were related to the stress and anxiety about doing well in graduate school.

Dan's therapy involved meeting with a counselor to discuss ways to manage the stress of graduate school and biofeedback training to deal specifically with his headaches. In biofeedback sessions, three small sensing devices, which monitored the activity of the forehead's frontalis muscle, were attached to Dan's forehead (**Figure 2.1**). The frontalis and certain muscles in the neck involuntarily contract during times of stress, which impedes blood flow to the head, resulting in a headache. Wires from the three sensors were connected to a biofeedback unit, which was placed on a table directly in Dan's view. Whenever Dan's frontalis muscle contracted, the biofeedback unit produced audible clicks. A very tense frontalis produced rapid clicks. A relaxed frontalis produced infrequent, irregular clicks.

Dan was instructed by his biofeedback therapist to try to reduce the number of clicks, a skill that required several training sessions to attain. Paradoxically, *not* trying to relax his frontalis produced the best results. The therapy proved successful. Dan seldom got headaches. And when he did, he could relieve them by relaxing the muscles in his forehead.

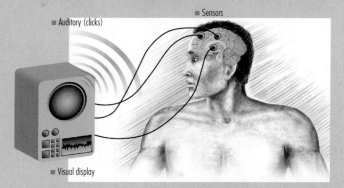

■ Auditory (clicks) ■ Sensors ■ Visual display

■ **Figure 2.1**

Biofeedback
The biofeedback device measures muscle tension in the head region. The speaker produces rapid audible clicks when muscles are tense, and infrequent and irregular clicks when head muscles are relaxed.

---

of nerves that regulate many of the body's physiological processes, such as heart rate, blood pressure, constipation, sweating, and incontinence (**Figure 2.2**). Centers in the brain, principally the brain stem and hypothalamus, receive information about the state of the body and, in response, activate the nerve fibers of the ANS to maintain appropriate physiological balance. For example, when you exercise, the ANS stimulates the heart's pacemaker cells to increase your heart rate, thus increasing the amount of blood pumped to moving muscles.

The autonomic nervous system derives its name from the fact that its activities normally operate without conscious control. Thus, you do not think about how fast your heart should beat or whether you should sweat to cool yourself when jogging. Even though the ANS functions without conscious control, the signals it sends to the body can be affected by thoughts and feelings. For example, nearly all students are familiar with the nervous stomach and sweaty palms that accompany taking an important exam. Realizing that it is possible to do poorly on an exam (a thought) leads to anxiety (an emotion), which activates the ANS to produce symptoms. Panic has an immediate effect on breathing and heart rate, and stress can constrict blood vessels, causing headaches or high blood pressure.

Many students live fast-paced, hectic lives that are full of time pressures and stress. Besides doing school assignments, many students work at jobs, and nearly all try to maintain harmonious social relationships with family and friends, which take time and attention. Moreover, the modern environment is filled with cell phones, the Internet, TV, video games, iPods, and other stimuli that compete for one's attention. Trying to accommodate all of life's demands produces near continuous physiologic arousal mediated by the sympathetic nerves of the ANS, causing, among other things, sleep disturbances, muscle tension, gastrointestinal symptoms, and an increased risk for cardiovascular disease.

Quieting the Autonomic Nervous System

It is possible to counteract ANS-mediated arousal by putting 20 to 30 minutes or more of quiet time into your life each day. (If you must, schedule it in your day-planner.) You can employ any of a number of techniques designed to lessen ANS arousal and create a sense of mind–body harmony (see Table 2.1). Or, you can find a quiet spot in a park or a room where you can comfortably and silently

TERMS

autonomic nervous system: the special group of nerves that control some of the body's organs and their functions

biofeedback: using an electronic device to "feed back" information about the body to alter a particular physiological function

Sympathetic

- Dilates pupils
- Inhibits salivation
- Dilates bronchi (lungs)
- Stimulates heartbeat
- Stimulates adrenal gland
- Inhibits digestion (stomach, pancreas, liver, spleen)
- Dilates bladder

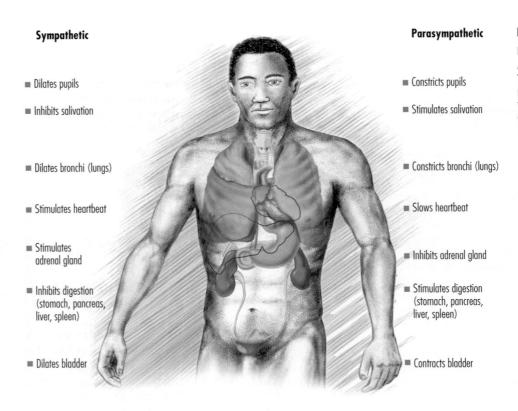

Parasympathetic

- Constricts pupils
- Stimulates salivation
- Constricts bronchi (lungs)
- Slows heartbeat
- Inhibits adrenal gland
- Stimulates digestion (stomach, pancreas, liver, spleen)
- Contracts bladder

■ **Figure 2.2**

Functions Controlled by the Autonomic Nervous System
The sympathetic nerves and the parasympathetic nerves regulate functions that normally are not under conscious control, such as breathing, digestion, and heart rate.

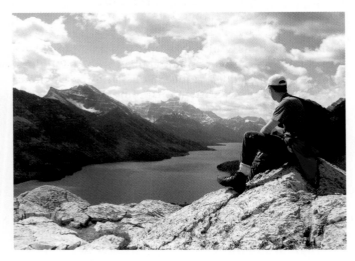

reflect on the good things in your life and let go, for a time, of the problems of the world and what you need to accomplish that day and in your life. Two methods with a body of research to support their effectiveness are the relaxation response and autogenic training.

The Relaxation Response

The **relaxation response** is an automatic physiological response that is the opposite of autonomic nervous system activation (Benson & Klipper, 2000). The relaxation response decreases oxygen consumption, respiratory rate, heart rate, blood pressure, and muscle tension. A variety of mind–body methods can produce the relax-

ation response, such as mantra meditation, progressive muscle relaxation, and guided imagery. For example, at the Harvard Medical School, patients are taught to sit quietly and silently repeat the word "one." Methods that elicit the relaxation response share these features:

- A quiet environment
- A focusing of the mind's attention, such as silently repeating a word or phrase, or focusing one's breathing
- A passive, accepting mental state
- A comfortable physical position

Autogenic Training

Autogenic training uses autosuggestion to establish a balance between the mind and body through changes in the autonomic nervous system. The method has been shown to be effective in relieving anxiety (Miu, Heilman, & Miclea, 2009) and improving the quality of life in people with chronic medical conditions (Sutherland, Anderson, & Morris, 2005).

Autogenic training involves learning to concentrate on one of six basic autogenic phrases for a few minutes each day over a week or more. After weeks or months of practice, one is able to attain a deep sense of relaxation, often within seconds, which can result in healthful physiological changes. The six basic autosuggestions are as follows:

- My arms and legs are heavy.
- My arms and legs are warm.
- My heartbeat is calm and regular.
- My lungs breathe for me.

Wellness Guide

Using Your Mind to Heal Your Body

Everyone has accidentally cut or burned his or her hand at one time or another. Perhaps you were chopping vegetables and the knife slipped, or perhaps you reached for a pan on the stove, forgetting that the handle was hot. The usual response to such accidents is anger at being careless or forgetful and anger at the sudden pain. We jump around, curse, and generally act in ways that exacerbate the injury and delay healing. A much better response to minor accidental injuries that do not require immediate medical attention is the following.

In case of a cut, place a clean cloth over the wound and press gently to help stop the bleeding. Then sit or lie down.

Close your eyes and allow yourself to become mentally and physically quiet. Visualize the injured part with your mind and see it as it was just *before* the accident. See the skin coming back together. Feel the pain recede. Notice that there is no bleeding. Continue doing this for five minutes or longer until you feel calm. If the accident caused a burn, place an ice bag or cool, wet cloth over the wound. Then lie down and visualize the skin becoming cooler and looking like the normal skin around the burn.

By immediately calming the mind after an injury, inflammation and other harmful physiological reactions in the area are reduced. Healing processes begin immediately when you send positive, calming thoughts and images to the injured area. Continue to visualize healing in the injured area.

- My abdomen is warm.
- My forehead is cool.

The exact phrasing of any autogenic suggestion is not critical to its effectiveness. The words carry no particular power. Any suggestion can be rephrased so that it becomes comfortable, believable, and acceptable to the practitioner's mind.

Hormones

Besides the autonomic nervous system, the mind can affect physiology via the endocrine (hormone) system. **Hormones** are chemicals produced by special organs and tissues in the body. Each hormone regulates specific biological functions (**Figure 2.3**). Hormones notify the body of changes outside and inside the body that must be responded to in order to maintain health.

Many hormones respond to changes in thoughts and feelings. For example, if the mind interprets a situation as threatening or frightening, regardless of whether the danger is real or imagined, adrenalin and several other hormones are released into the blood that make the body alert and ready for action. The hormones bring about an increased heart rate and mobilize stored nutrients to supply energy for dealing with the danger.

The Immune System

Besides the ANS and endocrine system, the mind communicates with the body via the immune system. The immune system (discussed in detail in Chapter 12) is responsible for combating infections and ridding the body of foreign organisms and toxic substances. Immune system cells, tissues, and organs are located throughout the body. The immune system can be influenced by the mind via the nervous and endocrine systems. Nerves of

the sympathetic nervous system connect to certain immune tissues. Many immune cells respond to the presence of the hormone cortisol as part of the stress response (see Chapter 3). Moreover, the immune system releases special chemicals called cytokines, which can affect the nervous and endocrine systems.

That the mind can affect the workings of the immune system is illustrated in a study of the effects of mindfulness meditation on immune function in a work environment with healthy employees (Davidson et al., 2003). Volunteers were trained in mindfulness meditation for eight weeks, and at the end of training they were vaccinated with influenza vaccine. Compared to nonmeditating volunteers, antibody levels to the influenza vaccine were higher among meditators, demonstrating that mindfulness meditation produces measurable effects on the immune system.

The Mind Can Create Illness or Wellness

That thoughts and feelings can alter physiological processes means that individuals have the power to influence their health for ill or for well-being.

TERMS

autogenic training: the use of autosuggestion to establish a balance between the mind and body through changes in the autonomic nervous system

hormones: chemicals produced in the body that regulate body functions

relaxation response: the physiological changes in the body that result from mental relaxation techiques

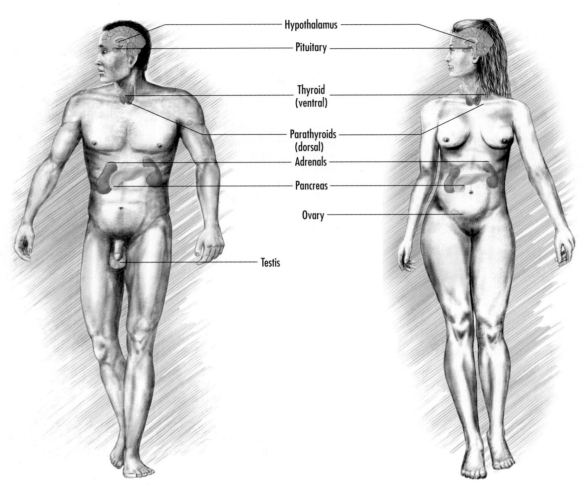

Hypothalamus
Pituitary
Thyroid (ventral)
Parathyroids (dorsal)
Adrenals
Pancreas
Ovary
Testis

■ **Figure 2.3**

Where Hormones Are Released
Hormones are released from different glands throughout the body. The synthesis and release of these hormones are regulated by the mind and autonomic nervous system. Hormones carry chemical messages that tell organs in the body how to respond to stimuli.

Psychosomatic Illnesses

The power of the mind to cause illness is borne out by a long list of **psychosomatic illnesses** (**Figure 2.4**). These conditions are caused, in large measure, by mental states and attitudes such as persistent anxiety, depression, and stress that produce unhealthy physiological changes. That is why these illnesses are called psychosomatic, a term derived from the Greek (*psych*, mind; *soma*, body).

Many people believe that psychosomatic means imaginary, that "it's all in the head." This is not the case. The damage to the gastrointestinal tract in someone with stress-related irritable bowel syndrome is just as real as the damage caused by an infection or injury. Psychosomatic means that thoughts and feelings are at the root of the physiological abnormalities causing the symptoms.

Modern medicine (see Chapter 19) tends not to treat psychosomatic illnesses directly. Physicians prefer to use drugs that suppress symptoms, but rarely do they address the underlying mental states that cause the illness. This is caused in part by their training, which focuses on biological causes of disease, and in part by doctors not having time to probe the lifestyle of a patient with a psychosomatic illness; also, the patient's health insurer is not likely to pay for the doctor to do so.

Somatization Disorders

Somatization refers to the occurrence of physical symptoms without the presence of medically detectable injury or disease. Psychological and social problems such as depression or anger may cause pain, fatigue, nausea, diarrhea, and sexual problems. It is estimated that 25% to 75% of all patients who visit primary care physicians suffer from somatization disorders. These are difficult to treat, time-consuming for physicians to diagnose, and expensive for the health care system. The diagnostic criteria for a somatization disorder are shown in **Table 2.2**; the chief complaint is pain of long duration in several parts of the body that cannot be explained by any medical condition or injury.

The lives that many people choose to live or are forced to live by financial or family circumstances can cause mind–body disruption that eventually produces pain and sickness. People suffering from somatization disorders are not feigning sickness; they have lost mind–body harmony to a serious degree.

The Mind Can Create Wellness

The power of the mind to create wellness is illustrated by studies that show that positive emotions are associated with healthful biological changes. For example, a

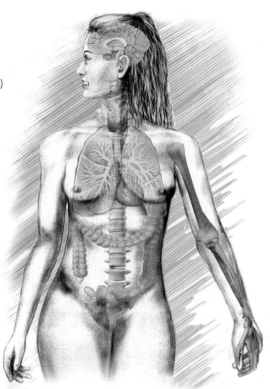

- Tension headaches

- Bruxism (grinding of teeth)

- Hyperactive thyroid

- Bronchial asthma

- Essential hypertension

- Erection problems in men/menstrual problems in women

- Eczema

- Tinnitus (ringing in one or both ears)

- Acne

- Back pain

- Ulcerative colitis

- Irritable bowel syndrome

- Rheumatoid arthritis

■ **Figure 2.4**

Psychosomatic Illnesses
Many diseases and disorders of the body are partly caused by thoughts and feelings.

Table 2.2

Diagnostic Criteria for Somatization Disorder

A. History of physical complaints begins before age 30, lasts for several years, and results in the request for treatment or in significantly impaired social, occupational, or other types of functioning.

B. Each of these four criteria must be met, with individual symptoms occurring at any time:

   1. History of pain related to at least four sites or functions

   2. History of at least two gastrointestinal symptoms other than pain

   3. History of at least one sexual or reproductive symptom other than pain

   4. History of at least one symptom or deficit suggesting a neurologic condition not limited to pain (a conversion symptom, a dissociative symptom, or loss of consciousness other than fainting)

C. One of these two criteria must be met:

   1. Symptoms in B cannot be explained by a medical condition or the effects of a substance.

   2. When there is a related medical condition, the physical complaint or the resulting social or occupational impairment is in excess of what would be expected from the history, physical examination, or laboratory findings.

D. Symptoms are not intentionally produced or feigned.

Source: American Psychiatric Association. (1994). *Diagnostic and statistical manual of mental disorders* (4th ed.). Washington, DC: Author. Copyright 1994, American Psychiatric Association. Reprinted with permission.

Wardle, & Marmot, 2005). Those with the highest happiness ratings showed the lowest heart rate and stress hormone levels (there was no effect of happiness on blood pressure).

Humor also can have a positive effect on health (Christie & Moore, 2005). Humor increases comfort levels and decreases stress and anxiety in patients with cancer. Humor has a positive effect on the immune system by elevating levels of natural killer cells (Bennett et al., 2004). Humor also improves pain thresholds, perhaps by activating endorphin (a hormone) release in the brain.

The importance of humor on health was recognized as far back as ancient Greece. Plato was a strong advocate of humor as a means to lighten the burdens of the soul and to improve one's state of health. From medieval court jesters to circus clowns, humor has long been a factor influencing mind–body healing. Only now is medical science learning what people have known intuitively for centuries—laughter is good medicine.

TERMS

psychosomatic illnesses: physical illnesses brought on by negative mental states such as stress or emotional upset

somatization: occurrence of physical symptoms without any bodily disease or injury being present

group of English civil service workers were asked to rate their state of happiness several times during a typical work day while researchers measured blood pressure, heart rate, and stress hormone (cortisol) levels (Steptoe,

Mind–Body Healing

Placebo Effect

The **placebo effect** is the lessening of symptoms or curing of disease by believing in the healing powers of a make-believe medicine or "sugar pill." Although the curative powers of placebos are based on the recipient's belief in their power, that is not to say that the placebo effect is not real. Placebos act on the mind, which brings about physiological changes.

The placebo effect is so common and powerful that the U.S. Food and Drug Administration requires that a new drug undergo a *double-blind, placebo-controlled* trial. This means comparing one group of patients' responses to a new drug with a different, matched group's responses to a placebo (the control group). So as to minimize bias, people in the test-drug group and the placebo group do not know which substance they are receiving; that is, they are "blind." Furthermore, none of the scientists administering the test drug or the placebo knows what the patients are receiving; that is, they also are "blind." Only the project administrator knows who is receiving what. The efficacy of the new drug is determined by its performance compared to the placebo.

The placebo effect has been found to be effective in the treatment of ulcers, postoperative pain, seasickness, headache, coughs, rheumatoid arthritis, hay fever, hypertension, warts, and other diseases. The number of people responding to placebos for any symptom ranges from 30% to 70%; most drug studies report about a 50% response to a placebo. Thus, for almost any disease or symptom, a person has about a 50% chance of improvement simply by *believing* in the power of the treatment, whether or not it has any specific biological effect.

Depression is a condition in which the placebo effect can account for as much as 75% of any relief experienced. **Figure 2.5** shows the results of a study comparing two antidepressant drugs with a placebo pill. Notice that during the first three weeks of the study, depressed individuals got almost as much relief from the placebo as from the antidepressant drugs. Why the benefits of the placebo did not increase after that time could be a result of differences in the rates at which the antidepressants and the placebo were eliminated from the body or subtle chemical effects in the brain produced by the antidepressant drugs. Nevertheless, as demonstrated in this study, the placebo effect accounted for 60% to 70% of the relief.

To determine how the placebo effect could be operating to relieve depression, researchers used positron emission tomography (a PET scan) to visualize the activity in different regions of the brain when depressed individuals received antidepressant medication or placebo (Mayberg et al., 2002). The results showed that the pattern of brain activity of patients receiving

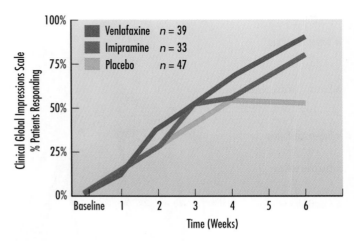

■ **Figure 2.5**

Placebo Study

A double-blind, placebo-controlled study comparing two antidepressant drugs, venlafaxine and imipramine, with placebo in reducing the symptoms of clinical depression. (*n* is the number of patients in each group.) For at least one month, just as many patients experienced relief of their symptoms with a placebo as with either antidepressant drug.

placebo was almost the same as those receiving antidepressants. Apparently, the expectation that their symptoms would improve caused biological changes in the brain that contributed to relief of depression.

Pain responds exceptionally well to the placebo effect (**Figure 2.6**). As with depression, pain relief from placebo can occur from biological changes in the brain. For example, researchers used functional magnetic resonance imaging (fMRI) to map changes in blood flow in the brains of volunteers (Wager et al., 2004). The volunteers were subjected to harmless but occasionally painful electric shocks or heat. When they believed an antipain cream had been applied to their arm, they rated the pain as less intense. Moreover, placebo pain relief was related to decreased brain activity in pain-sensitive brain regions and was associated with increased activity during anticipation of pain in other brain regions, providing evidence that placebos alter the experience of pain.

Other studies show that placebo-induced pain relief likely occurs because the expectation of relief might change the body's manufacture or release of its own internal pain-relieving chemicals, called endorphins (Benedetti, 2007). For example, after having wisdom teeth removed, adults were given morphine or placebo for pain relief; about 33% of those receiving placebo experienced pain relief. Then, a chemical that blocks the effects of morphine and endorphins, called naloxone, was given to any patient who had experienced pain relief, either from morphine or placebo. All patients receiving naloxone experienced return of their

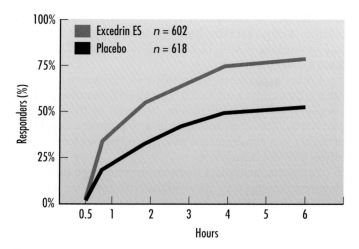

■ Figure 2.6

Double-blind, placebo-controlled study comparing Excedrin and placebo in relieving the pain of migraine headache. A responder is a patient with moderate or severe pain whose pain was reduced to mild or none following treatment. Note that more than half of over 600 patients with migraine headache had mild or no pain after taking a placebo pill.

pain. Thus, it would appear that the expectation of pain relief can stimulate the manufacture and release of endorphins.

Why, if placebos are so effective in healing, are they not used more by physicians in treating patients? One reason is an ethical dilemma for physicians: A placebo might work for one patient but not for another. Although the same could be true for a prescribed drug, the physician is protected legally by prescribing a drug that has been clinically tested and approved by the FDA. However, no legal protection exists for a physician prescribing a placebo if the patient decides to sue, claiming that the treatment did not meet accepted medical standards.

Yet another reason that placebos are not part of medical practice is that placebos can be dangerous, just as drugs can be dangerous. Patients can become addicted to placebo pills used for pain relief and suffer withdrawal symptoms when they stop using them. Also, like prescription drugs, placebo pills can cause side effects. In one experiment, 40 volunteer asthmatic patients were asked to inhale a placebo spray, which they were told contained an allergen. Twelve of the volunteers had full-blown asthma attacks, and seven had lesser symptoms. The asthma attacks were reversed by inhalation of another placebo spray, which they were told would relieve the symptoms.

Words can produce a placebo effect in the same way as a pill. Because of this fact, you should always seek out health practitioners whom you trust and who use positive, constructive healing suggestions and who encourage you to become involved in self-healing prac-

tices. Avoid health practitioners who voice negative and pessimistic recommendations. No one needs to hear negative suggestions such as "You'll probably have to take these pills for the rest of your life," or "I doubt that you'll be able to move around much after an accident like that." In the presence of a physician, many patients become very open to suggestions, both positive and negative, because their minds are intently focused on what the doctor is saying. Such a focused state of mind is similar to that obtained in meditation or hypnosis. It is more helpful to practice being alert and critical when discussing your health concerns or diagnostic test results with a health professional. Of course, this is not always easy to do, especially when the information being conveyed causes distress or fear.

A tragic, but dramatic, example of mind–body communication and the power of a negative placebo effect involved a patient who died apparently from reading a single word (Hewlett, 1994). This person had a history of chronic lymphatic leukemia, a form of blood cancer that usually is easily controlled with drugs. The patient had been well for more than three years with only intermittent need for medication. However, he had never actually been informed of the original diagnosis of his condition.

One day he was in his physician's office on a routine visit and happened to read the physician's notes, which were lying on the desk. He saw the word *leukemia* in his file. He missed his next scheduled office visit and shortly thereafter showed up in the hospital's emergency room. Within three weeks he died in the hospital. No cause of death could be discovered at autopsy, and his leukemia was still in remission. The patient apparently *believed* that he had terminal cancer just from seeing the word *leukemia* in his medical records. The mind *does* heal; the mind *does* kill.

Faith and Healing

Thousands of years ago the priest–healers of ancient civilizations and the shamans of native tribes used the beliefs of their people to heal by incantation, to exorcise evil spirits, and to vanquish demons who were thought to cause disease. The existence of shamans, faith healers, and medicine men and women in cultures throughout human history suggests that their healing methods must have been generally successful. Egyptian papyri

TERMS

placebo effect: healing that results from a person's belief in a treatment that has no medicinal value

show that although the priest–physicians of ancient Egypt prescribed herbs and performed surgeries, their treatments relied on the belief of the people in the healing power of the gods. Priests would put patients into a trance in a temple and tell them that when they awakened, they would be healed. And often they were.

The Greeks and Romans also had gods, oracles, and temples of healing. Their priests also used trance and sleeplike mental states to impart healing suggestions to receptive minds. Sometimes "miraculous cures" resulted. Greek and Roman emperors and priests also healed by the "laying on of hands"; people were healed because they believed that their rulers had divine powers. King Pyrrhus of Epirus is reputed to have cured sick patients solely by the touch of his big toe.

> Faith. You can do little with it and nothing without it.
>
> *Samuel Butler*

All religions teach that divine persons have the power to heal. The New Testament recounts many examples of the healing power of Jesus.

> Is any sick among you? Let him call for the Elders of the church and let them pray over him, anointing him with oil in the name of the Lord; and the prayer of faith shall save the sick.
>
> —*James 5:14–15*

> That evening they brought him many who were possessed with demons, and he cast out the spirits with a word, and healed all who were sick.
>
> —*Matthew 8:14*

> And he said to her, "Daughter, your faith has made you well; go in peace and be healed of your diseases."
>
> —*Mark 5:34*

Over the centuries, faith and prayer have healed many people. Some ascribe healing to the power of God; others explain it simply by the power of belief to produce a placebo effect.

Today's patients have faith in the knowledge of their physicians and the drugs they prescribe just as people of ancient civilizations believed in their priests and herbs. The improvement in any patient's condition probably is a combination of faith in the healer and the efficacy of the treatment.

For years, scientists have attempted to evaluate the power of prayer to heal either oneself or others. Because there is no experimental way to measure the effects of personal prayer on a person's condition, studies focus on the therapeutic effects of *intercessory prayer*, in which groups of people pray for the health and recovery of patients either with or without the patients' knowledge. Some studies have claimed that prayer does help healing; other studies have found no effect. To try to resolve whether intercessory prayer has a positive effect on healing others, six major U.S. hospitals participated in a large-scale experiment. In this study, some patients about to undergo coronary artery bypass surgery (see Chapter 14) were told that they would be prayed for; another group of patients were not informed that they were being prayed for. The conclusion of this study was that intercessory prayer had no effect on recovery or complications from the bypass surgery (Benson et al., 2006). Will this scientific study resolve the question of whether prayer benefits health? It cer-

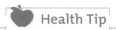 **Health Tip**

Repeating This Phrase May Improve Your Health

In the early 1900s, a French pharmacist named Emile Coué (1857–1926) became famous for using autosuggestion to cure people of all kinds of ailments. His most famous autosuggestion, which millions of people recited to themselves, was: "Every day, in every way, I'm getting better and better."

Try this autosuggestion or make up one of your own to fit a particular situation you want to improve. Repeat the suggestion in your mind as often as feels comfortable. Do it without effort or expectation. Autosuggestion is a powerful tool for improving health and for healing.

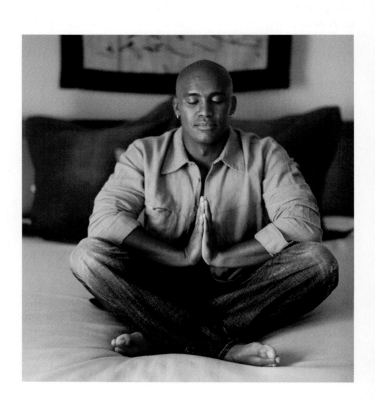

tainly will not shake the convictions of people of faith who believe in the power of prayer.

Spirituality, Religion, and Health

Many people believe that spirituality—finding meaning, hope, comfort, and inner peace through religion, a connection with Nature or some force larger than oneself—plays a role in health and illness. One study (MacLean et al., 2003) found that 66% of individuals want their physicians to be aware of their spiritual or religious beliefs. However, most individuals do not want their physicians to be directly involved in their health-related spiritual experiences. For example, only about 20% want their doctors to pray with them in routine office visits; about 50% want their doctors to pray with them in a hospitalized, near-death situation. A survey of doctors showed that 95% believed a patient's spiritual outlook was important to handling health difficulties, and 68% believed that physicians should ask patients about spiritual and religious issues (McCauley et al., 2005), although few physicians believe that it is appropriate for them to recommend prayer and religious activities to patients (Sloan et al., 2001).

Many people believe in the healing power of prayer and the capacity of faith to help them prevent and recover from illness. For example, people who attend religious services at least monthly were found to have a 30% to 35% reduced risk of death compared to a control group of people who did not attend church (Gillum et al., 2008). The positive effect on health of religious attendance is associated with healthier lifestyles (especially engaging in physical activity), increased social relationships, and stable marriages (Strawbridge et al., 2001). These factors may be responsible for the finding that weekly religious attendance is associated with a healthy immune system (Lutgendorf et al., 2004).

For centuries, science and religion provided separate ways of understanding the world. By definition, religious experience or the claims of religions cannot be tested by science because they are not subject to experimentation or reproducibility. With the development of new brain imaging techniques, however, spiritual experiences and brain electrical activity have become accessible to scientific investigation. The new field, called neurotheology, has shown that in brains of persons deep in prayer or meditation, visible biological changes occur (Lutz et al., 2008). When people experience a "cosmic unity, loss of self, or perception of God," brain activity is altered, particularly in a region called the temporal lobe. On reflection, it is not surprising that a strong spiritual experience is reflected in altered brain activity, just as a strong emotional experience is. What probably will never be answered is whether brain activity *creates* the mystical experience or whether the mystical experi-ence has a reality of its own that occasionally is perceived by a human brain. As the Buddhist koan asks, "If a tree falls in the forest and no one hears it, does the fallen tree make a sound?"

Spiritual experiences tend to engender feelings of compassion and empathy; peace of mind; relatedness and communion with a force, power, or set of values larger than oneself; and harmony with the environment. These feelings are believed to be a cornerstone of health because they represent a balance between the inner and outer aspects of human experience. For some, the spiritual dimension of life is embodied in the practice of a specific religion. For others, the spiritual dimension is nonreligious and simply part of a personal philosophy. Many practices can help people experience the spiritual realms of existence—prayer, meditation, yoga, musical and artistic endeavors, and helping others are but a few common ones.

Becoming more spiritually aware, regardless of the chosen path, can lead to a healthier life. Being in touch with your spiritual feelings helps you handle life's ups and downs with understanding and compassion for yourself and others. You become open to love in the highest sense of its meaning, which is acceptance and tolerance. You begin to love yourself despite your problems and hang-ups. You love your family and friends when relations are strained. You see beauty and harmony in more and more aspects of living. And occasionally—however fleetingly—you may experience the truly wondrous feeling of being completely and joyfully alive.

Hypnosis and Healing

The modern use of hypnosis as a medical technique began with the Viennese physician Franz Anton Mesmer, who practiced in the late eighteenth and early nineteenth centuries. History has preserved the term *mesmerism* for the trancelike state that Mesmer produced in his patients. Many years later, a Scottish physician, James Braid, introduced the term *hypnosis* (from the Greek *hypnos*, meaning sleep) and began to practice **hypnotherapy**, the use of hypnosis to cure sickness.

Mesmer called his technique for healing "animal magnetism" because he had his patients hold onto metal rods that supposedly transmitted healing energy while the patients were in trance. Mesmer was so successful that other physicians in Vienna forced the authorities to order him to stop using his unorthodox

TERMS

hypnotherapy: the use of hypnosis to treat sickness

> We do not see things as they are. . . . We see things as we are.
>
> *Talmud*

methods. In 1778, Mesmer moved to Paris, where he again was successful in attracting patients. Eventually, the French authorities appointed a scientific panel, which included Benjamin Franklin (U.S. ambassador to France at the time), to investigate Mesmer and his methods. The panel concluded that there was no scientific basis to animal magnetism and that Mesmer was a fraud. This conclusion was reached even though the panel did not dispute Mesmer's success in curing many patients. Discredited by physicians and scientists, Mesmer died in obscurity in 1815.

Despite being officially discredited, mesmerism (now called hypnotism) flourished throughout England, Europe, and the United States in the nineteenth century. In 1847, J. W. Robbins, a Massachusetts physician, reported using hypnotherapy to treat eating disorders and to help people stop smoking. Dr. Robbins used aversive suggestions while patients were in trance and also gave them posthypnotic suggestions. Many of the same procedures are used today in treating these and other behavioral disorders.

In the late nineteenth century, two French physicians showed that healing could be accomplished solely by suggestion and that cures resulted from the patient's expectation of being cured. Hippolyte-Marie Bernheim, who used hypnotherapy successfully with thousands of patients, argued that almost all healing resulted from suggestions he gave receptive patients while they were in trance.

Effective use of suggestion in healing seems to depend on the degree of mental relaxation involved. For reasons that are not entirely clear, a mind engaged in the conscious thoughts of daily living is not as open to suggestion as one that is internally relaxed by hypnosis, meditation, or other mental relaxation techniques.

Understanding Hypnosis May Help You Relax

To study hypnosis, researchers must have a way of measuring the hypnotic state. A series of suggestibility tests that consist of a 12-point scale was developed by psychologists at Stanford University in the 1950s. A low score means that the subject does not enter a state of hypnosis; a high score means that the subject is highly susceptible to hypnosis. Most people score between 5 to 7 on the Stanford test, which is still used by researchers today (Nash, 2001).

Many people have fears about being hypnotized, and many myths about hypnosis still exist. Perhaps the greatest fear people have is that they can be forced to do something terrible or evil if they are hypnotized. This view was greatly reinforced by the popular film *The Manchurian Candidate,* which showed hypnotized people who were programmed to kill when given a verbal command by the hypnotist. Other people feel that they

will lose their moral values if they become hypnotized, but this also is not true. Some of the misconceptions and apprehensions about hypnosis are summarized in **Table 2.3**.

Hypnotherapy is potentially a valuable adjunct to medical practice and has a long and successful history. It is not used widely because of time constraints and the almost universal belief that the right pill will cure everything. Physicians have to take time to develop a rapport with patients and be willing to take as much time as necessary to answer all questions and make sure the patient is comfortable with being hypnotized. Modern medical practice does not allow for this in an age of managed care and HMOs (see Chapter 19). Time is money in modern medical practice.

Virtual Reality Therapies

It has been known for many centuries that *distraction* is a very effective treatment for pain. That is why meditation, hypnotherapy, prayer, and other methods that focus the mind's attention on something other than pain or other symptoms are so effective. Many Buddhist monks and devout individuals of many faiths learn to focus their attention so completely on a mantra, mandala, breathing, or exalted inner state that they are, quite literally, "out of their bodies." Modern medical researchers are using this aspect of mind to create **virtual reality therapies (VRT)** to treat burns, pain, phobias (e.g., fear of flying, insects, or heights). A very important use of VRT is in the treatment of posttraumatic stress disorder (PTSD; see Chapter 3), which was experienced by many survivors of the 9/11 attack in New York and more recently by soldiers who served in Iraq (Thacker, 2003). Examples of environments simulated are virtual Iraq, virtual airplane, virtual nicotine, and virtual 9/11. Patients using VRT can manipulate the virtual environments to lessen their fears and stress. Some manage to reduce their overall anxiety and arousal response so that they become relatively free of PTSD.

Anyone who has seen the film *Matrix* or plays video games knows that virtual reality involves focusing one's attention on a computer-generated imaginary world. A medical application of VRT exposes burn patients to virtual realities of glaciers, ice, snow, snowmen, and other features of a cold, cold world to distract them from their pain. Another application is to expose a person with a fear of flying to virtual reality flight experiences (Hoffman, 2004). While in the fearful virtual world patients are, at the same time, safe in their therapist's office and know that they can remove the headset at any time. Because part of their mind knows they are safe, patients can confront their fears in the virtual world and learn to overcome them.

The software for virtual reality therapies is costly to develop, and so is the equipment to deliver the therapeu-

🧘 Managing Stress

Progressive Muscle Relaxation

In the technique called progressive relaxation, you lie on your back in quiet, comfortable surroundings with your feet slightly apart and palms facing upward. Before beginning the exercise, allow the thoughts of the day and any worries to leave your mind. Then you are ready to begin.

1. Close your eyes; squeeze your lids shut as tightly as you can. Hold them shut for a count of five, then slowly release the tension. Notice how your eyes feel as they relax. Keep your eyelids lightly closed; breathe slowly and deeply.

2. Turn your palms down. Bend your left hand back at the wrist, keeping your forearm on the floor. Bend your hand as far as it will go until you feel tension in your forearm muscles. Hold for a count of five, then release the tension. Notice the warm, relaxed sensation that enters your wrist. Repeat with your right hand.

3. With palms up, make a tight fist in your left hand by tightening the muscles of the arm and fingers. Hold for a count of five; release the tension. Notice the tingling, relaxed sensation in your hand and arm. Repeat with your right hand.

4. Focus your attention on your left leg; slowly bring the top of your foot as far forward as you can while keeping your heel on the floor. Notice the tension in the muscles of your lower leg. Hold for a count of five; release the tension. Repeat with your right leg.

5. Point the toes in your left foot away from you as far as you can. Notice the tension in your calf muscles. Release the tension slowly. Repeat with your right foot.

Similar exercises can be performed to tense and relax other muscles.

Table 2.3

Myths and Facts About Hypnosis

Myth: Hypnotized subjects are faking being in a trancelike state.
Fact: Brain wave measurements and physiological responses show that subjects are not faking and are in an altered state of consciousness.

Myth: You must be quiet and relaxed to be hypnotized.
Fact: It helps but is not necessary. Long-distance runners and people exercising vigorously sometimes enter a hypnotic state.

Myth: Hypnosis is a sleeplike state.
Fact: Not true. Hypnotized subjects are fully aware of what they are saying or doing, unless they accept a suggestion to go to sleep.

Myth: People with certain personalities are easier to hypnotize than others.
Fact: There is no correlation between personality type and hypnotizability. Some people accept suggestions more readily than others and are more open to being hypnotized.

Myth: Hypnotized subjects can be made to do or say anything.

Fact: Not true. Subjects will refuse to do things that they find embarrassing or immoral. They can also terminate the hypnotic state at any time.

Myth: Under hypnosis people remember past events more accurately.
Fact: Often the opposite is the case. The testimony of hypnotized subjects remembering what happened at a crime scene or after being attacked is often inaccurate.

Myth: Hypnotized subjects do not remember what they did or said while hypnotized.
Fact: If subjects accept a suggestion that they will forget what they have said or done while hypnotized, subjects will usually say they cannot remember. This suggestion is usually used in stage hypnosis acts to impress an audience.

Myth: Hypnotized subjects can be made to commit an evil or criminal act.
Fact: Absolutely not. Peoples' fundamental values or beliefs cannot be overridden by hypnosis.

> Meditation is not what you think.
> *Krishnamurti*

tic treatments. Nevertheless, virtual reality therapy has enormous potential to help people overcome a variety of fears and symptoms of fear.

Meditation

Meditation has been associated with both Eastern and Western religions for centuries. Meditation is simply focused awareness. If you examine what is going on in your mind at any given moment, odds are you will find it flitting from one thought to another: "Did I remember to turn off the stove before I left the house?" "My feet are killing me; I shouldn't have worn these shoes." "I wonder what mood she's going to be in tonight?" "Did the kids say something about going to a sleepover this weekend?" Our minds are generally constantly active and often involved in worrying or thinking about emotional upsets, financial concerns, or the pressures of daily activities.

TERMS

virtual reality therapy (VRT): use of computer programs to create virtual worlds that engage the mind in order to overcome pain and fear and to treat symptoms of posttraumatic stress disorder

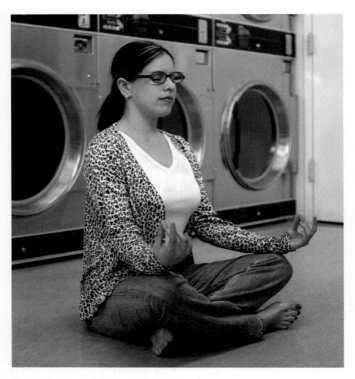

Meditation can be done anywhere, any time.

🍎 Health Tip

Make Up Your Own Mantra for Changing Behaviors

Use the power of a mantra to change some aspect of performance or behavior. Choose some behavior or activity that you would like to change or improve. Then create your own mantra. It should not be something complicated, but a small thing that you feel you can achieve. It should be as specific as possible. For example:

Sports: I feel my body getting stronger.
              I feel my body moving more swiftly through the water.
              I become less tired each time around the track.

Behaviors: I will stop eating when I feel full.
              I will not speak until the anger passes.
              My mind will stay alert during classes and exams.

Be creative in designing your own mantra and spend time each day reciting it internally while in a quiet state. You can be a skeptic and the mantra will still work.

Quieting the mind is healthy, and meditation is a way to accomplish that. Focused awareness can be achieved in a number of ways, and there are many different kinds of meditation. *Zen meditation* (zazen) involves sitting still with legs crossed while trying to empty the mind of its chatter. *Transcendental meditation* teaches practitioners to focus on a particular phrase (called a **mantra**) that is repeated internally; focusing the mind's attention on a single phrase excludes other random thoughts. *Insight meditation* (Vipassana) teaches meditators simply to observe the flow of thoughts that pass through the mind with detachment. Buddhists, especially Tibetan Buddhists, often meditate by focusing their attention on a religious image (called a **mandala**). Prayer is a form of meditation in that it focuses awareness on God. Thus, meditation is something that everyone has experienced even if they have not called it meditation.

Meditation does not have to be done in a religious setting, nor is it complicated. To begin meditating, follow these simple suggestions:

- Choose a quiet place in your home or outside.
- Find a comfortable sitting position with your back straight. (Lying down is not recommended because it is strongly associated with sleep.)
- Be sure that you have at least 10 to 30 minutes during which you will not be disturbed.
- A good way to begin meditation is to focus your attention on breathing. Begin by becoming aware of the way you are breathing. Is it slow and deep? Is it quick and shallow? Is it through one nostril or both?

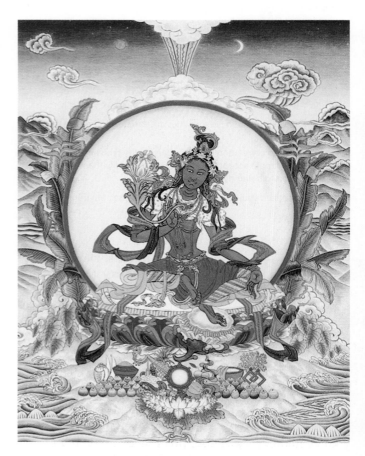

A mandala is a complex visual image used to focus attention and facilitate meditation. ("Green Tara," an original painting by Maile Yawata)

🧘 Managing Stress

Relaxation with Music

Many people know that listening to or playing music can be relaxing. Music can focus the mind just as meditation, hypnosis, and prayer do. Thus, listening or playing music can reduce stress. In medical settings, music can help patients lessen anxiety and stress. One study found that patients undergoing surgery were just as likely to be calmed by music as by sedative drugs (Berbel, Moix, & Quintana, 2007). Music can help reduce the chronic pain that accompanies rheumatoid arthritis, herniated discs, or fibromyalgia. Music can help those who have experienced stroke, Alzheimer's, and other neurological diseases.

The kind of music that people find helpful varies according to individuals' preferences. In general, soft music is preferred to loud; gentle rhythms and moderate beats that approximate the heart rate (65–75 beats per minute) are preferred to vigorous or complex rhythms and fast beats. The "background music" found in doctors' and dentists' offices is known to reduce heart and breathing rates and reduce anxiety.

To use music as a therapy for insomnia, pain, stress, anxiety, or other problem, use the following guidelines:

- Choose music that you enjoy and find relaxing. Many types of classical music, soft jazz, Celtic and Native American music, and chants are suitable. Most people prefer music with flowing rhythms.
- Pick a time and place where you will not be disturbed and can let go of daily concerns. Plan to spend at least an hour in a relaxed state.
- You can listen at low volume or may feel more comfortable using ear-cupping headphones that reduce outside noise and distractions.
- Consider consulting a music therapist for additional advice and help.

Gradually try to breathe by using your stomach muscles to move your diaphragm. Some people recommend the 4/7/8 pattern of breathing—inhale through the nose for a count of 4, hold for a count of 7, and exhale for a count of 8 through pursed lips. If this sequence is not comfortable, make up your own and focus on taking each breath the same way.

Practice this meditation twice a day, particularly if you are upset, tired, or in pain. Once you are comfortable with a breathing meditation, you may want to explore other forms of meditation. Meditation has many documented health benefits—lowered blood pressure, decreased heart rates, less stress, increased blood flow, reduced pain, and relief of many chronic conditions such as asthma, arthritis, and irritable bowel syndrome.

The faster the world becomes, the more we need to slow down.

The Power of Suggestion

Any time the mind becomes focused and relaxed, it also becomes more open to suggestion. This can be very beneficial or it can create problems, depending on the kind of suggestions being received by the mind. Suggestions given as warnings, especially to children who are particularly vulnerable to suggestion, can affect behaviors and cause health problems throughout life. For example, here are some common admonitions given to children that can cause health problems because young children *believe* what they are told.

- Put on your boots when you go out in the snow or you will catch cold.
- If you keep eating cookies, you'll get fat.
- If you don't try harder, you'll be a failure in life.
- If you climb those trees, you'll fall and get hurt.
- If you go out at night, the ghosts will get you.

Each of these suggestions predicts a negative outcome. To a child's mind, which is usually in a trancelike, suggestible state, these negative suggestions become fixed in the unconscious mind and may have a harmful effect even many years later.

The mind can be made more open to suggestion by many things we are exposed to in daily life. For example, movies and television focus attention with both images and sound. As a consequence, they can induce a trancelike state and cause us to cry, laugh, and become angry or upset; they can actually manipulate our emotions through light and sound. No one dies on a movie screen, but we often react as if they did. The violence and horror people watch in movies and on TV often do affect both physical and emotional states. As a result of watching some frightening scene, people may actually become sick days, weeks, or years later when something reminds the subconscious mind of the scene and brings back the fear.

Advertisers know how to take advantage of viewers' suggestible, hypnotic states of mind. Television programs usually are interrupted at an emotional peak in the story by advertising a product while viewers are still in a suggestible state of mind. Many people believe they are not influenced by advertising, but marketing studies indicate otherwise. Most advertisers try to persuade people to buy products they usually do not need. It is important to become more aware of how suggestible you are and to

TERMS

mandala: an artistic, religious design used as an object of meditation

mantra: a sound or phrase that is repeated in the mind to help produce a meditative state

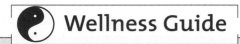

Wellness Guide

Using Your Mind to Improve Health

- Become more aware of the power your mind has to improve health, hasten healing, and help you perform better in school and in other activities. Belief in yourself, in prayer, or in a particular treatment can facilitate healing and help prevent sickness.

- Use mental images that feel right to you to reduce exam anxiety and to improve performance in sports or other activities. Avoid negative mental images and thoughts such as "I feel lousy," or "I'm too tired to run," or "I just know I can't

do that." Use your mind to create positive images and thoughts. You can reverse what seems to be a "bad" day by suggesting to yourself that things are going to change and improve.

- Practice a daily mental relaxation technique in a place that is comfortable and quiet. Use the time to "talk" to your body to promote healing or to change behaviors. Visualize scenes from the past or the future that you know are healthy and constructive. As you become more adept at using your mind, you will find new ways to use mental relaxation in all aspects of your life. (*Notice how we inserted a positive suggestion.*)

protect yourself from both obvious and subtle suggestions that can damage your health and peace of mind.

Image Visualization

One of the most effective ways to promote wellness and change undesirable behaviors is through the use of **image visualization.** Many mind–body healing techniques employ some form of image visualization. For example, frightening scenes from the past, especially from early childhood, can be reexperienced while a person is in a state of mental relaxation brought on by hypnosis or some other technique. As the scenes and emotional upsets are visualized in the mind, they can be reinterpreted and reprogrammed to change their negative effects on health and behaviors. Mental imagery can also be used to reduce pain; hasten healing; improve performance in sports; change smoking, drinking, or eating behaviors; and help control compulsive urges to gamble. At one time or another in our lives, we all daydream or run an "internal movie," fantasizing our hopes and fears. During such fantasies we visualize experiences and create feelings. Image visualization can change body temperature, blood flow, heartbeat, breathing rate, production of hormones, and other body processes regulated by the brain.

Most psychologists who work with athletes to improve physical performance use image visualization. The so-called inner games of tennis, golf, skiing, and skating are based on image visualization. Baseball players in a batting slump use relaxation and visualization to "see" themselves getting hits. Basketball players use the technique to "see" their free throws going cleanly through the hoop.

Image visualization is also the secret to improved sexual responses and enjoyment. Sexual arousal begins in the mind, and negative thoughts or fears can stifle the sexual responses. The sex organs are particularly sensitive to images generated in the mind. Most sex therapists use relaxation techniques and image visualization to help clients improve their sexual experiences. Tension related to sexual performance is usually the

main reason for not experiencing the desired sexual sensations. In all areas of your life, begin to use your mental powers more to enhance health and improve performance in daily tasks.

Taking Time Out to Quiet the Mind

Most of us live pretty hectic lives that are full of time pressures and mental stress. Most young people either go to school, work at a job, or do both. In addition to school and work, students engage in extracurricular activities, sports, concerts, cell phone conversations, computer chat rooms, video games, movies, television—the list goes on and on. To do all these things requires a healthy mind and body. Usually, health is something young people take for granted until it disappears. But staying healthy, even when you are young, means finding time to be quiet, to silence stressful thoughts, and to alleviate tensions in the body.

There are many ways to quiet down, and some suggestions and techniques have been presented in this chapter. But the best ones are the ones that you discover for yourself. Find a quiet spot in a park or in your yard where you can sit and reflect on the good things in your life. Forget for a time the problems of the world and what you need to accomplish in life. Just notice things around you, especially the small things. Watching an ant carry a bit of food twice its size is a good thing to do. Looking at the pattern of stars in the night sky is a good thing to do. Experiencing the freshness of new snow and the taste of rain is a good thing to do. Just be quiet as often as you can. It's good for your mental and physical health.

TERMS

image visualization: use of mental images to promote healing and change behaviors

Critical Thinking About Health

1. Identify one time in your life when you have been seriously ill (not counting colds or minor injuries). Describe the nature of the illness and the time it took to become well again. Discuss all of the factors that you think may have contributed to your becoming sick, including stress, emotional problems, poor nutrition, and so forth. Then discuss all of the factors that you believe contributed to your becoming well again, including medical care, prayer, alternative medicines, and other factors. What were the most important factors that led to your becoming sick? What were the most important ones in the healing process?

2. Find a selection of medical journals in the library and look at the drug company advertisements. Try to locate ones that show a comparison of the drug's effectiveness with a placebo. Determine how effective the placebo was from the data given (usually shown in a graph). Then compare the effectiveness of the drug with the placebo. If the placebo was effective, explain why you think it was so effective in this instance. Give your views on whether doctors should prescribe a placebo pill for some conditions before prescribing an active drug.

3. What is the role of religion/spirituality in health? To what degree should religion/spirituality be part of the clinical encounter between patient and physician?

4. Describe any experiences you have had with meditation, hypnosis, yoga, *qigong*, image visualization, or any other form of mental focusing and relaxation. Describe how you became involved with this activity and for what purpose you used it. Did it help you solve a particular health or emotional problem? Would you recommend this technique to others?

Health in Review

- The human mind can cause changes in body chemistry through thoughts and feelings, which may have a positive or negative effect on your health.
- Optimal health is achieved when the mind and body communicate harmoniously.
- The unconscious regulation of all vital processes in the body is called homeostasis.
- Disease can be regarded as disruption of homeostasis or disruption of the harmonious interaction of mind and body.
- The mind and organs of the body communicate continuously via the autonomic nervous system, which maintains vital body functions such as heart rate, level of blood sugar, and temperature.
- Psychosomatic illnesses are physical symptoms caused by stress, anxiety, and emotional upsets.
- Somatization disorders are caused by psychosocial problems.

- The placebo effect often is almost as powerful as drugs in treating symptoms of illness.
- Religious activity is often associated with a healthier lifestyle.
- Hypnosis and meditation can play a positive role in healing illnesses.
- Belief, faith, and suggestion all have the power to heal because the mind can change disturbed body functions and reestablish homeostasis.
- A key to maintaining or improving health and wellness is to learn and practice a mental relaxation technique.
- Image visualization can be used to reduce anxiety and stress, modify behaviors, and enhance performance.
- Virtual reality therapies use computer software to treat phobias and severe pain.

Health and Wellness Online

The Web contains a wealth of information about health and wellness. By accessing the Internet using Web browser software, you can gain a new perspective on many topics presented in *Health and Wellness,* Tenth Edition. Access the Jones and Bartlett Publishers Web site at **health.jbpub.com/hwonline.**

References

Astin, J. S., et al. (2003). Mind–body medicine: State of the science, implications for practice. *Journal of the American Board of Family Practice, 167,* 131–147.

Bennett, M. P., et al. (2004). The effect of mirthful laughter on stress and natural killer cell activity. *Alternative Therapies in Health and Medicine, 9,* 38–45.

Benson, H., & Klipper, M. (2000). *The relaxation response.* New York: HarperCollins.

Benson, H., et al. (2006). Study of the therapeutic effects of intercessory prayer (STEP) in cardiac bypass patients: A multicenter randomized trial of uncertainty and certainty of receiving intercessory prayer. *American Heart Journal, 15,* 934–942.

Christie, W., & Moore, C. (2005). The impact of humor on patients with cancer. *Clinical Journal of Oncologic Nursing, 9,* 211–218.

Davidson, R. J., et al. (2003). Alterations in brain and immune function produced by mindfulness meditation. *Psychosomatic Medicine, 65,* 564–570.

Hewlett, C. (1994). Killed by a word. *Lancet, 344,* 695.

Hoffman, H. G. (2004, August). Virtual reality therapy. *Scientific American,* 58–65.

Lutgendorf, S. K., et al. (2004). Religious participation, interleukin-6, and mortality in older adults. *Health Psychology, 23,* 465–475.

MacLean, C. D., et al. (2003). Patient preference for physician discussion and practice of spirituality. *Journal of General Internal Medicine, 18,* 38–43.

Mayberg, H. S., et al. (2002). The functional neuroanatomy of the placebo effect. *American Journal of Psychiatry, 5,* 728–735.

Mayo Clinic. (2008). Biofeedback: Using your mind to improve your health. Retrieved January 30, 2009, from http://www.mayoclinic.com/health/biofeedback/SA00083

McCauley, J., et al., (2005). Spiritual beliefs and barriers among managed care practitioners. *Journal of Religion and Health, 44,* 137–146.

Nash, M. R. (2001, June). The truth and hype of hypnosis. *Scientific American,* 37–54.

Sloan, R. P., et al. (2001). Should physicians prescribe religious activities? *New England Journal of Medicine, 342,* 1913–1916.

Steptoe, A., Wardle, J., & Marmot, M. (2005). Positive affect and health-related neuroendocrine, cardiovascular, and inflammatory processes. *Proceedings of the National Academy of Sciences, 102,* 6508–6512.

Strawbridge, W. J., et al. (2001). Religious attendance increases survival by improving and maintaining good health behaviors, mental health, and social relationships. *Annals of Behavioral Medicine, 23,* 68–74.

Sutherland, G., Andersen, M. B., & Morris, T. (2005). Relaxation and health-related quality of life in multiple sclerosis: The example of autogenic training. *Journal of Behavioral Medicine, 28,* 249–256.

Thacker, P. D. (2003). Fake worlds offer real medicine. *Journal of the American Medical Association, 290,* 2107–2112.

Wager, T. D., et al. (2004). Placebo-induced changes in fMRI in the anticipation and experience of pain. *Science, 303,* 1162–1167.

Suggested Readings

Benedetti, F. (2007). Placebo and endogenous mechanisms of analgesia. *Handbook of Experimental Pharmacology, 17*, 393–413.

Berbel, P., Moix, J., & Quintana, S. (2007). Music versus diazepam to reduce preoperative anxiety: A randomized controlled clinical trial. *Revista Española de Anestesiología y Reanimación, 54*, 355–358.

Christensen, D. (2001, February 3). Medicinal mimicry. *Science News,* 74–78. Describes some of the experiments aimed at understanding placebo effects and discusses some of the concerns about their use.

Cohen, K. S. (1997). *The way of qigong.* New York: Ballantine. The definitive guide to *qigong*—what it is, how it works, and what it can do for you.

Dalai Lama. (2005). *The universe in a single atom: The convergence of science and spirituality.* New York: Morgan Road Books. The spiritual head of one of the world's oldest religions, Buddhism, explains why he does not see any conflict between spirituality and science.

Gillum, R. F., et al. (2008). Frequency of attendance at religious services and mortality in a U.S. national cohort. *Annals of Epidemiology, 18*, 124–129.

Hendricks, G. (1995). *Conscious breathing.* New York: Bantam Books. Explains the benefits of breathing meditations and describes many advanced techniques for practicing conscious breathing.

LeShan, L. (1999). *How to meditate.* Boston: Back Bay Books. A good introduction to the practice of meditation and its benefits.

Ludwig, D. S., & Kabat-Zinn, J. (2008). Mindfulness in medicine. *Journal of the American Medical Association, 300*, 1350–1352. The authors review studies showing the beneficial effects of meditation on health and healing.

Lutz, A., et al. (2008). Regulation of the neural circuitry of emotion by compassion meditation: Effects of meditative expertise. *PLoS ONE, 3*, e1897.

Miu, A. C., Heilman, R. M., & Miclea, M. (2009). Reduced heart rate variability and vagal tone in anxiety: Trait versus state, and the effects of autogenic training. *Autonomic Neuroscience, 145*, 99–103.

Nash, M. R. (2001, June). The truth and hype of hypnosis. *Scientific American,* 37–54. A good introduction to our scientific understanding of hypnosis.

Thacker, P. D. (2003). Fake worlds offer real medicine. *Journal of the American Medical Association, 290*, 2107–2112. How virtual reality therapy is being used to treat medical problems.

Thompson, G. (2005). *The placebo effect and health: Combining science and compassionate care.* Amherst, NY: Prometheus Books. The author provides a comprehensive examination of the placebo effect.

Recommended Web Sites

Please visit **health.jbpub.com/hwonline** for links to these Web sites.

Audio Relaxation Cassettes
Dr. Emmett E. Miller presents articles on mental well-being and sells audiocassettes on image visualization, self-hypnosis, and many aspects of wellness and healing.

Meditation
Descriptions of several kinds of meditation practices.

Study Help
The University of Toronto's suggestions for mastering academic skills and reducing stress from classes and studying.

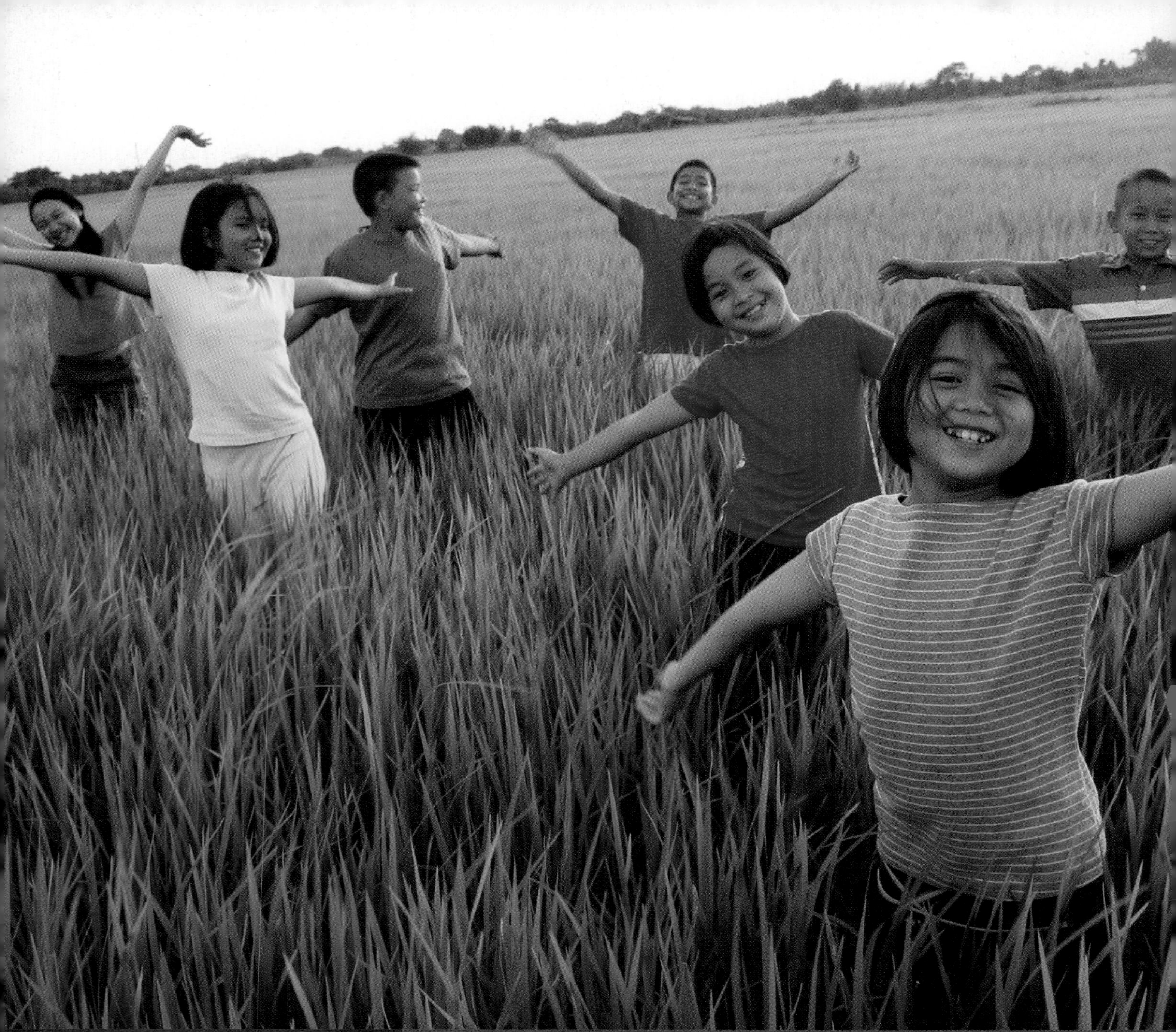

Health and Wellness Online: health.jbpub.com/hwonline

Study Guide and Self-Assessment

3.1 My Stressors
3.2 My Stress Reactions
3.3 How Susceptible Am I to Stress?
3.4 Warning Signs of Stress
3.5 My Life Changes and Stress
3.6 Prioritizing Tasks: First Things First
3.7 Time Audit for Time Management
3.8 Are You a Procrastinator?
3.9 Minimizing In-Class Listening Errors
3.10 Image Visualization for Exam Anxiety

Chapter Three

Managing Stress: Restoring Mind–Body Harmony

Learning Objectives

1. Define the terms *stress, stressor, eustress,* and *distress.*

2. Describe the environmental, mental, and emotional components of stress.

3. Describe the physiological components of stress.

4. Describe four ways that stress causes illness.

5. Define problem-focused and emotion-focused coping.

6. Explain how college students can manage overload and practice time management and test management.

Health Instructor (to class): What stresses you?

Student 1: Not enough money.

Student 2: My relationship. It's like a 5-unit class.

Student 3: Econ pop quizzes.

Student 4: No, all tests.

Student 5: All of that!

College students are very familiar with stress, its associated feelings of being overwhelmed, anxiety, frustration, anger, and depression, and the sleeplessness, fatigue, gastrointestinal upset, headache, muscular tension, increased susceptibility to infections, and the invitations to engage in unhealthy behaviors (e.g., smoking, drinking) stress can engender.

> She would rather light a thousand candles than curse the darkness.
>
> *Adlai Stevenson (Eulogy for Eleanor Roosevelt)*

Stress is a disruption in one's psychobiological balance and sense of harmony within oneself and/or with the social and physical environments. The experience of stress is unpleasant, so when we become stressed, we try to regain psychological and physical balance. If we are successful, not only do we feel better, but we also gain confidence in our ability to handle stress in the future. If we are not successful, however, and stress is prolonged or severe, we may fee helpless become fatigued, worn out, and sick (**Table 3.1**).

In this chapter we discuss stress and suggest ways to reduce it.

How Stress Occurs

Stress results from the interplay of environmental situations and life events and the mental (cognitive), emotional, and physical reactions to those occurrences (**Figure 3.1**). Stress experts define stress as "a relationship between the person and the environment that is

Table 3.1

Disorders That Can Be Caused or Aggravated by Stress

Gastrointestinal disorders	*Musculoskeletal disorders*
Constipation	Rheumatoid arthritis
Diarrhea	Low back pain
Duodenal ulcer	Migraine headache
Ulcerative colitis	Muscle tension
Respiratory disorders	*Metabolic disorders*
Asthma	Hyperthyroidism
Hay fever	Hypothyroidism
Tuberculosis	Diabetes
Colds	Overweight
Flu	Metabolic syndrome
Skin disorders	*Cardiovascular disorders*
Eczema	Coronary artery disease
Pruritus	Essential hypertension
Urticaria	Congestive heart failure
Psoriasis	*Menstrual irregularities*
Eating disorders	*Cancer*
Depression	*Accident proneness*

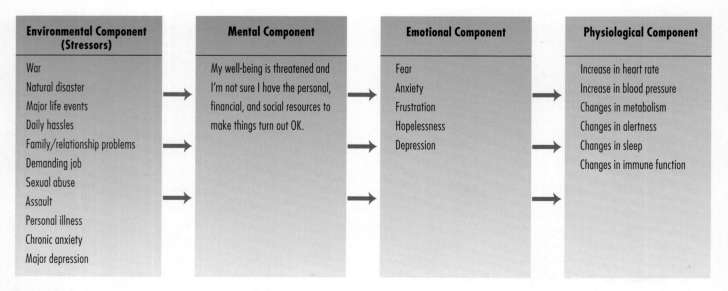

Environmental Component (Stressors)	Mental Component	Emotional Component	Physiological Component
War	My well-being is threatened and I'm not sure I have the personal, financial, and social resources to make things turn out OK.	Fear	Increase in heart rate
Natural disaster		Anxiety	Increase in blood pressure
Major life events		Frustration	Changes in metabolism
Daily hassles		Hopelessness	Changes in alertness
Family/relationship problems		Depression	Changes in sleep
Demanding job			Changes in immune function
Sexual abuse			
Assault			
Personal illness			
Chronic anxiety			
Major depression			

■ **Figure 3.1**

The Components of Stress

Stress results from the interplay of potentially stressful environmental situations and life events and the mental (cognitive), emotional, and physiological reactions to those occurrences.

appraised by the person as taxing or exceeding his or her resources and endangering his or her well-being" (Folkman, 1984). In other words, stress comes from thinking, "This situation puts my well-being at risk and I'm not sure I have the personal, social, economic, or physical resources to meet this challenge and come out OK."

The Environmental Component of Stress

The environmental component of stress consists of situations and events that bring about stress, which are called **stressors.** They can be the day-to-day hassles and complexities that block the efficient and timely accomplishment of daily life tasks, family problems, unpleasant interactions with other people, job/school problems, major external events (war, flood, famine), and major life changes and events (see the Wellness Guide feature "Assessing Life Changes") that become obstacles to achieving desired life goals, or positive experiences, such as starting a new love relationship or graduating from college, which, although positive, can be taxing. In general, stressful situations can be classified into these types:

> **Harm-and-loss situations,** which include death of a loved one, theft or damage to one's property, physical injury or loss of a body part, physical assault, or loss of self-esteem.
>
> **Threat situations,** which are perceived as likely to produce harm or loss whether any harm or loss actually occurs. The experience is one of continually watching for and warding off potential dangers.
>
> **Challenge situations,** which are perceived as opportunities for growth, mastery, and gain. The stress that comes from challenging situations is called **eustress** (positive stress), as opposed to **distress** (negative stress) that accompanies harm, loss, and threat.

The Mental Component of Stress

The mental component of stress consists of (1) the appraisal of a situation as absolutely or potentially damaging to one's physical or psychological well-being or a threat to one's survival, and (2) believing that one's personal resources are insufficient to ward off or overcome the threat to one's well-being. The situation can be real, such as breaking up in a relationship, or imagined, such as the possibility of a pop quiz that may or may not happen.

The degree to which a situation is appraised as stressful depends on an individual's psychological makeup. Everyone interprets the world and events differently. Thus, a situation that is upsetting and stressful to one person may not even bother another.

The Emotional Component of Stress

The emotional component of stress consists of unpleasant emotions that arise from one's appraisal of

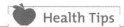 Health Tips

Warning Signs of Stress

Although stress is pervasive in the life of a college student, it is not always easy to recognize when stress has become a threat to physical or mental health. If you experience any of these signs of stress, it's time to make some changes in your life, and perhaps seek professional help to reduce the stress.
- Trouble falling asleep
- Difficulty staying asleep
- Waking up tired and not well rested
- Changes in eating patterns
- Craving sweet/fatty/salty ("comfort") foods
- More headaches than usual
- Short temper or irritability
- Recurring colds and minor illness
- Muscle ache and/or tightness
- Trouble concentrating, remembering, or staying organized
- Depression

a situation as harmful or threatening and that one's resources for protection are limited or uncertain. These emotions are anxiety, fear, frustration, anger, and depression.

Factors Affecting the Experience of Stress

Several factors influence the degree of stress a person experiences. Among them are predictability, personal control, belief in the outcome, and social support.

Predictability Knowing when a stressful situation will occur produces less stress than not knowing. This is because knowing when a stressful event will occur (like taking an exam) allows a person to relax in the interim, whereas not knowing puts a person on constant alert (like having to face pop quizzes). For example, people whose employment status is secure have less stress than people who must worry constantly about losing their jobs

TERMS

challenge situations: positive events that may involve major life transitions and may cause stress

distress: stress resulting from unpleasant stressors

eustress: stress resulting from pleasant stressors

harm-and-loss situations: stressful events that include death, loss of property, injury, and illness

stress: the sum of physical and emotional reactions to any stimulus that disturbs the harmony of body and mind

stressor: any physical or psychological situation that produces stress

threat situations: events that cause stress because of a perception that harm or loss may occur

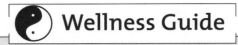

Wellness Guide

Assessing Life Changes

Stress researchers have developed methods to identify and measure the potential for life experiences to cause stress. One such method is the Recent Life Changes Questionnaire (RLCQ), which contains a list of 74 life events that are common stressors among Americans (**Table 3.2**). Each life event on the

RLCQ is associated with a number of life change units (LCUs), which represent the relative amount of psychological and physiological adjustment required to meet the challenge of the particular life event. Accumulation of 300 LCUs within six months or 500 LCUs within one year indicates a high degree of recent life stress and an increased risk of illness or injury.

Table 3.2

The Recent Life Changes Questionnaire

Life event	Life change units		Life event	Life change units	
	Women	Men		Women	Men
Death of son or daughter	135	103	Moderate illness	47	39
Death of spouse	122	113	Loss or damage of personal property	47	35
Death of brother or sister	111	87	Sexual difficulties	44	44
Death of parent	105	90	Getting demoted at work	44	39
Divorce	102	85	Major change in living conditions	44	37
Death of family member	96	78	Increase in income	43	30
Fired from work	85	69	Relationship problems	42	34
Separation from spouse due to marital problems	79	70	Trouble with in-laws	41	33
Major injury or illness	79	64	Beginning or ending school or college	40	35
Being held in jail	78	71	Making a major purchase	40	33
Pregnancy	74	55	New, close personal relationship	39	34
Miscarriage or abortion	74	51	Outstanding personal achievement	38	33
Death of a close friend	73	64	Troubles with coworkers at work	37	32
Laid off from work	73	59	Change in school or college	37	31
Birth of a child	71	56	Change in your work hours or conditions	36	32
Adopting a child	71	54	Troubles with workers whom you supervise	35	34
Major business adjustment	67	47	Getting a transfer at work	33	31
Decrease in income	66	49	Getting a promotion at work	33	29
Parents' divorce	63	52	Change in religious beliefs	31	27
A relative moving in with you	62	53	Christmas	30	25
Foreclosure on a mortgage or a loan	62	51	Having more responsibilities at work	29	29
Investment and/or credit difficulties	62	46	Troubles with your boss at work	29	29
Marital reconciliation	61	48	Major change in usual type or amount of recreation	29	28
Major change in health or behavior of family member	58	50	General work troubles	29	27
Change in arguments with spouse	55	41	Change in social activities	29	24
Retirement	54	48	Major change in eating habits	29	23
Major decision regarding your immediate future	54	46	Major change in sleeping habits	28	23
Separation from spouse due to work	53	54	Change in family get-togethers	28	20
An accident	53	38	Change in personal habits	27	24
Parental remarriage	52	45	Major dental work	27	23
Change residence to a different town, city, or state	52	39	Change of residence in same town or city	27	21
Change to a new type of work	51	50	Change in political beliefs	26	21
"Falling out" of a close personal relationship	50	41	Vacation	26	20
Marriage	50	50	Having fewer responsibilities at work	22	21
Spouse changes work	50	38	Making a moderate purchase	22	18
Child leaving home	48	38	Change in church activities	21	20
Birth of grandchild	48	34	Minor violation of the law	20	19
Engagement to marry	47	42	Correspondence course to help you in your work	19	16

Source: Adapted from Miller, M. A., and Rahe, R. H. (1997). Life changes scaling for the 1990s. *Journal of Psychosomatic Research, 43,* 279–292, with permission from Elsevier Science.

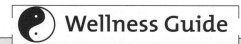 **Wellness Guide**

The Powerful General and the Monk

The powerful general and his army arrived at the border of a neighboring country. Scouts were sent into the countryside to reconnoiter. After a time a scout returned. Throwing himself off his horse, he knelt at the powerful general's feet and bowed his head.

"What is your report?" barked the powerful general.

"Master," replied the scout. "Hearing that your magnificent and powerful armies have landed, all for miles around have fled."

The powerful general stood proudly and smiled. The scout looked up ever so meekly and continued, "Except the monk."

"What?!?"

"Yes, sire, except the monk. He has not fled."

"Where is this foolish monk?" bellowed the powerful general.

The scout looked up. "In the village, sire, not 15 minutes' ride from here. He is in his hut at the top of the hill."

The powerful general, by now enraged, strapped on his sword and armor, mounted his massive white horse, and galloped south along the coast road. At the village he sped up the hill and quickly dismounted in front of the monk's hut. Drawing his sword from its scabbard, the powerful general burst into the hut. There, a small man in clean but tattered robes, with a shaved head, was sitting on a cushion, meditating.

The powerful general placed the tip of his sword at the monk's throat, and in his deepest, most commanding voice said, "You dare not flee before my powerful armies? Do you realize I could run you through with my sword without blinking an eye?"

The monk opened his eyes, looked at the general, and said, "Do you realize that I could let you run me through with your sword without blinking an eye?"

The powerful general thought for a moment. Then he put the sword back in its scabbard, bowed to the monk, and rode away.

---

have (Ferrie et al., 2005). During World War II, London was bombed every night, but the London suburbs were not. Londoners had fewer ulcers than suburbanites, presumably because they knew when bombings would occur.

Personal Control Individuals who believe they can influence the course of their lives are likely to experience less stress than are individuals who believe that their fate is determined by factors outside of their control. The crucial factor is belief in one's ability to control situations and not whether control is actually possible. For example, people who have jobs that involve a lot of pressure to perform but allow them little opportunity for deciding how the tasks are to be accomplished have more stress than workers who have more control over decisions have (Orth-Gomér, 2007).

Belief in the Outcome People who believe that things are likely to improve (optimists) experience less stress than do people who believe that things will get worse (pessimists).

Social Support Having someone to talk to and believing that the person can help manage a stressor by providing physical, emotional, or intellectual help lessens stress (Graham et al., 2007). For example, heart attack patients experience less stress if they have social support (Lett et al., 2007). Also, patients who talk to their surgeons about their fears of an impending surgery have a smaller stress response than patients who go through such procedures feeling uninformed and unsupported do.

The Physiological Component of Stress

The physiological component of stress consists of automatic physiological responses to real or imagined situations that are considered damaging or threatening. One physiological response to stress is called the **fight-or-flight response (Figure 3.2)**. Its purpose is to prepare an individual to deal with a stressor by confronting it (fight) or running away or avoiding it (flight). The fight-or-flight response involves the coordinated activation of the autonomic nervous system and the release of adrenaline (also called epinephrine) from the adrenal glands (located in the thorax above the kidneys). Stress activation of the autonomic nervous system elevates the heart rate and blood pressure (to provide more blood to muscles), constricts the blood vessels of the skin (to limit bleeding if wounded), dilates the pupil of the eye (to let in more light, thereby improving vision), increases activity in the reticular formation of the brain (to increase the alert, aroused state), liberates glucose and free fatty acids from body storage sites (to make energy available to the muscles, brain, and other tissues and organs), and activates certain immune cells to prepare to defend the body if it is wounded.

A second physiological response to stress is activation of the **hypothalamo-pituitary-adrenal (HPA) axis (Figure 3.3)**. The thought that one is in a stressful situation causes the hypothalamus of the brain to release a hormone called corticotrophin releasing factor (CRF).

> ## TERMS
>
> **fight-or-flight response:** a defensive reaction that prepares the organism for conflict or escape by triggering hormonal, cardiovascular, metabolic, and other changes
>
> **hypothalamo-pituitary-adrenal (HPA) axis:** a coordinated physiological response to stress involving the hypothalamus of the brain and the pituitary and adrenal glands

■ **Figure 3.2**

The Fight-or-Flight Response
All humans display this response when confronted with challenges they interpret as frightening or threatening.

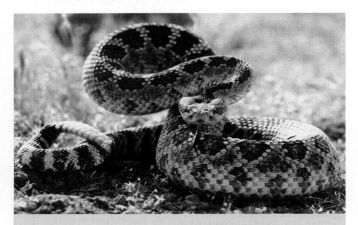

Heart	**Intestines**
Increases in heart rate and force of contractions	Decreased motility and relaxation of sphincters
Blood	**Skin**
Constriction in abdominal viscera and dilation in skeletal muscles	Contraction of pilomotor muscles and contraction of sweat glands
Eye	**Spleen**
Contraction of radial muscle of iris and relaxation of ciliary muscle	Contraction
	Brain
	Activation of reticular formation

This hormone stimulates the pituitary gland (located at the base of the brain) to release a hormone called ACTH into the bloodstream. ACTH circulates in the blood and stimulates the pair of adrenal glands to release into the blood yet another hormone called cortisol. In the immediate (acute) response to stress, this hormone circulates in the blood, causing tissues to respond to the stressor, generally by providing energy for confrontation (fight) or avoidance (flight), for fighting infection, and for healing wounds. However, in the extended (chronic) response to stress, this hormone alters metabolism, contributing to overweight and type 2 diabetes; suppresses the immune system, thereby increasing susceptibility to infections and cancer; weakens bones; impairs memory; and worsens depression (Dhabhar & McEwan, 2007).

The fight-or-flight response and activation of the HPA axis are designed for short-term (minutes to hours) management of a stressful situation. If the individual can think differently or do something to change the perception that the situation is overwhelmingly threatening, stress activation of the nervous system and the secretion of stress hormones stop and the person's mind and body return to balance. This can be accomplished by attempting to change the stressful situation, changing one's interpretation of it, or thinking that the situation is manageable rather than overwhelming. If nothing changes, however, and the stress response continues, then a person can feel anxious, depressed, irritable, fatigued, and burned out, and the risks of becoming both mentally and physically ill increase.

■ **Figure 3.3**

The Hypothalamo-Pituitary-Adrenal Axis
Stressful thoughts trigger the release of a hormone called corticotrophin releasing factor (CRF) from the hypothalamus of the brain. CRF flows in the bloodstream to the pituitary gland, where it stimulates the release of the hormone ACTH. ACTH flows in the bloodstream to the adrenal glands, where it stimulates the release of cortisol and other stress hormones. In acute stress, cortisol helps prepare the body for fight, flight, wound healing, and infection. In chronic stress, cortisol unbalances metabolism and suppresses the immune system.

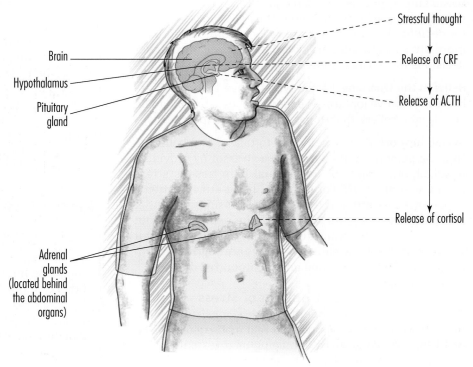

🌐 Global Wellness

Overwork Causes Death in Japan

Stress not only can increase a person's susceptibility to infections and sickness, but also can cause death, as recognized in Japan. Many people in Japan work long hours and sometimes are asked to take on more work than they can handle. The stress from overwork can raise blood pressure, lower immune system functioning, and cause changes in some people's bodies that result in sudden death. In Japan, sudden death from overwork is called *karoshi*.

In 1987 the Japanese Labor Ministry officially recognized karoshi (overwork) as a cause of death. Between 2002 and 2005, the ministry reported approximately 300 cases of karoshi, but the actual number of deaths from overwork is thought to be about 10,000. Families who have lost someone to karoshi can sue the employer who imposed the stressful workload. In 2006, for example, one of Toyota's top automotive engineers who was working on the Camry hybrid died from a heart attack. In June 2008, a Japanese labor court ruled that he died of karoshi and that his family was entitled to compensation.

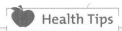

🍎 Health Tips

Worry, Worry, Worry: How to Stop Stressful Thoughts

If you have the same worrisome thought over and over, try this:

1. *Stop the thought* when you realize you are having it. Say to yourself, "There's that worry again. Stop!"
2. *Replace the thought* with a more positive thought.

Here's an example: A student realizes that when he looks at his watch to see how much time remains on a test, he immediately has the thought "There's not enough time." This thought comes over and over again, stressing him and disrupting his focus. He learns thought-stopping. The next time this occurs, he *stops.* He puts down his pencil, closes his eyes, takes a deep breath, and says to himself, "There's that thought again. I'm going to relax and stop it." A few seconds later the thought is gone, his mind is clear, and he returns to the exam.

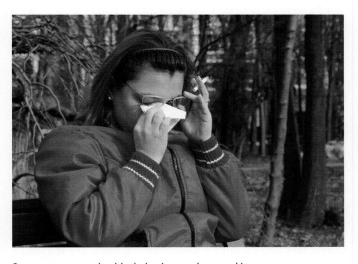

Stress can cause unhealthy behaviors, such as smoking.

How Stress Contributes to Illness

Stress contributes to illness by (1) causing the mind and body to become exhausted, worn down, and damaged, (2) weakening immunity, and (3) motivating unhealthy behaviors in an attempt to deal with stress (**Figure 3.4**). Some people who have been exposed to a life-threatening, traumatic experience, such as a car crash or combat, can develop posttraumatic stress disorder (PTSD), unpleasant and often debilitating symptoms that persist for months and years after the traumatic experience (discussed later in this chapter).

> Heavy thoughts bring on physical maladies; when the soul is oppressed so is the body.
> *Martin Luther*

The General Adaptation Syndrome

Continual physiological response to stressors can bring about a three-stage biological response called the **general adaptation syndrome (GAS)** (**Figure 3.5**).

1. *Stage of alarm:* A person's ability to withstand or resist any type of stressor is lowered by the need to deal with the stressor, whether it is a burn, a broken arm, the loss of a loved one, the fear of failing a class, or losing a job.
2. *Stage of resistance:* The body adapts to the continued presence of the stressor by producing more epinephrine, raising blood pressure, increasing alertness, suppressing the immune system, and tensing muscles. If interaction with the stressor is prolonged, the ability to resist becomes depleted.
3. *Stage of exhaustion:* When the ability to resist is depleted, the person becomes ill. Because many

TERMS

general adaptation syndrome (GAS): a three-phase biological response to stress

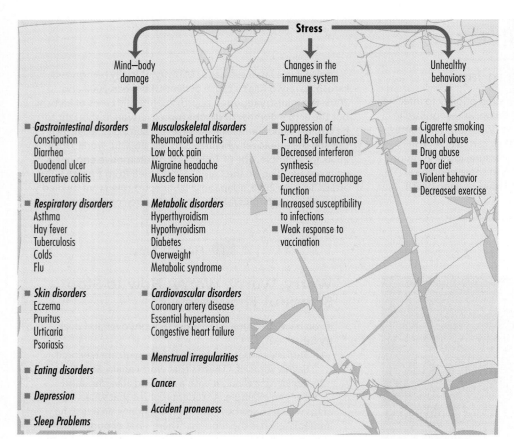

■ **Figure 3.4**

The Stress–Illness Relationship
Stress contributes to illness by causing the mind and body to become exhausted, worn down, and damaged; by weakening immunity; and by fostering unhealthy behaviors.

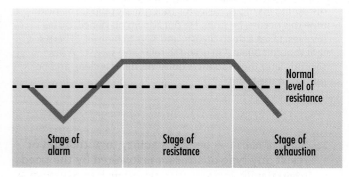

■ **Figure 3.5**

The General Adaptation Syndrome
In the stage of alarm, the body's normal resistance to stress is lowered from the first interactions with the stressor. In the stage of resistance, the body adapts to the continued presence of the stressor and resistance increases. In the stage of exhaustion, the body loses its ability to resist the stressor any longer and becomes exhausted.

months or even years of wear and tear may be required before the body's resistance is exhausted, illness may not appear until long after the initial interaction with the stressor.

Stress Weakens Immunity

A variety of studies have shown that stress can impair the functions of the immune system (Kiecolt-Glaser et al., 2002; Rabin, 2007). For example, students who experience considerable stress prior to taking exams show

reduced blood levels of immune system cells (e.g., natural killer cells, T-cells; see Chapter 12), thus making exam stress a risk factor for colds and flu. Stress also slows the body's ability to mount an immune response to a vaccine (Wetherell & Vedhara, 2007). Furthermore, stress impairs immune functioning in people who have lost their jobs, recently experienced the death of a loved one, or are unhappily married, never married, or recently divorced.

Stress-related impairment of the immune system is mediated by stress hormones, particularly cortisol, which bind to immune system cells and alter their functions. Stress activation of sympathetic nervous system fibers that connect to immune system tissues also alters immune functioning.

> The man who fears suffering is already suffering from what he fears.
>
> *Montaigne*

Unhealthy Behaviors

Stress can contribute to ill health by fostering unhealthy behaviors. To manage stressful feelings, some people smoke cigarettes, overeat, undereat, overwork, or drink alcohol and use other drugs. Among U.S. college students, for example, overconsumption of alcohol is commonly employed to reduce stressful feelings (Park, Armeli, & Tennen, 2004). Furthermore, people with high levels of stress may not engage in health-promoting

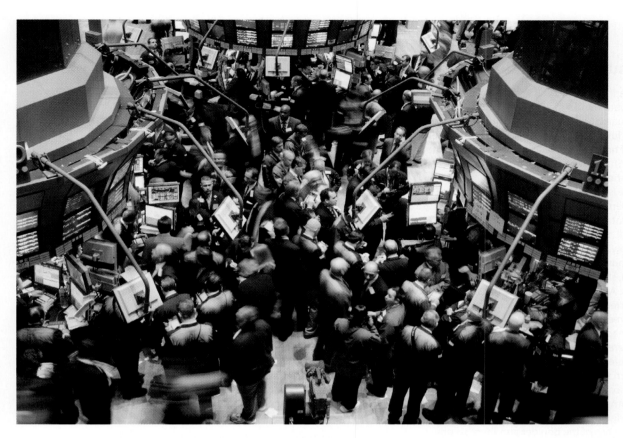

Several heart attacks occur every year on the floor of the New York Stock Exchange, making it one of the highest-density heart attack zones in the United States. The exchange has installed a defibrillator near the bank of phones used to place orders for stock trading, and it has trained workers to use the defibrillator and perform CPR when a heart attack occurs.

activities, such as exercising regularly, eating properly, or getting enough sleep.

Posttraumatic Stress Disorder

Some forms of stress are so severe that they produce a serious, long-lasting condition called **posttraumatic stress disorder (PTSD).** This condition can result from witnessing or being confronted with events that involve death or serious injury or a threat to the physical or psychological integrity of oneself or others. In such traumatic situations, the person experiences intense fear, helplessness, or horror. The most common source of PTSD in American men is combat in war; in American women, rape and sexual molestation (see Chapter 23). Other sources of PTSD are living through a natural disaster, experiencing a severe car or plane crash, physical assault, repeated psychological abuse, or a life-threatening illness. About 4% of the U.S. population is estimated to have PTSD.

Some of the diagnostic criteria for PTSD include (1) flashbacks to the traumatizing event(s) or recurrent unbidden thoughts and dreams of the experience; (2) persistent avoidance of cues that symbolize the traumatizing event(s); (3) difficulty sleeping, outbursts of anger, and being hyperalert and easily startled; and (4) having little interest in daily activities, feeling cut off from others, and a sense of having a limited future.

Although not known by its current medical name, the symptoms of PTSD were long recognized as an outcome of exposure to combat in war. The Vietnam war ushered in the current concept of PTSD because nearly 50% of returning soldiers had clinically significant symptoms of PTSD (Grinage, 2003). About 10% of military personnel returning from the Iraq war have a diagnosis of PTSD (Hoge et al., 2006).

How the traumatic stress of combat, natural disasters, and physical and sexual assault produces the symptoms of PTSD is not understood. Because not everyone exposed to a traumatic situation develops PTSD, researchers suspect that some people are more susceptible, perhaps because of some aspect of temperament,

TERMS

posttraumatic stress disorder (PTSD): physical and mental illnesses resulting from severe trauma

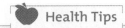

Health Tips

Image Visualization Reduces Stress

Image visualization is telling yourself a story and "seeing" the images in your mind's eye. An attorney in Los Angeles uses image visualization once in a while during the first few minutes of her lunch break. She closes the door to her office, takes off her shoes, and sits on the floor with her back against a wall. She closes her eyes and takes a few deep breaths. Then she imagines . . .

. . . that she is standing at the edge of a meadow that is filled with golden wildflowers. The sun is shining and the air is a very pleasant temperature. On the far side of the meadow is a hill. She imagines herself slowly walking across the meadow toward the hill on a path that has been worn down by previous walks through the flowers. When she reaches the hill, she begins to walk on a gently winding path toward the top. As she walks, she hears the sounds of birds and a nearby stream. Along the side of the path she sees bushes, small trees, a few flowers, and a few stones. Finally, she reaches the top of the hill, where there is a lovely stand of tall trees. There's a clearing in the trees, and on one side of the clearing there's a fallen log. She sits on the log and enjoys the warm sun filtering through the branches of the tall trees. She closes her eyes and rests. After a few minutes, it's time to return, so she opens her eyes, rises, and walks across the clearing to a very large, smooth, white boulder. She looks on the top of the boulder and there's a private message written just for her. She reads the message and then begins to walk down the path to the meadow, still hearing the sounds of the birds and the stream, and still feeling the warm sun. Eventually she reaches the meadow, retraces her path through the golden flowers, and then . . .

. . . she opens her eyes and embarks on the rest of her work day.

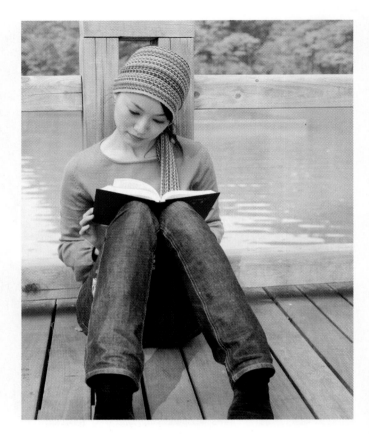

Taking time to relax helps eliminate stress.

prior stressful experiences, or a history of anxiety or depression. For example, children born to some New York women who were pregnant during the 9/11 attacks, and developed PTSD because of them, show PTSD stress hormone patterns, indicating a possible susceptibility to PTSD later in life (Yehuda et al., 2005). Treatment of PTSD includes psychological therapy and one of a variety of drugs that stabilize mood.

> If you don't learn to laugh at trouble, you won't have anything to laugh at when you are old.
>
> *Will Rogers*

Managing Stress

The best ways to manage stress are to replace stressful ways of living with beliefs, attitudes, and behaviors that promote peace, joy, and mind–body harmony. That does not mean you must become reclusive or try to eliminate all sources of conflict and tension in your life. People need challenges to be creative and grow psychologically and spiritually. It may mean, however, changing some self-harming ways of thinking and behaving.

Living healthfully is fundamental to limiting stress. By eating properly, stretching and exercising regularly, getting sufficient sleep, limiting consumption of tobacco, caffeine, alcohol, and other drugs, and taking "quiet time" to be contemplative, creative, and joyful, you establish a strength of mind–body–spirit that can help buffer the twists, turns, and pulls of stress. When very busy, it's tempting to put off taking care of oneself ("There isn't time; I'll do it later."), so if you must, schedule time for healthful living as you do a class or other regular activity.

Besides living healthfully, managing stress also involves **coping,** which refers to efforts to manage a stressful situation regardless of whether those efforts are successful. In general, there are three types of coping processes (Folkman et al., 1986):

Problem-Focused Coping The stressful situation is appraised as changeable and a plan for changing something to improve things is devised and attempted. The key feature of **problem-focused coping** is the belief that one can change things for the better (optimism). Even if it turns out that change is not possible, believing it to be so lessens stress. Believing that one cannot change a *changeable* situation for the better (pessimism) creates a sense of helpless, which can lead to giving up and depression.

Some ways to practice problem-focused coping include the following:

- Limit or eliminate interaction with the stressor. Be assertive with an annoying roommate, say "no" to unreasonable requests, use earplugs to block out noise, change jobs, change your major.
- Alter your perception of a stressful situation (called cognitive reappraisal). By perceiving a situation as less challenging, you lessen the chance of feeling overwhelmed. Ask yourself: "Am I seeing this situation realistically? And even if I am, is it really that threatening?"
- Change beliefs and goals. Winning may be an athlete's highest goal, but worrying about losing can make one sick. The solution is not to give up sports but to change priorities, perhaps by emphasizing the joy of participation rather than the outcome of competition.
- Have confidence in your ability to lessen stress. Give yourself credit for things you have done to lessen stress rather than believing that it was blind luck. This enhances the belief and confidence that you can master many situations that you encounter. Remember that stress is a function of one's belief about managing a challenging situation.
- Seek social support. Talk to friends, family members, counselors, teachers—anyone who you believe can understand, lend a sympathetic ear, and offer sound feedback and advice if you request it (see Chapter 4). Remember: A problem shared is a problem halved.
- Reduce physical tension. Take a walk, ride a bike, jog, or do yoga, progressive muscle relaxation, or t'ai chi—any physical activity that can release muscle tension and focus your mind on something other than your problems.
- Keep your sense of humor. Laughter and joy are beneficial to the spirit and immune system (Moore, 2005) (see Chapter 2).

Emotion-Focused Coping The stressful situation is appraised as not immediately changeable and one decides to accept and work with the reality of the situation, perhaps by waiting for an opportunity to take action or by looking for the good in the bad ("a learning experience"). To facilitate acceptance, one might seek solace and comfort in religion, social contact, being with Nature, or perhaps becoming more involved in helping others.

Some ways to practice **emotion-focused coping** include the following:

- Ease your mind. Employ any of a variety of methods that can stop the physiological stress response and produce instead the "relaxation response" (see Chapter 2). These include meditation, image visualization, guided imagery, journal writing, and prayer. Making one of these methods work for you requires practice and persistence. After learning about the methods, choose one to experiment with almost daily over the course of a week. When you find one or two that you like, make doing them a regular part of your life.
- Let go. Even if only for a few minutes, stop carrying problems in your mind. Give yourself a break from stress by "leaving it at the river" (see the Managing Stress feature: "Two Monks and the River").

Denial/Distancing/Giving Up The stressful situation is appraised as not amenable to change, and rather than accepting that reality, one chooses not to think about it (denial), to undertake escapist activities (oversleeping, overeating, using drugs and alcohol, or increased TV watching or Web surfing), or to become fatalistic and helpless (give up).

In general, problem-focused coping is best for dealing with practical problems and situations that can be resisted or overcome with one's personal efforts. Emotion-focused coping is best for dealing with situations not amenable to change but which must be faced, such as the death of a loved one, illness, or coping with a natural disaster. Denial and avoidance tend to be ineffective coping strategies.

College Student Stress

Being in college can be both rewarding and intense. In college you get the opportunity to learn a variety of interesting things, meet new people, prepare yourself for a rewarding job/career, become an honorable person and good citizen, and identify your values, abilities, and preferences. On the other hand, college life has the potential to be stressful (**Table 3.3**). Students are challenged daily to perform academic tasks, some of which are new (that's why it's called learning) and thus raise doubts about oneself and one's abilities. The college experience is rife with change and unfamiliarity: new classes, new teachers, new people, new living situations. Because college is not home and the people are not family, there may be little support. And, to top it off,

> ■ T E R M S ■
>
> coping: efforts to manage a stressful situation regardless of whether those efforts are successful
>
> emotion-focused coping: appraising and accepting a stressful situation as not immediately changeable and adopting an attitude that lessens anxiety and brings comfort
>
> problem-focused coping: appraising a stressful situation as changeable and making and attempting a plan for changing something to improve things

Table 3.3

Examples of College Student Stressors

Academic
Competition
Schoolwork (difficult, low motivation)
Exams and grades
Poor resources (library, computers)
Oral presentations/public speaking
Professors/coaches (unfair, demanding, unavailable)
Choosing and registering for classes
Choosing a major/career

Time
Deadlines
Procrastination
Waiting for appointments and in lines
No time to exercise
Late for appointments or class

Environment
Others' behavior (rude, inconsiderate, sexist/racist)
Injustice: seeing examples or being a victim of
Crowds/large social groups
Fears of violence/terrorism
Weather (snow, heat/humidity, storms)
Noise
Lack of privacy

Social
Obligations, annoyances (family/friends/girl-/boyfriend)
Not dating
Roommate(s)/housemate(s) problems
Concerns about STDs

Self
Behavior (habits, temper)
Appearance (unattractive features, grooming)
Ill health/physical symptoms
Forgetting, misplacing, or losing things
Weight/dietary management
Self-confidence/self-esteem
Boredom

Money
Not enough
Bills/overspending
Job: searching for or interviews
Job/work issues (demanding, annoying)

Tasks of daily living
Tedious chores (shopping, cleaning)
Traffic and parking problems
Car problems (breaking down, repairs)
Housing (finding/getting or moving)
Food (unappealing or unhealthful meals)

rather than getting paid for all their hard work, students do the paying. Furthermore, college students are on their own, and they may not always make the wisest, safest, and healthiest choices.

A healthy lifestyle—eating properly, exercising regularly, getting sufficient restful sleep, having daily quiet time and regular creative relaxation (reading, socializing, art, music)—is fundamental to dealing with college stress. Unfortunately, with so many demands and time pressures, it is tempting to put off choices for living healthfully.

Overload

If they were to occur sequentially, individual stressors in college, such as taking a test, going through a rough time with a romantic partner, or moving to a new residence, although unpleasant, would be generally manageable. However, in college, many challenges and changes occur virtually simultaneously. For example, at the end of a semester, a student could face having to write two final papers, take five finals, deal with a bad cold, and move to a new apartment. And the next semester, there would likely be a new set of challenges (an ill parent, a course that makes no sense) along with some of the usual ones (final papers and exams and problematic social relationships).

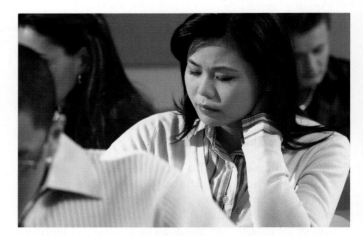

Academic pressures and test taking can produce anxiety and stress.

Being confronted with too many challenges and changes can lead to **overload**—the feeling that there are too many demands on your time and energy. Your life consists of zipping from here to there to attend to all of your tasks, but what you really want is a week off to hang with your friends and "veg." And if overload grows to feeling overwhelmed, a student might drop a class or two, drop out of school, get depressed, or use alcohol or drugs.

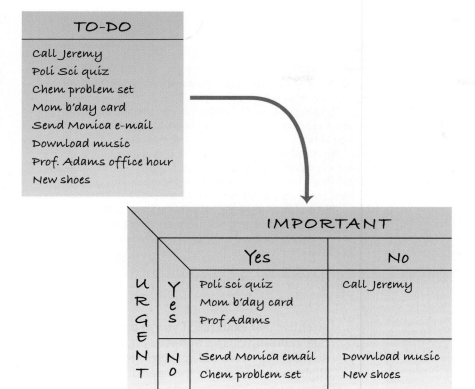

■ Figure 3.6

Prioritizing Tasks

Classify tasks from your to-do list according to their *urgency* and *importance* and do them in this order: (1) urgent and important; (2) not urgent and important; (3) urgent but not important; and (4) not urgent or important. Move tasks labeled "urgent and not important" to other categories because urgency is a state of mind and makes things seem important even if they are not.

intentions. Ask yourself, "What do I want/need to make happen today?" "What do I need to do to keep my mind, body, and spirit healthy and well?" Don't think only of accomplishing tasks but also the effects your behaviors will have on yourself and others.

4. *Prioritize tasks.* First things first. Classify tasks according to their urgency and importance (**Figure 3.6**), and do them in this order: (1) urgent and important; (2) not urgent but important; (3) urgent but not important; and (4) not urgent or important. Distinguishing the urgent/important tasks from the urgent/not important ones is often difficult because urgency is a state of mind and makes everything seem important. Before prioritizing items on your to-do list, take a few minutes to become mentally and physically quiet. This will allow you to place truly urgent and important items at the top of your to-do list.

5. *Don't sweat the small stuff.* Eliminate unimportant tasks from your list. Don't do, think about, or worry about anything that doesn't match your most important values and long-term goals. "Keep your eyes on the prize."

At the heart of overload is the sense of lacking personal control. Individuals who believe they can influence the course of their lives (internal locus of control) are likely to experience less stress than individuals who believe that their fate is determined by factors outside of their control (external locus of control) (Schmitz et al., 2000). Thus, although it is tempting to focus on things outside of yourself to explain feelings of overload and overwhelm, it is more productive to look at yourself. Which is good, because you have more control over yourself than you do over things in your environment.

Here are some antidotes to overload:

1. *Plan ahead.* Knowing when a stressful situation will occur produces less stress than not knowing does. For example, most of the time, you will know at the beginning of a semester when major assignments are due. Plan for them.

2. *Keep a to-do list.* At the beginning of each day, or the night before, write down all the things you have to do.

3. *Clarify intentions.* Before you begin each day, take a few moments to be quiet and still and clarify your

6. *Schedule downtime.* Even if it's only a few moments a day, take time for activities that you find meaningful and fun, or just chill.

7. *Sleep.* Not sleeping enough reduces performance and efficiency on tasks by as much as 50%, which makes tasks take longer and contributes to the sense of overload.

8. *Don't "Just do it."* "Just do it" is a slogan for selling sports shoes, not living a life. Students often erroneously believe that the solution to overload is to put in more effort ("just do it"). Because they already are maxed out, putting in more effort cannot succeed, although a list of undone tasks can contribute to a loss of confidence and self-esteem.

TERMS

overload: the feeling that there are too many demands on one's time and energy from being confronted with too many challenges

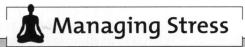

Managing Stress

Two Monks and the River

Two monks set out on their last day's journey to their monastery. At midmorning they came upon a shallow river, and on the bank there stood a beautiful young maiden.

"May I help you cross?" asked the first monk.

"Why, yes, that would be most kind of you," replied the maiden.

So the first monk hoisted the maiden on his back and carried her across the river. They bowed and went their separate ways.

After an hour or two of walking, the second monk said to the first monk, "I can't believe you did that! I just can't believe it! We take vows of chastity, and you touched a woman. You

even asked her! What are we going to tell the abbot when we get home? He's going to ask how our journey was, and we can't lie. What are we going to say?"

Another couple of hours passed and the second monk erupted again. "How could you do that? She didn't even ask. You offered! The abbot's going to be incredibly angry."

By late afternoon the two were nearing their home, and the second monk, now filled with anxiety, said, "I can't believe you did that! You touched a woman. You even carried her on your back. What are we going to tell the abbot?"

The first monk stopped, looked at the second monk and said, "Listen, it's true that I carried that maiden across the river. But I left her at the river bank hours ago. You've been carrying her all day."

Table 3.4

Time Diary

Time	Activity
6:00 A.M.	Wake up
6:15 A.M.	Shower/dress/eat
7:00 A.M.	Go to school
8:00 A.M.	Chem lecture
9:30 A.M.	Hang out in library/snack
10:30 A.M.	Psych lecture
12:00 P.M.	Work
5:00 P.M.	Go home

Directions: Record your activities for three representative days. Enter data two to three times a day. For example, at noon, record your activities since awakening; at 5:00 P.M., record your activities since noon; at bedtime, record your activities since 5:00 P.M. Calculate the average daily hours awake, asleep, at school, studying/schoolwork, at work, with family, with friends, with self, commuting, other.

Time Management

A major cause of college student stress is the sense that there's too much to do and not enough time to do it. Because you can't make more time, the way to ease this pressure is to make the best use of the time you have. Here are some tips for time management:

- *Perform a time audit.* For at least three representative days in your week (a whole week is better), write down everything you do during each of the 24 hours. Make a chart (**Table 3.4**). Identify windows of time that could be put to better use and alter your activities accordingly.
- *Be energy efficient.* Schedule important activities for the times of the day when you are most alert and

attentive. For example, if you're a morning person, take morning classes and study in between them. Schedule exercise and socializing for the afternoon. Night people might do the opposite.
- *Resist multitasking.* Try to do only one thing at a time Multitasking appears to be time efficient, but it also creates a sense of urgency, which produces anxiety and stimulates the secretion of stress hormones, thus contributing to stress.
- *Control interruptions.* Discourage drop-in visiting; don't answer the pager, the phone, or instant messages (if it's important, the person will try again); stay away from TV, computer games, and the Internet.
- *Tame any tendencies toward perfectionism.* Don't waste time trying to make everything perfect. Every task has a point of diminishing returns—when the time and energy you put in is out of proportion to what you can reasonably hope to get back.
- *Understand any tendencies to procrastinate.* Procrastination often grows out of the fear of failure or exposure (people seeing you or your work and judging it harshly). When you hear your litany of excuses for not working at a task, ask yourself what you fear. Be your own best friend and encourage yourself to move ahead. Rather than focus on the end product of your efforts, do *one thing* that will move you ahead. If you have not begun to study for an upcoming exam, don't think about the exam. Instead, promise yourself that you will take your textbook out of your backpack today. That's all. Tomorrow, promise yourself you will open it. Remember: "The journey of a thousand miles starts with the first step."

Test Anxiety

It is a rare college student who does not get nervous when taking tests. People in American society equate educational success, academic degrees, and professional licenses with the attainment of important life goals, particularly financial ones. As a consequence, competition among students at all levels is intense. Students believe that grades and exam scores will determine how successful their lives will be in terms of jobs, careers, and money.

Many students experience health problems because of academic pressures and anxiety about exams. They may suffer from headaches, stomach and bowel problems, disordered eating, recurrent infections, and other symptoms of stress. Students whose exam anxiety affects their health need to make personal adjustments to reduce the anxiety while they pursue their goals.

Test anxiety is a sense of unease and apprehension—frequently accompanied by physiological symptoms such as upset stomach, restlessness, sleep problems, irritability, and "nervous" eating—that precede the taking of an exam. Besides creating physical illness, test anxiety can make it difficult to concentrate, which increases the likelihood of forgetting (blocking) and making "careless" errors.

Test anxiety is a form of performance anxiety, which can occur in any activity in which someone cares about the outcome of her or his performance. (If the person didn't care about the outcome, then he or she would not be nervous about it.) Students, athletes, musicians, actors, and people who interview for jobs are all familiar with performance anxiety.

Being somewhat nervous about how well you are going to do leads to performing well. Unfortunately, being too nervous reduces performance on the task (**Figure 3.7**). With regard to tests, being a little nervous can motivate you to study prior to the test and to focus your attention while taking the test. Being too nervous prior to the test can lead to procrastination and during the test can distract you from the test.

Whenever you are performing a task (and you care about the outcome), your goal is to be just nervous enough to be at peak performance but not so nervous that you panic. The only way to know where this peak is for you is by experience. This is why, after having taken dozens of tests, students become expert test-takers. And this is why during the first couple of years of college, many students are petrified of tests.

Test anxiety is caused by a test-taker's internal mental messages, or self-talk, which focuses on imaginary "terrible" outcomes of doing poorly on the exam. Some examples include the following:

- *Exaggerating the importance of the test:* "If I do poorly on this test, I'll do poorly in the class. If I do poorly

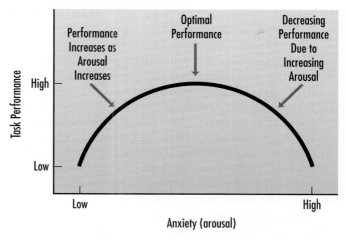

■ **Figure 3.7**

Performance Is Affected by Anxiety/Arousal
Performance on a task is affected by how anxious a person is about how well she or he is going to do. Being somewhat anxious leads to better performance until an optimum level of performance is reached. Being too anxious distracts the mind and reduces performance.

in the class, I won't get into law school. If I don't get into law school, I'll be a failure and die of shame."
- *Fear of autonomy and exposure:* "If I do well, everyone will notice me and I will be embarrassed."
- *Fear of abandonment:* "If I do poorly, my friends and family will dislike me."
- *Confusing one's performance on an exam with one's self-worth:* "If I do poorly on the exam, it will prove that I'm worthless."

Solutions to Text Anxiety Acknowledge that you get nervous before tests and try to become aware of the roots of your test anxiety. Keep a journal of pretest feelings and symptoms. Be attentive for the images and negative messages in your internal self-talk. If you tell yourself, "You're not smart enough to do well," perhaps respond by saying to yourself, "That's your opinion. Mine is that I know I can do this." Remember: If you don't prepare adequately for the exam by studying, and you care about your performance, then it's realistic to feel anxious about the possibility of doing poorly.

Here are some other suggestions for managing test anxiety:
- Realistically appraise the importance of an exam. Remind yourself that a test is only a test and not a measure of your self-worth.
- Remind yourself that focusing on the grade will distract you from learning the material.
- As part of test preparation, give yourself periods of quiet time in which to relax and visualize yourself taking the test (see the Health Tips features "Image

Visualization Reduces Stress" and "Visualization Reduces Exam Anxiety"). In your image, see yourself taking the exam confidently and masterfully. See yourself coming across a difficult question and taking that experience in stride and moving on to another question that you can respond to with confidence.

- Focus your awareness on the test by getting your test-taking materials together before test time. Sharpen your pencils and get your Scantron or blue book and write your name on it. Arrive at the exam 5 to 10 minutes early and let yourself relax.
- Don't get into a frenzy before the test. Don't cram. That only increases anxiety.
- Get a good night's sleep. Eat a balanced meal (protein and complex carbohydrate; not sugary/fatty snacks) one or two hours before the exam.
- Once in the test situation, stop worrying. Try to flow. If you block, put down your pencil, put your feet flat on the floor, close your eyes, and focus your awareness on your breathing. After 20 to 30 seconds, when you're ready, go back to the exam.
- Realize that test-taking is a skill only partially related to how much one knows and understands. Like any skill, one improves with practice.

What You Can Do About Stress

In the fast-paced, competitive world we live in, it's almost impossible not to experience stress and its many physiological and psychological manifestations. When stressed, we generally identify its causes as the hassles, obstacles, time pressures, unpleasantnesses in generally pleasant relationships, interactions with unpleasant others, and other situations that disrupt our feelings of inner harmony. What we often fail to recognize, however, is that we often contribute to our stress by how we think about and respond to what we experience. It is not always possible to avoid or escape stressful situations. Neither is it generally possible to change others so that they behave in ways we desire. In the face of stress, a wise course is to become mindful of how your thoughts contribute to feeling stressed. Becoming increasingly aware of how your mind works can help you decrease the time your mind swirls around in the throes of stress.

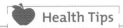 Health Tips

Visualization Reduces Exam Anxiety

The following exercise can reduce the stress and anxiety of taking exams. It can result in improved scores and a reduction in symptoms produced by stress.

1. Find a comfortable place in your house or room and a time when you will not be disturbed by other people. Sit in a comfortable chair or lie down on a couch or floor. The main thing is to get physically comfortable. If music helps you relax, play some of your favorite music softly.
2. Close your eyes and ask your mind to recall a place and time where you felt contented. It might be a vacation time, being with someone, or being alone in a beautiful environment. Use your imagination and memory to reconstruct the scene where you felt happy and healthy. Notice that you had no concerns there at that time. Let yourself become involved with the scene. The process is similar to having a daydream or a fantasy. While your mind is focused on pleasurable memories, your body automatically relaxes.
3. When you feel quite relaxed, refocus your mind on the upcoming exam. See yourself taking the exam while feeling relaxed and confident. Because your mind and body are relaxed and comfortable, your mind automatically associates the same feelings with the image of taking the exam. Visualize the exam room, the other students, yourself answering the questions; let your mind focus on as many details as possible.
4. Now project your mind into the future to the actual day and place of the exam. Notice how relaxed you feel as you take the exam; the anxiety you used to experience seems to have vanished. Continue with the visualization until you see yourself turning in the exam and feeling confident and pleased with your performance.
5. Do this exercise for several days prior to any exam that causes anxiety. You will be surprised at the absence of nervousness and stress on exam day. You will be even more pleased at the improvement in your grades.

Critical Thinking About Health

1. Three groups of people were vaccinated against a test substance (one that could not make anyone sick). Group 1 consisted of students during final exams; group 2, people complaining of loneliness; group 3, people whose spouse had cancer. Each group was further subdivided into two subgroups. One subgroup in each major group was given six weeks of weekly support group meetings plus education about reducing the stress of their circumstance. The other subgroup in each major group was given no support or education. The accompanying figure shows the results of the strength of the immune response to the test vaccine.

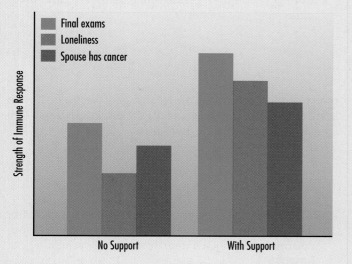

a. Explain the results of the experiment.
b. Suggest a hypothesis to explain the results of the experiment.
c. What do the results suggest about how you can better deal with stress in your life?

2. Johann Wolfgang von Goethe (1749–1832), the German author of *Faust* and other literary works, once wrote: "Things which matter most must never be at the mercy of things which matter least."
a. What is your interpretation of Goethe's idea?
b. How does letting things which matter most be at the mercy of things which matter least contribute to stress?
c. How susceptible are you to stress from letting things which matter most be at the mercy of things which matter least? What could you change to reduce that stress?

3. Offer an explanation for the following: In the 1980s, researchers studied the health of adults living in two communities that were separated by a river. North River was a prosperous suburb, and South River was an industrial region in which the major employer, an auto plant, had shut down. The research showed that after the auto plant closed, children living in South River had many more doctor visits for infections and allergies than did children in North River. Also, adults in South River had more motor vehicle accidents and colds and flu during winter months than adults in North River did.

4. On the Recent Life Changes Questionnaire, the death of a child, spouse, sibling, or parent carries the highest LCU values.
a. Offer a hypothesis to explain that result. In your hypothesis, take into account the nature of those kinds of relationships and what is lost when someone dies.
b. Given that the loss of a loved one is associated with the highest LCU values, how should someone who experiences that kind of loss navigate life so as to reduce his or her stress and the risk of becoming ill?
c. What is the best way to cope with the loss of a loved one?

5. Do you experience test anxiety to such a degree that you become physically or emotionally upset before or after taking an exam? If so, describe your symptoms and feelings. If you have an exam that makes you anxious coming up in the next few weeks, try the exercise described in the Managing Stress box entitled "Visualization Reduces Exam Anxiety" for at least a week before taking the exam. After the exam, describe your experience in detail and indicate whether you performed better than you expected on the exam.

Health in Review

- Stress is the disruption of mind–body harmony brought about by trauma, threats to life, or obstacles to carrying out daily tasks, accomplishing life goals, or achieving desired changes in life.
- Stressors are situations and circumstances that cause stress.
- The mental component of stress consists of the interpretation of a situation as threatening and the appraisal that one's personal resources are insufficient to meet the demands of dealing with the stressful situation.
- The physiological components of stress are the fight-or-flight response and activation of the hypothalamo-pituitary-adrenal axis, with consequent secretion of stress hormones, especially cortisol.

- Stress contributes to illness by wearing down the mind and body (general adaptation syndrome), impairing immunity, and fostering unhealthy behaviors.
- Posttraumatic stress disorder is a serious medical condition resulting from exposure to traumatic events and near-death experiences.
- Stress can be reduced by disengaging from stressors and/or by altering perceptions and goals, thereby reducing the potential for stress-related illness.
- Stress can be reduced by techniques that produce a peaceful state of being, such as image visualization, meditation, exercise, yoga, and just taking it easy.
- College student stress includes overload, time pressures, and test anxiety.

Health and Wellness Online

The Web contains a wealth of information about health and wellness. By accessing the Internet using Web browser software, you can gain a new perspective on many topics presented in *Health and Wellness,* Tenth Edition. Access the Jones and Bartlett Publishers Web site at **health.jbpub.com/hwonline**.

References

Dhabhar, F. S., & McEwan, B. S. (2007). Bi-directional effects of stress on immune function. In Robert Ader (Ed.), *Psychoneuroimmunology* (4th ed.). Boston: Elsevier Academic Press.

Ferrie, J. E., et al. (2005). Self-reported job insecurity and health in the Whitehall II study: Potential explanations of the relationship. *Social Science and Medicine, 60,* 1593–1602.

Folkman, S. J. (1984). Personal control and stress and coping processes: A theoretical analysis. *Journal of Personality and Social Psychology, 46,* 839–852.

Folkman, S., et al. (1986). Dynamics of a stressful encounter: Cognitive appraisal, coping, and encounter outcomes. *Journal of Personality and Social Psychology, 50,* 992–1003.

Graham, J. E., et al. (2007). Close relationships and immunity. In Robert Ader (Ed.), *Psychoneuroimmunology* (4th ed.). Boston: Elsevier Academic Press.

Grinage, B. D. (2003). Diagnosis and management of post-traumatic stress disorder. *American Family Physician, 68,* 2401–2408.

Hoge, C. W., et al. (2006). Mental health problems, size of mental health services, and attrition from military service after returning from deployment to Iraq or Afghanistan. *Journal of the American Medical Association, 295,* 1023–1032.

Kiecolt-Glaser, J. K., et al. (2002). Emotions, morbidity and mortality: New perspectives from psychoneuroimmunology. *Annual Review of Psychology, 53,* 83–107.

Lett, H. S., et al. (2007). Social support and prognosis in patients at increased psychosocial risk recovering from myocardial infarction. *Health Psychology, 26,* 418–427.

Miller, M. A., & Rahe, R. H. (1997). Life changes scaling for the 1990s. *Journal of Psychosomatic Research, 43,* 279–292.

Moore, C. W. (2005). The impact of humor on patients with cancer. *Clinical Journal of Oncology Nursing, 9,* 211–218.

Orth-Gomér, K. (2007). Job strain and risk of recurrent coronary events. *Journal of the American Medical Association, 298,* 1693–1694.

Park, C. L., Armeli, S., & Tennen, H. (2004). The daily stress and coping process and alcohol use among college students. *Journal of Studies of Alcohol, 65,* 126–135.

Rabin, B. (2007). Stress: A system as a whole. In Robert Ader (Ed.), *Psychoneuroimmunology* (4th ed.). Boston: Elsevier Academic Press.

Schmitz, N., Neumann, W., & Oppermann, R. (2000). The relationship of burnout, stress and locus of control in nurses. *International Journal of Nursing Studies, 37*, 95–99.

Wetherell, M. A., & Vedhara, K. (2007). Stress-associated immune dysregulation can affect antibody and T-cell responses to vaccines. In Robert Ader (Ed.), *Psychoneuroimmunology* (4th ed.). Boston: Elsevier Academic Press.

Yehuda, R., et al. (2005). Transgenerational effects of posttraumatic stress disorder in babies of mothers exposed to the World Trade Center attacks during pregnancy. *Journal of Clinical Endocrinology and Metabolism, 90*, 4115–4118.

Suggested Readings

Ader, R. (Ed.). (2007). *Psychoneuroimmunology* (4th ed.). Boston: Elsevier Academic Press. A complete and thorough discussion of all aspects of psychoneuroimmunology.

Cohen, S., et al. (2007). Psychological stress and disease. *Journal of the American Medical Association, 298*, 1685–1687. Discusses recent research on the relationship of psychological stress to illness.

Davis, M. (2008). *The relaxation and stress reduction workbook*. Oakland, CA: New Harbinger. Offers many self-assessment tools and calming techniques to help overcome anxiety and promote physical and emotional well-being.

de Kloet, E. R., et al. (2005). Stress and the brain: From adaptation to disease. *Nature Reviews in Neuroscience, 6*, 463–475. Discusses the biological mechanisms that cause stress.

Kiecolt-Glaser, J. K., et al. (2002). Emotions, morbidity and mortality: New perspectives from psychoneuroimmunology. *Annual Review of Psychology, 53*, 83–107. A review of the scientific research on the effects of emotions on the immune system and consequent risks of disease.

Levey, J., Levey, M., & Green, E. (2003). *The fine arts of relaxation, concentration and meditation: Ancient skills for modern minds*. New York: Wisdom Publications. A presentation of several techniques for releasing stress and tension.

McEwan, B., & Lasley, E. L. (2003). *The end of stress as we know it*. Washington, DC: John Henry Press. A world-famous neurobiologist explains stress and offers suggestions for reducing it in one's life.

Recommended Web Sites

Please visit **health.jbpub.com/hwonline** for links to these Web sites.

Anchoring
An online tutorial on how to quiet your mind, by Eric Golanty, PhD, coauthor of *Health and Wellness* and professor of health at Las Positas College.

College Student Stress
The University of Chicago's list of online resources.

Health Psychology Resources: Stress-Related Links
A compilation of many authoritative Web resources on stress, maintained by health psychologist Fuscia M. Sirois.

Mind/Body Health Stress
Explains stress and offers methods for lessening it; from the American Psychological Association.

Stress Resources
U.S. National Library of Medicine.

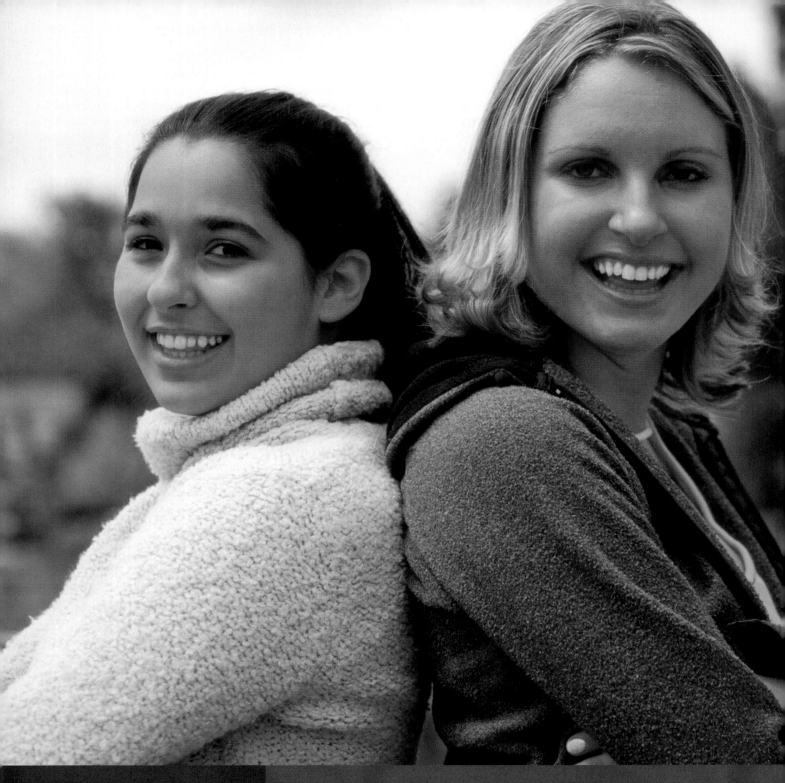

Chapter Four

Mental Health and Mental Illness

Learning Objectives

1. Describe Maslow's hierarchy of needs and its role in mental health.
2. Explain the role of positive emotions in mental and physical health.
3. List and describe strategies for coping with emotional distress.
4. Define defense mechanisms.
5. List and describe four common anxiety disorders.
6. List five signs of depression.
7. Discuss anger and dealing with it constructively.
8. Describe adult attention deficit hyperactivity disorder.
9. Discuss the importance of sleep for well-being.
10. List and describe seven facets of sleep hygiene.
11. Identify characteristics of schizophrenia.

Your state of mind is fundamental to your health and well-being. If your mind is relaxed, you are at peace with yourself, and you live harmoniously within your social and physical environment, you are more likely to feel good and enjoy good health than if you are chronically angry, frightened, tense, depressed, and at odds with your surroundings.

> Forgiveness benefits the forgiver much more than the forgiven.
>
> *Vusi Mahlassela, South African musician*

The term *mind* refers to the totality of brain functions that produce thoughts, feelings, and intentional behaviors. **Mental health** is when your mental functions produce a sense of optimism, vitality, and well-being, and when your intentional behaviors lead to productive activities (including healthy behaviors), fulfilling relationships with others, and the ability to adapt to change and to cope with adversity (U.S. Department of Health and Human Services, 1999).

Mental illness refers to alterations in thinking, emotions, and/or intentional behaviors that produce psychological distress and/or impaired functioning. Because mental functions are carried out by the brain, very often mental illness is associated with disease, infection, drug/toxin-induced alterations in brain biology, and abnormal physical conditions and biological changes in the brain. Mental illness accounts for more than 15% of the burden of disease in developed countries, which is greater than that from all cancers. Mental illness is the second leading cause of disability and premature mortality in the United States. One in five children and adolescents shows signs and symptoms of a mental illness during the course of a year.

Some Mental Illnesses Have Their Origins in Biology

What causes severe mental illnesses such as depression, schizophrenia, bipolar disorder, and addiction? Some argue that most mental illness is caused by environmental factors, for example, physical and psychological abuse, neglect, emotional trauma, and recreational drug use. Others argue that mental illness is rooted in biology—genes that cause abnormal biological development either in a fetus or early in childhood while the brain is still developing. These biological changes, in turn, create a susceptibility to mental illness. Which idea is right? It now appears that mental illnesses are caused by both environmental and genetic effects on development (Saey, 2008).

Some of the evidence comes from studying identical twins. Identical (monozygotic) twins have the same genes, so, if mental illness were largely due to a person's genes, you would predict that if one twin of an identical pair had depression or schizophrenia, the other twin would also be affected. But in only about half of identical twin pairs do both twins suffer from the same mental illness. So, although their genes are identical, one twin of an identical pair may become mentally ill while the other twin remains well. This suggests that inheriting a particular gene can only account for about half of the cases of mental illness; the other half must be due to environmental factors. Or, more likely, both inherited genes and environmental factors are involved to varying degrees in any given case of mental illness.

Scientists have begun to identify some of the non-hereditary biological factors that cause or affect mental illnesses. These involve alterations in the chemical structure of genes but not the genetic information, or the sequence of letters in DNA, a process that is called *epigenetic change*. Imagine that the letters in this paragraph are the code of inheritance in DNA. Now imagine that the punctuation or spacing on the page is changed. Information is carried in the words, but without punctuation and spacing, it is likely to be nonsense. In cases of mental illness, hereditary information that is encoded in the chemical structure of DNA may be normal, but it functions abnormally due to the epigenetic changes. These epigenetic modifications can be introduced by environmental factors such as nutrition, drug use, stress, physical abuse, and other insults.

Inherited changes in genes that cause genetic diseases are, for the most part, irreversible. But epigenetic changes may be reversible to some degree. This may explain why some mental illnesses respond to drugs or disappear on their own over time. It also may explain why mental illnesses sometimes reoccur years after a remission. Understanding the epigenetic changes that alter brain functions may lead to strategies for preventing mental illnesses and to better ways to treat them.

Basic Needs and Mental Health

Much of human behavior is motivated by basic human needs. When individuals succeed in meeting their basic needs, they experience pleasant emotions, such as joy, pleasure, satisfaction, and contentment. When they do not, however, they experience unpleasant emotions, such as frustration, anger, sadness, grief, and shame.

Although basic needs are intrinsic to humans, the ways in which people satisfy them are not. Everyone may need to eat, but not everyone obtains food in the same way. Neither does everyone choose to eat the same kind of food. Similarly, people engage in a variety of activities, occupations, relationships, and recreational pursuits to meet their needs.

Infants have a limited need-fulfilling repertoire. A child can cry when wanting to be fed or comforted and can smile or coo to invite touch and play. Beginning in childhood, individuals learn to understand the nature of their needs and develop strategies for interacting with the environment to meet them.

There are two types of basic human needs: **maintenance needs** involve physical safety and survival; **growth needs** involve social belonging, self-esteem, and mental, psychological, and spiritual stimulation. Mental and emotional health are functions of how successfully a person meets her or his basic needs and deals with circumstances in which these needs are not met. Thoughts, beliefs, and attitudes that help us appropriately interpret and respond to internal needs, as well as environmental challenges, are involved. We should have emotional experiences that accurately help us interpret the environment and our interactions with it, as well as a biologically healthy brain and nervous system, not one that is undernourished, diseased, or disequilibrated with drugs or alcohol.

According to psychologists, there is a **hierarchy of needs.** These include physiological needs, safety, love, self-esteem, and self-actualization (**Figure 4.1**). When the needs for food, clothing, and shelter have been met, less urgent needs become a priority. As people meet their needs, they move up the hierarchy. A person attains **self-actualization** (the highest level), by living to the fullest. People who are self-actualized have met their basic needs and reached their full human potential (Maslow, 1970).

To be mentally healthy, we do not have to be like everyone else. Being true to ourselves leads to greater satisfaction in life than social conformity does. Also, being mentally healthy does not mean that we never feel angry, anxious, lonely, depressed, confused, or overwhelmed. These are normal human emotions. Furthermore, being mentally healthy does not mean that we never need support, advice, or other kinds of help. In fact, inner strength is being able to recognize our limits and to seek and accept help so we can restore harmony when our mental and emotional resources are taxed.

Thoughts, Emotions, and Mental Health

One foundation of mental health is seeing the world realistically. This perspective helps people devise appropriate strategies to meet their needs.

How we see the world is determined by the mental process called **cognition** (from the Latin *cognito*, meaning "I know"). Cognition includes the following mental processes:

- *Perception:* interpreting data gathered by the senses (sight, smell, hearing, taste, touch, movement)
- *Learning:* integrating new perceptions with previous ones and storing them in memory as values, beliefs, and attitudes
- *Reasoning and problem solving:* formulating plans of action

Some thoughts, beliefs, attitudes, and emotions are **conscious,** which means that an individual can be aware of them. Others are **unconscious,** which means that they are not in our everyday awareness. Unconscious

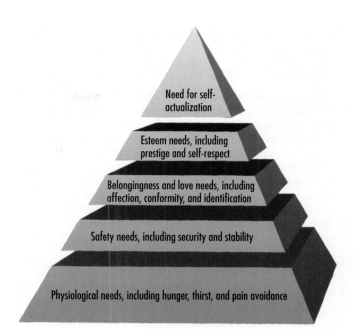

■ Figure 4.1

Maslow's Hierarchy of Human Needs

thoughts can be accessed through hypnosis, dreams, fantasies, and various forms of creative experience.

Cognition is usually associated with emotions. Emotions are patterns of neuronal activity in the brain

---

TERMS

cognition: the act or process of knowing

conscious: being aware of one's thoughts, beliefs, and emotions

growth needs: human needs that include social belonging, self-esteem, and spiritual growth

hierarchy of needs: a progression of human requirements, including physiological needs, safety, love, self-esteem, and self-actualization

maintenance needs: human needs that include physical safety and survival requirements, such as food and water

mental health: a sense of optimism, vitality, and well-being, and intentional behaviors that lead to productive activities, fulfilling relationships with others, and the ability to adapt to change and to cope with adversity

mental illness: alterations in thinking, emotions, and/or intentional behaviors that produce psychological distress and/or impaired functioning

self-actualization: a state in which a person has achieved the highest level of growth in Maslow's hierarchy of needs

unconscious: mental activities outside of conscious awareness

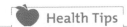 Health Tips

Tips for Emotional Wellness

People who have a positive self-image
. . . are not incapacitated by their emotions of fear, anger, love, jealousy, or guilt.
. . . can take life's disappointments in stride.
. . . have a tolerant attitude toward themselves and others; they can laugh at their shortcomings and mistakes.
. . . respect themselves and have self-confidence.
. . . are able to deal with most situations that come along.
. . . get satisfaction from simple, everyday pleasures.

People who feel positive about other people
. . . are able to give love and accept others the way they are.
. . . have personal relationships that are satisfying.
. . . expect to like and trust others and take it for granted that others will like and trust them.
. . . respect the many differences they see in people.
. . . do not need to control or push other people around.
. . . feel a sense of responsibility to friends and society.

People who are able to meet life's demands
. . . do something about their problems as they arise.
. . . accept their responsibilities.
. . . shape their environment whenever possible; otherwise, they adjust to it.
. . . plan ahead but do not fear the future.
. . . welcome new ideas and experiences.
. . . use their natural capacities and talents.
. . . set attainable and realistic goals for themselves.
. . . get satisfaction from what they accomplish.

that can arise spontaneously or in response to cognitive evaluations of what we experience, have experienced, or believe we may experience. Emotions provide a sense of what is pleasant or unpleasant, which helps us evaluate an experience. This sets the stage for appropriate behavior. Emotions also provide the energy or motivation for behavior, and they play a part in evaluating the outcome of behavior. In general, the function of unpleasant emotions (e.g., anger, fear, anxiety, disgust, guilt, and shame) is avoiding threats to one's well-being or survival. The function of pleasant emotions (e.g., joy, interest, contentment, and love) is the pursuit of novel, creative, enjoyable activities (Fredrickson, 1998).

Here is an example of how cognition and emotions affect behavior. An exam is scheduled in an economics course. If a student believes that success on the exam is beneficial (i.e., doing well meets a need), she is likely to feel challenged and anxious. These emotions motivate her to study. If she does well on the exam, she is likely to feel happy. If she attributes her success to the fact that she studied, she is likely to study for the next exam and feel good about herself and her ability to master schoolwork.

Another student in the same economics class believes that performance on the exam will determine

all future success in school and in life. This erroneous belief is likely to produce anxiety that is so intense that he is unable to concentrate; he may even be sick or psychologically incapacitated on the day of the test (see Chapter 3). This experience may be so unpleasant that he may drop economics or even drop out of school. He might have helped himself by changing his belief about the significance of the test, which would have altered his emotional experience. This could have produced a different set of behavioral choices. With a different perspective, he might have done quite well on the exam.

Positive Thoughts and Emotions Contribute to Health

Much research shows that negative thoughts, stress, and unpleasant emotions, such as fear, anxiety, anger/hostility, and depression, can damage health (see Chapters 2 and 3). It is also likely that positive thoughts and emotions, such as joy, interest, contentment, and love, can promote health (Rozanski & Kubzansky, 2005). For example, researchers analyzing early-in-life personal writings of 180 elderly American nuns found that those whose writings had the highest degree of positive emotional content lived the longest (**Figure 4.2**) (Danner, Snowdon, & Friesen, 2001). Another study showed that positive emotions such as joy and contentment lessened the risk of developing a cold, most likely because of enhanced immune response to cold viruses (Doyle, Gentile, & Cohen, 2006). Higher degrees of hope and curiosity were found to be associated with a decreased likelihood of having or developing hypertension, diabetes, and respiratory tract infections (Richman et al., 2005).

One major way positive thoughts and emotions are believed to influence health and illness is by fostering healthy behaviors and avoidance of unhealthy ones. Living healthfully requires action based on accurate knowledge. Action has the components of goals, strategies for attaining goals including managing obstacles, and expectations of whether you will be successful (called outcome expectancies).

Goals A goal can be something you want or something you want to prevent or avoid. There are short-term goals ("I want to get a good night's sleep") and long-term goals ("I want to get my degree"). Goals can be clearly defined ("I'm going to study this Friday night instead of partying") or fuzzy ("I want to do better at school").

Goals reflect a person's or a culture's values, which are beliefs about what is important. Two values that affect health are valuing oneself (**self-esteem**) and valuing the physical and social environments in which one lives. When you value yourself, you are more likely to engage in healthful behaviors and have a high degree of

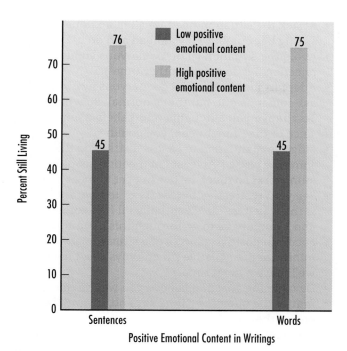

■ **Figure 4.2**

Percentage Survival at Age 80 of Nuns with Low or High Degree of Emotional Content in Writings in Early Life
Source: Danner, D. D., Snowdon, D. A., & Friesen, W. V. (2001). Positive emotions in early life and longevity: Findings from the nun study. *Journal of Personality and Social Psychology, 80,* 804–813.

psychological well-being (Adler & Stewart, 2004). When you value your physical and social environments, you are more likely to contribute to making them clean, healthy, and supportive, that is, to be helpful to others in attaining their goals.

Strategies for Action Strategies involve your ability to generate plans for attaining your goals and your attitudes about your ability to carry out those plans. Generating plans involves research, critical thinking, and creativity. You want to seek the knowledge and experiences of others, and you want to evaluate it critically to be sure it is authoritative and authentic. For example, when using the Internet to obtain health information, you must determine the authoritativeness of the source of the information and ask yourself in whose interest is this information posted on the Web, yours or parties who want you to act on their behalf. The creative aspect of planning involves generating a variety of possible paths (brainstorming) and evaluating the ones with the greatest likelihood for success.

Besides planning what to do, people assess whether they can carry out the actions required to accomplish a goal. This belief is called **self-efficacy.** Self-efficacy is associated with confident, encouraging inner self-talk, such as "I can do it," and "I won't give up."

Slogans like "Just do it," although seemingly encouraging self-efficacy, can undermine it because they ignore the fact that not every goal is realistic or attainable and

no one can do everything no matter how hard they try. Generating false hopes to accomplish the impossible damages one's sense of self-efficacy and self-esteem.

Agency is the belief that one can influence the nature and quality of one's life, rather than believing that one's fate is determined by reacting to circumstances not in one's control. People exhibit agency when they develop intentions and motivations for manifesting them; act on their own behalf in accordance with their values and goals, and evaluate the consequences of their actions in terms of their original goals and strategies. Agency means acknowledging that obstacles to accomplishing one's goals are ever present, and thus not a cause to become stressed. In the face of obstacles, one is flexible and is willing to change goals and strategies that are not working rather than letting discouragement become defeat. Repeated success at accomplishing goals leads to confidence and vitality rather than insecurity and passivity. It also leads to strengthening hope, the general expectation that one will experience good outcomes in life.

Expectations for Success People pursue goals with expectations about the outcomes of their efforts. **Optimism**—imagining a high probability of attaining your goal—motivates, whereas **pessimism**—imagining a low probability of attaining your goal—stifles. Optimism is associated with perceiving negative events as specific, temporary obstacles to be overcome, whereas pessimism is associated with explaining negative events as self-caused (it's my fault), stable (it will last forever), and global (it's going to ruin everything). A pessimistic explanatory style is associated with a greater degree of illness and a shorter life expectancy (Giltay et al., 2004) because pessimists are more likely (1) to be anxious and depressed, (2) to believe that living healthfully or getting help from others when ill won't make things better, and (3) to experience a state of chronic stress and its negative physiological and immune consequences (see Chapter 3).

> ┌─ TERMS ─┐
>
> **agency:** the belief that one can influence the nature and quality of one's life, rather than believing that one's fate is determined by reacting to circumstances not in one's control
>
> **optimism:** the thought process of imagining a high probability of attaining a goal
>
> **pessimism:** the thought process of imagining a low probability of attaining a goal
>
> **self-efficacy:** the belief that one can carry out the actions required to accomplish a goal
>
> **self-esteem:** the judgment one places on one's self-worth

Optimism also is associated with the tendency to perceive oneself as being able to move toward a desired goal and/or away from an undesirable goal. Optimism is associated with inner self-talk that is encouraging and hopeful ("I'll find a way to solve this problem"). On the other hand, the self-talk associated with pessimism is anxious ("I'm not sure what to do"; "I'm not sure it will work out") and self-critical ("I'm inept"). Optimism has been shown to be associated with consuming fresh vegetables and fruits and low-fat foods, whereas pessimism has been associated with low-fiber diets and greater consumption of fat and alcohol (Giltay et al., 2007).

Developing Coping Strategies

There are times in life when everything seems to be going well, and it is possible to experience reasonably long periods of great joy. Change is a fact of life, however, and satisfaction is rarely permanent. Even if all your physical needs are met, you live in harmonious relationships, and your work is meaningful and fulfilling, you still probably experience some degree of frustration and conflict because you initiate changes in your life in the pursuit of new and enriching experiences to satisfy your growth needs.

Coping strategies are ways to deal with the emotional distress that comes from not having your needs met. In general, there are three categories of coping strategies: You can alter (1) the interaction with the cause of the distress, (2) thoughts and beliefs regarding the significance of the need that is not being met, or (3) the distressing feeling, without changing the situation or how you think about it.

To reduce emotional distress by changing your interaction with the situation, you could do any of the following:

- Attack the situation head-on ("I'm anxious about asking her out, but I'll go ahead and do it").
- Avoid the situation ("I'm too nervous about possible rejection. I'll do it some other time").
- Adapt to the situation ("I get nervous every time I ask someone out, but that's normal. So what?").

To change your thoughts and beliefs about the significance of the unmet need, you could:

- Judge your situation to be less distressing than someone else's ("At least I'm meeting people. Poor John works so much he doesn't get to meet anyone").
- See your distress as necessary or temporary ("This is the way it is," or "Eventually I'll find somebody and I won't have to go through this anymore").
- Focus on positive aspects of a situation and minimize the negative ("If she says yes, I'm sure we'll have a great time").
- Devalue the goal and believe you will do fine no matter the outcome ("If he says no, it won't be the end of the world").

Reducing emotional distress by changing or reducing the intensity of the feeling itself could involve releasing emotional energy through an alternative activity:

- Exercise helps with frustration and anger.
- Meditation helps with sadness and anger.
- Talking to a receptive and empathic person can help with grief, shame, and anxiety.

Defense Mechanisms

Defense mechanisms are strategies people use to distort the perception and awareness of reality to avoid unpleasant thoughts, memories, emotions, and situations (**Table 4.1**). A common defense mechanism is denial, which is not believing a truth. An example of denial is a smoker not believing she is at risk for lung cancer even though she knows that smoking causes cancer. This person denies reality to prevent awareness of the truth, possibly to avoid the fear of death.

 Managing Stress

Do It the "Write" Way

When we're stressed and troubled, quite often we get so caught up in our emotions that we lose perspective on what's going on. We only know that we're distressed. This is where writing down thoughts and feelings can help.

Research has shown that writing about one's traumatic experiences can lessen stress, improve immune functioning, and foster health and well-being. Apparently, writing about psychologically painful experiences releases the stress and anxiety associated with trying to keep painful unpleasant feelings out of conscious awareness. Writing about trauma helps one sort, understand, and put the experience into the past.

You don't have to experience a trauma to benefit from writing out your thoughts and feelings. Doing so can help you clarify why you feel a certain way and how your thoughts, perceptions, and reactions to situations are affecting your life. Writing forces you to look at your life honestly. Also, writing lets you express yourself privately without concern about someone else's reaction.

"Write for health" by making regular entries in a *journal,* which is similar to a diary except you express thoughts and feelings instead of record daily events.

- Use a special notebook for your journal.
- Write in a quiet place.
- Keep your journal private so you can be honest with yourself.
- Write continuously. Don't worry about grammar or spelling.
- Be expressive. Don't worry about making sense.

Table 4.1

Common Defense Mechanisms

Defense	Description	Example
Denial	Absolute rejection of a truth or of objective reality	A college student who drinks a six-pack of beer a day but believes that he has no problem with alcohol
Repression	Keeping distressing thoughts and feelings unconscious	A rape victim who has no memory of the assault
Projection	Attributing one's own thoughts and feelings to someone else	A student dislikes her roommate but believes the roommate dislikes her
Displacement	Diverting an emotion from the original target or source to another	You are angry with your parents but yell at your best friends
Reaction formation	Believing and experiencing the opposite of how you truly feel	You are friendly with someone you dislike
Rationalization	Creating a plausible but false reason for your behavior	Believing that failing a course was due to the teacher's poor teaching and not your ineffective studying
Identification	Imagining that someone's or some group's attributes are your own	Feeling superior because one's favorite sports team is successful
Isolation and dissociation	Compartmentalizing thoughts and feelings in different parts of awareness	A successful professional negotiator frequently feuds with his neighbors

Defense mechanisms protect us from thoughts and beliefs that we find threatening; we distort reality to feel safe. Strategies for meeting needs that are based on a faulty foundation generally result in needs not being met. This may lead to disappointment, depression, self-blame, and withdrawal or avoidance of involvement in similar situations.

Distorting reality is not always bad. Sometimes it is necessary because of feeling overwhelmed, trauma, or abuse. In such instances, denial helps a person cope with what would otherwise be a highly stressful psychological situation. Other times, denial can be a way to take a mental vacation. From the perspective of mental health, however, the key is knowing when you are "on a fantasy trip" and when you are not and not letting certain defensive ways of thought become habitual. You can do this by learning to observe how your mind works. Such self-knowledge is a goal of meditation, yoga, modern psychotherapies, and other practices that help to focus on awareness and engage one's consciousness.

Facilitating Coping

Even when emotions make us aware that something in our lives is not going well, we do not always know what the problem is, what is the best way to deal with it, or how to overcome fear of change or longstanding inertia. People should not suffer in silence or believe themselves to be flawed or "crazy." Support and advice are available from trusted family members, friends, teachers, clergy, and mental health professionals, such as counselors, psychotherapists, and physicians. Reaching out to such people helps those in distress gain a new perspective on their problems and to see a workable solution.

Psychotherapists are professionals who have undergone considerable training to help people deal with their emotional distress. Whether a person has

feelings of inferiority, is troubled by painful dependency in a love relationship, or is immobilized by fear, a psychotherapist can facilitate change that can make a person's life better. The change comes about not only by talking, but also by helping the distressed person adopt new behaviors and attitudes. It is one thing to know intellectually the source of a personal problem and even what to do about it, but it may be quite another to face unpleasant emotions and adopt new behaviors ("the map is not the road").

The value of psychotherapy, regardless of the method, is that the distressed person has faith in the professional's ability to facilitate change. This faith produces a situation of trust that enables the distressed person to be honest about himself or herself and to disclose painful and unflattering thoughts, memories, and emotions that would not likely be shared with a friend or relative.

Social Support Contributes to Health

Social support refers to the resources that one receives from others, particularly people in one's immediate social network with whom one has emotional bonds

> **TERMS**
>
> coping strategies: ways people devise to prevent, avoid, or control the emotional distress of unfulfilled needs
> defense mechanisms: mental strategies for avoiding unpleasant thoughts and emotions
> social support: resources that one receives from others, particularly people in one's immediate social network with whom one has emotional bonds and/or social ties

and/or social ties, such as family, friends, schoolmates, coworkers, fellow church members, and professional helpers within one's community. There are several kinds of social support, including the following:

- Emotional support, including reassurance, acceptance, love, trust, and intimacy. When you feel cared for, accepted, and understood, you feel less alone, your self-esteem is enhanced, and you feel more confident and optimistic about managing your life. When you offer emotional support, you feel trustworthy and derive the pleasure and satisfaction of helping another.
- Instrumental support, including tangible help and material and financial assistance. Sometimes you need someone to take you to the doctor, bring you a meal, or loan you some money.
- Informational support, including specific information and knowledge of resources in the environment. Lack of information can block decision making, leading to ruminating and worry about your situation instead of acting.
- Appraisal support, including help with decision making. Sometimes you aren't sure what course of action to take, so you ask knowledgeable and trusted others for their opinions and advice.
- Inclusional support, including encouraging feelings of belonging to the community or a group and access to social contacts and group activities. Belonging to groups alleviates loneliness and provides opportunities for fun, recreation, and the giving and receiving of help.

Numerous studies have shown that people with abundant social support live longer and more healthfully (Uchino, 2005). For example, a study showed that a close friendship, whether with a spouse, friend, or lover, reduced the risk of a second heart attack by as much as 50% (Dickens et al., 2004). Apparently, social support and encouragement from another helped patients carry out rehabilitative activities and lessened the propensity to worry about their medical situation.

Social support contributes to health in several ways. First, social support encourages people to live healthfully. When you decide to exercise regularly, eat less junk food, or stop smoking, the encouragement, advice, and support from family and friends can help you stay on track with your plans. Also, when you are stressed or sick, social support can help you take care of yourself, including obtaining help from health professionals and following medical instructions. Second, social support can make you feel good. When others care about you, you feel good about yourself, you are more optimistic about accomplishing your goals, and you are less lonely, anxious, and depressed. All of these factors contribute to better health. Third, social support diminishes the body's stress responses and strengthens the immune system, thus lessening your risk of illness (Bachen et al., 2007).

People differ in their willingness to seek and accept social support. Some prefer to meet challenges on their own, seeking help only when absolutely necessary, whereas others are more inclined to offer and accept the support of others. In either case, believing that support is available if needed, called **perceived social support,** contributes to feeling valued and able to meet life's stresses without becoming overwhelmed, whether or not support actually exists. Indeed, perceived social support is a better predictor of a sense of well-being and the ability to cope with stress than actual social support is (Lett et al., 2007).

In many ways, social support is reciprocal. People get as they give. Thus, you become a worthy recipient of social support when you are a willing giver of it. There are times in life when you become removed from your established sources of social support, for example, when going away to college or relocating for a job. These are times for making an effort to reestablish a supportive network. One proven strategy for developing a supportive social network is to become involved in activities, groups, and organizations that interest you at campus or within the community. For example, join an exercise class or a hobby group; volunteer at a hospital, museum, church, or community center; or get involved in a cause that you believe in. Groups are always happy for new members, and you will be meeting and doing things with people with interests similar to yours. Some of the most rewarding activity is that which helps others.

Fears, Phobias, and Anxiety

Everybody experiences fear at some time or another. Fear is a powerful emotion that arises in situations that are interpreted as dangerous. The purpose of fear is to alert you to take protective action—usually to fight, flee, or seek assistance. For example, if you were hiking in the woods and encountered a snake, you would naturally interpret this situation as dangerous, which would produce the emotion of fear, which, in turn, would motivate some self-preserving behavior—probably an attempt to escape. If, however, you recognize that the snake is harmless, interpreting the situation as dangerous and thus triggering the emotion of fear would be erroneous. Notice how important the cognitive act of interpretation is in experiencing fear.

A **phobia** involves an intense, irrational fear. The word *phobia* comes from the Greek *phobos,* meaning "to take flight." Thus, a phobia causes us to avoid the object or situation that we fear—to flee from it both metaphorically and actually. The phobia can be a fear of anything: spiders, worms, snakes, bees, roses, a color, flying, boats, darkness—the list of phobias is very long. Some common phobias are *acrophobia* (fear of heights), *mysophobia* (fear of dirt and germs), *ophediophobia* (fear of snakes), and *zoophobia* (fear of animals). A particularly disabling phobia is *agoraphobia,* which is a fear of open spaces. People with agoraphobia are often so fear-

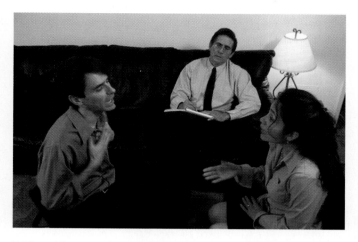

Talking with a counselor can help solve emotional problems.

stricken that they are unable to leave their homes to even run an errand or go shopping.

A person with a phobia almost always knows that the fear is irrational and illogical, yet is unable to control the feelings of anxiety even when thinking about the feared object or situation. Phobias often are triggered in childhood by a frightening event that may or may not be consciously remembered. For example, being stung by a bee while sniffing a rose in the garden at age four may result years later in fear produced by the smell of roses or an exaggerrated fear of bees.

Specific phobias, including agoraphobia, can be treated by a variety of image visualization techniques, with hypnotherapy to uncover the unconscious sensitizing event or events, and by systematic desensitization therapy. Because a phobia exists only in the mind, the mind is where the healing must take place. Imagination is a powerful tool. By imagining the thing that is feared while safe and relaxed at home or in the therapist's office, the mind gradually learns to be comfortable with the object or situation that evokes fear. For example, a person with agoraphobia might begin at home by lying down and visualizing opening the door and looking out. After several days of open-door visualization, he or she might further imagine walking down the stairs, and so on, until he or she can visualize going to the corner while feeling safe and comfortable. After imagining the trip outside, the next step is to actually open the door and step outside. The key to systematic desensitization is to monitor the anxiety and only take the step that feels safe. A trusted counselor or friend is essential in this process.

If fear is the response to a situation interpreted as threatening, **anxiety** is the response to an *imaginary situation*—usually something in the future that has not yet happened—that is interpreted as threatening. The purpose of anxiety is to warn you of *potentially* threatening situations and can take many forms. For example, anxiety about encountering a snake while on a hike, while heightening your awareness of this potential danger, could make the hike very unpleasant or

prevent the hike from taking place at all, even if there were no snakes to encounter.

Anxiety is a normal part of life. It helps us anticipate and prepare for life's challenges. As discussed in Chapter 3, some degree of anxiety can increase performance on a task, because it can help focus attention and motivate preparation. However, some people experience anxiety to a degree that impairs normal, daily functioning and health (**Figure 4.3**). This kind of anxiety tends to be more physiologically and psychologically intense than common anxiety is, and it can seem out of proportion, or even unrelated, to a specific situation. More than 19 million adult Americans experience one or another of the major types of anxiety disorder (**Table 4.2**).

Social anxiety disorder is characterized by an ongoing, pervasive fear of being observed and evaluated by others in all social situations most of the time. Individuals diagnosed with social phobia are constantly apprehensive that they will do or say something to embarrass or humiliate themselves. They compensate for these feelings by avoiding most social situations or interactions with others or, if unavoidable, enduring them with great anxiety and stress. Affected persons typically have few friends, drop out of school, have difficulty in work environments or in holding jobs, drink alcohol or use drugs to dull the anxiety, and often develop other psychological problems.

Social anxiety disorder affects about 6% of Americans. It should be emphasized that a diagnosis of social anxiety disorder entails more than just being shy or nervous in personal interactions at work or in social settings. It usually involves isolating oneself from even simple kinds of interactions: being unable to talk to authority figures such as a teacher or boss, avoiding informal interactions with coworkers, not accepting social invitations, and being unable to talk even in small groups. However, drug company advertisements would have you believe that almost any form of shyness means you suffer from social anxiety disorder and need to take their drug. It might be wise to shy away from such advertisements.

Panic disorder is a condition that involves sudden, terrifying *panic attacks* that generally occur without warning. Panic attacks tend to affect otherwise healthy

TERMS

anxiety: the fear of an imaginary threat

panic disorder: severe anxiety accompanied by physical symptoms

perceived social support: believing that support from one's social network is available if needed

phobia: a powerful and irrational fear of something

social anxiety disorder: fear of being observed and evaluated by others in social situations

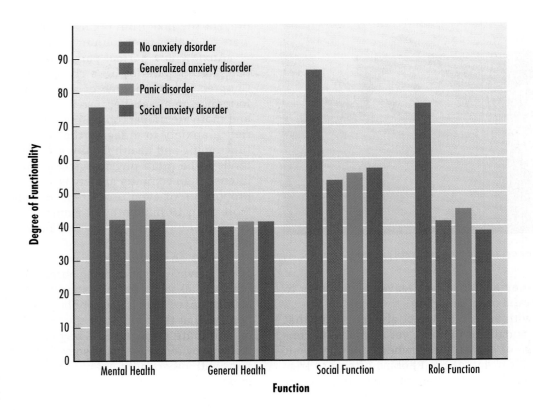

■ **Figure 4.3**

Degree of Functionality with Various Anxiety Disorders

Functionality is assessed by scores on the Medical Outcomes Study Short Form-20, which measures physical, mental, and general health. Role function includes ability to work, do household tasks, or engage in other activities without having to rest and to the degree desired. Social functioning includes engaging in normal social activities without limitations due to decrements in physical and/or emotional health.

Source: Modified from Kroenke, K., et al. (2007). Anxiety disorders in primary care. *Annals of Internal Medicine, 146,* 317–325.

Table 4.2

Kinds of Anxiety Disorders

Condition	Description
Social anxiety disorder (social phobia)	Persistent, intense, and chronic fear of being watched and judged by others and being embarrassed or humiliated by their own actions, an overwhelming and excessive self-consciousness in everyday social situations such as speaking in formal or informal situations, eating or drinking in front of others or, in its most severe form, being around other people for any reason. Fear may be so severe that it interfers with work, school, and other ordinary activities. Accompanying physical symptoms include blushing, profuse sweating, trembling, nausea, and difficulty talking.
Panic disorder	Unexpected and repeated episodes of intense fear accompanied by physical symptoms that my include chest pain, nausea, hear palpitations or pounding, shortness of breath, abdominal distress, and feeling sweaty, weak, faint, dizzy, flushed, or chilled. Feelings of terror may strike suddenly and repeatedly with no warning. The hands may tingle or feel numb. There may be smothering sensations, a sense of unreality, or fear of impending doom or loss of control.
Generalized anxiety disorder	Chronic anxiety and exaggerated worry and tension, even when there is little or nothing to provoke it. Anxiety is often accomanied by fatigue, headaches, muscle tension, muscle aches, difficulty swallowing, trembling, twitching, irritability, sweating, and hot flashes.
Obsessive-compulsive disorder (OCD)	Recurrent, unwanted thoughts (obsessions) and/or repetitive behaviors (compulsions) such as handwriting, counting, checking, or cleaning, often performed with the hope of preventing obsessive thoughts or making them go away. Performing these rituals provides only temporary relief, and not performing them markedly increases anxiety.
Posttraumatic stress disorder (PTSD)	Persistent, frightening thoughts and memories of a prior traumatic experience in which grave physical harm occurred or was threatened and feeling emotionally numb, especially with people to whom one was once close. People with PTSD may experience sleep problems, feel detached or numb, or be easily startled.

Source: Modifed from American Psychiatric Association. (1994). *Diagnostic and statistical manual of mental disorders: Primary care version* (4th ed.). Washington, DC: Author.

young adults; they are characterized by the sudden appearance of intense fear, pounding heart, shortness of breath, paralyzing terror, sweating, and fear of dying or losing control. Because of these symptoms, panic disorder was formerly known as irritable heart or hyperventilation syndrome. Because the antecedents of a panic attack are often not identifiable, it is very unlike a phobia (fear of specific things such as snakes or air travel) or other kinds of anxiety disorder.

Panic disorder affects about 7% of healthy adult Americans and seriously disrupts their quality of life. Persons with panic disorder often wind up in hospital emergency rooms suffering from dizziness, bowel distress, and symptoms of a heart attack. In the case of a panic disorder, all medical diagnostic tests are negative for disease, but the symptoms reoccur. Although the cause of panic disorder is still unknown, research suggests that a disturbance of neurotransmitters in the brain is responsible, which may be the reason that some people with panic disorder are helped by medications.

Because of the unexpected suddenness and intensity of panic attacks, people with panic disorder often are helped simply by learning that they have an illness and are not crazy. This knowledge opens the way to adopting other helpful measures, including identifying thoughts and situations that might trigger a panic attack (e.g., an upcoming exam, family problems, or noticing a strong heart beat or shallow breathing, which could suggest the onset of a panic attack).

One of the most effective ways to control a panic attack is through deep, abdominal breathing that can prevent hyperventilation and other related symptoms. Yoga breathing techniques are a good way to begin, or one can consult a breathing specialist who can teach techniques that help an affected person avoid shallow, rapid breathing. The fact that panic disorder appears at certain periods of life, that no biological or genetic cause is known, and that it is effectively relieved by psychotherapy or placebo should encourage people to focus on lifestyle changes that will free them of the serious and debilitating consequences of panic disorder (Barlow et al., 2000).

Generalized anxiety disorder is characterized by persistent and excessive worry and feelings of anxiety. The condition is distinct from phobia, panic disorder, or social anxiety disorder (see Table 4.2), with its own set of diagnostic criteria:

- Excessive worry and anxiety over work or school performance that has continued for at least six months.
- The patient is unable to control or cope with the anxiety and feels that it interferes with performance at work or other aspects of daily life.
- The anxiety must be accompanied by at least three of the following: restlessness or being on edge, fatigue, difficulty concentrating, irritability, muscle tension, and problems sleeping.

- The anxiety is not caused by the effects of any drug (legal or illegal) and is not caused by a physiological condition (e.g., hyperthyroidism).

Where does normal worry end and excessive anxiety begin? There does not seem to be any clear or easy answer to this question. For example, many people have ongoing worries (generalized anxiety) about being able to pay their bills, keep their jobs, or get good grades in school. Anxious people may have trouble sleeping or be on edge most of the time. Is one person mentally ill and another mentally well depending on how anxious they are about their money, job, or school problems? This is the dilemma for psychotherapists who treat people with ongoing worries.

Obsessive-Compulsive Disorder

Obsessive-compulsive disorder (OCD) is characterized by persistent, unwelcome thoughts or images (*obsessions*) that often are accompanied by an uncontrollable, urgent need to engage in certain rituals (*compulsions*). Rituals such as handwashing, counting, checking, or cleaning are often performed in hope of preventing obsessive thoughts or making them go away. Performing these rituals, however, provides only temporary relief, and not performing them markedly increases anxiety. OCD affects about 2% of the U.S. population. The condition typically begins during adolescence or late childhood. It is sometimes accompanied by depression, eating disorders, substance abuse, attention deficit hyperactivity disorder, or other anxiety disorders. Symptoms of OCD can also coexist and may even be part of a spectrum of neurological disorders, such as Tourette's syndrome. OCD likely has a neurobiological basis and is not caused by family problems or by attitudes learned in childhood, such as an inordinate emphasis on cleanliness or a belief that certain thoughts are dangerous or unacceptable. Treatments for OCD involve medications and behavioral therapy.

Depression

In the course of their lifetime, about 17% of Americans experience an episode of **major depression,** characterized by feelings of helplessness, hopelessness, reduced

---

TERMS

generalized anxiety disorder: persistent and often nonspecific worry and anxiety

major depression: a mental state characterized by feelings of helplessness, hopelessness, and self-recrimination

obsessive-compulsive disorder: persistent, unwelcome thoughts or images and the urgent, uncontrollable need to engage in certain rituals

interest in previously enjoyable activities, and a variety of other symptoms (Table 4.3). If asked how they feel, depressed people usually say something like, "Life's a drag" or "What's the use of doing anything?" One hallmark of depression is a helpless/hopeless attitude.

The American College Health Association (2008) reports that nearly half of college students feel sufficiently depressed at some point during the school year that they have trouble functioning; about 16% are depressed enough to require treatment. College students with depression experience most of the same symptoms other American adults, do, including some specific to students:

- Withdrawal from formerly pleasurable social activities
- A drop in grades
- Inability to concentrate on schoolwork; reading material becomes overwhelming
- Sleep disturbances (sleeping much more or less soundly than usual) not related to studying or cramming for tests
- Consuming more alcohol than usual

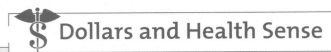

$ Dollars and Health Sense

Drugs for Coping with Everyday Life

A TV advertisement for a prescription drug shows a woman in her kitchen with dirty dishes in the sink, toys on the floor, and food on the counters waiting to be prepared. Viewers hear the woman's inner voice anxiously complaining about all the things she has to do and how hard it is to cope. No doubt about it, she's stressed. The ad tells viewers that overreactions to life's challenges could be a sign of an anxiety disorder and to see a doctor about getting medication. The ad closes with a shot of the same woman in the same kitchen, now clean and neat. Instead of complaining, her inner voice is singing. All thanks to the drug being advertised.

The makers of this ad are using the strategy of defining normal aspects of living as illnesses to increase sales of a prescription medication. This strategy has also been applied to shyness. In each case, the drugs being advertised were initially approved for treatment of a recognized illness. However, the marketing of the drug focuses on symptoms that are part and parcel of everyday life and for which drugs are inappropriate because they do not resolve the issues causing the problem, and their side effects, and in some cases addiction potential, pose health risks.

Here is another example of "medicalizing" a common experience to sell a drug intended for something else. The prescription drug modafinil (Provigil) was approved by the FDA for treatment of narcolepsy, a serious medical condition characterized by sudden and unintentional falling asleep during wakeful activity, and to ameliorate a specific kind of sleep disturbance in some shift workers. However, until the FDA told its manufacturer to stop, advertising for modafinil claimed that the drug was suitable for fatigue, tiredness, sleepiness, decreased activity, or lack of energy—symptoms characteristic of a large percentage of American college students and many people with legitimate psychological disorders such as depression. People who are drowsy while awake because they cheat on sleep do not have a disease; they are experiencing the predictable consequences of a choice. Rather than taking a drug and risking side effects and possible permanent alterations in brain biology, drowsy people would feel better if they turned off their TVs and computers and got more sleep.

Always remember: Pharmaceutical companies are massive corporations with the goal of making money. Your health is their concern only insofar as it enhances profits. You are the one responsible for your health. Until manipulation is no longer a part of drug company advertising, you are better off ignoring it.

Table 4.3

Common Symptoms of Depression

Psychological symptoms	Behavioral symptoms	Physical symptoms
Depressed mood	Crying spells	Fatigue
Irritability	Interpersonal confrontation	Reduced or too much sleep
Anxiety/nervousness	Anger attacks/outbursts	Decreased or increased appetite
Reduced concentration	Avoidance of anxiety-provoking situations	Weight loss/gain
Lack of interest/motivation	Social withdrawal	Aches and pains
Inability to enjoy things	Workaholism	Muscle tension
Reduced interest in sex	Tobacco/alcohol/drug use or abuse	Heart palpitations
Hypersensitivity to criticism/rejection	Self-sacrifice/victimization	Burning or tingling sensations
Indecisiveness	Suicide attempts/gestures	
Pessimism/hopelessness		
Feelings of helplessness		
Preoccupation with oneself		
Thoughts of death or suicide		

Often, a depressed student does not recognize that something is amiss. Instead, a parent, friend, roommate, or residence hall advisor may notice depressive symptoms and encourage the student to seek help.

Depression can occur as a normal response to the loss of something that a person values or is attached to, such as a loved one, a job, good health, or self-esteem (e.g., when a person does not succeed at a task she or he deems important). When individuals experience a loss, it is normal to feel sad and depressed, and to grieve the loss. Sadness and grief are the human spirit's way to heal the hurt of loss and open the way for new attachments. When normal depression is associated with a loss, the depressed individual may be simultaneously aware that the experience is transitory and, along with grief, feel that there is hope for the future. This kind of depression tends to lift after the grieving ends.

In contrast to the normal depression that may accompany loss, some people experience a long-lasting depressive state or periodic episodes of deep depression that are not self-limiting and may hinder and even jeopardize a person's life. These depressions may be a response to stress, severe psychological trauma, injury, disease, biological malfunctions of some part of the brain, or a combination of factors. In some persons, major episodes of depression are accompanied by periods of excited euphoria (*mania*), resulting in a condition referred to as **bipolar disorder**.

Some individuals are susceptible to depression during the winter months because a lack of sunlight disturbs the production of neurotransmitters in the brain that affect mood. This **seasonal affective disorder** (SAD) is sometimes remedied by increased exposure to stronger-than-normal indoor lighting that mimics sunlight or relocation to southern latitudes where there is more light.

Depression can also accompany the experience of being very sick or injured. In such cases, depression results from a combination of factors, such as grieving the loss of health; coping with the stress of being sick; lack of exercise and normal routine; disruption of regular social activities; or alterations in physiology that may change brain chemistry. Medications may also make one susceptible to depression. Some people experience a mild form of depression called **dysthymia**. Like major depression, dysthymia is associated with disturbances in sleep, appetite, and the ability to concentrate.

One of the characteristics of severe depression is a considerable degree of negative thinking, characterized by severe self-criticism; negative views about the self, the world, and the future; and a variety of logic errors in assessing the self and the world. Some of these logic errors include the following:

- *All-or-none thinking:* seeing things as polar extremes (e.g., all good and all bad)
- *Overgeneralizing:* interpreting one setback as evidence that *every* similar situation will *forever* turn out badly
- *Negative filtering:* focusing only on the negative while filtering out the positive
- *Disqualifying the positive:* transforming positive occurrences into negative experiences

Becoming aware of negative thoughts (often called *negative self-talk*) opens the way to adopting positive self-images and more realistic appraisals of the world. These, in turn, help to lessen the depressive state. Cognitive behavioral therapy is a very successful method for helping depressed people change their negative thought patterns.

Another characteristic of depression is that it can intensify itself, thus creating a depressive cycle. The depressed person's negative thoughts, social withdrawal, and loss of interest in pleasurable experiences serve to reinforce feelings of worthlessness, helplessness, gloom, and doom. Recovery from depression requires both interrupting the depressive cycle and correcting the life situation that brought on the depression. Recreational activity can divert attention from negative thinking and weaken the depression cycle.

One way to deal with depression is to get life moving again. This is accomplished by establishing and achieving simple, attainable goals that can be done in a brief period of time. The goals should involve movement that restores fundamental breathing and other mind–body rhythms, which may alter the chemistry of the brain to facilitate pleasant (instead of unpleasant) moods. Many a depressed person has found relief in taking up a regular exercise program.

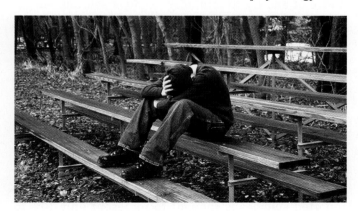

Many things may make us feel depressed temporarily.

TERMS

bipolar disorder: episodes of depression followed by episodes of mania

dysthymia: a long-lasting, mild form of depression

seasonal affective disorder: depressive symptoms that appear in autumn or winter and remit spontaneously in spring

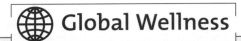
Global Wellness

Depression Is Worldwide

Missing my dear mother, as a son,
my liver and intestines are painfully broken!
Crying for my old mother, as a son,
my tears pour into my chest!
Thinking about my old mother, as a son,
to swallow food and tea is difficult!
Searching for my old mother, as a son,
I cannot sleep day and night!

Si-Lang, *Searching for Mother*
Tenth-Century Beijing Opera

Melancholy and depression know no geographic boundaries, as this thousand-year-old Chinese aria describing the physical aspects of depression shows. Depression has been documented in virtually all cultures, although its prevalence varies (World Health Organization, 2001). Depression in Asia, for example, is less prevalent than in North America and Europe (Table 4.4). Rates of depression in the United States even vary by cultural group: The lifetime prevalence of depression among people of African and Hispanic ancestry is about 12%; among people of European ancestry, it's 17%.

Besides prevalence rates, depression manifests differently among cultures. Several Native American cultures tend to experience depression as social loneliness. A typical Caucasian North American or European is likely to experience depression in terms of psychological symptoms, such as melancholy, moodiness, and lack of interest in pleasure. However, in Asian cultures, depression tends to be experienced as physical complaints (as in the Chinese aria above), such as fatigue, loss of appetite, and sleep problems.

Table 4.4
Prevalence of Depression in Selected Countries of the World

Country	Prevalence of depression (%)
Chile	29.5
United Kingdom	16.9
Netherlands	15.9
Brazil	15.8
France	13.7
Turkey	11.6
Germany	11.2
United States	6.3
Nigeria	4.2
China	4.0
Japan	2.6

Source: World Health Organization. (2001). World Health Report. Available: http://www.who.int/whr2001/2001/main/en/tables/table2.1.htm.

Help-seeking behavior for depression also varies among cultures. Latin American men and mainland Chinese tend not to seek help for depression, fearing that doing so will stigmatize them as weak. In Japan and Hong Kong, where depression tends to be experienced as a physical ailment, people tend to consult with a doctor for relief of physical symptoms. Latin American women and European Americans are more likely to consult mental health practitioners.

Also, depressed individuals should interact with people who offer support. Remaining in seclusion only reinforces feelings of loss and worthlessness. A depressed person should not engage in long conversations with friends and family about how lousy life is.

Several types of medication are available to treat depression. The most widely prescribed medications are *selective serotonin reuptake inhibitors* (SSRIs). Other medications include tricyclic antidepressants and monoamine oxidase inhibitors. Treatment of mild depression with SSRIs, although shown to be beneficial in clinical tests of the drugs, seems to be caused by a placebo effect rather than by any biological effects of the drugs (Kirsch et al., 2008). Because all drugs have side effects, and SSRIs in particular have been linked to an increased risk of suicide, particularly among young people, the risk of harm when taking these drugs must always be considered. In moderate to severe depression, SSRIs seem to be more helpful than placebo. That many medications for mild depression are no more effective than placebo shows that recovery from mild depression is more psychological than biological; belief that relief is at hand is a powerful healer of depression.

Because depression involves inactivity, withdrawal, hopelessness, and self-defeating thoughts and behaviors, it is often difficult for individuals to activate themselves on a program of self-healing. At such times, the encouragement of a caring friend or family member and the guidance of a therapist, counselor, or other helper can be invaluable. Others can help a depressed person confront the causes of the depression and become aware of and try to minimize negative self-talk—negative views about the self, the world, and the future; self-critical inner dialogue; and logic errors in the assessment of self and events.

Suicide

One of the most worrisome aspects of depression is the risk of suicide. Besides depression, the risk of suicide is associated with panic disorder, social phobia, PTSD, bipolar disorder, and adult attention deficit hyperactivity disorder. In the United States, suicide ranks among the 10 most frequent causes of death, accounting for approximately 30,000 deaths per year. The number of reported suicides is thought to represent only 10% to 15% of suicide attempts. People over age 65 make up the largest age group of suicides. Among young people (15

🧘 Managing Stress

If a Friend Is Considering Suicide

If you suspect that a friend is considering suicide, how can you help? You can take any of several possible courses of action. All involve you making a concrete intervention. Intervention is tough. It is much easier to tell yourself that things will get better, or tomorrow is another day. Rationalization and procrastination are not useful behaviors in a situation that involves depression or potential suicide. Let's look at some options available to you.

- Talk to your friend. Tell him or her that you are concerned. Describe the behavior that is causing you to worry. Ask if you can help (but don't give up if your friend says no).

- Ask your friend directly if he or she is thinking about suicide. You may be shocked if your friend answers yes, but remember, even someone who sees suicide as a potential solution always has a wish to live. If your friend admits thinking of suicide, ask if he or she has thought of a plan.

- Negotiate a "no-suicide" agreement before leaving your friend. Ask your friend to agree not to commit suicide at any

time. If your friend will not agree to this contract or tries to change it to a certain time, then he or she is at increased risk. Report this situation to a professional counselor (or even the police or fire department) at once. Stay with your friend or arrange for someone else to stay with him or her until professional help arrives.

- If your friend agrees to a "no-suicide" pact, go to your college health service or residence hall advisor, speak with a counselor or physician, and describe your friend's behavior. The professional will know the best way to handle the situation. And remember, even if you feel you are interfering or breaking a confidence, you may be saving a life. An intervention made now can prevent suicide.

- Talk to other friends, a residence hall advisor, or even a teacher—anyone who will assist you to verbalize your concerns and decide how to help. The most important action is to do something after you become aware of the potentially dangerous outcome.

---

to 24 years old), suicide ranks third behind accidents and murder as a cause of death.

Suicide is the second leading cause of death among college students, although the suicide rate among college students is half that of their noncollege age peers (7.5 per 100,000 vs. 15 per 100,000). About 10% of college students admit to having seriously thought about or attempted suicide within the prior 12 months (American College Health Association, 2008). Very often, these attempts occur on the same day or shortly after an acute life crisis. To help avert student suicides, campuses are developing and making students aware of helping services. Two risk factors for suicide to which college students are particularly susceptible are social isolation and feeling ineffective (Joiner, Brown, & Wingate, 2005). Until they can build an on-campus supportive social network, students away from home may feel lonely, insecure, and unworthy of others' attention, all of which can lead to feeling depressed. Furthermore, without a social network, they may be less able to find support when they are anxious and depressed. Feeling ineffective at school because of grade competition and a constant sense of not being able to keep up with coursework can result in feeling helpless, guilty, and ashamed.

Suicide is not a disease, nor is it a disorder that can be inherited. Suicides are not caused by the weather or a full moon. Generally people consider suicide because they feel overwhelmed and painfully distressed by life and they believe suicide to be their only option. Sometimes people attempt suicide not because they really want to die but because they want to express anger at others or signal others for help. In such instances, suicide attempts are characterized by limited self-destructive

acts, such as taking less than a lethal dose of sleeping pills or arranging that the attempt be discovered in time for the person to be saved.

Occasionally a person expresses thoughts of suicide to a friend or relative. This can be extremely distressing to the listener, who may react with disbelief, panic, or avoidance. In attempting to deal with his or her own uncomfortable feelings, a listener might say things like, "Cheer up, you've got a lot to live for," or "You're better off than I am," or "You can't be serious!" These and similar statements have the effect of denying the distressed person's feelings. Psychologists recommend instead that listeners speak directly to suicidal thoughts ("Tell me more about why you want to kill yourself"), offer the distressed person nonjudgmental sympathy and concern, and firmly but patiently direct the distressed person to professional help immediately.

Often suicidal individuals offer excuses for not seeing a professional and may even try to blackmail a friend into silence with threats ("I'll kill myself if you tell anyone"). The friend must hold firm and, if necessary, make an appointment with a counselor or psychiatrist at the student health center or hospital emergency room and deliver the distressed person there, or telephone a suicide prevention hotline.

At the time a person contemplates suicide, life seems absolutely hopeless. But few life problems are beyond solution. Life crises improve and distressing emotions pass. Time does heal many hurts. And the experience gained by working through a distressing time of life can bring confidence, insight, and understanding. Acquiring experience and understanding, a person is better able to cope with life's problems and is better able to help others deal with their challenges.

Adult Attention Deficit Hyperactivity Disorder (ADHD)

Adult attention deficit hyperactivity disorder (ADHD) is characterized by difficulty focusing on activities, organizing and finishing tasks, managing one's time, following instructions, and/or being overly restless, "on the go," and perceived as not thinking before acting or speaking. About 4% of adults are believed to have ADHD. Untreated ADHD in adults is associated with lower socioeconomic status, lower rates of professional employment, more frequent job changes, more work difficulties, and more spousal separations and divorce. Also, adults with ADHD have more automobile collisions, speeding violations, and driver's license suspensions. Moreover, adults with ADHD are likely to be distressed by the persistent discomfort of their symptoms and the personal and social problems that arise from them.

In many adults, ADHD persists from childhood, when they experienced difficulties in educational performance, discipline problems, and being labeled as intentional underachievers and lacking in intelligence. This blaming and lack of understanding and empathy often damaged self-esteem, creating another problem that contributed to difficulties in performance in adulthood.

ADHD is not intentional but most likely a consequence of biological conditions in the brain. Compared with other adults, those with ADHD show differences in brain dopamine and noradrenaline neurotransmitter systems and anatomical/functional differences in the frontal regions of the brain, which are responsible for attention and working memory (Biederman, 2005). That the effective medications for ADHD are ones that alter the balance of dopamine and noradrenaline in the brain suggest that brain biology is at the root of ADHD.

College students with undiagnosed ADHD generally struggle to complete school assignments, manage their time, get good grades, and even complete their degrees. With medications, coaching, and counseling, however, students with ADHD can learn to stay organized and manage the tasks of college (Table 4.5). Some adults with ADHD find ways to direct their bountiful energy, curiosity, and desire for novelty to achieve success in careers as physicians, journalists, attorneys, and salespeople.

Anger

Anger occurs when we've been attacked, blamed, hurt, or have experienced a loss; when we *imagine* we've been attacked, blamed, hurt, or have experienced a loss; when we imagine we *may* be attacked, blamed, hurt, or experience a loss; or when the pursuit of an important goal is blocked. Sometimes we get angry because we perceive something as threatening that really isn't. In this case, we make ourselves angry by what we think.

Anger is an excitatory emotion, providing the motivational energy to protect ourselves or things we care

Table 4.5
Success Strategies for Students with ADHD
Keep a day-planner and a to-do list.
Use a backpack as an organizer. Put pens and pencils in outside pockets, notebook in another pocket, and homework in another. Keep books inside.
Keep an assignment notebook. Daily, list all assignments, quizzes, and exams, and check them off when completed.
Create a two-pocket homework folder. Label one pocket "Work to Be Done" and put all assignment sheets therein. Label the other pocket "Work Completed" and put all finished assignments therein. Check the folder every day.
Help yourself pay attention in class. Sit close to the instructor to lessen distractions. Use a voice recorder for lectures and studying.
Let others help you. If friends and instructors know about your ADHD, they are more likely to help you stay organized and on top of your tasks.

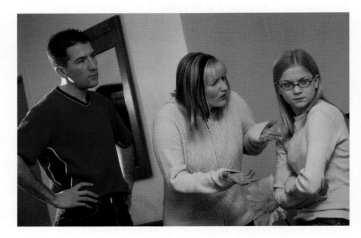

Family arguments disrupt the emotional well-being of parents and children.

about or to overcome obstacles to our goals. We use anger to stop physical or psychological abuse and to protect ourselves from the hurt of loss.

Whereas anger tends to be situational, **hostility** is a personal trait characterized by an ongoing mistrust of others, cynicism, a personal emotional style of anger mixed with disgust and contempt, and a tendency to act out those feelings with overt aggression, snide comments, or criticism. Studies show that hostility is related to an increased risk of heart disease (Smith et al., 2007).

One constructive way to work with anger is to understand the source of the emotion. For example, to deal with frustration you can reassess the merits of the goal you cannot attain or reconsider the strategy you've employed for attaining it. It may feel right to blame someone else for your troubles, but a reevaluation of how you contribute to the situation may be more productive.

Another strategy for dealing with anger is forgiveness. By forgiving, you are not saying that another's transgression is OK or even that you want to have a relationship with that person. When you forgive, you release yourself of the psychological weight and physio-

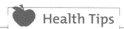 **Health Tips**

Some Tips for Dealing with Anger

Here are some suggestions for expressing anger constructively.

- *Acknowledge your anger.* Pay attention to anger in yourself when you become aware of it. Then take some time to determine which of your thoughts are causing it. Are you hurt, frustrated, frightened? What happened that made you angry?
- *Own your anger.* Try not to blame someone else for your angry feeling by means of thoughts or statements like "It's all your fault!" or "If it weren't for you," or "If only you'd have . . ." Don't put it onto someone else unless you're sure it belongs there.
- *Chill.* Even if you are very angry, try not to act immediately on those feelings. Instead, set aside a time to think about them and how best to express them.
- *Resolve the anger.* Try not to let anger build up over time. If you do, you may become resentful, which may cause you to distance yourself emotionally or physically or to displace the anger onto someone else, like a child or a coworker.
- *Don't ambush.* Attacking with anger when it's least expected is unfair and invites resentment or a counterattack, not reconciliation.
- *Be specific.* When you're talking about emotional conflicts, name exactly what's causing the anger and stick to that issue. Don't bring up past hurts. Don't discuss second and third topics until the first one is settled. If other issues arise, write them down so you can discuss them later. Make it a habit to keep pencil and paper handy when issues are discussed. Don't give in to the temptation to bring up secondary issues to retaliate for hurt feelings or as a way to avoid resolving the issue at hand.

- *Don't hit below the belt.* In an argument, don't attack the other person with a statement you know will hurt because you think you're losing the argument.
- *Attack the problem, not the other person.* Don't engage in character assassination with put-downs and accusations. Use "I" statements to communicate resentments. If someone attacks with a put-down, rather than retaliate, you can say, "Ouch, that hurt." This can be a cue to redress the attack and go on with the issue under discussion. If this doesn't happen, the discussion will probably be sidetracked from the main point to the put-down, and a fight about hurt feelings may ensue.
- *Be respectful and respectable.* When working to resolve an issue, try to maintain an attitude of respect. Try to understand the other's point of view. Ask the other person to respect you and your feelings, even though you disagree.
- *Take some time.* Sometimes you can sense that an anger-causing issue isn't getting resolved. It's all right to acknowledge that and to take a few hours or days to reconsider things, then discuss the issue again. Sometimes emotions are too intense and it's not possible to think clearly. Sometimes you just need time to reflect and figure things out.
- *Physical affection is acceptable.* Sex or any other affectionate behavior before an issue is resolved is acceptable, as long as it's not taken as a sign that the issue is resolved. Affectionate behavior shows that arguing about something can be accommodated within a caring relationship.
- *Both sides win.* After an issue has been discussed and the partners seem agreed on the outcome, if one or both feels a grudge, then the argument has produced a winner and a loser, and the relationship has been harmed. Holding a grudge is a sign that the issue is not resolved. Try again.

logical tension of internalized anger. You open the pathway to attaining psychological closure on the incident and the peace of mind that can follow. Furthermore, you contribute to your own health and well-being (Lawler-Row et al., 2008).

The next time you feel angry, take a "time-out" for a few seconds, minutes, or days if necessary. Ask yourself what you've experienced that's led you to be angry. Are you really being harmed or threatened or are you making yourself angry because you've interpreted a situation as such? If you feel frustrated about not being able to accomplish a goal, is your goal realistically attainable? Have you expected too much of yourself? Have you expected too much of someone else? Is your strategy for attaining your goal workable? Is something else better? Did you communicate your goals, needs, plans, and desires to people whose help you wanted or expected?

Sleep and Dreams

All living things exhibit cycles of rest and activity, which in humans are represented by the daily sleep–wake cycle. Everyone has a sleep–wake cycle that corresponds

to his or her optimal degree of physical, mental, and spiritual well-being. The optimum sleep for most adults is 7 to 8 hours per night, with some needing less sleep and others more. The duration of sleep is less significant than is whether an individual awakens feeling refreshed, vital, and able to function optimally. Nearly 60% of American college students report not getting enough

TERMS

adult attention deficit hyperactivity disorder (ADHD): difficulty focusing on activities, organizing and finishing tasks, managing one's time, following instructions, and/or being overly restless, "on the go," and perceived as not thinking before acting or speaking

hostility: a personal trait characterized by an ongoing mistrust of others, cynicism, a personal emotional style of anger mixed with disgust and contempt, and a tendency to act out those feelings with overt aggression, snide comments, or criticism

sleep on most days of the week to feel rested the next morning (American College Health Association, 2008).

Adequate sleep enhances attentiveness, concentration, mood, and motivation. Sleep deprivation, on the other hand, impairs a person's ability to be productive, good-humored, satisfied with life, and even to laugh at a joke! Lack of sleep can gravely impair judgment: Sleeplessness is second only to drunkenness as a cause of automobile accidents. Long-term sleep deprivation can be fatal.

Sleep is a basic biological function. Sleep centers in the brain control sleep behavior, much as appetite centers in the brain control eating behavior. When you don't get adequate sleep, your brain creates an urge to sleep, which can be irresistible if you are sufficiently sleep-deprived. Human sleep is composed of five stages, through which one cycles every 90 to 120 minutes during a sleep episode (**Figure 4.4**).

Good sleep requires diminished physiological and psychological arousal caused by heightened sympathetic nervous system activity (for example, caused by caffeine, a pre-bed-time cigarette, or anger, worry, and stress). Reading bedtime stories to children is a time-honored way to diminish their sympathetic nervous system arousal and provide a transition to sleep. Methods common to adults include reading before bedtime, prayer or meditation, taking a warm bath, and having a light snack. Drinking alcohol, while possibly contributing to drowsiness, actually impairs falling asleep and getting restful sleep.

Sleep researchers believe that a majority of Americans are sleeping 60 to 90 minutes a night less than the seven or eight hours that would leave them refreshed and energetic during the day (**Figure 4.5**). Individuals "cheat on their sleep" to create time for other things in their busy schedules that characterize modern life.

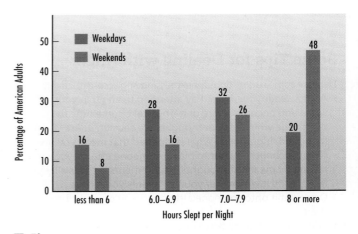

■ **Figure 4.5**

Number of Hours Slept per Night on Weekdays and Weekends by American Adults
Notice that many people are getting less than the recommended 7–8 hours a night on weekdays and are making up for it by sleeping more on weekends.

Source: Data from National Sleep Foundation. (2008). Sleep in America poll. Available: http://www.sleepfoundation.org.

Sleep is considered expendable, and not sleeping is considered a sign of ambition and drive. Furthermore, around-the-clock TV, radio entertainment, and the Internet can distract people from sleeping. Before the advent of the electric light bulb in the late 1800s, people tended to sleep about nine hours a night. When it got dark, people slept. Because sleep is so strongly linked to one's total state of well-being, focusing on healthy sleep habits can produce greater mind–body harmony.

College Students and Sleep

Deprive, deprive, deprive, deprive, crash. This is a very common sleep pattern among college students. During the week, students deprive themselves of sleep to complete their academic tasks, work, interact with electronic media, and socialize, and on the weekend they pay back their "sleep debt" with one or two extended episodes of sleep. Because this pattern is prevalent, it may seem normal, but it has drawbacks. For example, shortened sleep time, erratic sleep/wake schedules, and poor sleep quality are associated with lower academic performance, thus creating the irony that the motivation to sleep less to produce more is counterproductive (Wolfson & Carskadon, 2003). Sleeping only four to six hours a night can reduce the ability to pay attention, react to a stimulus, think quickly, not make mistakes, and multitask.

Many college students experience times of disturbed or nonrestful sleep (Forquer et al., 2008). They go to bed, but instead of falling asleep, they lie awake thinking about their to-do list, problems, an upcoming exam or speech, and just about anything else that enters their minds. Or they fall asleep, but after a few hours they awaken—ruminating—and cannot readily go

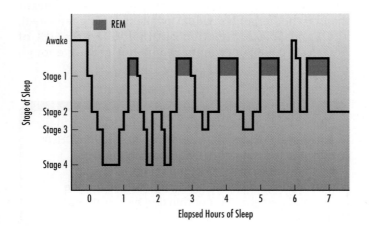

■ **Figure 4.4**

The Human Sleep Cycle
Sleep consists of moving through the five stages of sleep several times during a sleep episode.

Source: U.S. Coast Guard. (2004, January). *Crew Endurance News.*

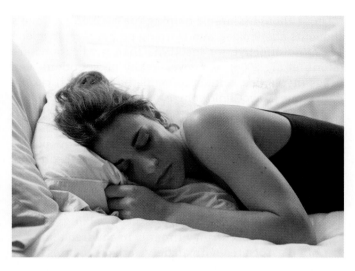

Sufficient sleep and dreams are essential to mental health.

back to sleep. Having not gotten a good night's sleep (or two or three), when awake they are irritable, depressed, tired, have low motivation (even for things they like), and diminished concentration. Frequently, when academic pressures relent and stress subsides, normal, restorative sleep returns. It is possible, however, that the factors producing disturbed sleep become habitual, causing chronic insomnia (see the following section).

Getting a Good Night's Sleep

Here are some suggestions for getting a good night's sleep.

- *Establish a regular sleep time.* Give your own natural sleep cycle a chance to be in synchrony with the day–night cycle by going to bed at the same time each night (within an hour more or less) and arising *without being awakened by an alarm clock.* This will mean going to bed early enough to give yourself enough time to sleep. Try to maintain your regular sleep times on the weekend. Getting up early during the week and sleeping late on weekends may upset the rhythm of your sleep cycle.

- *Create a proper (for you) sleep environment.* Sleep occurs best when the sleeping environment is dark, quiet, free of distractions, and not too warm. If you use radio or TV to help you fall asleep, use an autotimer to shut off the noise after falling asleep.

- *Wind down before going to bed.* About 20 to 30 minutes before bedtime, stop any activities that cause mental or physical arousal, such as work or exercise, and take up a "quiet" activity that can create a transition to sleep. Transitional activities could include reading, watching "mindless" TV, taking a warm bath or shower, meditation, or making love.

- *Make the bedroom for sleeping only.* Make the bedroom your place for getting a good night's sleep. Try not to use it for work or for discussing problems with your partner.

- *Don't worry while in bed.* If you are unable to sleep after about 30 minutes in bed because of worry about things in your life, get up and do some limited activity such as reading a magazine article, doing the dishes, or meditating. Go back to bed when you feel drowsy. If you cannot sleep because of thinking about all that you have to do, write down what's on your mind and let the paper hold onto the thoughts while you sleep. You can retrieve them in the morning.

- *Avoid alcohol, caffeine, and tobacco.* Some people have a glass of beer or wine before bed to relax. Large amounts of alcohol, although sedating, block normal sleep and dreaming patterns. Because caffeine remains in the body for several hours, people sensitive to caffeine should not ingest any after noon. Nicotine is a stimulant, so it should be avoided before bedtime.

- *Exercise regularly.* Exercising 20 to 30 minutes three or four times a week enhances the ability to sleep. You should not exercise vigorously within three hours of bedtime, however, because of the possibility of becoming too aroused to sleep.

Sleep Problems

Because of life's never-ending array of challenges, just about everyone has trouble sleeping once in a while. Experiences that commonly disrupt sleeping patterns include being sick, jet-lagged, nervous about an upcoming exam, or excited about something new; having consumed too much food, alcohol, or caffeine; or losing a loved one. Fortunately, most people tend to adjust to these situations, and their sleep rhythms return to normal (for them). A large percentage of Americans,

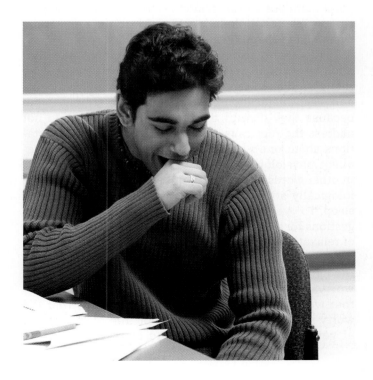

however, have problems with sleeping that last several weeks to years. The most common sleep problems are not sleeping enough (insomnia), sleeping during the day (excessive daytime sleepiness), and unusual activities associated with sleep (parasomnias).

Insomnia

The majority of people with long-term sleep problems have **insomnia**. They have trouble falling asleep or staying asleep, or they awaken after a few hours of sleep and cannot go back to sleep. The daytime results of insomnia are fatigue, the desire to nap, impaired ability to concentrate, impaired judgment, and a lack of zest for life. Although insomnia may be related to disease or injury in the brain's sleep centers, most often it is the result of a physical illness, chronic pain, stress, depression, anxiety, obsessive-compulsive ruminations, panic attacks, post-traumatic stress disorder, or drug or alcohol abuse.

Sometimes, as a result of insomnia, individuals have a difficult time staying awake during the day. They may feel sleepy most of the time, may nod off easily during a routine activity, or may nap at the slightest opportunity. Because they get insufficient sleep at night, about 20% of college students can fall asleep almost instantaneously if permitted to lie down in a darkened room. Extreme tendency to fall asleep during the day is called **narcolepsy.**

Insomnia is related to a variety of physical health problems, including more sick days, high blood pressure, type 2 diabetes, chronic respiratory disease, arthritis, pain, and headache. Insomnia increases the risks of depression, anxiety, and substance abuse. Because lack of sleep is a form of stress, and thus promotes the production of stress hormones, it tends to perpetuate itself. Furthermore, stress hormones may be responsible for the relationship of insomnia and being overweight (Chaput et al., 2008).

People with insomnia may try to improve their situation by going to bed early, staying in bed longer even though not sleeping, or trying to nap. Some try alcohol and sleep medications. In general, these strategies fail because they disrupt the biology of sleep and do not address the root causes of insomnia: negative expectations about one's ability to get to sleep and the consequent physiological arousal created by those thoughts. In other words, worry about not sleeping is psychophysiologically stimulating, and thus it defeats getting to sleep. To overcome insomnia, one must follow the suggestions for adequate sleep hygiene, practice some form of relaxation (e.g., meditation, progressive muscle relaxation), and become aware of and change one's negative thoughts about getting to sleep. For example, instead of worry, one acknowledges that one worries ("There's that worry, again") and then reminds oneself that the worry is both unnecessary ("It's not true that I will fail at getting to sleep again"), and counterproductive

("These thoughts aren't helping me"). Changing one's thoughts about sleep and learning proper sleep hygiene are more effective for insomnia than medications are (Morin et al., 2006). Moreover, many prescription sleep drugs (hypnotics, antidepressants, barbiturates) can be dangerous (MayoClinic.com, 2008).

Parasomnias

Parasomnias occur in many forms and have the potential to interrupt restful sleep. Common parasomnias include the following:

- *Nightmares*, dreams that arouse feelings of fear, terror, anxiety, or panic.
- *Somnambulism*, also known as sleepwalking. This is a condition occurring primarily in children and often associated with anxiety, fatigue, or stress. The person performs motor activity, usually leaving bed and walking around, while sleeping and has no memory of it on awakening. Other vigorous behaviors, such as punching, kicking, and night terrors (episodes that begin with a loud cry followed by rapid heart rate, sweating, and feelings of panic), will also interrupt sleep.
- *Sleep apnea*, in which breathing stops or gets very shallow for about 10 to 20 seconds and then resumes with a snort or choking sound. These pauses can occur 20 to 30 times or more an hour.
- *Restless legs syndrome* (RLS), characterized by a powerful urge to move the legs, often described as a creeping, crawling, tingling, or burning sensation. The urge to move and unpleasant feelings occur when resting and inactive, thus making it hard to fall asleep and stay asleep.

Because the majority of sleep problems represent some form of disharmony within ourselves or with our surroundings, restoring harmony is a way to return to our natural rest–activity cycle. This can be accom-

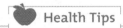 Health Tips

Wiped Out?

Fatigue is feeling tired, lacking energy, or acting weary. If you run a marathon, you are likely to be very tired afterward, but you will recover your strength and bounce back after you rest. If you are sick, you may feel lethargic and tired until you get better. However, if you are like many college students and day after day you don't get sufficient sleep or you live under constant stress, you are likely to feel unrelentingly worn out and bone tired. To feel spunky again, you need to establish good sleep patterns, take a little time each day to relax, eat properly, say "no" to invitations to overextend yourself, and stay away from tobacco, alcohol, and other drugs.

plished by employing mind–body health practices such as meditation, exercise, and proper nutrition. For extreme sleep disorders, professional help should be sought.

Understanding Your Dreams

We all dream while we sleep. Even animals dream. Although some people deny they dream, this is because they do not recall their dreams when awake. On the other hand, some people have vivid recall of the several dreams they have each night (a skill that can be learned).

Dreams tend to occur in the stage of sleep called **rapid eye movement (REM) sleep** (see Figure 4.4). REM sleep encompasses about 25% of sleep time, and it dominates sleep time in the last half of the night.

No one knows why we dream. Some researchers have suggested that REM sleep states are necessary for brain growth, daily information processing, and cellular rejuvenation. Others believe that dreams are the brain's way of processing and eliminating information and memories that are no longer useful. Whatever the reasons, dreams are necessary for health. Experimental subjects who were deprived of the chance to dream (they were awakened by experimenters during REM sleep) developed bizarre behaviors and psychotic symptoms. The individuals returned to normal after at least one night of catching up on the missed REM time.

For thousands of years dreams have been used in many cultures to restore mental and physical health. The temples of Asclepius were used by ancient Greeks for more than a thousand years as places where people went to have healing dreams and to have them interpreted by the priests and priestesses.

Indications that dreams can be healthy come from studies of the Senoi, a Malaysian tribe known as the "dream people." The Senoi live in a nonaggressive, noncombative, communal society. The tribe's members have a remarkable degree of mental and emotional health, which is attributed by some to the daily ritual of discussing and interpreting their dreams. Both children and adults gather each morning to recount their dreams to one another, singly and in groups. According to Senoi custom, the events, anxieties, and people in a dream are real and must be acknowledged and dealt with. Such behavior is similar to our custom of looking for meaning in dreams, especially as a component of psychotherapy.

Interpreting Your Dreams

In our culture, numerous theories of dream interpretation have been proposed. Perhaps the best known are those of Sigmund Freud and Carl Jung, who proposed universally applicable rules for uncovering the meaning of symbols and events in dreams. Most modern dream researchers do not believe in universal symbolism, however. Instead, they believe that the symbolism and meaning in a dream are unique to the dreamer. Dreams are private conversations with ourselves, communicated in a private language of images that often are bizarre, dramatic, emotional, and exaggerated.

Much dream research suggests that dreams are reflections of recent happenings, thoughts, and feelings that are not dealt with in our daily consciousness. Many people are too busy to attend to everything they experience, think, and feel. Sometimes, they purposely do not deal with reality because it is unpleasant. In a dream, however, you come clean with yourself. You bring forth subtle feelings and impressions that were not attended to while awake. You engage your innermost thoughts and feelings about fears, worries, conflicts, and problems that you chose not to deal with when awake. Thus, many problems (and sometimes their solutions!) are presented in dreams.

Dreams may also be a literal representation of reality that went unattended while awake. For example, if you dream of a mouse, perhaps you saw a mouse in your kitchen, or perhaps you noticed some movements out of the corner of your eye and thought of a mouse. In either case, your discomfort at the thought of a mouse in your house caused you to block the thought from consciousness.

Another way to find the message in a dream is to focus on the emotions in the dream and not on the dream's content. Although you may have dreamed of dancing an incredibly brilliant solo on a stage to an audience's wild applause, the actual emotion in the dream may have been fear. The dream, therefore, is probably about fear, not pride or accomplishment.

Mental Disorders

The brain, like all other body organs, is composed of molecules and cells whose functioning is controlled by biological processes. It is possible, therefore, for brain tissue to be affected by chemical imbalance, injury, infection, toxins, and genetic disorders. When brain injury or disease occurs, thoughts, mood, and behaviors can be impaired.

> **TERMS**
>
> **insomnia:** prolonged inability to obtain adequate sleep
>
> **narcolepsy:** extreme tendency to fall asleep during the day
>
> **parasomnias:** activities that interrupt restful sleep
>
> **rapid eye movement (REM) sleep:** stage of sleep in which dreams occur

Schizophrenia is a debilitating mental disorder characterized by hallucinations, delusions, an inability to maintain logical and coherent thought patterns, diminished emotional and social experience, and a diminished sense of purpose (**Table 4.6**). Typically, schizophrenia manifests in teenage years and progresses into adulthood. The disease occurs at the same rate (0.85%) in virtually all societies in the world; it is responsible for 2.5% of total U.S. health expenditures. The cause of schizophrenia is unknown, although scientists believe that biological (possibly inherited) factors are partially responsible. Although medications and psychosocial rehabilitation can help lessen symptoms, there is no cure. About one-third of schizophrenics become well spontaneously, but many individuals with a diagnosis of schizophrenia require ongoing medical and psychological support.

TERMS

schizophrenia: a mental disorder that involves a disturbance in thinking, in perceiving reality, and in functioning

Table 4.6

Signs of Schizophrenia

Aspect of life	Typical symptoms
Emotions	Inappropriate responses to stimuli
	Blunted or flat emotions
	Fear of warmth or closeness
	Erratic and negative feelings
Thought	Inability to tell real from unreal
	Delusions and hallucinations
	Disorganized and confused thoughts
	Tangential or circumstantial conversation
	Bizarre ideas and language
Interpersonal relationships	Thoughts only of self, autism
	Unpredictable responses when approached
	Social isolation
	Lack of response
	Withdrawal
	Impaired role functioning
Behavior	Deteriorated level of functioning, immobilization
	Inability to make decisions
	Poor judgment
	Bizarre or peculiar behavior
	Lethargy, loss of initiative
	Poor personal hygiene and grooming

Critical Thinking About Health

1. Dr. Razmataz's book, *30 Days to Exceptional Mental Health,* had been on the best-seller charts for 10 weeks, but after his appearance on TV's *Inside This Week,* sales went through the roof. Entertainers, business executives, professional athletes, and political leaders extolled the value of his program to lessen needless worry, improve sleep, and enhance mood, self-esteem, memory, and mental acuity.

    Dr. Razmataz based his program on 10 years of research he conducted as director of the Ersatz Mental Health Clinic. In his book and his media appearances, Dr. Razmataz explained that the type and severity of a particular mental illness were caused by either the over- or underactivity of the genes that controlled the production of the six basic neurotransmitter chemicals in the brain. The key to his method was determining a patient's genetic profile and matching it to one of six specific organic food diets. Questions:

    a. What factors are mentioned in the description above that might suggest to someone that Dr. Razmataz's method is credible and efficacious?

    b. Which of these factors do you find influence you when you are making a health decision?

    c. What additional information, if any, would you want before trying Dr. Razmataz's method yourself or recommending it to someone else? How would you find such information?

2. List five characteristics of a mentally healthy person. If you were a parent, how would you ensure that your child(ren) grow(s) up to manifest the five characteristics on your list? Also discuss how individuals can contribute to the mental health of people in their community.

3. John hasn't liked being Margie's supervisor since her first day of work. She just doesn't get it. And because she's the boss's niece, there is little he can do. In the past six months, whenever Margie is on John's shift-team, his finds himself so distressed that he doesn't want to go to work.

    a. The chapter describes several ways to cope with emotional distress, including (1) changing the situation that is causing the distress, (2) altering the significance one places on the distressing situation, and (3) lessening the distressing emotions. Discuss how John could employ each of these coping strategies to lessen his emotional distress. Also, describe the consequences for John of implementing each coping strategy.

    b. When you experience emotional distress, which of the three coping strategies do you employ most often? Do you notice situations in which one coping strategy works better than others?

4. Many people equate mental and emotional well-being with happiness. If they feel happy, they identify themselves as emotionally well. In your opinion, what is the relationship of emotional well-being and happiness? How do unpleasant emotions, such as sadness, grief, shame, guilt, and anger, affect one's sense of emotional well-being? Would you argue that the path to mental and emotional well-being is the pursuit of happiness? If not, in your view, what constitutes the path to mental and emotional well-being?

Health in Review

- Mental health is when your mental functions produce a sense of optimism, vitality, and well-being, and when your intentional behaviors lead to productive activities (including healthy behaviors), fulfilling relationships with others, and the ability to adapt to change and to cope with adversity.

- Mental illness refers to alterations in thinking, emotions, and/or intentional behaviors that produce psychological distress and/or impaired functioning.

- Mental and emotional health depend on how well individuals meet their maintenance and growth needs and cope with situations in which their needs are not met.

- People understand their needs by interpreting what they sense from the environment and in their bodies. As they mature, people develop ideas about and learn strategies to meet their emotional needs.

- Emotions tell us whether we are satisfied by, and the level of satisfaction from, our experiences, plans, and outcomes of behavior.

- Emotional distress occurs when needs are not met. People cope with emotional distress by changing their modes of interaction with the environment, changing the importance of their unmet needs, or changing the distressing feelings.

- Positive thoughts and emotions, including beliefs in one's worth (self-esteem) and abilities (self-efficacy and agency), motivate people to engage in healthy behaviors and to avoid unhealthy ones.

- Optimism is associated with perceiving negative events as specific, temporary obstacles to be overcome, whereas pessimism is associated with explaining negative events as self-caused, stable, and global.

- Counselors, therapists, and others can help clarify the source of emotional distress and find healthy ways to cope with it.

- Social support enables individuals to receive resources to help during difficult times.

- Phobias are exaggerated and often unrealistic fears.

- Anxiety disorders include social anxiety disorder, panic disorder, generalized anxiety disorder, and obsessive-compulsive disorder.
- Depression is often characterized by feelings of dejection, guilt, hopelessness, self-recrimination, loss of appetite, insomnia, loss of interest in sexual activity, withdrawal from friends, inability to concentrate, lowered self-esteem, and a focus on the negative.
- Suicide is the third leading cause of death among persons aged 15 to 24 years, of all races and both genders.
- Many of the signs of depression occur in someone suicidal. Many suicidal people talk about suicide when life appears hopeless.

- Adult attention deficit hyperactivity disorder is the result of conditions in the brain.
- Unresolved anger and hostility are risk factors for heart disease.
- Sleep and dreams are fundamental to human health. Sleep has five stages. REM sleep, during which dreams occur, happens during the cycle of sleep from deep to lighter stages.
- Many people use their dreams to help them understand and deal with distressing situations and confusing emotions.
- Schizophrenia is a mental disorder characterized by delusions, inability to think logically and coherently, diminished social and emotional experiences, and loss of sense of purpose.

Health and Wellness Online

The Web contains a wealth of information about health and wellness. By accessing the Internet using Web browser software, you can gain a new perspective on many topics presented in *Health and Wellness,* Tenth Edition. Access the Jones and Bartlett Publishers Web site at **health.jbpub.com/hwonline.**

References

Adler, N., & Stewart, J. (2004). Self-esteem. John D. and Catherine T. MacArthur Research Network on Socioeconomic Status and Health. Retrieved June 7, 2005, from http://www.macses.ucsf.edu/Research/Psychosocial/notebook/selfesteem.html

American College Health Association. (2008). National College Health Assessment. Retrieved April 10, 2008, from http://www.acha.org/projects_programs/assessment.cfm

Bachen, E. A., et al. (2007). Psychoneuroimmunology. In A. Baum et al. (Eds.), *Cambridge handbook of psychology, health and medicine.* Cambridge, UK: Cambridge University Press.

Basner, M., et al. (2007). American Time Use Survey: Sleep time and its relationship to waking activities. *Sleep, 30,* 1085–1095.

Biederman, J. (2005). Attention deficit/hyperactivity disorder: A selective overview. *Biological Psychiatry, 57,* 1215–1220.

Chaput, J. P., et al. (2008). The association between sleep duration and weight gain in adults: A 6-year prospective study from the Quebec Family Study. *Sleep, 31,* 517–523.

Danner, D. D., Snowdon, D. A., & Friesen, W. V. (2001). Positive emotions in early life and longevity: Findings from the nun study. *Journal of Personality and Social Psychology, 80,* 804–813.

Dickens, C. M., et al. (2004). Lack of a close confidant, but not depression, predicts further cardiac events after myocardial infarction. *Heart, 90,* 518–522.

Doyle, W. J., Gentile, D. A., & Cohen, S. (2006). Emotional style, nasal cytokines, and illness expression after experimental rhinovirus exposure. *Brain and Behavioral Immunity, 20,* 175–181.

Forquer, L. M., et al. (2008). Sleep patterns of college students at a public university. *Journal of American College Health, 56,* 563–565.

Fredrickson, B. L. (1998). What good are positive emotions? *Review of General Psychology, 2,* 300–319.

Giltay, E. J., et al. (2004). Dispositional optimism and all-cause and cardiovascular mortality in a prospective cohort of elderly Dutch men and women. *Archives of General Psychiatry, 61,* 1126–1135.

Giltay, E. J., et al. (2007). Lifestyle and dietary correlates of dispositional optimism in men. *Journal of Psychosomatic Research, 63,* 483–490.

Joiner, T. E., Jr., Brown, J. S., & Wingate, L. R. (2005). The psychology and neurobiology of suicidal behavior. *Annual Review of Psychology, 56,* 287–314.

Kirsch, I., et al. (2008). Initial severity and antidepressant benefits: A meta-analysis of data submitted to the Food and Drug Administration. *PLoS Medicine, 5,* e45. Retrieved from http://medicine.plosjournals.org/perlserv/?request=get-document&doi=10.1371%2Fjournal.pmed.0050045

Lawler-Row, K. A., et al. (2008). Forgiveness, physiological reactivity and health: The role of anger. *International Journal of Psychophysiology, 68,* 51–58.

Lett, H. S., et al. (2007). Social support and prognosis in patients at increased psychosocial risk recovering from myocardial infarction. *Health Psychology, 26,* 418–427.

Maslow, A. L. (1970). *Motivation and personality.* New York: Harper & Row.

MayoClinic.com. Prescription sleeping pills: What's right for you? Retrieved May 20, 2008, from http://www.mayoclinic.com/health/sleeping-pills/SL00010

Morin, C. M., et al. (2006). Psychological and behavioral treatment of insomnia. *Sleep, 29,* 1398–1414.

Rozanski, A., & Kubzansky, L. D. (2005). Psychological functioning and physical health: A paradigm of flexibility. *Psychosomatic Medicine, 67 (Supplement 1),* S47–S53.

Richman, L. S., et al. (2005). Positive emotion and health: Going beyond the negative. *Health Psychology, 24,* 422–429.

Saey, T. H. (2008, May 24). Epic genetics. *Science News,* 15–19.

Smith, T. W., et al. (2007). Hostile personality traits and coronary artery calcification in middle-aged and older married couples: Different effects for self-reports versus spouse ratings. *Psychosomatic Medicine, 69,* 441–448.

Uchino, B. N. (2005). *Social support and physical health: Understanding the health consequences of relationships.* New Haven, CT: Yale University Press.

U.S. Department of Health and Human Services. (1999). Mental health: A report of the Surgeon General. Retrieved May 7, 2005, from http://www.surgeongeneral.gov/library/mentalhealth/home.html

Wolfson, A. R., & Carskadon, M. A. (2003). Understanding adolescents' sleep patterns and school performance: A critical appraisal. *Sleep Medicine Reviews, 7,* 491–506.

World Health Organization. (2001). *Mental health: New understanding, new hope.* The World Health Report. Retrieved Nov 10, 2003, from http://www.who.int/whr2001/2001

Suggested Readings

Acocella, J. (2000, May 8). The empty couch—what is lost when psychiatry turns to drugs. *The New Yorker,* 82–118. A thoughtful article addressing the serious problems stemming from excessive use of therapeutic drugs in the treatment of mental disorders.

Belkmayer, R .H., & Agram, G. (2008). Major depressive disorder. *New England Journal of Medicine, 358,* 55–68. Discusses the roles of genetics, neurotransmitter biology, and stress biology on the development of severe clinical depression.

Bourne, E. J. (2005). *The anxiety and phobia workbook.* Oakland, CA: New Harbinger. Presents step-by-step guidelines, questionnaires, and exercises to help sufferers learn skills and make lifestyle changes to help them get relief from the most distressing symptoms.

Epstein, L., & Mardon, S. (2006). *The Harvard Medical School guide to a good night's sleep.* New York: McGraw-Hill. In-depth advice on how to maximize a night's sleep and energize your days.

Goleman, D. (2003). *Healing emotions: Conversations with the Dalai Lama on mindfulness, emotions, and health.* Boston: Shambhala. The world's leading Western physicians, psychologists, and meditation teachers discuss with the Dalai Lama contemporary research on the interrelationship between emotional states and physical well-being in the context of ancient Buddhist thinking.

Koerner, B. I. (2002, July/August). Disorders made to order. *Mother Jones,* 75. Retrieved May 17, 2005, from http://www.motherjones.com/news/feature/2002/07/disorders.html. Explains the marketing strategy of pharmamaceutical companies to define symptoms of everyday life as a new mental illness and then sell pills to cure it.

National Institute of Mental Health. (2008). *Suicide in the U.S.* (NIH Publication No. 06-4594). Retrieved from http://www.nimh.nih.gov/health/publications/suicide-in-the-us-statistics-and-prevention.shtml. A summary of suicide issues in the United States.

Saey, T. H. (2008, May 24). Epic genetics. *Science News,* 15–19. Discusses the hundreds of modified genes that now are thought to be at the root of serious mental illnesses such as depression, schizophrenia, bipolar disorder, and addictions.

Saul, H. (2002). *Phobias: Fighting the fear.* New York: Arcade. An examination of phobias from psychological and physiological viewpoints.

Uchino, B. N. (2005). *Social support and physical health: Understanding the health consequences of relationships.* New Haven, CT: Yale University Press. Reviews the research on social support and physical health, showing that social support is a causal factor influencing mortality.

Recommended Web Sites

Please visit **health.jbpub.com/hwonline** for links to these Web sites.

American Sleep Association
Information and resources on all aspects of sleep and sleep problems.

Depression Screening Tests
From the National Mental Health Association.

MedlinePlus on Mental Health and Behavior Topics
The National Library of Medicine's Web page of resources on a variety of mental health topics.

National Alliance on Mental Illnesses
900-960-6264
The nation's largest organization offering help to patients and families.

National Mental Health Consumers' Self-Help Clearinghouse
800-553-4539
Provides support for persons in search of self-help and advocacy resources.

National Sleep Foundation
Information and resources on all aspects of sleep and sleep problems.

National Suicide Prevention Lifeline
800-273-8255
This confidential hotline is staffed 24/7 by trained counselors.

PsychDirect
An extensive array of mental health information and resources maintained by the McMaster University Department of Psychiatry and Behavioral Sciences.

Part Two

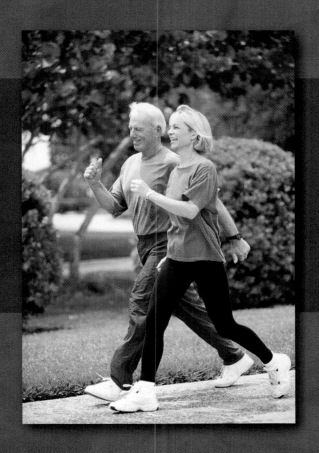

Eating and Exercising Toward a Healthy Lifestyle

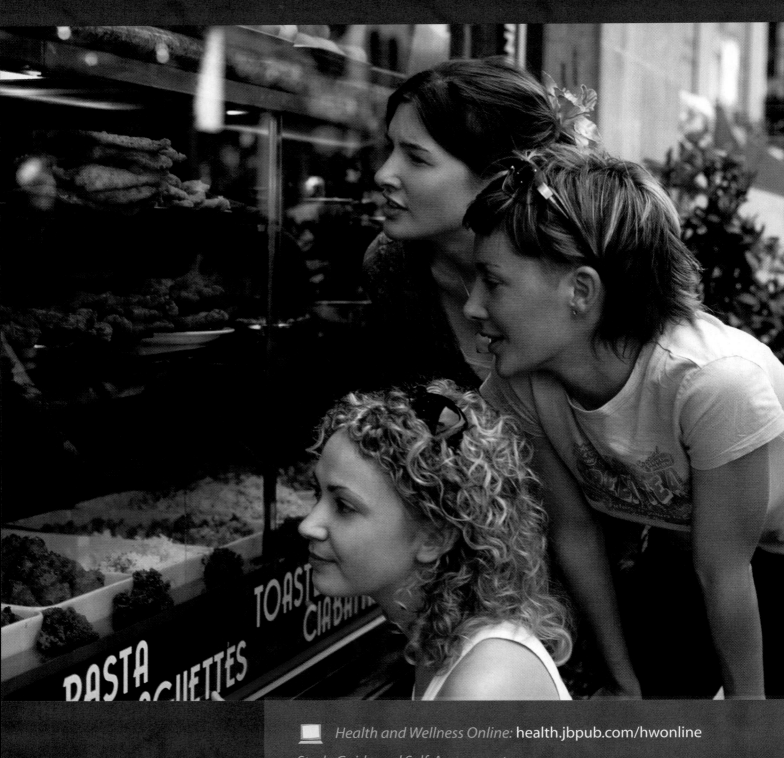

Chapter Five

Choosing a Nutritious Diet

Learning Objectives

1. List several factors that influence dietary choices.

2. Describe the dietary guidelines proposed by the U.S. government and health organizations.

3. Describe the Food Guide Pyramid and its recommendations.

4. Explain how to use the MyPyramid Web site.

5. Describe the ingredients and nutrition facts labels on manufactured foods.

6. Describe the three functions of food.

7. List the three functions of biological energy.

8. List the seven components of food, and identify common foods that contain each component.

9. Define and distinguish between dietary supplements used as food and as drugs.

10. Describe the three kinds of vegetarian diets and several reasons for vegetarianism.

Of the many things you can do to enhance your well-being, none is more important than maintaining proper nutrition. Many people are aware that good nutrition is essential and sincerely want to eat healthfully. But the plethora of claims and counterclaims about nutrition and health and the aggressive marketing of food products tend to confuse rather than enlighten. Indeed, one study found that about 40% of Americans are tired of hearing about what foods they should and shouldn't eat and have become skeptical of official dietary guidelines (Patterson et al., 2001).

> The destiny of a nation depends on the manner in which it feeds itself.
>
> *Jean Anthelme Brillat-Savarin (1755–1826)*

Moreover, many factors other than knowledge of nutrition influence a person's dietary choices—family, ethnic, and cultural eating patterns; social factors (eating what friends eat); food fads; and time pressures that limit thoughtful food shopping and meal preparation and make fast food and snacks attractive. Stress also influences food choices by encouraging consumption of foods high in fat and sugar to soothe jangled nerves and emotions ("comfort foods") (Lebel, Lu, & Dube, 2008).

Marketing and advertising also are major influences on American food consumption patterns. Food marketers are the nation's second largest advertisers (after automobiles), with around $30 billion per year in spending. About 70% of food advertising is for food products, principally packaged foods, snacks, and soft drinks. Another 28% is for food service (mostly fast food). McDonald's and Burger King spend over $1 billion a year on advertising. In contrast, advertising on fruits, vegetables, grains, and beans accounts for less than 2% of all food advertising. Most food advertising occurs on TV; for example, fast-food companies spend 95% of their advertising dollars on TV. In response to consumers' concerns, several purveyors of snack and fast foods have reduced or eliminated advertising of some of their products to children under age 12.

Dietary Guidelines for Eating Right

The $2 trillion-a-year U.S. food industry is a technological and marketing marvel. It contributes 13% to the gross domestic product and employs about 17% of Americans (Martinez, 2007). Compared with 100 years ago, when a large portion of a consumer's food dollar went to the farmer or grower, nowadays only 26% does. Food processing (9%), distribution (37%), and delivery to consumers via stores and restaurants (27%) make up the rest. Over the past 20 years, the food industry has become increasingly efficient, delivering more calories for less cost than at any time in U.S. history. Indeed, the food industry delivers 3,800 calories of food per day to the majority of American adults—about 1,500 more than are required for health, which is one reason for the current obesity epidemic.

Despite its massive presence in U.S. society, the food industry does not deliver healthy and safe foods to Americans in every instance. The American diet consists of too much saturated and trans fat, sugar, refined carbohydrate, and salt. A study found that sweets and desserts, sodas, and alcoholic beverages (principally beer) together contribute 25% of the average American's daily calories (Block, 2004). Salty snacks and fruit-flavored drinks contribute another 5%, whereas fruits and vegetables contribute only 10% of calories consumed. Poor nutrition increases the risks of heart disease, high blood pressure, some cancers, type 2 diabetes, and obesity.

Because it consists primarily of large, multinational conglomerates whose principal goal is profit, decisions within the U.S. food industry regarding the quality and healthfulness of food are secondary to considerations of manufacturing efficiencies and marketing food products (Nestle, 2007). This is the reason the U.S. government, the World Health Organization, and organizations such as the American Heart Association and the American Cancer Society (Table 5.1) promote guidelines for good nutrition. These guidelines are based on the latest scientific evidence for good nutrition, obtained by examining the biological effects of specific dietary components and by comparing dietary patterns and disease frequencies in different populations. For example, compared to the

Table 5.1

American Heart Association and American Cancer Society Dietary Guidelines

American Heart Association's dietary guidelines with your heart in mind

- Eat five or more servings of a variety of fruits and vegetables per day.
- Eat six or more servings of a variety of whole-grain products per day.
- Eat fat-free and low-fat milk products, fish, legumes (beans), skinless poultry, and lean meats.
- Use vegetable oils (canola, olive) and liquid or tub margarines.
- Balance the number of calories you eat with the number you utilize each day for living and physical activity. To lose weight, utilize more calories in physical activity than you consume in food.
- Be physically active. Walk or do other activities for 30 minutes on most days of the week.
- Limit intake of foods high in calories and low in nutrition.
- Eat less than 6 grams of salt (sodium chloride) per day (2,400 milligrams of sodium).
- Limit foods high in saturated fat, trans fat, and cholesterol, such as full-fat dairy products, fatty meats, tropical oils, partially hydrogenated vegetable oils, and egg yolks.
- Consume no more than one (women) or two (men) alcoholic drinks per day.

American Cancer Society's dietary guidelines for reducing your risk of cancer

- Eat five or more servings of a variety of fruits and vegetables each day.
- Eat other foods from plant sources, such as whole-grain breads, cereals, grain products, rice, pasta, or beans, several times each day.
- Choose foods low in fat.
- Limit consumption of meats, especially high-fat meats.
- Be at least moderately active for 30 minutes or more on most days of the week.
- Stay within your healthy weight range.
- Limit consumption of alcoholic beverages, if you drink at all.

common American diet, which is based on meats, refined-flour products, and industrial foods such as fast food and packaged fatty or sugary snacks and sweets, the diets of traditional Asian and Mediterranean societies, which are based on unprocessed grains (rice, whole-wheat flour), beans, fresh vegetables and fruits, and fish, are associated with less heart disease and several kinds of

cancer, apparently because they maintain healthy body weight, lessen inflammation and insulin resistance, and improve blood vessel functioning (Mitrou et al., 2007).

Periodically, the U.S. Department of Agriculture (USDA) issues dietary guidelines for the American people (USDA, 2005) (Table 5.2) designed to promote wellness and prevent illnesses that result from poor nutrition, including:

Table 5.2

2005 Dietary Guidelines for Americans: Key Recommendations for the General Population

Adequate nutrients within calorie needs
- Consume a variety of nutrient-dense foods and beverages within and among the basic food groups while choosing foods that limit the intake of saturated and trans fats, cholesterol, added sugars, salt, and alcohol.
- Meet recommended intakes within energy needs by adopting a balanced eating pattern, such as the U.S. Department of Agriculture (USDA) Food Guide or the Dietary Approaches to Stop Hypertension (DASH) Eating Plan.

Weight management
- To maintain body weight in a healthy range, balance calories from foods and beverages with calories expended.
- To prevent gradual weight gain over time, make small decreases in food and beverage calories and increase physical activity.

Physical activity
- Engage in regular physical activity and reduce sedentary activities to promote health, psychological well-being, and a healthy body weight.
  - To reduce the risk of chronic disease in adulthood: Engage in at least 30 minutes of moderate-intensity physical activity, above usual activity, at work or home on most days of the week.
  - For most people, greater health benefits can be obtained by engaging in physical activity of more vigorous intensity or longer duration.
  - To help manage body weight and prevent gradual, unhealthy body weight gain in adulthood: Engage in approximately 60 minutes of moderate- to vigorous-intensity activity on most days of the week while not exceeding caloric intake requirements.
  - To sustain weight loss in adulthood: Participate in at least 60 to 90 minutes of daily moderate-intensity physical activity while not exceeding caloric intake requirements. Some people may need to consult with a health care provider before participating in this level of activity.
- Achieve physical fitness by including cardiovascular conditioning, stretching exercises for flexibility, and resistance exercises or calisthenics for muscle strength and endurance.

Food groups to encourage
- Consume a sufficient amount of fruits and vegetables while staying within energy needs. Two cups of fruit and 2 1/2 cups of vegetables per day are recommended for a reference 2,000-calorie intake, with higher or lower amounts depending on the calorie level.
- Choose a variety of fruits and vegetables each day. In particular, select from all five vegetable subgroups (dark green, orange, legumes, starchy vegetables, and other vegetables) several times a week.
- Consume 3 or more ounce-equivalents of whole-grain products per day, with the rest of the recommended grains coming from enriched or whole-grain products. In general, at least half the grains should come from whole grains.
- Consume 3 cups per day of fat-free or low-fat milk or equivalent milk products.

Fats
- Consume less than 10% of calories from saturated fatty acids and less than 300 mg/day of cholesterol, and keep trans-fatty acid consumption as low as possible.
- Keep total fat intake between 20% to 35% of calories, with most fats coming from sources of polyunsaturated and monounsaturated fatty acids, such as fish, nuts, and vegetable oils.
- When selecting and preparing meat, poultry, dry beans, and milk or milk products, make choices that are lean, low fat, or fat free.
- Limit intake of fats and oils high in saturated and/or trans-fatty acids, and choose products low in such fats and oils.

Carbohydrates
- Choose fiber-rich fruits, vegetables, and whole grains often.
- Choose and prepare foods and beverages with little added sugars or caloric sweeteners, such as amounts suggested by the USDA Food Guide and the DASH Eating Plan.
- Reduce the incidence of dental caries by practicing good oral hygiene and consuming sugar- and starch-containing foods and beverages less frequently.

Sodium and potassium
- Consume less than 2,300 mg (approximately 1 teaspoon of salt) of sodium per day.
- Choose and prepare foods with little salt. At the same time, consume potassium-rich foods, such as fruits and vegetables.

Alcoholic beverages
- Those who choose to drink alcoholic beverages should do so sensibly and in moderation—defined as the consumption of up to one drink per day for women and up to two drinks per day for men.
- Alcoholic beverages should not be consumed by some individuals, including those who cannot restrict their alcohol intake, women of childbearing age who may become pregnant, pregnant and lactating women, children and adolescents, individuals taking medications that can interact with alcohol, and those with specific medical conditions.
- Alcoholic beverages should be avoided by individuals engaging in activities that require attention, skill, or coordination, such as driving or operating machinery.

Food safety
- To avoid microbial foodborne illness:
  - Clean hands, food contact surfaces, and fruits and vegetables. Meat and poultry should not be washed or rinsed.
  - Separate raw, cooked, and ready-to-eat foods while shopping, preparing, or storing foods.
  - Cook foods to a safe temperature to kill microorganisms.
  - Chill (refrigerate) perishable food promptly and defrost foods properly.
  - Avoid raw (unpasteurized) milk or any products made from unpasteurized milk, raw or partially cooked eggs or foods containing raw eggs, raw or undercooked meat and poultry, unpasteurized juices, and raw sprouts.

Note: The Dietary Guidelines for Americans 2005 contains additional recommendations for specific populations.
Source: From the U.S. Department of Agriculture, 2005. Available: http://www.healthierus.gov/dietaryguidelines.

- Heart disease, cancer of various organs, type 2 diabetes, and overweight from diets high in sugar and fat
- Cancer of the colon from consumption of too much red meat
- Diseases of the gastrointestinal tract from not consuming sufficient fiber
- High blood pressure from consuming too much salt
- Tooth decay and overweight from consuming too much sugar

The guidelines also stress the importance of physical activity in maintaining a healthy body weight.

Food Guide Pyramids

In 1992, the U.S. Department of Agriculture invented the **Food Guide Pyramid** to help people remember the composition of a healthful diet. The Food Guide Pyramid recommended that people construct a diet based on grains, fruits, and vegetables and to consume moderate to little saturated fat and cholesterol. The slogan "five-a-day" was coined to remind people to consume a total of five servings of fruits and vegetables per day.

In 2005, the U.S. Department of Agriculture revised the Food Guide Pyramid, which is now called **MyPyramid** (**Figure 5.1**). Like the original Food Guide Pyramid, MyPyramid recommends building a diet on grains, fruits, and vegetables and obtaining protein from nuts and meat and calcium from dairy products. It also acknowledges the role of vegetable oils in a healthy diet. Moreover, MyPyramid shows a figure walking a staircase to emphasize the importance of including physical activity in one's life. Unlike the original Food Guide Pyramid, MyPyramid does not recommend a number of daily servings from each food group. Instead, people are referred to a Web site (www.mypyramid.gov), where they can obtain food consumption recommendations suited for their age, sex, and amount of daily physical activity.

MyPyramid illustrates six basic concepts:
- Variety, symbolized by the six color bands representing the five food groups of MyPyramid plus oils. Foods from all groups are needed each day for good health.
- Moderation, represented by the narrowing of each food group from bottom to top. The wider base stands for foods with little or no solid fats, added sugars, or caloric sweeteners. These should be selected more often to get the most nutrition from calories consumed.
- Proportionality, shown by the different widths of the food group bands. The widths suggest how much food a person should choose from each group.
- Physical activity, represented by the steps and the person climbing them, as a reminder of the importance of daily physical activity.

- Gradual improvement, encouraged by the slogan "Steps to a Healthier You." Individuals can benefit from taking small steps to improve their diet and lifestyle each day. (See the Health Tip feature "Healthier Eating: One Step at a Time.")
- Personalization, demonstrated by the MyPyramid Web site. There, you can get a personalized recommendation of the kinds and amounts of food to eat each day.

The U.S. government's food pyramids were invented because the typical American's diet is laden with sugars, fats, and refined-grain foods (white bread, milled rice). Fiber and nutrient rich–whole grains (whole wheat, oats, bulgur), fruits, dark-green leafy and yellow vegetables, dry beans, fish, nuts, and low-fat dairy products are insufficiently consumed. Instead, the vegetable group is dominated by iceberg lettuce, potatoes (mostly french fries and potato chips), and tomato sauce (Putnam, Allshouse, & Kantor, 2003). Sugars come from sweeteners in processed foods ("high fructose corn syrup") and sugar added to sodas, candies, and pastries. Much of the fat is derived from manufactured trans fats added to commercial and restaurant foods. The amount of sugar and fat in the current American diet exceeds by 15% that of the average diet in 1985. It is no wonder that overweight and obesity have become significant health problems.

The U.S. government's food pyramids have been criticized because they accommodate politically powerful industries. For example, a box at the apex of the original Food Guide Pyramid was labeled "fats, oils, and sweets—use sparingly," which was meant to refer to fast and junk foods, yet, in deference to fast and junk food manufacturers, these items were not specifically named. In the revised MyPyramid, the "fats, oils, and sweets—use sparingly" box disappeared altogether. Meat, which can contain high percentages of saturated fat, is lumped together with beans and other legumes, which are high in fiber and contain little or no fat. Some products in the grain group are manufactured with considerable sugar and salt, but these additives are not reflected in the recommendations. In the grain group, little distinction is made between whole grains, which contain many nutrients and fiber, and products made with refined flour, which contain only nutrients added by the manufacturer and no fiber. In the vegetable group, no distinction is made between starchy (root) vegetables, such as

TERMS

Food Guide Pyramid: guidelines for a healthful diet based on grains, fruits, and vegetables

MyPyramid: an educational tool based on the 2005 Dietary Guidelines for Americans and other nutritional standards to help consumers make healthier food and physical activity choices

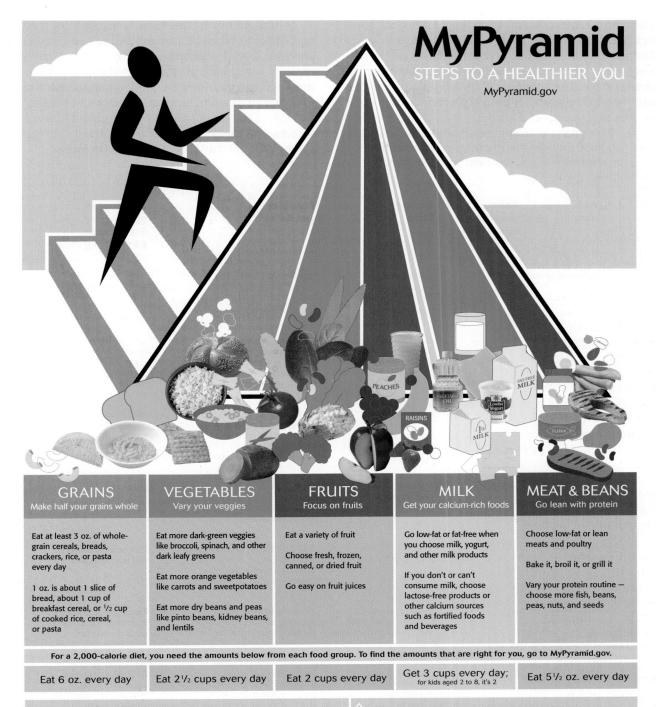

MyPyramid
STEPS TO A HEALTHIER YOU
MyPyramid.gov

GRAINS	VEGETABLES	FRUITS	MILK	MEAT & BEANS
Make half your grains whole	Vary your veggies	Focus on fruits	Get your calcium-rich foods	Go lean with protein

Eat at least 3 oz. of whole-grain cereals, breads, crackers, rice, or pasta every day 1 oz. is about 1 slice of bread, about 1 cup of breakfast cereal, or ½ cup of cooked rice, cereal, or pasta	Eat more dark-green veggies like broccoli, spinach, and other dark leafy greens Eat more orange vegetables like carrots and sweetpotatoes Eat more dry beans and peas like pinto beans, kidney beans, and lentils	Eat a variety of fruit Choose fresh, frozen, canned, or dried fruit Go easy on fruit juices	Go low-fat or fat-free when you choose milk, yogurt, and other milk products If you don't or can't consume milk, choose lactose-free products or other calcium sources such as fortified foods and beverages	Choose low-fat or lean meats and poultry Bake it, broil it, or grill it Vary your protein routine — choose more fish, beans, peas, nuts, and seeds

For a 2,000-calorie diet, you need the amounts below from each food group. To find the amounts that are right for you, go to MyPyramid.gov.

Eat 6 oz. every day	Eat 2½ cups every day	Eat 2 cups every day	Get 3 cups every day; for kids aged 2 to 8, it's 2	Eat 5½ oz. every day

Find your balance between food and physical activity
- Be sure to stay within your daily calorie needs.
- Be physically active for at least 30 minutes most days of the week.
- About 60 minutes a day of physical activity may be needed to prevent weight gain.
- For sustaining weight loss, at least 60 to 90 minutes a day of physical activity may be required.
- Children and teenagers should be physically active for 60 minutes every day, or most days.

Know the limits on fats, sugars, and salt (sodium)
- Make most of your fat sources from fish, nuts, and vegetable oils.
- Limit solid fats like butter, margarine, shortening, and lard, as well as foods that contain these.
- Check the Nutrition Facts label to keep saturated fats, *trans* fats, and sodium low.
- Choose food and beverages low in added sugars. Added sugars contribute calories with few, if any, nutrients.

■ **Figure 5.1**

MyPyramid

MyPyramid is an Internet-based educational tool that helps consumers implement the principles of the 2005 *Dietary Guidelines for Americans* and other nutritional standards.

Source: U.S. Department of Agriculture, www.MyPyramid.gov.

potatoes, and tomatoes and leafy vegetables, such as spinach, chard, and kale.

Despite these criticisms, MyPyramid provides many options to help people make healthy food choices and be physically active. The appendix at the end of this chapter contains helpful suggestions from MyPyramid.gov.

Although not in the form of a pyramid, the recommendations of the U.S. Department of Health and Human Services DASH (Dietary Approaches to Stop Hypertension) eating plan are similar to the food pyramids (**Figure 5.2**): Base your diet on whole grains, fresh fruits, and fresh vegetables and limit animal fats and sweets.

The DASH eating plan shown below is based on 2,000 calories a day. The number of daily servings in a food group may vary from those listed, depending on your caloric needs. Use this chart to help you plan your menus or take it with you when you go to the store.

Food Group	Daily Servings (except as noted)	Serving Sizes	Examples and Notes	Significance of Each Food Group to the DASH Eating Plan
Grains and grain products	7–8	1 slice bread 1 oz dry cereal* ½ cup cooked rice, pasta, or cereal	Whole wheat bread, English muffin, pita bread, bagel, cereals, grits, oatmeal, crackers, unsalted pretzels and popcorn	Major sources of energy and fiber
Vegetables	4–5	1 cup raw leafy vegetable ½ cup cooked vegetable 6 oz vegetable juice	Tomatoes, potatoes, carrots, green peas, squash, broccoli, turnip greens, collards, kale, spinach, artichokes, green beans, lima beans, sweet potatoes	Rich sources of potassium, magnesium, and fiber
Fruits	4–5	6 oz fruit juice 1 medium fruit ¼ cup dried fruit ½ cup fresh, frozen, or canned fruit	Apricots, bananas, dates, grapes, oranges, orange juice, grapefruit, grapefruit juice, mangoes, melons, peaches, pineapples, prunes, raisins, strawberries, tangerines	Important sources of potassium, magnesium, and fiber
Lowfat or fat free dairy foods	2–3	8 oz milk 1 cup yogurt 1½ oz cheese	Fat free (skim) or lowfat (1%) milk, fat free or lowfat buttermilk, fat free or lowfat regular or frozen yogurt, lowfat and fat free cheese	Major sources of calcium and protein
Meats, poultry, and fish	2 or less	3 oz cooked meats, poultry, or fish	Select only lean; trim away visible fats; broil, roast, or boil, instead of frying; remove skin from poultry	Rich sources of protein and magnesium
Nuts, seeds, and dry beans	4–5 per week	⅓ cup or 1½ oz nuts 2 Tbsp or ½ oz seeds ½ cup cooked dry beans peas	Almonds, filberts, mixed nuts, peanuts, walnuts, sunflower seeds, kidney beans, lentils	Rich sources of energy, magnesium, potassium, protein, and fiber
Fats and oils†	2–3	1 tsp soft margarine 1 Tbsp lowfat mayonnaise 2 Tbsp light salad dressing 1 tsp vegetable oil	Soft margarine, lowfat mayonnaise, light salad dressing, vegetable oil (such as olive, corn, canola, or safflower)	DASH has 27 percent of calories as fat, including fat in or added to foods
Sweets	5 per week	1 Tbsp sugar 1 Tbsp jelly or jam ½ oz jelly beans 8 oz lemonade	Maple syrup, sugar, jelly, jam, fruit-flavored gelatin, jelly beans, hard candy, fruit punch, sorbet, ices	Sweets should be low in fat

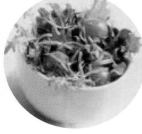
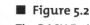

■ **Figure 5.2**

The DASH Eating Plan

*Equals ½–1¼ cups, depending on cereal type. Check the product's nutrition facts label.
†Fat content changes serving counts for fats and oils: For example, 1 Tbsp of regular salad dressing equals 1 serving; 1 Tbsp of a low-fat dressing equals ½ serving; 1 Tbsp of a fat-free dressing equals 0 servings.
Source: U.S. National Heart, Lung, and Blood Institute. Available: http://www.nhlbi.nih.gov/health/public/heart/hbp/dash/.

To address the deficiencies in U.S. government food pyramids, nutritionists at the Harvard University School of Public Health have developed the Healthy Eating Pyramid (**Figure 5.3**) (Nutrition Source, 2008a). The principal features of the Healthy Eating Pyramid include the following:

- Exercise daily, which helps control weight and maintain physical and mental health irrespective of weight control.
- Replace saturated fat and cholesterol in meats and whole-dairy foods and trans fats in manufactured and restaurant food with the polyunsaturated fats in canola, olive, sunflower, and corn oil.
- Replace refined grains (enriched flour, polished white rice, potatoes) with whole grains (oatmeal, whole-wheat baked goods, barley, bulgur, corn meal).
- Consume more than five servings a day of a variety of fruits and vegetables, especially dark-green leafy, yellow, orange, and red ones, and eat lots of beans.
- Eat fish, eggs, nuts, seeds, and beans instead of meats as a source of protein.

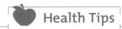 **Health Tips**

Healthier Eating: One Step at a Time

If you want to improve your diet, make *one* healthful change at a time. Here are some suggestions:
- Eat a breakfast consisting of at least a whole-grain product and a fruit.
- Substitute one daily serving of real fruit juice (not colored sugar water) for a soda.
- Substitute one daily serving of a fruit or nuts for a candy bar or a handful (or two) of chips.
- Substitute a lean meat sandwich with tomato on whole-wheat bread for a fast-food hamburger, fish entree, taco, or burrito.

- Consume one to two servings of low-fat dairy products per day to obtain calcium.
- Drink no more than one (women) or two (men) alcoholic beverages (a beer, a glass of wine, one mixed drink) per day.

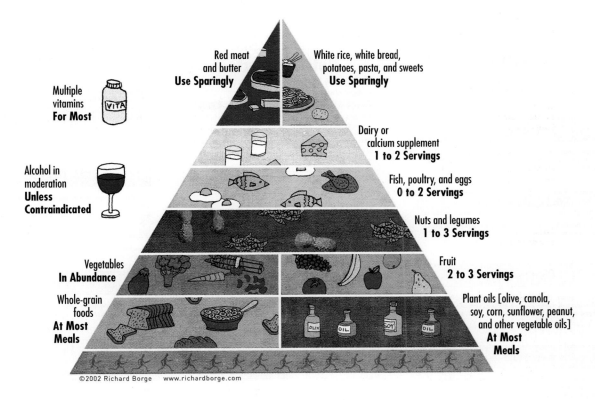

©2002 Richard Borge   www.richardborge.com

■ **Figure 5.3**

The Healthy Eating Pyramid

Unlike other pyramids, this one reminds you to think of exercise before you think of food so that you won't gain too much weight. Then be sure to consume polyunsaturated oils, instead of saturated animal fats, plenty of fresh fruits and vegetables instead of sweets and snacks, and whole-grain foods instead of those made with refined flour.

Copyright © 2008 Harvard University. For more information about the Healthy Eating Pyramid, please see The Nutrition Source, Department of Nutrition, Harvard School of Public Health, http://www.thenutritionsource.org, and *Eat, Drink, and Be Healthy*, by Walter C. Willett, M.D. and Patrick J. Skerrett (2005), Free Press/Simon & Schuster, Inc.

Food Labels

The U.S. government requires that all manufactured foods carry two food labels: the **ingredients label** (Figure 5.4) and the **nutrition facts label** (Figure 5.5). The ingredients label lists the chemical composition of the food, that is, all the substances that the manufacturer uses, including other foods (e.g., grains, eggs), natural and artificial sweeteners, natural and artificial fats, water, natural and artificial thickeners, natural and artificial flavorings, food colorings, and preservatives. The ingredients label lists substances in descending

Ingredients: Wheat flour, sugar, rolled oats, corn sweetener, molasses, partially hydrogenated safflower oil, salt, pantothenic acid, reduced iron, yellow No. 6, yellow No. 5, pyridoxine, ascorbic acid (vitamin C), BHT, riboflavin, folic acid.

■ **Figure 5.4**

The Ingredients Label

The government requires that food manufacturers list the substances within their products by weight from greatest to least.

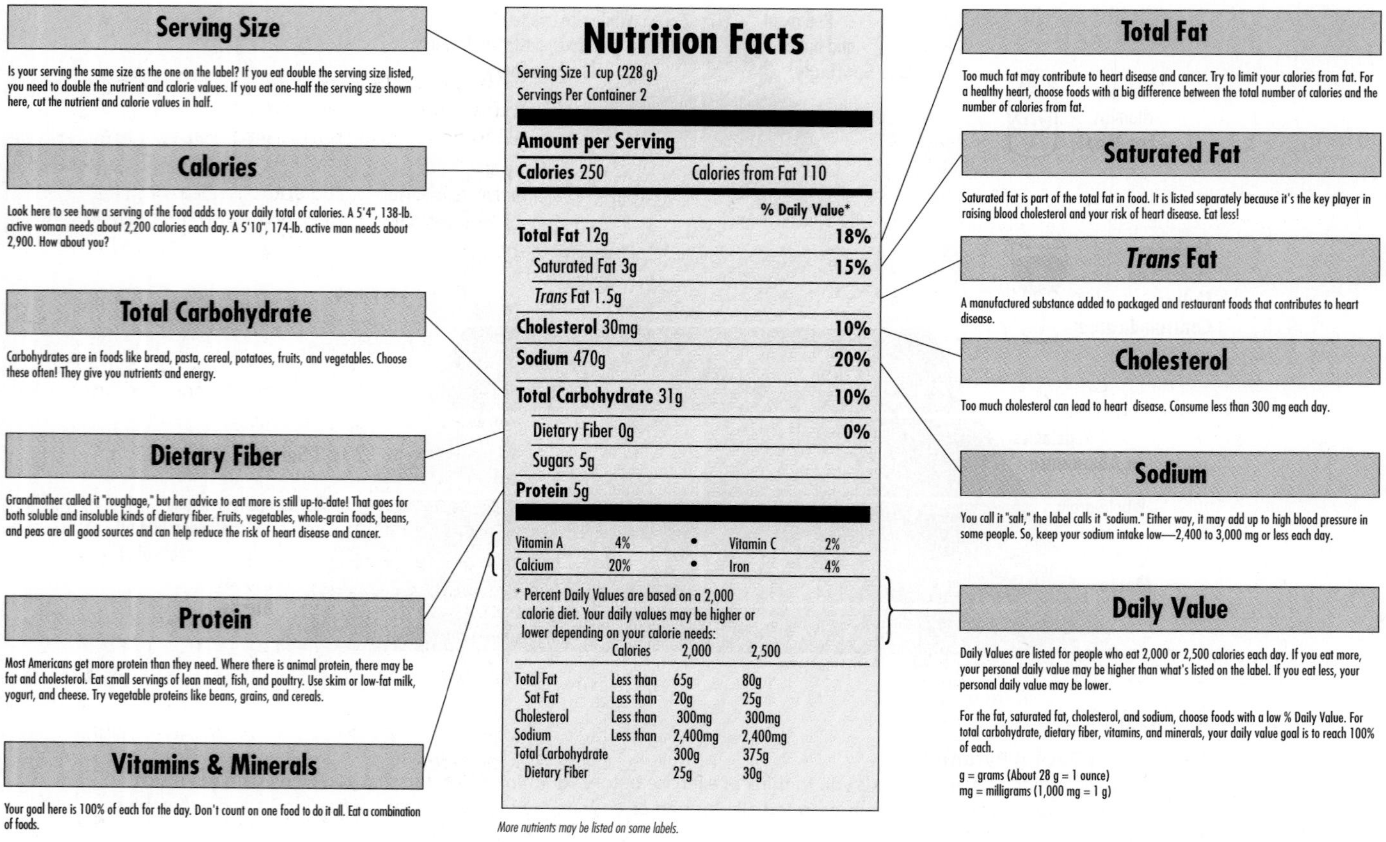

order by weight; the substance in the greatest amount is listed first and that in the least amount is listed last.

The ingredients label does not specify how much—either by weight or percentage—of an ingredient is in a food product, only its amount relative to the other ingredients. Also, by listing each individual substance, the ingredients label may not indicate the true relative amount of sugar or fat in the food. For example, a snack food's ingredients label could list separately sucrose, fructose, and corn sweetener, all of which are sugars.

Unlike the ingredients label, the nutrition facts label provides *quantitative* information on certain nutrients in the food (ones whose consumption should be monitored for good health) and the calorie content of the food. The amounts indicated for each nutrient and the calorie count are for a "serving," which is all or a portion of the food in the package, as determined by the manufacturer. The manufacturer's definition of a serving is given at the top of the nutrition facts label as the "serving size."

In addition to the actual amounts of nutrients and calories, the nutrition facts label lists the **percent daily value** (PDV) for each nutrient, which is the percentage of the recommended daily amount that is contained in the food. (The percent daily value on the nutrition facts

Serving Size

Is your serving the same size as the one on the label? If you eat double the serving size listed, you need to double the nutrient and calorie values. If you eat one-half the serving size shown here, cut the nutrient and calorie values in half.

Calories

Look here to see how a serving of the food adds to your daily total of calories. A 5'4", 138-lb. active woman needs about 2,200 calories each day. A 5'10", 174-lb. active man needs about 2,900. How about you?

Total Carbohydrate

Carbohydrates are in foods like bread, pasta, cereal, potatoes, fruits, and vegetables. Choose these often! They give you nutrients and energy.

Dietary Fiber

Grandmother called it "roughage," but her advice to eat more is still up-to-date! That goes for both soluble and insoluble kinds of dietary fiber. Fruits, vegetables, whole-grain foods, beans, and peas are all good sources and can help reduce the risk of heart disease and cancer.

Protein

Most Americans get more protein than they need. Where there is animal protein, there may be fat and cholesterol. Eat small servings of lean meat, fish, and poultry. Use skim or low-fat milk, yogurt, and cheese. Try vegetable proteins like beans, grains, and cereals.

Vitamins & Minerals

Your goal here is 100% of each for the day. Don't count on one food to do it all. Eat a combination of foods.

Nutrition Facts

Serving Size 1 cup (228 g)
Servings Per Container 2

Amount per Serving

Calories 250	Calories from Fat 110

	% Daily Value*
Total Fat 12g	**18%**
Saturated Fat 3g	**15%**
Trans Fat 1.5g	
Cholesterol 30mg	**10%**
Sodium 470g	**20%**
Total Carbohydrate 31g	**10%**
Dietary Fiber 0g	**0%**
Sugars 5g	
Protein 5g	

Vitamin A	4%	•	Vitamin C	2%
Calcium	20%	•	Iron	4%

* Percent Daily Values are based on a 2,000 calorie diet. Your daily values may be higher or lower depending on your calorie needs:

	Calories	2,000	2,500
Total Fat	Less than	65g	80g
Sat Fat	Less than	20g	25g
Cholesterol	Less than	300mg	300mg
Sodium	Less than	2,400mg	2,400mg
Total Carbohydrate		300g	375g
Dietary Fiber		25g	30g

More nutrients may be listed on some labels.

Total Fat

Too much fat may contribute to heart disease and cancer. Try to limit your calories from fat. For a healthy heart, choose foods with a big difference between the total number of calories and the number of calories from fat.

Saturated Fat

Saturated fat is part of the total fat in food. It is listed separately because it's the key player in raising blood cholesterol and your risk of heart disease. Eat less!

***Trans* Fat**

A manufactured substance added to packaged and restaurant foods that contributes to heart disease.

Cholesterol

Too much cholesterol can lead to heart disease. Consume less than 300 mg each day.

Sodium

You call it "salt," the label calls it "sodium." Either way, it may add up to high blood pressure in some people. So, keep your sodium intake low—2,400 to 3,000 mg or less each day.

Daily Value

Daily Values are listed for people who eat 2,000 or 2,500 calories each day. If you eat more, your personal daily value may be higher than what's listed on the label. If you eat less, your personal daily value may be lower.

For the fat, saturated fat, cholesterol, and sodium, choose foods with a low % Daily Value. For total carbohydrate, dietary fiber, vitamins, and minerals, your daily value goal is to reach 100% of each.

g = grams (About 28 g = 1 ounce)
mg = milligrams (1,000 mg = 1 g)

■ **Figure 5.5**

The Nutrition Facts Label

label is for someone who requires 2,000 calories of food energy per day; people with higher or lower calorie requirements have a larger or smaller PDV.) Near the bottom of the nutrition facts label is the recommended daily amount of nutrients, listed by weight (in grams) for 2,000- and 2,500-calorie diets.

To help consumers determine health-related claims on food labels, the U.S. government requires manufacturers to adhere to certain definitions (**Table 5.3**).

The Three Functions of Food

Food has three functions:

1. To provide the chemical constituents of the body
2. To provide the energy for life
3. To be pleasurable, including satisfying hunger; being appealing in its smell, taste, sight, and texture; and being associated with enjoyable social activities

Providing Chemical Constituents

Your body is made up of billions of atoms and molecules arranged in particular combinations and proportions.

Most of the atoms and molecules that now make up your body were not part of you even a few weeks ago because living things continually exchange their chemical constituents with the environment. Food provides the "raw materials" for your body's cells to manufacture the specific chemical substances that make you *you*.

Adequate amounts of 40 chemical substances, called the **essential nutrients** (**Table 5.4**), must be

> **TERMS**
>
> **essential nutrients:** chemical substances obtained from food and needed by the body for growth, maintenance, or repair of tissues; not made by the body; must be obtained from food
>
> **ingredients label:** label on a manufactured food that lists the ingredients in descending order by weight
>
> **nutrition facts label:** label on a manufactured food that lists the quantity of certain nutrients in the food and the percent daily value for those nutrients
>
> **percent daily value:** percentage of the recommended daily amount of a particular nutrient found in a food

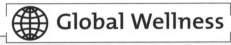

Global Wellness

The Mediterranean Diet

The Mediterranean diet is associated with longer life and reduced risk of heart disease and cancer. It's a diet based on whole grains, fresh fruits and vegetables, minimal animal and trans fat, and little red meat.

What is a Mediterranean diet?

- Meals based on whole-grain foods: breads, pasta, couscous, polenta, bulgur
- Abundant fresh vegetables and fruits
- Generous amounts of beans, nuts, and seeds
- Olive oil as the principal source of fat
- Use of garlic, onions, and herbs as condiments
- Moderate use of fish
- Moderate use of dairy
- Minimal use of red meat
- Low-to-moderate intake of alcohol

What makes the Mediterranean diet healthy?

- Low in saturated fat and cholesterol
- Energy supplied by unsaturated fat (in olive oil and nuts)
- No trans fats (artificial fats in packaged pastries and margarine)
- High in fiber
- High in antioxidants
- Low in refined sugar and flour
- High in plant-based vitamins and micronutrients

Researchers in France have determined that the Mediterranean diet lowers the risk of heart disease and many types of cancer.

Even though a large percentage of calories is derived from fat, mono- and polyunsaturated fats predominate, the kind that raise HDL (so-called good cholesterol). Almost absent are animal fats (saturated fats and cholesterol) and manufactured trans fats, which raise LDL (so-called bad cholesterol). The Mediterranean diet's high levels of antioxidants and other micronutrients reduce the risk of cardiovascular disease and cancer.

The typical American dinner, with a slab of meat in the center and one or two "sides," consisting of an overcooked vegetable and a butter-drenched potato, is a far cry from a typical Mediterranean dinner: pasta made of unrefined flour topped with a variety of minimally cooked vegetables (tomatoes, onions, peppers), some beans (peas, fava beans), and a sprinkle of hard cheese (Parmesan or Romano). For dessert, the Mediterranean diet calls for almonds and fresh fruit instead of cake, cookies, or ice cream.

It's too much to ask Americans to replace generations of dietary habits overnight. However, there are ways to incorporate some of the healthier aspects of the Mediterranean diet without radically changing customary eating patterns:

- Cut back on fast food, which is generally 50% saturated fat and cholesterol.
- Replace cake/ice cream desserts with fruit salad and nuts.
- Replace meat-centered meals with grain- and bean-centered ones.
- Replace doughnuts and sugar-laden snacks with fruit and mixed nuts.

Bon appetit!

Table 5.3

What Words on Product Labels Mean

Calorie free	Fewer than 5 calories per serving
Light (lite)	$1/3$ less calories or no more than $1/2$ the fat of the higher-calorie, higher-fat version; or no more than $1/2$ the sodium of the higher-sodium version
Fat free	Less than 0.5 g of fat per serving
Low fat	3 g of fat (or less) per serving
Reduced or less fat	At least 25% less fat per serving than the higher-fat version
Lean	Less than 10 g of fat, 4 g of saturated fat, and 95 mg of cholesterol per serving
Extra lean	Less than 5 g of fat, 2 g of saturated fat, and 95 mg of cholesterol per serving
Low in saturated fat	1 g saturated fat (or less) per serving and not more than 15% of calories from saturated fatty acids
Cholesterol free	Less than 2 mg of cholesterol and 2 g (or less) of saturated fat per serving
Low cholesterol	20 mg of cholesterol (or less) and 2 g of saturated fat (or less) per serving
Reduced cholesterol	At least 25% less cholesterol than the higher-cholesterol version, and 2 g (or less) of saturated fat per serving
Sodium free (no sodium)	Less than 5 mg of sodium per serving, and no sodium chloride (NaCl) in ingredients
Very low sodium	35 mg of sodium (or less) per serving
Low sodium	140 mg of sodium (or less) per serving
Reduced or less sodium	At least 25% less sodium per serving than the higher-sodium version
Sugar free	Less than 0.5 g of sugar per serving
High fiber	5 g of fiber (or more) per serving
Good source of fiber	2.5 to 4.9 g of fiber per serving

Table 5.4

The Essential Nutrients*

Amino acids	Fats	Water	Vitamins	Minerals
Isoleucine	Linoleic acid		Ascorbic acid (vitamin C)	Calcium
Leucine	Linolenic acid		Biotin	Chlorine
Lysine			Cobalamin (vitamin B_{12})	Chromium
Methionine			Folic acid	Cobalt
Phenylalanine			Niacin (vitamin B_3)	Copper
Threonine			Pantothenic acid	Iodine
Tryptophan			Pyridoxine (vitamin B_6)	Iron
Valine			Riboflavin (vitamin B_2)	Magnesium
Arginine†			Thiamine (vitamin B_1)	Manganese
Histidine†			Vitamin A	Molybdenum
			Vitamin D	Phosphorus
			Vitamin E	Potassium
			Vitamin K	Selenium
				Sodium
				Sulfur
				Zinc

*Must be obtained from food.
†Not essential for adults; needed for growth of children.

supplied continually to the body. Failure to do so can result in a nutritional deficiency disease, such as **goiter** from lack of iodine. Some forms of **anemia** result from insufficient dietary iron, and vitamin A deficiency is the most common cause of blindness in children worldwide.

Researchers have determined how much of the essential nutrients are required to prevent deficiency diseases. Many countries and the World Health Organization have produced dietary standards based on that research. In the United States, these requirements are called the **recommended [daily] dietary allowances,** or **RDA,** which lists values for protein, 11 vitamins, and 7 minerals. Nutrition scientists assume that if the listed nutrients are consumed in recommended amounts, all other necessary nutrients will be, too. The RDA also lists values for pregnant women, lactating women, and children. The RDA is set for people in reasonably good health, that is, not suffering from a major disease or under undue stress.

Surveys indicate that many Americans do not consume RDA amounts of calcium, vitamin B_6, magnesium,

zinc, copper, and potassium. People can determine whether their diets contain the RDA of particular nutrients by consulting tables and Web sites listing the composition of foods. Packaged food labels also carry information on the nutrient composition of the product.

Energy for Life

Food also provides energy to the body. The ultimate source of energy for complex organisms is sunlight, which is captured by green plants and converted to chemical energy that is stored as plant material. When humans eat plant matter or tissue from plant-eating animals, they obtain this stored chemical energy. Biological energy is used most efficiently when liberated in the presence of oxygen, which is one reason you breathe. In the process, the food material is converted to carbon dioxide, water, and other waste products and eliminated from the body in expired air, urine, feces, and sweat.

Energy transformations in living things are discussed in terms of calories. A **calorie** is the amount of heat energy required to raise 1 g of water from 14.5°C to 15.5°C. A **nutritional calorie,** which is what weight watchers watch, is 1,000 calories, or a **kilocalorie.** Books that discuss human nutrition and physical fitness frequently use the word "calorie" when actually referring to a kilocalorie. This book follows the same convention.

Energy from food is derived from the breakdown of carbohydrates, fats, and proteins. Carbohydrates and proteins

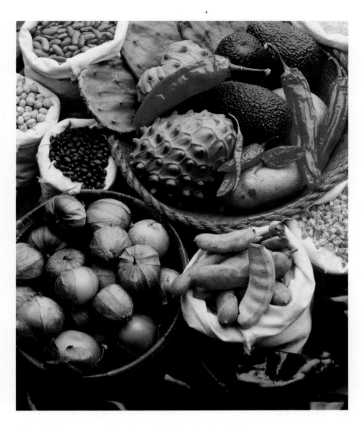

Natural, unprocessed foods provide the best nutrition.

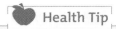 Health Tip

Eat! Eat! Breakfast, That Is

Even if you get by on only a few hours of sleep, when you wake up it's still been 5 to 10 hours since you last ate. Your biological gas tank is nearly empty. Before you dash to start your day, *break* your *fast* with a few hundred calories of food you like and that's reasonably healthy and nutritious. Although you can get a jolt from coffee and a pastry, whole-grain cereal (like oatmeal) or a whole-grain bread or bagel and some fruit or fruit juice is better. The whole grain pumps energy into your body slowly ("time release") so you aren't drowsy and ravenous in a couple of hours from low blood sugar and start craving *more* coffee and pastry. The fruit or fruit juice provides vitamins, minerals, phytochemicals, and a sweet taste.

Energy is also needed whenever the body produces more cells than are needed to replace ones that periodically die. Thus, all young people need additional energy for growth. Energy is also needed to produce new cells to repair wounds and injuries.

Energy requirements for individuals vary depending on a number of factors, including body size and composition; physical activity; growth needs during

supply approximately four calories per gram, and fats supply approximately nine calories per gram. Virtually every cell in the body is capable of the series of chemical transformations necessary to extract chemical energy from these nutrient molecules. The process of breaking down molecules to derive energy and to obtain material for the manufacture of cellular molecules is called **metabolism.**

Energy is needed to support three major processes: (1) **basal** (or resting) **metabolism,** which is the energy required to keep the body alive; (2) physical activity, the things you do when you're not completely at rest; and (3) growth and repair. The energy to support basal metabolism keeps cells functioning, maintains the body temperature within its normal limits, and keeps the heart, lungs, kidneys, and other internal organs functioning. The daily amount of energy required to support basal metabolism is called the **basal metabolic rate (BMR),** or resting metabolic rate (RMR). The BMR for adult women is about 1,100 calories per day, and 1,300 calories per day for adult men.

In addition to the energy you need for basal metabolism, you use energy in physical activity: walking, running, working, and so on. The amount of energy expended for these activities depends on how strenuous the activity is, how long it is engaged in, the body's size, and the environmental temperature. It takes more energy to be active in hot weather than in moderate temperatures, and it takes more energy to maintain body temperature when the weather is cold.

TERMS

anemia: a deficiency of red blood cells; often caused by insufficient iron

basal metabolic rate (BMR): the amount of energy needed per day to keep the body functioning while at rest

basal metabolism: the minimum amount of energy needed to keep the body alive

calorie: the amount of energy required to raise 1 g of water from 14.5°C to 15.5°C

goiter: an enlargement of the thyroid gland resulting from lack of iodine, causing a swelling in the front part of the neck

kilocalorie: unit of energy; the amount of heat needed to raise 1 kilogram of water 1°C, equivalent to 1,000 calories

metabolism: the process of obtaining energy and matter from the chemical breakdown of molecules obtained from food or from the body

nutritional calorie: unit of energy; often used interchangeably with the term *kilocalorie*

recommended [daily] dietary allowances (RDA): levels of nutrients recommended by the Food and Nutrition Board of the National Academy of Sciences for daily consumption by healthy individuals, scaled according to gender and age

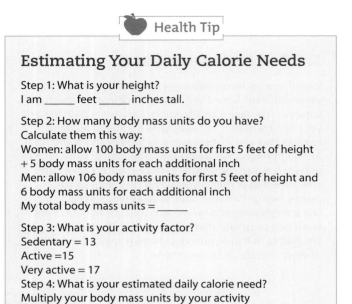

🍎 **Health Tip**

Estimating Your Daily Calorie Needs

Step 1: What is your height?
I am _____ feet _____ inches tall.

Step 2: How many body mass units do you have?
Calculate them this way:
Women: allow 100 body mass units for first 5 feet of height
+ 5 body mass units for each additional inch
Men: allow 106 body mass units for first 5 feet of height and
6 body mass units for each additional inch
My total body mass units = _____

Step 3: What is your activity factor?
Sedentary = 13
Active = 15
Very active = 17
Step 4: What is your estimated daily calorie need?
Multiply your body mass units by your activity
factor = _____

adolescence and young adulthood; pregnancy or breast-feeding; and injury or illness. The RDA for adult American men is 2,800 calories per day; for nonpregnant, nonlactating adult American women, it is 2,200. Nutritionists recommend that carbohydrates from whole grains, vegetables, and fruits be the principal source of energy, supplying about 50% of total calories consumed. Fats should make up no more than 30% of total calories consumed. Protein is generally not recommended as a source of energy, but only as a source of building blocks for the body's tissues and organs.

Pleasures of Eating

Everyone has experienced the feeling of hunger and its appeasement by eating something. But hunger is not the only reason for eating in our society. Most of the time we eat because it is "time to eat," because we have been presented with food, because it feels good to be eating something—especially something fatty or sweet—or because eating is an enjoyable social ritual. The ready availability of food is unique to modern societies; a hundred years ago there were no supermarkets, fast-food restaurants, or convenience stores on every block. Thus, we can consume food for a variety of reasons. Also, advertising encourages us to eat more and more often.

The Seven Components of Food

Food is composed of seven kinds of chemical substances: proteins, carbohydrates, lipids (fats), vitamins, minerals, phytochemicals, and water. Dietary proteins, most types of carbohydrates, and most lipids cannot be used by the body until they are broken down in the digestive system into smaller chemical units (**Figure 5.6**). In fact, only vitamins, minerals, a few kinds of carbohydrates, and water are absorbed into the body as is.

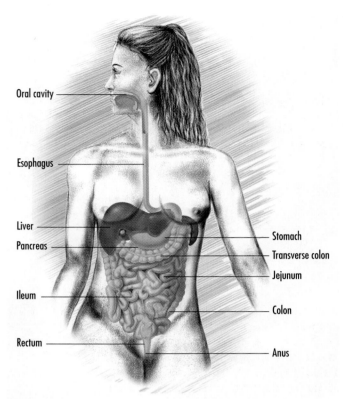

■ **Figure 5.6**

Human Digestive System
Teeth and glandular secretions in the mouth help break up food, which the esophagus transports to the stomach. The stomach breaks down some of the food molecules and passes the food to the rest of the digestive tube: the duodenum, jejunum, ileum, colon, and rectum. The pancreas secretes enzymes and fluid into the duodenum to help the digestive process. The liver controls release of absorbed nutrients into the body. Undigested material is eliminated from the body at the anus.

Proteins

About 20% of your body mass is **protein.** Much of the body's architecture and many of its vital functions are composed of or carried out by proteins.

Proteins are made up of chemical units called **amino acids,** which come in 20 different forms. Amino acids are classified as **essential** and **nonessential.** Adults require eight essential amino acids; those eight and two others are required by infants. Animal sources of protein include milk and milk products, meat, fish, poultry, and eggs. Plant sources include breads and cereal products, legumes, nuts, and seeds.

Amino acids are not stored in the body in any appreciable amounts; therefore, proper nutrition requires eating enough protein just about every day to meet the body's needs for essential amino acids. Adult women should consume about 45 grams per day and adult men about 55 to 60 grams. The average North American adult consumes about twice the recommended amount; the unneeded protein is broken down by the body and excreted in urine or stored as fat.

Because the amino acid composition of most animal protein is similar, people tend to acquire adequate

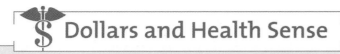

$ Dollars and Health Sense

The Food Industry: Profits, Not Health

Some of America's largest corporations are in the business of supplying consumers with less-than-healthy packaged foods, snack foods, sodas, and fast food. "Pouring rights" in public schools illustrate how the quest for profits can contribute to ill health.

To gain access to children and teens, a soda company gives a cash-strapped school money in exchange for the exclusive right to stock campus soda machines and the cafeteria with its products. Only milk and tap water can be offered as alternative beverages to the soda company's products. This may be good for company profits, but it is not particularly good for kids, for whom the sodas add extra empty calories. To support good nutrition, several school districts and some states have banned the sale of sodas on their campuses and have forbidden schools from entering into exclusive contracts with soda companies.

Some people are asking whether some food companies should bear some of the responsibility for the ill health caused by their products, just as tobacco companies have been (Mello, Studdert, & Brennan, 2006). Some advocate a "junk food tax" to deter consumption of sodas, candy, snack foods, and fast food (Jacobson & Brownell, 2000). Others advocate an approach reminiscent of the fight against smoking: lawsuits against junk and fast-food producers to recover health costs incurred from the consumption of their products. What do you think?

amounts and proportions of the essential amino acids from animal tissue, such as fish, meat, eggs, and dairy products. Most vegetable proteins, however, are deficient in one or more of the essential amino acids, so individuals who eat little or no meat or dairy products must eat foods in which an amino acid deficiency in one food is compensated for by an amino acid surplus in another. For example, wheat, rice, and oats contain very little lysine, but have large amounts of methionine and tryptophan. Soybeans and other legumes are relatively high in lysine, but are low in methionine and tryptophan. Meals consisting of both grains and legumes (e.g., rice and beans, corn and beans, wheat and soybeans) can supply adequate amounts of these essential amino acids.

Meat, dairy products, and eggs provide the essential amino acids, but they can be high in fat, and thus contribute to heart disease, cancer, and other fat-related health problems. For this reason, nutritionists recommend consuming nonfat or low-fat dairy products, using butter as a spread and not as an ingredient for cooking, being mindful of the amount of ice cream eaten, and limiting egg consumption to a few eggs per week. Nutritionists also favor trimming fat from meat before cooking, selecting meat with a low-fat content, and eating poultry (with skin removed because it contains fat) and fish, which have proportionately less fat than red meats. They also recommend using meat sparingly by adding it to grain- or bean-based dishes, rather than making it the center of the meal.

Another reason for avoiding a lot of meat is its association with colorectal cancer. People with the highest red and processed meat consumption have the highest rates of colon cancer (Santarelli et al., 2008). One reason for this is that commercially grown and distributed meats may contain cancer-causing or cancer-promoting pesticide residues (DDT), industrial chemicals (PCBs), growth hormones (DES), dyes for color enhancement, and preservatives, such as **nitrates** and **nitrites,** often found in hot dogs, ham, sausage, and other cured meats.

Another possibility is that bacteria in the colon convert substances necessary for the digestion of fats (bile acids) into cancer-causing agents. A third possibility is that charring meats in cooking converts substances in the meat into cancer-causing heterocyclic amines (HCAs).

> Vegetables aren't my meat and potatoes.
>
> *Yogi Berra*

Meat also is the vector for spongiform encephalopathy (mad cow disease) and a variety of bacteria and viruses that cause food poisoning. High-intensity meat production also is detrimental to the environment. The production of one pound of meat requires 15,000 to 20,000 gallons of water. Cattle are fed corn and soy, the excess production of which degrades the land and introduces pesticides into the food supply. The methane produced by cattle digestive processes contributes significantly to global warming.

TERMS

amino acids: compounds containing nitrogen that are the building blocks of protein

essential amino acids: amino acids that cannot be synthesized by the body and must be provided by food

nitrates: preservatives containing any salt or ester of nitric acid. Some individuals are sensitive to nitrates and may suffer from headache, diarrhea, or urticaria after ingesting them

nitrites: preservatives containing any salt or ester of nitrous acid

nonessential amino acids: eleven amino acids required for protein synthesis that are synthesized by humans and are not specifically required in the diet

protein: the foundation of every body cell; biological molecules composed of chains of amino acids

Wellness Guide

Are You a Sodaholic?

If you have one 12-ounce can of soda a day, here's what you're taking in (see **Table 5.5**):

- 40+ grams of sugar (about 10 teaspoons)
- 160 calories
- 40+ milligrams of caffeine

If you have two, three, or four sodas a day (or a 32-ounce "Big Gulp"), well, you do the math.

When you drink a soda, here's what's happening to you:

- The sugar adds non-nutritious (empty) calories.
- The sugar contributes to tooth decay.
- You probably drink less (or no) milk, so you get less calcium—bad for bones.
- Phosphate in soda weakens bones.
- Caffeine contributes to sleep problems.
- Caffeine is addicting.

In addition, the can may be one of the 45 billion a year that is not recycled and ends up in a landfill.

Alternatives: Poor Choices

Diet sodas. You cut out the sugar and its calories, but your bones, sleep, and the environment are still affected, and you are taking in 2 grams of aspartame, which may have some health risks in some people.

Table 5.5

Comparison of Sodas

Beverage	Quantity (oz)	Sugar (g)	Calories	Caffeine (mg)
Sunkist Orange Soda	12	52	190	41
Mountain Dew	12	46	184	55
Pepsi	12	41	164	37
Dr. Pepper	12	40	160	40
Coca-Cola Classic	12	39	156	34
7Up	12	39	156	0
Diet Coke	12	n/a	4	42
Red Bull	8	27	108	80
Jolt	8	27	108	71

Fruit drinks. These are colored, flavored sugar water—sodas without the fizz and caffeine. They often come in 20-ounce containers, so the amount of calories from the sugar is higher than from a regular 12-ounce can of soda.
Energy drinks. These are super-caffeinated sodas.

Alternatives: Healthful Choices

Water
Real fruit juice (not sugar-added "cocktails")
Noncaffeinated tea
Low-fat milk

Athletes are often encouraged to increase their intake of protein, sometimes to as much as 30% of total calories. Because body protein (that is, muscle tissue) can become a source of energy during exercise if carbohydrate and fat are not available, some endurance athletes may require more than the recommended amount of protein. A common recommendation for both endurance athletes and those involved in strength training is to consume 0.6 to 0.9 grams of protein per day per pound of body weight. That protein can come from lean meat, fish, poultry, vegetables, grains, and beans. It is not necessary to consume so-called high-protein liquids. Regular food will do.

Carbohydrates

Carbohydrates are a major source of the body's energy and also are used to manufacture some cell components, such as the hereditary material **deoxyribonucleic acid (DNA)**. Because the body can manufacture them from other substances, carbohydrates are not considered essential nutrients. However, not eating enough carbohydrates, recommended by some ill-conceived reducing diets, can force the body to break down muscle tissue to supply energy necessary for life functions.

Most animals have a "sweet tooth," and humans are no exception. That's why food manufacturers often add sugars and other sweeteners (such as high-fructose

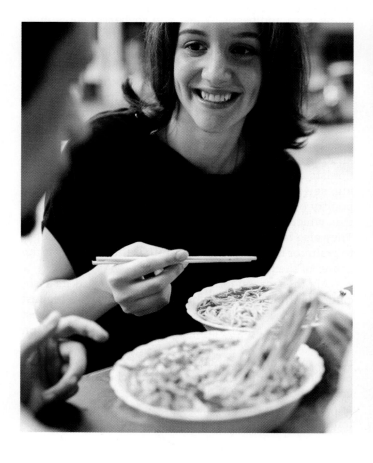

corn syrup) to their products. Indeed, many commercial breakfast cereals are 40% sugar by weight. Because added sugar provides calories but no essential nutrients, sugar is usually described as contributing "empty calories" to the diet. Excess calories from added sugar are converted to fat, which may contribute to overweight. Populations that consume large amounts of sucrose (refined beet or cane sugar) exhibit high rates of heart disease, obesity, diabetes, and dental caries. Sugar consumption in the United States averages about 156 pounds per person per year.

There are two principal types of carbohydrates: **simple sugars,** found predominantly in fruit, and **complex carbohydrates,** found in grains, fruit, and the stems, leaves, and roots of vegetables. Simple sugars contribute about 20% of total calories in the average American diet.

Glucose is the most common simple sugar; it is found in all plants and animals. Glucose circulates in the bloodstream and is commonly referred to as "blood sugar." Another simple sugar is fructose, which is found in fruits and honey. **Fructose** is one of the sweetest sugars, which means you can eat less fructose than other simple sugars and taste an equivalent amount of sweetness. High-fructose corn syrup is a common sweetener added to a variety of commercial food products.

Sucrose, which is common table sugar (the "refined" sugar added to many packaged foods), is a combination of glucose and fructose. Sucrose is digested by breaking down the glucose and fructose portions. Because fructose is sweeter than sucrose, you can reduce the amount of sugar in your diet without cutting out sweet tastes by replacing pastries with fresh fruit and table sugar with honey. Furthermore, you will be gaining other nutrients in the fruit and honey that are not present in refined sucrose.

Lactose, found principally in dairy products, is a sugar consisting of glucose combined with the simple sugar **galactose.** When lactose is digested, the glucose and galactose are separated and the galactose is converted to glucose. Whereas almost all babies have the capacity to digest lactose (it is the major sugar in mother's milk), many older children and adults, particularly of black and Asian heritage, are not able to digest it because they lack a required enzyme, **lactase,** which splits lactose into glucose and galactose. When lactase-deficient people consume dairy products, they experience gastrointestinal upset, diarrhea, and, occasionally, severe illness. These individuals can supplement their diets with products containing lactase (e.g., Lactaid) or by eating yogurt, cheese, and other dairy products in which the lactose has been broken down by the fermentation process. Because dairy products are a major source of calcium in the North American diet, people who avoid dairy products should consume calcium-rich vegetables (e.g., broccoli and peas) and possibly take calcium supplements.

Complex carbohydrates come primarily from grains (wheat, rice, corn, oats, barley); legumes (peas, beans); the leaves, stems, and roots of plants; and some animal tissue. There are two main classes of complex carbohy-

drates: **starch,** which is digestible, and **fiber,** which is not digestible.

Starch consists of many glucose molecules linked together. It is a way organisms store glucose until it is needed. In plants, starch is usually contained in granules within seeds, pods, or roots. Wheat flour, for example, is made by crushing wheat grain, which separates the outer husk (the bran) from the middle, starch-containing portion (the endosperm) and the inner germ. The white flour commonly used in baking is "70% extraction," which means that 70% of the original grain remains after crushing. In the milling of 70% extraction flour, many nutrients in the wheat grain are lost, so flour manufacturers add back several vitamins and minerals to produce "enriched flour." A "whole-grain flour," on the other hand, is 90% to 95% extraction and does not have to be enriched.

Bread made with whole-wheat flour is brown, but not all brown bread is whole-wheat bread. Some manufacturers add molasses or honey to white-flour dough to give it a brown color, and they are allowed to label the product "wheat bread." For this reason, it is important to read the package label before buying.

Starch is also found in potatoes, which have an undeserved reputation for being fattening. Potatoes are no more fattening than any other starchy food unless

TERMS

carbohydrates: the most economical and efficient source of energy; biological molecules consisting of one or more sugar molecules

complex carbohydrates: a class of carbohydrates called polysaccharides; foods composed of starch and cellulose

deoxyribonucleic acid (DNA): a substance occurring in cell nuclei; carrier of the genes; present in all body cells of every species

fiber: a group of compounds that make up the framework of plants; fiber cannot be digested

fructose: a simple sugar found in fruits and honey

galactose: a monosaccharide derived from lactose

glucose: the principal source of energy in all cells; also called dextrose

lactase: enzyme secreted by glands in the small intestine that converts lactose (milk sugar) into simple sugars

lactose: a molecule of glucose and galactose chemically bonded together; found primarily in milk

simple sugars: a class of carbohydrates called monosaccharides; all carbohydrates must be reduced to simple sugars to be digested

starch: complex chain of glucose molecules

sucrose: common refined table sugar; a molecule of glucose and a molecule of fructose chemically bonded together

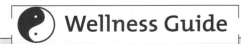

Wellness Guide

Taking Care of Your Teeth and Gums

Taking care of your teeth and gums means adopting practices for oral health that prevent tooth decay *(dental caries)* and gum disease *(gingivitis* and *periodontitis)*. Tooth decay and gum disease are caused by the action of a variety of bacteria that live in the mouth, which produce acids by breaking down the sugars in food. The acids attack the enamel of teeth, causing tooth decay. Other bacteria are involved in the conversion of sugars and some of the material in saliva into a gelatinous substance called *plaque,* which sticks to teeth and gums and fosters more bacterial growth and decay.

Tooth and gum disease could be prevented if (1) the bacteria responsible could be removed from the mouth, (2) the sugars and other substances bacteria use to produce acids and plaque were removed from the mouth, or (3) teeth were protected from the bacterial products.

It is not yet possible to keep all tooth and gum disease–causing bacteria from the mouth or to render them harmless. So, keeping the mouth free of sugar and plaque is the best way to prevent tooth and gum problems. You can accomplish this by doing the following:

- Not eating sugar and sugar-containing foods between meals
- Consuming sweets in liquid rather than solid form when possible
- Avoiding sticky or slowly dissolving sweets
- Brushing and flossing teeth after each meal
- Rinsing the mouth with warm water when unable to brush after a snack or meal
- Obtaining fluoride (to increase resistance to tooth decay) from toothpastes, mouthwashes, and drinking water
- Getting periodic dental checkups

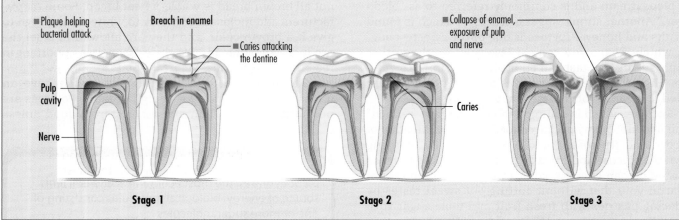

Stage 1   **Stage 2**   **Stage 3**

they are cooked in large amounts of fat or oil, which is used in making french fries and potato chips. One large potato has about 100 calories, less than a medium-sized soft drink. French fries made from a medium potato, however, contain over 300 calories.

Animals and humans produce a starch in muscle and liver tissue called **glycogen.** When energy is needed, the glycogen breaks down and its constituent glucose molecules are liberated. Athletes sometimes eat large quantities of carbohydrates the day before competition to build up their supply of glycogen, a practice known as *carbohydrate loading.* The practice of carbohydrate loading can be risky, particularly for diabetics.

Fiber is the second main class of complex carbohydrates. There are two kinds of fiber: **insoluble fiber,** which cannot dissolve in water, and **soluble fiber,** which can. Insoluble fiber is made up of **cellulose** and **hemicellulose,** substances that offer rigidity to plant material (wood; stems; the outer coverings of nuts, seeds, grains; the peels and skins of fruits and vegetables). Soluble fiber is composed of pectins, gums, and mucilages. The differences in insoluble and soluble fiber are not significant for health. Nutritionists recommend that individuals consume 20 to 35 grams of fiber daily, regardless of its type (**Table 5.6**).

Table 5.6

Fiber Content of Various Foods

Food	Amount	Fiber (g)
Whole-wheat bread	1 slice	1.6
Rye bread	1 slice	1.0
White bread	1 slice	0.6
Brown rice (cooked)	½ cup	2.4
White rice (cooked)	½ cup	0.1
Spaghetti (cooked)	½ cup	0.8
Kidney beans (cooked)	½ cup	5.8
Lima beans (cooked)	½ cup	4.9
Potato (baked)	Medium	3.8
Corn	½ cup	3.9
Spinach	½ cup	2.0
Lettuce	½ cup	0.3
Strawberries	¾ cup	2.0
Banana	Medium	2.0
Apple (with skin)	Medium	2.6
Orange	Small	1.2

Fiber adds bulk to the feces, thereby preventing constipation and related disorders, such as hemorrhoids and hiatal hernia, which can result from prolonged increase in intra-abdominal pressure while defecating. Fiber also facilitates the transport of waste material through the digestive tract, lessening the risk of appendicitis, diverticular disease (out-pocketings in the wall of the lower intestine), and cancer of the colon and rectum. High-fiber diets may also help to lessen the risk of heart disease and some cancers.

Because they contain complex carbohydrates, fiber, vitamins, and other nutrients, whole-grain foods are superior to manufactured and restaurant foods composed of refined grains (**Table 5.7**). Moreover, consumption of foods made of refined flour, which are nutrition-ally inferior, means that healthy whole-grain foods will not be consumed.

Lipids (Fats)

Lipids are a diverse group of substances that have the common property of being relatively insoluble in water. Some of these substances include **cholesterol** and **lecithin,** which are essential constituents of cell membranes; the steroid hormones produced by the reproductive organs and adrenal glands; vitamins A, D, E, and K; and bile acids, which aid the digestion of fats. Despite the current antifat trend, fats are an essential part of the diet. They supply calories, they provide flavor and texture to food, and digesting fat provides feelings of satiety and well-being. One kind of fat, **linoleic acid,** found in vegetable oils such as safflower, sunflower, and corn, is essential, and must be obtained in food. Deficiencies in this substance can produce skin lesions.

Much of the fat consumed in the diet is triglyceride, which is composed of **fatty acids.** These substances are further classified as **saturated, monounsaturated,** or **polyunsaturated,** depending on their chemistry. Saturation refers to the number of hydrogen atoms (and therefore the amount of energy) contained in a fatty acid. A

Table 5.7

Whole-Grain and Refined-Grain Foods

Whole-grain foods	Refined-grain foods
Brown rice	Cornbread*
Buckwheat	Corn tortillas*
Bulgur (cracked wheat)	Couscous*
Oatmeal	Crackers*
Popcorn	Flour tortillas
	Grits
Ready-to-eat breakfast cereals	
Whole-wheat cereal flakes	*Pasta*
Muesli	Noodles*
Whole-grain barley	Spaghetti
Whole-grain cornmeal	Macaroni
Whole rye	Pitas*
Whole-wheat bread	Pretzels
Whole-wheat crackers	
Whole-wheat pasta	*Ready-to-eat breakfast cereals*
Whole-wheat sandwich buns and rolls	Corn flakes
	White bread
Whole-wheat tortillas	White sandwich buns and rolls
Wild rice	White rice
Less common whole grains	
Amaranth	
Millet	
Quinoa	
Sorghum	
Triticale	

Note: Whole-grain foods contain the entire grain kernel: bran, germ, and endosperm. Refined-grain foods are foods in which the bran and germ are removed to produce a finer texture and longer shelf life; the refining process removes fiber, iron, and many B vitamins. Most refined grains are *enriched;* certain B vitamins (thiamin, riboflavin, niacin, folic acid) and iron are added back after processing. Fiber is not added back. Some food products are made from mixtures of whole grains and refined grains. Some grain products contain significant amounts of bran. Bran provides fiber, which is important for health. However, products with added bran or bran alone (e.g., oat bran) are not necessarily whole-grain products.

*Most of these products are made from refined grains. Some are made from whole grains. Check the ingredient list for the words "whole grain" or "whole wheat" to decide if they are made from a whole grain. Some foods are made from a mixture of whole and refined grains.

Source: U.S. Department of Agriculture. Available: http://www.mypyramid.gov/pyramid/grains.html.

TERMS

cellulose: a carbohydrate forming the skeleton of most plant structures and plant cells; the most abundant polysaccharide in nature and the source of dietary fiber

cholesterol: a fatlike compound occurring in bile, blood, brain, nerve tissue, liver, and other parts of the body

fatty acids: naturally occurring in fats, either saturated or unsaturated (monounsaturated or polyunsaturated)

glycogen: the form in which carbohydrate is stored in humans and animals

hemicellulose: substances found in plant cell walls that are composed of various sugars chemically linked together

insoluble fiber: cannot be dissolved in water

lecithin: an essential component of cell membranes

linoleic acid: an essential fat that must be obtained from food

lipids: fats such as cholesterol and triglycerides

monounsaturated fatty acid: carries one less than all the hydrogen atoms it possibly could

polyunsaturated fatty acid: carries at least two fewer hydrogen atoms than it would if saturated

saturated fat: generally solid at room temperature; comes from animal sources

soluble fiber: can be dissolved in water

saturated fatty acid carries all the hydrogen atoms it can. A monounsaturated fatty acid (MUFA) carries one less than all the hydrogen atoms it possibly could. A polyunsaturated fatty acid lacks two or more hydrogen atoms. A dietary fat is classified as saturated, monounsaturated, or polyunsaturated depending on the type of fatty acids it contains in greatest quantity.

Saturated fats are found in whole milk and products made from whole milk; egg yolks; meat; meat fat; coconut and palm oils; chocolate; regular margarine; and hydrogenated vegetable shortenings. Sources of monounsaturated fats include olive oil and some nuts. Polyunsaturated fats are found in safflower, cottonseed, corn, soybean, and sesame seed oils, and fatty fish (**Figure 5.7**).

Diets high in cholesterol and saturated fat increase the risk of heart disease, some cancers, and obesity. Many nutritionists recommend that adults consume no more than 300 mg of cholesterol per day and limit saturated fat intake to 10% or less of total calories. Conversely, polyunsaturated fats tend to lower blood cholesterol, which is why nutritionists recommend consuming vegetable oils, nuts, and fish.

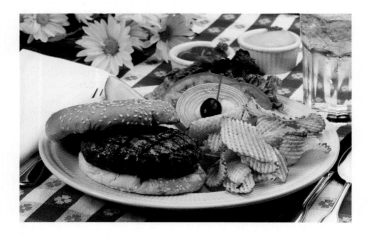

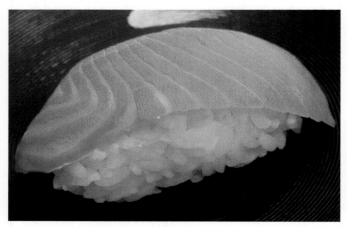

■ **Figure 5.7**
Unhealthy and Healthy Fats
Trans and saturated fats in fast and packaged food are less healthy than polyunsaturated fats found in fish, nuts, and vegetable oils.

Food manufacturers use a chemical process to transform natural polyunsaturated fatty acids derived from vegetable oils into artificial **trans-fatty acids**, or trans fats, which tend to be solid at room temperature. Chemically manufactured trans fats are also called *partially hydrogenated vegetable oils* (PHVO), industrial quantities of which are used to make crackers, candies, cookies, snack foods, baked goods, and other processed foods. The fast-food industry uses PHVO to cook french fries and other deep-fried products (a large order of french fries contains 6 grams of trans fat; a baked apple pie, 4.5 grams). Restaurants use it for cooking, frying, and baking.

Considerable research shows that trans fats are unhealthy (Booker & Mann, 2008). For example, one study found that women with the highest levels of trans fats in their blood have the highest risk of heart disease (Sun et al., 2007). To lessen the amount of trans fat in the American food supply, the state of California and cities such as New York and Philadelphia have banned trans fat from restaurants, and some fast-food corporations have begun to remove trans fats from their products.

Although you do not need to give up eating margarine, french fries, or doughnuts to be healthy, you need to practice moderation. The amount of trans fats in food products is listed on the product label. Intake of these artificial substances can be limited by using liquid vegetable oils that contain polyunsaturated fatty acids whenever possible. Moreover, vegetable oils are naturally devoid of cholesterol. Also, tell your school food service provider and favorite restaurants and bakeries that you prefer they use natural oils, such as canola, rather than artificial trans fats.

Artificial fats (olestra, Simplesse) are chemicals that are added primarily to packaged pastries and snack foods to provide the taste of fat without contributing calories. Ingesting these substances is not without risk, however, because they may both inhibit the absorption of fat-soluble vitamins from the gastrointestinal tract and cause diarrhea. The purported benefit of artificial fat—that it contributes to weight management—apparently is overstated because consumers tend to compensate for the lack of energy derived from fat by ingesting greater amounts of carbohydrates.

Vitamins

Vitamins are substances that facilitate a variety of biological processes. Vitamins do not provide building blocks for the manufacture of the body's tissues nor do they provide calories to fuel the body's functions. This is why the body requires much smaller amounts of vitamins than it does proteins, carbohydrates, and fats. The body cannot manufacture vitamins; they must be obtained from food (**Table 5.8**). Vitamins are classified as **water-soluble** or **fat-soluble**, depending on their chemistry.

Table 5.8

Water-Soluble and Fat-Soluble Vitamins

Water-soluble vitamin	Why needed?	Primary sources	Deficiency results in
Ascorbic acid (vitamin C)	Tooth and bone formation; production of connective tissue; promotion of wound healing; may enhance immunity	Citrus fruits, tomatoes, peppers, cabbage, potatoes, melons	Scurvy (degeneration of bones, teeth, and gums)
Biotin	Involved in fat and amino acid synthesis and breakdown	Yeast, liver, milk, most vegetables, bananas, grapefruit	Skin problems; fatigue; muscle pains; nausea
Cobalamin (vitamin B_{12})	Involved in single carbon atom transfers; essential for DNA synthesis	Muscle meats, eggs, milk, and dairy products (not in vegetables)	Pernicious anemia; nervous system malfunctions
Folacin (folic acid)	Essential for synthesis of DNA and other molecules	Green leafy vegetables, organ meats, whole-wheat products	Anemia; diarrhea and other gastrointestinal problems
Niacin	Involved in energy production and synthesis of cell molecules	Grains, meats, legumes	Pellagra (skin, gastrointestinal, and mental disorders)
Pantothenic acid	Involved in energy production and synthesis and breakdown of many biological molecules	Yeast, meats and fish, nearly all vegetables and fruits	Vomiting; abdominal cramps; malaise; insomnia
Pyridoxine (vitamin B_6)	Essential for synthesis and breakdown of amino acids and manufacture of unsaturated fats from saturated fats	Meats, whole grains, most vegetables	Weakness; irritability; trouble sleeping and walking; skin problems
Riboflavin (vitamin B_2)	Involved in energy production; important for health of the eyes	Milk and dairy foods, meats, eggs, vegetables, grains	Eye and skin problems
Thiamine (vitamin B_1)	Essential for breakdown of food molecules and production of energy	Meats, legumes, grains, some vegetables	Beri-beri (nerve damage, weakness, heart failure)
Fat-soluble vitamin	**Why needed?**	**Primary sources**	**Deficiency or excess results in**
Vitamin A (retinol)	Essential for maintenance of eyes and skin; influences bone and tooth formation	Liver, kidney, yellow and green leafy vegetables, apricots	Deficiency: night blindness; eye damage; skin dryness. Excess: loss of appetite; skin problems; swelling of ankles and feet
Vitamin D (calciferol)	Regulates calcium metabolism; important for growth of bones and teeth	Cod-liver oil, dairy products, eggs	Deficiency: rickets (bone deformities) in children; bone destruction in adults. Excess: thirst; nausea; weight loss; kidney damage
Vitamin E (tocopherol)	Prevents damage to cells from oxidation; prevents red blood cell destruction	Wheat germ, vegetable oils, vegetables, egg yolk, nuts	Deficiency: anemia, possibly nerve cell destruction
Vitamin K (phylloquinone)	Helps with blood clotting	Liver, vegetable oils, green leafy vegetables, tomatoes	Deficiency: severe bleeding

Vitamins A (and its dietary precursor, betacarotene), C, and E are classed as **antioxidants** because they have the capacity to neutralize the effects of chemicals called *free radicals*, which can damage biological structures via chemical oxidation. Antioxidant vitamins are found in a variety of fruits and vegetables (not beans) and can be obtained in vitamin supplements. Observational studies have shown that people who consume foods containing large amounts of antioxidant vitamins have less risk of cancer, heart disease, and cataracts than people who consume small amounts. However, in laboratory studies, antioxidant vitamins C, E, and betacarotene have not been shown to prevent cancer or cataracts (Bardia et al., 2008). In laboratory trials, large doses of vitamins A, C, and E were found to increase slightly the risk of death (Bjelakovic et al., 2008). Possible explanations of these discrepancies include the following: (1) Diets rich in fruits and vegetables contain beneficial substances (e.g.,

TERMS

antioxidants: substances that in small amounts inhibit the oxidation of other compounds

artificial fats: chemicals added to packaged foods to provide the taste and texture of fat but few or no calories

fat-soluble vitamins: soluble in fat; there are four fat-soluble vitamins

trans-fatty acid: also trans fat, an artificial fat manufactured by chemically modifying monounsaturated and polyunsaturated fatty acids

vitamins: essential organic substances needed daily in small amounts to perform specific functions in the body

water-soluble vitamins: soluble in water; there are nine water-soluble vitamins

$ Dollars and Health Sense

Functional Foods Increase Profits

When vitamins, minerals, herbs, or other substances are added to foods to allow the manufacturer to make health claims, the food is called a **functional food**. Americans have been eating functional foods since 1924, when iodine was added to salt to prevent goiter, a disease of the thyroid gland caused by iodine deficiency. For many years after that, some foods (such as enriched flour) were fortified with extra vitamins and minerals but without the manufacturer making health claims. That changed in 1993 when the FDA ruled that milk and yogurt, which contain high amounts of calcium, could carry labels claiming that the products helped prevent osteoporosis. Other food manufacturers quickly began adding calcium to other foods—orange juice, waffles, potato chips—so they, too, could make health claims.

Food companies have found that adding substances to foods in order to make health claims is good business, even if the added substances have not been shown scientifically to be helpful. Thus, we now have sodas with ginseng (for relaxation),

cereals with psyllium husk (to protect against heart disease or cancer), margarine with plant-derived sterols (to lower cholesterol), ice cream with echinacea (to help the immune system), and soups with St. John's wort (to combat depression). As people strive for better health, food companies have cashed in on the "health-conscious" market to the tune of about $60 billion per year (Consumer Reports on Health, 2007).

Neither the health claims nor the purity and amount of additives in functional foods are regulated or tested by the Food and Drug Administration (FDA). Herbs added to foods may be dangerous because amounts are not well controlled and, in some instances (e.g., St. John's wort), the herb can interfere with the action of certain medications. Some people may mistakenly believe that more is better and risk overdose with a vitamin, mineral, or plant product by ingesting both dietary supplements and a functional food. Moreover, functional foods often cost more, sometimes a lot more, than equivalent foods without supplements do.

---

phytochemicals) other than vitamins A, C, and E; (2) many clinical studies are carried out on people who already have cancer or heart disease or carry a high risk for such diseases (e.g., smokers); (3) to prevent cancer, antioxidant vitamins may require other plant substances that are not present in pills. With regard to antioxidant vitamins, the discrepancy in results from observational and laboratory studies illustrates (once again) that healthy nutrition is a matter of whole, fresh food choices rather than consuming large amounts of individual nutrients.

Folic acid (also called *folate* or *folacin*), a vitamin found in dark-green leafy vegetables, beans, and fruits, helps prevent spina bifida and other neural tube defects in newborn babies (see Chapter 15). The diets of most American women and elderly persons of both sexes are deficient in folic acid (on average, 200 micrograms per day are consumed; 400 micrograms are recommended), so the federal government requires that manufacturers of cereal-based foods (e.g., breads, breakfast cereals, pastas) fortify their products with it. There is debate whether the amount of folic acid in fortified foods is too low, so pregnant women are advised to ask their prenatal health care providers about taking folic acid supplements.

Folic acid also helps lower the body's manufacture of **homocysteine,** a substance derived from the essential amino acid methionine. High blood levels of homocysteine increase the risk of coronary artery disease and heart attack, so all individuals are advised to obtain adequate amounts of folic acid. The best way to do this is to eat beans and fruits, and possibly take supplements (not to exceed a total of 700 micrograms of folate per day because too much folate may be toxic).

Many people are deficient in vitamin D, which is made in the skin in response to the action of sunlight (Holick, 2007). People who live in northern or southern latitudes, who have dark skin, or who remain indoors for most of the day are most at risk for low levels of vitamin D. Vitamin D helps the body absorb and retain calcium and phosphorus, thus fostering strong bones. Vitamin D also helps maintain muscle strength, especially in the elderly. It enables the body to fight infections and some cancers, and may lessen the risk of heart disease. Adequate levels of vitamin D can be attained with 15 minutes' exposure of sunlight per day or by taking vitamin supplements (being mindful that too much vitamin D can be toxic).

Minerals

Many body functions require one or more inorganic elements called **minerals (Table 5.9)**. Sodium, potassium, and chlorine, for example, are essential for maintaining cell membranes, conducting nerve impulses, and contracting muscles. Magnesium, copper, and cobalt facilitate certain biochemical reactions; iron is essential for the oxygen-carrying function of hemoglobin; iodine is needed to produce thyroid hormone; and calcium and phosphorus make up bones and teeth. Selenium may reduce the risk of cancer, perhaps because of its activity as an antioxidant.

Minerals are found in almost all food, especially fresh vegetables. Women and young people are susceptible to iron deficiency, so they must eat iron-rich foods, such as eggs, lean meats, brans, whole grains, and green leafy vegetables. Most women and elderly people ingest too little calcium, which is found in dairy products and

Table 5.9

Essential Minerals

Mineral	Why needed?	Primary sources	Deficiency results in
Calcium	Bone and tooth formation; blood clotting; nerve transmission	Milk, cheese, dark-green vegetables, dried legumes	Stunted growth; rickets, osteoporosis; convulsions
Chlorine	Formation of gastric juice; acid–base balance	Common salt	Muscle cramps; mental apathy; reduced appetite
Chromium	Glucose and energy metabolism	Fats, vegetable oils, meats	Impaired ability to metabolize glucose
Cobalt	Constituent of vitamin B_{12}	Organ and muscle meats	Not reported in man
Copper	Constituent of enzymes of iron metabolism	Meats, drinking water	Anemia (rare)
Iodine	Constituent of thyroid hormones	Marine fish and shellfish, dairy products, many vegetables	Goiter (enlarged thyroid)
Iron	Constituent of hemoglobin and enzymes of energy metabolism	Eggs, lean meats, legumes, whole grains, green leafy vegetables	Iron-deficiency anemia (weakness, reduced resistance to infection)
Magnesium	Activates enzymes; involved in protein synthesis	Whole grains, green leafy vegetables	Growth failure; behavioral disturbances; weakness, spasms
Manganese	Constituent of enzymes involved in fat synthesis	Widely distributed in foods	In animals: disturbances of nervous system, reproductive abnormalities
Molybdenum	Constituent of some enzymes	Legumes, cereals, organ meats	Not reported in man
Phosphorus	Bone and tooth formation; acid–base balance	Milk, cheese, meat, poultry, grains	Weakness; demineralization of bone
Potassium	Acid–base balance; body water balance; nerve function	Meats, milk, many fruits	Muscular weakness; paralysis
Selenium	Functions in close association with vitamin E	Seafood, meat, grains	Anemia (rare)
Sodium	Acid–base balance; body water balance; nerve function	Common salt	Muscle cramps; mental apathy; reduced appetite
Sulfur	Constituent of active tissue compounds, cartilage, and tendon	Sulfur amino acids (methionine and cysteine) in dietary proteins	Related to intake and deficiency of sulfur amino acids
Zinc	Constituent of enzymes involved in digestion	Widely distributed in foods	Growth failure

some green leafy vegetables such as broccoli and turnip greens (Table 5.10). Because sodas tend to replace milk—and therefore calcium—in the diet, nutritionists recommend that soda consumption be limited (if not elimi-

nated) in the diets of children and adolescents to strengthen bones in both early and later life.

Many people consume too much sodium, which may contribute to high blood pressure. The amounts of sodium naturally present in almost every kind of food pose no problem; excess sodium comes from manufactured and restaurant food, to which salt is added to increase flavor, and from the overuse of table salt. Some people consume as many as 20 grams of sodium per day, which is about 10 times the 2 grams per day the body needs.

Table 5.10

Calcium in Various Foods

The recommended daily value for adults is 1,000 mg.

Food	Serving size	Milligrams (mg) calcium
Tofu, calcium processed	$\frac{1}{3}$ cup	581
Yogurt, plain	8 oz container	411
Milk, skim and low fat	1 cup	301
Sesame seeds, whole roasted	1 oz	297
Cheese, Swiss	1 oz	288
Cheese, cheddar	1 oz	216
Cheese, mozzarella	1 oz	194
Soybeans, cooked	$\frac{1}{2}$ cup	131
Turnip greens, cooked	$\frac{1}{2}$ cup	116
Blackeyed peas, cooked	$\frac{1}{2}$ cup	115
All-bran cereal	$\frac{1}{2}$ cup	106
Collard greens	$\frac{1}{2}$ cup	101
Sardines, canned	1 oz	105
Salmon, canned (with bones)	1 oz	59

TERMS

functional food: a food to which additional vitamins, minerals, herbs, or other substances are added to allow the manufacturer to make health claims

homocysteine: a substance derived from the amino acid methionine; high blood levels increase the risk of heart disease; blood levels are reduced with adequate intake of folic acid

minerals: inorganic elements found in the body both in combination with organic compounds and alone

The Institute of Medicine recommends that Americans limit sodium intake to 1,500 mg per day, or about half a teaspoon (the amount in a can of soup). This can be done not by tossing out the dinner table salt shaker but by cutting back on restaurant (especially fast) food and avoiding processed and manufactured foods. It takes a few weeks for the palate to adjust from a high-salt diet to a lower-salt one. Once this occurs, foods that formerly tasted "good" tend to taste salty.

Athletes are often advised to take salt tablets to replace body salt lost in sweat; this advice is misguided. Except in cases of severe fluid loss, which more often accompanies medical therapies involving diuretics than sports, salt is readily replaced by eating food.

Phytochemicals

Many vegetables and fruits contain chemical substances, referred to as **phytochemicals,** that are not nutrients per se but that positively affect human physiology (**Table 5.11**). Phytochemicals may help the body destroy and eliminate toxins acquired from the environment or tissue-damaging by-products of metabolism, such as oxygen free radicals. For example, cruciferous

vegetables (e.g., broccoli, kale, cauliflower, brussels sprouts, cabbage, mustard greens) are rich in the cancer-preventing phytochemicals *sulforaphane* and *isothiocyanates.* Tomatoes and tomato products (ketchup, tomato sauce), pink grapefruit, papaya, peaches, and watermelon contain a phytochemical called *lycopene,* which protects against oxidative damage and reduces the risk of cancer and heart disease. *Lutein,* found in dark leafy and brightly colored vegetables, reduces the risk of heart disease and the eye disease of age-related macular degeneration. Green and black tea, onions, apples, and grapes contain a family of phytochemicals called *flavonoids,* which also protect against cancer and heart disease. Dates, figs, and other dried fruits contain *polyphenols,* which are powerful antioxidants.

Water

Water is the principal constituent of blood and is the major component of all cells. Water provides the medium in which all cell chemical activities take place.

Body water is maintained at a relatively constant level by the nervous, endocrine, and urinary systems. If body water volume is low, a person experiences thirst, which motivates drinking. A low volume of body water activates hormonal mechanisms that reduce the production of urine. Excess body water volume activates hormonal mechanisms that increase the output of urine. Increasing output is the function of diuretics, often given to reduce blood pressure, fluid volume after a heart attack, or feelings of bloatedness. The popular maxim that you should drink eight glasses of water a day is partially correct. The average adult loses about that much body water through sweat, moisture in expired air, urine, and feces. This loss is partly offset by drinking water and obtaining water in other fluids and foods.

Body water should be replaced by consuming pure water, milk, or real juice. So-called enhanced waters are not pure. They contain a few grams of sugar, a small amount of vitamins, and often caffeine. Soda also is a poor substitute for water. A study found that physically active teenage girls who drank sodas were 4 to 5 times more likely to have had bone fractures than girls who did not drink sodas, possibly because sodas contain phosphoric acid, which affects calcium metabolism and bone mass. Another possibility is that young people may replace milk in their diets with sodas, giving their bodies less calcium with which to strengthen bones. Liquids containing caffeine (coffee, tea, sodas) and alcohol are diuretics, which means that some of the fluid ingested is lost in additional urine output.

Many people drink bottled water in the belief that it is more healthful than tap water. Not all bottled water comes from "natural" sources as the name of the product may suggest. The source of some bottled water products is a municipal water tap. One should look on the product label to ascertain the source of the water inside.

Table 5.11

Phytochemicals in Fruits and Vegetables and Their Possible Benefits

Food	Phytochemicals	Possible benefits
Berries Blueberries, strawberries, raspberries, blackberries, currants, etc.	Anthocyanidins, ellagic acid	Antioxidants Cancer prevention
Chili peppers	Capsaicin	Possible antioxidant Topical pain relief
Citrus fruits Oranges, grapefruit, lemon, limes, etc.	Flavanones (tangeretic, nobiletin, hesperitin) Carotenoids	Antioxidants
Cruciferous vegetables Broccoli, kale, cauliflower, brussels sprouts, cabbage, mustard greens	Indoles Isothiocyanates Sulforaphane Carotenoids	Antioxidants Anticancer properties
Garlic family Garlic, onions, shallots, leeks, chives, scallions	Allylic sulfides Flavonoids (quercetin)	Anticancer properties
Soy	Daidzein, equol, genestein, enterolactone, and other plant estrogens	Reduce risk of breast, prostate cancer; reduce risk of heart disease

$ Dollars and Health Sense

The Marketing of Dietary Supplements

For the last 50 years "effectiveness" meant that there'd be scientific evidence to demonstrate that something worked. Now, effectiveness is measured by how quickly something moves off the shelves.

David Kessler, MD
former FDA Commissioner

In 1906, and again in 1938, the U.S. Congress passed the Pure Food and Drug Act to ensure that foods are safe and medicines are both safe and effective. The federal agency that enforces the law is the Food and Drug Administration (FDA), which requires rigorous testing of drugs before they can be marketed.

In 1994, however, Congress passed a separate law that defines the FDA's regulatory powers over the dietary supplement industry. This law was enacted to prevent the FDA from regulating dietary supplements with the same rigor it does drugs and food additives. However, the agency still can ban a product if it is found to be harmful after being used by the general public. This means that manufacturers and distributors of dietary supplements are able to sell substances that may be worthless or even harmful until they are caught— which usually means a number of people first have to get sick or die.

Proponents of the law opposed government regulation of substances they believed to be safe (often because they were "from plants," "nonmedical," or "natural"). Moreover, they believed that such regulation would limit the variety of products people could take and would drive up the cost of

vitamins. Also, people feared that FDA regulation would stop the dietary supplement industry from being a viable alternative to conventional medicine and prescription drugs.

Opponents of the law argued that without independent scientific testing, consumers cannot be assured that a supplement is safe or effective. They feared people could be harmed by impurities in a product or a product's unknown actions or by outright fraud.

Dr. David Kessler, the former head of the FDA, has stated that the lobbying for passage of the law was the most intense he had ever seen. The supplement industry told consumers that if the law did not pass, they would need a prescription to buy vitamins—if they could get them at all! Millions of frightened people contacted their elected representatives. The lobbying effort was a huge success; the law passed unanimously in Congress.

With more than 25,000 supplements on the market, and with its current budget, the FDA cannot possibly oversee all of the advertising claims made by supplement manufacturers or test even a small fraction of the products. Proponents of an unregulated supplement industry point out that only a handful of people die each year from ingesting supplements, compared to many thousands who die each year from taking prescription medications. Because there is no government oversight, one must be a wise consumer before using a supplement or herbal product. Read a product's label to learn about ingredients and doses. ConsumerLab.com is an independent laboratory that tests many supplements to verify their contents.

Dietary Supplements

More than 25,000 products are available in the United States as **dietary supplements**. In the strictest sense, dietary supplements are ingested to provide one or more of the 40 essential nutrients, such as a particular vitamin, mineral, or amino acid (see Table 5.4). For example, someone might take a multivitamin pill every day to ensure that an adequate amount of all vitamins is obtained (Nutrition Source, 2008).

Besides vitamins, however, dietary supplements include a variety of minerals, enzymes, amino acids, herbs, hormones, and nucleic acids (DNA and RNA), the use of which is intended to alter one or more of the body's biological systems to produce a specific physiological or psychological effect. For example, someone might take capsules containing omega-3 fatty acids (fish oil) to try to prevent a heart attack (or *another* heart attack) or stroke by lowering serum lipids. Or, someone may drink herbal tea to feel energized. A dietary supple-

ment intended to prevent or treat an illness or disease is called a **nutraceutical**.

When a dietary supplement is used to augment the nutritional quality of the diet, it is considered a food. When a dietary supplement is used to bring about a particular biological change, it is considered a drug. About 100 million Americans spend a total of $22 billion each year on dietary supplements.

> **TERMS**
>
> **dietary supplements:** products that provide one or more of the 40 essential nutrients or nonessential vitamins, minerals, enzymes, amino acids, herbs, hormones, and nucleic acids
>
> **nutraceutical:** a dietary supplement intended to prevent or treat an illness or disease
>
> **phytochemicals:** chemicals produced by plants

Dietary Supplements as Food

A varied diet that conforms to the recommendations of MyPyramid or the Healthy Eating Pyramid (Figure 5.3) is likely to provide most people with sufficient essential nutrients for good health. For these people, a nutritional dietary supplement is probably unnecessary, although some may want to take one as a form of "dietary insurance."

People who suspect that their diets are nutritionally inadequate may benefit from taking a daily multivitamin and mineral supplement. For example:

- People who skip meals and eat a lot of processed and fast food
- People who consume an unusual or low-calorie diet for weight loss
- People who consume nutritionally inadequate diets for reasons of economic hardship
- Athletes who are concerned about body size
- People who consume large amounts of coffee and/or alcohol

Others who may benefit from dietary supplements include strict vegetarians, who may need vitamin B_{12} because that vitamin comes primarily from animal tissue; people who are lactose intolerant (have difficulty digesting dairy products); and women of childbearing age who tend to consume insufficient amounts of folic acid and iron. When supplementing the diet with vitamins and minerals, remember that more is not necessarily better. In high doses, vitamins A, D, K, B_3 (niacin), and B_6 (pyridoxine) may be toxic.

Supplements containing enzymes, other proteins, and nucleic acids are not absorbed intact from the digestive tract; instead, they are broken down into smaller subunits. When a supplement is intended for use in the digestive tract, such as lactase, this is of little concern because the substance acts prior to being digested. However, an enzyme or nucleic acid will not be absorbed intact into the body, so using them is a waste of money.

Whether a substance is natural or synthetic makes no difference chemically as long as the manufacturer has taken care to be sure that the product is pure. In 1990, thousands of Americans became ill and more than 30 died from consuming a supplement of the amino acid tryptophan because of manufacturing impurities in the product. Moreover, just because a product is labeled "natural" or "comes from plants" does not mean it is safe or effective. A "natural" or "plant" product can have a large number of impurities and may be toxic.

Dietary Supplements as Drugs

Besides being intended to augment the nutritional quality of the diet, many dietary supplements are touted by manufacturers as preventatives or cures for ailments, stress, moods, and recreational drug use. A few supplements that act as drugs have been scientifically tested and found to be safe and effective for certain conditions (**Table 5.12**).

Table 5.12

Dietary Supplements That Have Been Scientifically Tested and Found to Be Effective

Supplement	Use
Glucosamine	Reduce symptoms of arthritis
Echinacea	Enhance immune functioning
Garlic	Reduce risk of heart disease
Gingko biloba	Slow the progression of some forms of dementia
Omega-3 fatty acids	Prevent heart disease and stroke
S-adenosyl methionine (SAM-e)	Relieve mild to moderate depression
St. John's wort	Relieve mild to moderate depression
Saw palmetto	Treat prostate disease

Unlike prescription and over-the-counter medicines, dietary supplements do not have to be tested before going on the market, so consumers have no assurance of a supplement's contents, that it has no impurities, that it is not harmful, or that it actually does anything beneficial. Some examples of supplement problems are as follows.

Uncertain or impure contents: Independent tests of a variety of supplements (e.g., folic acid, St. John's wort, dihydroepiandrostenedione [DHEA]) have shown that they may not contain the amounts of active ingredients listed on the product labels. For example, an analysis found that only 49% of samples of echinacea obtained in supermarkets, drug stores, and health food stores contained the labeled amount of echinacea; 6% had none (Gilroy et al., 2003). Other analyses have found supplements to be contaminated with lead, glass, pesticides, or bacteria. The FDA requires supplement manufacturers to abide by "current good manufacturing standards" to ensure that supplements are free of contaminants or impurities and that they are labeled accurately.

Harmful supplements: Products containing ephedra (also called *ephedrine* or *ma huang*) were marketed for weight loss and enhancement of athletic performance and energy. In 2003, an FDA analysis revealed 16,000 reports of adverse reactions from consuming ephedra-containing products, including seizures, panic attacks, and several strokes and heart attacks. Several people, including some college and professional athletes, have died from taking ephedra-containing products. Eventually, ephedra-containing products were removed from the market.

Because St. John's wort did not undergo rigorous testing before being marketed, it was not known that the herb could stimulate the liver, which inactivates toxic chemicals and drugs. Thus, taking St. John's wort can

Wellness Guide

Rules for Organic Labeling

In 2002, after many years of discussion, the U.S. Department of Agriculture (USDA) set standards for foods labeled "organic." Foods labeled "100% organic" and "organic" cannot be produced using sewage sludge, ionizing radiation, artificial growth hormones, genetically modified crops, and most synthetic fertilizers and pesticides. The labeling requirements apply to both fresh products and processed foods. Foods that are sold, labeled, or represented as organic have to be produced and processed in accordance with the USDA standards, and they may carry the "USDA Organic" seal.

The labeling requirements are based on the percentage of organic ingredients in a product. Foods and food products labeled "100% organic" must contain (excluding water and salt) only organically produced ingredients. Products labeled "organic" must consist of at least 95% organically produced ingredients. Any remaining ingredients must consist of nonagricultural substances approved on the national list of products that are not commercially available in organic form.

Processed products that contain at least 70% organic ingredients can use the phrase "made with organic ingredients" and list up to three of the organic ingredients or food groups on the product label. For example, soup made with at least 70% organic ingredients and only organic vegetables may be labeled either "soup made with organic peas, potatoes, and carrots" or "soup made with organic vegetables." Processed products that contain less than 70% organic ingredients cannot use the term "organic" anywhere on the principal display panel. However, they may identify the specific ingredients that are organically produced under ingredients on the information panel.

Source: USDA National Organic Program. Available: http://www.ams.usda.gov/nop/.

inadvertently cause the breakdown of medicines taken for other reasons. For example, St. John's wort can lessen body levels of anti-AIDS drugs, immunosuppressant drugs in heart transplant patients, antiseizure medication, breast cancer drugs, and oral contraceptive (birth control) pills. A number of women taking oral contraceptives and St. John's wort became pregnant, which provided the clue to the undesired effects of the herb.

Food Additives

Almost all manufactured foods contain chemicals that are added during production to alter their texture, stability, color, and flavor. For example, vitamins and minerals are added to highly processed white flour to replace nutrients lost in its production. Many so-called functional foods (see the Dollars and Health Sense feature on p. 112) contain added substances that claim (often without supporting scientific evidence) to enhance health.

Many food additives are nutritionally unnecessary, and some may adversely affect health. For example, sugar and salt are added to many foods to intensify taste and thereby increase sales. Unfortunately, overconsumption of sugar and salt can have severe health consequences (see Chapters 6, 13, and 14). The FDA estimates that 350,000 Americans are intolerant to the food dye FD&C Yellow No. 5 (*tartrazine*), increasing their risk of hives, allergies, asthma, and other health problems.

The U.S. Food and Drug Administration, the European Food Safety Authority, and many international agencies monitor the safety of chemicals added to food. Some chemical additives, such as food colorings, must be tested for safety by the manufacturer prior to being approved for use in foods. On the other hand, many kinds of food additives are not tested rigorously for safety before entering the food supply; safety issues arise only after an additive has been in use and a deleterious effect on consumers' health is suspected. At that point the suspect chemical can undergo rigorous testing, and if found harmful, food safety agencies can order that it be removed from food products. Food safety regulations refer to untested additives that have been in use for a long time and are not suspected of causing harm as *generally regarded as safe* (GRAS). A suspected or potentially harmful chemical additive can be considered generally safe if it is present in foods in very low amounts, referred to as *acceptable daily intake levels* (ADI).

Preservatives

About 20% of the world's food supply is lost to spoilage each year. Common preservatives include BHA (butylated hydroxyanisole), BHT (butylated hydroxytoluene), and sodium nitrite. Each of these substances can be toxic and damaging to humans if consumed in excess; however, in amounts commonly present in food, they are presumed safe.

Sulfites in the form of sulfur dioxide, sodium sulfite, sodium or potassium bisulfite, and sodium or potassium

TERMS

sulfites: used as preservatives for salad, fresh fruits and vegetables, wine, beer, and dried fruit; in susceptible individuals, especially those with asthma, they can cause a severe reaction

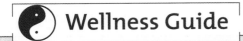

Guidelines for Food Safety

When Purchasing Food

1. Purchase meat and poultry products after all other groceries have been selected and keep packages of raw meat and poultry separate from other foods, particularly foods that will be eaten without further cooking. Consider using plastic bags to enclose individual packages of raw meat and poultry.
2. Make sure meat and poultry products—whether raw, prepackaged, or cooked from the deli—are refrigerated when purchased.
3. USDA strongly advises against purchasing fresh, prestuffed whole birds.
4. Canned goods should be free of dents, cracks, or bulging lids.
5. Take food straight home to the refrigerator. If travel time will exceed one hour, pack perishable foods in a cooler with ice and keep groceries and cooler in the passenger area of the car during warm weather.

When Storing Food at Home

1. Verify the temperature of your refrigerator and freezer with an appliance thermometer—refrigerators should run at 40°F or below; freezers at 0°F. Most foodborne bacteria grow slowly at 40°F, which is a safe refrigerator temperature. Freezer temperatures of 0°F or below stop bacterial growth.
2. At home, refrigerate or freeze meat and poultry immediately.
3. To prevent raw juices from dripping on other foods in the refrigerator, use plastic bags or place meat and poultry on a plate.

4. Wash hands with soap and water for 20 seconds before and after handling any raw meat, poultry, or seafood products.
5. Store canned goods in a cool, clean, dry place. Avoid extreme heat or cold, which can be harmful to canned goods.
6. Never store any foods directly under a sink and always keep foods off the floor and separate from cleaning supplies.

When Getting Food Ready to Prepare

1. The importance of hand washing cannot be overemphasized. This simple practice is the most economical, yet often forgotten, way to prevent contamination or cross-contamination.
2. Wash hands (gloved or not) with soap and water for 20 seconds: (a) before beginning preparation; (b) after handling raw meat, poultry, seafood, or eggs; (c) after touching animals; (d) after using the bathroom; (e) after changing diapers; and (f) after blowing the nose.
3. Don't let juices from raw meat, poultry, or seafood come in contact with cooked foods or foods that will be eaten raw, such as fruits or salad ingredients.
4. Wash hands, counters, equipment, utensils, and cutting boards with soap and water immediately after use. Counters, equipment, utensils, and cutting boards can be sanitized with a chlorine solution of 1 teaspoon liquid household bleach per quart of water. Let the solution stand on the board after washing, or follow the instructions on sanitizing products.
5. Thaw meat in the refrigerator, *never on the counter*. It is also safe to thaw in cold water in an airtight plastic wrapper or bag, changing the water every 30 minutes

---

metabisulfite are added to many foods to kill bacteria and to slow the food's chemical breakdown. Sulfites are commonly added to wine and to dehydrated soups, vegetables, and dried fruit (apples, apricots, raisins, pears, and peaches). To keep vegetables looking fresh, they are also used in restaurant salad bars. Some individuals, particularly those with asthma, may be extremely sensitive to sulfite and may experience nausea, diarrhea, respiratory distress, and skin eruptions. Such problems have led to banning the use of sulfites in restaurants.

Consumers concerned about additives should read product labels. Manufacturers must list all the additives in the order of their relative proportions in the food. Do not assume that the words "natural," "organic," or "health food" mean that foods are free from additives or extra sugar and salt. The only way to be certain of the contents of a food is to know how it was produced.

Artificial Sweeteners

Artificial sweeteners are chemicals capable of producing the sensation of sweetness far more effectively—from 200 to 10,000 times more, depending on the chemical—

than sucrose, fructose, glucose, and other natural sugars. Five chemicals are approved for use as artificial sweeteners in North America: aspartame, saccharin, acesulfame-K, neotame, and sucralose. Although many thousands of food products contain artificial sweeteners, their main source in the food supply is so-called diet sodas.

Although touted as aids to weight control, diabetes management, and moderating tooth decay, artificial sweeteners have yet to be shown to promote health in any way. Indeed, consumption of artificial sweeteners may be harmful to some individuals. For example, aspartame (Nutrasweet) has been associated with mood changes, insomnia, seizures, compromised learning, and emotional functioning (Humphries, Pretorius, & Naudé, 2008). Animal studies suggest that ingestion of large amounts of aspartame may increase the risk of cancer (Huff & LaDou, 2007). Many people who consume considerable amounts of diet soda may be inadvertently harming themselves because the soda is replacing more nutritious beverages in the diet. Diet soda manufacturers are no doubt pleased at the popularity of the myths that diet sodas aid in weight control and that milk makes one fat.

until meat is thawed; or thaw in the microwave and cook the product immediately.

6. Marinate foods in the refrigerator, *never on the counter*.

7. The USDA recommends that if you choose to stuff whole poultry, you must use a meat thermometer to check the internal temperature of the stuffing. The internal temperature in the center of the stuffing should reach 165°F before removing it from the oven. If you don't have a meat thermometer, cook the stuffing outside the bird. Also, don't put hot stuffing into a frozen bird. By the time it thaws, it will be contaminated inside.

When Cooking

1. Always cook thoroughly. If harmful bacteria are present, only thorough cooking will destroy them; freezing or rinsing the foods in cold water is not sufficient to destroy bacteria.

2. Use a meat thermometer to determine if your meat, poultry, or casserole has reached a safe internal temperature (145°F for roasts and steaks, 180°F for whole poultry, 160°F for ground meat, and 165°F for leftovers). Check the product in several spots to assure that a safe temperature has been reached and that harmful bacteria, such as *Salmonella* and certain strains of *E. coli*, have been destroyed.

3. Avoid interrupted cooking. Never refrigerate partially cooked food to later finish cooking on the grill or in the oven. Meat and poultry products must be cooked thoroughly the first time, and then they may be refrigerated and safely reheated.

4. When microwaving foods, carefully follow the manufacturer's instructions. Use microwave-safe containers, cover, rotate, and allow for the standing time, which contributes to thorough cooking.

When Serving

1. Wash hands with soap and water before serving or eating food.

2. Serve cooked products on clean plates with clean utensils and clean hands. Never put cooked foods on a dish that has held raw products unless the dish is first washed with soap and hot water.

3. Hold hot foods above 140°F and cold foods below 40°F.

4. Never leave foods, raw or cooked, at room temperature longer than two hours. On a hot day with temperatures at 90°F or warmer, this time decreases to one hour.

When Handling Leftovers

1. Wash hands before and after handling leftovers. Use clean utensils and surfaces.

2. Divide leftovers into small units and store in shallow containers for quick cooling. Refrigerate within two hours of cooking.

3. Discard anything left out too long.

4. Never taste a food to determine if it is safe.

5. When reheating leftovers, reheat thoroughly to a temperature of 165°F, or until hot and steamy. Bring soups, sauces, and gravies to a rolling boil.

6. If in doubt, throw it out.

Source: U.S. Department of Agriculture, Food Safety and Inspection Service.

Health-conscious consumers should be aware of the artificial sweeteners used in the products they ingest.

Food Safety

Outbreaks of food poisoning in the United States from bacterial and viral contamination of commercial beef, poultry, and fruit and vegetables have raised concerns about the safety of the food supply. In the United States, there are 76 million cases of foodborne illness annually, resulting in 325,000 hospitalizations. Four pathogens—*Salmonella, Escherichia coli* O157:H7, *Campylobacter,* Norwalk-like virus, and *Toxoplasma*—account for most of the infections and approximately 1,600 deaths each year (**Table 5.13**). Symptoms of bacterial food poisoning are headache, nausea, fever, abdominal cramps, and diarrhea.

The foods most likely to be contaminated with infectious microorganisms are raw meat and poultry, raw eggs, unpasteurized milk, and raw shellfish. Foods that mingle the products of many individual animals, such as bulk raw milk, pooled raw eggs, or ground beef, are particularly hazardous because a pathogen present in an individual animal can contaminate the entire mix. For example, a single hamburger may contain meat from hundreds of animals. A single restaurant omelet may contain eggs from hundreds of chickens. A glass of raw milk may contain milk from hundreds of cows.

Besides animal products, uncooked fruits and vegetables also carry pathogenic microorganisms. Often contamination is the result of improper handling and processing, for example, using contaminated water to wash fresh produce after it is harvested. Another source of contamination is fresh manure used to fertilize food crops. Unpasteurized fruit juice can also be contaminated if there are pathogens in or on the fruit that is used to make it.

The Food and Drug Administration's and the U.S. Department of Agriculture's inspectors oversee nearly 60,000 food manufacturers and processors and billions of tons of imported food—clearly a monumental task. That's why it's imperative for consumers to follow food safety guidelines when they purchase, store, and prepare food (see the Wellness Guide).

Table 5.13

Pathogens That Cause Foodborne Illness

Pathogen	Found	Transmission	Symptoms
Campylobacter jejuni	Intestinal tracts of animals and birds, raw milk, untreated water, and sewage sludge.	Contaminated water, raw milk, and raw or undercooked meat, poultry, or shellfish.	Fever, headache, and muscle pain followed by diarrhea (sometimes bloody), abdominal pain, and nausea. Symptoms appear 2 to 5 days after eating; may last 7 to 10 days.
Clostridium botulinum	Widely distributed in nature; in soil, water, on plants, and in intestinal tracts of animals and fish. Grows only in little or no oxygen.	Bacteria produce a toxin that causes illness. Improperly canned foods, garlic in oil, vacuum-packed and tightly wrapped food.	Toxin affects the nervous system. Symptoms usually appear 18 to 36 hours after eating, but can sometimes appear as few as 4 hours or as many 8 days after eating; double vision, droopy eyelids, trouble speaking and swallowing, and difficulty breathing. Fatal in 3 to 10 days if not treated.
Clostridium perfringens	Soil, dust, sewage, and intestinal tracts of animals and humans. Grows only in little or no oxygen.	Called "the cafeteria germ" because many outbreaks result from food left for long periods in steam tables or at room temperature. Bacteria destroyed by cooking, but some toxin-producing spores may survive.	Diarrhea and gas pains may appear 8 to 24 hours after eating; usually last about 1 day, but less severe symptoms may persist for 1 to 2 weeks.
Escherichia coli O157:H7	Intestinal tracts of some mammals, raw milk, unchlorinated water; one of several strains of *E. coli* that can cause human illness.	Contaminated water, raw milk, raw or rare ground beef, unpasteurized apple juice or cider, uncooked fruits and vegetables; person to person.	Diarrhea or bloody diarrhea, abdominal cramps, nausea, and malaise; can begin 2 to 5 days after food is eaten, lasting about 8 days. Some, especially the very young, have developed hemolytic-uremic syndrome (HUS), which causes acute kidney failure. A similar illness, thrombotic thrombocytopenic purpura (TTP), may occur in adults.
Listeria monocytogenes	Intestinal tracts of humans and animals, milk, soil, leafy vegetables; can grow slowly at refrigerator temperatures.	Ready-to-eat foods such as hot dogs, luncheon meats, cold cuts, fermented or dry sausage, and other deli-style meat and poultry, soft cheeses, and unpasteurized milk.	Fever, chills, headache, backache, sometimes upset stomach, abdominal pain and diarrhea; may take up to 3 weeks to become ill; may later develop more serious illness in at-risk patients (pregnant women and newborns, older adults, and people with weakened immune systems).
Norwalk-like virus	Human intestinal tract	Person to person.	Nausea, vomiting, diarrhea, resolving in 1 to 2 days.
Salmonella (more than 2,300 types)	Intestinal tracts and feces of animals; *Salmonella enteritidis* in eggs.	Raw or undercooked eggs, poultry, and meat; raw milk and dairy products; seafood; and food handlers.	Stomach pain, diarrhea, nausea, chills, fever, and headache usually appear 8 to 72 hours after eating; may last 1 to 2 days.
Shigella (more than 30 types)	Human intestinal tract; rarely found in other animals.	Person to person by fecal–oral route; fecal contamination of food and water. Most outbreaks result from food, especially salads, prepared and handled by workers using poor personal hygiene.	Disease referred to as *shigellosis* or bacillary dysentery. Diarrhea containing blood and mucus, fever, abdominal cramps, chills, and vomiting; 12 to 50 hours from ingestion of bacteria; can last a few days to 2 weeks.
Staphylococcus aureus	On humans (skin, infected cuts, pimples, noses, and throats).	Person to person from improper food handling. Multiply rapidly at room temperature to produce a toxin that causes illness.	Severe nausea, abdominal cramps, vomiting, and diarrhea occur 1 to 6 hours after eating; recovery within 2 to 3 days—longer if severe dehydration occurs.

Source: U.S. Department of Agriculture. Food safety education: Foodborne illness—What consumers need to know. Available: http://www.fsis.usda.gov/OA/pubs/fact_fbi.htm.

One method of protecting food involves exposing it to **gamma irradiation** to destroy fungi, bacteria, and other microorganisms. Some opponents of food irradiation argue that the method has not been proven safe in all instances. Their concern is that irradiation may produce cancer-causing or toxic by-products or mutant strains of toxic, radiation-resistant microorganisms. Furthermore, vitamins can be destroyed by irradiation. Nonetheless, the U.S. government allows irradiation for sterilizing insects, extending shelf life, controlling pathogens and parasites, and inhibiting the sprouting of vegetables. Irradiation also is approved for red meat, poultry, pork, fruits and vegetables, some spices, seeds, herbs and seasonings, eggs, and wheat. At approved doses, irradiation does not eliminate toxins, prions (agents that cause mad cow disease), and many types of viruses. Irradiation does not prevent subsequent contamination of food by food-service workers or consumers, a major source of bacterial and viral contamination.

Keep in mind that irradiation *does not* make food radioactive and therefore consumers are not at risk from radiation. The U.S. government requires a written radia-

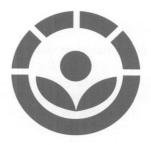

■ **Figure 5.8**
The Radura Symbol
The radura symbol is used internationally to indicate that a food has been treated with irradiation.

tion disclosure statement on the label of irradiated foods; the use of the radura symbol (**Figure 5.8**), however, is optional.

Fast Food

Grabbing a fast-food meal is integral to the fast-paced life in America today. Each day approximately 46 million people, or 20% of the U.S. population, eat fast food. Nearly one-third of American children aged 3 to 19 years eat fast food daily. Compared to nonregular fast-food consumers, those who regularly consume fast food ingest between 150 to 200 excess calories per day, which can contribute to a gain of several pounds in a year. Moreover, the large amounts of salt, fat, and sugar in fast food set these consumers on a course for high blood pressure, type 2 diabetes, heart disease, and blocked arteries. On any given day, one-third of children younger than 2 years consume no fruits or vegetables (Devaney et al., 2004). Instead, each day 20% have french fries, and 40% have a sugary fruit drink. Convenience notwithstanding, fast-food items must be chosen carefully because many contain high quantities of saturated fat, cholesterol, and salt; few complex carbohydrates; and low levels of vitamins A and C (**Table 5.14**). The major fast-food companies have responded to consumers' concerns about nutrition by offering salads, baked potatoes, roast beef, and broiled chicken. Roast beef has less fat than hamburger, and broiled chicken breast has less fat than deep-fried chicken. Be cautious, though. Fish, a low-fat food, if breaded and fried, may be 50% fat. Salads and baked potatoes can be carriers of high-fat toppings.

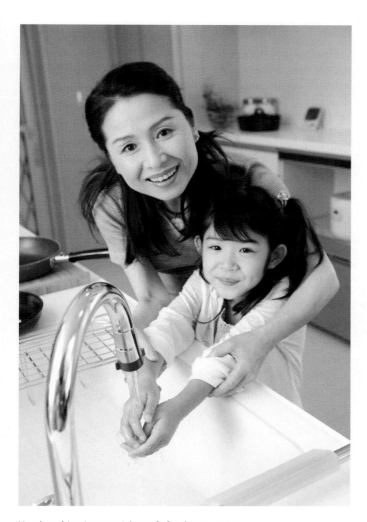

Hand washing is essential to safe food preparation.

TERMS

gamma irradiation: nonchemical method of food preservation

Vegetarian Diets

Vegetarianism has existed as long as humankind has and has been advocated by such famous people as Leonardo da Vinci, George Bernard Shaw, Mahatma Gandhi, and Albert Einstein. People choose to be vegetarians for various reasons, including the following:

1. To avoid killing animals—either killing them oneself or killing by others. Some people, who have a strong affection for other animals and feel a certain biological and spiritual kinship with them, object to killing them for food.

2. To contribute to the more efficient utilization of world protein supplies. It takes approximately 10 pounds of livestock feed, usually corn or soybeans, to produce one pound of meat. Obviously, the 10 pounds of corn or soybeans could feed more people than one pound of meat can. With the population of the earth doubling approximately every 30 years, some people feel a moral obligation to avoid overconsuming food resources in the hope that ways will be found to distribute the world food supply more equitably.

3. To live longer and healthier lives. In many cases, health benefits result from a combination of vegetarianism and nondietary lifestyle factors. Vegetarians, in comparison to nonvegetarians, tend to be leaner, to exercise more, to not smoke cigarettes, and to not abuse alcohol. Vegetarians have a reduced risk for heart and blood vessel disease and for colorectal cancer because of a reduced intake of cholesterol and animal fat. Their increased fiber intake also contributes to the reduced colorectal cancer risk.

There are three kinds of **vegetarian** diets: strict or **veganism**, which excludes all animal products, including milk, cheeses, eggs, and other dairy products; **lacto-vegetarianism**, which excludes meat, poultry, fish, and eggs, but includes dairy products; and **lacto-ovo-vegetarianism**, which excludes meats, poultry, and seafood, but includes eggs and dairy products. Properly planned vegetarian diets can meet the body's nutritional needs, especially by combining sources of protein to assure adequate intake of the essential amino acids. Vegans may need vitamin B_{12} (cobalamin) supplements.

How Food Affects the Brain

The brain requires nutrients to function properly. For example, the amount of the neurotransmitter serotonin in the brain is influenced by levels in the blood of the amino acid tryptophan and by the amount of carbohydrate recently eaten. A meal containing tryptophan (derived from dietary protein) and high in carbohydrate increases brain levels of serotonin. Brain levels of the amino acid tyrosine, the precursor of the neurotransmitters dopamine, norepinephrine, and epinephrine, increase after the ingestion of tyrosine-containing protein in a meal. Ingesting choline, a component of lecithin (found in egg yolks, liver, and soybeans), increases the level of the neurotransmitter acetylcholine.

To some degree, moods, feelings of vitality, and sleep patterns may depend on the amount of neurotransmitter molecules ingested and therefore depend indirectly on meals. The habit of eating cookies and milk at bedtime may be a way someone increases brain serotonin to help bring about a peaceful night's sleep. Some preliminary experiments indicate that tyrosine may help to relieve depression and cho-

> Don't buy much from the center aisles of the supermarket. Avoid packaged food with more than five ingredients and anything with a cartoon on it.
>
> *Marian Nestle*
> What to Eat

Table 5.14

Partial Composition of Selected Fast-Food Items

Food	Total calories	Total fat (grams)	Calories from fat	Cholesterol (milligrams)	Sodium (milligrams)
Big Mac (beef)	600	33	300	85	1050
Burrito Supreme	440	18	170	45	1220
French fries (medium/salted)	450	22	200	00	290
Turkey sub sandwich	330	5	50	40	1510
Fried chicken breast	380	19	170	145	1150
Pizza (slice)	300	14	120	25	610
Caesar salad (no dressing)	300	26	230	15	690
Caesar salad (with dressing)	450	42	540	55	930
Chocolate shake (medium)	600	18	160	70	470
Starbuck's chocolate Frappuccino Blended Crème, Grande	530	19	170	55	420

Source: Fast food facts. Available: http://www.foodfacts.info.

line may help to modify certain postural and motor disturbances.

The thoughts, moods, and body sensations of some individuals are sensitive to the amount of fat and sugar they ingest. We all know of individuals who use certain foods—chocolate, fatty, and sugary foods ("comfort foods")—to lessen the experience of stress or emotional upset or for consolation when feeling sad, lonely, or fatigued. Some individuals experience anxiety, fatigue, weakness, depressed mood, and an inability to concentrate shortly after consuming a couple of doughnuts or a candy bar. This response, called **reactive hypoglycemia,** is often the result of a sharp drop in blood sugar when insulin is secreted; this drop, in turn, is produced in response to the large load of sugar in the blood. Something akin to reactive hypoglycemia may be at the root of an eating pattern common to many: consumption of a high-sugar food at breakfast, followed two hours later by a reactive blood sugar low, which motivates a midmorning sugar "hit." The cycle is repeated at noon and midafternoon, and at dinner and late in the evening. To break this cycle, it helps to consume complex carbohydrates with protein and some fat, thereby moderating the rate at which simple sugars enter the body.

The brains of developing fetuses and children can be adversely and permanently affected by exposure to malnutrition in early life. Maternal starvation during pregnancy is associated with an increased risk in children of schizophrenia, antisocial personality, and affective disorders (Kyle & Pichard, 2006).

TERMS

lacto-ovo-vegetarian: one who excludes meats, poultry, and fish, but includes eggs and dairy products

lacto-vegetarian: one who excludes meat, poultry, fish, and eggs, but includes dairy products

reactive hypoglycemia: occurring after the ingestion of carbohydrate, with consequent release of insulin

vegan: one who excludes all animal products from the diet, including milk, cheese, eggs, and other dairy products

vegetarian: one who consumes no meat, poultry, or fish

Chapter 5 Appendix

Table A5.1

Playing with Pyramid Portions

Your favorite sports can help you visualize MyPyramid portion sizes.

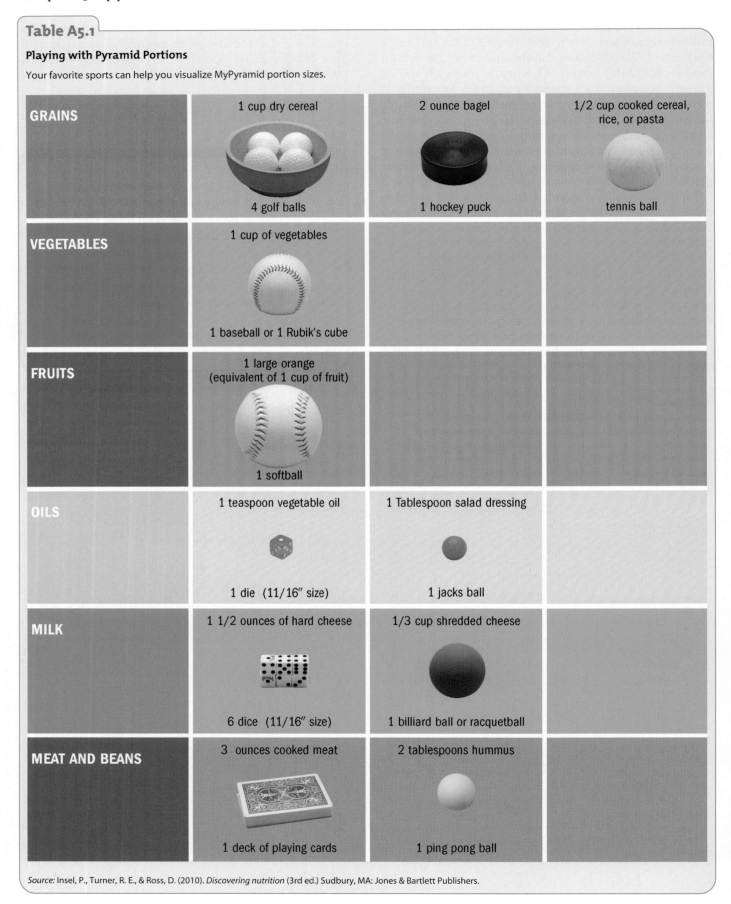

GRAINS	1 cup dry cereal	2 ounce bagel	1/2 cup cooked cereal, rice, or pasta
	4 golf balls	1 hockey puck	tennis ball
VEGETABLES	1 cup of vegetables		
	1 baseball or 1 Rubik's cube		
FRUITS	1 large orange (equivalent of 1 cup of fruit)		
	1 softball		
OILS	1 teaspoon vegetable oil	1 Tablespoon salad dressing	
	1 die (11/16″ size)	1 jacks ball	
MILK	1 1/2 ounces of hard cheese	1/3 cup shredded cheese	
	6 dice (11/16″ size)	1 billiard ball or racquetball	
MEAT AND BEANS	3 ounces cooked meat	2 tablespoons hummus	
	1 deck of playing cards	1 ping pong ball	

Source: Insel, P., Turner, R. E., & Ross, D. (2010). *Discovering nutrition* (3rd ed.) Sudbury, MA: Jones & Bartlett Publishers.

Sample Menus for a 2000 Calorie Food Pattern

Averaged over a week, this seven day menu provides all of the recommended amounts of nutrients and food from each food group. (Italicized foods are part of the dish or food that preceeds it.)

MyPyramid.gov
STEPS TO A HEALTHIER YOU

Day 1

BREAKFAST

Breakfast burrito
1 flour tortilla (7" diameter)
1 scrambled egg (in 1 tsp soft margarine)
1/3 cup black beans*
2 tbsp salsa
1 cup orange juice
1 cup fat-free milk

LUNCH

Roast beef sandwich
1 whole grain sandwich bun
3 ounces lean roast beef
2 slices tomato
1/4 cup shredded romaine lettuce
1/8 cup sauteed mushrooms (in 1 tsp oil)
1 1/2 ounce part-skim mozzarella cheese
1 tsp yellow mustard
3/4 cup baked potato wedges*
1 tbsp ketchup
1 unsweetened beverage

DINNER

Stuffed broiled salmon
5 ounce salmon filet
1 ounce bread stuffing mix
1 tbsp chopped onions
1 tbsp diced celery
2 tsp canola oil
1/2 cup saffron (white) rice
1 ounce slivered almonds
1/2 cup steamed broccoli
1 tsp soft margarine
1 cup fat-free milk

SNACKS

1 cup cantaloupe

Day 2

BREAKFAST

Hot cereal
1/2 cup cooked oatmeal
2 tbsp raisins
1 tsp soft margarine
1/2 cup fat-free milk
1 cup orange juice

LUNCH

Taco salad
2 ounces tortilla chips
2 ounces ground turkey, sauteed in 2 tsp sunflower oil
1/2 cup black beans*
1/2 cup iceberg lettuce
2 slices tomato
1 ounce low-fat cheddar cheese
2 tbsp salsa
1/2 cup avocado
1 tsp lime juice
1 unsweetened beverage

DINNER

Spinach lasagna
1 cup lasagna noodles, cooked (2 oz dry)
2/3 cup cooked spinach
1/2 cup ricotta cheese
1/2 cup tomato sauce tomato bits*
1 ounce part-skim mozzarella cheese
1 ounce whole wheat dinner roll
1 cup fat-free milk

SNACKS

1/2 ounce dry-roasted almonds*
1/4 cup pineapple
2 tbsp raisins

Day 3

BREAKFAST

Cold cereal
1 cup bran flakes
1 cup fat-free milk
1 small banana
1 slice whole wheat toast
1 tsp soft margarine
1 cup prune juice

LUNCH

Tuna fish sandwich
2 slices rye bread
3 ounces tuna (packed in water, drained)
2 tsp mayonnaise
1 tbsp diced celery
1/4 cup shredded romaine lettuce
2 slices tomato
1 medium pear
1 cup fat-free milk

DINNER

Roasted chicken breast
3 ounces boneless skinless chicken breast*
1 large baked sweetpotato
1/2 cup peas and onions
1 tsp soft margarine
1 ounce whole wheat dinner roll
1 tsp soft margarine
1 cup leafy greens salad
3 tsp sunflower oil and vinegar dressing

SNACKS

1/4 cup dried apricots
1 cup low-fat fruited yogurt

Day 4

BREAKFAST

1 whole wheat English muffin
2 tsp soft margarine
1 tbsp jam or preserves
1 medium grapefruit
1 hard-cooked egg
1 unsweetened beverage

LUNCH

White bean-vegetable soup
1 1/4 cup chunky vegetable soup
1/2 cup white beans*
2 ounce breadstick
8 baby carrots
1 cup fat-free milk

DINNER

Rigatoni with meat sauce
1 cup rigatoni pasta (2 ounces dry)
1/2 cup tomato sauce tomato bits*
2 ounces extra lean cooked ground beef (sauteed in 2 tsp vegetable oil)
3 tbsp grated Parmesan cheese
Spinach salad
1 cup baby spinach leaves
1/2 cup tangerine slices
1/2 ounce chopped walnuts
3 tsp sunflower oil and vinegar dressing
1 cup fat-free milk

SNACKS

1 cup low-fat fruited yogurt

Source: U.S. Department of Agriculture. http://MyPyramid.gov.

Sample Menus for a 2000 Calorie Food Pattern

Averaged over a week, this seven day menu provides all of the recommended amounts of nutrients and food from each food group.
(Italicized foods are part of the dish or food that preceeds it.)

MyPyramid.gov
STEPS TO A HEALTHIER YOU

* Starred items are foods that are labeled as no-salt-added, low-sodium, or low-salt versions of the foods. They can also be prepared from scratch with little or no added salt. All other foods are regular commercial products which contain variable levels of sodium. Average sodium level of the 7 day menu assumes no-salt-added in cooking or at the table

Day 5

BREAKFAST

Cold cereal
1 cup puffed wheat cereal
1 tbsp raisins
1 cup fat-free milk
1 small banana
1 slice whole wheat toast
1 tsp soft margarine
1 tsp jelly

LUNCH

Smoked turkey sandwich
2 ounces whole wheat pita bread
1/4 cup romaine lettuce
2 slices tomato
3 ounces sliced smoked turkey breast*
1 tbsp mayo-type salad dressing
1 tsp yellow mustard
1/2 cup apple slices
1 cup tomato juice*

DINNER

Grilled top loin steak
5 ounces grilled top loin steak
3/4 cup mashed potatoes
2 tsp soft margarine
1/2 cup steamed carrots
1 tbsp honey
2 ounces whole wheat dinner roll
1 tsp soft margarine
1 cup fat-free milk

SNACKS

1 cup low-fat fruited yogurt

Day 6

BREAKFAST

French toast
2 slices whole wheat French toast
2 tsp soft margarine
2 tbsp maple syrup
1/2 medium grapefruit
1 cup fat-free milk

LUNCH

Vegetarian chili on baked potato
1 cup kidney beans*
1/2 cup tomato sauce w/ tomato tidbits*
3 tbsp chopped onions
1 ounce lowfat cheddar cheese
1 tsp vegetable oil
1 medium baked potato
1/2 cup cantaloupe
3/4 cup lemonade

DINNER

Hawaiian pizza
2 slices cheese pizza
1 ounce canadian bacon
1/4 cup pineapple
2 tbsp mushrooms
2 tbsp chopped onions
Green salad
1 cup leafy greens
3 tsp sunflower oil and vinegar dressing
1 cup fat-free milk

SNACKS

5 whole wheat crackers*
1/8 cup hummus
1/2 cup fruit cocktail (in water or juice)

Day 7

BREAKFAST

Pancakes
3 buckwheat pancakes
2 tsp soft margarine
3 tbsp maple syrup
1/2 cup strawberries
3/4 cup honeydew melon
1/2 cup fat-free milk

LUNCH

Manhattan clam chowder
3 ounces canned clams (drained)
3/4 cup mixed vegetables
1 cup canned tomatoes*
10 whole wheat crackers*
1 medium orange
1 cup fat-free milk

DINNER

Vegetable stir-fry
4 ounces tofu (firm)
1/4 cup green and red bell peppers
1/2 cup bok choy
2 tbsp vegetable oil
1 cup brown rice
1 cup lemon-flavored iced tea

SNACKS

1 ounce sunflower seeds*
1 large banana
1 cup low-fat fruited yogurt

Source: U.S. Department of Agriculture. http://MyPyramid.gov.

Sample Menus for a 2000 calorie food pattern

Averaged over a week, this seven day menu provides all of the recommended amounts of nutrients and food from each food group.
(Italicized foods are part of the dish or food that preceeds it, which is not italicized.)

Food Group	Daily Average Over One Week		
GRAINS	Total Grains (oz eq)	6.0	
	Whole Grains	3.4	
	Refined Grains	2.6	
VEGETABLES *	Total Veg* (cups)	2.6	
FRUITS	Fruits (cups)	2.1	
MILK	Milk (cups)	3.1	
MEAT & BEANS	Meat/ Beans (oz eq)	5.6	
OILS	Oils (tsp/grams) 7.2 tsp/32.4 g		

*Vegetable subgroups   (weekly totals)

Dk-Green Veg (cups)	3.3
Orange Veg (cups)	2.3
Beans/ Peas (cups)	3.0
Starchy Veg (cups)	3.4
Other Veg (cups)	6.6

Nutrient	Daily Average Over One Week
Calories	1994
Protein, g	98
Protein, % kcal	20
Carbohydrate, g	264
Carbohydrate, % kcal	53
Total fat, g	67
Total fat, % kcal	30
Saturated fat, g	16
Saturated fat, % kcal	7.0
Monounsaturated fat, g	23
Polyunsaturated fat, g	23
Linoleic Acid, g	21
Alpha-linolenic Acid, g	1.1
Cholesterol, mg	207
Total dietary fiber, g	31
Potassium, mg	4715
Sodium, mg*	1948
Calcium, mg	1389
Magnesium, mg	432
Copper, mg	1.9
Iron, mg	21
Phosphorus, mg	1830
Zinc, mg	14
Thiamin, mg	1.9
Riboflavin, mg	2.5
Niacin Equivalents, mg	24
Vitamin B6, mg	2.9
Vitamin B12, mcg	18.4
Vitamin C, mg	190
Vitamin E, mg (AT)	18.9
Vitamin A, mcg (RAE)	1430
Dietary Folate Equivalents, mcg	558

* Starred items are foods that are labelled as no-salt-added, low-sodium, or low-salt versions of the foods. They can also be prepared from scratch with little or no added salt. All other foods are regular commercial products which contain variable levels of sodium. Average sodium level of the 7 day menu assumes no-salt-added in cooking or at the table.

MyPyramid.gov
STEPS TO A HEALTHIER YOU

Source: U.S. Department of Agriculture. http://MyPyramid.gov.

Tips for Eating Healthy When Eating Out

- As a beverage choice, ask for water or order fat-free or low-fat milk, unsweetened tea, or other drinks without added sugars.

- Ask for whole-wheat bread for sandwiches.

- In a restaurant, start your meal with a salad packed with veggies, to help control hunger and feel satisfied sooner.

- Ask for salad dressing to be served on the side. Then use only as much as you want.

- Choose main dishes that include vegetables, such as stir fries, kebobs, or pasta with a tomato sauce.

- Order steamed, grilled, or broiled dishes instead of those that are fried or sautéed.

- Choose a "small" or "medium" portion. This includes main dishes, side dishes, and beverages.

- Order an item from the menu instead of heading for the "all-you-can-eat" buffet.

- If main portions at a restaurant are larger than you want, try one of these strategies to keep from overeating:

  - Order an appetizer or side dish instead of an entrée.

  - Share a main dish with a friend.

  - If you can chill the extra food right away, take leftovers home in a doggy bag.

  - When your food is delivered, set aside or pack half of it to go immediately.

  - Resign from the "clean your plate club"—when you've eaten enough, leave the rest.

- To keep your meal moderate in calories, fat, and sugars:

  - Ask for salad dressing to be served on the side so you can add only as much as you want.

  - Order foods that do not have creamy sauces or gravies.

  - Add little or no butter to your food.

  - Choose fruits for dessert most often.

- On long commutes or shopping trips, pack some fresh fruit, cut-up vegetables, low-fat string cheese sticks, or a handful of unsalted nuts to help you avoid stopping for sweet or fatty snacks.

Source: U.S. Department of Agriculture. http://MyPyramid.gov.

MyPyramid Worksheet

MyPyramid.gov
STEPS TO A HEALTHIER YOU

Check how you did today and set a goal to aim for tomorrow

Food Group	Tip	Goal Based on a 2000 calorie pattern.	List each food choice in its food group*	Estimate Your Total
GRAINS	Make at least half your grains whole grains	**6 ounce equivalents** (1 ounce equivalent is about 1 slice bread, 1 cup dry cereal, or ½ cup cooked rice, pasta, or cereal)		ounce equivalents
VEGETABLES	Try to have vegetables from several subgroups each day	**2 ½ cups** Subgroups: Dark Green, Orange, Starchy, Dry Beans and Peas, Other Veggies		cups
FRUITS	Make most choices fruit, not juice	**2 cups**		cups
MILK	Choose fat-free or low fat most often	**3 cups** (1 ½ ounces cheese = 1 cup milk)		cups
MEAT & BEANS	Choose lean meat and poultry. Vary your choices—more fish, beans, peas, nuts, and seeds	**5 ½ ounce equivalents** (1 ounce equivalent is 1 ounce meat, poultry, or fish, 1 egg, 1 T. peanut butter, ½ ounce nuts, or ¼ cup dry beans)		ounce equivalents
PHYSICAL ACTIVITY	Build more physical activity into your daily routine at home and work.	At least **30 minutes** of moderate to vigorous activity a day, 10 minutes or more at a time.		minutes

Write in Your Choices for Today

*Some foods don't fit into any group. These "extras" may be mainly fat or sugar—limit your intake of these.

How did you do today? ☐ Great   ☐ So-So   ☐ Not so Great

My food goal for tomorrow is: _____

My activity goal for tomorrow is: _____

Source: U.S. Department of Agriculture. http://MyPyramid.gov.

Critical Thinking About Health

1. Everyone aboard the Zoracian space vehicle XTA-9781 was thrilled when their ship's sensors indicated life forms on a small planet orbiting a medium-sized star in the Milky Way galaxy. To make contact with and explore the planet, a landing party of six underwent molecular rearrangement to take on human form both to survive on Earth and communicate and interact with any Earthlings they encountered.

   "When you reach the surface," explained the mission commander, "you will have about eight of their time segments before you must refuel. Energy packets can be obtained in large, stationary pods the locals call supermarkets."

   The crew of the landing party nodded. It seemed similar enough to refueling on their home planet of Zorax not to cause confusion.

   "Except for one thing," the commander cautioned. "There are thousands of kinds of energy packets, from which you will have to choose the appropriate ones."

   "Appropriate ones?" asked the assistant crewchief.

   "Yes. None of the fuel packets are efficient. You will have to sort and select."

   The crew shifted nervously.

   "Do not worry," said the commander, handing each member of the crew a copy of the Food Guide Pyramid. "Their leaders have prepared refueling guidelines. Take these and use them when the time comes."

   a. How would you explain to the Zoracian landing party why, with the great abundance of food choices in American supermarkets, the U.S. government advises its citizens how to eat properly?
   b. From the Zoracians' point of view, the American food supply, although abundant with many kinds of foods, is inefficient with regard to refueling. Explain why the American food supply is so diverse yet nutritionally inefficient.
   c. What factors influence your food selection?

2. A crusading nutrition journalist points out that the food label on a soup company's best-selling product indicates that the product has 6 grams of fat. Fearing that consumers will stop buying the product, the company responds, and within weeks the label indicates that the product has 3 grams of fat. The company has changed nothing in the product.
   a. Why does the label show that the product contains half the fat?
   b. What limits, if any, would you advocate be placed on what food manufacturers can put on product labels? Where would you draw the line between free enterprise, *caveat emptor* (buyer beware), and the public good?
   c. How much attention do you pay to what is written on food product labels?

3. Explain how an herbicide (weed-killing chemical) could wind up in the breast milk of a woman living hundreds of miles away from the site of herbicide application. Are you concerned about pesticides and additives in the food supply? Why or why not?

Health in Review

- The U.S. government and a variety of health organizations have created dietary guidelines to help people make nutritional choices to prevent heart disease, cancer, and other diseases based on the consumption of whole grains, fruits, and vegetables while limiting the consumption of meats, whole-fat dairy products, and fatty, sugary snacks and sweets.
- MyPyramid emphasizes exercise and the consumption of polyunsaturated fats, fruits, and vegetables rather than refined-grain products, meats, and sweets.
- The ingredients label on a food product lists the components of the product in descending order by weight.
- The nutrition facts label provides information on the amounts of certain nutrients in a food product.
- Food has three functions: to provide chemical constituents of the body, energy, and pleasure.
- Food is composed of seven components: protein, carbohydrate, fat, water, vitamins, minerals, and phytochemicals.
- Dietary supplements are unregulated substances that are used to augment the nutritional adequacy of the diet and as drugs to heal or prevent illness.
- Manufactured foods contain a variety of additives that alter their texture, flavor, color, and stability. Preservatives keep foods from spoiling through the use of sulfites.
- One nonchemical method of food preservation involves exposing food to gamma irradiation to destroy microorganisms.
- Artificial sweeteners are widely used, most commonly in diet soft drinks.
- There are several reasons for being a vegetarian, including increased interest in health, ecology, and world issues; economical issues; and the philosophy of not killing animals. A strict vegetarian, or vegan, diet eliminates all animal products, including milk, cheese, eggs, and other dairy products.

Health and Wellness Online

The Web contains a wealth of information about health and wellness. By accessing the Internet using Web browser software, you can gain a new perspective on many topics presented in *Health and Wellness*, Tenth Edition. Access the Jones and Bartlett Publishers Web site at **health.jbpub.com/hwonline.**

References

Bardia, A., et al. (2008). Efficacy of antioxidant supplementation in reducing primary cancer incidence and mortality: Systematic review and meta-analysis. *Mayo Clinic Proceedings, 83,* 23–34.

Bjelakovic, G., et al. (2008). Antioxidant supplements for prevention of mortality in healthy participants and patients with various diseases. *Cochrane Database Systematic Reviews.* April 16. DOI: 10.1002/14651858 .CD007176. Retrieved May 29, 2008, from http:// www.cochrane.org/reviews/en/ab007176.html

Block, G. (2004). Foods contributing to energy intake in the US: Data from NHANES III and NHANES 1999–2000. *Journal of Food Composition and Analysis, 17,* 439–447.

Booker, C. S., & Mann, J. I. (2008). Trans fatty acids and cardiovascular health: Translation of the evidence base. *Nutrition, Metabolism, and Cardiovascular Diseases, 18,* 448–456.

Consumer Reports on Health. (2007, February). Functional—or dysfunctional—foods.

Devaney, B., et al. (2004). Nutrient intakes of infants and toddlers. *Journal of the American Dietetic Association,* 104(1 suppl 1), s14–21.

Gilroy, C. M., et al. (2003). Echinacea and truth in labeling. *Archives of Internal Medicine, 163,* 699–704.

Holick, M. F. (2007). Vitamin D deficiency. *New England Journal of Medicine, 357,* 266–281.

Huff, J., & LaDou, J. (2007). Aspartame bioassay findings portend human cancer hazards. *International Journal of Occupational and Environmental Health, 13,* 446–448.

Humphries, P., Pretorius, E., & Naudé, H. (2008). Direct and indirect cellular effects of aspartame on the brain. *European Journal of Clinical Nutrition, 62,* 451–462.

Jacobson, M. F., & Brownell, K. D. (2000). Small taxes on soft drinks and snack foods to promote health. *American Journal of Public Health, 90,* 854–857.

Kyle, U. S., & Pichard, C. (2006). The Dutch famine of 1944–1945: A pathophysiological model of long-term consequences of wasting disease. *Current Opinion in Clinical Nutrition and Metabolic Care, 9,* 388–394.

Lebel, J. L., Lu, J., & Dube, L. (2008). Weakened biological signals: Highly-developed eating schemas amongst women are associated with maladaptive patterns of comfort food consumption. *Physiology and Behavior, 94,* 384–392.

Martinez, S. (2007). *The U.S. food marketing system* (U.S. Department of Agriculture, Economic Research Service Report No. 42). Retrieved May 22, 2008, from http://www.ers.usda.gov/publications/err42/err42.pdf

Mello, M. M., Studdert, D. M., & Brennan, T. A. (2006). Obesity—The new frontier in public health law. *New England Journal of Medicine, 354,* 2601–2610.

Mitrou, P. N., et al. (2007). Mediterranean dietary pattern and prediction of all-cause mortality in a US population: Results from the NIH-AARP Diet and Health Study. *Archives of Internal Medicine, 167,* 2461–2468.

Nestle, M. (2007). *Food politics: How the food industry influences nutrition and health.* Berkeley: University of California Press.

Nutrition Source. (2008a). The Healthy Eating Pyramid. Retrieved May 27, 2008, from http://www.hsph.harvard .edu/nutritionsource/what-should-you-eat/pyramid/ index.html

Nutrition Source. (2008b). Vitamins. Retrieved May 31, 2008, from http://www.hsph.harvard.edu/ nutritionsource/what-should-you-eat/vitamins/index .html

Patterson, R. E., et al. (2001). Is there a consumer backlash against the diet and health message? *Journal of the American Dietetic Association, 101,* 37–41.

Putnam, J., Allshouse, J., & Kantor, L. S. (2003). Per capita food supply trends: More calories, refined carbohydrates, and fats. *FoodReview* 25(3), 2–15.

Santarelli, R. L., et al. (2008). Processed meat and colorectal cancer: A review of epidemiologic and experimental evidence. *Nutrition and Cancer, 60,* 131–144.

Sun, Q., et al. (2007). A prospective study of trans fatty acids in erythrocytes and risk of coronary heart disease. *Circulation, 115,* 1858–1865.

U.S. Department of Agriculture. (2005). Dietary guidelines for Americans (6th ed). Retrieved May 6, 2005, from http://www.healthierus.gov/dietary guidelines

Suggested Readings

Consumer Reports. (2004, May). Dangerous supplements: Still at large. *Consumer Reports*. Identifies and discusses 12 dangerous dietary supplements.

Entis, P. (2007). *Food safety: Old habits and new perspectives*. Washington, DC: ASM Press. An investigation of the workings—and nonworkings—of the American food safety system.

Nestle, M. (2007). *Food politics: How the food industry influences nutrition and health*. Berkeley: University of California Press. A noted professor of nutrition analyzes how the food industry, in its search for profits, contributes to ill health.

Nestle, M. (2007). *What to eat*. San Francisco: North Point Press. A noted professor of nutrition shows how to navigate supermarket aisles healthfully by resisting marketers' attempts to influence the purchase of unhealthy foods and using common sense to make healthy choices.

Pollan, M. (2006). *The omnivore's dilemma*. New York: Penguin Press. Describes in vivid detail the modern industrial food chain from the ground to the human body.

Sabate, J. (Ed.). (2001). *Vegetarian nutrition*. Boca Raton, FL: CRC Press. Expert summaries of all aspects of plant-based, meatless diets.

Schlosser, E. (2001). *Fast food nation*. New York: Houghton Mifflin. Everything you ever wanted to know (and not know) about fast food: Its history, role in the economy, and contribution to the epidemic of obesity.

Shapin, S. (2006, May 15). Paradise sold. *The New Yorker Magazine*. A discussion of the intricacies of America "going organic."

Silver, L., & Bassett, M. T. (2008). Food safety in the 21st century. *Journal of the American Medical Association, 300,* 957–959. Officials at the New York City Department of Health argue that the American food supply is tainted with too much salt, sugar, and fat (especially trans fat) and is therefore unhealthy.

Willett, W. C., & Skerrett, P. J. (2005). *Eat, drink and be healthy*. New York: Free Press. Two prominent nutritionists explain healthy eating.

Willett, W. C., & Stampfer, M. F. (2003, January). Rebuild the Food Pyramid. *Scientific American,* 64–71. Prominent nutritionists discuss the problems with the current Food Guide Pyramid and offer an alternative guide to healthy eating.

Recommended Web Sites

Please visit **health.jbpub.com/hwonline** for links to these Web sites.

American Cancer Society
Discusses the importance of nutrition in cancer prevention.

American Dietetic Association
Provides information and daily tips.

American Heart Association
Provides information on the association's eating plan.

Herbs and Botanical Information
Provides scientific information on more than 130 botanical agents used in health and disease.

MyPyramid.gov
Use this online tool to determine the food pattern that is optional for you.

Nutritional Analysis Tool (NAT)
Allows analysis of foods for various nutrients.

Nutrition.gov
Provides easy access to all online federal government information on nutrition, including healthy eating, physical activity, and food safety.

Nutrition Source
The Department of Nutrition at the Harvard School of Public Health provides a comprehensive Web site designed to inform and educate the public, journalists, and nutrition professionals about the latest news and issues concerning diet and health.

Quackwatch
Offers information on safety and health issues of dietary supplements.

U.S. Department of Agriculture Food Safety and Inspection Service
Includes consumer advice on foodborne illnesses.

U.S. Department of Agriculture National Organic Program
Provides information on organic food.

U.S. Food and Drug Administration Center for Food Safety and Applied Nutrition

Provides information on food safety, food additives, dietary supplements, and food biotechnology.

U.S. Food and Drug Administration Food Labeling Publications Page

Labeling requirements for prepared foods such as breads, cereals, canned and frozen foods, snacks, desserts, drinks, etc.

Vegetarian Resource Guide

Dos and don'ts of vegetarian eating.

What To Eat

Professor Marion Nestle of the Department of Nutrition at New York University blogs about nutrition, the food industry, and health.

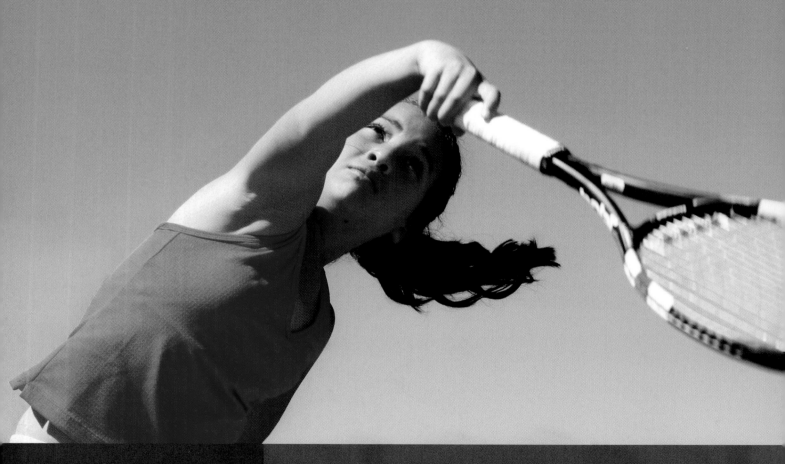

Health and Wellness Online: **health.jbpub.com/hwonline**

Study Guide and Self-Assessment

6.1   My Body Weight
6.2   Managing My Weight
6.3   My Body Image

Chapter Six

Managing a Healthy Weight

Learning Objectives

1. Describe the extent and causes of overweight in American society.

2. Describe the significance of body mass index (BMI) to health.

3. Describe the body's energy-control system and factors affecting it.

4. Explain why calorie-restriction weight-loss regimens fail.

5. List the features of sensible weight management.

6. Discuss the advantages and disadvantages of medical treatments for overweight.

7. Describe common weight-loss fads and fallacies.

8. Define anorexia nervosa, bulimia, and binge eating disorder.

Overweight has become a monumental health problem in the United States and the world. Approximately 130 million American adults—about 66% of the population—are considered overweight (**Figure 6.1**). Seventeen percent of U.S. children between the ages of 6 and 19 also

> There is no sincerer love than the love of food.
>
> *George Bernard Shaw*

are considered overweight. The World Health Organization estimates that 300 million people in the world are overweight, an increase from 200 million since 1995.

Many people consider overweight to be primarily a cosmetic issue. Although feeling attractive is important, overweight is a serious health issue. Overweight individuals are predisposed to a variety of illnesses (**Figure 6.2**), including heart disease and type 2 diabetes, which can result in blindness, kidney failure, and nonhealing skin ulcers, the leading cause of nontraumatic amputation in the United States. Because of their large body size, overweight individuals tend to have more job-related injuries and an increased risk of becoming disabled from arthritis, gait disturbances, back pain, and general instability (Gregg & Guralnik, 2007). Overweight also predisposes individuals to the *metabolic syndrome,* which is characterized by high body fat primarily located around the abdomen, high blood sugar and triglycerides, high blood pressure, and the inability to respond to insulin (see Chapter 14). People who are overweight live several years less than healthy-weight age peers. Annually, about 120,000 Americans die prematurely from complications of being overweight (Flegal et al., 2007). Annual U.S. health care costs related to overweight are $120 billion.

The percentage of Americans who are overweight has been increasing steadily since about 1970 (**Figure 6.3**). The reasons for this increase in overweight include the following:

- An overconsumption of calorie-dense foods in relation to energy expenditure. Between 1971 and

2000, average daily energy intake per American man rose from 2,450 calories to 2,618 calories (168 more per day), and per American woman rose from 1,542 calories to 1,877 calories (335 more per day) without a compensatory increase in calorie use through physical activity (U.S. Centers for Disease Control, 2004).

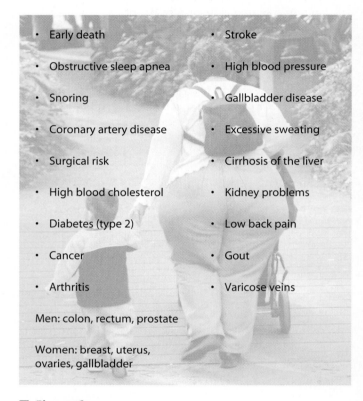

■ **Figure 6.2**

Health Consequences of Overweight
Overweight and obese people have a greater likelihood of developing certain health problems than do people of normal weight.

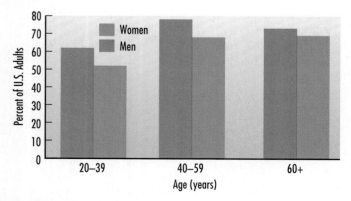

■ **Figure 6.1**

Prevalence of Overweight in the United States
Overweight is defined as a body mass index (BMI) greater than 25.0.

Source: Centers for Disease Control and Prevention, National Center for Health Statistics.

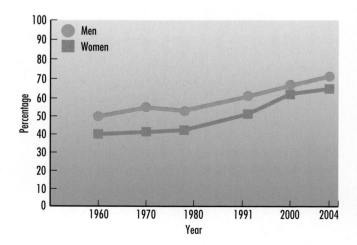

■ **Figure 6.3**

Overweight in the United States
The percentage of adult Americans who are overweight (BMI > 25), by year.

- An abundance (and relentless marketing) of inexpensive, palatable foods that contribute to weight gain (highly processed foods and snack foods, sodas, and fast food). Fast-food consumption (more than twice per week) is strongly associated with weight gain (Rosenheck, 2008). The prevalence of overweight is proportional to the number of residents per fast-food restaurant and the number of fast-food restaurants in a community (Mehta & Chang, 2008).
- An increase in portion sizes; for example, in the past 25 years a "regular" soft drink increased in size from 10 to 16 ounces. A supersized soda contains 64 ounces. Also in that time period, the energy content of a typical burger and fries and a serving of Mexican food has increased by 150 calories. Despite calls in recent years to do so voluntarily, major fast-food companies have not lessened the portion sizes of many of their products, and in some instances, portion sizes have increased (Young & Nestle, 2007).
- A reduction in jobs that require physical labor.
- A decrease in the amount of leisure-time physical activity. One study found that each additional hour spent in a car per day was associated with a 6% increase in the likelihood of obesity and each

additional kilometer walked per day was associated with a 4.8% reduction in the likelihood of obesity (Frank, Andresen, & Schmid, 2004).
- An increase in suburban living, with an associated reliance on automobile travel rather than walking or bicycling.
- Reductions in school physical education and after-school physical activities.
- An increase in time spent watching TV, using the computer, and playing video games.
- An increase in the pace of life, which creates a demand for prepackaged and fast food.
- An increase in the stress of life, which fosters eating high-fat, high-sugar "comfort foods" and alters metabolism that can lead to weight gain as part of the metabolic syndrome (Dallman, Pecoraro, & la Fleur, 2005).

Among American college students, about 22% of women and 39% of men have body weights that exceed recommendations for people of their height (Wharton, Adams, & Hampl, 2008). Some of these students may have been overweight when they entered college, whereas others gained weight during freshman year, referred to by many on campus as the "freshman 15"—meaning a gain in weight of 15 pounds—which research shows

 ## $ Dollars and Health Sense

Junk Food Marketing and the Childhood Obesity Epidemic

Approximately 18% of American children between the ages of 6 and 19 are overweight, a tripling in prevalence since 1980 (see accompanying figure). Although a variety of social factors have been offered to explain it, a report from the United States Institute of Medicine (IOM), a division of the U.S. National Academy of Sciences, concludes that the marketing of high-calorie, low-nutrient "junk" food to kids is a major contributor to this disturbing trend (McGinnis et al., 2006).

The IOM report shows that 30% of the calories in an average child's diet come from sweets, salty snacks, fast food, and sodas, which together account for 10% of the average daily calories ingested. Beverage companies spend millions of dollars per year to market their products to youth via TV (American children see between 10 and 20 food-related TV commercials per day). Many, many more marketing dollars are spent on getting products into TV shows as props (e.g., a character consumes a particular brand of soda), product-related toys, games, Web sites, special events sponsorship, and the licensing of popular characters to sell products. Studies show that children prefer foods that are associated with a particular character or brand, even if equivalent alternatives are offered (Robinson, 2007).

The IOM report points out that numerous firms, on behalf of advertising agencies and food manufacturers, conduct extensive research to elucidate the psychological factors that

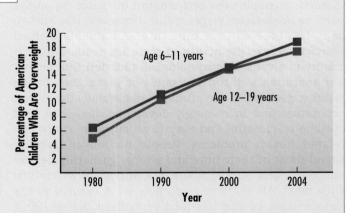

Prevalence of Overweight Among American Children, 1980–2004
Source: U.S. National Center for Health Statistics.

influence children's food choices and their strategies for obtaining the foods they desire.

Some advertisers and food companies have promised to limit advertising of a few unhealthy foods to children under 12. This promise offers little peace of mind to parents and health care professionals who still must battle with marketers whose principal goal is to undermine their efforts to provide children with healthy food alternatives.

actually to be closer to the "freshman 3 or 4" (Racette et al., 2008). Some reasons for weight gain in college include the following:

- Being away from home and thus having greater independence in food choices (which may not always be the healthiest)
- Fragmented schedules that promote skipping meals and the resultant consumption of high-calorie snacks and fast food when hungry
- Little time invested in physical activity due to academic and paid work responsibilities
- Exposure to factors that promote food consumption, for example, soda and snack vending machines on campus, unlimited access to dorm/dining facility food, and academic and social stress

Judging from the number of books and magazine articles extolling various "surefire" weight-loss methods and of TV infomercials peddling dietary supplements and exercise gear, it would appear that the U.S. national pastime is weight control. Indeed, about half of adult women and one-fourth of adult men are on so-called reducing diets ("so-called" because they generally fail to reduce weight in the long run).

Concern about body weight (more typically, body *fatness*) fuels a $40 billion industry of weight-reduction machines and programs, special foods, and dietary supplements, most of which are useless and costly in the long run.

With all the passion for being slim, it is no wonder that many people view any amount of visible fat on the body as something to get rid of. However, the human body has evolved over time in environments of food scarcity; hence, the ability to store fat easily and efficiently is a valuable physiological function that served our ancestors well for thousands of years. Only in the last few decades, in the primarily industrially developed economies and increasingly developed ones, has food become so plentiful and easy to obtain as to cause fat-related health problems. People no longer have to spend most of their time and energy gathering berries and seeds and hoping that a hunting party will return with meat. All we have to do nowadays is drive to the supermarket or the fast-food restaurant, where for a very low cost we can obtain nearly all of our daily calories (Table 6.1).

Body weight issues are not solely about food intake, but also are about food intake in relation to a number of other factors, including the following: a sedentary lifestyle and lack of movement activities, heredity, advertising that promotes food products, lack of guidance regarding proper nutrition, confusing information about the effects of food on health and well-being, the custom of using body shape as a measure of social desirability, and a hectic, stressful lifestyle. In such a complex environment, the overavailability of food allows it to be used for a variety of reasons other than to provide nutrients and energy for life.

Table 6.1

Percentage of Daily Calories Provided by Typical Fast-Food Meals

Meal	Percentage of daily calories for three different daily calorie levels		
	1,600 calories/day	2,000 calories/day	2,500 calories/day
Quarter Pounder French fries Milkshake	73	58	47
Whopper French fries Diet soft drink	66	54	43
Two slices of pizza Diet soft drink	33	25	20

Many people whose body weight does not predispose them to health problems still may be weight conscious, primarily for cosmetic reasons. Their goal is to achieve a body size and shape that meets society's standards of "perfection" (generated by the fashion and advertising industries). Most "body-conscious" persons want to lose weight. These individuals seem to be in a continual battle with the same 5, 10, or 20 pounds, which they struggle to shed to look youthful and attractive.

In contrast to those who wish to lose weight, some—almost always men—want to gain weight. Although not unhealthy, they perceive themselves to be less attractive and masculine and desire to gain several pounds of muscle. Interestingly, men who want to gain weight imagine that women prefer men who are much more muscular than these men perceive themselves to be. However, studies show that women prefer men with ordinary body sizes without added muscle (Pope et al., 2000). There are biological limits to how muscular one can become. One can try to maximize one's potential for muscularity by engaging in strength training (see Chapter 7) and consuming healthy foods to support that activity. Special diets of "superfoods" and supplements in and of themselves will not produce increased muscularity, advertising claims notwithstanding. And drugs that are purported to bring about weight (muscle) gain are either worthless (chromium, creatine, protein powders) or dangerous (ephedra, anabolic steroids).

What Is Healthy Weight?

In most instances, concerns about being overweight are really concerns about being *overfat*. There is a difference. Some professional male athletes, for example, weigh much more than the recommended weight standards for persons of similar height. Yet as little as 1% of their body weight may be fat. Most of the nonwater body weight of a well-conditioned athlete is muscle and bone.

Female body builders, who are the leanest of all female athletes, have about 8% to 13% of their total body weight as fat. This probably represents the lower limit of fat for a healthy woman.

Body fat is composed of two parts: **essential fat**—fat necessary for normal physiological functioning, such as nerve conduction—and **storage fat.** Essential fat constitutes about 3% to 7% of body weight in men and about 10% to 12% of body weight in women. This sex difference, which is presumably caused by hormones, is due to the deposition of greater amounts of fat on the hips, thighs, and breasts in females. Storage fat, also called depot fat, constitutes only a small percentage of the total body weight of lean individuals and 5% to 25% of the body weight of the majority of the population. **Obesity** is the medical term for storage fat exceeding about 30% of body weight.

Social standards for the most "desirable" or "ideal" body weight or body composition (fat percentage) vary. For example, in some cultures, women with significant storage fat are considered physically attractive and sexually desirable, and fatness in children is considered a sign of robust health. In the United States, attitudes about desirable body configuration fluctuate and are often keyed to fashion trends. During the 1950s, for example, large body size, characterized by "full-figured" women and "he-men," was considered desirable, whereas today "slim is in."

Healthy body weight is determined by the **body mass index (BMI)**, which is calculated by dividing a person's weight in kilograms by his or her height in meters squared (**Table 6.2**). Studies show that good health is associated with weighing no more than 5% below or 20% (for men) and 30% (for women) above the weight-for-height standards, or having a BMI between 19 and 25 (**Figure 6.4**). Above the upper limits of these measures, people have higher risks for type 2 diabetes, gallbladder disease, varicose veins, arthritis, heart disease, stroke, high blood pressure, breathing problems, and accident proneness (because of a large body). People who are extremely overweight often face stigmas, such as job discrimination, and lower social acceptance, and they tend to have lower self-esteem.

TERMS

body mass index (BMI): a measure of body fatness, calculated by dividing body weight (in kilograms) by the square of height (in meters)

essential fat: necessary body fat required for normal physiological functioning

obesity: storage fat exceeding 30% of body weight

storage fat: also called depot fat; energy stored as fat in various parts of the body

---

Table 6.2

Body Mass Index (BMI) Table

BMI	19	20	21	22	23	24	25	26	27	28	29	30	31	32	33	34	35
Height								Weight (in pounds)									
4'10" (58")	91	96	100	105	110	115	119	124	129	134	138	143	148	153	158	162	167
4'11" (59")	94	99	104	109	114	119	124	128	133	138	143	148	153	158	163	168	173
5' (60")	97	102	107	112	118	123	128	133	138	143	148	153	158	163	168	174	179
5'1" (61")	100	106	111	116	122	127	132	137	143	148	153	158	164	169	174	180	185
5'2" (62")	104	109	115	120	126	131	136	142	147	153	158	164	169	175	180	186	191
5'3" (63")	107	113	118	124	130	135	141	146	152	158	163	169	175	180	186	191	197
5'4" (64")	110	116	122	128	134	140	145	151	157	163	169	174	180	186	192	197	204
5'5" (65")	114	120	126	132	138	144	150	156	162	168	174	180	186	192	198	204	210
5'6" (66")	118	124	130	136	142	148	155	161	167	173	179	186	192	198	204	210	216
5'7" (67")	121	127	134	140	146	153	159	166	172	178	185	191	198	204	211	217	223
5'8" (68")	125	131	138	144	151	158	164	171	177	184	190	197	203	210	216	223	230
5'9" (69")	128	135	142	149	155	162	169	176	182	189	196	203	209	216	223	230	236
5'10" (70")	132	139	146	153	160	167	174	181	188	195	202	209	216	222	229	236	243
5'11" (71")	136	143	150	157	165	172	179	186	193	200	208	215	222	229	236	243	250
6' (72")	140	147	154	162	169	177	184	191	199	206	213	221	228	235	242	250	258
6'1" (73")	144	151	159	166	174	182	189	197	204	212	219	227	235	242	250	257	265
6'2" (74")	148	155	163	171	179	186	194	202	210	218	225	233	241	249	256	264	272
6'3" (75")	152	160	168	176	184	192	200	208	216	224	232	240	248	256	264	272	279

Directions: Find your height in the left column. Go across the row to find your weight. Go up the column to the top row to find your BMI. Healthy BMI = 18–24.99. Overweight BMI = 25–29.99. Unhealthy BMI ("obese") = 30+.

Source: NIH/National Heart, Lung, and Blood Institute (NHLBI).

Another health-related index of body size is the waist-to-hip ratio, which is calculated by dividing the circumference of the waist by the circumference of the hips. For example, someone with a 28-inch waist and 37-inch hips would have a waist-to-hip ratio of 0.75. Health problems are less likely in women whose waist-to-hip ratio is less than 0.8 and in men whose waist-to-hip ratio is less than 0.95. In other words, it is healthier for a body to be pear-shaped than apple-shaped, and it's healthier *not* to have a beer belly (**Figure 6.5**). Doctors sometimes use only the waist circumference as an indicator of health risks associated with being overweight. A waist circumference greater than 40 inches in men and 35 inches in women is associated with greater health risk.

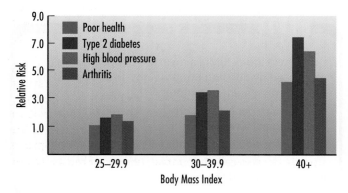

■ **Figure 6.4**

Relative Health Risks of Various Body Mass Indexes
The risks for poor health, type 2 diabetes, high blood pressure, and arthritis increase as body mass index increases. Relative risk means that the risk for each BMI is standardized to the BMI range of 18.5 to 24.9, which is considered normal.

Source: Adapted from Mokdad, A. H., et al. (2003). Prevalence of obesity, diabetes, and obesity-related health risk factors, 2001. *Journal of the American Medical Association, 289,* 76–79.

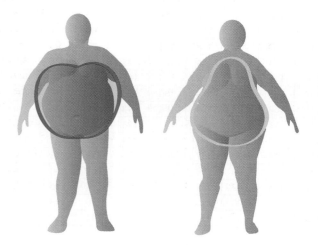

■ **Figure 6.5**

Apple or Pear?
Apple-shaped people carry much of their body fat above the waist. Pear-shaped people carry their body fat on the hips and thighs. Studies show that it's healthier to be pear-shaped than apple-shaped.

The Regulation of Body Fat

The main principle of healthy weight maintenance is that you will store fat if you take in more calories than you expend. Calories enter the body as food: four calories per gram of protein or carbohydrate, seven calories per gram of alcohol, and nine calories per gram of fat. Calories leave the body as energy expended to fuel basal (resting) metabolism, physical activity, growth, injury repair, and to maintain body temperature. Calories from food that are not used right away are stored either as glycogen, a complex carbohydrate that is found in liver and muscle, or as **triglyceride,** a fat that is found in adipose tissue located on the body in all-too-familiar places. At nine calories per gram, fat is the most efficient form of energy storage (one pound of fat will fuel a 40-mile walk), and fat has other biological advantages: it's lightweight, compact, spongy, and a good thermal insulator.

The body has an extremely complex energy-control system, designed to provide efficiently the nutrients and energy required for life. This system is centered in a region of the hypothalamus of the brain. The body sends messages to the brain about its nutrient and energy status via nerves and hormones. Upon receiving these messages, the brain alters hunger, appetite, and eating behaviors accordingly. When your body needs nutrients or energy, nerves and hormones signal the brain and you feel hungry and turn your attention and behavior to eating. After you have eaten sufficiently, nerves and hormones signal the brain and you feel full and stop eating.

Besides levels of nutrients and energy in the body, the brain also responds to food-related thoughts and emotions that are independent of hunger. For example, you can walk into the mall and smell freshly baked chocolate chip cookies and not resist consuming one or more even if you have just eaten and are full. Or, you can go to a restaurant with friends or eat dinner with your family at "dinnertime" even if you are not hungry. On the other hand, you could be hungry, but you really dislike the pizza toppings your friends have ordered and you lose your appetite. Or, you invite a new love interest to dinner and are too distracted by your emotions to eat.

As long as you are generally healthy, your energy-control system is working properly, *and you are paying attention to it,* you are unlikely to develop a weight (fat) problem because your calorie intake will pretty much equal your calorie output; this is called being in a state of **energy balance.** However, you only have to exceed energy balance a little bit to develop a weight problem over time. Consider this example:

Marci is a 26-year-old woman of normal weight with a BMI of 23 who recently changed jobs. Previously the office manager in a small real estate company, she now works as an executive assistant in a much larger firm. Two consequences of this change are (1) Marci now spends more time sitting at her desk typing and answering the phone than in her former job, where she moved around for *every* office task, and (2) she now goes to lunch with office mates. The combination of less movement and fast-food lunches has increased Marci's daily calorie intake over expenditure an average of 10%.

What's 10%? That's about 160 calories per working day, or 3,200 calories a month. At 3,500 calories per pound, that's enough for Marci to gain about 10 pounds per year. You can see what a few years at this job might do to Marci's waistline. When the office crew goes to lunch, often their intention is to socialize and get away from the stress of the office; they don't intend to consume a big lunch. However, the desire to be social, the smell of food, and the size

> The trouble with Italian cooking is that after five or six days you're hungry again.
> *Henry Miller, author*

of the portions served to them make it easy to ignore satiety signals from the brain and to overeat.

Of course, Marci could prevent gaining those 10 pounds a year by being more mindful of her lunchtime eating behaviors and walking a few minutes more each day. By eating one less cookie or half of a 12-ounce soda, she would consume 80 fewer food calories per day. Also, if she parked her car a 10-minute walk from her workplace, she would utilize 80 calories more than usual. Eating 80 calories less and walking off 80 calories more would stop the accumulation of 160 calories of fat per day and those 10 extra pounds each year. If she doesn't eat less and exercise more, however, her body is likely to store those excess calories as fat, and in a couple of years she is likely to find

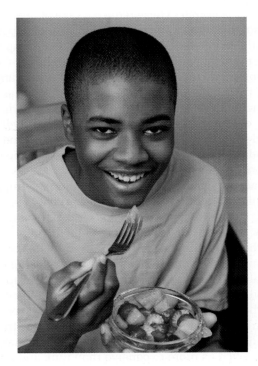

If you have to snack, choose healthy foods such as fruits and vegetables.

herself with a BMI near 30 and in need of a new wardrobe. If that happens and she decides to lose that extra fat, she's likely to discover—as many of us do—that it will take a permanent change in exercise and eating habits to lose and then keep the lost weight (fat) from returning.

That's because the body doesn't like to let go of fat it has accumulated, or as scientists say, the body defends against fat loss. Remember that the body is designed to store fat easily, in case you ever have to go without food for several days as your ancient ancestors did. Of course, that almost never happens to economically advantaged modern people, but those built-in, efficient fat-storage mechanisms are still present. So once fat is deposited, it's very hard to lose.

One reason it is hard to lose fat is that a decrease in body fat triggers an increase in the efficiency with which the body uses energy. The resting metabolic rate decreases, and the efficiency with which muscles do work increases.

Generally, the best weight-loss efforts produce a 5% to 10% reduction in body weight (fat) over the first six months of trying, with no further weight loss after that. This is the reason that people are encouraged not to gain weight in the first place. Fortunately, even a 3% reduction in body weight (fat) can significantly improve health status even though reduction in body size is not significant.

Diets Don't Work

To a nutritionist, the word *diet* means what an individual usually eats and drinks. To almost everyone else, the word *diet* means restricting calories or eating unusual foods to lose weight, as in "I'm on a diet."

It's logical to think that consuming less food than usual will produce weight loss because overeating is generally identified as the reason for weight gain. Although logical, unfortunately, consuming fewer calories than usual works only when people are in a continuous state of near starvation, for example, in environments where food is chronically scarce. When living in an environment in which food is plentiful, however, people are unable *not* to eat what they want for very long because—as pointed out earlier—semistarvation turns on biological mechanisms designed to conserve both body fat and energy expenditure, and being hungry and craving your favorite foods is no fun. Whereas calorie-restricting diets initially tend to be moderately successful, resulting in a loss of a

> **TERMS**
>
> energy balance: when energy consumed as food equals the energy expended in living
> triglyceride: a storage form of fat

few pounds in a week or two, within several weeks after the diet begins the body resists further weight loss even if the calorie-restriction diet is maintained (**Figure 6.6**).

Besides the fact that the body defends against weight (fat) loss, calorie-restriction diets fail because of the following reasons:

- Dieters focus on food and not on increasing physical activity. Increasing energy expenditure, rather than decreasing energy intake, is the key to successful weight loss and long-term healthy weight management (Slentz et al., 2004).

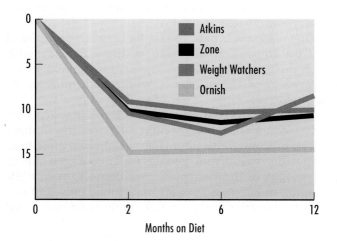

■ Figure 6.6

Weight Loss from Adherence to Several Popular Diet Programs
Source: Data from Dansinger, M. I., et al. (2005). Comparison of the Atkins, Ornish, Weight Watchers, and Zone diets for weight loss and heart disease risk reduction. *Journal of the American Medical Association, 293,* 43–53.

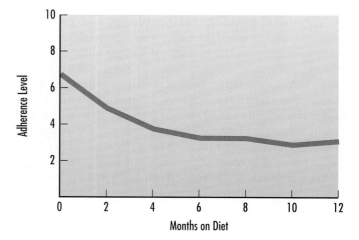

■ Figure 6.7

Adherence to Popular Weight-Management Diets
Dieters' self-reports show a gradual decline in adherence to a weight-management diet over 12 months. This pattern is similar for the Atkins, Zone, Weight Watchers, and Ornish diets.

Source: Data from Dansinger, M. I., et al. (2005). Comparison of the Atkins, Ornish, Weight Watchers, and Zone diets for weight loss and heart disease risk reduction. *Journal of the American Medical Association, 293,* 43–53.

- Because continued adherence to a calorie-restricting plan does not produce commensurate reduction in weight loss, dieters become disillusioned and discouraged and stop following the plan (**Figure 6.7**). Moreover, any weight lost while on the diet tends to be regained. Among those who lose weight by restricting calories, about 50% regain the lost weight within one year after stopping the diet, and nearly all regain the lost weight within four years.
- Dieters become bored eating the same required foods. This is especially true of diets recommending principally one kind of food (e.g., liquid diet programs, grapefruit, steak, papaya, cottage cheese).
- Dieters become frustrated not being able to eat the kinds and quantities of foods they like.
- Dieters are constantly hungry. They become obsessed with food. They even dream about food.
- Prepackaged, special diet foods can be expensive.

Popular Weight-Loss Programs

Popular weight-loss programs generally are of the following types:

Low-calorie: These reduce portion size to limit calories consumed. Examples are Weight Watchers, Zone, Jenny Craig, LA Weight Loss, Medifast, and eDiets. The benefit of these programs are that they are balanced nutritionally. The drawbacks are that they produce at best a modest loss of weight (5% to 10% of prediet weight) and the reduction in calories makes people hungry and thus leads to discontinuation of the program.

Low-carbohydrate: These reduce intake of breads, rice, pasta, potatoes, sweets, snack foods, and, depending on the plan, vegetables and fruits. To make up for the exclusion of carbohydrate, the programs recommend foods high in protein and fat. Examples are the Atkins and South Beach programs. The benefit of this kind of eating plan is that it reduces the consumption of refined complex carbohydrates and simple sugars found in packaged, fast, and junk foods. Also, protein and fat tend to reduce appetite more effectively than *refined* carbohydrate does. The disadvantage of a low-carb diet is the consumption of high amounts of fat and cholesterol, which are risk factors for heart and blood vessel disease.

Low fat: These diets recommend high complex carbohydrate and little fat. An example is the Ornish diet. A major benefit is that the diet is "heart healthy." A drawback is that in our present food environment, calories from unhealthy refined carbohydrate products are plentiful and heavily marketed, whereas complex carbohydrates from whole grains, fruits, vegetables, and beans are perceived as more expensive than junk and fast food and more difficult to obtain.

When diet programs work, it is generally because they reduce the number of calories consumed and not because of the types and proportions of food consumed. For example, the Atkins diet, Weight Watchers program, and the Ornish diet each deliver about 1,450 calories per day (Freedman, King, & Kennedy, 2001). This represents about a 500- to 700-calorie per day difference between calories ingested and calories expended, which produces a loss of about a pound a week until the body's weight-loss-resistance mechanisms kick in.

Sensible Weight Management

If calorie-restricting diets by themselves do not produce lasting weight loss, what does? Results from studies in the National Weight Control Registry show that American adults who lost weight and kept it off for several years did so by engaging in an hour of moderate physical activity daily; consuming five small high-carbohydrate, low-fat meals or snacks; regularly monitoring their weight and exercise activities; and virtually never eating fast food (National Weight Control Registry, 2008). In a different study, over 1,000 overweight American adults lost an average of 15 pounds by walking or exercising about 30 minutes a day and following the recommendations of the DASH diet, which is based on consumption of whole-grain foods, at least five servings of fruits and vegetables per day, and limited high-salt, high-calorie fast and junk food (see Chapter 5) (Svetkey et al., 2008).

Rather than adopting unusual weight-loss regimens in the search for the "ideal" body size, sensible and successful weight-losers live healthfully and let their bodies find the weight that is right for them, which involves the following:

- *Forget slim, go for health.* Images in media and advertising suggest that a healthy body is slim and muscular. However, a variety of body sizes, shapes,

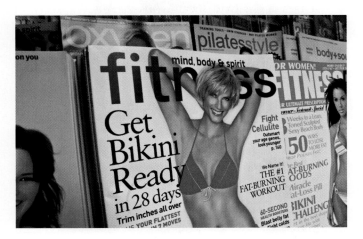

Although most people want to feel good about their bodies, advertisements often portray unrealistic images that can lead to unhealthy diets and eating habits.

and fat compositions are healthy. For example, someone who is 5 feet 4 inches tall can weigh between 110 pounds (BMI = 19) and 148 pounds (BMI = 25) and still have a healthy body weight.

- *Set realistic goals.* A major obstacle to weight loss is setting a goal of attaining one's youthful, former, slim body size—and quickly. Because the body resists fat loss, with patient adherence to a sensible plan, most people can expect to lose about 5% to 10% of their body weight, which, although probably not sufficient to return them to their former body size, nevertheless will lessen risks for heart and other serious diseases, and result in feeling better. Everyone must realize that stereotypes of attractiveness can be very difficult to attain without a predisposing genetic makeup or a visit to the cosmetic surgeon. Sensible weight management involves being aware of social pressures toward unattainable goals and not succumbing to advertising and fashion trends.

- *Eat only when hungry and don't overeat.* Pay attention to hunger and satiety signals from your body. Be aware of habits and customs that influence your eating behavior: Do you eat at predetermined times of day (mealtime, between classes, on the way to work) regardless of your state of hunger? Do you eat *everything* on your plate? Do you work or study while eating and vice versa? Be aware of satiety signals from your body. Say to yourself, "That's enough for now."

- *Eat healthy foods.* Base your diet on whole-grain foods, beans, nuts, and fresh fruits and vegetables. This will add nutrients to your diet and limit the consumption of calorie-laden, nutritionally inferior fast and junk food.

- *Exercise.* Move your body around for at least 20 minutes per day, three to four times a week. You don't have to work out in a gym or engage in any activity in which you breathe hard and sweat (**Table 6.3**). The goal is simply to expend energy by moving your body. Even nonexercise movements such as standing, toe-tapping, walking from room to room, talking, and fidgeting can utilize significant amounts of energy during the day (**Figure 6.8**). (Levine et al., 2005). And don't subscribe to the myth that exercising will increase appetite and food

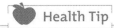 Health Tip

Walk the Walk

Count the number of steps you take each day using a pedometer, a pager-sized device you clip to your clothes. Shoot for 10,000 steps per day (about 5 miles)—15,000 steps is even better.

Table 6.3

Nongym Ways to Increase Physical Activity

Take stairs whenever possible.

Count steps with a pedometer; aim for 10,000 steps a day (15,000 is better).

When feasible, park your car so that you walk 10 minutes to and from your final destination.

Get off of public transportation and walk 10 minutes to your destination.

Walk 20–30 minutes on lunch break.

Exercise/walk with friends or in a group.

Stretch for 5 minutes while on a break at work or before bed.

Strengthen muscles (isometrics, push-ups) 2–3 times a week.

consumption. In fact, except for individuals who expend enormous amounts of energy (e.g., lumberjacks, football players), the opposite is true. Appetite and food consumption tend to decrease as physical activity increases.

- *Limit mindless snacking.* Mindless snacking is the kind we do when we are ravenously hungry, stressed, or zoned-out watching TV. We wish that bag of chips were bottomless. TV advertisers encourage mindless snacking. They know that when you're watching TV you're in a state of autohypnosis, and they bank on your susceptibility

to their images of beer, snack foods, candy, and soft drinks. Instead of mindless snacking, it's better to focus on the food you are eating.

- *Consume little or no alcohol.* Alcohol contains seven calories per gram (about 100 calories per 12-ounce beer, 4-ounce glass of wine, or one shot of distilled liquor). A couple of beers per day without a compensatory reduction in food intake or increase in exercise could lead to an excess of body fat rather quickly.

- *Be aware of eating triggers.* Many of us are susceptible to environmental cues that trigger eating. For example, some people cannot pass a candy or soft-drink machine without feeding it money in exchange for it feeding them. At some worksites, well-meaning supervisors and coworkers provide pastries and candy for staff members, who may have a difficult time resisting, especially when stressed or fatigued.

- *Don't feed your feelings.* Stress, anxiety, loneliness, boredom, fatigue, and anger can motivate overeating. Many people derive emotional comfort from food. One possible explanation is that as children, we learn to associate eating (particularly nursing as infants) with receiving love, affection, and comfort. Another possibility is that when we consume certain foods, particularly those containing sugar and fat, they alter brain chemistry and contribute to feelings of calm.

NEAT stands for *nonexercise activity thermogenesis.* This is energy you use while doing regular activities such as sitting, talking on the phone, walking, and doing a hobby. While doing their daily activities, some people more than others have a propensity to move parts of their bodies. They fidget, wiggle, tap their fingers and toes, take breaks to move and stretch. It turns out that these folks can utilize several hundred calories of energy doing these NEAT movements, and they rarely have a weight problem.

The propensity for NEATness is probably biological, but it is something that a non-NEAT person can pick up easily. Modifying an environment is one way to force people to move rather than sit, ergo, the NEAT desk, designed by Dr. James Levine and his colleagues at the Mayo Clinic. It can be used with a treadmill, exercise bike, standing, or regular chair. It has see-through panels that let in light and allow a person to stay visually connected with the rest of the room. Using the NEAT desk at 1 mile per hour (mph) uses about 100 calories per hour. Dr. Levine recommends walking 15 minutes every hour and during all phone calls. In an average 8-hour workday, this would result in expending more than 200 calories, which, without equivalent energy intake, would produce a loss of 1 to 1.5 pounds a month.

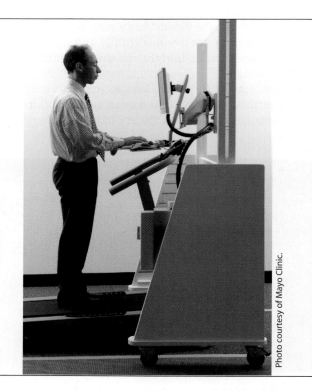

Photo courtesy of Mayo Clinic.

■ **Figure 6.8**

A NEAT Desk

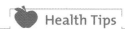 Health Tips

Mindful Eating

Eating should be a relaxed, pleasurable activity but is rarely that in our hectic daily lives. We eat on the run or take only enough time to grab a bite. Most teenagers polish off a full plate of food in a couple of minutes. Just as taking time for physical activity is important for your body, so is taking time with your meals. You can begin to break the habit of wolfing down your food by practicing "mindful eating."

Start by choosing a very small piece of food, perhaps a grape, slice of carrot, or a piece of dried fruit. Sit quietly and slowly place the food in your mouth. Pay attention to its texture and flavor.

Begin to chew it very slowly and notice the response in your mouth—how your saliva starts to flow and how your jaw is moving. Chew until you feel ready to swallow; pay attention to the process of swallowing. Practice this mindful eating exercise every day until you feel that you have become more aware of your food and the nourishment you receive from it.

When you eat a meal, focus all of your attention on the food and the satisfaction of eating. Do not read or watch TV while eating. Make eating a quiet, pleasurable occasion. Do not bring problems or arguments to the table. By eating slowly and quietly you also will hear the message from your stomach when it is full. Listen to the message and stop eating.

Mindful eating can be a powerful technique in weight control and limiting food consumption that your body does not need.

The energy equivalent of one pound of body fat is 3,500 calories. If you want to adopt a weight-reducing program that results in a loss of one pound a month, plan your dietary and physical activities so you can produce a net daily deficit of 120 calories. Walk a little more each day or cut out a soft drink or a couple of cookies. If you want to lose one pound a week, plan for a net daily deficit of 500 calories that includes at least a 300-calorie expenditure per day of exercise (**Table 6.4**). The number of calories is not nearly as important as *making a plan to which you can realistically adhere over the long haul*. Here are some other suggestions:

- Keep a diary of your weight-loss activities and modify things in your plan that do not work.
- Keep faith with your intention to attain a healthful weight. Don't let the inevitable setbacks demoralize you.
- Don't count calories or constantly weigh yourself; focus on developing healthy behaviors and feeling good.
- Ignore weight-loss and exercise-machine advertising.

Besides being good for individuals, altering your lifestyle to maintain a healthy body weight is also good for the planet. Instead of driving or riding in a car for short trips, if all Americans between the ages of 10 and 64 walked or biked for 30 minutes a day, not only would they collectively shed 3 billion pounds and eliminate the current epidemic of overweight, but also annual carbon dioxide emissions in the United States would be lessened by 64 million tons, and 6.5 billion gallons of gasoline would be saved (Higgins & Higgins, 2005).

The Medical Management of Overweight

Managing body weight is principally a matter of adopting healthful living habits: eating whole-grain foods and fresh fruits and vegetables, limiting consumption of fast foods and junk foods, and increasing movement. Still, some people cannot successfully manage weight on their own, and they may benefit by seeking the help of a health professional. Methods that health professionals employ to help people reduce and maintain body weight include psychological counseling, hypnotherapy, medications, and surgery.

Counseling and Hypnosis

Counseling for weight loss involves helping individuals examine the reasons for their unhealthful eating and exercise behaviors and developing ways to behave more healthfully. Hypnosis has been shown to increase the benefits of counseling. Counseling for weight loss and maintenance focuses on the following (Levy et al., 2007):

- Increasing one's self-awareness of the inner dialogue that contributes to the weight problem, for example, changing the thought "I've had a bad day so I deserve a treat; I'll have some fries" to "I deserve a treat; I'll take a soothing bath"

Table 6.4

Approximate Energy Expenditures During Various Activities

Light exercise (4 calories per minute)		
Cycling 5 mph	Slow dancing	Table tennis
Walking 3 mph	Volleyball	Yoga
Canoeing	Softball	T'ai chi ch'uan
Housecleaning	Golf	
Moderate exercise (7 calories per minute)		
Tennis	Basketball	Snowshoeing
Fast dancing	Swimming 30 m/min	Walking 4.5 mph
Cycling 9 mph	Heavy gardening	Roller skating
Heavy exercise (10 calories per minute)		
Jogging	Mountain climbing	Skiing
Climbing stairs	Cycling 12 mph	Ice skating
Football	Handball and racquetball	

🧘 Managing Stress

Treating the Underlying Emotional Causes of Obesity

Mrs. Johnson made an appointment with a psychologist to discuss being overweight. She is 40 years old, 5 feet 5 inches tall, and weighs 180 pounds. She works as a nurse at a community hospital and has no serious medical problems. She is married, her husband is unemployed, and she has three teenage children at home. Her take-home pay is modest, and the family has difficulty paying bills. She eats mostly junk food from fast-food restaurants and does not exercise.

Because appropriate weight depends on *both* a healthy diet *and* exercise, the counselor must look for barriers to those two goals. The counselor must help the patient discover the causes of stress and negative emotions that underlie the weight problem. These generally include job or family stressors, depression, anger, loneliness, or boredom. Sometimes adult obesity has its roots in childhood sexual abuse (i.e., having a large body makes one sexually unattractive and is therefore protective).

Social aspects of being overweight also have to be explored. What are the barriers to obtaining healthy food? Does the job require a lot of travel time or sitting for extended periods? How can exercise be incorporated into the daily lifestyle?

In Mrs. Johnson's case, she has a high-stress, low-paying job, a bad marriage, and children at a difficult stage of development. Her lifestyle is out of control. With the counselor's help, Mrs. Johnson adopted a low-fat diet and began walking—and later jogging—in the morning before work. Later, she added weight training to her exercise program. After a few months she obtained a better-paying job with regular hours. She and her husband went to a marriage counselor and eventually decided to divorce. After about a year, Mrs. Johnson's weight stabilized at 130 pounds. She has maintained her low-fat diet and continues to exercise. She has found new friends and has begun going out on dates.

Many overweight people have problems similar to Mrs. Johnson's. Counseling, diet changes, exercise, and social support can help most overweight people who are willing to make the effort to change their lives.

- Keeping records of eating and exercise activities in order to assess current behavior and target personal and environmental changes
- Changing the environmental factors that trigger overeating and underexercising, for example, not having a full cookie jar on the kitchen counter or not going out for fast food with friends when the goal is socializing rather than sating hunger
- Education about healthy nutrition and physical activity
- Setting realistic weight-management goals and adopting feasible plans for accomplishing them
- Teaching about "feeding one's feelings" and the tendency to eat when feeling stressed
- Providing social support for weight-management activities
- Identifying and managing mental health issues, such as depression and anxiety, that may be associated with weight issues

Psychological counseling is generally effective in facilitating weight loss of about a pound a week and a significant percentage of the initial body weight, and it promotes weight-loss maintenance for several months after treatment ends (Jones, Wilson, & Wadden, 2007).

Medications

Medications to produce weight loss include appetite suppressants—agents that alter certain neurotransmitters in the brain (norepinephrine or serotonin) to make one feel less hungry—and a drug that blocks the absorption of fat from the intestines (orlistat). Drugs alone cannot produce significant weight loss, and generally any weight lost is regained when the drug is no longer taken (Rucker et al., 2007). This is why health professionals consider medications to be an adjunct to lifestyle modification (diet, exercise, and greater awareness of eating habits) and not to be used alone to achieve weight loss.

Surgery

Weight-reduction (bariatric) surgery is for people with a BMI over 40 or with a BMI between 35 and 40 who have severe weight-related medical conditions, such as heart disease or type 2 diabetes, and who have not responded to supervised diet and exercise regimens or drug therapy. There are several methods of weight-loss surgery. Some involve constricting the stomach, which makes the person feel full after having consumed small amounts of food. Other methods involve surgically restructuring the gastrointestinal tract so that only a fraction of the food ingested in a meal is absorbed into the body and the activities of some of the nerves and hormones that control eating and metabolism are altered. Weight-loss surgery does not return a person to a slim body shape; rather, it reduces the amount of body fat to a degree that the adverse health effects of extreme overweight are reduced. Weight-loss surgery carries a 1% risk of death, so it requires serious thought.

Liposuction

Liposuction is the surgical removal by suction of fat stored under the skin and is not recommended as a substitute for proper diet, exercise, and counseling for weight loss and weight management. It is for shaping the body. Indeed, after the surgery, without attention to diet and exercise, fat may appear on other parts of the body, and in time, patients actually may gain weight.

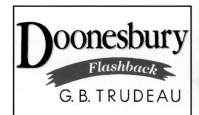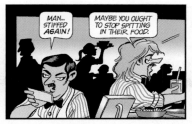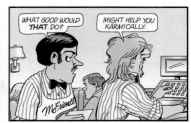
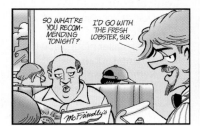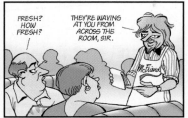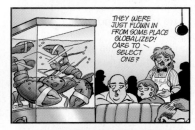
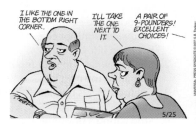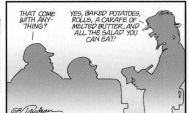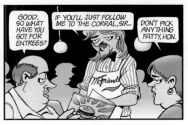

Source: Doonesbury © 2008 G. B. Trudeau. Reprinted with permission of Universal Press Syndicate. All rights reserved.

Annually, more than 450,000 liposuction procedures are performed in women and men in the United States by plastic surgeons, dermatologists, and other physicians (see Chapter 8). Liposuction is currently the most common cosmetic surgical procedure performed. Liposuction is surgically risky, and anyone considering it should investigate the procedure thoroughly. Although rare, deaths have occurred from liposuction.

Weight-Control Fads and Fallacies

"Lose weight effortlessly, even as you sleep!" "New diet discovery lets you lose excess pounds in just one week!" So claim advertisements for products and eating regimens that are directed to chronic dieters and others concerned about being overfat. Some products, such as "diet rings" and weight-loss soaps, are clearly worthless, but some overweight people are so desperate they will try anything.

> If slaughterhouses had glass walls, everyone would be a vegetarian.
>
> *Paul McCartney*

Unfortunately for consumers, nearly all of the claims made by heavily advertised weight-control regimens and products are exaggerated and misleading. The U.S. Federal Trade Commission estimates that weight-loss scams are the most prevalent types of fraud, affecting nearly 5 million Americans per year. By themselves, these are not likely to produce a significant reduction in body fat over any long-term period.

Although totally ineffective, these products are advertised in reputable magazines and newspapers, on TV, and on the Internet, which contributes to their credibility. Something to consider: If any of the products advertised for rapid, effortless weight loss really worked, surely every overweight person would use them and the obesity epidemic would be history. The best, and so far only proven, ways to reduce body fat are to eat healthfully and moderately and engage in exercise of some type; weight-loss surgery can be an option for a small percentage of very obese people who cannot lose weight otherwise.

Some popular and largely ineffective weight-loss schemes include body wraps and chemicals and supplements, which are described below.

Body Wraps

Body wraps are hot linens, blankets, saran or plastic sheets, elastic or rubber waist belts, or whole-body garments that are applied in spas or at home, often in combination with herbal compounds, minerals, amino acids, and other substances. Commonly, body wraps promise to open pores to let fat and other toxins escape the body. A wrap designed for just one part of the body (such as the waist or hips) is supposed to reduce the size of just that body region ("spot reducing").

TERMS

liposuction: surgery used to remove fat under the skin to reshape parts of the body

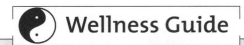

Wellness Guide

Weight-Management Suggestions

Control your home environment in these ways:

1. Do all at-home eating at the kitchen or dining room table.
2. Eat without reading or watching TV.
3. Keep tempting foods out of sight; make them hard to reach and bothersome to prepare.
4. If you must snack, have low-calorie foods accessible, visible, easy to reach, and ready to eat.
5. Store tempting foods in containers that are opaque or difficult to open.
6. Give other family members their own snack-food storage areas.
7. Don't do non-food-related activities in the kitchen; stay out of the kitchen as much as possible.

Control your work environment in these ways:

1. Do not eat at your desk or while working. Eat at some place designated (by you) for eating only.
2. Do not keep tempting food near your workplace.
3. Prepackage low-calorie snacks and take them with you to work.
4. Carry no change to use at vending machines.
5. Use exercise instead of food when you need to take a break from work.
6. If you eat in a cafeteria, plan your order in advance and bring only enough money to cover your order.

Manage your daily food sources:

1. Do not shop when hungry.
2. Shop from a list prepared beforehand.
3. Shop quickly.
4. Avoid buying large sizes of hard-to-resist high-calorie foods.
5. Prepare foods during periods when your control is highest.

6. Try to prepare several meals at once (lunches with dinners).
7. Remove leftovers from sight as soon after mealtime as possible (use opaque storage devices).

Control your mealtime environment:

1. Do not keep serving bowls at the table.
2. Use smaller plates, bowls, glasses, and serving spoons.
3. Remove the plate from the table as soon as you finish eating.
4. Practice polite refusal when extra food is offered to you.

Eat slowly:

1. Put down the eating utensil, sandwich, drink, or chicken leg between bites.
2. Swallow what is in your mouth before preparing the next bite.
3. Cut food as it is needed rather than all at once.
4. Stop eating a few times during the meal to control your eating rhythm.
5. Make each second serving only half as large as the usual amount.

Control snacking:

1. Instead of snacking, do an activity incompatible with eating.
2. Instead of snacking, do something you like to do or a small task around the house or office.
3. Instead of snacking, do a short burst of intense activity or a relaxation exercise.
4. Brush your teeth or use mouthwash to curb the urge to eat.
5. Make snacks difficult to get.
6. Drink a large glass of water before snacking.
7. Have low-calorie snack foods on hand rather than high-calorie foods.

Source: J. Waltz. (1978). *Food habit management.* Seattle, WA: Northwest Learning Associates.

Body wraps do result in weight loss and a reduction in body size. The catch is that the weight lost is body water and not body fat. The lost body water is quickly regained and so is the lost body weight. Because these products cause a loss of body water, they make dehydration a potential danger. Some athletes have died from exercising while using body wraps.

Chemicals and Supplements

A number of products that contain drugs and "natural" substances are sold as weight-loss remedies. Often these products are used in conjunction with dieting, modification in eating behavior, and exercise programs, so they appear effective to the naive consumer. However, no

single product by itself has been shown to reduce weight safely and permanently. Several types of popular, generally ineffective weight-loss products are listed here:

Appetite suppressants/energy boosters. If they actually contain the ingredients listed on the label (because they are unregulated there is no guarantee that they do), these products contain chemicals that act as central nervous system (CNS) stimulants such as ephedra (*ma huang*), synephrine (bitter orange), and caffeine (guarana, yerba mate). Ingestion of sufficient quantities of a CNS stimulant can result in short-term loss of a couple of pounds. However, these substances have side effects, especially ephedra, which increases the risk of psychiatric,

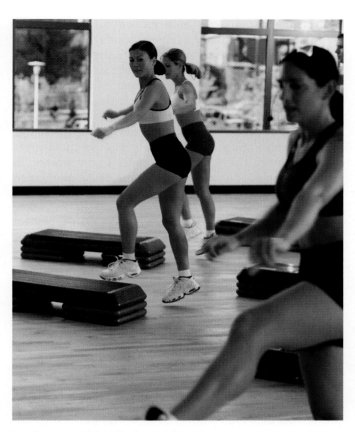

Exercise is essential to effective weight management.

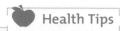

Inform Yourself: Don't Buy Worthless Weight-Loss Products

Dietary supplements are unregulated. Before you take anything, check out what the experts have to say about it. Use the Web. Don't do a general search because you are likely to be inundated with Web sites that sell stuff rather than inform. Start with these authoritative Web sites:
- Herbs and Botanical Information (http://www.mskcc.org/aboutherbs)
- National Center for Complementary and Alternative Medicine (http://nccam.nih.gov)
- U.S. Food and Drug Administration (http://www.fda.gov)

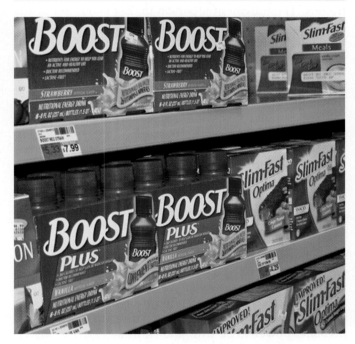

People take hundreds of different herbs, supplements, and other pills to lose weight.

temperature-control, and gastrointestinal problems, and these products have been associated with several deaths. Do not risk your life to lose a few pounds. A related product, *hoodia gordonii*, a South African plant, is purported to be a nonstimulant appetite suppressant. It is supposed to act in the hypothalamus to produce a feeling of fullness. No scientific studies have yet found hoodia to be effective. Products containing triatricol, or "triac," a thyroid hormone–like substance, are marketed as "metabolic accelerators." Because it can cause heart attacks and strokes, the FDA has warned consumers not to take supplements containing "triac." However, triac-containing products are still sold on the Internet along with other thyroidlike chemicals.

Fat burners/fat blockers. These products claim to oxidize ("chemically burn") stored body fat or stop the production of body fat. They contain chemicals such as hydroxycitric acid (HCA), conjugated linoleic acid (CLA), green tea, licorice, pyruvate, vitamin B, and L-carnitine. All of these are generally ineffective. Chitosan, derived from chitin found in crustaceans, is supposed to bind fat in the digestive tract. Studies indicate that this also is ineffective.

Bulk-producing agents. These include methyl-cellulose, psyllium, and agar. They are supposed to produce a sense of fullness in the gastrointestinal tract, thus suppressing appetite. These agents swell when mixed with water and are much more effective as laxatives than as weight reducers. Glucomannan, a bulk-producing starch derived from konjac tubers, is often touted by health food enthusiasts as a "natural" weight-loss method. There is no evidence that glucomannan or any other bulk producer aids weight loss.

Vitamins, minerals, and amino acids. Vitamins, minerals, and some amino acids (including arginine, ornithine, tryptophan, and phenylalanine) are occasionally sold as weight-loss agents. For example, spirulina, a product made from blue-green algae, is claimed to be effective in reducing weight because it contains the amino acid phenylalanine, which supposedly regulates the body's appetite. Chromium (generally listed on product labels as chromium picolinate) is supposed to alter carbohydrate metabolism and thus result in weight loss. No studies have ever confirmed this hypothesis. Vitamins, minerals, and amino acids have not been shown to be effective in causing weight loss. And in very high doses, some of these substances, although "natural," can be harmful.

Body Image

Body image is a person's mental picture of her or his body. Nearly everyone has a body image. Nearly everyone judges that image as good or less good by comparing her or his body image to a standard of the "ideal body" communicated to individuals by their culture and people who are important to them, such as lovers, family, and friends. The judgment a person makes about her or his body image is called *body esteem*. Individuals with a positive body image tend to have higher body esteem than do individuals with a less positive body image.

Many women are excessively concerned about their body image and tend to have low body esteem because they believe themselves to be overweight. Books, films, TV, and popular magazines (especially women's magazines) consistently send messages that our society esteems thin women and disdains heavy ones. Whereas maintaining appropriate body size is associated with good health, attempting to achieve an unrealistic ideal of slimness is oppressive to many women. Failure to meet unrealistic standards leads many women to judge themselves as unattractive and lowers their self-esteem.

The current emphasis on slimness is partly fad—there have been times when thinness was associated with being sickly and a full body was a sign of health and sexual attractiveness—and partly desire to be healthy and fit. A lean body is associated with high status, sexual attractiveness, youthfulness, and a demonstration of the personal power to be trim and fit in a culture in which sedentary habits and overeating are common.

Body dysmorphic disorder is a preoccupation with an imagined defect in one or more of one's body parts, which causes considerable personal and social distress and occupational impairment. Males tend to be concerned with their muscularity (*muscle dysmorphia*, or "bigorexia") and height, genitals, and thinning hair. Females tend to be concerned about their body size, buttocks, breasts, thighs, facial features, and body hair (Hunt, Thienhaus, & Ellwood, 2008). The preoccupation with imagined physical defects leads to seeking medical procedures such as cosmetic ("aesthetic") surgery, cosmetic dentistry, or cosmetic dermatology (skin abrasions, Botox). Males may engage in extreme body building activities, excessive consumption of ineffectual sports supplements, abnormal eating patterns, and ingestion of various illegal drugs. Females are at high risk for anorexia nervosa (see the following section). Almost always, efforts to change the identified defect do not produce mind–body harmony. Cognitive behavioral therapy and certain medications can help individuals reduce their preoccupation with their imagined defects and help them establish a more realistic attitude about their bodies.

For the most part, standards of attractiveness and a healthful appearance are set by companies seeking to sell products and increase profits. Advertisements try to convince women that they fall short of an ideal and that by purchasing a product, dieting, or exercising to change their body size and shape, they can improve themselves and their lives. These messages cause many women to judge themselves on how they look and cause many men to judge women largely by their physical appearance. Overconcern about body image and weight can have adverse health consequences, including the following:

- Depression from low body esteem and low self-worth
- Poor nutrition from extensive dieting
- Inadequate calcium and iron intake from undernutrition
- Anorexia or bulimia
- Musculoskeletal injuries from overexercising
- Risks associated with cosmetic surgery
- Cigarette smoking to reduce body weight

Eating Disorders

Eating disorders are complex psychophysiological conditions that manifest as compulsive, unusual eating behavior. Three of the most common eating disorders are anorexia nervosa, a voluntary refusal to eat; bulimia, binge eating and immediate purging of the ingested food either by vomiting or by using laxatives or intense exercise; and binge eating disorder, episodes of binge eating without subsequent purging. Occasionally, anorexia involves purging as well. The lifetime prevalence of eating disorders among American adults is approximately 5%. About 90% of those affected with anorexia nervosa or bulimia are women; nearly half of those with binge eating disorder are men. Eating disorders are anchored in tightly held, biologically inaccurate, and perfectionistic core beliefs, such as "You can never be too thin," "Any fat is bad," "I'm too fat," and "Anything I eat immediately turns to fat that everyone else can see" (Yager, 2007). Striving to adhere to these core beliefs fosters compulsive disordered eating and purging behaviors (e.g., excessive exercise). In some instances, individuals hold so tightly to these beliefs and their associated behaviors that they reject any suggestions that they are at risk and must change or face serious health consequences and even death.

Compared to the general population, eating disorders are more prevalent among athletes, particularly among those whose bodies are exposed to view (swimmers, runners, gymnasts, dancers) or those whose performance may be affected by body weight (wrestlers, swimmers, divers, gymnasts) (Reinking & Alexander, 2005). Among athletes, attitudes and behaviors to lessen body weight, such as overexercising, dieting, or using

🌐 Global Wellness

Eating Disorders Are a Worldwide Concern

Eating disorders among women are becoming a worldwide problem. They used to be common only in North America and Europe, but now have spread to other regions of the world, including Saudi Arabia, China, Russia, Latin America, and Asia.

The growing prevalence of eating disorders is caused, experts say, by young women trying to emulate advertising models and actors that they see on TV, in films and magazines, and on the Internet. These media present images of "ideal" women as unrealistically thin, which causes some women to lose social and psychological confidence in themselves; they attempt to regain it by disordered eating behaviors. For example, after the introduction of TV to the island of Fiji in 1995, the number of teenage girls with eating disorders rose from 3% to 15%. Fiji has only one TV station, which broadcasts shows from the United States, Australia, and the United

Kingdom. Whereas the increase might be attributable to something other than TV, researchers believe that the dramatic jump in the prevalence of eating disorders after the introduction of TV is the most plausible explanation.

In Argentina, aggressive advertising by the diet and cosmetic industries is generally recognized as contributing to an epidemic of eating disorders. Major newspapers distribute discount coupons for diet and liposuction clinics. And Argentine clothing manufacturers—out of step with international standards—size women's clothes much too small (e.g., a "medium" T-shirt that is more suitable for a preadolescent than an adult), reinforcing the idea that a woman must be extremely thin to be normal. The Argentine government and health establishment instituted a large media campaign of their own to educate young women on the dangers of believing what they see on TV, in the movies, and in magazines with respect to eating, body size, and cosmetic surgery.

---

drugs to lessen weight, are often considered normal and are even valued. Unfortunately, "thinner is better" activities rob the body of strength and energy, so they lead to decreased performance and occasionally illness. Also, acceptance of disturbed eating behaviors, overexercising, and compulsive attempts at perfecting performance can attract people to certain sports who are vulnerable to developing an eating disorder. Women athletes who expend many more calories than they consume risk developing the **female athlete triad**: cessation of menstruation (*amenorrhea*), disordered eating, and weak bones from osteoporosis.

Anorexia Nervosa

Anorexia nervosa is characterized by a relentless pursuit of thinness resulting in progressive weight loss and metabolic disturbances. Most of those affected are young women. Anorexia is not caused by any known disease-causing agent but by self-induced starvation, which can lead to serious illness and even death.

Elizabeth Barrett Browning (1806–1861), one of England's most famed poets, is thought to have had anorexia nervosa. As a teenager, Elizabeth was nagged by her parents to eat and gain weight, yet she stubbornly refused to eat much more than toast. When she met her future husband, poet Robert Browning, she weighed only 87 pounds. Apparently, the Barrett family possessed characteristics found in other families with an anorectic member: overprotectiveness, overinvolvement with each other, and inability to express or resolve intrafamilial conflict.

Persons with anorexia nervosa are likely to defend their emaciated appearance as normal and will insist that weight gain makes them feel fat. Besides distortions in normal body image, people with anorexia nervosa tend to be preoccupied with food. They may spend

an inordinate amount of time planning and preparing elaborate meals for others, while they themselves eat only a few bites and claim to be full. Often they will not eat in the presence of others; when they do, they may dawdle over their food. Some anorectic persons resort to self-induced vomiting or frequent use of diuretics or laxatives to reduce their body weight. These practices may lead to severe depletion of body minerals, which can precipitate abnormal heart rhythms and even cardiac arrest. Despite the low intake of calories, anorectic persons are remarkably energetic.

Persons with anorexia may see themselves as responding to demands of others rather than taking initiative in life. Young people with anorexia tend to be obedient, dutiful, helpful, and excellent students. Some psychologists interpret the intense preoccupation with weight loss as an expression of an underlying fear of incompetence. Control of eating and body weight becomes a way of demonstrating general control and competence.

TERMS

anorexia nervosa: disorder occurring most commonly in adolescent females, characterized by abnormal body image, fear of obesity, and prolonged refusal to eat, sometimes resulting in death

body dysmorphic disorder: a preoccupation with an imagined defect in one or more of one's body parts

body image: a person's mental image of his or her body

female athlete triad: combination of disordered eating, cessation of menstruation (amenorrhea), and weakened bones (osteoporosis)

That anorexia nervosa affects predominantly young women suggests that its roots lie in our society's preoccupation with slimness as a prerequisite to social success. Anorexia may also reflect an attempt to remain a child who is cared for and fed by others, who can be stubborn and obstinate, and who has no sexual identity or desires. Anorexia may also be a manifestation of a struggle for a sense of identity and personal effectiveness through controlling the environment; the resulting stubborn, rejecting behavior then becomes reinforced by the attention received from others. The family of the anorectic person becomes so engrossed with the symptoms that they avoid dealing with conflicts among themselves.

Three goals characterize the treatment of anorexia nervosa: (1) weight gain, (2) changed attitudes toward food and eating, and (3) resolution of underlying personal and family conflicts. Unfortunately, therapeutic intervention is not always successful and the condition may persist for years. Anorexia nervosa has a 15% to 20% mortality rate.

Bulimia

Bulimia is marked by a voluntary restriction of food intake followed by a binge–purge cycle: extreme overeating, usually of high-calorie junk foods, immediately followed by self-induced vomiting, use of diuretics or laxatives, or intense exercise. Like anorexia nervosa, bulimia occurs primarily in young women with a morbid fear of becoming fat, who pursue thinness relentlessly. Most bulimic persons are model individuals: good students, athletes, extremely sociable, and pleasant. Fearing discovery of their bulimic behavior, they frequently carry out their binge–purge episodes in private. Bulimic persons usually are aware that their binge–purge behavior is abnormal; however, they are unable to control it. Many feel guilty and depressed about their problem, which leads to a tendency to hide the behavior. Bulimia can pose a serious risk to health for many of the same reasons that anorexia does.

Several theories have been proposed to explain bulimia. One is that bulimia is a maladaptive way of dealing with anxiety, loneliness, and anger. Another suggests that bulimia is a manifestation of the drive to become the "ideal" woman, achieving the societal norm of slimness. Bulimic persons tend to have low self-esteem and a weak sense of identity.

Recovering from bulimia includes stopping binge–purge cycles and regaining control over eating behavior. Persons with bulimia must also establish more appropriate ways to handle unpleasant feelings and discomfort with close relationships, and their self-esteem must be improved. Often psychological counseling is helpful.

Binge Eating Disorder

Binge eating disorder is characterized by an uncontrolled consumption of large quantities of food in a short period of time, even if the person does not feel hungry. During binge episodes, food is consumed much faster than usual, and frequently the person is alone to avoid embarrassment about the amount of food eaten. A binge episode is often followed by feelings of disgust, depression, and guilt.

About 2% of adults in the United States (about 4 million people) have binge eating disorder, and most of them are overweight. About 10% to 15% of people who are mildly obese and who try to lose weight on their own or through commercial weight-loss programs have binge eating disorder. The disorder is even more common in people who are very overweight.

Many people with binge eating disorder have a history of depression and impulsive behavior (acting quickly without thinking). Many people who are binge eaters say that being angry, sad, bored, or worried can cause them to binge eat. People with binge eating disorder tend to be malnourished because they consume large amounts of fat and sugar, which have few essential nutrients.

Most people with binge eating disorder have tried to control it on their own, but are unable to control it for very long. People with binge eating disorder should get help from a health professional, which could include instruction in how to keep track of and change unhealthy eating behaviors, identifying social factors that contribute to the problem, psychological counseling, and medications.

It's in Your Hands

Successful weight management involves reducing intake of calories (often by recognizing the social and psychological reasons that cause overeating) and increasing the level of physical activity. Heavily advertised reducing schemes, such as body wraps, diet pills, and fad diets, are almost totally ineffective in producing permanent fat reduction and weight loss.

The primary reason that people are overfat is that their lifestyles do not include sufficient physical activity to use up the calories ingested in food. You can begin today to consciously watch what you eat and how much you exercise. When offered a cookie, decline. When you have the choice between the elevator and stairs, take the stairs. These efforts, which appear to be small, can make a difference when made daily and over an extended period of time.

> **▌TERMS▌**
>
> **binge eating disorder:** an uncontrolled consumption of large quantities of food in a short period of time, even if the person does not feel hungry
>
> **bulimia:** serious disorder, especially common in adolescents and young women, marked by excessive eating, often followed by self-induced vomiting, purging, or fasting

Critical Thinking About Health

1. Jordana couldn't stand herself anymore, so she went to the campus health center's peer nutrition counseling program for help.

   "I disgust myself," she told her counselor. "I'm fat, fat, fat and no matter what I do I can't change it. I jog, I don't eat ice cream. I suck."

   Jordana's BMI calculated out to 28.4. "It's a little on the high side," said the counselor, "but you're not in the danger zone."

   "Tell that to my Dad," Jordana snapped. "And my boyfriend. When they look at me, their eyes go right to my stomach. It's like that's all I am—a stomach on legs!"

   a. What expectations regarding body size and shape do you experience as a member of your sex?

   b. How were these expectations transmitted to you and by whom (or by what social institution)?

   c. How are these expectations enforced in your peer group, and what are the social penalties for not meeting such expectations?

   d. To what lengths do people go to meet these expectations? Are any of these practices extreme or unhealthy?

2. **Sam:** Oh, man, not Roni. She's too wide!

   Mick: No, she's not. She's real nice. Call her.

   Sam: Nah.

   Mick: You're a dweeb, sucker. You didn't like Nan because her face was too round. You didn't like Carla because she was too tall. You didn't like Evy because . . . why didn't you like Evy, anyway? I forget.

   Sam: Thunder thighs.

   Mick: You're going to wind up one lonely dude.

   a. Is Sam really destined to be lonely or is he being smart to wait for someone who matches his ideal of the perfect body?

   b. In your peer group, are there examples of people being attracted to people who do not resemble the ideal? Can you explain that discrepancy?

   c. What is the social purpose of an ideal body size and shape?

3. It is likely that in the near future there will be many drugs that are moderately effective in producing weight (fat) loss. It is also likely that these drugs will carry some risks to health.

   a. Do you think that such drugs should be made available to anyone who wants them, or should such medications be restricted to people whose weight puts them at serious risk for health problems and premature death?

   b. Besides potential harm from side effects, is it appropriate for people to depend on drugs for weight maintenance instead of modifying dietary and exercise habits and learning to reduce stress?

4. How have eating disorders touched your life?

Health in Review

- Approximately two-thirds of the U.S. population is overweight and at risk for a variety of illnesses, including heart disease, type 2 diabetes, hypertension, and gallbladder disease.

- Obesity is defined as having a body weight 20% (for men) and 30% (for women) over recommended weight for height or a body mass index greater than 30.

- Health problems are less likely when the waist-to-hip ratio is less than 0.8 (women) or 0.95 (men).

- Body fatness is maintained by neural and hormonal signals acting on the brain, which controls feelings of hunger and satiety. Many physiological, psychological, social, and environmental factors affect the brain and thus body weight.

- People eat for reasons other than hunger, such as social interaction, recreation, and relief from stress.

- Successful weight control involves changing eating and exercise habits.

- Healthy body weight corresponds to having a body mass index between 19 and 25. There are a variety of ways to achieve a healthy body weight. Starvation dieting is not one of them.

- Counseling, surgery, and medications can help some overweight people lose body fat and maintain a healthy body weight.

- There are three major ineffective weight-control schemes: body wraps, diet pills, and diet programs.

- Three common eating disorders are anorexia nervosa, bulimia, and binge eating disorder.

Health and Wellness Online

The Web contains a wealth of information about health and wellness. By accessing the Internet using Web browser software, you can gain a new perspective on many topics presented in *Health and Wellness,* Tenth Edition. Access the Jones and Bartlett Publishers Web site at **health.jbpub.com/hwonline.**

References

Dallman, M. F., Pecoraro, N. C., & la Fleur, S. E. (2005). Chronic stress and comfort foods: Self-medication and abdominal obesity. *Brain, Behavior, and Immunity, 19,* 275–280.

Flegal, K. M., et al. (2005). Cause-specific excess deaths associated with underweight, overweight, and obesity. *Journal of the American Medical Association, 298,* 2028–2037.

Frank, L. D., Andresen, M. A., & Schmid, T. L. (2004). Obesity relationships with community design, physical activity, and time spent in cars. *American Journal of Preventive Medicine, 27,* 87–96.

Freedman, M. R., King, J., & Kennedy, E. (2001). Popular diets: A scientific review. *Obesity Research, 9,* 1S–5S.

Gregg, E. W., & Guralnik, J. M. (2007). Is disability obesity's price of longevity? *Journal of the American Medical Association, 298,* 2066–2067.

Higgins, P. A. T., & Higgins, M. (2005). A healthy reduction in oil consumption and carbon emissions. *Energy Policy, 33,* 1–4.

Hunt, T. J., Thienhaus, M. D., & Ellwood, A. (2008). The mirror lies: Body dysmorphic disorder. *American Family Physician, 78,* 217–222.

Jones, L. R., Wilson, C. I., & Wadden, T. A. (2007). Lifestyle modification in the treatment of obesity: An educational challenge and opportunity. *Clinical Pharmacology and Therapeutics, 81,* 776–779.

Levine, J. A., et al. (2005). Interindividual variation in posture allocation: Possible role in human obesity. *Science, 307,* 584–586.

Levy, R. L., et al. (2007). Behavioral intervention for the treatment of obesity. Strategies and effectiveness data. *American Journal of Gastroenterology, 102,* 2314–2321.

McGinnis, J. M., et al. (2006). *Food marketing to children and youth: Threat or opportunity?* Washington, DC: National Academies Press.

Mehta, N. K., & Chang, V. W. (2008). Weight status and restaurant availability: A multilevel analysis. *American Journal of Preventive Medicine, 34,* 127–133.

Mokdad, A. H., et al. (2003). Prevalence of obesity, diabetes, and obesity-related health risk factors, 2001. *Journal of the American Medical Association, 289,* 76–79.

National Weight Control Registry. (2008). NWCR facts. Retrieved June 12, 2008, from http://www.nwcr.ws/Research/default.htm

Pope, H. G., et al. (2000). Body image perception among men in three countries. *American Journal of Psychiatry, 157,* 1297–1301.

Racette, S. B., et al. (2008). Changes in weight and health behaviors from freshman through senior year of college. *Journal of Nutrition Education and Behavior, 40,* 39–42.

Reinking, M. F., & Alexander, L. E. (2005). Prevalence of disordered-eating behaviors in undergraduate female collegiate athletes and nonathletes. *Journal of Athletic Training, 40,* 47–51.

Robinson, T. N. (2007). Effects of food branding on young children's taste preferences. *Archives of Pediatric and Adolescent Medicine, 161,* 792–797.

Rosenheck, R. (2008). Fast food consumption and increased caloric intake: A systematic review of a trajectory towards weight gain and obesity risk. *Obesity Reviews, 9,* 535–547.

Rucker, D., et al. (2007). Long term pharmacotherapy for obesity and overweight: Updated meta-analysis. *British Medical Journal, 335,* 1194–1199.

Slentz, C. A., et al. (2004). Effects of the amount of exercise on body weight, body composition, and measure of central obesity. *Archives of Internal Medicine, 164,* 31–39.

Svetkey, L. P., et al. (2008). Comparison of strategies for sustaining weight loss. *Journal of the American Medical Association, 299,* 1139–1148.

U.S. Centers for Disease Control. (2004). Trends in intake of energy and macronutrients—United States, 1971–2000. *Morbidity and Mortality Weekly Report, 53,* 80–82.

Wharton, C. M., Adams, T., and Hampl, J. S. (2008). Weight loss practices and body weight perceptions among U.S. college students. *Journal of American College Health, 56,* 579–584.

Yager, J. (2007). Assessment and determination of initial treatment approaches for patients with eating disorders. In Joel Yager and Pauline S. Powers (Eds.), *Clinical manual of eating disorders.* Washington, DC: American Psychiatric Publishers.

Young, L. R., & Nestle, M. (2007). Portion sizes and obesity: Responses of fast-food companies. *Journal of Public Health Policy, 28,* 238–248.

Suggested Readings

Bray, G. A. (2003). Low carbohydrate diets and the realities of weight loss. *Journal of the American Medical Association, 289*, 1853–1855. A noted researcher and physician explains weight-loss dynamics and how low-carbohydrate diets affect them.

Brownell, K. D. (2000). *The LEARN program for weight management* (10th ed.). New York: American Health Publishing. This is the most widely used weight-control manual in the world.

Eckel, R. H. (Ed.). (2003). *Obesity: Mechanisms and clinical management*. Philadelphia: Lippincott Williams & Wilkins. Addresses the development of obesity and its clinical management and discusses the worldwide epidemic of obesity in adults and children.

Fletcher, A. M. (1994). *Thin for life*. Boston, MA: Houghton Mifflin. Reports on the successful weight-loss/maintenance strategies of people in the National Weight Control Registry.

Ornish, D. (2000). *Eat more, weigh less: Dr. Dean Ornish's Advantage Ten program for losing weight safely while eating abundantly*. New York: Quill. You can eat more and weigh less if you know what to eat.

The truth about dieting. (2002, June). *Consumer Reports*, 26–31. A valuable report on weight loss.

Weil, A. (2000). *Eating well for optimum health: The essential guide to food, diet and nutrition*. New York: Knopf. The well-known physician describes his nutritional formula for supplying the basic needs of the body for calories and nutrients, reducing risks of disease, and fortifying the body's defenses and intrinsic mechanisms of healing.

Yager, J., & Anderson, A. E. (2005). Clinical practice: Anorexia nervosa. *New England Journal of Medicine, 353*, 1481–1488. An up-to-date review of the topic.

Recommended Web Sites

Please visit **health.jbpub.com/hwonline** for links to these Web sites.

American Obesity Association
Education, information, and advocacy on overweight and obesity.

Overweight and Obesity
Data and health recommendations from the U.S. Centers for Disease Control and Prevention.

Weight Control Information Network
The U.S. National Institutes of Health provides science-based information on overweight and weight control.

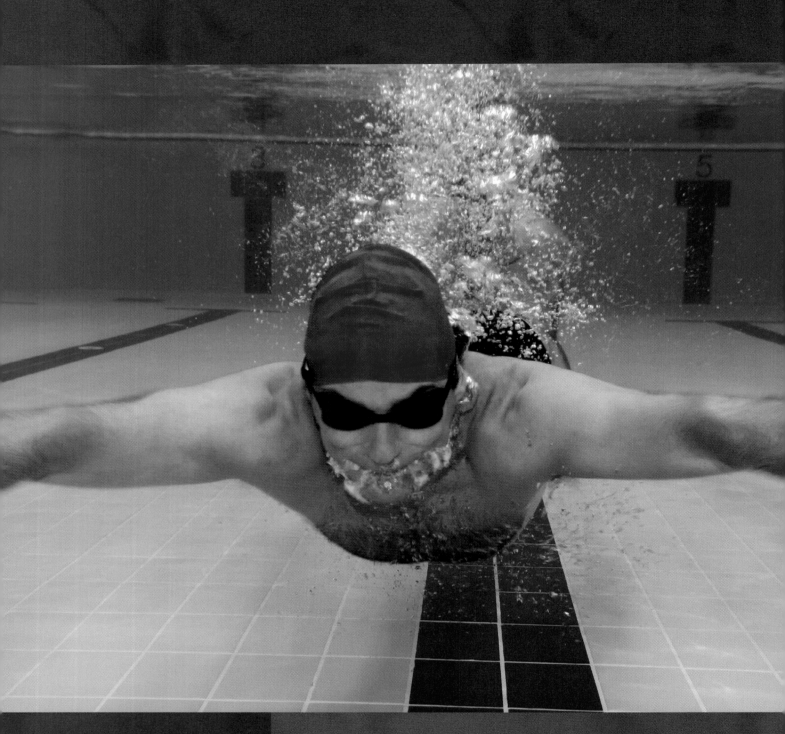

Chapter Seven

Physical Activity for Health and Well-Being

Learning Objectives

1. Define *sedentary lifestyle* and identify reasons for its current prevalence.

2. List the four categories of physical activity: household tasks, work-related movement, leisure-time activities, and performance-based activities.

3. Explain three different measurements of physical activity: calories per minute, METs, and PAL.

4. Describe levels of physical activity for health.

5. List the six components of physical activity: motivation, cardiorespiratory fitness, body strength, endurance, flexibility, and body composition.

6. Describe guidelines for integrating physical activity into one's life.

7. Discuss the types of performance-enhancing substances.

8. Define *overuse injuries*.

9. Discuss exercising in hot and cold weather.

Everyone knows that regular physical activity is good for health, helping the mind and body to function best and in harmony. Conversely, a lack of regular physical activity, or a **sedentary lifestyle** (from the Latin *sedere*, meaning to sit), contributes to ill health, including an increased risk of heart disease, overweight, type 2 diabetes, high blood pressure, osteoporosis, some forms of cancer, and other illnesses (U.S. Department of Health and Human Services, 1996). A sedentary lifestyle is also associated with nearly 15% of premature deaths among Americans, particularly deaths related to heart disease and overweight (Mokdad et al., 2004; see Chapter 1).

Worldwide, nearly 60% of adults lead sedentary lives (many people work while sitting), which contributes to hundreds of millions of cases of chronic disease and millions of premature deaths each year (World Health Organization, 2004). About 50% of American adults, including college students, do not get recommended amounts of physical activity, which means they exercise at home, school, work, or during leisure time for less than 30 minutes a day on most days of the week.

A sedentary lifestyle is a new dimension in human history. For 99% of the many thousands of years that humans have inhabited the earth, adults have had to walk, run, lift, bend, and carry in order to find and raise their own food, provide themselves with shelter, raise children, and protect themselves. However, starting about 200 years ago and accelerating greatly in the twentieth century, people began using machines to carry out all manner of activities (**Table 7.1**). Now, most of the North American labor force works in occupations that involve sitting at a desk, standing behind a counter, or occasionally walking a few steps while tending to others' needs and requests.

Regardless of the type of work, over 90% of Americans travel to their jobs while sitting in a car (Purcher & Renne, 2003). Furthermore, when they get home, even if they have few household tasks to do, many people watch TV, play video games, or interact with the Internet rather than move their bodies (other than to go to the refrigerator). It is estimated that people living in modern, industrialized societies expend almost half as much energy each day carrying out the tasks of living than ancient humans did (Booth et al., 2002) (**Table 7.2**).

Although it has freed people from considerable physical labor, the integration of work-saving machines into the fabric of modern life has had the inadvertent consequence of increasing risks to health from too little physical activity. Thus, to prevent a decline in health from physical inactivity in daily life, people *must* engage in some form(s) of movement during nonpaid/nonhousehold work time—not an easy assignment for those whose schedules are overfull with tasks and other responsibilities or who hate the word *exercise* and disdain anything that causes them to breathe hard and sweat.

Recognizing that physical inactivity is detrimental to health, many countries, communities, health professionals, public health organizations, schools, employers, and religious organizations are seeking ways to encourage people to be more physically active, as the following illustrate:

- The U.S government, the European Union, the World Health Organization, and other governmental bodies have made engaging in physical activity national goals and are developing

Table 7.1

Twentieth-Century Innovations That Contribute to Reduced Physical Activity

Year	Innovation
1900	Modern escalator invented
1901	Vacuum cleaner invented
1903	Airplane invented by the Wright brothers
1904	Tractor invented
1906	First Mack trucks built
1908	Ford begins to mass produce and sell Model T automobile
1923	Frozen food invented
1923	Television invented
1950	First automatic elevators
1951	First computers sold commercially
1954	First McDonald's
1956	Establishment of U.S. Interstate Highway System
1976	Apple home computer invented
1981	First IBM PC sold
1990	World Wide Web/Internet protocol and language created

Source: Transportation Research Board, Institute of Medicine. (2005). *Does the built environment influence physical activity?* Washington, DC: National Academy of Sciences.

Table 7.2

Activities Contributing to Total Energy Expenditure (TEE) Among American Adults

Activity	Percent Contribution to TEE
Driving a car	10.9
Job: Office work, typing	9.2
Watching TV/home theater	8.6
Taking care of child/baby	8.4
Activities performed while sitting/lying	5.8
Eating (implied sitting)	5.3
Household activities	3.9
Talking/visiting (phone/in-person)	3.8
Job: Industrial/factory (assembly line)	3.8
Food preparation	2.9
Total	62.3

Source: L. Dong et al. (2004). Activities contributing to total energy expenditure in the United States. *International Journal of Behavior, Nutrition, and Physical Activity, 1,* 4–10.

programs that encourage individuals to devote 30 minutes a day to some sort of movement activity.

- Employees receive company-supplied training and time at work to engage in various types of physical activities.
- New housing developments are required to include inviting public spaces, parks, walking and biking paths, and close access to public transportation and shopping to minimize driving.
- Walking during work hours is encouraged by placing parking lots some distance from buildings, giving employees pedometers, resetting elevators to run slowly, and making staircases wide, carpeted, brightly painted, and with picture windows.
- Communities designate and maintain "safe walking" routes for schoolchildren and adult walkers.
- Colleges, universities, churches, and other organizations offer programs that encourage walking and other types of physical activity.

The Defintion of Physical Activity

Physical activity is anything you do when you are not sitting or lying down, from clicking your computer's mouse to running a marathon. Among Americans and residents of developed countries, physical activity occurs in the following contexts (**Table 7.3**):

- *Doing household tasks*, such as washing the floor, being with and taking care of children, and gardening
- *Work-related movement*, for example, walking from a desk to the elevator, being a server in a restaurant, or working in construction

- *Leisure-time activities*, such as taking a walk or engaging in recreational exercise such as dancing, running, swimming, or tennis
- *Skill-based performance activities*, for example, exercising the body (or specific body regions) in order to excel at a particular activity or sport

Physical activity is scientifically defined in terms of the amount of energy expended to produce movement. Movement occurs when energy derived from food is utilized by muscles that are connected to bones to shorten (*concentric contraction*) or lengthen (*eccentric contraction*). When muscles shorten or lengthen, the bones they are attached to move, and so do you (**Figure 7.1**).

Energy for movement is derived principally from carbohydrate and fat—and on occasion the amino acids in protein, but not vitamins and minerals—which the body acquires from food and can store until needed (see Chapter 5). There are four calories of energy in a gram of carbohydrate and protein, and nine calories of energy in a gram of fat. Energy can be derived from food with or without the addition of oxygen. Oxygen-absent energy production is called **anaerobic**; oxygen-present energy production is called **aerobic**. Compared with oxygen-

TERMS

aerobic: biological energy production using oxygen
anaerobic: biological energy production without using oxygen
sedentary lifestyle: a pattern of living that lacks physical activity sufficient for good health

Table 7.3

Comparison of Energy Used in Various Physical Activities

Context	Moderate intensity (4–7 calories/minute, 3–6 METs)	Vigorous intensity (7+ calories/minute, 6+ METs)
Household	Gardening	Shoveling snow
	Scrubbing a floor	Pushing a lawn mower
	Carrying a child	Active play with a child
Work	Sawing with a power saw	Hand sawing hard woods
	Waiting tables	Firefighting
	Packing boxes for shipping	Loading/unloading a truck
Leisure	Walking 3–4 miles per hour	Jogging/running
	Yoga	Circuit weight training
	Dancing (most kinds)	Tennis (singles)
Performance	Weight training	Circuit weight training
	Shooting baskets	Football practice
	Skateboarding	Long-distance running

METs, metabolic equivalents.
Source: U.S. Centers for Disease Control and Prevention. General physical activities defined by level of intensity.
Available: http://www.cdc.gov/nccdphp/dnpa/physical/everyone/measuring/index.htm. Note: This source lists values for dozens of activities.

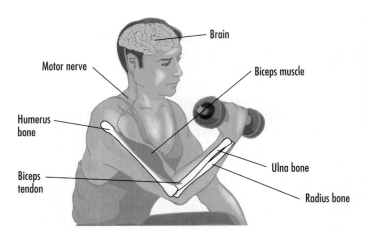

Figure 7.1

The Human Movement System
The human movement system consists of muscles, bones, tendons (which attach muscles to bones), and ligaments (which attach bones to bones). Movement occurs when the brain sends a signal via a specific nerve connecting it to a specific muscle. If the nerve signal directs a muscle to shorten, the two bones it connects move toward each other. If the nerve signal directs the muscle to lengthen, the two bones it connects move away from each other.

absent, oxygen-present energy production is nearly 20 times more efficient, which is the major reason you breathe.

Oxidation is the chemical term for the process of oxygen-present energy production. *Burning* is another term for the process of oxidation. When biological material is burned in a fire, oxidation generates very little useful energy and considerable heat. When carbohydrate and fat are burned in cells, oxidation is controlled to capture the energy for useful work and to minimize energy lost as heat. So, when you hear the expression "burn calories," it means extracting energy to fuel cellular processes and not melting fat with heat.

The nervous system controls movement by signaling muscles to contract. Some movements are *reflexive*, meaning they do not require a conscious decision, for example, when quickly pulling your hand from a hot stove. A *voluntary movement* involves both decision and movement-control centers in the brain, which send nerve signals to specific muscles, resulting in movement.

Physical activity is measured in terms of calories used per minute, metabolic equivalents, or physical activity level, as follows:

- *Calories used per minute.* A nutritional or movement calorie is scientifically defined as the energy equivalent of the amount of heat energy required to raise a kilogram of water from 15.5 to 16.5. Muscles do not use heat as an energy source; energy is chemically extracted from carbohydrate and fat within muscle cells and provided directly to the tissue that creates movement. A calorie can fuel about 25 steps of walking. The calories utilized in various physical activities are presented in Table 7.3

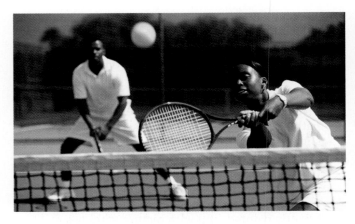

Tennis is an excellent form of exercise at any age.

- *Metabolic equivalents (METs).* **Metabolic equivalents,** or **METs,** are per-minute multiples of the amount of energy used while sitting or lying still, which is defined as 1 MET. For people of average size, 1 MET is about 1.2 calories. Moderate physical activity utilizes 3 to 6 METs; vigorous physical activity utilizes more than 6 METs (see Table 7.3).
- *Physical activity level (PAL).* **Physical activity level (PAL)** is a measure of the amount of energy expended per day over and above that required for *basal* or *resting* metabolism, which is the energy needed to fuel basic life functions (i.e., heart beat, breathing, kidney and brain function, etc.) (see Chapter 5). A person is considered sedentary if the PAL is less than 1.4, that is, the daily energy expended to fuel all forms of movement is less than 1.4 times the energy expended in basal metabolism. PAL values between 1.4 and 1.7 indicate a moderate level of physical activity. PALs greater than 1.7 indicate a vigorous level of physical activity (**Figure 7.2**).

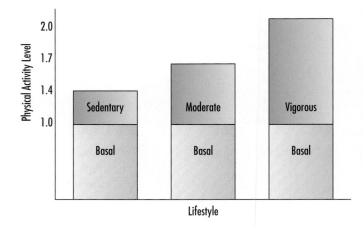

Figure 7.2

Physical Activity Levels
Physical activity level (PAL) is the amount of daily energy expended over and above a person's basal or resting metabolism, which is the energy required to fuel basic life functions while at rest.

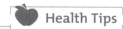 Health Tips

Incorporate Exercise in Your Daily Activities

- At school or work, take fitness breaks by walking or doing desk exercises instead of taking food breaks. If you are the social type, take a friend on a talk-walk.
- Exercise while watching TV (for example, use hand weights, a stationary bicycle, treadmill, or stair climber, or stretch).

Any movement or activity can be discussed in terms of the following (FITT) dimensions:

- **F**requency: how often the movement or activity occurs
- **I**ntensity: the energy required to render the movement or activity
- **T**ime: how long the movement or activity takes place
- **T**ype or mode: the kind of movement or activity

For example, you can walk (*type*) for 10 minutes (*time*) to a particular class three times a week (*frequency*) at a pace utilizing 4 calories per minute (*intensity*). Thus, each walk to class utilizes 40 calories of energy, with a resulting expenditure of about 120 calories per week (10 minutes × 4 calories per minute).

Physical Activity for Health

Many studies show that moderate amounts of regular physical activity, whether it is household, work-related, leisure-time, or performance-enhancing, counteracts the deleterious effects of sedentariness and contributes to health and well-being in a variety of ways (**Table 7.4**). A moderate amount of physical activity expends between 1.4 and 1.7 times the energy required for basal metabolism, which for most people amounts to 120 and 300 calories per day of activity, or a total of about 600 to 1,500 calories per week.

The scientifically based finding that moderate levels of physical activity are beneficial to health stands in stark contrast to the exhortations of the health club, exercise equipment, dietary supplement, and fashion industries, as well as the advertising, popular magazines, and TV infomercials that support them, which would have people believe that physical activity for health requires considerable time, energy, special equipment and clothing, painful effort, and sweating a lot in order to attain a svelte, lean body (and for men one that is highly muscular or "cut")—appearances more suited to computer-enhanced images than real people. You do not have to run like an Olympic athlete or look like a model in a fitness advertisement to be healthy.

An efficient way to attain a moderate level of physical activity is to walk briskly for 30 to 45 minutes on

Table 7.4
Health Benefits of Physical Activity
Puts into life the good feelings and enjoyment that come from body movement
Increases the ability to cope effectively with stress
Increases endurance in daily activities and lessens fatigue
Increases longevity
Strengthens the heart muscle
Decreases the heart rate
Increases blood flow to the heart
Maintains normal blood pressure and reduces high blood pressure
Increases blood levels of high-density lipoproteins (good) cholesterol
Reduces blood levels of low-density lipoproteins (bad) cholesterol
Reduces blood levels of triglycerides (fats)
Boosts the immune system, thus lessening the risk of colds and other infections
Enhances sleep
Maintains a healthy body weight
Improves food choices
Increases bone mass and reduces the risk of osteoporosis
Prevents and alleviates chronic low back pain
Lessens the desire to smoke cigarettes and consume alcohol and drugs
Lessens depression
Enhances self-image, self-esteem, and creativity

most days of the week. Your pace should be such that your heart and breathing rates increase slightly but not so much that you could not carry on a conversation while walking; for most people, this pace is about 3 to 4 miles per hour. Also, you should experience a light to moderate increase in **relative perceived exertion**, which is awareness of one's relative response to exercise (sensations of effort and muscular force, breathing rate, and body and skin temperature).

Although it seems tame in comparison to running on a treadmill, walking is nevertheless excellent for health (Murphy et al., 2007). It strengthens the heart and skeletal muscles, increases breathing ability, clears and quiets the mind, reduces stress, uses calories (weight maintenance), and causes few injuries, if any. Other

TERMS

metabolic equivalents (METs): per-minute multiples of the amount of energy used while lying still

oxidation: the chemical term for the process of oxygen-present energy production

physical activity level (PAL): a measure of the amount of energy expended per day over and above that used for basal metabolism

relative perceived exertion: awareness of one's relative response to exercise

than appropriate shoes, walking requires no special clothing or equipment, and with a little preplanning, can be worked into any busy schedule; you can break up the total walking time into several small parts and attain the same health benefits. Walk stairs instead of riding an elevator, park the car 10 minutes from your destination and walk the rest of the way, take a dog for a walk twice a day (Fido will be forever grateful), do a walk-talk with a friend, family member, or spouse (good for relationship maintenance and also fun), and make it a habit to walk around while you talk on your mobile phone.

Many people find that counting their daily steps with a **pedometer**, a pager-size device that clips to the waist, leg, or shoe, helps keep them focused on walking (Bravata et al., 2007). An average-sized person takes 2,000 steps to walk a mile. Health experts recommend taking a total of 10,000 steps per day in all one's activities combined—15,000 if possible—and keeping a step-count diary that records not only the number of steps you take but also any obstacles that prevented you from walking as much as you wanted to.

People who enjoy vigorous physical activities (e.g., running, swimming laps, singles tennis) should do them at least three days a week for 20 minutes each time. Vigorous activities have PALs of between 1.7 and 2.5. They utilize seven or more calories per minute, make you breathe hard and sweat, and are sufficiently intense that you could not talk to anyone while doing them. Compared with moderate physical activity, vigorous physical activity provides slightly greater heart-health benefits and longevity (O'Donovan et al., 2005) (**Figure 7.3**). However, it also carries a higher risk of physical injury and psychological burnout, either of which can curtail activity for weeks or even months.

Besides direct effects on health, both moderate and vigorous physical activity can provide time and attention for you. Many people feel overwhelmed by the demands of school, jobs, and family. Just taking a few minutes several days a week to move your body can give you a chance to relax, reflect, and indulge your imagination. Also, physical activity can improve mental functioning and contribute to enhanced work performance (Hillman et al., 2008).

Components of Physical Activity

Although your whole being responds to movement, it is possible to identify the following six components of physical activity:

1. *Motivation:* the willingness to focus attention and energy on movement
2. *Cardiorespiratory fitness:* the body's ability to obtain and utilize fuel and oxygen efficiently during sustained, effortful physical activity
3. *Body strength:* the ability to lift or move an object (including your body, as when you walk or climb stairs)
4. *Endurance:* the ability to move an object (including yourself) without becoming quickly fatigued
5. *Flexibility:* the ability to move a joint (where two bones meet) through its anatomical range of motion
6. *Body composition:* the body's relative amounts of water, bone, fat, and tissue

These six components and activities that promote them are discussed in the following subsections.

Motivation

Your ancient ancestors did not require specific motivation to be physically active. Because they had to move their bodies to acquire food and avoid environmental dangers, hunger and fear were motivation enough for movement. Most modern humans can eat and be safe without much daily movement; indeed, many occupations require little movement. Thus, to gain the health benefits from movement, other motivations must come into play, including the following:

- Being paid, such as in an employer-sponsored exercise class
- Desiring to be healthy
- Desiring to "look good"
- Enjoying socializing while engaged in a movement activity
- Accomplishing a personal goal, such as losing weight, climbing a mountain, running a distance race, or biking 50 miles

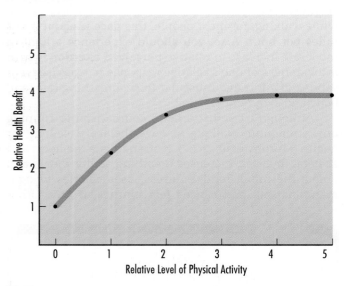

■ Figure 7.3

Relative Health Benefit of Physical Activity

The graph is a composite from many studies that demonstrate the positive effect of physical activity on health. Notice that the graph is not linear; the largest benefit comes from changing from a sedentary lifestyle to one with low-to-moderate levels of physical activity. High levels of physical activity do not produce corresponding gains in health. Health benefits include lessened risk of morbidity and mortality from cardiovascular disease, cancer, hypertension, and type 2 diabetes. Each level of physical activity (e.g., walking, running, cycling) corresponds to between 500 and 1,000 calories per week of activity.

Regardless of the motivation, it is important that one's chosen physical activities be enjoyable, or at the very least, not objectionable. Doing enjoyable activities promotes continuing with them. If what you do is unpleasant, however, you won't do it for very long. This might mean experimenting with several types of activities in order to find ones that you are likely to make a regular part of your life. It might mean engaging in more than one activity to break up monotony and boredom. **Cross-training** is incorporating more than one activity into your regular activity plan, for example, walking four days a week and doing strength training or cycling two days a week (and resting one day).

Also, it is important to realize that obstacles to accomplishing one's movement goals arise frequently. Regardless of your motivation and dedication, there may be weeks or even months when getting your desired level of physical activity is a challenge. Perhaps you get sick or injured. Perhaps your schedule is very tight and there seems to be no time for anything but work. Perhaps you lose interest in former activities. At such times it is important not to become so discouraged that you give up wanting physical activity in your life. Realize that obstacles are to be expected and that they will pass in time. When they do, you can resume your desired activities or replace them with better alternatives.

Cardiorespiratory Fitness

Cardiorespiratory fitness is the degree to which the body can supply sufficient fuel (carbohydrate, fatty acids, and oxygen) to produce sustained, effortful physical activity—in other words, the degree to which someone is "in shape." Exercise physiologists define cardiorespiratory fitness in terms of the maximum amount of oxygen the body can utilize in physical activity, called VO_2 *max* ("volume of oxygen maximal"). Studies show that higher fitness levels, defined by VO_2 max, are associated with a lower risk of death from cardiovascular disease (O'Donovan et al., 2005). It is not known how cardiorespiratory fitness reduces the risk of heart disease; one suggestion is that it lowers blood levels of total and bad cholesterol and triglycerides, which are progenitors of heart disease (see Chapter 14). Cardiovascular fitness also lowers the heart rate.

Because modern lifestyles do not require vigorous physical activity in the carrying out of daily life tasks, attaining high levels of cardiorespiratory fitness requires planned bouts of sustained, high-intensity, vigorous activity, called **aerobic training**.

Aerobic Training

Aero is derived from Greek, meaning air. With regard to physical activity,

- *Aerobic* means requiring oxygen.
- *Aerobic exercise* is any activity that requires the body to use more oxygen than it does in usual activities.
- *Aerobic capacity* is the extent to which an individual can perform aerobic exercise.

- *Aerobic training* is engaging in aerobic exercises *on a regular basis* to increase the amount of oxygen the body can process in a given time. Aerobic training requires that the heart and lungs work harder than usual to provide oxygen to exercising muscles. In this way, they become more efficient in acquiring and delivering oxygen to the body, both during exercise and at rest.

Three to four days of exercise per week are sufficient to produce a training effect. Two days per week may suffice for people already in good condition. One day a week does little to improve fitness and may increase the chances for injury. Also, exercising more than five days a week does little to increase fitness. It does expend calories, but it also makes one susceptible to injuries.

When aerobic training is carried out over a period of time, the resultant physiological changes in the heart, lungs, and muscles are called the **training effect**. You induce the training effect by exercising such that the heart rate during exercise increases to between 60% and 80% of its theoretical maximum. This is called your **target heart rate**. To determine your target heart rate:

- Calculate your theoretical maximum heart rate (MHR) by subtracting your age from 220.
- Multiply your MHR by 60% and 80% to determine the upper and lower limits of your target heart rate, called the *target zone* or *target heart rate zone*.

For example, for a 20-year-old, the MHR is 200 (220 – 20), and the lower and upper limits of the target zone are 120 (60% × 200) and 160 (80% × 200) heart beats per minute (see **Table 7.5**).

A session of aerobic exercise should begin with about 10 minutes of warm-up activity during which heart rate gradually increases (**Figure 7.4**). As the intensity of activity increases, the target zone heart rate is attained and maintained for 20 to 30 minutes. This is followed by a cool-down period during which the heart rate returns to preexercise levels. You can obtain your heart rate with a heart rate monitor, a device you strap to your chest or

---

TERMS

aerobic training: exercise that increases the body's capacity to use oxygen

cardiorespiratory fitness: the degree to which the body can supply sufficient fuel and oxygen to produce sustained, effortful physical activity

cross-training: incorporating more than one activity into a regular activity plan

pedometer: a step-counter

target heart rate: the heart rate during strenuous exercise associated with inducing the training effect

training effect: beneficial physiological changes as a result of aerobic exercise

Table 7.5

Maximum and Target Heart Rates Predicted from Age

Take your pulse for 15 seconds immediately after exercising, and multiply by 4. If heart rate is in the target range for your age, optimal training benefits have been obtained. If below target range, step up activity. If above the maximum, take it easier during workouts and gradually increase intensity.

Age (in years)	Predicted maximum heart rate (in beats per minute)	Target heart rate range (in beats per minute)
20	200	120–160
25	200	117–156
30	194	114–152
35	188	111–148
40	182	108–144
45	176	105–140
50	171	102–136
55	165	99–132
60	159	96–128
65	153	93–124

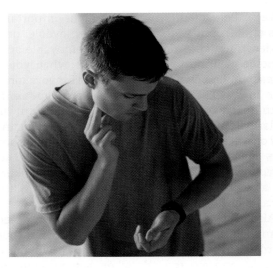

■ **Figure 7.5**

Measuring Your Heart Rate
Place your index and middle finger below the base of the thumb or at the side of the throat (Adam's apple). Press firmly until you feel the pulsations. Count the beats for 15 seconds. Multiply by 4 to get heart rate in beats per minute.

wrist, or by counting your heart beats at your wrist or carotid artery (**Figure 7.5**).

Body Strength

Body strength is the ability of a muscle or group of muscles to move an object, including your body. Whereas it often conjures up images of supermuscular body builders lifting heavy weights, body strength for health requires minimal, if any, change in body size and lifting of weights. The goal is to have sufficient strength to carry out normal tasks (work, lifting packages, walking stairs, shoveling snow) and participate in physical activities without injury. Two popular ways to increase body strength are strength training and Pilates.

Strength Training

Strength training (also called resistance training) involves building muscle and bone strength by repetitively moving individual muscles or muscle groups against resistance, commonly applied by weights, such as barbells, dumbbells, and exercise machines, and also by pushing against an immovable object (**isometric training**). Some of the benefits of strength training include the following:

- Enhanced ability to combat fatigue in everyday activities
- Improved fitness
- Preventing and rehabilitating orthopedic (musculoskeletal) injuries
- Reduction in body fat

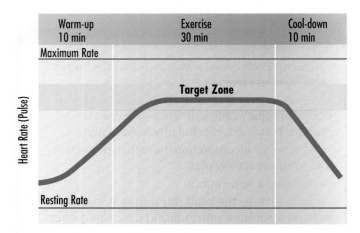

■ **Figure 7.4**

Heart Rate Pattern for a Typical Exercise Routine
A diagram of heart rate during warm-up, aerobic exercise, and cool-down.

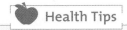 Health Tips

Weight Training Dos and Don'ts

Do
- Use spotters when trying major lifts
- Keep your back straight when lifting
- Use proper lifting technique
- Wear shoes with good traction
- Use equipment that is in good condition
- Follow safety rules

Don't
- Hyperventilate or hold your breath—breathe out when you press
- Continue if you feel pain; ice the painful region
- Lift if you feel lightheaded
- Exercise a set of muscles more than three times per week
- Cheat on technique to lift heavier weights

- Increased basal metabolic rate
- Decreased blood pressure
- Lower risk for cardiovascular disease
- Lessen low back pain

Many people imagine that the goal of strength training is to enlarge greatly the size of the body's muscles. This is an image proffered by the media (and advertising to sell dietary supplements) that idealizes a muscular body as a sign of attractiveness. Many men believe that a large, muscular body is the definition of masculinity (Pope, 2001). However, from a health point of view, the goal of strength training is stronger muscles, not necessarily bigger ones. Strength training for health means having the strength to participate without hindrance in activities of daily living (lifting packages, walking stairs, shoveling snow) and the ability to move muscles over a period of time (endurance). Strength training to increase muscle size is a very specialized activity (*body building*).

To engage in strength training for health and fitness, the American College of Sports Medicine (2002) recommends the following for healthy adults:

- Follow a specific activity plan (workout) two to three times a week.
- Perform 8 to 10 resistance exercises per workout.
- Exercise all major muscle groups.
- Repeat each exercise 8 to 12 times ("reps").
- Use an amount of weight that can be moved the desired number of times.
- Breathe normally while exercising.
- Move a muscle or muscle group through the full range of motion.
- Warm up prior to and cool down after an exercise session.

Whereas gyms and health clubs can supply all manner of strength training equipment, one needs only a few 5- or 10-pound dumbbells and a simple training program to derive considerable health benefits from strength training.

Strength training can involve progressive increases in the time, intensity, and amount of weight moved. Muscle strength is built by moving heavy weights a few times per set, whereas endurance is built by moving smaller weights through many repetitions. Also, in an extended training program, the repetitions, number of sets, amount of weight, and other exercise variables should vary (called periodization). To avoid injury (see the Health Tip "Weight Training Dos and Don'ts"), it is imperative that one receive professional assistance in the design of a strength training program and professional instruction in strength training methods.

Compared with most aerobic exercise, strength training produces only a modest improvement in cardiovascular fitness. The time spent exercising is insufficient to increase the heart rate long enough to produce a training effect. The energy expended during strength training is about four calories per minute, nearly the same as for walking or swimming at a comfortable pace.

A common myth associated with strength training is that consuming high-protein foods and special vitamin

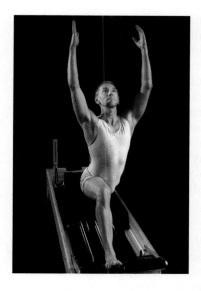

The Pilates method strengthens core muscles.

supplements will increase muscle mass. This assumption is incorrect. Muscle tissue responds to the demands of work, not to food. In a progressive strength training regimen, sufficient protein to build new muscle tissue will be obtained in a well-balanced diet. Excess protein and vitamins are simply excreted.

Pilates

Pilates is a widely used method of body conditioning developed by Joseph H. Pilates (pronounced Puh-lah-tees) in the 1920s. Pilates was born in Germany in 1880 and was a frail child with asthma and rickets who was determined to be strong. He was interned in England during World War I because of his German citizenship. While in England, he became a nurse and began designing exercise apparatus for immobilized hospital patients. The devices and exercises became the foundation for his method of body conditioning and strengthening. In 1926, he moved to New York City and opened his first Pilates Studio. The body building and fitness regimen he developed became widely used all over the world by dancers, actors, sports teams, spas, and fitness enthusiasts. Dancers such as Martha Graham and George Balanchine were among the first to adopt his fitness techniques. Today, his exercises are recommended by physical therapists, chiropractors, and others.

The Pilates method consists of hundreds of stretching and strengthening exercises that are performed on a mat

TERMS

isometric training: a type of strength training

Pilates: a system of stretching and strengthening exercises

strength training: the use of resistance to increase one's ability to exert or resist force for the purpose of improving performance with or without Pilates rings and other devices used to assist in strengthening muscles. Many of the exercises are designed to strengthen the back, abdomen, and buttocks; Pilates believed that these regions were the core of strength and the basis of good posture. Like yoga, the Pilates method emphasizes a balance of mind, body, and spirit. Rather than performing many repetitions of exercises, Pilates advocated intense mental concentration on performing each exercise with precision and awareness. Although developed many years ago, the Pilates exercises are still widely used to improve strength and performance and for overall body conditioning.

Endurance

Endurance is the ability to move an object, including yourself, without becoming quickly fatigued. Endurance is a combination of fitness, strength, and motivation. The fitness aspects of endurance relate to the body's ability to acquire and utilize oxygen, carbohydrate, and fat to fuel movement for an extended period of time. The strength aspect of endurance involves having sufficiently strong muscles to carry out an activity for an extended period without damage. The motivational aspect of endurance is the will to carry on with an activity even though you feel fatigued.

Endurance develops by extending yourself past former limits of physical activity. In this way, the anatomy and physiology of the heart, lungs, muscles, and energy-supplying and energy-utilizing systems, and your own expectations of your ability to persevere, gradually adapt to meet the challenges of extended activity. Endurance training generally involves both aerobic and strength training activities.

Flexibility

Flexibility is the degree to which you can rotate, bend, and twist a part of your body. Rotating, bending, and twisting occur where bones meet, an anatomical structure called a *joint*. For example, your elbow is a joint at which the two lower arm bones attach to the upper arm bone, allowing you to bend your arm. Imagine how difficult arm movement would be if you had no elbow joint.

Joints are held together by ligaments and tendons, which are elastic, fibrous bands of *connective tissue*. Flexibility is determined by the pliability of a joint's connective tissue and associated muscles. Every joint has a **range of motion**, which is the amount of rotating, bending, or twisting that the anatomy of the joint allows. Satisfactory flexibility is being able to move a joint through its full range of motion. Satisfactory flexibility contributes the following health benefits:

- Lessens the effort in carrying out physical tasks, such as lifting a package or bending to pick up something
- Fosters good balance, which aids mobility and reduces the risk of falling

- Reduces bodily and psychic tension resulting from stress
- Lessens the risk of low back pain
- Reduces exercise-associated soreness
- Improves blood flow to muscles
- Lessens the risk of activity-related injuries

Movement at a joint can increase its flexibility; lack of movement can reduce it. That is one reason that exercisers feel "loose" after activity, whereas sedentary people tend to feel stiff and have difficulty bending. Flexibility at a particular joint can be fostered by specific stretching exercises (**Figure 7.6**). Each joint's flexibility is independent of other joints; that is, you can be more flexible at one joint than you are at another. Activities such as yoga and tai chi ch'uan, which are discussed next, help increase flexibility at many joints simultaneously.

Yoga

Yoga is a system of exercises formulated in India thousands of years ago to unite one's mind and body. The word *yoga* means to join or yoke together. Of the several kinds of yoga, the most common is *hatha yoga*, which uses body postures, called poses or *asanas*, breathing techniques *(pranayama)*, and meditation to bring the body, mind, and spirit into healthy harmony (see Appendix A, Exercise 4). In yoga practice, one pays attention to the physical, mental, and spiritual effects of doing each posture (called *observing*). Also, yoga's breathing techniques increase a sense of positive energy and minimize negative inner self-talk.

Yoga is best learned in a class taught by an experienced practitioner. The method is generally practiced for 30 minutes at a time, two or more days a week. A combination of postures, called the Sun Salute, can be done daily to increase flexibility and bring the mind and body into harmony (**Figure 7.7**). The principal physical benefits of yoga are enhancing muscular fitness and body flexibility; the exercises are not sufficiently strenuous to produce significant cardiovascular benefit. Nevertheless, yoga can help reduce risk factors for cardiovascular disease, high blood pressure, and diabetes. It also helps reduce symptoms of osteoarthritis.

TERMS

endurance: the ability to move an object without becoming quickly fatigued

flexibility: the degree to which one can rotate, bend, and twist a part of the body

range of motion: the amount of rotating, bending, or twisting allowed by the anatomy of a joint

yoga: a system of exercises formulated in India thousands of years ago to unite one's mind and body

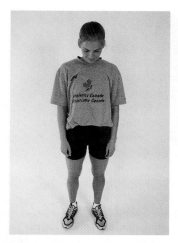

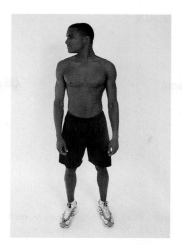

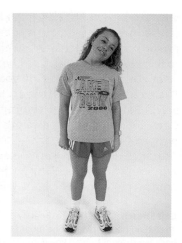

Neck   Drop your chin to your chest. Turn your head as far right as you can without moving your shoulders and hold. Repeat to the left. Tilt your head toward the left ear without bending your torso or hunching your shoulders and hold. Repeat to the right.

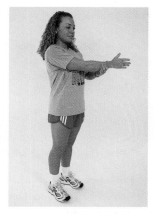

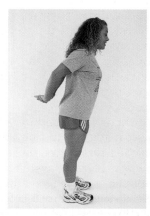

Shoulder Stretch 1   With your left hand, grasp your right elbow and pull your arm across your chest, keeping it bent at a 90° angle. Alternate arms.

Shoulder Stretch 2   Standing, grasp both arms behind your back and raise them up as far as you can.

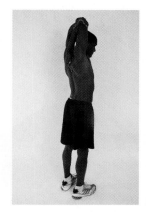

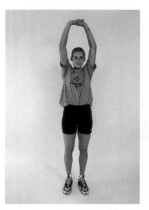

Triceps Stretch   Grasp the opposite elbow and pull the arm behind the head and down until a stretch is felt in the back of the arm. Hold and then repeat for the other arm.

Upper-back Stretch   Clasp your hands in front of your body, and press your palms forward.

(*continued on next page*)

■ **Figure 7.6**

Flexibility Exercises

It is best to do stretching exercises when the muscles are warm. You should stretch to the point of *mild* discomfort, but stop immediately if you experience pain—particularly in the lower back or knees. Hold all stretches for 15 to 30 seconds, rest for 30 to 60 seconds, and then repeat the stretch, trying to go a little further. For all standing stretches, legs should be hip-width apart, with knees slightly bent, back straight, and weight evenly distributed from the front to the back of the feet. To view a video of the exercises, visit **health.jbpub.com/hwonline.**

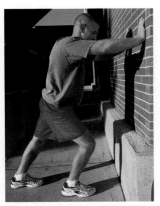

Calf Stretch   Stand approximately 2 to 3 feet away from a wall, tree, or stretching partner. Move one foot in close to the wall, while keeping the back leg straight behind you with the foot and heel flat on the ground. Slowly move your hips forward, bending the forward knee and keeping the back foot on the ground. You should feel a slight stretch in your calf muscles. Repeat with the opposite leg.

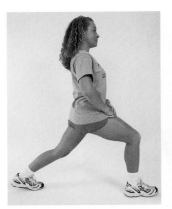

Lunge Stretch   Step forward and bend your forward knee, keeping it directly above your ankle. Stretch your other leg back behind you but don't lock your knee. Press your hips forward and down to stretch. Your arms can be at your sides, on top of your knee, or on the ground for balance. Repeat on the other side.

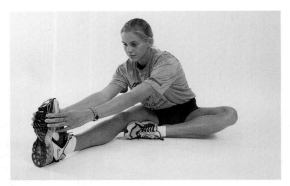

Modified Hurdler   Sit with your right leg straight out in front of you and your left leg tucked close to your body. Reach toward your right foot as far as possible. Do not curve your back. Go only as far as you can with a straight back. Repeat for the other leg.

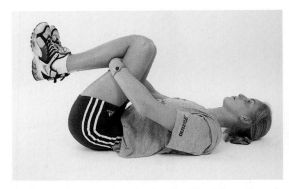

Lower-back Stretch   Lie on your back and pull both knees in to the chest. Keep your lower back on the floor.

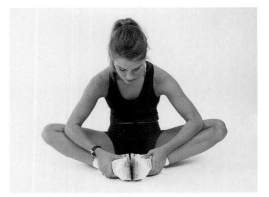

Groin Stretch   Sit with your back straight (don't slouch; you may want to put your back against a wall) and bend your legs, with the soles of your feet together. Try to get your heels as close to your groin as is comfortably possible. For a passive stretch, push your knees to the floor as far as you can (you may use your hands to assist but do not resist with the knees) and hold them there. This can be hard on the knees so please be careful. Now, keep your knees where they are, and then exhale as you bend over, trying to get your chest as close to the floor as possible.

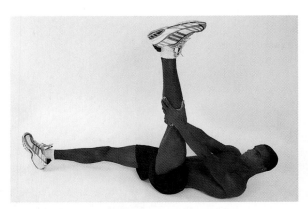

Supine Hamstring Stretch   Lie on your back and pull one leg up to a stretched position. The leg should remain as straight as possible. The opposite leg should be bent with the heel on the floor; keep your lower back on the floor. Alternate legs.

■ **Figure 7.6**

Flexibility Exercises (*continued*)

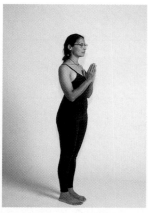

Position 1 Stand erect with your feet hip-width apart and palms together in front of your chest. Inhale and exhale slowly and calmly.

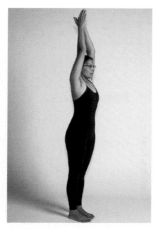

Position 2 Inhaling, raise your arms above your head, palms facing in. Lengthen through the spine, but do not arch your back.

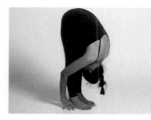

Position 3 Exhaling, bend forward from the hips, keeping your arms extended and your head hanging loosely between them. Keep your legs slightly bent and relax your neck and shoulders.

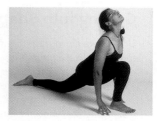

Position 4 Inhaling, bend both knees and place your palms flat on the floor by the outsides of your feet. Extend your left leg back. Stretch your chin toward the ceiling.

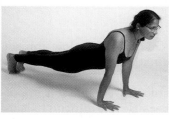

Position 5 Continue while holding the breath if you can—don't strain. Reach your forward leg back next to the other leg. Hold your body straight, supported by your hands and toes, with ankles, hips, and shoulders in a straight plane.

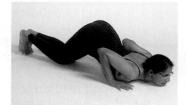

Position 6 Exhaling, lower your knees, chest, and chin or forehead to the floor, keeping your hips up and toes curled under.

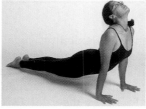

Position 7 Inhaling, bring the tops of your feet to the floor, straighten your legs, and come up to straight arms, opening the chest and stretching your chin toward the ceiling. Be careful not to overarch your lower back.

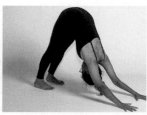

Position 8 Exhaling, curl your toes under and raise your hips into an inverted "V." Push back with your hands and lengthen your spine by reaching your hips upward. Keep your head hanging loosely.

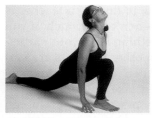

Position 9 Inhaling, lift your head and bring your left leg between your hands, keeping the right leg back. Raise your chin toward the ceiling.

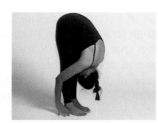

Position 10 Exhaling, bring your left foot forward so your feet are together. Bend forward from the hips, keeping your legs slightly bent and your upper body relaxed. If you can, touch your head to your knees and place your palms beside your feet.

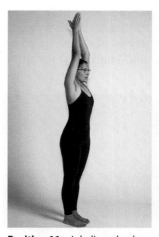

Position 11 Inhaling, slowly straighten up with your arms extended above your head. If you have any lower back pain, be sure to bend your knees.

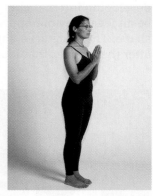

Position 12 Exhaling, bring your hands together in front of you. Close your eyes for a moment and feel the sensations in your body.

■ **Figure 7.7**

The Sun Salute

This hatha yoga exercise is a series of 12 postures, or asanas, intended to be done in one flowing routine. Each of the 12 postures is held 3 seconds.

Wellness Guide

Getting into Shape

Undertake a program to increase aerobic conditioning by following these guidelines.

1. *Frequency:* You should exercise three to five times a week.
2. *Intensity:* You should exercise within 60% to 80% of your exercise heart rate.
3. *Time:* You should exercise within your target zone for 20 to 60 minutes each time.
4. *Type of exercise:* Appropriate exercises are rhythmic and continuous and use the large muscles of the legs and hips. Such exercises include walking, jogging, bicycling, swimming, cross-country skiing, and aerobic dancing.
5. *Warm-up and cool-down:* It is optimal to raise the body's core temperature about 1°F to 3°F by doing the warm-up and stretching activities before the aerobic workout. After the aerobic workout, you should slow your heart rate and

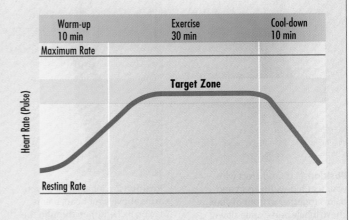

cool down for 30 to 60 minutes. Optimal time to stretch is when the muscles are warmed (i.e., after aerobic exercise).

Besides building strength and flexibility, yoga enhances well-being, mood, attention, mental focus, and stress tolerance. It can lessen sleep problems. Yoga is a beneficial, low-risk, low-cost adjunct to the treatment of stress, anxiety, posttraumatic stress disorder (PTSD), depression, stress-related medical illnesses, substance abuse, and rehabilitation of criminal offenders (Brown & Gerberg, 2005).

T'ai Chi Ch'uan

T'ai chi chuan comes from China and is based on a system of martial arts. In practicing t'ai chi, the individual concentrates on moving the joints of the body freely and developing internal energy. The practice of t'ai chi can be an ideal way of improving your health and staying in shape. There are several major styles of t'ai chi (named after the families that founded them) and great variation

within each style. All t'ai chi forms are low impact, improve balance and coordination, increase mobility, and reduce stress.

If you are interested in studying t'ai chi, it is important that you find a teacher because it is difficult to learn from a book or video. Find a teacher who practices the martial aspects of t'ai chi, which can include self-defense applications of movements from the t'ai chi form, push-hands and boxing, and weapons forms. Though you need not become a great fighter to benefit from practicing t'ai chi, you can gain a greater understanding of the form and the health-giving aspects of t'ai chi by studying the martial aspects.

A second guideline to follow in finding a teacher is to go to a class and participate—don't just watch. If you feel that you have learned something from your participation and feel the teacher and other students are sincere in their efforts to learn, then you have probably found a good class and teacher. Like any activity that you enjoy and engage in fully, practicing t'ai chi can offer immediate benefits, but it takes many years to become highly skilled. Beware of teachers who say that they have secrets or shortcuts, for there is no such thing. It is your own diligent practice that will bring you the full benefits of t'ai chi. The teacher is there to show you the way.

Body Composition

Body composition refers to the relative amounts of the body's major constituents, that is, water, protein (called the *fat-free mass*), minerals (including the calcium and phosphate in bones), and essential and storage fat. Two health concerns relating to body composition are body fat percentage and bone density.

T'ai chi exercises help maintain physical fitness and mind–body harmony.

Body Fat Percentage As pointed out in Chapters 5 and 6, the body has two kinds of fat: essential fat to carry out life functions and storage fat to supply energy. The healthy range for the amount of storage fat for nonathletic, young adult males is between 10% and 20% of the total body weight. Because of differences in sex hormone biology, the healthy range for the amount of storage fat for nonathletic, young adult females is 15% to 30% of the total body weight. Greater or lesser body fat percentages can be a risk to health.

Bone Density From a health perspective, one wants bone density of about 4% of total body weight; low bone density, such as in osteoporosis (see Chapter 22), increases the risk of falls and bone fracture. Healthy bone density is achieved by engaging in regular weight-bearing exercise, consuming adequate amounts of calcium and phosphate, and consuming little or no phosphate-containing sodas. Bone density is largely determined when one is young, which is the reason young people are encouraged to exercise, consume dairy foods, and not to consume sodas.

Physical Activity Among College Students

According to the American College Health Association (2008), about 60% of North American college students acquire less than the recommended amounts of physical activity. Like many in the general adult population, North American college students carry out most of their daily tasks while sitting—in lectures, at libraries, and studying. Many student jobs involve sitting at desks or standing behind counters (restaurant servers who walk a lot are exceptions). During nonschool/nonwork leisure time, many students watch TV, listen to music, play video games, or involve themselves in the Internet. Travel is generally by car.

Most college students know they should be more physically active, but they encounter a variety of barriers to doing so. For example, many students believe that health-promoting physical activity should be vigorous, frequent, and prolonged; they mistakenly imagine that physical activity for health requires hour-long workouts at a gym or running nearly every day—a serious time investment that many cannot realistically make. Moreover, whereas many college students were active in sports while in high school, they find exercise for its own sake to be boring and even unpleasant. Furthermore, if exercise facilities are crowded or otherwise uninviting, or the campus community is perceived as unsafe, students are less likely to go out to exercise. Perceiving these barriers as insurmountable, students give up on putting physical activity in their lives altogether.

So, if you actively participate in sports or are otherwise moving your body around for at least half an hour a day on most days of the week in any way you can, keep doing it. If not, find ways to do so and not necessarily by taking up a sport or exercising vigorously. A "just do it" attitude, buying new exercise clothes and shoes, and going to a gym several times a week (especially at odd hours) are unnecessary and unlikely to be maintained for very long. It's better to get into the habit of walking for 30 minutes almost every day. Remember, moderate amounts of physical activity are sufficient to promote health and reduce stress. Your goals are to find activities that you enjoy, that you can work into your schedule, and that you can make a regular part of your life.

Integrating Physical Activity in Your Life

Some individuals are habitual exercisers; they simply enjoy movement. Others, however, are not so inclined. In order to gain its health benefits, they must find other ways to integrate physical activity in their lives. This is especially true for those whose lifestyles are sedentary. Anything they can do to increase their amount of movement each day produces multiple rewards. Indeed, the greatest health gains derive from going from a sedentary to a moderate degree of daily physical activity.

Here are some guidelines for incorporating physical activity into your life.

1. *Define specific goals.* Goals can be general or specific. For example, "I want to be in shape" or "I want to lose weight" are general goals. "I want to run 2 miles, three times a week" or "I want to lose 20 pounds" are specific goals. Include among your goals that you want to do activities that you enjoy and that you want to make a regular part of your life for the long term. If you are unsure about your exercise goals, then set as a goal to make some more specific goals by experimenting with three kinds of activity to see what each offers.

2. *Research.* Consult books, magazines, the Internet, or teachers, coaches, and health professionals to determine ways to accomplish your goals. Be sure to assess the authoritativeness of the information you acquire; you do not want to undertake an

---

TERMS

body composition: the relative amounts of the body's major components

t'ai chi ch'uan: a Chinese martial arts system of movements that enhances freedom of movement and focus of mind

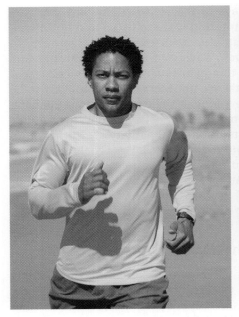 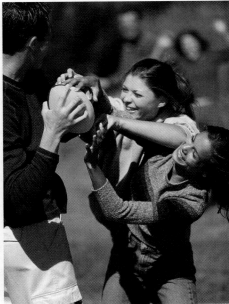 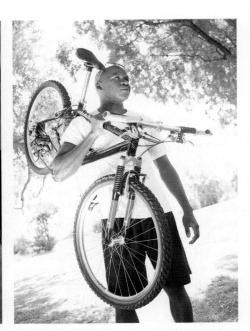

When choosing an exercise, pick one that's fun and convenient for you.

injurious activity or set an unattainable goal and have a failure experience. Because they are not experts, consulting friends may be of limited usefulness.

3. *Make a plan.* Having defined your goals and acquired information on how to accomplish them, make a realistic and feasible plan for putting and maintaining physical activity in your life. Be sure your activity plan fits into your schedule; use a time audit to identify times of the week during which you can exercise (see Chapter 3). Also, choose activities that are interesting (or likely to be) and enjoyable. That way you are more likely to want to do them. Write down your plan; perhaps discuss it with a coach, teacher, or health professional. Even better, take a class. That way you will learn proper technique, have a built-in schedule, and will have the enjoyment of being with others.

4. *Get a physical checkup.* Consult a health professional if you have been inactive for many months or have concerns about your body's ability to perform at the level you want.

5. *Progress slowly.* Deliberate progress enables you to assess the feasibility of your choices and also to integrate them into your normal life routine. Try not to let your enthusiasm for beginning your plan stimulate you to take on too much too soon. You don't want to get sore or injure yourself.

6. *Track progress.* Keep a diary of your activity. For each activity day, record the time you spent doing the activity, what you experienced doing the

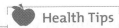
Health Tips

Walking in Balance

Native Americans have an expression that helps when trying to understand our place in the physical world. The expression "walking in balance" means engaging your body with your mind in the natural world, feeling a sense of connectedness with nature. Walking in balance suggests that we combine the powers of the mind and body to become more aware of ourselves in our environment.

During your next workout try this: While you dress and warm up, remind yourself that you are taking time away from your problems and worries—a mini vacation, if you will, from daily responsibilities. The mission during this exercise period (preferably walking or running) is to see where you are exercising as if you were seeing it for the first time. Notice the trees, the birds, the clouds in the sky, and so on. Try to feel that you are a part of nature by noticing as much about the natural world as you can.

activity, any obstacles that prevented you from carrying out a day's activity, and strategies for overcoming any obstacles.

7. *Evaluate.* Each week, ask yourself if your plan is working to accomplish your goals. If so, continue. If not, identify the obstacles and make course corrections, for example, by changing the choice of activities, the time devoted to them, and perhaps even your goals themselves.

Performance-Enhancing Substances

The saying "Better living through chemistry" aptly describes the intentions of those who use any of a variety of substances, or **ergogenic aids**, to increase strength and endurance, enhance athletic performance, or bulk up or "body sculpt" to feel better about their physical appearance (see Dollars and Health Sense). Performance-enhancing substances include stimulants to increase alertness and "energy" and to "burn fat," muscle enlargers, and endurance enhancers. They come in the form of dietary supplements, herbals, over-the-counter and prescription-only pharmaceuticals, and illegal drugs.

Many people mistakenly assume that because herbs and dietary supplements are marketed as "natural" they are safe. Before taking any kind of herbal or dietary supplement, keep in mind that the U.S. government does not regulate dietary supplements, so consumers cannot be certain that any product conforms to information on the product label. For example, frequently the actual amount per serving (dose) is not as indicated on the label. Also, although manufacturers promise to adhere to manufacturing standards, they are not compelled to, so products may contain impurities and other chemicals not listed on the label. If one eats and exercises healthfully, any kind of ergogenic aid is unnecessary.

Stimulants

Stimulants commonly used as performance enhancers include amphetamine and similar chemicals, ephedra (*ma huang*), synephrine (hoodia, bitter orange) and similar chemicals, and caffeine. These substances can induce euphoria, increase alertness, combat fatigue, and in some instances, reduce appetite. They also increase the risk of heart attack, seizures, and psychotic episodes. Because of their harmful effects, amphetamines are legally controlled, and ephedra has been banned for sale in dietary supplements.

Energy drinks generally contain a variety of substances purported to increase alertness and endurance and to combat fatigue, including caffeine (and caffeine-like substances such as theophylline), the herb guarana, which contains caffeine, taurine, ginseng, ginkgo, creatine, carnitine, glucuronolactone, and lots of sugar. There is no doubt that high doses of caffeine are stimulatory; however, the effects of caffeine on physical performance remain in question (George, 2005).

Muscle Enlargers

Muscle enlargers include protein and amino acid dietary supplements, androgenic anabolic steroids, and human growth hormone. Although new muscle tissue is made of protein, ingesting protein or certain amino acids will not produce new muscle tissue. Muscles grow in response to work, not food. Anyone consuming a balanced diet obtains sufficient protein and amino acids to meet the demands of nearly any kind of exercise; body builders or athletes who need to build considerable strength are exceptions.

Androgenic anabolic steroids (testosterone and similar substances) are used to build muscle strength in women and men. They are legal only by prescription for medical reasons. Androstenedione ("andro") is a "prohormone" that is converted in the body to testosterone. Prior to 2005, androstenedione and similar substances could be purchased legally as dietary supplements. However, in 2005, the U.S. Food and Drug Administration banned the sale of andro and other testosterone prohormones because they are dangerous. Potential long-term consequences of testosterone use in men include infertility, erection problems, breast development (gynecomastia), heart disease, liver disease, and cancer. In women, steroids can cause male pattern baldness, deepening of the voice, increased facial hair, and abnormal menstrual periods. Children and young adults who use steroids are at risk for early onset of puberty and premature cessation of bone growth.

Human growth hormone (HGH or GH) is manufactured by the pituitary gland and secreted into the bloodstream. Although reputed to enhance athletic performance by increasing energy and/or building muscle mass, scientific evidence of any ergogenic effects is lacking. Despite unscrupulous advertising claims to the contrary, HGH cannot be taken orally because it is broken down in the digestive system. There is no evidence that so-called HGH precursors or "secretogogues" are effective as ergogenic aids (Juhn, 2003).

Endurance Enhancers

Endurance enhancers include B vitamins (see Chapter 5), creatine, and erythropoetin.

Creatine, a natural substance in muscle tissue required for muscle contraction, can be purchased as a nutritional supplement. Some, but not all, studies show that creatine supplementation might enhance short-burst activity, such as weight lifting or sprinting. It is not helpful for endurance activities. In doses commonly in

---

TERMS

androgenic anabolic steroids: synthetic male hormones used to increase muscle size and strength

creatine: a natural substance in skeletal muscle tissue required for muscle contraction, which can also be purchased at as dietary supplement

ergogenic aids: substances used to increase strength and endurance

human growth hormone: a naturally occurring pituitary hormone

$ Dollars and Health Sense

Caveat Emptor: The Business of Sports Supplements

Everyone has heard of professional, Olympic, and other high-level athletes who have been punished for taking banned—and often illegal—substances (i.e., steroids, hormones, and other drugs). Apparently, in a world where winning is everything, some elite athletes are willing to risk their careers and their health to gain a competitive edge.

Unfortunately, a significant number of high school athletes, college athletes, nonathletes, and people who just want to "look good" also take drugs to gain a competitive edge. Among athletes, the edge might be enhanced athletic performance. Or it may be solidifying one's identity as an athlete or gaining recognition as an athlete among one's peers. Among the "body conscious," the edge is generally sculpting the body to compete socially for friends and sexual and intimate partners.

The dietary supplement industry is masterful at catering to concerns about competing athletically and socially. Advertising of supplements supports a variety of "fitness" magazines and a host of e-commerce "sports supplement" or "sports nutrition" Web sites that lure potential consumers with information of dubious authoritativeness, all with the intention to sell them something. For example, a body building Web site tells visitors about the ban on testosterone prohormones but not to worry because "we have a number of other products that work just as well." The banner of a "sports nutrition" Web site shows a cluster of several nearly naked, "buff" college-age men and women, offering a plethora of generally worthless products to enhance performance, increase energy, lose weight (and look just like the models in the banner). Advertisements depicting muscular, "fit" models influence people to view their own bodies as inferior (Leit, Gray, & Pope, 2002).

The dietary supplement industry is estimated at $15 billion a year and is largely unregulated. A federal law in 1994 made it possible for manufacturers of dietary supplements not to adhere to the same testing for safety, efficacy, and purity as required for prescription and over-the-counter medications. With over 25,000 dietary supplements on the market, U.S. government agencies cannot investigate the purity and safety of every batch of a particular supplement, nor can claims made in the advertising of every supplement be evaluated for truthfulness. In the world of dietary supplements, the watchword is *caveat emptor:* Let the buyer beware.

use (three to five grams per day), creatine is apparently not harmful. However, because herbs and other nutritional supplements are unregulated, one cannot be sure of the purity or dose of any such product.

Erythropoetin is a hormone that increases the number of red blood cells, thus increasing the body's ability to carry oxygen to tissues. Erythropoetin is a prescription medication given to people whose bodies cannot produce sufficient blood cells, such as people undergoing cancer treatment. It is used illegally by athletes to increase endurance, especially at high elevations. The drug can be very dangerous, causing heart attacks and strokes.

Sports Injuries

Regardless of type, physical activity and sports participation carry some risk of injury, whether it's working up a blister while walking in new shoes, pulling a leg muscle while cycling, or jamming a finger in a volleyball game (see Chapter 21). When an injury occurs, one should apply first aid in the form of **RICE** (rest, ice, compression, and elevation; see the Wellness Guide "First Aid for Sports Injuries: RICE"). When an injury heals, one should endeavor to prevent the injury (and others) from occurring again (see the Health Tips box).

> Long ago when men cursed and beat the ground with sticks, it was called witchcraft. Today it's called golf.
>
> *Will Rogers*

About half of injuries in physical activity occur because some part of or the entire body is being exercised beyond its biological limits. Such injuries are referred to as **overuse injuries.** Commonly, overuse injuries affect the skin and muscles, tendons, ligaments, and joints, which are constructed of fibrous bands of protein (Table 7.6). These fibers can be torn if they are overworked, as when lifting a heavy weight or running farther or faster than one should, or when forced to perform when fatigued. Damage can also occur by repeated small injuries that lead over time to a more serious problem. The common causes of overuse injuries are excessive exercising, faulty technique, and poor equipment.

Table 7.6

Common Overuse Injuries

Strain	Commonly referred to as "pulled muscles" or "pulled tendons." Caused by overstretching, tearing, or ripping of a muscle and/or its tendon
Tendonitis	Inflammation of a tendon caused by chronic, low-grade strain of a muscle–tendon unit
Bursitis	Inflammation of the lubricating sac that surrounds a joint (*bursa*) caused by repeated low-grade strain of the joint's supporting tissues
Sprain	Overstretching or tearing of ligaments
Blisters	Fluid-filled swellings on the skin caused by undue friction from the rubbing of skin against shoes, clothing, and equipment

All bodies are not anatomically capable of the same degree of physical exertion, especially the high performance exhibited by marathon runners or triathletes. The architecture of the body, the alignment of the legs, the capacity of the lungs, the size and strength of the bones and muscles, and other anatomical factors set limits on an individual's physical ability. Few people have the biological endowment to perform at championship levels. Physical activity can be much more enjoyable when you respect, accept, and appreciate your body's biological limits.

Don't ask your muscles to do more than they can. Relishing the pain of overexertion—"going for the burn"—is dangerous. Pain is the body's message that something is wrong, not that the exerciser is lazy. If you want to increase your performance, progress slowly, following a supervised regimen. Injuries are more likely if equipment such as weights and other kinds of apparatus is used improperly or is in disrepair.

Most people participate in physical activity because they want to have fun, they want to gain a sense of accomplishment by doing something well, and they want to feel physically and psychologically better. While pursuing these goals, no one wants to be hurt. It turns out that maximizing the "have fun, do well, feel good" aspects of physical activity and minimizing the potential for injury go together.

Physical Activity in Cold and Hot Weather

Your body is designed to maintain its operating temperature at 37°C (about 98°F). Because heat always moves toward cold, your body loses heat in cold environments and absorbs heat in warm environments. Moreover, exercised muscles produce heat, which can elevate body temperature. Sweating is the evaporation of body water to rid the body of excess heat.

Cold Stress

Overexposure to cold, windy/wet weather may lead to an abnormally low body temperature (hypothermia). Symptoms of hypothermia include shivering, muscle weakness, numbness, drowsiness, and occasionally unconsciousness. In instances of cold stress, get out of the cold environment and seek protection from the wind. Gently remove wet clothes and replace them with dry ones. Rewarm the body by immersion in warm (105–110°F) water and wrapping in warm blankets. Do not consume alcohol "to warm up" because alcohol dilates arteries and causes heat loss. Seek medical attention as soon as possible.

Frostbite is the freezing of tissues with the formation of ice crystals in the fluid around cells and blood vessels. Frostbitten skin may become white or grayish-yellow. The onset of frostbite is usually painful, but pain generally diminishes and the region becomes cold and numb. Gently rewarm a frostbitten region and seek medical attention as soon as possible.

To prevent cold stress during exercise follow these recommendations:

- Dress appropriately for cold weather. Wear no more than three layers of clothing; be sure all layers can be opened if necessary to cool the body overwarmed by vigorous exercise.

TERMS

erythropoetin: a hormone that increases the number of red blood cells, thus increasing the body's ability to carry oxygen to tissues.

overuse injuries: injuries to muscles, tendons, ligaments, and joints resulting from too much exercise

RICE: an acronym for rest, ice, compression, elevation; the first aid measures for sports injuries

---

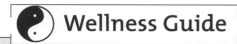 Wellness Guide

First Aid for Sports Injuries: RICE

Most sports injuries involve the release of fluids and other substances from damaged tissues. Immediate treatment of a sports injury, therefore, requires limiting any swelling and internal bleeding by administering RICE—rest, ice, compression, and elevation.

Rest: Resting and possibly immobilizing an injured region prevent additional tissue damage and limit internal bleeding.

Ice: Cool an injured region immediately with crushed ice or ice cubes wrapped in a towel (to avoid frostbite), a cold pack, or a bag of frozen peas or corn. The cold reduces swelling, internal bleeding, and pain. Cool for 30 minutes. Allow the region to warm for 15 minutes, and then cool again.

Compression: Wrap the injured region with an elastic bandage to control swelling. Be careful not to wrap so tight as to turn the skin pale or cause lack of sensation.

Elevation: Raise the injured region to limit swelling and internal bleeding.

- Wear mittens rather than gloves to allow the fingers to insulate each other.
- Wear appropriate thermal head covering.
- Keep the feet warm and dry.
- Be prepared to change into warm, dry clothes quickly.

Heat Stress

Heat stress results from the loss of considerable body water and minerals from sweating, from dehydration, and the unavailability of sufficient body water to cool the body through sweating. Types of heat stress include the following:

Heat cramps: painful, constant contraction of one or more muscles. Stop activity, replace water and minerals by drinking water or dilute fruit juice; massage and stretch the cramping muscle(s); and rest and cool the body before returning to activity.

Heat exhaustion: weakness, nausea, dizziness. Stop activity; lie down and elevate the legs 12 to 18 inches; replace water and minerals by drinking water or dilute fruit juice; and cool the body with wet cloths and going to a cool room. Rest for several days before returning to activity. Consult a physician.

Heat stroke: high body temperature (105°F), disorientation, alteration in normal mental status, unconsciousness. Stop activity, remove clothes, cool the body with cold water or ice packs. Replace water and minerals by drinking water or dilute fruit juice. Seek medical attention immediately.

To prevent heat stress during exercise follow these recommendations:

- Acclimate to exercising in hot, humid environments by gradually increasing the level of physical activity over the span of several days.

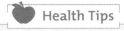 Health Tips

Preventing Sports Injuries

- Strengthen muscles.
- Be physically fit and improve endurance.
- Don't overwork the body.
- Improve body flexibility with stretching exercises before and after activity.
- Be aware of how the body is functioning.
- Be aware of hazards in the environment; use facilities designed for sports activity.
- Use state-of-the-art equipment, particular athletic shoes, and protective gear.
- Participate only when weather conditions are safe.
- Improve running or playing form; get expert coaching.
- Rehabilitate injuries adequately before returning to activity.

- Be wary of overexertion in hot/humid conditions. Heat stress may occur rapidly.
- Drink lots of fluid (water, dilute fruit juice, or sports drinks) before activity and regularly during extended activity. Do not rely on thirst to signal fluid loss or high body temperature.
- Wear light-fitting, light-colored clothing made of breathable fabric and a light-colored cap and sunscreen to limit sun exposure.
- Exercise during the coolest times of the day (morning and evening) and in the shade.

A Plan for Fitness

Here are some guidelines to keep in mind when incorporating any kind of physical activity into your life.

1. **Have a plan.** Before beginning any physical activity program, you need to develop a plan and commit yourself to it for a reasonable amount of time. To make a plan that will help you achieve your personal goals, you can consult a high school or college coach, attend an exercise class, or follow the plan in one of the how-to books or authoritative Web sites that have been written for almost every activity.

2. **Get a physical checkup.** If you have been inactive for many months or have concerns about your body's ability to perform at the level you would like, you may want to have a physician check you over.

3. **Accomplish goals.** The goal of any physical activity program is attainment of complete mind–body harmony. It is customary in our culture to measure progress by "how far" and "how fast." Such goals might be suitable for competitive athletes, but they are unsuitable for people who engage in physical activities for the purpose of receiving greater enjoyment from living. For most of us, personal goals based on such questions as "Does this level of activity make me feel good?" or "Does this help me toward my goal of losing weight?" make more sense than blind adherence to a stopwatch.

4. **Progress slowly.** Slow, deliberate progress gives you the opportunity to integrate your physical activity into your normal life routine. Begin slowly; don't impulsively try to run a long distance the first day.

5. **Warm up and cool down.** All physical activity should be preceded by a brief period of stretching, breathing, and relaxation to prepare your mind and body to receive the utmost benefit and pleasure from the activity. This is a good time to focus attention on how your body feels. When you have finished your physical activity, it is a good idea to let your body cool down slowly. If you

have been involved in strenuous aerobic exercise, slowly reduce the pace of your activity until your heart rate and breathing return to almost normal. By reducing your activity level slowly, you help prevent muscle cramps that sometimes occur when strenuous activity is suddenly stopped. You can prevent later muscle stiffness by doing a few stretching exercises to loosen the muscles that have worked hard during exercise. While cooling down, try to focus your attention on the sensations that your body work has brought you.

Critical Thinking About Health

1. Another Christmas day at Grandma's. Well, almost. After everyone had eaten all they possibly could and all the children had ripped open their Christmas gifts, Suzanne's Uncle Ron sat next to her on the couch.

   "I understand that you're taking a health class at school," he said.

   "That's right," Suzanne replied.

   "Then tell me," Uncle Ron continued, "What's the best exercise? My New Year's resolution is to get back in shape, and I want to do it right this time. I'm joining the gym on January 2. What workouts do you recommend?"

   a. What advice should Suzanne give her uncle? Take into account that Uncle Ron has tried working out before, apparently without success. Uncle Ron is a 39-year-old telecommunications engineer who works long hours at a computer terminal when he's at his office. His job also requires him to travel, so he eats a lot of fast food. He is married and has three young children.

2. What are the effects on society and on organized sports of athletes using performance-enhancing drugs, even when such substances are legal?

3. How far? How fast? How much? How might questions such as these affect a person's attitude and approach to physical activity for health (i.e., not competition)? List a new set of questions that illustrate a noncompetitive perspective on physical activity for health.

Health in Review

- Many people live sedentary lives because machines carry out most of the physical labor of living. Sedentariness is associated with a variety of risks to health, which is the reason governments and social institutions are seeking ways to help individuals increase the amount of physical activity in their lives.
- Physical activity is any kind of movement, including doing household tasks, work-related movement, leisure-time activities, and performance-based activities.
- Physical activity is measured as calories of energy expended per minutes, metabolic equivalents (METs), and physical activity level (PAL).
- Moderate, rather than vigorous, amounts of physical activity are sufficient for health. Experts recommend walking briskly for 30 minutes on most days of the week.

- Physical activity has six components: motivation, cardiorespiratory fitness, body strength, endurance, flexibility, and body composition.
- Guidelines for integrating physical activity into life involve goal setting, developing and carrying out a plan, and tracking and evaluating progress.
- Performance-enhancing substances include stimulants (e.g., amphetamines, caffeine), muscle enlargers (e.g., androgenic anabolic steroids), and endurance enhancers (e.g., creatine).
- The most common cause of sports injury is exercising a body part or the entire body beyond its biological limit to the point of injury. Common injuries include strain, tendonitis, bursitis, sprain, and blisters.
- Exercising in hot or cold weather requires taking special precautions to prevent injury and illness.

Health and Wellness Online

The Web contains a wealth of information about health and wellness. By accessing the Internet using Web browser software, you can gain a new perspective on many topics presented in *Health and Wellness,* Tenth Edition. Access the Jones and Bartlett Publishers Web site at **health.jbpub.com/hwonline.**

References

American College Health Association. (2008). National college health assessment. Baltimore: American College Health Association. Retrieved July 1, 2008, from http://www.acha-ncha.org/index.html

American College of Sports Medicine. (2002). Strength, power, and the baby boomer. *Current Comment.* Retrieved August 12, 2005, from http://www.acsm.org/health+fitness/comments.htm

Booth, F. W. (2002). Exercise and gene expression: Physiological regulation of the human genome through physical activity. *Journal of Physiology, 543,* 399–411.

Bravata, D. M., et al. (2007). Using pedometers to increase physical activity and improve health. *Journal of the American Medical Association, 298,* 2296–2304.

Brown, R. P., & Gerbarg, P. L. (2005). Sudarshan kriya yogic breathing in the treatment of stress, anxiety, and depression: Part II—Clinical applications and guidelines. *Journal of Alternative and Complementary Medicine, 11,* 711–717.

George, A. J. (2005). Central nervous system stimulants. In David R. Mottram (Ed.), *Drugs in sport.* London: Routledge.

Hillman, C. H., et al. (2008). Be smart, exercise your heart: Exercise effects on brain and cognition. *Nature Reviews Neuroscience, 1,* 58–65

Institute of Medicine. (2007). *Adequacy of evidence for physical activity guidelines development.* Washington, DC: National Academies Press.

Juhn, M. S. (2003). Popular sports supplements and ergogenic aids. *Sports Medicine, 33,* 921–939.

Leit, R. A., Gray, J. J., & Pope, H. G., Jr. (2002). The media's representation of the ideal male body: A cause for muscle dysmorphia? *International Journal of Eating Disorders, 31,* 334–338.

Mokdad, A. H., et al. (2004). Actual causes of death in the United States. *Journal of the American Medical Association, 291,* 238–245.

Murphy, M. H. (2007). The effect of walking on fitness, fatness, and resting blood pressure. *Preventive Medicine, 44,* 377–385.

O'Donovan, G., et al. (2005). Changes in cardiorespiratory fitness and coronary heart disease risk factors following 24 weeks of moderate- or high-intensity exercise of equal energy cost. *Journal of Applied Physiology, 98,* 1619–1625.

Pope, H. G. (2001, March). Unraveling the Adonis complex. *Psychiatric Times, 63.* Retrieved August 10, 2005, from http://www.psychiatrictimes.com/p010353.html

Purcher, J., & Renne, J. L. (2003). Socioeconomics of urban travel: Evidence from the 2001 NHTS. *Transportation Quarterly, 57,* 49–77.

U.S. Department of Health and Human Services. (1996). *Physical activity and health: A report of the Surgeon General.* Atlanta, GA: Centers for Disease Control.

World Health Organization. (2004). Move for health. Retrieved July 3, 2008, from http://www.who.int/moveforhealth/en/

Suggested Readings

American Heart Association. Start! A free tool that helps people make positive lifestyle changes through walking and eating better; includes a way to track your progress as part of the Start! Walking Program. Available: http://www.americanheart.org/presenter.jhtml?identifier=3053031

Anderson, B. (2000). *Stretching*. New York: Shelter Publications. Easy-to-follow exercises and drawings.

Benaugh, B. (2006). *Yoga for stress relief*. Yoga-instructor Barbara Benaugh teams with the Dalai Lama on this DVD that teaches how to practice this ancient mind–body method for modern stresses.

Capouya, J. (2003, June 16). Real men do yoga. *Newsweek, 141*, 78–79. Describes yoga and how it contributes to health and well-being.

Institute of Medicine Committee on Physical Activity, Health, Transportation, and Land Use. (2005). *Does the built environment influence physical activity?* Washington, DC: National Academies Press. Public health officials, city and regional planners, and transportation experts report on the contribution of land use and travel patterns to the epidemic of physical inactivity.

Juhn, M. S. (2003). Popular sports supplements and ergogenic aids. *Sports Medicine, 33*, 921–939. An extremely thorough and comprehensive discussion.

PilatesInsight.com (http://www.pilatesinsight.com/). All about Pilates.

Pope, H. G. (2001, March). Unraveling the Adonis complex. *Psychiatric Times, 63*. Available: http://www.psychiatrictimes.com/p010353.html. Discussion of reasons muscularity has become an important sign of masculinity.

U.S. National Institutes of Health. (2007). Walking: A step in the right direction. Available: http://www.niddk.nih.gov/publications/walking.htm

Yau, M. K. (2008). T'ai Chi exercise and the improvement of health and well-being in older adults. *Medicine and Sport Science, 52*, 155–165. Review of research showing the many health benefits of t'ai chi.

Recommended Web Sites

Please visit **health.jbpub.com/hwonline** for links to these Web sites.

American Society of Sports Medicine
Information on exercise and exercise equipment.

National Center for Chronic Disease Prevention and Health Promotion
Information and education about making physical activity a part of your life.

Pilates Studio
Information about the Pilates method and its creator.

The President's Council on Physical Fitness and Sports
Information on exercise.

Part Three

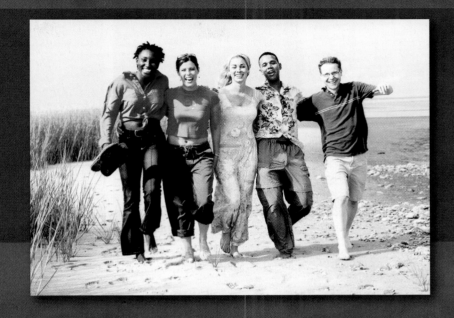

Building Healthy Relationships

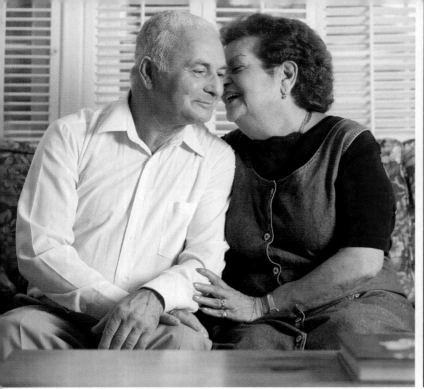
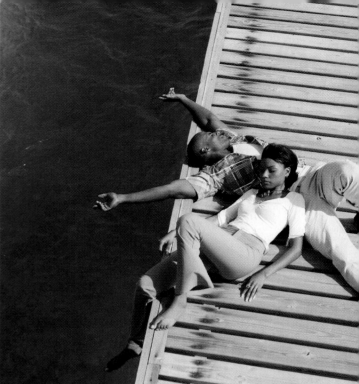
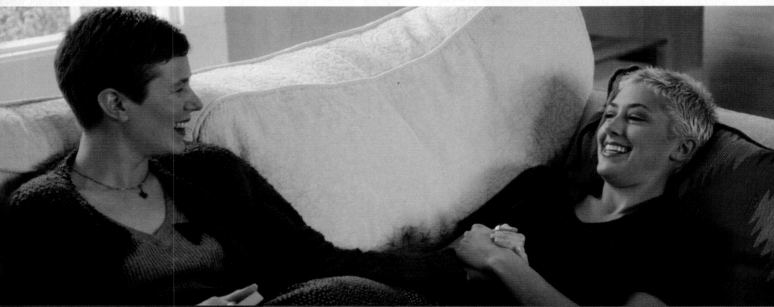

Chapter Eight

Sexuality and Intimate Relationships

Learning Objectives

1. List and define the major dimensions of human sexuality: physical, psychological, orientation, behavioral, and relationship.

2. Describe female and male sexual anatomy.

3. Describe the menstrual cycle and name three common menstrual difficulties.

4. Define *sexual orientation*.

5. List and describe the phases of the sexual response cycle.

6. Describe common sexual difficulties.

7. Describe the stages of development in intimate relationships.

8. Identify and describe the essential components of good communication.

Sexuality represents a truly holistic aspect of living, for it involves the simultaneous expression of mind, body, and spirit—the whole self. Although sexuality is commonly represented in advertising and other media as having to do solely with physical gratification, most people are aware that sexuality involves much more than the stimulation of the body's sex organs. Sexuality has several dimensions, including the following:

> *Love is a great exaggeration of the worth of one individual over the worth of everybody else*
>
> *George Bernard Shaw*

1. *The physical dimension:* those parts of the body that define a person as a female or male, contribute to sexual experiences, and are involved in reproduction
2. *The psychological dimension:* values, beliefs, attitudes, and emotions that influence a person's sexual thoughts and behaviors
3. *The orientation dimension:* the tendency to feel attracted to, and the desire to emotionally bond with, a member of the same or other sex
4. *The behavioral dimension:* physical and social activities intended to meet one's sexual wants and needs
5. *The relationship dimension:* aspects of sexuality that interface and integrate with intimate relationships

From the standpoint of personal health, sexuality is an area over which you have considerable individual control. You choose when and with whom you wish to have sex, and which feelings you wish to express in sexual ways. With some fundamental knowledge of sexual biology, you can conduct your sexual life responsibly, thus avoiding unnecessary illness and exercising a choice of whether and when to have children.

Sexuality: The Physical Dimension

One of the fundamental functions of sexuality is biological reproduction. Males produce reproductively capable sperm and deposit them in the female reproductive tract during sexual intercourse. Females provide reproductively capable eggs, called **ova,** and a safe, nutrient-filled environment in which the fetus develops for the nine months of pregnancy.

Male and female sexual biology are genetically determined at conception. The fusion of an X-bearing egg with the X-bearing sperm produces a female (XX); fusion with the Y-bearing sperm produces a male (XY). Once the chromosome pattern is set, the development of the sexual anatomy follows from the precise instructions of the genes contained in the chromosomes. A particular chromosome set determines whether the as yet immature sex cells that appear at about the fifth week of development will eventually produce sperm or ova. The sex chromosomes determine whether the fetus will ultimately develop the male sex organs—testes, sperm ducts, semen-producing glands, and penis—or the female organs—ovaries, fallopian tubes, uterus, vagina, and external female genitals.

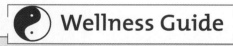 Wellness Guide

Attend to Your Sexual Health

Women: Regular Gynecological Exams
The gynecological exam is a medical examination of a woman's reproductive system—the internal and external pelvic organs and the breasts. The internal exam (called a *pelvic exam*) includes examination of the vagina and cervix, the bladder, the ovaries, and the fallopian tubes for any abnormality in size and shape. A urine test, a blood test for iron deficiency, a test for sexually transmitted diseases (STDs), and a Papanicolaou (Pap) test can also be part of the gynecological exam. The Pap test (or Pap smear) is a screening test for cancer of the cervix. A few cells are taken from the cervix and observed for abnormalities. The Pap test does not screen for sexually transmitted diseases. STD tests must be requested.

Women who are or have been sexually active, or have reached age 18, should have Pap tests and physical exams annually.

Men: Testicular Self-Examination
Because testicular cancer is the most common cancer in men aged 15 to 35 years, young men are encouraged to check their testes about once a month for the appearance of any abnormal lumps or swellings—possible signs of testicular cancer. Men who examine themselves regularly become familiar with the way their testicles normally feel.

Testicular self-examination should be performed after a warm bath or shower. The heat relaxes the scrotum, making it easier to find anything unusual.

1. Stand in front of the mirror. Look for any swelling on the skin of the scrotum.
2. Examine each testicle with both hands. The index and middle fingers should be placed under the testicle while the thumbs are placed on the top. Gently roll the testicle between the thumbs and fingers. It's normal for one testicle to be larger than the other.
3. Find the epididymis (the soft, tubelike structure at the back of the testicle that collects and carries the sperm). Do not mistake the epididymis for an abnormal lump.

If you find a lump, contact your doctor right away. Testicular cancer is highly curable, especially when treated promptly.

The genetic determination of sexual biology also specifies the pattern of male or female steroid hormone production, which in turn affects the **secondary sex characteristics** that distinguish males and females: the extent and distribution of facial and body hair; body build and stature; and appearance of breasts (**Figure 8.1**).

Female Sexual Anatomy

A woman's internal sexual organs consist of two **ovaries**, which lie on either side of the abdominal cavity, the **fallopian tubes**, the **uterus**, and the **vagina**; together these structures make up a specialized tube that goes from each ovary to the outside of the body (**Figure 8.2**). The function of the ovaries, which are about the size and shape of almonds, is to produce fertilizable ova as well as sex hormones, which control the development of the female body type, maintain normal female sexual physiology, and help regulate the course of pregnancy. The fallopian tubes gather and transport the ova that are released from the ovaries (about one each month). The two fallopian tubes connect to the uterus, an organ about the size of a woman's fist, which is situated just behind the pelvic bone and the bladder (**Figure 8.3**). The uterus is part of the passageway for sperm as they move from the vagina to the fallopian tubes to effect fertilization; after fertilization, it provides the environment in which the fetus grows. It is the inner lining of the uterus that is shed each month in menstruation.

TERMS

fallopian tubes: the usual site of fertilization; a pair of tubelike structures that transport ova from the ovaries to the uterus

ova: female eggs (singular, *ovum*)

ovaries: a pair of almond-shaped organs in the female abdomen that produce egg cells (ova) and female sex hormones

secondary sex characteristics: anatomical features appearing at puberty that distinguish males from females

uterus: the female organ in which a fetus develops

vagina: a woman's organ of copulation and the exit pathway for the fetus at birth

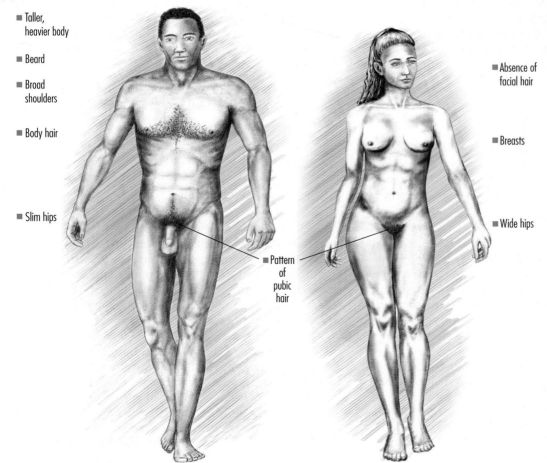

■ **Figure 8.1**

Secondary Sexual Characteristics of Men and Women

■ Taller, heavier body

■ Beard

■ Broad shoulders

■ Body hair

■ Slim hips

■ Absence of facial hair

■ Breasts

■ Wide hips

■ Pattern of pubic hair

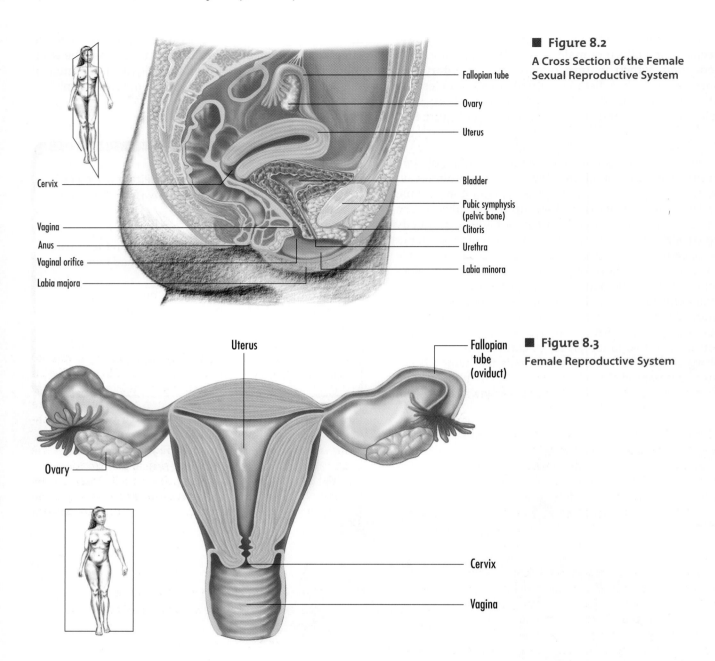

■ **Figure 8.2**

A Cross Section of the Female Sexual Reproductive System

Fallopian tube

Ovary

Uterus

Bladder

Pubic symphysis (pelvic bone)

Clitoris

Urethra

Labia minora

Cervix

Vagina

Anus

Vaginal orifice

Labia majora

■ **Figure 8.3**

Female Reproductive System

Uterus

Fallopian tube (oviduct)

Ovary

Cervix

Vagina

The lower part of the uterus is the **cervix,** and the cavity of the uterus is connected to the vagina by means of a small opening called the cervical os. The cervix secretes mucus, which changes in consistency depending on the phase of the menstrual cycle. Some women learn to estimate the time of **ovulation** (ovum release) by examining their cervical mucus (see Chapter 10).

The vagina is a hollow tube that leads from the cervix to the outside of the body. The sexually nonaroused vagina is approximately 3 to 5 inches long. Normally, the vaginal tube is rather narrow, but it can readily widen to accommodate the penis during intercourse, a tampon during menstruation, the passage of a baby during childbirth, or a pelvic examination. The vagina possesses a unique physiology that is maintained by the secretions that continually emanate from the vaginal walls. These secretions help regulate the growth of microorganisms that normally inhabit the vagina, and they also help to cleanse the vagina. Because the vagina is a self-cleansing organ, it is usually unnecessary to employ any extraordinary cleansing measures, such as douching. Very often douching merely upsets the natural chemical balance of the vagina and increases the risk of developing vaginal inflammation, called **vulvovaginitis** or *vaginitis*. Symptoms of vulvovaginitis include irritation or itching, redness or swelling of the vagina and vulva, unusual discharge, discomfort or a burning sensation when urinating, and, sometimes, a disagreeable odor.

Vulvovaginitis is commonly referred to as a "yeast infection." Whereas yeast (typically *Candida albicans*) can

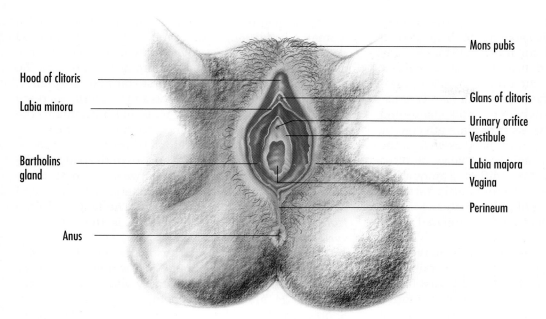

External Female Sexual Reproductive Organs

Mons pubis

Hood of clitoris

Labia minora

Glans of clitoris

Urinary orifice

Vestibule

Bartholins gland

Labia majora

Vagina

Perineum

Anus

cause vulvovaginitis, other microorganisms, such as the protozoan *Trichomonas vaginalis,* bacteria, and viruses, also cause it. Even irritation from vaginal sprays, spermicidal products, and other chemicals can produce symptoms of vulvovaginitis. Anyone with symptoms of vulvovaginitis should see a health practitioner to obtain an accurate diagnosis and treatment.

A number of factors increase susceptibility to vulvovaginitis, including the use of antibiotics, emotional stress, a diet high in carbohydrates, hormonal changes caused by pregnancy or birth control pills, chemical irritants, intercourse without adequate lubrication, and heat and moisture retained by nylon underwear and pantyhose.

The **vulva** encompasses all female external genital structures—pubic hair, the folds of skin, the **clitoris,** and the urinary and vaginal openings (**Figure 8.4**). The smaller, inner pair of folds are called the **labia minora,** and the larger, outer pair are called the **labia majora.** The clitoris, a highly sensitive sexual organ, is situated above the vaginal opening.

The opening of the **urethra,** which is the exit tube for urine, is located at the vaginal region just below the clitoris. The fact that the urethra is only about one-half an inch long and located close to the vagina makes it susceptible to irritation and infection, called **urethritis,** characterized by a burning sensation during urination and usually by the frequent urge to urinate. Occasionally, bacteria introduced into the urethra migrate the short distance to the bladder and produce a bladder infection called **cystitis.** The symptoms of cystitis are similar to those of urethritis. The occurrence of urethritis or cystitis is often referred to as a **urinary tract infection,** or **UTI.**

The most frequent causes of a UTI are irritation from sexual intercourse and the introduction of bacteria (prin-

cipally, *E. coli*) from the anal region into the vaginal region and into the urethra. To prevent UTIs care should be taken not to introduce anal bacteria into the vaginal region during sexual activity (manually or with the penis). It is recommended that a woman urinate immediately after having sex, wear absorbent cotton underpants or underpants with a cotton crotch, and wipe the urethra in the front-to-back direction after urinating.

The risk of urethritis or cystitis can be lessened by drinking a lot of fluids to wash the bacteria from the urinary tract and by drinking cranberry juice to prevent

TERMS

cervix: the lower, narrow end of the uterus

clitoris: erotically sensitive organ located above the vaginal opening

cystitis: inflammation of the bladder

labia majora: a pair of fleshy folds that cover the labia minora

labia minora: a pair of fleshy folds that cover the vagina

ovulation: release of an egg (ovum) from the ovary

urethra: a tube that carries urine from the bladder to the outside

urethritis: an irritation or infection of the urethra caused by bacteria

urinary tract infection (UTI): inflammation and/or infection of the urethra and/or bladder, usually by bacteria

vulva: the female external genital structures

vulvovaginitis: inflammation of the vaginal region

bacteria from clinging to the cells lining the urinary tract. If a UTI occurs, it is advisable not to drink alcohol or ingest caffeine or spices, for these substances may irritate an already inflamed urinary tract. If pain is severe or if there is blood in the urine, consult a physician. UTIs can be successfully treated with medications.

The **breasts** consist of a network of milk glands and milk ducts embedded in fatty tissue and are affected by pregnancy, nursing, or birth control pills, as well as the different phases of the menstrual cycle. The variation in breast size among women is due to differing amounts of fatty tissue within the breasts. There is little variation among women in the amount of milk-producing tissue; thus, a woman's ability to breastfeed is unrelated to the size of her breasts.

The breasts are supplied with numerous nerve endings, which are important in the delivery of milk to a nursing baby. These nerves also make the breast highly sensitive to touch, and many women find certain forms of tactile stimulation to be sexually pleasurable. Sexual arousal, tactile stimulation, and cold temperatures can cause small muscles in the nipples to contract, resulting in erection of the nipples.

The Fertility or Menstrual Cycle

Approximately monthly, a woman usually produces a single ovum that can be fertilized. These periods of ovum production are referred to as the woman's **fertil-**ity cycle (**Figure 8.5**). During the fertility cycle, a woman's body undergoes several hormonally induced changes to prepare her body for pregnancy. One of these changes is the thickening of the lining of the uterus, the **endometrium,** to support the first stages of pregnancy. In addition, special blood vessels in the uterus increase in size. Their role is to bring maternal nutrients to the embryo and, later in pregnancy, to the fetus. If conception does not occur, the endometrium and the special blood vessels are sloughed off and leave the body via the vagina. This is **menstruation.** Between 15 to 45 milliliters (about 2 to 3 teaspoons) of material are discharged over the span of three to six days. The length of time from one menstruation to another is the **menstrual cycle.**

The length and regularity of the menstrual cycle vary from woman to woman. Most women experience cycles of approximately 28 days, with cycle lengths between 24 and 35 days being the most common. Shorter and longer cycles are possible. Irregular cycles, in which the number of days between menstruations varies from cycle to cycle, can occur. Irregular cycles are common when females first begin to menstruate and also when they stop producing ova later in life.

The menstrual cycle is controlled by a number of hormones. Hormones from the hypothalamus in the brain influence the release of two hormones from the pituitary gland, **follicle-stimulating hormone** (FSH) and

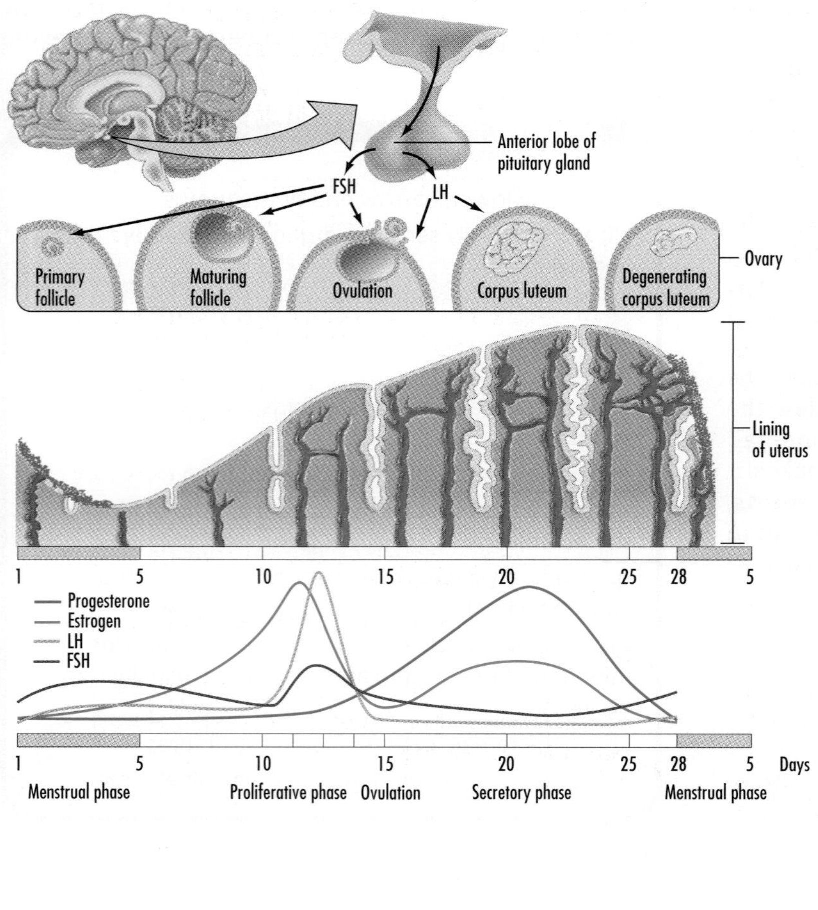

■ Figure 8.5

The Menstrual Cycle

Menstrual phase (days 1–5): The beginning of a cycle is marked by the first day of menstrual bleeding. Proliferative phase (days 6–14): Hormones from the hypothalamus trigger the release of follicle-stimulating hormone (FSH) from the pituitary gland, which circulates through the blood to the ovaries and stimulates the production of estrogen and the maturation of an egg. Estrogen stimulates the proliferation of the lining of the uterus and uterine blood vessels. Ovulation phase (days 14–15): The egg is released from the ovary. Secretory phase (days 16–25): Hormones from the hypothalamus trigger the release of luteinizing hormone (LH) from the pituitary gland, which circulates through the blood to the ovaries and stimulates the production of progesterone from a structure called the corpus luteum. Progesterone stimulates the development of nutrient-producing glands in the lining of the uterus. Next menstrual phase: If pregnancy does not occur, hormone levels drop, the uterine lining breaks down, and menstruation ensues.

luteinizing hormone (LH). These hormones circulate throughout the woman's bloodstream and induce the secretion of estrogen and progesterone from the ovaries, which help prepare a woman's body for pregnancy. If fertilization does not occur, the hormonal support of the endometrium stops, and the uterine tissue is lost in a menstrual discharge.

For some women, menstruation may be accompanied by unpleasant symptoms. For example, it is estimated that half of women experience abdominal pain, commonly referred to as "cramps" and medically referred to as **dysmenorrhea,** usually during the first day or so of menstruation. Although psychological, anatomical, and hormonal factors can contribute to menstrual cramps, in most cases they occur because naturally occurring substances called prostaglandins induce strong contractions of the uterine muscle tissue. The prostaglandins are formed when the uterine lining breaks down; they likely function to promote removal of menstrual tissue from the body. In some instances dysmenorrhea is the result of medical problems such as endometriosis, pelvic inflammatory disease (PID), uterine fibroids, and tumors in the pelvic cavity.

In many instances, the severity of cramps is lessened or eliminated by taking nonsteroidal antiinflammatory drugs (e.g., ibuprofen) or if no ovum is released, which is why women who take combination oral contraceptives ("the pill") often experience relief of cramps. Other ways to lessen menstrual cramps include having a flexible body, practicing meditation or other mental relaxation exercises, or taking medications that reduce levels of prostaglandins.

Another menstrual difficulty is changes in feelings and disposition as the time of menstruation approaches and during the first day or two of menstrual flow. As many as 70% of women report having these or other premenstrual symptoms at some time in their lives (Yonkers, O'Brien, & Eriksson, 2008). These symptoms may include headache, backache, fatigue, feeling bloated, breast tenderness, depression, irritability, unusual aggressive feelings, and social withdrawal. With the onset of menstruation, the symptoms virtually vanish. In about 5% of women, premenstrual symptoms are severe enough to cause **premenstrual dysphoric disorder (PMDD),** which is characterized by a combination of marked mood swings, depression, irritability, and anxiety.

Relief from premenstrual symptoms can be achieved by reducing the intake of caffeine, sugar, and salt around the time of menstruation, increasing exercise, increasing the intake of vitamin B$_6$ (50–100 mg), and having an adequate intake of calcium (1,200 mg a day).

Another common menstrual difficulty is **amenorrhea,** defined as the interruption or cessation of regular menstrual periods. The most common reason periods stop is pregnancy, but the list of factors that can interfere with normal menstruation is quite long. Some factors are psychological stress, depression, marital or sexual problems, fatigue, ingestion of opiate drugs, medications for depression, anxiety, hormonal imbalances, nutritional abnormalities such as severe calorie-restriction diets, anorexia nervosa, and extreme physical activity.

Menopause

Menarche is the first menstruation a young woman experiences. The average age for menarche is between 12 and 13 years, although it can occur as early as 10 years or as late as 19 years. **Menopause** is the gradual cessation of ovulation and menstruation.

Menopause is a time when the ovaries stop producing ova and the ovaries' production of hormones wanes considerably. Therefore, the two principal biological consequences of menopause are that a woman no longer is capable of becoming pregnant, and that her body may undergo changes from the diminished production of estrogen. Many women experience menopause between ages 50 and 52; however, it can occur as early as age 35 and as late as age 55. The age at which menopause occurs may be affected by hereditary, social, and nutritional factors. There is no relation between the age at which menopause occurs and the age at which a woman first begins to menstruate.

TERMS

amenorrhea: cessation of menstruation

breasts: a network of milk glands and ducts in fatty tissue

dysmenorrhea: abdominal pain during menstruation ("menstrual cramps")

endometrium: the inner lining of the uterus

fertility cycle: the near-monthly production of fertilizable eggs

follicle-stimulating hormone: stimulates ovaries to develop mature follicles (with eggs); the follicle produces estrogen

luteinizing hormone: stimulates the release of the ovum (egg) by the follicle; the follicle produces progesterone

menarche: the beginning of menstruation

menopause: the cessation of menstruation in midlife

menstrual cycle: the period of time from one menstruation to another

menstruation: the regular sloughing of the uterine lining via the vagina

premenstrual dysphoric disorder (PMDD): premenstrual symptoms severe enough to impair personal functioning

Because menopause signifies the end of a woman's reproductive capacity, some people believe that it necessarily means the end of her sexual interest and abilities. Whereas this belief is not supported by biological fact, nevertheless, it can have a powerful effect on a woman's (and her partner's) mind and body. Women who accept menopause as a normal part of life can continue to be sexually active.

Although menopause brings biological changes, some of which may be uncomfortable for a while, it is important that menopause not be viewed as a disease (NIH Consensus Panel, 2005). The tendency among women and their health care providers to medicalize menopause led to more than 30 years of replacement therapy with estrogen (hormone replacement therapy), which was thought to be safe but ultimately was shown to increase the risk of heart disease and cancer. Now, replacement therapy with hormones is intended only for women with specific symptoms related to menopause. Some women find relief of menopausal symptoms from nondrug alternatives, such as soy products and the herb black cohosh.

Male Sexual Anatomy

Male sexual anatomy consists of two **testes**, the sites of sperm and sex hormone production; a series of connected sperm ducts that originate at the testes, course through the pelvis, and terminate at the urethra of the penis; glands that produce seminal fluid; and the **penis** (**Figure 8.6**).

The testes are located in a flesh-covered sac, the **scrotum**, that hangs outside the man's body. In the embryo, the testes develop inside the body, but just before birth they descend into the scrotum. Inside the scrotum, the testes are kept at a temperature a few degrees cooler than the internal body temperature, a condition necessary for the production of reproductively capable sperm. Normally, the scrotum hangs loosely from the body wall, although cold temperatures, fear, excitement, or sexual stimulation may cause it to move closer to the body. One testis is usually a little higher than the other.

When a man ejaculates, sperm are propelled through the sperm ducts and out of the penis by contractions of the smooth muscle that lines the sperm ducts and the muscles of the pelvis. As they move out of the body, the sperm mix with secretions of seminal fluid from the **seminal vesicles**, **prostate gland**, and **Cowper's glands** to form **semen**. The semen, which is the gelatinous milky fluid emitted at ejaculation, contains a mixture of about 300 million sperm cells and about 3 to 6 milliliters of seminal fluid. The seminal fluid contributes 95% or more of the entire volume of semen.

The penis is normally soft, but when a man becomes sexually aroused, its internal tissues fill with blood and the penis enlarges and becomes erect. All

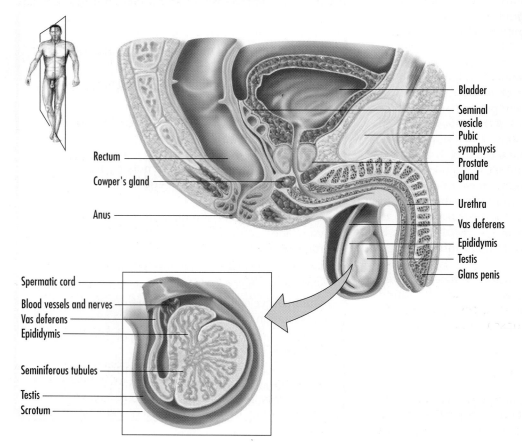

■ **Figure 8.6**
Male Reproductive Organs

Bladder
Seminal vesicle
Pubic symphysis
Prostate gland
Urethra
Vas deferens
Epididymis
Testis
Glans penis

Rectum
Cowper's gland
Anus

Spermatic cord
Blood vessels and nerves
Vas deferens
Epididymis
Seminiferous tubules
Testis
Scrotum

men are born with a fold of skin, the **foreskin,** that covers the end of the penis. In the United States today, parents of male infants can elect to have the foreskin removed surgically within hours after a child's birth. Removal of the foreskin is called **circumcision.** Muslim and Jewish traditions call for the circumcision of all males. Although circumcision may lessen the risk of adult penile cancer and the transmission of sexual infections to sex partners, the American Academy of Pediatrics does not recommend routine neonatal circumcision (American Academy of Pediatrics, 2005). Removal of the foreskin does eliminate the buildup of **smegma,** a white, cheesy substance that can accumulate under the foreskin. The belief that circumcision leads to an increase in sexual arousal because it exposes the glans, and the related belief that circumcision produces an inability to delay ejaculation, are myths. For most men, circumcision has no effect on sexual arousal and sexual activity.

Sexuality: The Psychological Dimension

The psychological dimension of sexuality consists of one's emotions—most frequently joy, excitement, pleasure, love, and affection—and the conscious and unconscious beliefs that guide the interpretation of experience and generate behaviors designed to meet one's sexual and relationship needs. These include an assessment of one's social and sexual attractiveness, one's self-worth, and appropriate attitudes and behaviors for members of each sex (gender roles).

They also include beliefs about what is "natural," beautiful, and good, the behaviors considered "proper" for sexual activity, when and where sexual activity may take place, and who may legitimately have sex with whom. Some beliefs are specific to an individual, such as the willingness to engage in "casual sex," and others are shared among a group, such as the disapproval of having sexual relationships with someone other than one's spouse. Occasionally a society's shared beliefs are codified into law, such as the prohibition of prostitution.

Beliefs are acquired through **socialization,** the process by which a social group confers attitudes and behavioral expectations upon individuals. It is through socialization that individuals learn what sexuality means for members of their group. Socializing influences include parents, family, school, peer groups, religion, employment setting, and mass media.

Sexuality: The Orientation Dimension

Sexual orientation is the propensity to be sexually and romantically attracted to members of a particular sex. People with a same-sex orientation are referred to as

homosexual; people with an other-sex orientation are referred to as *heterosexual.* People whose orientation is for either sex are referred to as *bisexual.* It is estimated that 5% to 10% of adults are exclusively homosexual. Some surveys indicate that about 50% of the population have had some same-sex sexual experience, often occurring in childhood and adolescence when sexual experimentation is common. Many people say they are erotically aroused by individuals of their sex but have no desire to act on those feelings.

Traditionally our culture has forbidden same-sex sexual and intimate relationships, asserting that they are wrong, immoral, unnatural, or indicative of psychological illness. Neither the American Psychological Association nor the American Psychiatric Association considers same-sex orientation to be a mental illness. Scientific studies have failed to uncover any inherited, hormonal, or metabolic abnormalities that account for same-sex orientation. The neuropsychological mechanisms underlying the development and patterning of sexual orientation are unknown. One thing that is certain is that sexual orientation is rarely a choice; to each individual, it seems "natural."

By and large, same-sex intimate relationships are similar to other-sex ones, with the possible exception that they involve less gender-specific stereotypical behaviors. Some same-sex relationships are casual and do not involve long-term commitments, whereas others involve a deep and lasting emotional commitment and

---

TERMS

circumcision: a surgical procedure to remove the foreskin from the penis

Cowper's glands: small glands secreting drops of alkalinizing fluid into the urethra

foreskin: a fold of skin over the end of the penis

penis: the male's organ of copulation and urination

prostate gland: gland at the base of the bladder providing seminal fluid

scrotum: the sac of skin that contains the testes

semen: a whitish, creamy fluid containing sperm

seminal vesicles: glands that secrete a fluid that is a component of semen

sexual orientation: the propensity to be sexually and romantically attracted to a particular sex

smegma: a white, cheesy substance that accumulates under the foreskin of the penis

socialization: the process by which social groups confer attitudes and expectations upon individuals

testes: a pair of male reproductive organs that produce sperm cells and male sex hormones

sexual exclusivity. Sexual orientation in itself does not affect the desire to love and be loved and to be involved in committed, caring relationships.

Sexuality: The Behavioral Dimension

The behavioral dimension of sexuality includes activities intended to produce a sexual experience. Although sexual activity is generally thought of in terms of genital stimulation, genital responses, and orgasm, in reality it also involves one's mind, spirit, and relationship with one's partner.

Generally, sexual activity requires that a person be interested in creating a sexual experience. The propensity to be interested in sexual experiences can be likened to interests in anything else. Some people are very interested in playing tennis and others are less so. Although in our society people are expected to be highly and frequently interested in sex, in reality the desire for sexual activity varies among individuals and couples, changes over time, and is influenced by interpersonal and psychological factors. For example, many couples report a higher degree of sexual desire at the beginning of their relationship than after the relationship has matured. Alternatively, couples who have been together for many years may experience an increase in sexual interest when the childrearing phase of the family life cycle is completed. Various physical and psychological situations can affect sexual interest as well. For example, many women report a transient loss of sexual interest during the first few weeks after childbirth. Depression and physical illness are also often associated with loss of interest in sex.

Having sexual desire does not necessarily mean that a person will behave sexually. Human sexual behavior is not "reflexive"; sexual activity does not occur automatically whenever one feels "horny" or one is presented with a sexual opportunity. Instead, sexual activity is the result of a decision (except in instances of sexual coercion and assault) that is based on desire to conform to social norms, personal values, and physical and psychological needs.

Creating a sexual experience involves two kinds of decision. The first concerns context, that is, the social situation in which sexual activity takes place. Societies have rules and norms that govern sexual activity. Individuals are not permitted to have sex with just anyone or in any social setting.

The second type of decision concerns participation in a sexual episode. Even in a situation or relationship in which sexual activity is acceptable and opportunities to have sex are present, a person can decide "yes," "no," "not yet," or "maybe" whenever a sexual opportunity occurs. The decision is made by evaluating how one feels physically and emotionally at the time, one's per-

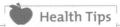

Health Tips

Alcohol: The Risky Social/Sexual Lubricant

How many people do you know say they need to drink to have a good time? Probably lots. Many students say they use alcohol to quell their nervousness about going to parties or other social gatherings, or that they need alcohol to feel less nervous or inhibited about sex. The problem with using alcohol to reduce anxiety is that it reduces other physical processes and inhibitions that often protect us from danger. So if you need to get tipsy or drunk before you can say "yes" to sex, consider the following:

- Alcohol can suppress the body's ability to respond sexually, thus impairing erection, lubrication, and orgasm.
- Being drunk can impair your ability to feel pleasure or even be aware of what you are doing.
- You might have sex with someone you would not otherwise be involved with ("beer goggles").
- You create a situation for sexual assault.
- It's easy to get unintentionally pregnant.
- You may forget to practice safer sex and thereby increase the risk of HIV/AIDS or another sexually transmitted disease.

sonal criteria for being sexual within the presenting situation, and one's expectation of how having sex at that time will affect one's self-esteem and the relationship.

Sexual Arousal and Response

There is no formula for creating sexual arousal. Everyone has preferences. In situations and circumstances that they deem appropriate for sex, most people respond sexually to being touched in certain ways. Certain regions of the body are highly sexually sensitive in nearly all people. These are the erogenous zones—the genitals, the breasts, the anus, the lips, the inner thighs, and the mouth.

When a person becomes sexually aroused, the brain and nervous system prepare the body for sexual activity. Impulses from the brain are transmitted by the spinal nerves to various parts of the body and cause physiological changes. These changes include the tightening of many skeletal muscles (**myotonia**); changes in the pattern of blood flow (**vasocongestion**), especially in the pelvis; increases in heart rate, blood pressure, and respiratory rate; increase in the general level of excitement; and increase in erotic feelings.

Increased pelvic blood flow in the male produces erection of the penis. The penis enlarges because the spongy tissues within it fill with blood. In the female, increased pelvic blood flow produces lubrication of the vagina and swelling of the clitoris and vaginal lips. Vaginal lubrication is produced by the release of fluids from

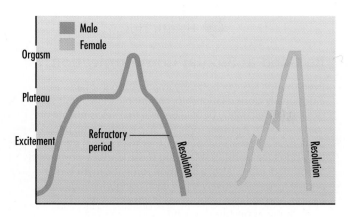

■ **Figure 8.7**
Sexual Response Cycle

the walls of the vagina. Swelling of the clitoris and vaginal lips is caused by the filling with blood of spongy tissues within them. In some women the changes in blood flow caused by sexual arousal also produce a swelling of the breasts.

Regardless of the type of sexual stimulation, the physiological response in both men and women is similar and follows a pattern called the **sexual response cycle,** which consists of four phases (**Figure 8.7**):

- *Phase 1:* Excitement, in which the person experiences sexual arousal from any source and the body responds with specific changes, including erection of the penis in males and vaginal lubrication and swelling of the clitoris and genitalia in females.
- *Phase 2:* Plateau, in which the physiological changes of the excitement phase level off, although subjective feelings of sexual arousal tend to increase.
- *Phase 3:* Orgasm, in which the tensions that build during excitement and plateau are released.
- *Phase 4:* Resolution, in which the body returns to the physiologically nonstimulated state. Resolution may include a *refractory period,* a period of time (from minutes to days) during which orgasm and ejaculation cannot occur.

There is considerable variation in the extent and duration of the sexual response cycle among individuals of either sex. There is even variation in the nature of the response in the same person because each sexual encounter is different.

Orgasm

When sexual arousal builds to a certain point, the associated sexual tensions are released in an **orgasm.** The orgasmic response in both women and men frequently is associated with rhythmic contractions of the pelvic muscles; tightening of the muscles of the face, hands, and feet; and feelings of pleasure. Most commonly, men

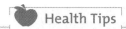 **Health Tips**

Tips for Enhancing Sexual Experience

- Create pleasure by stimulating the whole body, not just the genitals.
- Vary the manner and intensity of stimulation. Allow sensations to build and wane.
- Try not to make sex = work.
- Set aside time that is free of intrusions and distractions. Disconnect the phone; lock the door to ensure privacy.
- Make yourself an open, effective channel for sexual arousal before sexual activity begins. Satisfying sex is not a mechanical activity involving only bodies, but a blending of mind–body energies. Remove sex-negative energies such as hunger, fatigue, and anger, and focus your energy on sex through deep breathing or other relaxing activity.
- Be aware of differences between you and your partner in the state of readiness for sexual activity. Try to synchronize both partners' states of sexual arousal through talking, light touching, dance, massage, and so on, before sexual activity begins.
- Address concerns about birth control and STDs prior to sexual experience.
- Take your time. Go slowly.
- Communicate likes and dislikes to your partner either verbally or nonverbally.
- Do not focus just on orgasms. Learn to appreciate the many sexual sensations from touching all parts of the body.
- Either partner may reach orgasm through manual, oral, or other means of stimulation before or after intercourse.
- Sexual activity need not stop after one partner reaches orgasm. If a couple chooses, lovemaking can continue until both wish to stop.
- Neither individual may desire an orgasm during a particular sexual episode. Physically expressing love and caring does not require orgasm.

ejaculate during orgasm, although it is possible for males to experience orgasm without ejaculation and vice versa. The media have perpetuated the myth that during male or female orgasm, bells ring, the earth shakes, lights flash, and moans and groans are elicited, but often orgasms are quiet.

TERMS

myotonia: muscle tension

orgasm: the climax of sexual responses and the release of physiological and sexual tensions

sexual response cycle: the four-phase physiological response to sexual arousal in both men and women

vasocongestion: the engorgement of blood in particular body regions in response to sexual arousal

Orgasmic experiences vary greatly from person to person and from one encounter to another. For all persons there are "big orgasms" and "little orgasms" depending on the level of arousal. Sometimes, if a person is not sufficiently aroused, or too tired, tense, or ill, there may be no orgasm.

Our society is oriented toward achievement, and it has become common to apply measures of success to sex, especially orgasm. For example, many people believe that "success" is determined by the number of orgasms a woman has during a sexual episode. By this standard, a successful male is someone who can delay ejaculation until his partner has experienced at least one orgasm and preferably more, whereas a successful female is someone who can have more than one orgasm in every sexual encounter. Men and women who cannot "manufacture" the appropriate number of orgasms may be erroneously labeled "inadequate" by themselves and others. When people become overly concerned with "succeeding" or "performing well," they can become psychologically detached from the activity. Rather than abandon themselves completely to sexual experience, they withdraw their attention and observe their actions. This is called **spectatoring**.

Masturbation

Masturbation is self-stimulation to produce erotic arousal, usually to the point of orgasm. Although social and religious attitudes in many cultures consider it improper, immoral, or perverse, masturbation is nevertheless practiced widely throughout the world and even among other animal species.

Many people find masturbation a rewarding variation in their sex lives. People masturbate for many of the same reasons that they have partner sex: to experience erotic pleasure; to relieve physical tensions; to produce a sense of relaxation; to induce sleep; and, when done with a partner, to create feelings of intimacy and bonding. Often, people find masturbation to be a way to understand what pleases them sexually.

A number of personal harmful effects have long been rumored to result from masturbation. Among them are hair loss, insanity, pimples, warts, unhappy personal relations, and the inability to have children. There is no evidence that any of these claims are true. Physically, masturbation is harmless as long as it is not injurious to the stimulated organs.

Sexual Abstinence

> It's been so long since I made love, I can't remember who gets tied up.
>
> *Joan Rivers*

Although someone may have interest in and desire for sex, he or she may choose to abstain from sexual activity. For religious reasons certain people practice lifelong sexual abstinence (sometimes

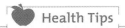
Health Tips

Be Good at Sexual Communication

Even though sex can be a very important part of an emotionally close relationship, communicating about sex can be difficult. Many people believe that sex is private or "dirty" and not a proper topic for discussion. Some people don't have a sexual vocabulary other than sexual slang, and they don't feel comfortable using those kinds of words with an intimate other. Also, a common romantic myth is that people in love intuitively know each other's feelings and desires, and so talking about sex is unnecessary.

Sometimes gestures, touches, and glances can communicate sexual messages, but such nonverbal cues run the risk of being missed or misunderstood. Verbal communication lessens the risk of misunderstandings and hurt feelings. Talking about sex in the early part of a relationship can prevent the development of negative patterns, especially the unspoken assumption that it's not OK to talk about sex.

If talking about sex is difficult for you, it might help to share with your partner your unease: *"The sexual aspects of our relationship are important to me, but I'm nervous [uncomfortable, shy, etc.] about talking about this subject"* or *"There's something I want to talk about, but it's hard for me. I'd like to try, but before I do I'd like to be sure that at first you'll just listen and not comment."*

Then, you can share your personal and family history about sexuality and sex talk. You can describe how sexual topics were dealt with in your family and peer group, how you learned sexual words, and your current attitudes about talking about sex. Eventually you will develop sufficient comfort to talk about specific sexual aspects of your relationship.

called **celibacy,** which literally means remaining unmarried). Some individuals refrain from sexual intercourse until they marry. Still others avoid sexual interaction because they fear the closeness and intimacy implied by sex or they have strong negative feelings regarding sex.

Individuals not wishing to practice lifelong sexual abstinence may nevertheless benefit from a sex "time out." For example, recovery from a physical or emotional illness may include sexual abstinence. No sex is a sure way to avoid an unintended pregnancy or a sexually transmitted disease. Some people find abstaining helpful while recovering from the breakup of a love relationship. The healing of the emotional wound seems to proceed more smoothly without the emotional intensity that often accompanies sexual interaction.

Sexual abstinence can also provide an opportunity to develop a new set of personal and relational experiences. By avoiding the intimacy that often accompanies sex, abstinence provides a way to discover new dimensions in interpersonal relationships. Without the diver-

Table 8.1

Factors Contributing to Sexual Difficulties

Types of factors	Examples
Organic factors	Illness of any kind
	Hormonal, vascular, and neurological illness
	Fatigue or psychoendocrine stress
	Medications and recreational drugs
Values, beliefs, and attitudes	*Negative values about sex*
	Sex is dirty; sex is sinful
	Genitals (especially female) are dirty
	Women are not supposed to enjoy sex
	Men are supposed to always be interested in sex
	Men are supposed to always be capable of sex
	Narrow definition of sex
	Sex = penis-in-vagina intercourse
	Goal orientation (sex = orgasm)
	Performance expectations
Personality and experiences	Low self-esteem
	Emotional difficulties (anxiety, depression, grief)
	Prior incidence of sexual abuse
	Poor body image
Relationship factors	Discomfort with intimacy
	Relationship problems
	Fear of pregnancy or sexually transmitted disease
	Sexual orientation

sion of sex (or the search for sex partners) an individual can focus on self-development, career, or school and put energy into friendships. New romantic relationships can develop without the pressure for sex early in the relationship, thus permitting the partners to develop trust and caring before becoming sexual.

Sexual Difficulties

Many individuals expect sex always to be exciting and satisfying; anything less is cause for concern. Life is full of changes, however, and the demands of career or parenting or occasional illness can sometimes produce a temporary loss in interest in sex or the ability to engage in sex (Table 8.1). Such changes in sexual interest and ability are normal and usually resolve themselves. Persistent difficulties with sex may signal that consulting a health professional would be helpful.

Lack of Interest Therapists and counselors refer to the lack of interest in sex as hypoactive sexual desire or sexual aversion, and note that it can result from the following:

1. *Underlying sexual difficulty.* One or both partners may have some physical difficulty engaging in sex: A man may be unable to gain or maintain an erection, or a woman may experience pain during intercourse. Such problems can make sexual activity unpleasant for either or both partners, and they eventually lose sexual interest.

2. *Failure to communicate likes and dislikes.* One partner may find some aspects of sex unsatisfying and not communicate this information to the other partner. Resentment and displeasure may subsequently build up to the point that interest in sex is lost.

3. *Boredom.* Like anything else that becomes predictable and routine, sex can become boring if it is always done in the same way and at the same time. As with other activities, the old cliché is true: "Variety is the spice of life."

4. *Stress, fatigue, and depression.* Being emotionally drained by work or other responsibilities or being "low" or "blue" can interfere with sexual desire.

5. *Alcohol and other drugs.* Frequent ingestion of alcohol and other drugs can lower sexual desire. Drug use can also turn off a partner who does not want to make love to someone who is drunk or on drugs. Some medications can also lessen interest in sex.

6. *Pregnancy and children.* During pregnancy and child raising, the increase in responsibilities and the decrease in private time can lower interest in sex. Busy couples must make an effort to schedule time to be together (for sex and other activities).

7. *Hostility and anger.* Unresolved conflicts are a common cause of lost sexual interest. It may be difficult to feel intimate with someone with whom you are angry.

8. *Change in physical appearance.* Once they are in a relationship, some people stop caring about their appearance, which may lessen a partner's sexual interest.

9. *Physical illness.* Physical illnesses can cause some people to believe they shouldn't have sex. For example, the man who has a heart attack may be afraid to have sex because he fears another heart attack.

Erection Problems Difficulty in attaining or maintaining an erection can result from vascular disease in the pelvic region, being sick or injured, and being stressed or depressed. It can also result from smoking and the use

---

TERMS

celibacy: sexual abstinence

masturbation: self-induced sexual stimulation

spectatoring: observing one's own sexual experience rather than fully taking part in it

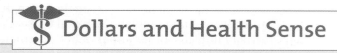

$ Dollars and Health Sense

Sex Sells

Many people are concerned about their sex lives. This is one reason that Viagra and similar drugs for the treatment of erection problems are widely advertised to healthy young men *without* erection problems who are looking for a sexual enhancer (Delate, Simmons, & Motheral, 2004). Prescription drugs for the treatment of male erection problems have become big money-makers.

The successful selling of sex drugs to men prompted an attempt by pharmaceutical companies to come up with sex-enhancer drugs for women. Company-sponsored conferences brought together scientists (all of whom were paid) to produce definitions for "female sexual dysfunction" that suggested a need for drug treatment (Moynihan, 2003). Most often, the "dysfunction" under consideration was diminished sexual desire, and the drugs suggested to "treat" the condition included the same ones for male erection problems and various types of androgens (male sex hormones). These drugs were found to have minimal therapeutic effects in women and were not approved for treatment of female sexual problems.

Some sexual difficulties are sometimes amenable to drug treatment. It is one thing to provide a legitimate treatment, however, and quite another to suggest that a deviation from an ideal is a disease. For example, the expectation that a woman (or man) should be continuously interested in and willing and able to engage and respond passionately in sexual relations is unrealistic. Life is full of challenges, changes, and circumstances that affect sexual desire and activity. But if lack of interest in sex, anxiety about sexual performance, and difficulties with vaginal lubrication can be diagnosed as medical problems, drug companies stand to make huge profits.

---

of alcohol, marijuana, opiates, other recreational drugs, and some medications, including those for neurological disease and high blood pressure. Erection problems also result from fear of sexual performance (including anxiety about one's ability to get an erection), fear of pregnancy or contracting an STD, or the wish not to be sexual with a particular partner. Counseling and/or drugs that increase blood volume in the penis (e.g., *Viagra*) are common treatments.

Rapid Ejaculation Rapid or "premature" ejaculation is persistent or recurrent ejaculation before a man or his sexual partner wishes it. Rapid ejaculation is reported to occur in 25% of American men, most commonly between the ages of 20 and 40. Because it is a reflex activity, with practice, a man can learn to control ejaculation voluntarily just as he does with bladder function. The key to controlling ejaculation is awareness of the bodily sensations that signal the onset of ejaculation, followed by modulation of sexual arousal according to one's desires. A variety of counseling techniques can help men learn to control ejaculation. Other methods include lessening penile sensations (condoms, topical anesthetics) or using selective serotonin reuptake inhibitors (SSRIs), which cause ejaculatory delay (Waldinger, 2008).

Painful Intercourse In women, painful intercourse can be caused by vaginal infections, insufficient vaginal lubrication before intercourse (usually the result of not being sufficiently sexually aroused), and anxiety-produced spasms of the muscles surrounding the vagina, which makes vaginal penetration painful. Another source of pain associated with intercourse is a deep, aching sensation in the pelvis for women or in the scrotum ("blue balls") for men. This condition is caused by the congestion of blood in the pelvic region brought about by sexual arousal. Orgasm often reverses the con-

gestion, but lack of orgasm can cause blood to remain and cause discomfort and pain.

Orgasm Difficulties Both men and women can have difficulty experiencing orgasm. Most often this difficulty is the result of insufficient sexual arousal, perhaps because of aversion to a particular partner, fear of pregnancy or sexually transmitted diseases, fear of letting go emotionally, lack of trust, or negative attitudes about sexual pleasure.

Sexuality: The Relationship Dimension

The relationship dimension of sexuality consists of the tendency to behave sexually in interpersonal relationships characterized by feelings of love, intimacy, and emotional closeness. Most people find that sexual activity influences—and is influenced by—these kinds of relationships because, by its very nature, sex is an intimate act. Sexually relating individuals share themselves with each other in special ways that they do not share with friends, even close ones. They expose their bodies to each other; they touch each other; they create powerful emotions; their bodies join physically.

Intimacy is a feeling of closeness, trust, and openness with another person that tells us that our innermost self can be shared without fear of attack or emotional hurt and that we are understood in the deepest sense possible.

Intimate relationships can have an enormous impact on one's sense of vitality and well-being. When an intimate relationship is flowing smoothly, it can produce rich emotional satisfaction unparalleled by any other experience. Those who are involved in genuinely supportive and caring relationships tend to feel confident about the potential of life to be harmonious and

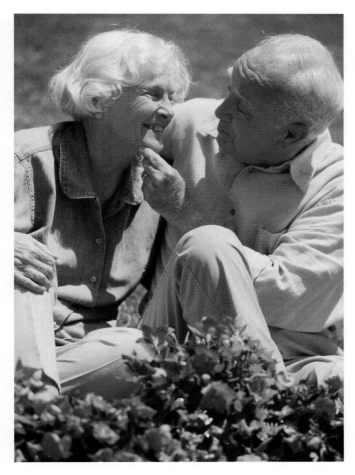

Intimacy is a basic human need at every age.

find intimate relationships to be distracting or psychologically threatening. In some instances, previous life experiences can leave an individual fearful of emotional closeness, which can block the establishment of intimacy. In some of these instances, there are repeated attempts to form relationships; however, without the element of intimacy, these relationships can fail.

Factors that influence the choice of intimate partners include the following:

- *Proximity.* People are most likely to become intimate with someone with whom they are in physical proximity.
- *Similarity.* Similar age, religion, race, education, social background, attitudes, values, and interests affect the possibility for intimacy in two ways: They influence proximity, and they reflect social norms for permissible peer intimacies. Note, for example, biases against interracial and older–younger intimacies. Colleges and universities provide students with relatively easy access to a "pool of eligibles" because they bring together individuals of similar age, intelligence, expectations, and values.
- *Physical appearance.* Physical appearance provides cues that indicate who among the pool of eligibles is a desirable intimate partner. Those who are judged "attractive" tend to be thought of as kind, understanding, and affectionate ("what is beautiful is good"). Pairing with someone who is considered physically attractive enhances one's social status and self-esteem.

Developing Intimacy

Most people want their intimate relationships to develop feelings of closeness, positive regard, warmth, and familiarity with the other's innermost thoughts and feelings. This deep knowledge of each other comes from sharing the most important and often secret aspects of one's personality—one's goals, aspirations, strengths, weaknesses, and physical and sexual desires. The sharing of such private information is called **self-disclosure.**

When relationships begin, little intimate information is usually disclosed. People talk about the weather,

> The question that women casually shopping for perfume ask more than any other is this: "What scent drives men wild?" After years of intense research we know the definitive answer. It is bacon.
>
> *John Lanchester, The New Yorker*

beautiful. On the other hand, when an intimate relationship is not going well, those involved can be overwhelmed by moroseness and unable to think of anything but their misery. They can be angry, depressed, anxious, or distraught, sometimes to the point of being unable to function at work or at school.

Many people mistakenly equate genuine intimacy with sexual intercourse. This happens because love and affection are feelings associated with intimacy. But intimacy is a feeling, not an act. It is the *quality* of a relationship between two people—a shared experiencing of their personal lives. People who have an intimate relationship may or may not choose to express their intimate feelings with sex.

The Life Cycle of Intimate Relationships

Intimate relationships tend to develop through the stages of (1) selecting a partner, (2) developing intimacy, and (3) establishing commitment. Before an intimate relationship can develop, however, the partners have to be psychologically open to entering and maintaining it. Some individuals choose not to be involved in an intimate relationship, perhaps because they wish to devote energies to school, work, or self-development, or they

TERMS

self-disclosure: sharing personal experiences and feelings with someone

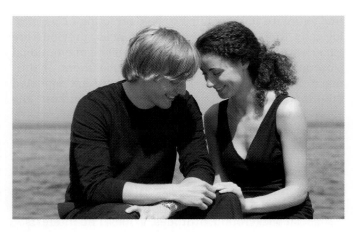

Intimacy begins by doing fun things together.

sports, TV, or politics. They gossip about professors, students, or other people they know. And they ask each other the classic leading questions: Where are you from? What do you do? What's your major? People face these questions so many times that they become adept at revealing as much or as little about themselves as feels comfortable. It is when they begin to talk about their personal history, current life problems, hopes and aspirations, and fears and personal failures that they begin to disclose important information—important because disclosing it makes them feel vulnerable. Most people discuss their deepest feelings only with those in whom they have developed considerable trust.

Intimacy develops through a progressive, mutual revealing of innermost thoughts. Psychologists compare people's personalities to onions—having many layers, from an outer surface to an inner core. As acquaintances gain more and more knowledge about each other, they penetrate deeper and deeper through the layers of the other's personality, which establishes their intimacy. Another view compares intimate development to the peeling of an artichoke. Resistance and barriers to sharing information about oneself are like the leaves of the artichoke; as intimacy progresses, intimates peel away the leaves to get to the other's "heart."

Self-disclosure leads to the development of intimacy in two ways. First, you tend to be affected either positively or negatively by the information that is disclosed. If you make a positive judgment, you are likely to want to continue interacting with that person, for you believe that future interactions will be equally or even more positive. The same logic applies to negative assessments. If your reaction is unfavorable, you are likely to terminate the relationship, or perhaps maintain it on a lesser level of intimacy.

The second way that self-disclosure leads to intimacy is the *act* of self-disclosure, which, regardless of the information offered, often leads to reciprocal self-disclosure. By sharing important information, you communicate that you trust the other person, and usually that person accepts your trust and becomes more willing to disclose information. In this way intimacy progresses by a cycle of self-disclosure leading to trust, which brings about self-disclosure, which leads to more trust, and so on.

Establishing Commitment

After a period of self-disclosure, individuals may sense that their relationship has progressed to a state of "us-ness," that it has become a special friendship, a love relationship, or a marital-type relationship. This state of "us-ness" is one of commitment, which has three aspects:

- *An action, pledge, or promise:* One makes a promise and thus announces one's intention explicitly, even if it is only to the partner. Various social values and norms regarding keeping promises and the guilt and loss of self-esteem that come with breaking promises are among the "push" factors that keep a person committed. If the promise involves a social ritual (i.e., marriage ceremony, getting pinned), then family, friends, and the state become additional "push" factors.
- *A state of being obligated or emotionally compelled:* This state involves a cluster of emotions such as love, comfort, caring, and relief from separation anxiety and loneliness.
- *An unwillingness to consider any partner other than the current one:* The rewards of the current relationship outweigh the costs of exploring other opportunities for intimacy.

Endings

Everything in the universe (even the universe itself!) has a beginning and an end. Close relationships have a beginning and an end also. Sometimes a relationship lasts for only a few minutes; sometimes it lasts until one of the partners dies (and even then the relationship may still be "alive" in the imagination of the surviving partner). Sometimes the structure of a close relationship persists but the closeness and the dynamism wane, creating a "shell" relationship without vitality. Sometimes a relationship goes through cycles of birth and death within the structure of its ongoingness. When a close relationship ends, some or all of its structure, exchange of resources (e.g., love, caring, financial support), and feelings of attachment and emotional bondedness end also.

Endings occur for a variety of reasons. Partners' feelings of attachment and bondedness may be absent or weak. Life goals, values, or interests may no longer be shared. One or both partners may be unwilling or unable to invest personal resources such as greater time shared with the partner, or to commit to an exclusive relationship. Whether partners continue in a relationship also is affected by their assessment of other options, such as another potential partner or singlehood. Without suitable alternatives, leaving a relationship may seem difficult, unwise, or impossible.

Another reason ongoingness stops is that the partners, either individually or as a dyadic unit, are unable to move the relationship into its next stage. For example, some couples cannot navigate the transition from being idealistic, passionate lovers to realistic, companionate lovers. In nonmarital close relationships, a partner may not be considered suitable as a potential marital partner, even in the presence of considerable love, attachment, and liking.

Another factor associated with endings is lack of support, or even hostility, from the partners' social network. Families may not accept a son's or daughter's choice of a dating or marital partner. Interracial, disabled, and same-sex relationships are still heavily stigmatized in our society.

Occasionally the seeds of an ending are sown into a relationship at its beginning. For example, partners may seek closeness as a way to cope with or avoid personal problems. They may feel rejected and lonely because of the breakup of a previous relationship. They may feel that they cannot take care of themselves. They may be afraid of leaving home or school. If, as often happens, a partner or relationship does not turn out to be the solution to a personal problem, a disappointed, angry, or frustrated partner may seek alternative ways of coping. These alternatives, such as drug or alcohol abuse, extra-relationship affairs, or physically or emotionally abusing the partner (or other family members) (see Chapter 23), may very well be destructive to the relationship.

When a breakup does occur, individuals may feel tired, lethargic, lonely, sad, depressed, angry, resentful, and guilty. They may be unable to sleep or eat, may miss class, or be unable to work. They may withdraw from friends. They may find concentrating difficult because they are continually thinking about the partner and what happened in the relationship. They may feel helpless ("What will become of me?") and hopeless ("I'll never find a true love") or skeptical and cynical ("Love can never work out").

Some partners feel relaxed, hopeful, and relieved that what they identify as a bad or going-nowhere relationship has ended and they are free to pursue personal goals or find a relationship partner who is better suited to them. Sometimes individuals feel euphoric and self-confident. They say that the separation was for the best, and they become more active and outgoing. This positive outlook may alternate with emotional distress.

When a person is emotionally (and sometimes physically) wracked with the pain of an ending, he or she may have difficulty seeing any good in that experience, but often endings mark the start of a new and better future. A study of remarried people showed that many had learned a lot about themselves and the nature of close relationships from a previous marriage(s) and found that their current marriage was much more satisfying. Guiding principles for enhanced relationships are patience and experience.

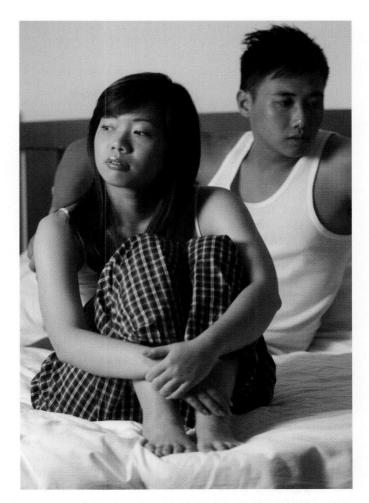

When communication breaks down, stress and tension can occur.

Communicating in Intimate Relationships

Communication is a symbolic process of creating and sharing meaning. At the heart of communication is an individual act that involves imparting a message to another person to share information or feelings, to coordinate behavior with an individual or group of people, or to persuade someone to do something.

A communication act begins as a mental image; an idea, a wish, or a feeling (or some combination of these). If humans were capable of mind reading, people could impart mental images directly to each other. Few people can read minds, however, so communication requires that thoughts be transformed into symbols that can carry information. Those symbols make up the message. The most common symbols in communication are

> Start every day with a smile and get it over with.
> *W. C. Fields*

- *Words:* spoken or printed
- *Visual images:* paintings, sculpture, photos

- *Posture or body language:* gaze, touch, smile, physical proximity, folding arms, frowning, turning away
- *Objects:* flowers, gifts, food
- *Behaviors:* doing a favor, giving a kiss, ignoring an appointment

Encoding a mental image into the symbols that make up a message is only half of a communication act. The other half is taking in the symbols that make up the message and decoding them into mental images. Thus, a communication act requires two transformations: in the sender, the transformation of mental images into symbols; in the receiver, the transformation of symbols into mental images.

Consider this example of a communication act between Beth and Ron one rainy morning. Beth doesn't want Ron to get wet in the rain, so she decides to use spoken words as the symbols to encode her thoughts. Beth says, "Ron, it's raining." Ron hears Beth's words, and decodes them into a mental image of the weather that day, and he picks up his umbrella.

In this communication act Beth accomplished her goal. But a different outcome could have occurred if one or more of the steps in the communication act had been distorted, weakened, or blocked completely. For example, if Beth had said "it's raining" in a tone of voice that Ron didn't appreciate, or if her words had been misunderstood, the communication process would have been distorted.

Every communication act carries two types of message or potential meaning. The first is the **literal message**, which is the message conveyed by the symbols themselves, as in the words "it's raining." The second is the **metamessage** (*meta* is the Greek word for "beyond," "additional," or "transcendent"), which carries implicit messages about the reason for the communication, how the message is to be interpreted, and the nature of the relationship of the sender and receiver.

When Beth said to Ron, "it's raining," not only did she send a literal message about the weather, but she also sent several metamessages, including "I care about you" and "an expectation in our relationship is that we help each other out."

After Beth had told Ron that it was raining, if Ron had kissed Beth and said, "Thanks, honey, for looking out for me," he would have been responding to one of the metamessages in the communication. If Ron had interpreted the metamessage as "Ron, you're terribly childlike and I have to make decisions for you"—even though Beth didn't intend to impart that message—Ron might have responded angrily with something like "Beth, I can look out for myself!" Her feelings may then have been hurt and possibly they would have had an argument. Acknowledging and responding to metamessages can sometimes be much more important than dealing with the literal ones.

Sending Clear Messages

A clear message is one in which the symbols represent as closely as possible the sender's intent. Clear messages are best delivered with **I-statements**; these are sentences that begin with (or have as the subject) the pronoun "I." I-statements clearly identify the sender as the source of a thought, emotion, desire, or act: I think . . . I feel . . . I want (need) . . . I did (will do). . . .

You-statements, which begin with (or have as the subject) the pronoun "you," as in "You always . . .," "You never . . .," "You are . . .," or the interrogatives "Why don't you . . .?" or "How could you . . .?" often are put-downs or character assassinations. They imply that the receiver is not OK. Very often the not-OK message is explicit, as in "You're incompetent" or "You're stupid"—just about any negative adjective will do. People often respond to the metamessage in a you-statement, which is "I think you're no good," by feeling attacked, which can lead to hurt feelings and counterattacks or withdrawal.

Effective Listening

Effective communication requires both talking and listening. Effective listening is important because the listener not only takes in the speaker's message, but also helps establish the physical and emotional context for the communication. The listener also must communicate to the speaker that the message was received. This is called **feedback.** Some techniques for effective listening are giving the sender your full attention, making eye contact, listening, being empathic, being open for receiving the message, giving verbal feedback, acknowledging the sender's feelings, praising the sender's efforts, and being unconditional.

Give the Speaker Your Full Attention Don't fake it. If you can't pay attention because you are tired, hungry, distracted, angry, or whatever, tell the speaker how you feel and ask if it's OK to talk after you rest, or eat, or go to the bathroom, or just talk at another time. The speaker is likely to grant your request if immediacy is not an issue, because he or she wants your full attention.

Make Eye Contact Try to assume similar postures (i.e., both sitting or both standing) to create a sense of equal status. Making eye-to-eye contact allows the speaker to feel comfortable as well as conveying that you are listening to him or her and taking in the complete message.

Just Listen Don't interrupt until you have a signal that the speaker is finished or the speaker has asked for a response, unless you don't understand what is being communicated. You can acknowledge that you are actively listening with gestures, nods, and vocalizations like "uh-huh," "yes," "go on," "I see," and so forth.

Be Empathic Try to "hear" the speaker's feelings as well as the words. Be open to the speaker's intentions and motivations as well as her or his ideas. Ask yourself, "What is this person feeling right now?"

Be an Open Channel for Receiving a Message Don't judge or evaluate the speaker or the message while the speaker is talking. Try not to correct the speaker or, if the speaker is being critical of you, to think of a defense.

Give Verbal Feedback Don't mind read. Summarize in your own words your understanding of the speaker's thoughts and emotions. This way the speaker can find out if the message that was intended was actually received. If so, then you can respond. If not, then the speaker can try again. Ask for clarification if there's something you don't understand. You can say something like, "I don't think I understand everything you were saying about your mother. Can you tell me again, maybe in a different way?"

Acknowledge the Speaker's Emotions "It seems to me that you're feeling . . ." and if you're not sure, add "Do I have that right?" By acknowledging or providing feedback, you are sharing what you believe are the speaker's emotions. If you are incorrect, the speaker can relay that to you.

Praise the Speaker's Effort Acknowledge the speaker's efforts for investing the time, energy, and caring to communicate with you, especially if the communication was a difficult one.

Be Unconditional Let the speaker know that you respect him or her even if you are uncomfortable with the messages that are being communicated. Assure the speaker that even though things may be difficult, you are willing to continue talking and working through difficult feelings.

Expressing Anger Constructively

Disagreements and conflicts are inevitable in any close relationship. The notion that people in intimate relationships shouldn't fight because love makes them see eye to eye on everything and the idea that you can't possibly be angry with someone you love are romantic myths. By expressing anger constructively, intimates fight for the success of their relationship as well as for their individual needs.

In constructive fighting, there should be no "winner" and no "loser." Good fights are efforts of individuals to be heard and to improve the relationship. The best fights occur when the people involved feel that they have gained something.

Here are some suggestions for expressing anger constructively:

- Try not to let anger and resentment build up over time. Express feelings when you become aware of them.

- Agree on a time, a place, and the content for fights. It is certainly acceptable to get mad spontaneously if that is how you feel, but it is better to set aside a specific time for the resolution of an issue rather than trying to deal with it when you or your partner may not be psychologically or physically ready to argue. Be sure that the person you are angry with knows what the issue is before the fight.
- Be specific as to what you are angry about and stick to the issue. Don't bring up old hurts. Try not to discuss second and third topics, especially as a means of retaliation.
- Attack the problem, not each other. Don't denigrate the other's personal qualities. Use I-statements to communicate resentments. I-statements tell how you feel. You-statements are often received as personal attacks. At the same time, express appreciation for your partner as a person. This acknowledges that we can be angered by our partners' behaviors and feel loving toward them as people at the same time.
- Try to resolve the issue with an air of compromise and respect. Try to understand the other's point of view.
- Know when it is time to stop. Sometimes you can sense that the argument isn't getting resolved. It is okay to acknowledge that and to take a few hours or days to reconsider things and to discuss the issue again. Sometimes emotions are too high and it is not possible to think clearly. That may be the time to stop the fight until tempers cool.
- Engaging in sex or any other affectionate behavior before an issue is resolved should not be taken as a sign that everything is forgotten. Such behavior shows that the fight fits into what is believed to be a healthy relationship.
- Don't hold grudges.

TERMS

feedback: response of the receiver of a message to let the sender know the message was received

I-statements: statements beginning with "I"; positive communication skill

literal message: a message that is conveyed by symbols

metamessage: how the message is interpreted between sender and receiver

you-statements: statements beginning with "you"; negative communication skill

Critical Thinking About Health

1. Set aside some time to reflect on (and write down) your earliest learning experiences about sexuality. Were they open and positive or shrouded with secrecy and shame? How have these experiences shaped your adult sexual attitudes and behaviors? What, if anything, would you like to change?

2. Make a list of situations and relationships in which sexual activity is permissible for you personally. Would your list be different for your son or daughter? Explain.

3. In the United States when a boy is born, the parents are faced with the decision of whether to have him circumcised. Proponents of circumcision have any number of reasons for supporting it: religion, culture, health, or hygiene. Opponents of circumcision say that it is unnecessary surgery that brings with it unnecessary risk and pain to the child. What are your beliefs on circumcision? On what do you base your beliefs? Talk to someone who disagrees with you and see if your beliefs change or soften.

4. Communication is critical to negotiating condom use, whether for birth control or prevention of sexually transmitted diseases. There are many reasons why men and women do not want to use a condom, but you must be prepared in advance to respond thoughtfully and respectfully to ensure a condom will be used. Describe how you would respond to the following statements:

   Condoms are too expensive.
   Sex isn't pleasurable with a condom.
   I'm Catholic; I'm not allowed to use a condom.
   I can't believe that you think I have an STD.
   If you really loved me, you wouldn't ask me to use a condom.

5. List all the people (e.g., parents, siblings, friends, boyfriends or girlfriends, spouses) that you are currently "intimate" with. (Remember that "being intimate" does not mean "having sex.") Describe what each of those relationships means to you and discuss how they all contribute to your health and happiness.

Health in Review

- Sexuality has several dimensions: the physical (biological), psychological, orientation, behavioral, and relationship dimensions.
- One's sexual biology is determined by genetic makeup, which in turn determines the nature of sex organs: the testes, sperm ducts, semen-producing glands, and penis in the male; and the ovaries, fallopian tubes, uterus, vagina, and external genitalia in the female.
- One's sexual psychology is rooted in emotions and beliefs about sexuality.
- Sexual orientation is the tendency to feel attracted to, and the desire to emotionally bond with, a member of the same or other sex.

- Sexual arousal and response involves four phases: excitement, plateau, orgasm, and resolution.
- Sexual difficulties include lack of interest in sex, inability to attain or maintain an erection, lack of ejaculatory control, painful intercourse, and difficulties with orgasm.
- Intimate relationships involve sharing one's innermost self. They develop through three stages: selecting a partner, developing intimacy through self-disclosure, and commitment.
- Effective communication is crucial for developing and maintaining relationships.

Health and Wellness Online

The Web contains a wealth of information about health and wellness. By accessing the Internet using Web browser software, you can gain a new perspective on many topics presented in *Health and Wellness*, Tenth Edition. Access the Jones and Bartlett Publishers Web site at **health.jbpub.com/hwonline**.

References

American Academy of Pediatrics Task Force on Circumcision. (2005). Circumcision policy statement. *Pediatrics, 116,* 796.

Delate, T., Simmons, V. A., & Motheral, B. R. (2004). Patterns of use of sildenafil among commercially insured adults in the United States: 1998–2002. *International Journal of Impotence Research, 16,* 313–318.

Moynihan, R. (2003). The making of a disease: Female sexual dysfunction. *British Medical Journal, 326,* 45–47.

NIH Consensus Panel. (2005). Demedicalization of menopause. Retrieved October 7, 2005, from http://consensus.nih.gov/

Waldinger, M. D. (2008). Premature ejaculation. *Journal of Sex and Marital Therapy, 34,* 1–13.

Yonkers, K. A., O'Brien, P. M. S., & Eriksson, E. (2008). Premenstrual syndrome. *Lancet, 371,* 1200–1210.

Suggested Readings

The Boston Women's Health Book Collective. (2005). *Our bodies, ourselves for the new century: A book by and for women.* New York: Touchstone. This book reflects the vital health concerns of women of diverse ages, ethnic and racial backgrounds, and sexual orientation—a must-read for every woman.

Gottman, J. M. (2004). *The seven principles for making marriage work.* New York: Orion. A renowned couples researcher and professor of marital therapy shows how to maintain healthy intimate relationships.

Zilbergeld, B. (2000). *The new male sexuality.* New York: Bantam/Dell. The most comprehensive coverage of male sexuality available.

Recommended Web Sites

Please visit **health.jbpub.com/hwonline** for links to these Web sites.

Daily Reproductive Health Report
Daily news stories on human sexuality and reproduction, from the Kaiser Family Foundation.

Go Ask Alice!
A health (including sexuality, sexual health, and relationships) question-and-answer Internet service produced by the Columbia University Health Education Program.

MayoClinic.com
Sexual health: A discussion of healthy sexuality with Mayo Clinic specialist Dr. David Osborne.

Sex Information and Education Council of the United States (SIECUS)
Information and education about sexuality and responsible sexual choices.

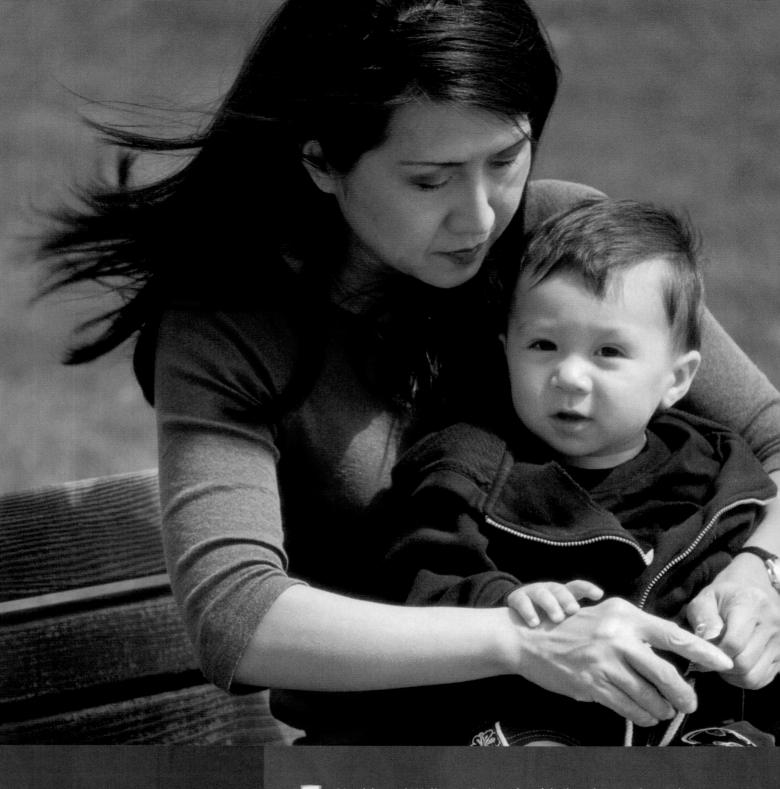

Health and Wellness Online: **health.jbpub.com/hwonline**

Study Guide and Self-Assessment

9.1   Parenthood and Me

Chapter Nine

Understanding Pregnancy and Parenthood

Learning Objectives

1. List and discuss reasons for becoming or not becoming a parent.

2. Describe the processes of fertilization and implantation.

3. Explain how pregnancy tests work.

4. Describe the major health habits in pregnancy.

5. Describe amniocentesis and chorionic villus sampling.

6. Describe the three stages of labor.

7. List the benefits of breastfeeding.

8. Discuss infertility and pregnancy options for infertile people.

This chapter is about one of the most profound life experiences: creating a child. Many people are awed by the idea that the union of one of their body's cells with a cell from their mate can bring forth a unique human being whose well-being is highly dependent on the physical and emotional foundations they provide. There is a tremendous responsibility in being the best kind of parent so that both the child and society benefit.

> You know what I did before I got married? Anything I wanted to.
>
> *Henry Youngman*

People want children for a variety of reasons, including the following:

- To create a social structure (family) to which one can belong
- To manifest a couple's sense of love and emotional bonding
- To improve a marriage
- To leave a legacy to the world
- To carry on the family name
- To accede to social and family pressure to have children
- To feel important, needed, loved, and proud
- To feel more feminine or masculine
- To add fun, excitement, love, and companionship to one's life

Choosing Whether to Be a Parent

Not everyone chooses to become a parent. About 5% of fertile American married couples do not become parents. Some see parenthood as infringing on their career goals or as an unnecessary or unwanted addition to their intimate partnership. Some may have doubts about their psychological or economic abilities to nurture or support children. Others may know or suspect that their children might inherit a genetic disease. Still others may feel that they do not want to contribute more children to an already overpopulated world.

Giving birth to and raising a child requires major adjustments in the parents' lives. The career plans of one or both parents and the distribution of family resources—time, energy, physical space, and money—may change. First-time parents may feel overwhelmed by their responsibilities. The decision to parent should not be taken lightly. The years of parenting are often intense. However, you will never experience such responsibility, hard work, and intimacy as that involved in the growth and development of another human being.

Children do not ask to be born. Parents make that decision. Therefore, before committing to this decision, potential parents must be as certain as they can that their decision is appropriate for their life goals and that they have the means to care for their children.

Becoming Pregnant

For most people, becoming a parent involves pregnancy—a 40-week period during which a fetus grows inside the mother's uterus and the mother's body undergoes changes to nurture the developing child. Every pregnancy begins with **fertilization**, which is the fusion of a father's sperm cell with a mother's ovum to form the first cell of their child, called the fertilized egg, or **zygote**. When a man ejaculates during sexual intercourse, hundreds of millions of sperm cells are released into the vagina. Propelled by the swimming motion of their long tails, these tadpolelike cells make their way through the uterus and into the fallopian tubes, the usual site of fertilization (**Figure 9.1**). Only one sperm cell fertilizes the egg. After fertilization, the zygote moves to the uterus, where it implants in the inner lining and develops as an **embryo**.

During each of a woman's menstrual cycles, usually one ovum, but sometimes two or more, is readied for fertilization. Once freed from the ovary at ovulation, an egg can survive for about 24 hours.

Sperm are produced in the testes in narrow, highly coiled, tubelike structures called **seminiferous tubules** (see Chapter 8). It takes about 70 days for an immature sperm cell to develop into a mature sperm. Once in the vagina, sperm can survive up to seven days.

The cervix is the gateway for passage from the vagina to the uterus (see Chapter 8). For most of the month, fluid produced by glands in the cervix is dense. This thick cervical mucus is a barrier to sperm and microorganisms. Near the time of ovulation, the cervical mucus becomes more fluid and has the consistency of egg white, and it becomes organized into channels that orient sperm movement toward the uterus.

Within seconds following ejaculation in the vagina, some sperm move through the cervix and uterus and into the fallopian tubes. The majority of sperm, however, become trapped in coagulated semen in the upper portion of the vagina. After about 20 minutes, the coagulated semen liquefies and sperm move into microscopic folds in the cervix. Weak or abnormal sperm are unlikely to move beyond the cervix. Healthy, motile sperm tend to be released into the uterus continuously throughout the ensuing 48 hours. Several hundred sperm capable of fertilization approach an ovum, but only one succeeds in penetrating the ovum's outer membrane.

During the first three days after fertilization, the cells of the embryo replicate at about daily intervals, and the embryo moves along the fallopian tube toward the uterus. By about the fourth day after fertilization, the embryo, now composed of between 50 and 100 cells, arranged as a fluid-filled sphere, enters the uterus. On about the sixth day after fertilization, the embryo attaches to the lining of the uterus; shortly thereafter, it implants in the uterus by eroding the uterine lining.

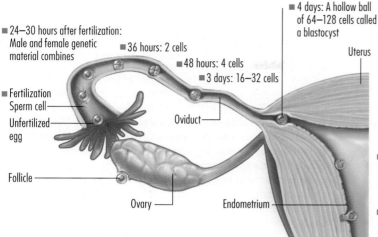

■ 24–30 hours after fertilization: Male and female genetic material combines

■ Fertilization Sperm cell

Unfertilized egg

Follicle

Ovary

■ 36 hours: 2 cells

■ 48 hours: 4 cells

■ 3 days: 16–32 cells

Oviduct

Endometrium

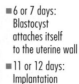

■ 4 days: A hollow ball of 64–128 cells called a blastocyst

Uterus

■ 6 or 7 days: Blastocyst attaches itself to the uterine wall

■ 11 or 12 days: Implantation of the embryo

■ **Figure 9.1**

Fertilization and Early Development of the Embryo

Joining of sperm and egg in fertilization. After fertilization, the zygote travels down the fallopian tube to the uterus. Implantation of the zygote begins approximately six days after fertilization.

menstrual period, occasional nausea and vomiting referred to as "morning sickness," enlarged and tender breasts, increased frequency of urination, fatigue, and enlargement of the uterus. Both clinical and home pregnancy tests are based on analyzing a woman's urine for the presence of HCG.

On rare occasions, the fertilized egg implants outside the uterus, usually in a fallopian tube where its passage is blocked by tubal malformation or scarring or twisting from a prior infection, often gonorrhea or chlamydia. A pregnancy in which the fertilized egg implants somewhere other than in the uterus is called an **ectopic pregnancy**. Implantation in a fallopian tube also is called a tubal pregnancy. If a tubal pregnancy remains undiscovered, the embryo will become too large for the fallopian tube sometime between the eighth and twelfth weeks of pregnancy and the tube will burst, creating internal bleeding and a critical situation that requires immediate medical intervention.

HCG in Serum

4   8   12   16   20   24   28   32   36   40

Weeks after Conception

■ **Figure 9.2**

Pattern of Human Chorionic Gonadotropin (HCG) Secretion During Pregnancy

Pregnancy

Soon after the embryo implants in the uterus, it secretes a hormone unique to pregnancy, called **human chorionic gonadotropin (HCG)**, into the maternal bloodstream (**Figure 9.2**). Under the influence of HCG, the mother's ovaries are stimulated to increase the production of estrogen and progesterone, which in turn forestalls the next menstrual period and permits the pregnancy to continue. Increases in the levels of estrogen and progesterone bring about the first noticeable signs of pregnancy: absence of the next

TERMS

ectopic pregnancy: a pregnancy occurring outside the uterus, usually in a fallopian tube

embryo: the developing infant during the first two months of conception

fertilization: the fusion of a sperm cell and an ovum

human chorionic gonadotropin (HCG): a hormone produced during the first stages of pregnancy; it is used as a basis for pregnancy tests

seminiferous tubules: convoluted tubules in the testicles that produce sperm

zygote: the first cell of a new person, formed at fertilization

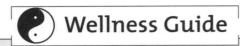

Wellness Guide

Home Pregnancy Testing

When a woman wants to know if she is pregnant, she can consult a health care provider or go to a family planning or public health clinic. Or, she can administer a pregnancy test herself. Several home pregnancy testing kits are available without prescription at low cost, and they are relatively easy to use.

Virtually all chemical tests for pregnancy—those carried out in clinics and the self-test kind—analyze a woman's blood or urine for the hormone of pregnancy, human chorionic gonadotropin (HCG).

Some brands of home pregnancy tests are not 100% accurate. Only rarely (about 3 times in 100) does the test indicate pregnancy when the woman is not pregnant. A "false positive" result is likely to be discovered when the woman seeks prenatal care.

Home tests for pregnancy are often wrong about 20% of the time, indicating that a woman is not pregnant when in fact she is. About half of these "false negative" results occur because the test has been administered too early in the pregnancy. About half of the false negatives are corrected if the test is readministered in about a week. However, about 10% of women who are pregnant still get the inaccurate test result that they are not pregnant. This is one of the most serious drawbacks of home pregnancy tests because the risks of complications in pregnancy and abortion rise the longer a pregnant woman waits to obtain professional care.

In spite of the possibility of inaccuracy, many physicians and family planning consultants believe home pregnancy testing to be useful. It enables women to take a more active part in their own health care, and it may help women who "would rather not think about it" confront the possibility that they are pregnant.

Fetal Development

The 9-month span of pregnancy is customarily divided into three 3-month segments called trimesters. Nearly all of the fetal body forms by the tenth week after fertilization. During the rest of pregnancy, the fetal body grows and many of the organs become functional; at birth the fetus weighs almost 3,000 grams (almost 7 pounds).

Fetal development and growth take place with the fetus enclosed in a fluid-filled membranous sac called the **amnion,** which forms during the second week of development. As it develops in the **amniotic fluid,** the fetus is able to grow unimpeded by the mother's internal organs. The amniotic fluid also protects the fetus from potentially damaging jolts when the mother changes her body position. The amnion ruptures just before birth, sometimes called "breaking of the bag of waters."

The growth and development of the fetus are supported by the **placenta,** an organ unique to pregnancy. The placenta manufactures many hormones needed to sustain pregnancy and is responsible for transporting oxygen and nutrients from the mother to the fetus and waste products from the fetus to the mother.

A number of changes occur in a pregnant woman's physiology (**Figure 9.3**). For example, the blood plasma increases in volume as much as 50% over her nonpregnant levels, the heart beats 10% faster and with 20% to 30% greater output per minute, the number of red blood cells increases, and breathing becomes deeper and slightly faster. One of the most striking changes during pregnancy is the growth of the uterus. The nonpregnant uterus is approximately 7 to 8 centimeters long (2¾ to 3½ inches) and weighs about 60 to 100 grams (2 to 3½ ounces). By the end of pregnancy, the uterus is approximately 30 centimeters long (12 inches) and weighs nearly 1,000 grams (2.2 pounds).

Sexual Interaction During Pregnancy

A woman's sexual interest and responsiveness may change throughout the course of her pregnancy because of the many psychological, emotional, and physical changes that influence her attitude toward and enjoyment of sex. In some pregnancies, sexual interest increases. In others, it decreases. Some of the most common reasons women give for decreasing sexual activity during pregnancy include physical discomfort, feelings of physical unattractiveness, and fear of injuring the unborn child.

It is now generally accepted that in pregnancies where there are no risk factors, sexual activity and orgasm may be continued, as desired, until the onset of labor. Unless her health care provider counsels a pregnant woman to the contrary, there is no physical reason to forgo sex during pregnancy.

Some couples find that pregnancy is a good time to explore new lovemaking positions—side by side, rear entry, or woman above are generally more comfortable at this time. Even if intercourse is not desired, pregnancy can also be a time to try other sensual and sexual pleasures, such as oral sex, mutual masturbation, massage, or just total body touching and holding.

Health Habits During Pregnancy

Every child deserves to be born as healthy as possible. It is only fair to the unborn child—who did not ask to be conceived—that all the genetic potential to develop a healthy body and mind be given the opportunity to be fully expressed. Few of us are as careful about maintaining proper health habits as we could be. Most people live with whatever risk might be associated with nonhealthy

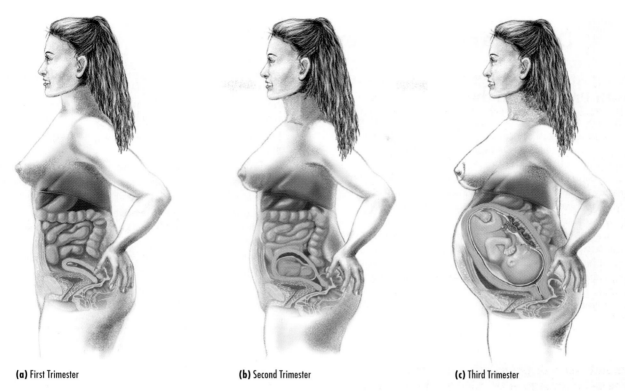

(a) First Trimester   **(b)** Second Trimester   **(c)** Third Trimester

■ **Figure 9.3**

Changes in a Woman's Body During Pregnancy
Through the three trimesters, the shape of the pregnant woman's body changes dramatically.

behaviors and are presumably willing to accept the consequences of those behaviors. But when a woman is pregnant, disregarding fundamental health practices endangers her child as well as herself, and perhaps more so, because the developing baby's body and mind are extremely vulnerable to damage. A mother-to-be must make every effort to practice good health habits. If her developing baby could talk, he or she might say, "Mom, my lifelong health and well-being are in your hands now. I know nine months is a long time to have to be concerned about what you eat and drink, but it's important to me that you do the right things for both of us. Not only will that give me the chance to become the best person I can be but will also keep you healthy so we can share a lot of good times after I'm born." The factors that deserve a pregnant woman's attention to ensure her own health and that of her baby are proper nutrition, obtaining professional prenatal care, getting enough exercise, refraining from smoking and consuming alcohol or other drugs while pregnant, and accepting and dealing with emotional and sexual feelings that may be different from those experienced when not pregnant.

Nutrition

Throughout pregnancy, the fetus's cells and physiological capacities are developing. Perhaps more than at any other time of life, an ample supply of nutrients is required

so that the formation of new cells and the development of organs proceed optimally. All fetal nutrients come from the mother by way of the placenta. Therefore, a pregnant woman directly influences the nutritional status of her baby, and she must be aware that she must "eat for two," meaning that she must be sure her diet contains adequate nutrients for herself and for her baby. Mothers-to-be who eat highly nutritious diets during pregnancy are more likely to give birth to healthy babies than are mothers whose diets are nutritionally poor. Pregnant women should increase their intake of essential nutrients and calories (**Table 9.1**). For some women it is advisable to supplement a generally well-balanced diet with extra iron and folic acid.

TERMS

amnion: the inner membrane that forms a fluid-filled sac surrounding and protecting the embryo and fetus

amniotic fluid: fluid in the amniotic sac

placenta: the flat circular vascular structure within the pregnant uterus that provides nourishment to and eliminates wastes from the developing embryo and fetus and is passed as afterbirth after the baby is born

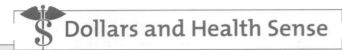

Dollars and Health Sense

Buying At-Home Pregnancy (and Other) Health Products on the Internet

Shopping on the Internet is a marvel. You can buy anything, including unapproved at-home pregnancy test kits. The Food and Drug Administration (FDA) approves some at-home diagnostic kits, but not all. Some tests kits are approved only for health clinics and not for home use. Ads for some at-home pregnancy test kits promise in-home results, but most tests should be followed with a second, more sophisticated laboratory test to confirm the results.

If you want to buy a test kit over the Internet, avoid products that claim to test for more than one thing, such as pregnancy and HIV infection, are made in a country other than the United States, or are made by only one laboratory and sold directly to the public. If you have any doubts, check whether the FDA has approved the product for use at home (1-888-INFO-FDA

[1-888-463-6332]). The FDA offers these general precautions for buying health care items on the Internet:

- Don't be fooled by a professional-looking Web site. Anyone can hire a Web page designer to create an appealing site.
- Avoid Web sites with only a post office box number and no telephone number.
- Avoid Web sites that use the words "new cure" or "miracle cure."
- Avoid products with impressive-sounding terminology that is used to deceive.
- Avoid products that claim the government, medical profession, or research scientists have conspired to suppress the product.
- Beware of claims that the test complies with all regulatory agencies.
- Beware of tests labeled for export only. This usually means that the test is not cleared or approved for sale in the United States.

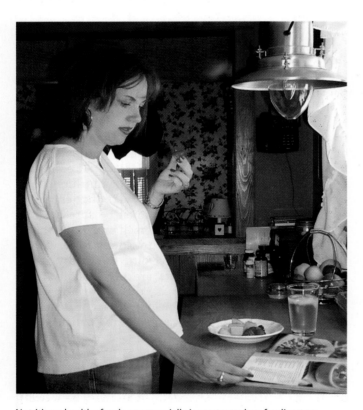

Nutritious, healthy foods are especially important when feeding two.

Table 9.1

Recommended Daily Dietary Reference Intakes (DRI) for Nonpregnant, Pregnant, and Lactating Women, Ages 25–50

	Nonpregnant	Pregnant	Lactating
Protein (g)	46	71	71
Carbohydrate	130	175	210
Vitamin A (µg)	700	770	1300
Vitamin D (µg)	5	5	5
Vitamin C (mg)	75	85	120
Thiamine (mg)	1.2	1.1	1.4
Riboflavin (mg)	1.1	1.4	1.6
Niacin (mg)	14	18	17
Vitamin B_6 (mg)	1.3	1.9	2.0
Folate (mg)	400	600	500
Vitamin B_{12} (mg)	2.4	2.6	2.8
Calcium (mg)	1000	1000	1000
Phosphorus (mg)	700	700	700
Iron (mg)	18	27	9
Zinc (mg)	8	11	12
Iodine (mg)	150	220	290

Source: Data from Food and Nutrition Board, Institute of Medicine, National Academies of Sciences. (2004). *Dietary reference intakes.*

Many pregnant women are concerned with the amount of weight they gain. Although it is never good to weigh too much, current obstetric practice allows a mother-to-be to gain about 28 to 30 pounds by the end of pregnancy, most of which comes in the last two-thirds of pregnancy. About 7 of these pounds are con-tributed by the fetus. The enlarged uterus accounts for another 2 pounds, and the placenta and amniotic fluid contribute 1 pound each. About 4 to 8 pounds of fluid are added to the maternal system as extra blood and extracellular fluid, and the mother may gain about 4 pounds of body fat.

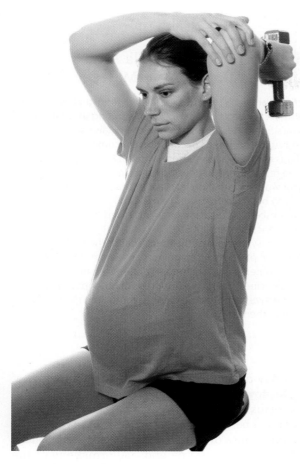

Staying physically active during pregnancy has many benefits.

Table 9.2		
Safe Physical Activity During Pregnancy		
Safe even for beginners	Safe for experienced exercisers	Unsafe*
Walking	Running	Downhill snow skiing
Swimming	Racquet sports	Contact sports
Cycling	Strength training	Scuba diving
Low-impact aerobics		
Prenatal yoga		

*Avoid exercises that increase the risk of falling, involve extra weight bearing, and, after the first three months of pregnancy, that involve lying on the back.

The degree of physical activity a pregnant woman engages in depends on her desires and abilities (**Table 9.2**). Some athletic women engage in sports almost to the day of delivery. Women who are not routinely athletic are wise to begin a program early in pregnancy that involves exercises to maintain correct posture, strengthen abdominal muscles, and improve their breathing and ability to relax.

Emotional Well-Being

Pregnancy can be a time of intense feelings, not only for the mother-to-be but also for her partner and others who are close to her. Enthusiasm, excitement, anticipation, fear about the baby's condition, uncertainties about one's suitability as a parent, and a desire for more (or less) love, affection, and sex are all natural. Recognizing that intense feelings are normal in pregnancy and accepting them with patience and understanding are the keys to a rewarding experience.

Perhaps the best way to deal with intense feelings at any time in life, including pregnancy, is to take time each day to quiet the mind and body with meditation, yoga, or other relaxation methods. Massage is also beneficial, and it fulfills some of the desires of those who feel more sensual during pregnancy.

Prenatal Care

Pregnancy involves several profound biological changes. Not only does the fetus develop from a single cell to a 7- or 8-pound newborn infant (composed of many millions of cells), but the mother's body also undergoes a number of anatomical and physiological changes to support fetal development. Moreover, the fetal–maternal relationship is maintained by the placenta, an organ that develops only during pregnancy and is expelled from the mother's uterus after the baby is born. Any rapidly changing system is vulnerable to errors and problems, and so it is with pregnancy and fetal development. That is why it is recommended that mothers-to-be receive professional prenatal care. A number of studies have shown that the more prenatal care a woman receives, the fewer problems she will have during pregnancy and

Physical Activity and Exercise

There are benefits to being physically active during pregnancy. Some women feel lethargic during pregnancy. In just a few weeks, their bodies take on unfamiliar proportions and they have to carry up to 20% more weight than when they are not pregnant. They may feel uncomfortable, unattractive, and clumsy. Through movement and exercise, a pregnant woman can become accustomed to the temporary changes in her body and accept pregnancy as a positive and fulfilling time of her life. Physical activity also helps prepare the mother's body for childbirth, which is often physically demanding. By keeping active, a pregnant woman can improve her circulation and thereby reduce swelling and formation of varicose veins in the lower legs, which can be common in pregnancy. Well-conditioned women who engage in aerobics or run regularly tend to have (as a group) shorter labors and fewer cesarean deliveries. Exercise during pregnancy can tone a woman's muscles so that her body returns more quickly to its prepregnant shape after delivery. Perhaps the greatest benefit from physical activity during pregnancy is maintaining the habit of being active.

childbirth and the more likely that her infant will be born healthy. Professional prenatal care can help a mother-to-be avoid the consequences of a number of pregnancy-specific illnesses, such as high blood pressure (preeclampsia), pregnancy-induced diabetes, and infection. These illnesses can threaten both the mother's health and the proper development and delivery of her baby. Professional prenatal care can also help manage problems resulting from a malfunctioning placenta and can educate a mother about proper nutrition and advise her on how smoking at any time during pregnancy can adversely affect her baby's development, as can consumption of alcohol. Maternal infections that are harmful to the fetus, such as rubella (German measles), syphilis, gonorrhea, toxoplasmosis, herpes, and HIV, can be detected and managed. Another reason for prenatal care is to be sure the maternal and fetal blood cells are immunologically (Rh factor) compatible.

Risks to Fetal Development

A variety of factors can adversely affect an embryo or fetus during development. Although the placenta prevents some kinds of bacteria and viruses from passing into the fetal blood system, many others are able to cross the placenta, including the AIDS virus. Furthermore, many substances ingested by the mother, such as drugs, alcohol, and nicotine and other chemicals from tobacco, easily cross the placenta and damage the developing fetus.

Drugs

Any drug ingested by a pregnant woman potentially can harm her fetus, resulting in birth defects or possibly even fetal death. All illegal psychoactive drugs, such as heroin, methamphetamine, and cocaine, pose dangers to a developing fetus because they may cause neurological abnormalities and addiction. Alcohol and tobacco also are dangerous (see the following sections), as are prescription and over-the-counter medicines and many dietary supplements. For her own health and the health of her child, a woman should avoid all drugs during pregnancy except those deemed necessary by a health care provider.

Alcohol

When alcohol crosses the placenta, it reaches a level in the fetus equal to that in the body of the mother. Because the body of the fetus is small and its detoxification system immature, alcohol remains in fetal blood long after it has disappeared in the woman's blood. Thus, drinking alcohol can harm the fetus, and the risk of damage increases as the quantity and frequency of maternal alcohol consumption increases. The fetus is at risk of developing fetal alcohol syndrome (FAS) if the mother drinks six or more

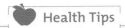 **Health Tips**

Environmental Chemicals Affect Genital Development in Males

Endocrine disruptors (see Chapter 24) are industrial and agricultural chemicals that alter the functioning of some of the body's hormones. Phthalates are chemicals used in hundreds upon hundreds of common consumer products. Phthalates are known to interfere with the functions of the hormone testosterone in developing male fetuses. Pregnant women with high levels of phthalates in their bodies may be at risk for having a male child with a small penis, undescended testicles, or an increased risk for testicular cancer (Swan, 2008).

It is not easy to avoid phthalates because they are ubiqitous—in plastic food containers and wraps, funiture polish, perfumes, soaps, shampoos, detergents, time-release medicines, paint, and hundreds of other products—but prospective parents should endeavor to limit their exposure to them.

drinks per day during her pregnancy. The symptoms of FAS include growth retardation, facial malformations, and central nervous system dysfunctions, including mental retardation and behavioral dysfunctions. FAS is the third most common cause of mental retardation in the Western world, after Down syndrome and malformations of the nervous system. This is particularly distressing because FAS can be prevented.

Cigarette Smoking

Maternal smoking increases the chances of spontaneous abortion and of complications that can result in fetal or infant death. Smoking reduces the amount of oxygen in the bloodstream, which can adversely affect the fetus by slowing its growth. Infants of mothers who smoked during pregnancy often weigh less and are in poorer general condition than are infants of nonsmoking mothers. Smoking may be teratogenic, causing cardiac abnormalities and anencephaly (absence of a cerebrum). Maternal smoking appears to be a significant factor in the development of cleft lip and palate.

> When I was a kid my parents moved a lot . . . but I always found them.
> *Rodney Dangerfield*

How Birth Defects Are Detected

Tests may be performed if there is reason to suspect that there may be fetal abnormalities. Circumstances in which tests may be beneficial include pregnant women over age 35, parents who have previously given birth to a child with birth defects, and parents with a history of genetic or chromosomal disorders who may want to confirm the absence of birth defects in an unborn child (see Chapter 15).

Amniocentesis

A reliable and accurate test, known as an **amniocentesis,** can be performed between the fourteenth and eighteenth week of pregnancy. The procedure consists of inserting a hollow needle with the assistance of ultrasonographic imagery through the woman's abdominal wall and into the uterine cavity to draw out a sample of the amniotic fluid (fluid surrounding the fetus), which contains fetal cells that have been sloughed off in the normal course of development. The procedure can detect several hundred fetal abnormalities and biochemical defects.

The test can be performed during any trimester if enough fluid is present. If done during the first trimester, it is usually for genetic studies; in the second trimester, for Rh isoimmunization studies; and in the third trimester, for assessing fetal lung maturity.

Chorionic Villus Sampling

Chorionic villus sampling (CVS) is used during the first trimester of pregnancy to detect biochemical disorders and chromosomal abnormalities. Chorionic villi are threadlike protrusions on a membrane surrounding the fetus that are composed of fetal cells. This test involves inserting a thin catheter with the assistance of ultrasonographic imagery through the abdomen or vagina and cervix into the uterus, where a small sample of chorionic villi is removed for analysis. This procedure has an advantage over amniocentesis because it can be done as early as the eighth week after the last menstrual period.

Childbirth

For the parents, the moment of childbirth can bring a mixture of feelings that might include great joy, relief that the nine months of waiting are over, and surprise at the baby's appearance. All in attendance may experience concern for the condition of the mother and baby and awe and wonder at the miracle of new life.

Childbirth Preparation

A variety of programs and organizations provide education for parents-to-be in preparation for the childbirth experience and parenthood. These are usually six- to eight-week courses, sometimes called "natural childbirth," "Lamaze," or simply childbirth preparation. Childbirth preparation classes can enhance the intimate relationship of the expectant couple and increase their confidence and self-esteem. In addition, women who participate in childbirth preparation are likely to have less pain and discomfort in childbirth, to require less

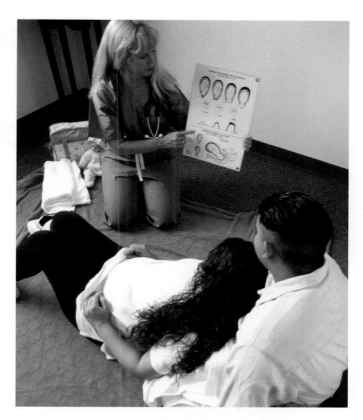

Childbirth preparation classes help ensure a healthy baby.

medication, and to have fewer complications. Prepared parents are also more likely to have positive attitudes toward childbirth and parenting. Fathers who attend childbirth preparation classes tend to feel more comfortable about sharing the birth experience with their partners and about helping them during it. They are also more likely to be interested and involved in parenting after the baby is born.

Almost all childbirth preparation courses teach prospective parents the basic biology of pregnancy and childbirth. They also teach breathing and relaxation exercises, and some teach imagery and affirmations, all intended to make the delivery of the baby proceed smoothly and comfortably. While attending these courses, parents-to-be meet other expectant couples with whom they can share their feelings and experiences. The classes also address birthing options.

TERMS

amniocentesis: a procedure that involves aspiration of amniotic fluid from the uterus to detect certain abnormalities in the fetus

chorionic villus sampling (CVS): a method to detect biochemical disorders and chromosomal abnormalities in the fetus

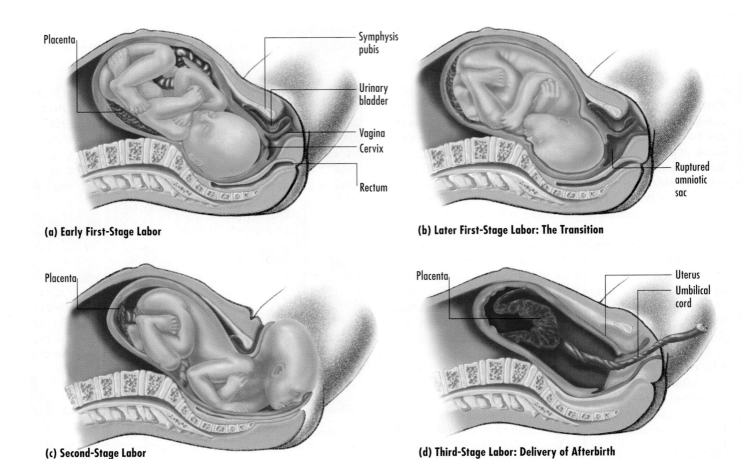

(a) Early First-Stage Labor

(b) Later First-Stage Labor: The Transition

(c) Second-Stage Labor

(d) Third-Stage Labor: Delivery of Afterbirth

■ **Figure 9.4**

Childbirth

The stages of labor. (a) Early first stage: The cervix is dilating. (b) Late first stage (transition stage): The cervix is fully dilated, and the amniotic sac has ruptured, releasing amniotic fluid. (c) Second stage: The birth of the baby. (d) Third stage: Delivery of the placenta (afterbirth).

Because childbirth preparation courses reflect the biases of those who teach them, prospective parents are likely to gain more complete information about birthing options by consulting additional sources (e.g., books, Web sites, and other parents).

Studies have shown that continuous emotional support during labor can shorten labor time, give the woman in labor greater perception of control, decrease her need for pain medication, and, overall, lead to fewer complications that affect the baby. On the other hand, labor can be slowed or stopped if the woman feels uncomfortable, anxious, frightened or experiences performance pressure because of others' expectations about how the labor should be proceeding.

Giving Birth

A few weeks before the onset of childbirth, or **labor,** the fetus becomes positioned for birth by descending in the uterus, a process called **lightening.** When this happens the pressure on some of the mother's internal organs is relieved and she may find it easier to breathe, stand,

and digest food. In about 95% of all births the fetus is in a head-down position. When not head-down, the fetus may be head-up, referred to as a *breech position.* In nearly all instances, the fetus's legs are tucked up against its abdomen in the "fetal position."

Throughout much of pregnancy, the uterus contracts intermittently, tightening in waves that sometimes are so gentle that the woman is unaware of them. During the last half of pregnancy, a woman may at times feel her abdomen becoming hard or otherwise perceive the uterine contractions as they prepare her body for the true labor. Health professionals refer to these as **Braxton-Hicks contractions.** They can be distinguished from true labor by their occurrence at irregular intervals and their rather short duration.

There are three generally recognizable stages in the process of childbirth (**Figure 9.4**). Before the first stage begins, the cervix has already effaced (flattened and thinned) and dilated slightly. The **first stage** of labor starts with the beginning of uterine contractions and lasts until the cervix is fully dilated. Another indication of first-stage labor may be the "bloody show," the discharge of the mucous plug from the cervix. The first stage is the longest of the three stages, usually lasting 10 to 16 hours for the first childbirth and 4 to 8 hours in subsequent deliveries. This stage lasts until the cervix is dilated about 10 centimeters.

The **second stage** of labor begins when the cervix is fully dilated and the infant descends farther into the birth canal (normally, head first). This stage lasts from 30 minutes to 2 hours. During this time the woman can actively push with each contraction until the infant is expelled. The remaining amniotic fluid gushes out. The infant is cleaned and its vital signs, such as breathing and color, are quickly checked. The umbilical cord is clamped several inches from the navel, and the baby soon begins to breathe.

The **third stage** of labor lasts from the time of birth until the delivery of the placenta, or **afterbirth.** With one or two more uterine contractions, the placenta usually separates from the uterine wall and is expelled from the vagina, generally within 30 minutes after the baby is born.

Medical Interventions

Options for Controlling Discomfort

Intense discomfort or pain can accompany labor, especially in the later phases of the first stage and the early stages of the second. The intensity of feeling is caused by stretches and strains on the uterine muscle tissue, effacement of the cervix, and stretching of the perineum. Pain relief methods include relaxation techniques, deep breathing, acupuncture, hypnosis, massaging and supporting of the perineum by the birth attendant, medications that block pain awareness (analgesia), and medications that block the pain sensations (anesthesia). The most common anesthesia used during labor is a regional anesthetic to diminish sensation only in the pelvic region. This leaves the mother conscious during labor so that she can actively "bear down" to help push the baby out. General anesthesia (complete unconsciousness) is used only in cases of difficult births and interventions, such as cesarean sections.

Social and psychological support also contribute to lessening labor pain and discomfort. Women who expect to be able to manage childbirth successfully generally have less discomfort and require less pain medication than those who are fearful (Leeman et al., 2003). This is one reason pregnant women are encouraged to take childbirth preparation classes. Also, women who have continuous emotional support during childbirth generally need less pain medication. Support can come from a husband or other family member, a trained labor assistant called a *doula,* a nurse, or other obstetric professional. Giving birth in a homelike setting and with caregivers in attendance who the mother knows also contribute to a more successful birthing experience.

Induction of Labor

Induction of labor involves medically stimulating uterine contractions and, hence, the onset of labor. Induction of labor now occurs in about 20% of American childbirths, a doubling in percentage since 1990. The main reasons for labor induction include extended pregnancy (41–42 weeks), toxemia (elevated maternal blood pressure), premature rupture of the amniotic sac, and an excessively large baby (macrosomia).

The most common methods of inducing labor are administering prostaglandins to the cervix, breaking the amnionic sac, and giving the hormone oxytocin (Pitocin). A centuries-old method of labor induction involves a birth attendant stimulating a laboring woman's breasts to produce the release of oxytocin from the mother's posterior pituitary gland, as would occur when the mother later nurses her infant. Other nonmedical methods for labor induction include herbal compounds, castor oil, hot baths, enemas, acupuncture, acupressure, and sexual intercourse (Tenore, 2003).

Episiotomy

Episiotomy is an incision in the perineum from the vagina to the anus which can be performed during the first stage of labor to enlarge the vaginal opening. Not long ago, episiotomies were routine obstetrical procedures because it was believed they lessened tearing of the vaginal tissues and aided postbirth healing after delivery. It is now known, however, that episiotomies increase the risk of injury and do not aid significantly in

---

TERMS

afterbirth: placenta and fetal membranes

Braxton-Hicks contractions: normal uterine contractions that occur periodically throughout pregnancy

episiotomy: an incision in the perineum to facilitate passage of the baby's head during childbirth, while minimizing injury to the woman

first-stage labor: the beginning of labor during which there are regular contractions of the uterus

labor: the process of childbirth

lightening: the positioning of the fetus for birth by descent in the uterus

second-stage labor: the stage during which the baby moves out through the vagina and is delivered

third-stage labor: the stage during which the afterbirth is expelled

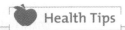 Health Tips

Pregnancy and Childbirth: Belly-Breathing Exercise

In Lamaze classes, expectant mothers (and fathers) are taught to place the emphasis of their breathing on the lower stomach or diaphragm. During the several hours of labor and the actual delivery, this breathing skill is employed to ease the pain of childbirth. What is taught and practiced in the stressful event of childbirth is now taught and practiced in several other stressful situations as well.

Each breathing cycle is composed of four distinct phases:

Phase I: Inspiration, taking the air into your lungs through the passage of your nose or mouth

Phase II: A very slight pause before exhaling the air out of your lungs

Phase III: Exhalation, releasing the air from your lungs and through the passage it entered

Phase IV: A very slight pause after exhalation before the next inhalation is initiated

These phases can be enhanced when the breathing cycle is exaggerated by taking a very slow and comfortable deep breath. When trying this technique, try to isolate and recognize these four phases by identifying them as they occur. Remember not to hold your breath at any one time during each phase. Rather, learn to regulate your breathing by controlling the pace of each phase in the breathing cycle. Remember that diaphragmatic breathing is not the same as hyperventilation: This style of breathing is slow, relaxed, and as deep as feels comfortable. The most relaxing phase of breathing is the third phase, exhalation. In this phase the chest and abdominal areas relax, producing a relaxing effect throughout the body. When focusing on your breathing, feel how relaxed your whole body becomes during exhalation, especially your chest, shoulders, and abdominal region.

An Energy Breathing Exercise

There are three phases to this exercise, and you can use this technique either sitting or lying down.

1. First get comfortable, allowing your shoulders to relax. If you choose to sit, try to keep your legs straight. As you breathe in, imagine that there is a circular hole at the top of your head. As the air enters your lungs, visualize energy in the form of a beam of light entering the top of your head. Bring the energy down from the crown of your head to your abdomen as you inhale. As you exhale, allow the energy to leave through the top of your head. Repeat this 5 to 10 times, trying to coordinate your breathing with the visual flow of energy. As you continue to bring the energy down to your stomach area, allow the light to reach all the inner parts of your upper body. When you feel comfortable with this first phase, you are ready to move on to the second phase.

2. Now, imagine that in the center of each foot there is a circular hole through which energy can flow in and out. Again think of energy as a beam of light. Concentrating on only your lower extremities, allow the flow of energy to move up from your feet into your abdomen as you inhale from your diaphragm. Repeat this 5 to 10 times, trying to coordinate your breathing with the flow of energy. As you continue to bring the energy up into your stomach area, allow the light to reach all the inner parts of your lower body.

3. Once you have coordinated your breathing with the visual flow of energy through your lower extremities, begin to combine the movement of energy from the top of your head and your feet, bringing the energy to the center of your body as you inhale air from your diaphragm. Then, as you exhale, allow the flow of energy to reverse. Repeat this 10 to 20 times. Each time you move the energy through your body, feel each body region—each muscle, organ, and cell—become energized. At first it may be difficult to visually coordinate the movement of energy coming from opposite ends of your body, but this will become very easy with practice.

---

postbirth healing (Hartmann et al., 2005). Episiotomies should be performed only when medically necessary and not routinely.

Cesarean Birth

When a normal vaginal delivery is considered dangerous or impossible, a fetus is removed through an incision made in the abdominal wall and uterus, in a surgical procedure called a **cesarean section,** or **C-section.** Cesarean births may be recommended in a variety of situations, including a fetal head that is too large for the mother's pelvic structure, maternal illness, active herpes infection

in the vagina, fetal distress during labor, birth complications such as breech fetal presentation (feet or bottom coming out of the uterus first), or previous C-section.

For both mother and baby, cesareans are less safe than uncomplicated vaginal deliveries, and they cost more. In the United States today, nearly 28% of births are cesarean. In 1970, only 5% of births were cesarean. Among the reasons offered for this increase are the parents and/or physician wanting a convenient labor and the doctor and hospital not wanting to risk a difficult labor that might harm the baby, which might trigger an expensive lawsuit. Parents understandably expect their newborn to be healthy and well. If a birth is difficult and a child is harmed, parents may blame the physician for not performing a cesarean or not performing one quickly enough to avoid trouble. Along with this blame can come a malpractice lawsuit. Obstetrical malpractice judgments are the largest among medical subspecialties, and obstetrical liability insurance is the highest among primary care practitioners. Thus, it is in the doctor's, the hospital's, and the malpractice insurance company's interests to encourage a mother to have a cesarean rather than risk difficulties during childbirth.

The Postpartum Transition

After the child is born, the mother goes through several weeks of postpartum transition called the **puerperium.** During this time, the physiological changes of pregnancy slowly reverse and the vagina and the surrounding structures recuperate from labor. Uterine tissue that is no longer needed is discharged for the first month or so after childbirth. The discharge, called *lochia*, at first resembles a heavy menstrual flow, then typically tapers off after a week or two. Following delivery, estrogen and progesterone levels, which were high during pregnancy, drop rapidly, reaching almost zero about 72 hours after birth.

During this period the mother and her partner begin to adjust to their often demanding new life situation. Childbirth and infant care are exhausting. Many women experience the "baby blues," which are transitory mood changes involving tiredness, depression, loneliness, or fear. These feelings usually abate in the weeks following childbirth, but about 13% of women experience postpartum depression severe enough to be disabling and to require professional help (Musters, McDonald & Jones, 2008). Postpartum mood changes are so common that experts suggest they may be related to the massive changes in hormone levels that accompany childbirth. Others, although not denying the effects of hormonal changes, point out that childbirth is a life transition that brings many changes and psychological adjustments for the woman, her partner, and other family and household members.

It is recommended that couples refrain from intercourse for several weeks following childbirth to allow the uterus and vagina to return to prepregnancy states. Intercourse is usually physically safe within three to four weeks after delivery, but this all depends on the mother's desire and comfort.

Breastfeeding

The preparation of the breasts for nursing begins in the early weeks of pregnancy with an increase in the number of milk ducts and the deposit of fat in the breast tissue.

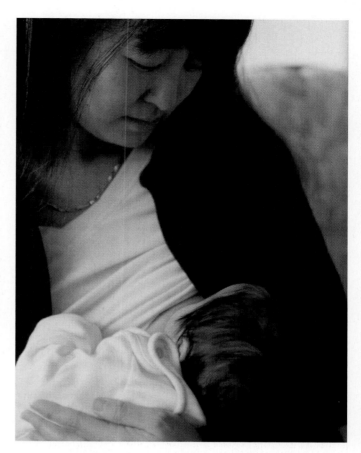

Breast milk provides a baby with essential nutrients and helps prevent infections.

This growth causes breast tenderness early in pregnancy. In addition to the increase in breast size, the nipples enlarge and often deepen in color. About midway into pregnancy, the breasts begin to manufacture **colostrum,** a yellowish precursor to actual mother's milk. For the first few days after birth, colostrum is the major substance emitted from the breasts. As the newborn nurses, colostrum is drained from the breasts and is replaced by mother's milk. Colostrum contains nutrients and is especially high in antibodies that protect the infant against infection. Mother's milk contains specific milk proteins, antibodies, lactose, fat, and water. The synthesis of milk is

> ### TERMS
>
> cesarean section (C-section): delivery of the fetus through a surgical opening in the abdomen and uterus
>
> colostrum: yellowish liquid secreted from the breasts; contains antibodies and protein
>
> puerperium: the six weeks after childbirth, also called postpartum period

🌐 Global Wellness

Infant Mortality

The first year of any infant's life can be risky, especially if there is an insufficient health care system to intervene when a pregnant woman, an infant, or an infant's mother gets sick. The worldwide infant mortality rate (the rate at which babies die before their first birthday) is 42 deaths per 1,000 live births. This means that worldwide, 7.1 million infants die each year.

There is an enormous disparity in infant mortality among countries (**Table 9.3**). Singapore has the lowest infant mortality rate, at 2.30 deaths per 1,000 live births; Afghanistan is among the highest, at 154 deaths per 1,000 live births.

When mothers and babies have access to good health care, infant mortality is caused by serious birth defects, preterm delivery and low birth weight, automobile accidents, sudden infant death syndrome (SIDS), and infections, including HIV. When mothers and babies do not have access to health care, infants die because of complications surrounding childbirth, malnutrition, infection (e.g., HIV and malaria), unsanitary conditions, and absence of the mother or other caretaker.

The overall U.S. infant mortality rate is 6.3 deaths per 1,000 live births. The U.S. rate is higher than in other industrialized countries because many Americans do not have access to health care. The U.S. infant mortality rate varies by race. The rate for non-Hispanic Caucasians is 5.76 deaths per 1,000 live births; African Americans, 13.63; Hispanics, 5.8; American Indians and Alaskan natives, 4.9; and Asian/Pacific Islanders, 8.06.

To reduce the rate of infant mortality in the world, the World Health Organization wants to increase the availability of health services to all mothers. To reduce the rate of infant mortality in the United States, the Department of Health and Human Services wants to increase the proportion of mothers getting early prenatal care; decrease the incidence of SIDS; lessen the percentage of pregnant women who smoke cigarettes, drink alcohol, and take other drugs; and reduce the number of low-birth-weight infants.

Table 9.3

Infant Mortality Rate (Deaths per 1,000 Live Births) in Various Countries

Country	Rate	Country	Rate
Sweden	2.75	Panama	13.40
Japan	2.80	China	21.16
France	3.36	Indonesia	31.04
Germany	4.03	World	42.09
United Kingdom	4.93	Bolivia	49.09
New Zealand	4.99	Pakistan	66.94
Canada	5.08	Chad	100.36
United States	6.30	Afghanistan	154.67
Chile	7.90	Angola	182.31

Source: U.S. Central Intelligence Agency World Fact Book, 2008. Available: http://www.cia.gov/library/publications/the-world-factbook/rankorder/2091rank.html. Retrieved September 22, 2008.

controlled by the pituitary hormone **prolactin,** the levels of which rise tremendously during pregnancy and are maintained as long as the mother continues to nurse.

Milk is delivered from the breast through the coordinated activity of the mother and infant. Inserting the nipple into the baby's mouth activates the baby's sucking reflex. When the baby sucks, nerve impulses that stimulate the release of the hormone oxytocin are transmitted from the breast to the mother's brain. Oxytocin circulates through the mother's bloodstream to the breasts, where it causes the muscle cells that line the milk ducts to contract and eject milk from the nipple. Oxytocin also stimulates contractions of the uterus, so breastfeeding helps return the uterus to its prepregnant size.

A mother can nurse for many months. As long as the baby is sucking and the breasts are regularly drained of milk, the hormonal stimulation of milk production will continue. Without such stimuli, milk production stops. The many advantages of breastfeeding include the following:

- It is economical, readily available, and eliminates the effort involved in purchasing, preparing, and heating bottles and formula.
- It transfers immunity (protection against infections) from the mother to the infant, and breast milk itself and the act of nursing stimulate the development of the infant's own immune defenses.
- Breast milk promotes development of the infant's digestive system.
- Breastfed babies have fewer allergies, less diarrhea, fewer dental problems, and less colic (stomachache).
- Breast milk is nutritionally balanced for human infants; formulas containing cow's milk are not nutritionally identical to human milk, although they are nutritionally adequate.
- Breastfeeding may increase the psychological attachment between mother and infant.
- The hormones involved in the production and release of milk cause uterine contractions, which help the uterus return to its normal size. During the first week or so after childbirth these contractions may be intense and even painful. Thereafter some women describe them as pleasurable, sensual, or erotic.

Many women find that breastfeeding offers them a relaxing, pleasurable experience with their babies. Often the pleasurable feelings of breastfeeding will have an erotic tone, possibly producing genital sensations and even occasionally orgasm. These feelings and responses are normal and natural, and a woman need not feel guilty or distressed by them.

The many advantages of breastfeeding do not mean that bottle feeding is not wholesome. Many healthy, well-adjusted people were bottle-fed infants. Some women are physically unable to reastfeed. Some mothers choose not to breastfeed because work, family, and other responsibilities make it inconvenient. Breastfeeding in public or at work is, unfortunately, still not acceptable in many communities or places of employment. Some women choose not to breastfeed because they fear that changes in the shape of their breasts will decrease their sexual attractiveness.

Some women breastfeed their infants for several weeks or months and then gradually substitute bottle feedings for breast feedings until the child is completely **weaned,** that is, has stopped nursing altogether. More important than whether the milk comes from the breast or a bottle is the physical contact and loving the infant receives while being fed.

Infertility

Approximately one in five of all American married couples of childbearing age is **infertile,** which means that they are unable to become pregnant after a year of trying. Male factors are responsible for infertility in about 40% of infertile couples; female factors are responsible in another 40% to 50%. In about 10% of infertile couples, no cause can be determined. With professional help, about half of all infertile couples can eventually have children. A significant percentage of couples medically determined to be infertile eventually have children without medical interventions. Permanent infertility is called **sterility.**

> The reason grandparents and grandchildren get along so well is that they have a common enemy.
>
> *Sam Levenson*

In both sexes, infertility can be caused by a variety of conditions that adversely affect the functioning of an otherwise normal reproductive system. For example, ill health, cigarette smoking, chronic alcohol use, marijuana and other drug abuse, exposure to radiation or toxic chemicals, malnutrition, anxiety, stress, and fatigue can lessen a person's reproductive capabilities. Medical treatments or changes in lifestyle can often restore fertility. Age also plays a role. Women in their 20s conceive more readily than women in their late 30s and early 40s.

Because sperm and ovum production and the functions of the male and female reproductive tracts are absolutely dependent on adequate hormone production, hormonal problems are a common cause of infertility in both men and women. Infertility can result from undersecretion of the hypothalamic hormone GnRF and from the pituitary hormones FSH and LH. Infertility also can be caused by abnormal synthesis or release of testosterone from the testes and estrogen and progesterone from the ovaries. Fertility often can be restored by augmenting low levels of hormones with either natural or synthetic hormones such as clomiphene or pergonal. Use of such "fertility drugs," however, increases the chance of multiple births.

Infertility can also be caused by anatomical abnormalities or damage to the male or female reproductive systems. A common cause of damage is scarring and subsequent blocking of the fallopian tubes and, less frequently, the epididymis by gonorrhea or chlamydia infections (see Chapter 11). The scar tissue from such diseases blocks the tubes and prevents the passage of sperm and ova. Growths and tumors in the reproductive tract can also block the passage of sperm and ova. Sometimes surgical repair of blocked or damaged tubes can restore fertility.

Problems with insemination and sperm delivery and transport can also cause infertility. For example, a man may have difficulty getting and maintaining an erection or ejaculating into the vagina. A woman may produce very thick or voluminous cervical mucus, which can block entry of sperm into the uterus. Sometimes a couple has trouble conceiving because they are not having intercourse near the time of ovulation.

Enhancing Fertility Options

A variety of medical interventions is available to help infertile couples become pregnant. For example, conception is unlikely if fewer than 20 million healthy sperm are deposited in the vagina. If a man produces too few healthy sperm in a single ejaculate, sperm from several ejaculates may be combined and introduced into the woman's reproductive tract with a syringe; this procedure is called **artificial insemination.** If the male partner cannot produce sufficient numbers of healthy sperm

---

■ T E R M S ■

artificial insemination: introduction of semen into the uterus or oviduct by other than natural means

infertile: unable to become pregnant or to impregnate

prolactin: a hormone produced by the anterior lobe of the pituitary gland that stimulates milk secretion

sterility: the state of permanent infertility

wean: to discontinue breastfeeding, using other means to provide nutrients

🌐 Global Wellness

Boy or Girl—Should Parents Have the Right to Choose?

American parents can opt for "family balancing" by choosing the sex of their next child. Although controversial, sex selection is regarded as an ethical decision by the American Society for Reproductive Medicine. Techniques currently available that allow parents to have a child of a desired sex are *in vitro* fertilization (IVF) and sperm sorting.

IVF: In vitro fertilization can guarantee the birth of a baby of the chosen sex. Several eggs are surgically collected from the prospective mother and fertilized in the laboratory with the father's sperm. A single cell is removed from the developing embryo and analyzed to see if the chromosomes are XX (girl) or XY (boy). One or two embryos of the desired sex are then implanted into the uterus of a woman who has been hormonally prepared for pregnancy. If the pregnancy is successful, one (or two) babies of the desired sex will be born. IVF is most commonly used to prevent a couple with known genetic defects from having a genetically handicapped child. In addition to sex, the embryo can be tested for the presence of specific genetic defects and only embryos without abnormal genes are implanted. IVF is particularly useful for preventing sex-linked traits, such as hemophilia and some forms of muscular dystrophy, from being inherited.

Sperm sorting: Sperm sorting separates sperm carrying an X chromosome from those carrying a Y chromosome. A woman can be artificially inseminated with sperm that will produce an embryo of the desired sex. This technique is far simpler and less traumatic to the woman than IVF, but its success rate is only about 90% for females and 75% for males. So, a couple has to be prepared to accept a child that is not of the desired sex if the sperm sorting method is used.

Sex selection has been condemned partly because in countries such as India and China, sex selection has been used to abort female fetuses because male offspring are more desirable. In India, mobile ultrasound scanners would be taken from village to village, and, for a small fee, a woman could have the sex of her fetus determined. If it were a girl, often she would seek an abortion. In India, this practice has skewed the normal male-to-female ratio of 106:100 to 130:100. Both India and China have banned the use of ultrasound scans for purposes of sex selection. In the United States, there is no evidence that ultrasound scans are used for sex selection and abortion of an undesired fetus.

Others argue that sex selection is a form of sexism—that people regard one sex as being inferior to the other. But so far, in the United States sex selection has been used for family balancing: A couple with one or more children of one sex want to have a child of the opposite sex.

Another worry is that sex selection will lead to selection of traits other than sex as more genetic tests become available. A couple might want their child to be tall, intelligent, muscular, or musical. Opponents of the new reproductive technologies argue that they open the door to "designer babies" in which parents choose the traits they desire in their children. This concept raises the specter of eugenics (selective breeding for "good" genes) as practiced by the Nazis, who introduced reproductive policies in the 1930s in which people with certain traits were encouraged to reproduce and others, such as Jews, Gypsies, and persons with disabilities, were exterminated.

Controversy over the use of new reproductive technologies and genetic testing for desired traits is certain to increase in the future.

---

even for artificial insemination, the couple may become pregnant by artificial insemination with semen from a donor. Each year in the United States, about 10,000 babies are conceived by artificial insemination.

Another way to try to overcome infertility is **in vitro fertilization (IVF),** which is employed when a woman's fallopian tubes do not function properly and for other reasons, for example, to avoid passing an inherited disorder to a child.

In vitro fertilization involves the following steps:

- Surgically removing several ova (usually 2–12) that are ready for fertilization
- Obtaining healthy sperm from the male partner or male donor
- Fertilizing the eggs in a laboratory dish until at least one embryo develops to the four- to eight-cell stage

- Administering hormones to the woman to prepare her body for pregnancy
- Inserting several embryos into the woman's uterus (several are implanted to increase the chance of pregnancy; remaining embryos are frozen and stored for future use if necessary)

The first baby to be conceived by IVF was born in England in 1978. Since then, more than 1 million babies worldwide have been conceived using IVF. Despite the widespread use of IVF, the procedure is not without risk, and it fails more often than it succeeds.

One major problem with IVF is increased risk of multiple births. To increase the chances of pregnancy, several embryos are inserted into the prospective mother's uterus. In about 35% of IVF procedures, two embryos develop, thus producing fraternal twins. In about 4% of IVF procedures, three embryos develop. Multiple births are associated with lower birth weights and higher rates of congenital defects. Multiple births also endanger the prospective mother by increasing her risks of high blood pressure, anemia, premature labor, and cesarean section. Multiple live births also pose financial and psychological burdens for many parents.

The success rate for IVF ranges between 20% to 40% depending on many factors such as the woman's age, the experience of the medical professionals conducting the procedure, and the number of embryos inserted into the uterus. Even when only a single child is conceived by using IVF, the chance of delivering a low-birth-weight baby or one with congenital defects is about twice that for a baby conceived through sexual intercourse.

GIFT (gamete intrafallopian transfer) and ZIFT (zygote intrafallopian transfer) are similar to *in vitro* fertilization. With GIFT, the ova are placed in equal numbers in each of the fallopian tubes, and semen is introduced directly into the tubes. With ZIFT, eggs are fertilized *in vitro* and an embryo is placed in the fallopian tube. These procedures are successful between 10% and 20% of the time.

For some couples, the prospect of not being able to have a child is devastating. Many of these couples embark on lengthy efforts, which may cost thousands of dollars and consume much of their emotional energy, to become pregnant and have a healthy baby. Such couples may be asked to keep careful records of the woman's fertility cycle and to time intercourse for maximum likelihood of conception. They may be counseled to have intercourse at certain times after hormone treatments. They may make repeated visits to fertility clinics to undergo IVF or other medical interventions.

About 40,000 infertile couples in the United States attempt to have a child using IVF techniques each year. However, for most of these couples repeated attempts to conceive end in failure. For women under age 35, the success rate is approximately 20%; for women over age 40, the success rate is under 10%. In addition to the poor success rate, couples can pay several thousand dollars for each attempt to become pregnant, and health insurance generally does not cover any IVF costs.

Adoption

There are many reasons why adults may want to raise children who are not biologically their own. They may be partially motivated by a concern with overpopulation and a desire to give homeless children love and security. Another common reason is that a couple is unable to

have children because of infertility. One alternative for couples, or even single people and gay couples, is adoption. Many adoptions bring the anticipated happiness to otherwise childless couples.

There are three avenues to pursue when couples would like to adopt a child. Most commonly, adoptions are handled through state-licensed *private* or *public adoption agencies*, usually nonprofit social services, which handle approximately 70% of all adoptions. An agency adoption may be the best option for adopting an older child or a child with special needs, although agencies also help in the adoption of infants and children from other countries. Signing up with an adoption agency can be a lengthy process, often lasting several years.

Another way to adopt a child is through an *independent* or *private adoption*. The individuals wishing to adopt a child make arrangements with a woman who wants to give up custody of her child, often with an attorney, physician, or cleric serving as an intermediary. Every state has its own laws concerning independent adoption, and the prospective parents should know the laws in their state as well as the state of the birth mother. In all independent adoptions, the birth parents can give consent for adoption only after the birth of the child.

A third avenue to pursue is an *international adoption*. This is becoming an increasingly popular avenue for prospective parents. Both state and federal requirements must be met in international adoptions; however, the waiting period is not as lengthy as it is in private or public adoptions.

> **T E R M S**
>
> *in vitro* fertilization (IVF): a procedure in which an egg is removed from a ripe follicle and fertilized by a sperm cell outside the human body; the fertilized egg is allowed to divide in a protected environment for about two days and then is inserted into the uterus

Critical Thinking About Health

1. "Hmmmm," muttered Dr. Johnson, the hospital's new chief of medicine, as he pored over the hospital's recent birthing statistics. Dr. Johnson's curiosity and concern were piqued by data showing a wide variation in the rates of labor induction among the medical practitioners at the hospital: Dr. Smith, 7%; Dr. Anderson, 12%; Dr. Tompkins, 45%; and Dr. Hastings, 74%. Dr. Johnson knew that the U.S. national rate was 20%, and at the hospital he managed prior to this assignment the rate was 12%.

   Following a hunch, Dr. Johnson checked the hospital's computerized records to determine the days and times of the births at the hospital for the previous four months. He discovered that Dr. Tomkins had only one weekend delivery during that time period, and Dr. Hastings had no weekend deliveries and only two after 2 A.M.

   Dr. Johnson investigated the medical records further and discovered that Dr. Hastings had noted in several patients' medical records that the women had requested labor induction for reasons of personal convenience. Although Dr. Johnson personally disagreed with the practice of inducing labor for reasons of convenience, he nevertheless believed that if something went wrong, compared to nights and weekends when the hospital was not fully staffed, weekday births were financially less risky for the hospital.

   Should Dr. Johnson do anything to change the labor induction practices at the hospital? If so, what should he do? If not, why not?

2. We know that drugs, alcohol, and smoking are dangerous to a developing fetus. Imagine that you are working as a server in a restaurant.
   a. What would you say or do if a customer who was pregnant ordered a glass of wine?
   b. What would you say or do if a customer who was pregnant was smoking a cigarette?

3. Comment on this point of view: People have been having babies for thousands of years. Nowadays, the entire process is way too medicalized with birthing classes, hospital delivery rooms, anesthesia, fetal monitoring, episiotomy, labor induction, cesareans, circumcision of male infants, and bottle feeding.

Health in Review

- Conception, pregnancy, and childbirth are important and meaningful life experiences. The decision to become a parent requires psychological and physical preparation so every child can have parents prepared to meet its needs.
- Fertilization is followed by cleavages of the embryo as it moves into the uterus. About the sixth day after fertilization, the embryo implants in the lining of the uterus, and for the next 266 days or so the fetus develops. After 40 weeks of pregnancy a baby is born.
- Health habits during pregnancy such as good nutrition, seeking prenatal care, exercise and physical activity, and emotional well-being contribute to a successful pregnancy.
- Taking drugs, consuming alcohol, and smoking cigarettes during pregnancy can cause fetal damage or birth defects. Tests, such as amniocentesis or chorionic villus sampling, are available to determine whether birth defects are present.
- Optimal childbirth can be achieved by attending childbirth preparation classes, ensuring emotional support for the mother during childbirth, and making wise choices about medical interventions, such as episiotomy and pain management.
- Childbirth is divided into three stages. The first stage starts with the beginning of labor and lasts until the cervix is fully dilated. The second stage is the birth of the baby. The third stage is the delivery of the placenta.
- The period after childbirth may involve breastfeeding and resumption of sexual activities.
- Approximately 20% of American married couples are infertile. Some of these couples can be medically assisted to become pregnant; pregnancy also may occur with *in vitro* fertilization or artificial insemination.
- Adoption is an alternative for childless couples. Children can be adopted through a private or public adoption agency, in an independent or private adoption, or an international adoption.

Health and Wellness Online

The Web contains a wealth of information about health and wellness. By accessing the Internet using Web browser software, you can gain a new perspective on many topics presented in *Health and Wellness*, Tenth Edition. Access the Jones and Bartlett Publishers Web site at **health.jbpub.com/hwonline**.

References

Hartmann, K., et al. (2005) Outcomes of routine episiotomy: A systematic review. *Journal of the American Medical Association, 293*, 2141–2148.

Leeman, L., et al. (2003). The nature and management of labor pain: Nonpharmacological pain relief. *American Family Physician, 68*, 1109–1112.

Musters, C., McDonald, E., & Jones, I. (2008). Management of postnatal depression. *British Medical Journal, 337*, a736.

Swan, S. H. (2008). Environmental phthalate exposure in relation to reproductive outcomes and other health endpoints in humans. *Environmental Research, 108*, 177–186.

Tenore, J. L. (2003). Methods for cervical ripening and induction of labor. *American Family Physician, 67*, 2123–2128.

Suggested Readings

Boston Women's Health Book Collective. (2008). *Our bodies, ourselves: Pregnancy and birth*. New York: Touchstone. A comprehensive, accessible, up-to-date book for expectant mothers.

Meadows, M. (2001, May/June). Pregnancy and the drug dilemma. *FDA Consumer*. Discusses the use of medications during pregnancy. Available: http://www.fda.gov/fdac/features/2001/301_preg.html

Murkoff, H., Eisenberg, A., & Hathaway, S. (2002). *What to expect when you're expecting*. New York: Workman. This popular guide to pregnancy covers every aspect of the prenatal period, from developmental stages to nutrition.

Recommended Web Sites

Please visit **health.jbpub.com/hwonline** for links to these Web sites.

American Academy of Pediatrics
Information about immunizations, childhood illnesses, and child safety.

Healthy People 2010: Maternal, Infant, and Child Health
From the U.S. Department of Health and Human Services.

KidsHealth
Provides doctor-approved health information about children, from before birth to adolescence.

Motherisk Program at the Hospital for Sick Children, Toronto, Canada
Up-to-date information on the risk of medications on fetal development.

Parenthood.com
Tons of information about becoming pregnant, pregnancy, and parenthood.

ParentsPlace.com
Lots of information about pregnancy, including a detailed week-by-week pregnancy guide.

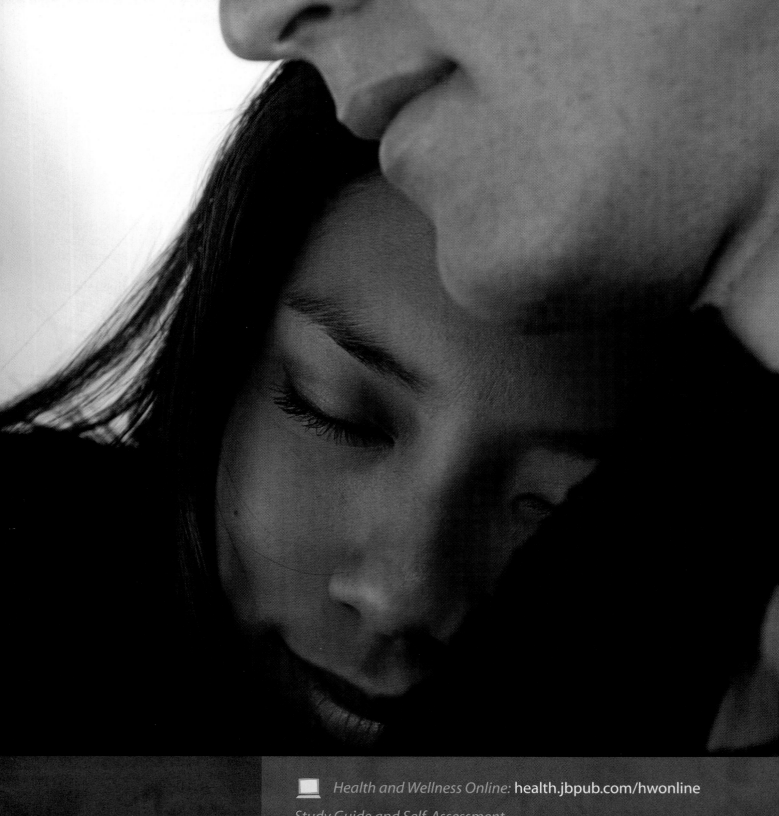

Chapter Ten

Choosing a Fertility Control Method

Learning Objectives

1. Define *contraceptive failure rate*.
2. Explain the drawbacks of withdrawal and douching.
3. Describe and list the advantages and disadvantages of combination and progestin-only hormonal contraceptives.
4. Explain how an IUD is used.
5. Describe barrier methods of contraception.
6. Describe five fertility awareness methods of contraception.
7. Describe male and female sterilization techniques.
8. Identify factors affecting fertility-control decision making.
9. Describe methods of medical and surgical abortion.

People have sexual intercourse for a variety of reasons other than to produce children (**Table 10.1**). Fortunately, knowledge of human reproductive biology and modern biotechnology have produced an array of relatively safe, reliable methods to help control fertility and reduce the risk of unintended pregnancy. Some fertility control techniques are preconception methods (contraceptives). They work by preventing the development or union of sperm and ova. Other techniques are postconception methods. They inhibit the development of the fertilized ovum or embryo.

> Whenever I hear people discussing birth control, I always remember I was the fifth.
>
> *Clarence Darrow*

In the United States each year, 6.3 million pregnancies occur. Nearly half (49%) of these pregnancies are unintended, and about half of these unintended pregnancies end in abortion. Of women who become pregnant unintentionally, about 50% are using some form of contraception at the time of conception. Pregnancy occurred, however, because the contraceptive method failed or it was being used incorrectly. Half of all American women aged 15–44 have experienced at leaast one unintended pregnancy (Trussell & Wynn, 2008).

When you consider the several methods of fertility control, keep in mind that sex without intercourse is a highly effective way to prevent pregnancy. Genital (penis-in-vagina) intercourse is not the only way to give and receive sexual pleasure. Touching, kissing, and stroking can bring intense sexual enjoyment and even orgasm to both partners.

Fertility Control Effectiveness

No fertility control method is perfect for everyone. Except for abstinence from sexual intercourse, no single method is 100% effective, 100% free of side effects, absolutely safe, financially available to everyone, and 100% reversible. Without a perfect contraceptive, avoiding an unintended pregnancy requires weighing the benefits and drawbacks of the various methods and choosing the one(s) that both partners are comfortable using and that they will use properly each time sexual intercourse takes place. Even the most technologically perfect contraceptive would fail if it were not used properly and consistently.

A fertility control method's effectiveness is measured in terms of its **failure rate,** which is the percentage of women who, on average, are likely to become pregnant using a particular method for a year. Each method has two failure rates: the **lowest observed failure rate,** a

Wellness Guide

A Comparison of Contraceptive Methods

Low effectiveness*

Method	Advantages	Disadvantages
Withdrawal	No health problems	Requires considerable ejaculatory control
Spermicides	No health problems; no prescription required	Must be used with each incidence of intercourse; messy
Fertility awareness	No health problems	Difficult to predict "safe" days; several days of abstinence may be required
Female condom	No prescription required	Vaginal irritation; must be used prior to intercourse

Moderate effectiveness†

Method	Advantages	Disadvantages
Male latex condom	No health problems; no prescription required	May break or tear
Diaphragm	No health problems	Must be used before intercourse; must be fitted by a clinician
Cervical cap	Can remain in place for up to 24 hours	Must be fitted by a clinician; cervical irritation

High effectiveness‡

Method	Advantages	Disadvantages
Combination hormonal methods (pills, patch, ring, injection)	Easy to use; not intercourse dependent	Side effects; serious risks to health in some users
Progestin-only methods (mini-pill, injection)	Easy to use; not intercourse dependent	Side effects
IUD	Not intercourse dependent	Side effects; irregular bleeding, heavy menstrual bleeding and cramps; increased risk of pelvic infection
Surgical sterilization (tubal ligation; vasectomy)	One-time procedure	Some postsurgical discomfort

*Low effectiveness: Failure rate greater than 20%.
†Moderate effectiveness: Failure rate between 6% and 19%.
‡High effectiveness: Failure rate between 0 and 5%.

Table 10.1

Some Common Reasons for Fertility Control

Reason	Explanation
Enhancing sexual pleasure	Anxiety about the possibility of pregnancy can divert a person's attention from the sexual experience and interfere with the flow of sexual feelings. Also, worry during intercourse can cause difficulties with erection and ejaculation in men and with vaginal lubrication and orgasm in women.
Family planning	Safe, reliable fertility control affords couples the opportunity to plan the size of their family and the timing of their children's births. Couples can have children when the family's financial resources are sound and the parents' relationship is ready for raising a child or children.
Increasing women's life choices	Fertility control allows women to choose when to devote time and energy to various life pursuits, including parenthood. In the not-too-distant past, when fertility control methods were unreliable, it was difficult for a woman to integrate her personal goals with parenthood because she had little control over the timing of the births of her children.
Health considerations	Fertility control helps couples reduce the risk of passing a hereditary disease to children. Fertility control also is advantageous to women for whom pregnancy and childbirth may be a significant health risk. Fertility control can prevent pregnancy in teenagers, who experience more pregnancy-related problems than older women.
World overpopulation	Some couples keep their families small because they want to take some responsibility for limiting the growth of the human population. Some people fear that overpopulation will create pressures for food, water, living space, energy, and other resources.

Table 10.2

Effectiveness Rates of Common Birth Control Methods

Method	Typical failure rate (%)	Lowest observed failure rate (%)
No method (chance)	85	85
Withdrawal	27	4
Combination birth control pill	8	0.3
Contraceptive patch	8	0.3
Vaginal ring	8	0.3
Hormonal injection	3	0.3
Progestin-only pill	3	0.5
Hormonal implants	0.05	0.05
Copper-T IUD	0.8	0.6
Hormonal IUD	0.2	0.2
Male latex condom	15	2
Female latex condom	21	5
Diaphragm	16	9
Sponge		
No prior births	16	9
Prior births	32	20
Spermicides	29	18
Fertility awareness	25	3–5
Tubal ligation	0.05	0.05
Vasectomy	0.15	0.1

Data are percentage of women becoming pregnant using a method for one year. *Typical failure rate* means the method was not always used correctly. *Lowest observed failure rate* means the method was nearly always used correctly and with every act of sexual intercourse.

Source: Data from J. Trussell and L. L. Wynn. (2008). Reducing unintended pregnancy in the United States. *Contraception, 77,* 1–5.

measure of how a method performs when used consistently and as intended, and the **typical failure rate,** a measure of how a method performs allowing for all of the errors and problems typically associated with a method (**Table 10.2**).

Withdrawal

The **withdrawal method** of fertility control (coitus interruptus) requires that the man withdraw his penis from the vagina before ejaculation. In theory, withdrawal prevents sperm from being deposited in the vagina and subsequently fertilizing an ovum. The male must exercise great control and restraint to withdraw the penis in time. Withdrawal is risky because a small emission may occur before ejaculation (pre-ejaculate), which may contain sperm, HIV, or other sexually transmitted bacteria or viruses. Even if no sperm are actually deposited in the vagina, pregnancy is possible if sperm are released near

the vagina and enter later, perhaps inadvertently, through body-to-body contact.

Withdrawal can diminish a couple's sexual pleasure. When the man must concentrate on withdrawing and the woman is concerned about whether he will withdraw in time, neither is free to fully experience the pleasure of sexual intercourse.

▌TERMS▌

failure rate: likelihood of becoming pregnant if using a birth control method for one year

lowest observed failure rate: likelihood of becoming pregnant if using a birth control method consistently and as intended

typical failure rate: likelihood of becoming pregnant considering all the potential problems associated with a birth control method

withdrawal method: removing the penis from the vagina just prior to ejaculation; also called coitus interruptus or pulling out

Douching

Douching (rinsing of the vagina with fluid) after sexual intercourse is a method of birth control that is almost totally ineffective. After ejaculation in the vagina, thousands of sperm move through the cervix and enter the uterus within a few seconds. There simply isn't time to flush out sperm from the vagina before a significant number enter the uterus. Furthermore, the force from the spray of the douche may propel sperm into the uterus, aiding conception rather than preventing it.

Hormonal Contraceptives

In 1960, the U.S. Food and Drug Administration approved the use of combination hormonal contraceptives for women. Since that time, millions of American women and hundreds of millions of women worldwide have adopted this form of fertility control because of its high effectiveness, reversibility, tolerable side effects, ease of use, and low cost.

Combination Hormonal Contraceptives

Combination hormonal contraceptives contain two kinds of synthetic hormones that are chemically similar to a woman's natural ovarian hormones, estrogen and progesterone. The ways these agents prevent pregnancy are shown in **Table 10.3**. Combination hormonal contraceptives are available as pills, a skin patch, a vaginal insert, and by injection.

Table 10.3

Mechanisms of Action of Estrogens and Progestogens Used in Oral Contraceptives

Hormone	Mechanisms of action
Estrogens	1. Inhibition of ovulation by suppressing the release of pituitary hormones FSH and LH
	2. Inhibition of implantation of the fertilized egg
	3. Acceleration of transport of the ovum in the fallopian tube
	4. Accelerated degeneration of the corpus luteum, which secretes progesterone, and consequent prevention of normal implantation of the fertilized ovum
Progestogens	1. Production of thick cervical mucus, which blocks sperm transport from the vagina to the uterus
	2. Change in the character of cervical mucus such that sperm are less able to effect fertilization
	3. Deceleration of ovum transport in the fallopian tubes
	4. Inhibition of implantation
	5. Interruption of the hormonal regulation of ovulation

Combination contraceptive pills (birth control pills) generally come in packets of 21, 24, or 28 pills. A 91-day, extended-use pill is also available, which has the advantages of fewer menstrual cycles per year and less opportunity to forget starting up a new packet of pills after a menstrual period. In the 21-pill packet, all the pills contain specific amounts of hormone. In the 24- and 28-pill packets, 21 of the pills contain hormones; the others (called "reminder pills") are inert or contain iron to help prevent iron-deficiency anemia. The first pill in a packet is taken on a predetermined day, and one pill is taken each day thereafter. Approximately two days after the last active pill is taken, a menstrual period occurs.

A pill should be taken at the same time each day to increase its effectiveness. It is recommended that pill taking be associated with a routine activity, such as going to bed or tooth brushing, to lessen the risk of forgetting. Forgetting near midcycle, when an egg is available for fertilization, can result in a pregnancy.

The effectiveness of combination pills may be lessened when they are taken simultaneously with St. John's wort and possibly other herbs or certain other medications, such as antibiotics, anticonvulsants, and a variety of pain relievers and anti-inflammatory drugs. Pill users should consult a health professional about this possibility.

Approximately half the women using combination oral contraceptives experience unwanted and unintended side effects. Most of the time the side effects present little long-term risk to health, and often they disappear after several cycles on the pill. The more common of the less serious side effects are nausea, weight gain, breast tenderness, mild headaches, spotty bleeding between periods, decreased menstrual flow, increased frequency of vaginitis, increased depression, and lowering of the sex drive. Some other frequent side effects are considered beneficial by many women. Among these are lessening of acne, diminution and even absence of menstrual cramps, decreased number of menstrual bleeding days, and absolute regulation of the menstrual cycle, which can be important for travelers and athletes.

Studies indicate that pill use may help prevent certain diseases. Compared with other women, women who take combination birth control pills have about one-third the chance of developing pelvic inflammatory disease, one-half the chance of developing benign (noncancerous) breast disease and ovarian cysts, nearly complete protection against ectopic pregnancy, and one-half the risk of developing iron-deficiency anemia. Data also indicate that combination birth control pills may protect against rheumatoid arthritis, endometrial cancer, and ovarian cancer.

There is no evidence that long-term fertility is lessened by using combination hormonal contraceptive pills, even after many years of use. Some women, however, experience menstrual irregularities in the first few

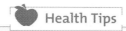 Health Tips

If You Forget to Take Your Pill

Being late or missing a pill (or two) can increase the risk of pregnancy. No matter what type of pill you take, if you take it late or miss taking it:

1. Contact your health care provider to ask what to do. You can also check the patient package insert, the pill manufacturer's Web site, or a book called *Physician's Desk Reference*.
2. Use a backup birth control method (e.g., diaphragm; sponge plus condom) for the rest of that pill cycle.

General Rules

Late pill taking

- More than 12 hours late: Take the "late" pill and use a condom for the next week.
- Between 12 to 24 hours late: Take the "late" pill as soon as you remember, and take the regular pill for that day at the scheduled time. Use condoms for the next week.

Combination pills

- Take the missed pill as soon as you remember, and take the next pill at the regular time, even if you take two pills in one day.
- If you miss any of pills 15 to 21, ask your doctor or pharmacist for special instructions. She or he may ask you to continue taking your pills but to start a new pack instead of taking the remaining pills.
- If you forget to take two or more pills, contact your health care provider for instructions. Depending on the type of pill, you may need to start a new pack or double up on pills for a while.

Progestin-only pill

- Take the missed pill as soon as you remember, and take the next pill at the regular time, even if you take two pills in one day. Use a backup method for the next two days.

Contraceptive patch

- The patch contains two days of extra hormone. If left on for more than nine days, use a backup method for the remainder of the cycle.

Contraceptive ring

- The ring contains a week's worth of extra hormone. Women should check the ring periodically to be sure it is in place and removed when required.

---

months after discontinuing the method. Even so, they can still become pregnant soon after discontinuing the pill. There is no association between pill use and subsequent birth defects in children born to pill users, unless a woman ingests pills while she is pregnant (e.g., becomes unintentionally pregnant while taking the pill). In this case, birth defects are possible because the hormones in the pills may damage the embryo and fetus.

For a small percentage of women, combination oral contraceptives present a risk of fatal blood clots and heart attack. Women most at risk are those who are over age 35 and those who smoke cigarettes. These women should consider using a birth control method other than the pill. Any pill user who experiences severe abdominal pain, chest pain, headaches, unusual eye problems (blurred vision, flashing lights, temporary blindness), or severe calf and thigh pain should consult a physician or family planning agency immediately. The risk of developing liver disease, gallbladder disease, high blood pressure, and stroke is also slightly greater for pill users. Users of combination oral contraceptives have no increased risk of developing breast cancer.

An alternative to hormonal contraceptive pills is a hormone-containing *skin patch*, which is applied to the lower abdomen, buttocks, or upper body (not the breasts) and releases hormones slowly. Each patch is worn continuously for one week and then replaced with a new patch on the same day of the week for a total of three weeks. The fourth week is patch free. This is when

menstruation occurs. In general, the patch is similar to the pill in effectiveness, side effects, and risks. Occasionally, the patch does not stay attached to the skin and contraceptive effectiveness is lost. Also, some women experience skin irritation and discontinue the patch. The product may be less effective in women weighing more than 200 pounds.

Another combination hormonal method is the *vaginal contraceptive ring*, a flexible device about two inches in diameter containing hormones that are similar to the active ingredients in combination contraceptive pills. A woman inserts the ring herself. After the ring is inserted, the hormones are continuously released. A ring is used for three weeks, then removed. After seven days, during which time a menstrual period occurs, a new ring is inserted. The ring is highly effective and has

TERMS

combination hormonal contraceptives: pills, a skin patch, a vaginal insert, and injections that contain two kinds of synthetic hormones that are chemically similar to a woman's natural ovarian hormones, estrogen and progesterone

douching: rinsing the vaginal canal with a liquid; not an effective means of birth control or STD prevention

the same side effects and risks as hormonal contraceptive pills. One additional caution is that the ring can be expelled before the three weeks are over. If the ring has been out of the vagina for more than three hours, an additional method of contraception (generally a barrier method) must be used until the ring has been back in place for seven days. Other side effects of the vaginal ring include vaginal discharge, vulvovaginitis, and irritation.

Progestin-Only Contraceptives

Progestin-only contraceptives are available as pills, implants, and injectables. Progestin-only contraceptives work by inhibiting ovulation and thickening the cervical mucus, making it more difficult for sperm to reach the egg. They also cause changes in the lining of the uterus that damage sperm and make implantation less likely to occur. Side effects may include menstrual irregularities, weight gain, depression, fatigue, decreased sex drive, acne or oily skin, and headaches. Progestin-only contraceptives are completely reversible. A woman returns to her previous level of fertility when she stops using any of the methods.

The **mini-pill** is a progestin-only pill containing 0.35 milligrams of progestogen or less. Twenty-one pills are taken one a day, and then pill taking stops for a week to allow for a menstrual period.

Progestin-only implantation methods (e.g., *Implanon*) involve inserting a 1.5-inch hormone-containing plastic rod under the skin, where it remains for three years. During this time the hormone continuously seeps into the user's bloodstream and brings about its contraceptive effects. Implantable methods are very effective, but their common side effects (irregular bleeding, prolonged bleeding, frequent bleeding, and absence of menstruation) are responsible for frequent discontinuation of the method.

Progestin-only injectable methods (e.g., *Depo-Provera*) involve injecting a 12-week supply of a hormone intramuscularly. The hormone is released at a steady rate. At the end of the 12 weeks, a replacement injection or another contraceptive must be obtained.

To stop using Depo-Provera, the woman does not get the next injection. Most women who get pregnant do so within 12 to 18 months of the last injection. This method can be used while breastfeeding, starting six weeks after delivery. The FDA warns that prolonged use of Depo-Provera can increase the risk of bone loss.

The Intrauterine Device

The **intrauterine device (IUD)** is a small device, containing copper or the hormone progesterone, inserted by a health care professional inside the uterus (**Figure 10.1**). A short string hangs into the vagina where it cannot be seen but where a woman can reach up and feel for its placement once a month. The most likely mechanisms

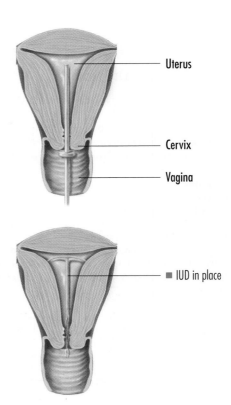

■ **Figure 10.1**

The IUD
The IUD is inserted past the cervix into the uterus. Prior to insertion the length of the uterus is measured with an instrument called a sound. Upon insertion the arms of the IUD gradually unfold. Once the inserter is removed, the threads attached to the IUD will be clipped to extend into the vagina through the cervical opening.

by which IUDs work include killing or weakening sperm and altering the timing of the ovum's or embryo's movement through the fallopian tube.

IUDs available in the United States are flexible plastic devices shaped like a T. One type is impregnated with hormone (progesterone or a synthetic progestin). Another type is wrapped with fine copper wire, which slowly dissolves and releases copper ions. Both the hormone and copper augment an IUD's effectiveness by damaging sperm and slowing sperm migration in the woman. Some IUD users experience heavier menstrual flow or menstrual cramps. IUD use is associated with an increased risk of pelvic inflammatory disease and uterine perforations with insertion, and ectopic pregnancy.

Barrier Methods

Barrier methods of fertility control involve devices that physically block the path of sperm movement in the female reproductive tract and usually bring sperm in contact with a sperm-killing (spermicidal) chemical, most often nonoxynol-9. Several contraceptive methods work on this principle, including the diaphragm; the cervical cap; the contraceptive sponge; spermicidal foams, jellies, and creams; and the condom.

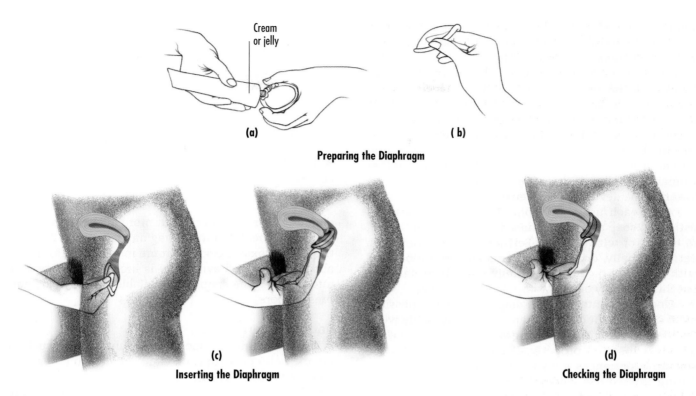

(a)

Cream
or jelly

(b)

Preparing the Diaphragm

(c)

Inserting the Diaphragm

(d)

Checking the Diaphragm

■ **Figure 10.2**

Procedure for Inserting a Diaphragm

(a) Before inserting the diaphragm, coat the rim and cup with a spermicidal cream or jelly. (b) Squeeze the rim of the diaphragm together between your thumb and index finger. (c) Insert the diaphragm into the vagina with the rim facing up and push it toward the small of your back. As you let go of the diaphragm, it will spring open; continue to guide it to your cervix with the tips of your fingers. (d) Be sure to check that the diaphragm completely covers the cervix.

The Diaphragm

The **diaphragm** is a dome-shaped latex cup, which is placed in the vagina to cover the cervix (**Figure 10.2**). A metal spring in the rim of the diaphragm holds the device snugly in place between the back wall of the vagina and the pubic bone in the front of the pelvis. In this position the diaphragm blocks the movement of sperm from the vagina to the uterus, although it does not fit snugly enough to keep all of the sperm out. Its primary purpose is to hold a spermicide in place next to the cervix. Correct usage requires that the rim and cup of the diaphragm be coated with a tablespoon or two of a spermicidal jelly or cream. The diaphragm should be left in place six to eight hours after intercourse. The spermicides used with the diaphragm also help prevent the transmission of some microorganisms responsible for genital infections.

One major advantage of the diaphragm is the absence of major medical problems associated with its use. A very few women or their partners may be allergic to the latex or the spermicide, and some develop urinary tract infections. Some women may experience discomfort with the diaphragm in place. Changing brands or getting a better-fitting diaphragm often solves these problems.

Another advantage is that the diaphragm can be inserted up to six hours before intercourse, so a couple does not have to interrupt sexual pleasuring to insert the device. If a diaphragm is inserted several hours before sexual activity, however, it is advisable to put an additional amount of spermicidal jelly or cream into the vagina before intercourse. The diaphragm must be left in place six to eight hours after last intercourse, but

TERMS

diaphragm: a soft, rubber, dome-shaped contraceptive device worn over the cervix and used with spermicidal jelly or cream

intrauterine device (IUD): a flexible, usually plastic, device inserted into the uterus to prevent pregnancy

mini-pill: a progestin-only contraceptive pill

progestin-only contraceptives: work by inhibiting ovulation and thickening the cervical mucus; completely reversible

progestin-only implantation methods: inserting a 1.5-inch hormone-containing plastic rod under the skin, where it remains for three years

progestin-only injectable methods: injection of a 12-week supply of hormone, which is released at a steady rate

should not be left in place longer than 24 hours because of the possible risk of toxic shock syndrome.

Each woman must be fitted (by a family planning professional or a physician) with a diaphragm that is the correct size for her. The need for proper fitting is one reason that diaphragms are available only by prescription. Any change in a woman's body size—a gain or loss of several pounds, pregnancy, or pelvic surgery—is reason to check the fit and have a new diaphragm prescribed if necessary. A woman should not use another woman's diaphragm because the fit might be wrong, lowering the device's effectiveness.

After each use the diaphragm should be washed with mild soap and water, rinsed thoroughly, and dried in the air or with a towel. Perfumed talcum powders, petroleum jelly, or scented creams should not be used with the diaphragm. Occasionally the rubber darkens, but this generally does not impair effectiveness.

One disadvantage of the diaphragm is the possibility of dislodgment during intercourse. Only rarely will a man feel the diaphragm during sexual intercourse if the device is inserted properly. If either the man or the woman experiences unusual sensations or discomfort during intercourse, then the diaphragm may not be inserted correctly, it may have become dislodged during intercourse, or it may be the wrong size. Another disadvantage of the diaphragm is an increased risk of toxic shock syndrome. Women with a history of toxic shock syndrome are advised to use a different method.

Periodically the diaphragm should be held against a light to check for tiny holes and weak spots (where the rubber buckles). With proper care a diaphragm will last a year or two.

The Cervical Cap

The **cervical cap** is a cup-shaped rubber device that snugly covers the cervix similar to the way a thimble fits on a finger (**Figure 10.3**). Like a diaphragm, a cervical cap needs to be coated with spermicide to be as effective as possible and remain in place for eight hours after last intercourse. Cervical caps come in several sizes and must be fitted for each woman. One difference between the diaphragm and the cervical cap is the fact that the cervical cap can be inserted up to 24 hours before intercourse.

The major disadvantages of the cervical cap are difficulty with insertion and removal, occasional discomfort during intercourse, dislodgment during intercourse, and possibly irritation of the cervix. The cervical cap should not be left in place for more than 48 hours.

The Contraceptive Sponge

The **contraceptive sponge** is a dome-shaped device made of a compressible, spongy material, which is inserted in the vagina to cover the cervix. The sponge contains **spermicide,** so it prevents pregnancy by blocking, absorbing, and destroying sperm. Once inserted, the sponge can be left in place for 24 hours. After use, it is discarded. The sponge is less effective than the

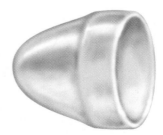

■ **Figure 10.3**
Cervical Cap

diaphragm or cervical cap but more effective than spermicides alone. If left in the vagina longer than 24 hours, the risk of toxic shock syndrome increases. Information about toxic shock syndrome is included with product information. The sponge is available without a doctor's prescription.

Vaginal Spermicides

When used alone, spermicidal chemicals, such as nonoxynol-9 or octoxynol, can provide some degree of contraception. The chemicals are available as foams, creams, jellies, and suppositories without a doctor's prescription. Spermicides are placed in the vagina immediately before intercourse and before every subsequent intercourse in a sexual episode. Although often displayed in stores with feminine hygiene products, vaginal spermicides are not to be confused with douches, deodorants, or vaginal lubricants, none of which are effective as contraceptives.

The effectiveness of all of the vaginal spermicides depends on a sufficient quantity of sperm-killing chemical bathing the cervix at the time of ejaculation. Users must put the spermicide in the vagina immediately before every act of intercourse and before each subsequent intercourse in the same sexual encounter.

Users of foam should be sure that the foam is frothy and bubbly, which is achieved by shaking the container about 20 times before filling the applicator. Because there is no way to know how much foam remains in a container, a spare container should be kept on hand.

Vaginal spermicides tend to be slippery, which occasionally can be a nuisance, but the moisture can augment a woman's natural vaginal lubrication and enhance sensation. In rare instances, someone may be allergic to a particular product. Changing brands may alleviate this problem. Some women experience irritation if a suppository has not dissolved completely before intercourse takes place. Spermicides do not cause birth defects.

Male Condoms

The male **condom,** or rubber, is a membranous sheath that covers the erect penis and catches semen before it enters the vagina. About 99% of male condoms are made of latex or polyurethane; the rest, so-called skin con-

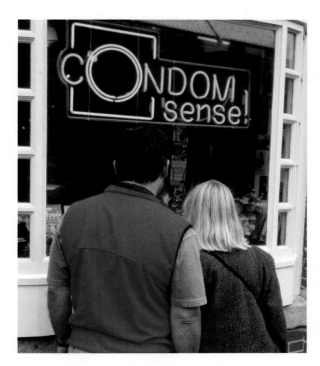

Condoms are an effective form of fertility control and provide protection against STDs. It's important that both partners take responsibility for using condoms.

doms, which are not effective against STDs, are manufactured from lamb intestines.

When stored in a cool, dry place, condoms retain their effectiveness for up to five years. Kept in a warm environment, such as in a wallet, in the back pocket of one's pants, or in the glove compartment of a car, the latex will deteriorate. To be most effective, condoms must be used with water-based lubricants, such as K-Y Jelly, because petroleum-based lubricants, such as Vaseline, destroy the latex.

A primary reason for condom failure in preventing pregnancy is error in use. Used in conjunction with another barrier method, such as a diaphragm or spermicidal foam, condoms are nearly 100% effective. Another advantage is that condoms help prevent the transmission of chlamydia, gonorrhea, herpes, HIV infection, and other kinds of infections.

Some people complain that the condom diminishes pleasurable sensations, but the device does not totally block genital feeling, which, in any event, is only one of many factors that contribute to sexual arousal and pleasure. A negative attitude about condoms may diminish pleasure far more than a thin layer of latex ever could. Instead of thinking about how condoms block sensations, it might enhance lovemaking to think of them as a fun way to help make lovemaking more pleasurable because of the protection they provide.

When using a condom, consider ways to incorporate putting on the device without interrupting lovemaking. For example, having a condom available before sexual activity begins makes breaking off contact to obtain one unnecessary. Before intercourse begins, either partner can put the condom on the erect penis while the couple continues to fondle, talk, or play.

Female Condoms

The female condom is a thin, loose-fitting polyurethane plastic pouch that lines the vagina. It has two flexible rings: an inner ring at the closed end, used to insert the device inside the vagina and hold it in place, and an outer ring that remains outside the vagina and covers the external genitalia. **Figure 10.4** shows the insertion and positioning of the female condom. Because the device is made from polyurethane, which is 40% stronger than latex, the female condom can be used with any type of lubricant without compromising the integrity of the device.

Two advantages of the female condom are that it warms up instantly to body temperature once it is inserted, thus enhancing sensation for both partners, and it provides protection from STDs (by covering both internal and external genitalia), including HIV, and prevents pregnancy. The female condom can be obtained in drugstores and supermarkets, and it can be used by people allergic to latex or spermicide.

A disadvantage of the female condom is that occasionally the outer ring may be pushed inside the vagina. Other problems include difficulties in insertion and removal; minor irritation; discomfort or breakage, which can be decreased by using enough lubrication; and that it costs more than male condoms.

Fertility Awareness Methods

Fertility awareness methods (also called natural family planning, the rhythm method, or periodic abstinence) attempt to determine when an ovum has been released

---

┃TERMS┃

cervical cap: small latex cap that covers the cervix, used with spermicidal jelly or cream inside the cap

condom: a latex or polyurethane sheath worn over the penis (male condom) or inside the vagina (female condom); can be both a barrier method of contraception and act as a prophylactic against sexually transmitted diseases

contraceptive sponge: a dome-shaped device coated with spermicide

fertility awareness methods: methods of birth control in which a couple charts the cyclic signs of the woman's fertility and ovulation, and/or uses basal body temperature, mucus changes, and other signs to determine fertile periods

spermicide: a chemical that kills sperm; particularly foams, creams, gels, and suppositories used for contraception

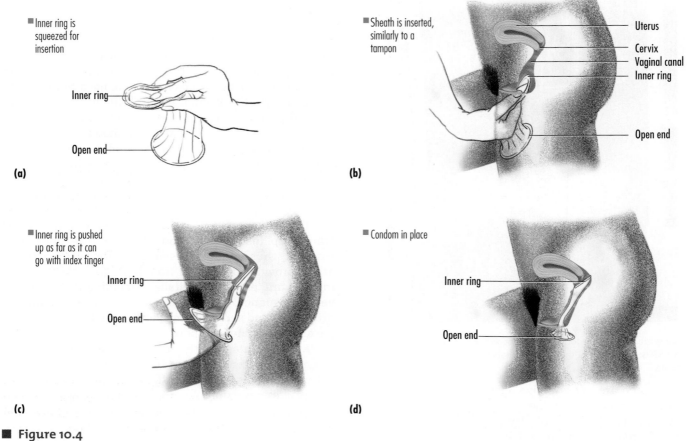

■ **Inner ring is**
squeezed for
insertion

Inner ring

Open end

(a)

■ **Inner ring is pushed**
up as far as it can
go with index finger

Inner ring

Open end

(c)

■ **Sheath is inserted,**
similarly to a
tampon

Uterus
Cervix
Vaginal canal
Inner ring

Open end

(b)

■ **Condom in place**

Inner ring

Open end

(d)

■ **Figure 10.4**

Female Condom Insertion and Positioning

from the ovary and is capable of being fertilized. In general, the time when a woman is most fertile occurs 14 days before her next menstrual period, or midcycle in a woman with a regular 28-day cycle.

Fertility awareness methods of birth control either estimate when ovulation is most likely to occur or indicate when ovulation has already taken place, thereby telling a couple the days in the menstrual cycle not to have unprotected intercourse. Those are referred to as "unsafe days." The days when a woman is not likely to be fertile are referred to as "safe days." On unsafe days, a couple should use an alternative method of birth control, such as condoms, a diaphragm, or spermicidal foam. Other options include enjoying ways of sexual pleasuring other than genital intercourse, or complete sexual abstinence.

Couples using fertility awareness methods should realize that, even on safe days, fertilization is still possible because of natural variations in a woman's reproductive processes. Therefore, safe days are really *relatively* safe days.

Fertility awareness offers the advantages of posing no health risks; furthermore, some people's religious convictions make fertility awareness the only acceptable

method of birth control. The effectiveness of fertility awareness is among the lowest of the common methods, about 25 pregnancies per 100 women per year. Failures occur because people do not keep careful records, they find the intervals of abstinence during the unsafe days too long, and they find having to plan sex only for the safe days a hindrance to spontaneous lovemaking.

Calendar Rhythm

Calendar rhythm is a way to estimate the most likely fertile, or unsafe, days in a woman's menstrual cycle by assuming that

1. Ovulation usually takes place 14 days (plus or minus 2 days) before the onset of the next menstrual flow.
2. An ovum is capable of being fertilized for 24 hours.
3. Sperm deposited in the vagina remain capable of fertilization for up to three days.

Using calendar rhythm effectively requires knowledge of the female fertility cycle and instruction in doing the calculations correctly (**Figure 10.5**). Family planning agencies, women's health clinics, books, and Web sites on fertility awareness methods can be helpful in learning the method.

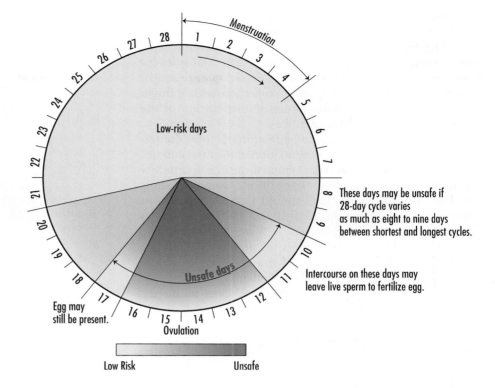

■ Figure 10.5

Calendar Rhythm Method
The calendar rhythm method is based on avoiding intercourse when sperm can fertilize an ovum. Unsafe days for intercourse in this chart are days 12 to 16.

The Temperature Method

The **basal body temperature (BBT)** is the lowest temperature in a healthy person during waking hours. In 70% to 90% of women, the BBT rises approximately one degree after ovulation, presumably because of changes in hormone levels. By keeping a daily record of the BBT, a woman can determine when ovulation has occurred and therefore the unsafe and safe days for intercourse

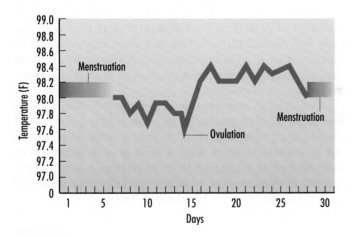

■ Figure 10.6

Basal Body Temperature Method of Contraception
A woman's body temperature rises about one degree during the days following ovulation. Once the BBT has risen for three consecutive days, assume that ovulation has taken place and that the rest of the days in that menstrual cycle are safe for unprotected intercourse. To use the BBT method, a woman must record her basal body temperature each morning before engaging in *any* activity. Temperature measurement should last at least five minutes.

between ovulation and the beginning of the next menstrual cycle. Because the BBT method cannot predict when ovulation will occur, a woman must still estimate with another fertility awareness method (calendar method, mucus method) the safe and unsafe days before ovulation.

Temperature measurements should take at least five minutes. Temperature measurements should be taken at the same time each day, and a record should be kept on a graph (**Figure 10.6**). Once the BBT has risen for three consecutive days, a woman can assume that ovulation has taken place and that the rest of the days in that menstrual cycle are safe for unprotected intercourse.

The Mucus Method

Certain hormone-sensitive glands in the cervix produce mucus that changes in amount, color, and consistency during different phases of the menstrual cycle. Learning to recognize the changes in cervical mucus can help

TERMS

basal body temperature (BBT) method: uses daily body temperature readings taken immediately after waking to identify the time of ovulation; approximately 24 hours after ovulation, the BBT increases

calendar rhythm: estimation of fertile, or unsafe, days to have intercourse

determine when ovulation occurs, and safe and unsafe days for intercourse can be planned accordingly.

The mucus method requires that cervical mucus be examined frequently during the cycle. Samples of mucus may be obtained with a finger, on toilet tissue, or from discharge on underpants. Collection with a finger is best because it permits direct determination of the amount and consistency of mucus.

Because douching, vaginal infections, semen, contraceptive foams and jellies, vaginal lubricants, medications, and vaginal lubrication from sexual arousal can interfere with the recognition of mucus patterns, women wishing to use the mucus method should obtain instructions from someone experienced with the method, a family planning clinic, or a health center. A woman should plan on charting her cervical mucus for at least a month to learn her individual pattern of mucus changes before relying on the method for fertility control.

The **sympto-thermal method** involves using the temperature and mucus methods simultaneously.

Chemical Methods

Chemical methods of fertility awareness measure the amount of **luteinizing hormone** (LH) in a woman's urine, which peaks at the time of ovulation. Ovulation predictor kits to measure the levels of LH can be purchased in pharmacies. Manufacturers claim that the kits have an accuracy rate of 85%.

Sterilization

Sterility is being permanently unable to have children. For people who are certain that they do not want children, or, as is more often the case, no more children, surgical methods that render a person sterile but have no effect on sexual arousal or activities may be the most desirable form of birth control. Indeed, for American married couples over age 30, "permanent fertility control" (sterilization of either the male or female partner) has become the most frequently chosen method of fertility control. The popularity of sterilization as a method of fertility control stems from its nearly 100% effectiveness, the relative safety of the procedure, and its relatively low one-time cost.

Male Sterilization

The sterilization of a man is called **vasectomy.** Approximately 500,000 men in the United States choose vasectomy every year. This procedure involves the cutting and tying of each of the two vasa deferentia, the sperm-transporting tubes between the testes (where sperm are made) to the penis (**Figure 10.7**). When these tubes are cut, sperm are no longer emitted upon ejaculation because their passage is blocked. Because the cut is made "upstream" from the organs that produce seminal fluid, a man still ejaculates, but the fluid contains no

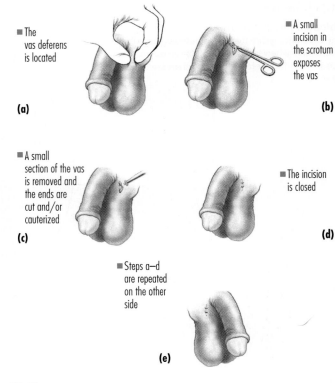

■ The vas deferens is located

(a)

■ A small incision in the scrotum exposes the vas

(b)

■ A small section of the vas is removed and the ends are cut and/or cauterized

(c)

■ The incision is closed

(d)

■ Steps a–d are repeated on the other side

(e)

■ **Figure 10.7**

Vasectomy

sperm. And because sperm make up only a small percentage of the total volume of the semen, neither a man nor his partner is aware of any change in their sex life, except that no other form of contraception is needed.

Although vasectomy should be considered a permanent form of contraception, it is sometimes possible to reverse the condition by rejoining the cut ends of the vasa deferentia. The success of vasectomy reversal as measured by the ability to have children again is about 50%, although some surgeons claim much higher reversal rates.

One of the reasons vasectomy is such a popular method of contraception is that it is uncomplicated and causes few problems. The procedure is usually carried out in a doctor's office with a local anesthetic in about 15 to 30 minutes. The incidence of postoperative complications is very low, and within a week most men can return to regular activities, including sex. About one-half to two-thirds of vasectomized men develop antibodies to sperm, but there is no evidence to suggest that this is harmful. A man can be fertile for several weeks after vasectomy, because the sperm pathway contains sperm present before the vasectomy. Once these are ejaculated, the man is sterile.

Female Sterilization

The principal sterilization procedure for women is **tubal ligation,** which involves blocking of the fallopian tubes by

(a) Side View

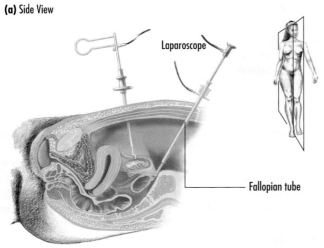

Laparoscope

Fallopian tube

(b) Front View

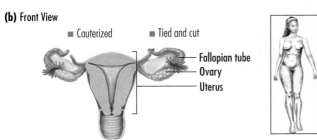

■ Cauterized   ■ Tied and cut

Fallopian tube
Ovary
Uterus

■ Figure 10.8

Tubal Ligation

Female sterilization by laparoscopic ligation. (a) Side view: The tubes are located using a laparoscope and cut, tied, or cauterized through a second incision. (b) Front view: The tubes after ligation.

cutting and tying, sealing, or closing them with clips, bands, or rings (**Figure 10.8**). Most tubal ligations are performed under local anesthesia in a clinic or doctor's office. The procedure involves entering the abdominal cavity and inflating the cavity (with carbon dioxide or nitrous oxide gas) so the surgeon can locate and block the tubes.

Usually one or two incisions about an inch long are made at the pubic hair line and/or belly button. Alternatively, an incision is made in the back of the vagina (*culpotomy*). The incidence of postoperative complications is very low; any complications that do occur are more to do with the skill of the surgeon rather than any inherent danger in the procedure itself.

Although tubal ligation is intended to be a permanent form of birth control, accidental pregnancies occur because a blocked tube spontaneously reopens. Surgical reversal of tubal blocking may be possible if a woman later decides that she wants to have children, with a success rate of 50% to 70%.

Another female sterilization technique is **hysterectomy,** the surgical removal of the uterus. Most experts do not recommend hysterectomy solely for sterilization

purposes because, when compared with tubal ligation, the chances for postoperative complications are 10 to 100 times greater, the operation is more expensive, and the negative psychological effect may be greater.

Choosing the Right Fertility Control Method

Most users of fertility control are principally concerned with two questions: How well does the method work? Is it safe? The efficacy of a fertility control method can be evaluated in terms of the lowest observed failure rate, which is how well the method performs if it is used consistently and as intended, and the typical failure rate, which is a measure of how well a method performs in actual use in a population. The typical failure rate takes into account improper, inconsistent, and careless usage.

Considerations about the safety of fertility control methods must take into account the health risks of a particular method, such as serious illness, the possibility of infection and its consequences, the risk of death, the risk of being unable to have children in the future, any effects on unborn children, and undesirable and unhealthful changes in the body.

Evaluation of a fertility control method's safety should also assess the physical and psychological consequences of an unintended pregnancy. These include the risks associated with terminating the pregnancy by abortion and the risks associated with carrying the pregnancy to term. Factors such as a woman's age, her physical health, whether she has had previous children, and her capacity to care for another child also need to be evaluated. Of course, the most serious risk associated with the use of any contraceptive is the risk of death, which is rare except for older pill users who smoke heavily.

TERMS

hysterectomy: surgical removal of the uterus

luteinizing hormone: anterior pituitary hormone that causes a follicle to release a ripened ovum and become a corpus luteum; in the male, it stimulates testosterone production and the production of sperm cells

sympto-thermal method: using both the basal body temperature and the mucus methods at the same time

tubal ligation: a surgical procedure in women in which the fallopian tubes are cut, tied, or cauterized to prevent pregnancy; a form of sterilization

vasectomy: a surgical procedure in men in which segments of the vas deferens are removed and the ends tied to prevent the passage of sperm

Responsibility for Fertility Control

Most people engage in sexual activity because they want a joyous, rewarding experience. Because an unintended pregnancy can cause enormous hardship, birth control is an important part of every sexual relationship. Denying the possibility of pregnancy by assuming "it can't happen to me" is just gambling against the odds.

The responsibility for fertility control has two components. First, a fertility control method must be chosen, taking into consideration the nature of an individual's sexual activities or a couple's sexual relationship, the frequency of intercourse, future plans regarding children, and personal and religious values. Second, the chosen method must be used consistently and correctly.

For both technological and sociological reasons, there has been a tendency to associate the responsibility for fertility control with the partner for whose body a particular method is designed. For example, in the late nineteenth century, when withdrawal and the condom were the principal methods of fertility control, and women were not supposed to be interested in sex, men were considered to be the ones responsible for fertility control (when it was used at all). In the late 1960s, when the pill and IUD were heralded as "perfect" contraceptives and women began to assert themselves socially and politically, the responsibility for fertility control shifted almost totally to women.

> If only one could tell true love from false love as one can tell mushrooms from toadstools.
>
> *Katherine Mansfield*

Today a large percentage of sexually active people believe that both partners in a sexual relationship should share the responsibility for fertility control. Yet, because so many methods are intended for use by the woman, in actual practice many women are left to manage fertility control on their own. Having to take total responsibility for fertility control can create resentment that blocks the feelings that many people wish to express with sex.

The responsibility for fertility control can be shared in a number of ways. The most important is to discuss it. In an ongoing relationship, there are many opportunities to talk about fertility control. Couples can go to fertility control clinics together, they can read and discuss information about the advantages and disadvantages of the different methods, and they can try out various methods to find out which are best suited for them. They can share the time and the financial costs of their chosen method, or they can divide responsibilities. For example, if a woman has to take time to go to a clinic or doctor, her partner could pay for the clinic visit and the contraceptives.

Partners can also share in using their chosen method. They can discuss any difficulties or concerns they have with their method of fertility control. Partners can even remind each other to use their chosen fertility control method. A man can learn how a diaphragm is used, a woman can learn about the condom, and they can incorporate into their lovemaking preparing to use these and other barrier methods. Furthermore, partners can share the responsibility of inserting, removing, and cleaning the woman's diaphragm or cervical cap. If a woman is using fertility awareness methods, a man can share the responsibility by helping to determine the safe and unsafe days and by sharing the responsibility for abstaining from sexual intercourse when necessary.

Partners who share the responsibility for fertility control are more likely to use their chosen method(s) properly, which makes fertility control more effective. And reducing the fear of pregnancy makes sex more enjoyable. Another benefit of sharing this responsibility is that it tends to enhance intimacy in a relationship. The discussion of fertility control and the mutual decision making involved in choosing and using a method lead to better communication.

It is always a good idea for you to have some method of fertility control with you if you anticipate that sexual intercourse might occur. For example, both men and women can carry a condom or spermicides with them on dates or to parties if they think that sexual activity is a possibility.

Talking About Fertility Control

A couple shares the responsibility for fertility control because both partners are responsible if an unintended pregnancy occurs. This fact alone is the most important reason for discussing fertility control. Although it is important to discuss fertility control before having sex, many individuals are embarrassed to do so. Talking about contraception implies that sex is going to take place, which may force an individual to face internal conflicts about engaging in sex. Many individuals subscribe to the myth that good sex should be spontaneous rather than planned. Therefore, sex and fertility control remain undiscussed. First-time partners may not discuss fertility control before sex because they fear spoiling a romantic mood.

Still, the best time to discuss fertility control is *before* sexual intercourse. A partner might say, "I would really like to make love (have sex) with you, and I want to be sure we're protected." That kind of introduction can be followed by a statement of preference and personal responsibility, such as, "I prefer to use condoms" or "I'm on the pill" or using a question such as "What birth con-

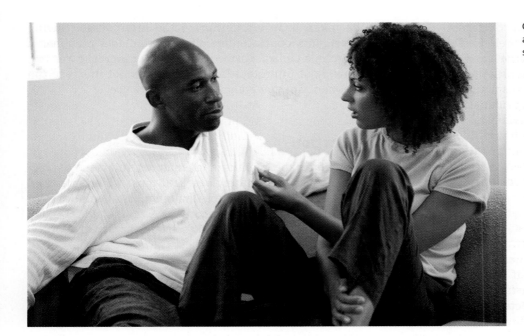

Choosing a fertility control method should be a decision made by both sexual partners and should be discussed before having sex.

trol method do you prefer?" or "What are we going to do about control?"

In some cases, even if a man is concerned about an unintended pregnancy and sexual diseases, he may not feel comfortable bringing up the topic, fearing embarrassment or appearing ignorant or weak. Many women, however, appreciate a man who initiates a discussion of birth control. Communication about birth control and other sexual matters, such as the role of sex in a relationship, likes and dislikes, and preventing STDs, is vital to a healthy sexual relationship.

Why People Do Not Use Fertility Control

About 10% of sexually active, fertile American women do not regularly use birth control despite being at risk for an unintended pregnancy (Wu et al., 2008). Contraceptive nonuse is responsible for half of the 3.1 million unintended pregnancies that occur each year in the United States. Some of the major reasons that people do not use fertility control, even if they wish to avoid pregnancy, include the following:

- *Low motivation:* People who have mixed feelings about avoiding pregnancy are less motivated to use fertility control. For example, a couple that has decided that they want to have a child "sometime in the near future" is less likely to be motivated to use fertility control than is a couple that is absolutely certain they do not want a child until some specified time, or at all.

- *Lack of knowledge:* Lack of knowledge about the process of conception and how to use fertility control effectively can lead to an incorrect perception of the risk of becoming pregnant. For example, some people believe the myths that pregnancy is not possible if a woman has an orgasm, if she urinates after intercourse, or if she is having sexual intercourse for the first time. Sometimes a method is believed to be more effective than it really is, or the chosen method is used incorrectly. For example, some people erroneously believe that a woman is most fertile during the bleeding days of the menstrual cycle and thus practice fertility awareness at the wrong time. Some couples lose, misplace, or run out of their primary method and do not have a backup method available.

- *Negative attitudes about fertility control:* Some people believe that fertility control is immoral, a hassle, unromantic, or harmful. One's own negative attitudes or the perceived negative attitudes of others, such as peers or parents, can inhibit one from obtaining contraceptives. People use these as excuses not to visit doctors or clinics, or they may shy away from obtaining over-the-counter contraceptives.

- *Relationship issues:* Individuals in committed relationships are better contraceptors than individuals who are not in such relationships. Involvement with a committed partner tends to lessen guilt associated with sexual activity and hence improves attitudes about contraceptive practice. People in a committed relationship tend to have sexual intercourse more often and regularly, which gives the couple opportunities to talk about contraception and to become adept at using method(s). Individuals with irregular sexual contact, either because of geographical separation or relationship problems, may have difficulties in establishing a birth control regimen. In new or casual sexual relationships, there is a tendency to use no method or a poor method at first.

Emergency Contraception

Emergency contraception ("the morning-after pill") is designed to prevent pregnancy if fertilization might have occurred. Situations that warrant emergency contraception include having unprotected intercourse, misusing a contraceptive (e.g., forgetting to take birth control pills; condom slipping off), or sexual assault. Emergency contraception is not intended to be a primary birth control method.

There are two forms of emergency contraception: hormonal and IUD insertion. Hormonal emergency contraception consists of taking the same kinds of hormones that are in birth control pills. One type contains both an estrogen and a progestogen. It is taken in two large doses 12 hours apart within 72 hours of unprotected intercourse. The other type consists of a progestin-only pill. Both methods are very effective, reducing the risk of pregnancy by 90%. Side effects include nausea and vomiting.

Emergency contraception with an IUD involves inserting a copper-T IUD up to five days after unprotected intercourse. This method is more effective than the hormonal methods, reducing the risk of pregnancy following unprotected intercourse by more than 99%. Emergency contraception has the potential to reduce the number of unintended pregnancies by 50% and the number of potential abortions by half, which equates to about 700,000 abortions in the United States each year (Steinauer, 2005).

Because of its safety and efficacy, emergency contraception is available without a prescription in many countries in the world. In the United States, emergency contraception pills are sold under the name Plan B and are available in licensed pharmacies to women 18 years of age or older without a prescription; women younger than 18 must have a doctor's prescription. A person 18 or older can buy multiple packages of Plan B at one time. Men can purchase Plan B, too. The World Health Organization recommends that women obtain an advance supply of emergency contraception pills because they must be taken soon after unprotected intercourse. Having emergency contraceptive pills on hand does not affect a woman's contraceptive use, does not increase her frequency of unprotected sex, and does not increase the frequency of emergency contraceptive use.

Abortion

Abortion is the intentional, premature termination of pregnancy. It is one of the oldest and most widely practiced methods of fertility control. Chinese medical writings from 2700 B.C. recommended abortion. A cross-cultural study found that all but one of 300 societies had used abortion to control the size of families. Currently in the United States, approximately 840,000 abortions are performed each year. This number represents about 25% of all pregnancies and about 50% of unintended pregnancies.

The most common method of abortion is **manual vacuum aspiration,** or MVA. A local anesthetic is given, the cervix is gradually widened, and the uterus is emptied with the gentle suction of a manual syringe. The procedure is extremely safe and effective. It can be performed from as soon as pregnancy is confirmed up to the tenth week after fertilization. The procedure takes about 10 minutes.

Abortion between the sixth and fourteenth week of pregnancy is carried out by dilation and suction curettage, called D&C or vacuum aspiration. As with MVA, anesthesia is used and the cervix is dilated. The uterus is then emptied with gentle, machine-operated suction. A curette (narrow metal loop) may be used to clean the walls of the uterus.

Dilation and evacuation (D&E) is performed after the fifteenth week of pregnancy. The cervix is dilated and the uterus is emptied with medical instruments, suction, and curettage. After the twentieth week, abortion is very rare.

Nonsurgical methods of abortion are called **medical abortions.** There are two kinds of medical (chemical) abortion, early and late.

Early medical abortion is carried out prior to the seventh or eighth week after fertilization. *Methotrexate* or *mifepristone* (also called *RU 486*) is given to a pregnant woman to block the action of the naturally occurring hormone progesterone, which is essential for successful implantation and pregnancy. Blocking progesterone's actions in the early phases of pregnancy causes a miscarriage. After the progesterone blockers, *misoprostol* (a type of hormone called a *prostaglandin*) is given to induce contractions of the uterus and expel the uterine contents within hours or days.

Early medical abortion can occur as soon as pregnancy is confirmed and is effective up to 63 days after

Global Wellness

Contraceptive Availability Reduces Abortions

The World Health Organization estimates that 125 million women in the world, mostly in developing countries, are not using contraception in spite of the desire to space or limit the number of children they have. The family planning needs of these women are unmet because of poor access to quality health services, limited availability of a variety of contraceptive methods, lack of birth control information, concerns about safety or side effects, and cultural factors such as social, religious, or partner disapproval.

Because so many women lack access to modern contraceptives, about 38% of all pregnancies worldwide are unintended, and about 60% of these result in an induced abortion. Moreover, about 20 million of these abortions are unsafe, that is, carried out by persons lacking the necessary skills or in an environment lacking the minimum medical standards, or both. Lacking quality care, about 80,000 women die of unsafe abortion every year, more than 200 per day.

The mortality rate from abortion is highest among developing nations; for example, 680 women die per 100,000 abortions in Africa, compared with 0.7 per 100,000 in developed regions. Obviously, when women have access to family planning services, the number of women both seeking abortions and dying as a result of them is low.

The World Health Organization and the World Bank estimate that $3.00 per person per year would provide basic family planning and maternal and neonatal health care to women in developing countries. Choosing when to become pregnant (and avoiding abortion) enhances a woman's health and well-being, which, in turn, enhances the health and well-being of her family and community.

---

the last menstrual period. Medical abortion with methotrexate is about 90% effective; with mifepristone (RU 486), between 92% and 95% effective. RU 486 should not be confused with Plan B. RU 486 is used to discontinue a pregnancy. Plan B is used to prevent a pregnancy from occurring.

> Tolerance implies no lack of commitment to one's own beliefs; rather, it condemns the oppression or persecution of others.
>
> *John F. Kennedy*

The procedure is overseen by trained medical personnel in a clinic over the course of a week, after which time a menstrual period occurs, which ends the pregnancy. Methotrexate and misoprostol can cause serious birth defects. The procedure carries a very small risk of toxic shock, which can be fatal (Cohen et al., 2007). If the medical abortion is unsuccessful, a surgical abortion usually follows.

Late medical abortion is carried out after the twelfth week of pregnancy. This method involves infusing saline (salty water), urea, or prostaglandin into the uterus. Saline and urea kill the fetus, and prostaglandin-induced uterine contractions empty the uterus.

Aftereffects of Abortion

Despite the fact that abortion in the United States is legal and that 840,000 American women annually receive them, the decision to terminate a pregnancy voluntarily is rarely an easy one. Most women are ambivalent about abortion, as are many men.

A variety of studies (Bradshaw & Slade, 2003) on women's psychological responses to legal abortion suggests that the time between the confirmation of pregnancy and receiving an abortion is generally emotion-

TERMS

abortion: the expulsion or extraction of the products of conception from the uterus before the embryo or fetus is capable of independent life; abortions may be spontaneous or induced

manual vacuum aspiration: the most common abortion method, in which the uterus is emptied with the gentle suction of a manual syringe

medical abortion: nonsurgical abortion using specific medications to stop pregnancy

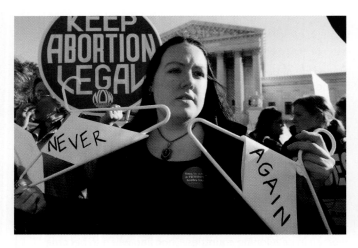

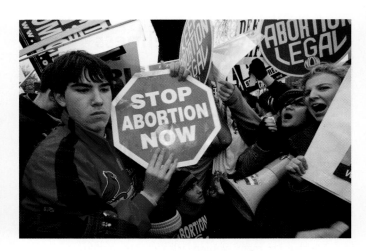

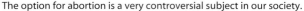

The option for abortion is a very controversial subject in our society.

ally trying, with most women experiencing anxiety and some women also experiencing depression. After the abortion, symptoms of anxiety or depression are less prevalent, although a woman may experience anger or disappointment. The predominant feeling of most women is relief that the abortion had been performed. Several months after their abortion, some women report upsetting feelings about the abortion and some continue to be troubled by the experience or consider it too upsetting to think about (Broen, 2005).

The Legal and Moral Aspects of Abortion

The propriety of abortion as a socially sanctioned method of fertility control has been debated in Western societies for centuries. More than 2,000 years ago, the Greek philosophers Aristotle and Plato recommended abortion, whereas Hippocrates, the founder of modern medicine, forbade it. Throughout the Middle Ages and the Renaissance, abortion was common, although various religious leaders objected to the practice on ethical grounds.

When the U.S. Constitution was ratified, and for several decades after, abortion was legal if it took place before the time of quickening—when a woman could feel fetal movements. Quickening usually occurs near the sixteenth week of pregnancy. The first statutes regulating abortion were enacted in the 1820s in Connecticut and New York. These laws prohibited abortion before the time of quickening, principally to protect women from what by modern standards were primitive and dangerous surgical techniques. By the end of the Civil War, more states had enacted restrictive abortion legislation, not only to preserve the health and life of a preg-

nant woman, but also to encourage American-born women to have children and to discourage nonreproductive sex. By 1900, abortion was illegal in all U.S. jurisdictions, and it remained so for more than 60 years.

Restrictive abortion laws did not stop women from having abortions, however. In the first decades of the twentieth century, millions of women obtained illegal abortions. Those with money could travel to other countries where abortion was legal and performed in a hospital with trained personnel, or they could obtain a clandestine abortion performed by an American physician who accepted the risk of prosecution in return for a high fee. Most women, however, had to obtain abortions from nonmedical people who often performed the procedure using coathangers, spoons, disinfectant, or lye. Many women were maimed or killed by such procedures. The psychological trauma even of successful procedures was enormous. By the 1950s, an estimated 200,000 to 1 million women were getting illegal abortions annually.

By the 1960s, people began to take into account the social and psychological costs of illegal abortion, and on January 22, 1973, the U.S. Supreme Court declared that states could not make laws prohibiting abortion on the ground that they violated a woman's right to privacy, in this case, the right to decide about the outcome of a pregnancy. This decision, known as *Roe v. Wade*, declared (1) that the decision to have an abortion during the first trimester (12 weeks) of pregnancy should be left entirely to the woman and her physician, and (2) during the second trimester, individual states could regulate the abortion procedure for only one purpose—to protect the woman's health.

Many people have mixed feelings about abortion. Because there is no universally accepted scientific definition of when a life begins, some individuals view abortion as murder. Some opponents of abortion believe that its availability encourages irresponsible sexual behavior. Some see abortion as a threat to family life. Even the staunchest proponents of abortion rights would prefer that abortions never occur, but they argue that women must have the right to control their bodies. They believe that abortion is a necessary last resort if contraception fails, if a woman becomes pregnant because of rape or incest, if the child may suffer a serious birth defect, or if the woman's life and health are jeopardized by pregnancy or childbirth.

Critical Thinking About Health

1. "Oh, not again," said a disgusted Janet Haley, chief of research at Leeward Pharmaceuticals, as she waved the hard copy of an e-mail in the air at her group's weekly staff meeting. "Every five years someone gets the bright idea that we need to develop a contraceptive for men. They just don't get it."

   "It could be done, you know," said Richard Duval, one of the company's newest and brightest researchers. "Sure, hormonal methods are no good, but there's lots more we can do with metabolic inhibitors, sperm viability, semen composition . . ."

   "No offense, Richard, but you aren't getting it either. Even if we had a method for men, who'd buy it? Can't you just see a woman asking, "Did you take your pill today, honey?"
   a. Do you agree that developing a contraceptive pill for men would be an unsound business decision? Explain your reasoning.
2. When choosing a method of contraception, a couple decided to base their decision on a method's lowest observed/theoretical failure rate. Explain why it would be better for them to use the typical/actual failure rate.
3. The placard read "Not paying for your playing." Students from the Committee for Fairness took turns holding the placard on the steps of the Student Health Center, talking to anyone who would stop, especially reporters from the campus newspaper and the local TV station. The CFF students were objecting to the fact that contraceptives were available at the Student Health Center. "They're not medicines," they argued. "We don't think our health center fees should pay for sexual partying."
   a. Do you agree or disagree with this point of view?
   b. What are the advantages and disadvantages to any institution or community of making fertility control methods available to anyone who wants them?

Health in Review

- A variety of safe, reliable, and effective fertility control methods is available. These include combination and progestin-only hormonal contraception, barrier methods (condom, diaphragm, cervical cap, and spermicides), fertility awareness methods, the IUD, and sterilization.
- A contraceptive's effectiveness is measured in terms of lowest observed and typical failure rates.
- Although most fertility control methods are designed for use in the woman's body, both partners share the responsibility for fertility control. Communication and cooperation are keys to shared responsibility.
- People who say they do not want to have a baby, yet do not practice fertility control, tend to have low motivation, lack of knowledge of human reproduction and fertility control methods, negative attitudes toward fertility control, or are in relationships that hinder correct fertility control practice.
- Medical and surgical abortions are available.
- Abortion became legal in the United States in 1973 with the Supreme Court's *Roe v. Wade* decision.

Health and Wellness Online

The Web contains a wealth of information about health and wellness. By accessing the Internet using Web browser software, you can gain a new perspective on many topics presented in *Health and Wellness*, Tenth Edition. Access the Jones and Bartlett Publishers Web site at **health.jbpub.com/hwonline**.

References

Bradshaw, Z., & Slade, P. (2003). The effects of induced abortion on emotional experiences and relationships: A critical review of the literature. *Clinical Psychology Reviews, 7,* 929–958.

Broen, A. N., et al. (2005, December 12). The course of mental health after miscarriage and induced abortion: A longitudinal, five-year follow-up study. *BMC Medicine.* Retrieved September 25, 2008, from http://www.biomedcentral.com/1741-7015/3/18

Cohen, A. L., et al. (2007). Toxic shock associated with *Clostridium sordellii* and *Clostridium perfringens* after medical and spontaneous abortion. *Obstetrics & Gynecology, 110,* 1027–1033.

Steinauer, J. (2005). A new era of contraception. *Johns Hopkins Advanced Studies in Medicine, 6,* 285–293.

Trussell, J., & Wynn, L.L. (2008). Reducing unintended pregnancy in the United States. *Contraception, 77,* 1–5.

Wu, J., et al. (2008). Contraceptive nonuse among U.S. women at risk for unplanned pregnancy. *Contraception, 78,* 284–289.

Suggested Readings

Blumenthal, P. D., & Edelman, A. (2008). Hormonal contraception. *Obstetrics & Gynecology, 112,* 670–684. A thorough update of the various forms of hormonal contraception.

Hatcher, R. A., et al. (2008). *Contraceptive technology* (19th ed.). New York: Thompson Reuters. The most comprehensive discussion of contraception and abortion available, written by world-renowned experts in the field.

Trussell, J., & Raymond, E. G. (2008). Emergency contraception. Available: http://ec.princeton.edu/questions/ec-review.pdf. Provides a detailed academic review of the medical and social science literature about emergency contraception.

Recommended Web Sites

Please visit **health.jbpub.com/hwonline** for links to these Web sites.

Birth Control Guide
The U.S. Food and Drug Administration's descriptions of the major birth control methods.

The Emergency Contraception Web site
All about emergency contraception, from Princeton University.

Family Planning Information
Compiled by the Emory University School of Medicine.

Planned Parenthood
All there is to learn about family planning.

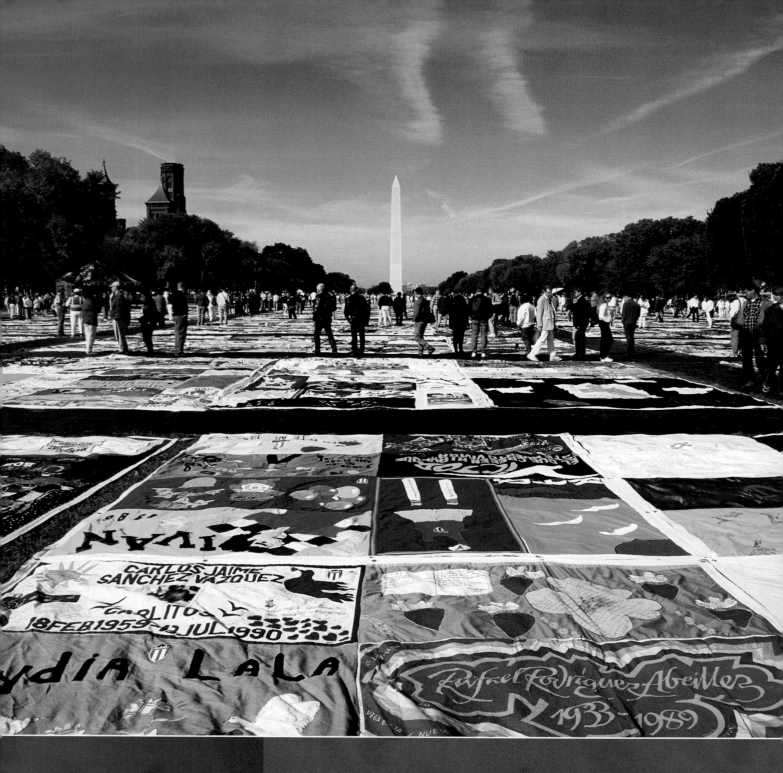

Chapter Eleven

Protecting Against Sexually Transmitted Diseases and AIDS

Learning Objectives

1. Describe the impact of sexually transmitted diseases (STDs) on society.

2. List the risk factors for contracting an STD.

3. Identify the causative agent, symptoms, and treatment for the following diseases: trichomoniasis, chlamydia, gonorrhea, syphilis, genital herpes, genital warts, pubic lice, scabies, and AIDS.

4. Describe the importance of testing for HIV infection and the proper testing procedures.

5. Identify several "safer sex" practices.

6. Describe the importance of effective communication in reducing the risk of STDs and AIDS.

Throughout the world, about 25 different infectious diseases can be passed from person to person through sexual contact; 11 are common in North America (**Table 11.1**). These infections are called **sexually transmitted diseases (STDs)** or sexually transmitted infections (STIs). The World Health Organization estimates that 250 million people in the world acquire an STD each year; in the United States, the number is about 16 million (**Figure 11.1**). About half of these infections occur in people under age 25 (Weinstock, Berman, & Cates, 2004).

> Women need a reason to have sex. Men just need a place.
>
> *Billy Crystal*

Sexually transmitted diseases have been afflicting humans for thousands of years. Ancient Chinese medical writings describe diseases of the genitalia that were probably syphilis. The ancient Egyptians described genital diseases that were probably gonorrhea. Old Testament and Talmudic writings describe a condition called "ziba," which was associated with the emission of fluid, referred to then as "issue," from the nonerect penis or the vagina. "Ziba" was probably gonorrhea, and "issue" was probably the discharge associated with gonorrhea. Many famous historical figures are thought to have had sexually transmitted diseases (**Table 11.2**).

The human and social costs of STDs are enormous. In the United States, the direct and indirect economic costs of the major STDs and their complications total $20 billion a year. The human suffering and economic costs wrought by AIDS are also well known. Less well known are the disappointment and suffering of thou-

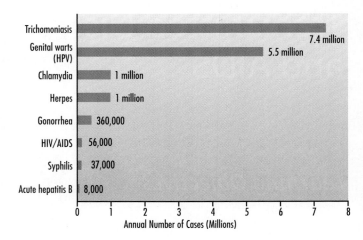

■ Figure 11.1

Estimated Yearly Number of STDs in the United States

Table 11.1

Common Sexually Transmitted Diseases (STDs)

STD	Symtoms	Treatment
HIV/AIDS	Flulike symptoms followed by any of a number of diseases characteristic of immunodeficiency	New drugs may retard viral reproduction temporarily; opportunistic infections can be treated to some degree
Chlamydia	Usually occur within three weeks: Infected men have a discharge from the penis and painful urination; women may have a vaginal discharge, but often are asymptomatic	Antibiotics
Genital warts	Usually occur within one to three months: small, dry growths on the genitals, anus, cervix, and possibly mouth	Podophyllin
Gonorrhea	Usually occur within two weeks: discharge from the penis, vagina, or anus; pain on urination or defecation or during sexual intercourse; pain and swelling in the pelvic region; genital and oral infections may be asymptomatic	Antibiotics
Hepatitis B	Low-grade fever, fatigue, headaches, loss of appetite, nausea, dark urine, jaundice	Rest, proper nutrition; vaccination for hepatitis B
Genital herpes	Usually occur within two weeks: painful blisters on site(s) of infection (genitals, anus, cervix); occasionally itching, painful urination, and fever	None; acyclovir relieves symptoms
Molluscum contagiosum	Smooth, rounded, shiny, whitish growths on the skin of the trunk and anogenital region	Surgical
Pubic lice	Usually occur within five weeks: intense itching in the genital region; lice may be visible in pubic hair; small white eggs may be visible on pubic hair	Gamma benzene hexachloride
Scabies	Tiny, itchy lesions caused by mites burrowing into the skin	Topical insecticides
Syphilis	Usually occur within three weeks: a chancre (painless sore) on the genitals, anus, or mouth; secondary stage, skin rash (if left untreated); tertiary stage includes diseases of several body organs	Antibiotics
Trichomoniasis	Yellowish-green vaginal discharge with an unpleasant odor; vaginal itching; occasionally painful intercourse	Metronidazole

Table 11.2			
Famous People with an STD			
No one knows for sure, but historians say these famous people were infected with an STD.			
Abraham	Job	Dürer	Gauguin
Sarah	King David	Schubert	Boswell
Julius Caesar	Cleopatra	Molière	Goethe
Charlemagne	Napoleon	Van Gogh	Oscar Wilde
Henry VIII	Columbus	Nietzsche	Goya
The Greats: Peter and Catherine			

sands of women who are left infertile after a serious STD-related pelvic infection. Women who acquire a human papillomavirus (HPV) infection (genital warts) are predisposed to cervical cancer. And the million people who acquire genital herpes each year will be potentially infectious for their entire lives.

What Is an STD?

An STD is an infection that is transmitted by sexual behavior. An infection occurs when one or more biological agents inhabit parts of the body they are not supposed to and acquire nutrients from the body so they can survive and reproduce. Human STDs are caused by viruses, bacteria, protozoa, worms, and insects.

STD-causing agents can enter the body (1) through breaks in the skin, (2) through the mucous membranes of the body's orifices—nose and mouth, penis, vagina, urethra, and anus, and (3) the blood, either by injection or during sexual activity, by means of tiny microscopic abrasions on the penis or in the vagina or mouth. Some STD-causing agents enter body cells by attaching to specific sites, called receptors, on a body cell's surface. Once inside the body, the infectious agents reproduce and their population grows in numbers.

In general, STDs are not transferred by air, water, or contact with doorknobs, toilet seats, and other inanimate objects. In the case of insects, however, contact with any surface on which the organisms, their larvae, or eggs might be present may cause an infection.

A certain number of STD-causing agents must be transferred to cause an infection. This number varies according to how well the recipient's body can defend itself and a variety of specific host–parasite factors. For chlamydia and gonorrhea, the transfer of about 1,000 organisms is sufficient to cause an infection, and the risk of becoming infected with one exposure is about 60% to 90% in men and 20% to 35% in women. With syphilis, the requisite number of infecting organisms is about 100.

STD Risk Factors

Several factors increase the risk of contracting an STD. Being aware of these factors can help you decrease your risk of infection and help you to support STD prevention efforts in your community.

Multiple Sexual Partners

About 20% of unmarried adults have more than one sex partner in a year. About 27% of American college students have more than one sexual partner in a year (American College Health Association, 2008). Also, many people in supposed sexually exclusive relationships have sex outside the relationship, generally without the "exclusive" partner's knowledge. Individuals who are unaware that their partners are sexually active with other people have higher rates of STDs than do individuals who do know their partners are sexually active with others (Drumright, Gorbach, & Holmes, 2004).

False Sense of Safety

Using hormonal contraceptives tends to decrease the use of condoms, which help prevent transmission of STDs. The availability of antibiotics makes many people less afraid of sexually transmitted diseases. They erroneously believe that there is a cure for every STD.

Absence of Signs and Symptoms

Some STDs have very mild or no symptoms, so that the infection can worsen and may be unknowingly passed on to others. One study showed that approximately 8% of college students were infected with chlamydia and did not know it. Another 1.5% were infected with gonorrhea and did not know it. People infected with HIV can have mild or no symptoms for years, yet still be infectious.

Untreated Conditions

Some individuals lack sufficient knowledge of the signs and symptoms of STDs to know that they are infected. Those who are not accustomed to seeking health care, or who financially cannot afford it, are less likely to seek treatment for an infection. Furthermore, many individuals with STDs do not comply with treatment regimens. When medications are not taken for the required length of time, an infection may not be completely eradicated even though symptoms may disappear. People who do not complete treatment may still be infectious.

Impaired Judgment

The use of drugs, including alcohol, can increase the risk of transmitting STDs because people with alcohol-impaired judgment are less likely to use condoms. Also,

TERMS

sexually transmitted diseases (STDs): infections passed from person to person by sexual contact

people in a drugged condition may be more likely to have sex with someone they do not know; they may know nothing of their partner's past sexual and drug history.

Lack of Immunity

Some STD-causing organisms, such as HIV and herpesvirus, can escape the body's immune defenses, causing individuals to remain infected and transmit the infection. This may permit reinfection and also makes the development of effective vaccines difficult or impossible (see Chapter 12).

Body Piercing

Piercing of the body, particularly the genitals, increases the risk of transmission of STDs. The wound from piercing gives organisms direct access to the bloodstream, and pierced genitals may impede proper use of condoms. Moreover, people with nipple, tongue, and lip jewelry may have a higher risk of infection via oral sex. People who have their bodies pierced should follow after-care instructions faithfully to prevent infection and should abstain from sexual contact in the pierced region until the hole is completely healed, which takes three to six months.

Value Judgments

Unlike nearly all other kinds of infections, STDs are associated with sinfulness, dirtiness, condemnation, shame, guilt, and disgust. These negative attitudes keep people from getting checkups, contacting partners when an STD has been diagnosed, and talking to new partners about previous exposures. In the nineteenth century, when syphilis was a scourge of Europe, rather than trying to prevent its spread (effective treatments had not yet been invented), countries blamed the disease on the weak character or immorality of their neighbors: The English referred to syphilis as the "French disease," and the French called it the "Spanish disease." Prejudice and scapegoating helped spread the disease.

> If love is the answer, could you please rephrase the question?
>
> *Lily Tomlin*

Denial

With respect to contracting an STD, many people think, "It can't happen to me," or "He is too nice to have an STD," or "She isn't the type of person who would have an STD." Because there are no vaccinations against most of the infectious agents that cause STDs, the only way to prevent them is for sexually active individuals who are not in lifelong single-partner (monogamous) sexual relationships to assume responsibility for protecting themselves and their partners. This means becoming aware of the signs and symptoms of the common STDs and seeking treatment when such signs

occur. It means that sexually active people who have more than one partner within a year should obtain periodic (about every six months) STD checkups. It also means knowing about and practicing "safer sex."

Common STDs

The most common STDs in the United States and Canada can be categorized according to the type of organism causing them (**Table 11.3**). Organisms that cause STDs are viruses, bacteria, protozoa, and insects. The distinction is important medically because there are no cures for viral diseases, whereas there are drugs that can eradicate bacteria, protozoa, and insects from the body.

Trichomoniasis

Although not commonly thought of as sexually transmitted diseases, vaginal infections caused by the protozoan *Trichomonas vaginalis* can be transmitted during intercourse. Symptoms tend to occur only in women (vaginal itching and a cheesy, odorous discharge from the vagina), but the organisms can survive in the urethra of the penis and under the penile foreskin. A man who harbors these organisms can infect other partners or even reinfect the partner who transmitted the organisms to him.

About 7 million new cases of trichomonas are diagnosed each year. Clinically, a diagnosis is made by collecting fluid from the vagina and testing for the presence of *Trichomonas* organisms. Medications are effective in treating these infections. An infected woman's male partner(s) should also undergo treatment.

Table 11.3

Agents That Cause Common STDs

Infectious agent	Disease
Bacteria	
Chlamydia trachomatis	Chlamydia
Neisseria gonorrhoeae	Gonorrhea
Treponema pallidum	Syphilis
Viruses	
Herpes simplex virus, types 1 and 2	Genital herpes
Human papillomavirus	Anogenital warts
Human immunodeficiency virus (HIV)	AIDS
Hepatitis virus B	Hepatitis
Molluscum contagiosum virus	Molluscum contagiosum
Protozoa	
Trichomonas vaginalis	Trichomoniasis (vaginitis)
Insects	
Phthirus pubis	Lice ("crabs")
Sarcoptes scabiei	Mites ("scabies")

Bacterial Vaginosis

The vagina normally contains a variety of bacteria that support a healthy vaginal environment. However, overgrowth of certain types of bacteria (generally *Gardnerella vaginalis*) can cause an infection called **bacterial vaginosis (BV),** which can be sexually transmissible through intercourse. Symptoms of BV include vaginal discharge, which may have a "fishy" smell, particularly after intercourse. Sometimes BV has no symptoms.

Chlamydia

Chlamydia is caused by the microorganism *Chlamydia trachomatis,* which specifically infects certain cells lining the mucous membranes of the genitals, mouth, anus, rectum, the conjunctiva of the eyes, and occasionally the lungs. The chlamydial microorganisms bind to surfaces and induce the host cells to engulf them. After gaining entrance to the cell, these organisms resist a host cell's defenses and eventually "steal" from the host cell the biochemical compounds required for their own survival. The chlamydial organisms use the stolen nutrients to reproduce and multiply, and ultimately the host cell dies.

In the United States and other Western countries, chlamydia is the most commonly reported STD. Each year approximately 1 million Americans contract chlamydia. In as many as one-third of all cases, chlamydia occurs simultaneously with gonorrhea. Newborns also are susceptible to chlamydial infection if their mothers are infected at the time of delivery. The most common complications of chlamydial infection in newborns are conjunctivitis (eye infection) and pneumonia.

One reason that chlamydial infections are so common is that 75% of infected women and 50% of infected men often have extremely mild or no symptoms. Thus, infected individuals can unknowingly transmit the infection to new sex partners. When symptoms do occur, they include pain during urination in both men and women (dysuria) and a whitish discharge from the penis or vagina. Symptoms generally appear within 7 to 21 days after infection.

Chlamydia can be treated with antibiotics. Left untreated, the chlamydial bacteria can multiply and cause inflammation and damage of the reproductive organs in both sexes. In men, untreated chlamydia can result in inflammation of the epididymis (**epididymitis**), characterized by pain, swelling, and tenderness in the scrotum and sometimes by a mild fever. Damage to the tissues in the epididymis can eventually lead to sterility. In women, chlamydial infections affect the cervix, uterus, fallopian tubes, and peritoneum. Often chlamydial infections of the reproductive tract produce no symptoms until the infection is advanced. A woman may then experience chronic pelvic pain, vaginal discharge, intermittent vaginal bleeding, and pain during intercourse. Infection of the fallopian tubes can produce scar tissue that damages the tubes' lining and partially or completely blocks the tubes. These effects may increase the risk of ectopic pregnancy or render a woman infertile; in fact, about 10,000 cases of female infertility per year result from fallopian tube damage from chlamydia.

Chlamydial infections induce an immune response in the host, but for unknown reasons infected individuals do not gain immunity to future chlamydial infections. This means that treated individuals can be reinfected upon exposure to chlamydia.

Gonorrhea

Gonorrhea, also known as "the clap," is caused by the bacterium *Neisseria gonorrhoeae.* Gonorrheal organisms specifically infect the mucous membranes of the body, most often the genitals, reproductive organs, mouth and throat, anus, and eyes. *N. gonorrhoeae* cannot survive on toilet seats, doorknobs, bedsheets, clothes, or towels. Transmission in adults almost always occurs by genital, oral, or anal sexual contact; infection of the eyes occurs by hand (often through self-infection). Each year, hundreds of thousands of American adults are infected with gonorrhea.

Newborn babies exposed to gonorrheal organisms in the mother's birth canal may develop gonorrhea of the eyes. Most states require that antibiotics or a few drops of silver nitrate be put into the eyes of babies immediately after birth to kill the gonorrhea bacteria and prevent possible blindness.

Although the bacteria causing them are different, the symptoms of gonorrheal and chlamydial infections are very similar. Like chlamydia, many people infected with gonorrheal organisms do not develop symptoms and their infections go unnoticed. If the infection progresses, men may develop epididymitis and women may develop infections of the uterus, fallopian tubes, and pelvic region. Such infections may cause sterility. When symptoms appear, they include painful urination in both sexes and a yellowish discharge from the penis or vagina. Occasionally there is pain in the groin, testes,

---

TERMS

bacterial vaginosis (BV): a bacterial infection of the vagina

chlamydia: a sexually transmitted disease caused by the bacterium *Chlamydia trachomatis*

epididymitis: inflammation of the epididymis, a structure that connects the vas deferens and the testes

gonorrhea: sexually transmitted disease caused by gonococcal bacteria (*Neisseria gonorrhoeae*)

or lower abdomen. The first symptoms of gonorrhea usually appear within 7 to 10 days after exposure.

Gonorrhea can be treated with antibiotics. However, new antibiotic-resistant strains of the organism are constantly evolving. In nearly half of all cases of gonorrhea, chlamydia also is present. Individuals undergoing diagnosis for gonorrhea should also be tested for chlamydia.

Syphilis

Syphilis is caused by a spiral-shaped bacterium called *Treponema pallidum*. These organisms are transmitted from person to person through genital, oral, and anal contact, as well as being acquired from infected blood. Syphilis can also be transmitted from a mother to her unborn fetus, perhaps as early as the ninth week of pregnancy.

The first noticeable sign of syphilis is a painless open sore called a **chancre** ("shanker"), which can appear any time between the first week and third month after infection. If the infection is not treated within that period, the chancre will heal and the disease will enter a secondary stage, characterized by a skin rash, hair loss, and the appearance of round, flat-topped growths on most areas of the body. Left untreated, the signs of the secondary stage also disappear, and the infection enters a symptomless (latency) period, during which the syphilis organisms multiply in many other regions of the body. In the final, tertiary stage, the disease eventually damages vital organs, such as the heart or brain, and can cause severe symptoms or death. Syphilis can be treated with antibiotics at any stage of the infection.

Genital Herpes

Herpes infections of the genital region are caused by either of two strains of herpes simplex virus (HSV): HSV-1, which is associated primarily with cold sores on the mouth ("fever blisters"), and HSV-2, associated primarily with lesions on the penis, vagina, or rectum. As many as 50 million American adults have been infected with HSV-1 or HSV-2. Each year up to 1 million American adults acquire a genital herpes infection.

Infections with HSV-2 are often asymptomatic. Indeed, 90% of people infected with HSV-2 do not know it. Nevertheless, they are infectious and may contribute to the spread of the disease by having unprotected sex. If they appear, symptoms of a genital herpes infection are evident within 2 to 20 days after contact with the virus.

The major symptoms of a genital herpes infection are the presence of one or more blisters, which eventually break to become wet, painful sores that last about two or three weeks; fever; and occasionally pain in the lower abdomen. Eventually these initial symptoms disappear, but the herpes virus remains dormant in certain of the body's nerve cells, permitting periodic recurrences

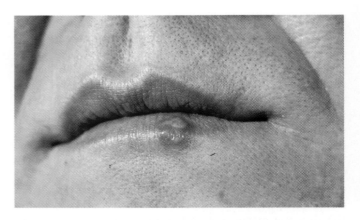

"Cold sores" on the lip or inside the mouth are a common occurrence in people who are infected by the herpes simplex virus. The sores usually heal in a week or so but can flare up again because the viral infection is permanent.

of symptoms at or near the site(s) of the initial infection. It is thought that stress, anxiety, poor nutrition, sunlight, and skin irritation can bring on recurrences.

Recurrences are usually mild and last only about a week. They may be telegraphed by a tingling feeling or itching in the genital area, or pain in the buttocks or down the leg. For some people, these early symptoms can be the most painful and annoying part of an episode. Sometimes, only the tingling and itching are present, and no visible sores develop. At other times, blisters appear that may be very small and barely noticeable, or they may break into open sores that crust over and then disappear. Herpes is extremely contagious when a sore is present. People with open lesions should avoid sex with others until the lesions disappear. Even if no sore is present, transmission is possible, although much less likely, through the "shedding" of virus particles from the skin.

Whereas genital herpes infections are caused most frequently by HSV-2 and oral herpes infections are caused most frequently by HSV-1, both HSV-2 and HSV-1 can cause genital and oral infections with identical symptoms. Thus, people with oral herpes can transmit the infection to partners via oral sex. They can also transmit it to themselves through masturbation. Occasionally, sores also appear on other parts of the body where the virus has entered through broken skin.

Herpes simplex also can infect the eyes, leading to impaired vision and even blindness. If the virus is present in the birth canal, newborn babies can be infected, often resulting in brain damage and abnormal development. In the United States, about 500 babies are born each year with herpes, and two-thirds of infected babies who are not treated die. Pregnant women who have had a prior genital herpes infection should tell their physicians to prevent transmission of HSV to their babies.

There is no cure for herpes, and individuals remain infected for life. Drugs such as acyclovir can minimize

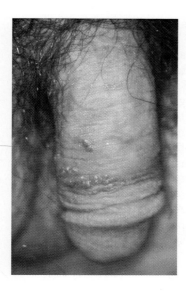

Genital warts on the penis are caused by infection of the skin by papilloma viruses. Genital warts can be removed by a variety of treatments but sometimes recur.

the duration and severity of the symptoms of an initial infection or a recurrence.

Human Papillomavirus and Anogenital Warts

Human papillomaviruses (HPV) are a group of more than 100 types of viruses, about 30 of which can be passed from person to person through sexual contact. About 5.5 million Americans are infected with HPV each year through sexual activity. The prevalence of HPV infection among all American women aged 14 to 59 is 27%; the prevalence among women aged 14 to 19 is about 44% (Dunne et al., 2007). The majority of HPV infections are symptomless and go away on their own. However, persistent infections with one or more of 10 types of HPV can cause cervical cancer in women.

Some types of HPV may cause visible warts (*Condylomata acuminata*) on or around the genitals or anus within three months of contact with an infected person. Other types of HPV do not cause visible **anogenital warts,** although they infect the vagina, cervix, penis, and the mouth and larynx (as a result of oral sex with an infected person). The types of HPV that cause visible warts on hands and feet are different from those that cause growths in the genital region.

Visible anogenital warts usually are raised or flat, single or multiple, small or large, sometimes cauliflower shaped, soft, moist, pink, or flesh-colored swellings. They can appear on the vulva, in or around the vagina or anus, on the cervix, and on the penis, scrotum, groin, or thigh. The warts are contagious. Anogenital warts can be removed by self-applied medications (imiquimod cream, podophyllin or podofilox solutions). Also, they can be removed by a health care provider. Clinician-applied treatments include applying 10% to 25% podophyllum resin, trichloroacetic acid, or bichloroacetic acid; physically excising the wart; cryosurgery (freezing), electrocautery (burning), or exposure to laser. Treatments remove the warts but not HPV in cells, so warts can reap-

pear after treatment. Without treatment, warts may disappear or they may grow more numerous, or larger.

Many genital HPV infections do not cause visible warts. The virus lives in the skin or mucous membranes and usually causes no symptoms. A health practitioner can detect invisible infections in either of several ways: (1) applying vinegar (acetic acid) to suspected infected regions and looking for infected cells to whiten; (2) viewing the vagina and cervix with a magnifying instrument (culposcopy); (3) removing a small amount of tissue (biopsy) for analysis of HPV DNA, and (4) performing a Pap smear to look for abnormalities in cervical cells associated with HPV infection.

High-risk HPV infections are invisible; they are associated with cancer of the cervix, vulva, vagina, anus, penis, or larynx. Low-risk HPV infections cause visible warts and may cause minor Pap test abnormalities, but not cancer. Because the Pap smear is such a common procedure, cervical cancer has decreased. Nevertheless, about 11,000 American women develop cervical cancer each year; about 4,000 die each year of the disease.

The types of HPV that infect the genital area are spread primarily through genital contact. Because most HPV infections have no signs or symptoms, most infected persons are unaware they are infected, yet they can transmit the virus to a sex partner. Rarely, a pregnant woman can pass HPV to her baby during vaginal delivery.

There is a vaccine against two types of HPV that cause about 70% of cervical cancers and two types of HPV that cause about 90% of genital warts. The vaccine is given in a series of three injections over a six-month period. The vaccine is highly effective in preventing HPV infection in young women who have not yet been exposed to HPV. Indeed, it is recommended that all young women be vaccinated against HPV before they reach the age at which they are likely to become sexually active. Other ways to prevent HPV infection are to

TERMS

anogenital warts: hard growths caused by an infection with human papillomavirus (HPV) that appears on the skin of the genitals or anus

chancre: the primary lesion of syphilis, which appears as a hard, painless sore or ulcer, often on the penis or vaginal tissue

herpes: sexually transmitted disease caused by herpes simplex virus (HSV)

human papillomavirus (HPV): a genus of viruses including those causing papillomas (small nipplelike protrusions of the skin or mucous membrane) and warts

syphilis: a sexually transmitted disease caused by spirochete bacteria (*Treponema pallidum*)

avoid skin-to-skin contact with an infected person, avoid sexual contact if warts are visible, and male use of latex condoms.

Hepatitis B

Hepatitis B is a disease of the liver caused by infection by hepatitis B virus (HBV), one of several types of hepatitis viruses (see Chapter 12). Compared with other hepatitis viruses, which tend to be transmitted in fecally contaminated food, HBV is transmitted sexually and by blood, in a manner similar to HIV, the AIDS virus. Hepatitis B virus is sexually transmitted 100 times more effectively than HIV.

The symptoms of hepatitis B infection include low-grade fever, tiredness, headaches, loss of appetite, nausea, dark urine, and jaundice (i.e., yellowing of the white of the eyes and the skin). The first symptoms, which are flulike, tend to occur 14 to 100 days after infection. Signs of liver disease (e.g., dark urine, jaundice) appear later. No specific therapy exists for HBV infection. Rest, proper nutrition, and avoidance of substances harmful to the liver (e.g., alcohol and drugs) are required for recovery, which may take many months. Long-term liver damage is possible, including liver cancer and death.

> Sex is like air . . .
> It's not important
> unless you aren't
> getting any.
> *Anonymous*

A vaccine against HBV exists and everyone is advised to be vaccinated, especially children, health workers, and others who are at high risk of exposure (see Chapter 12).

Molluscum Contagiosum

Molluscum contagiosum is caused by a virus of the same name. Fewer than 100,000 infections occur in the United States each year. The infection is characterized by the appearance of freckle-sized, smooth, rounded, shiny, whitish growths on the skin of the trunk and anogenital region. Generally, there are no associated symptoms. The lesions may resolve spontaneously, but it is best to have them removed by a health care provider; otherwise, they may be transmitted to others or reoccur.

Pubic Lice

Pubic lice (*Phthirus pubis*), also known as "crabs," are barely visible insects that live on hair shafts primarily in the genital-rectal region and occasionally on hair in the armpits, beard, and eyelashes. The organisms' claws are specifically adapted for grasping hairs with the diameter of pubic and axillary hair, which differs in diameter from the shafts of scalp hair. Thus, pubic lice are not usually found on the head. (Scalp hair is the ecological niche of the head louse, *Pediculus humanus capitis*.)

Lice feed on blood taken from tiny blood vessels in the skin, which they pierce with their mouth. Some people are sensitive to the bites and may experience itching, which is often the main symptom of infestation. The lice can also be seen; they look like small freckles. The eggs of lice are enclosed in small white pods (called nits), which attach to hair shafts. The presence of nits is also a sign of infestation.

Transfer of lice is through physical—usually sexual—contact. They can also be transmitted through contact with objects on which eggs might have been laid, such as towels, bed linens, and clothes. An infestation of pubic lice can be eliminated by washing the pubic hair with liquids or shampoos containing agents that specifically kill lice (e.g., pyrethrins, piperonyl butoxide, and gamma benzene hydrochloride). All of an infected person's clothes, towels, and bed linens should also be washed with cleaning agents made specifically for killing lice.

Scabies

Scabies is an infestation of certain regions of the skin by extremely small (invisible to the naked eye) mites, *Sarcoptes scabiei*. The mites burrow into the skin, where they live and lay eggs. The tiny lesions produced by the mites often cause intense itching, which is the major sign of a scabies infection. The mites produce tiny burrows across skin lines, which often go unnoticed. Occasionally, an infestation will produce small round nodules. The mites tend to live in the webs between the fingers, on the sides of fingers, and on the wrists, elbows, breasts, abdomen, penis, and buttocks. Rarely do mites live on the face, neck, upper back, palms, and soles.

Scabies can be transmitted both sexually and nonsexually. All that is required is close personal contact. The itching and physical symptoms often take several weeks to appear. Scabies can be treated with topical agents that kill the mites and their eggs.

Acquired Immune Deficiency Syndrome (AIDS)

AIDS is caused by **human immunodeficiency virus,** or **HIV** (see Chapter 12). HIV infection causes disease by destroying immune system cells and weakening the body's immune system. Destruction of the body's immune system makes HIV-infected individuals susceptible to a variety of bacterial, viral, and fungal infections that a person with an intact immune system could readily ward off. HIV infection in the brain leads to loss of mental faculties (AIDS dementia).

HIV is mainly transmitted by blood, semen, or vaginal fluids of infected people (Table 11.4). When individuals become infected with HIV, their immune systems are still intact and they produce copious antibodies to HIV. The mounting of an immune response in the early phases of an HIV infection provides the basis for HIV testing. Nearly all of the tests for HIV infection detect antibodies to HIV. A positive result (seropositive) indicates that a person has been exposed to sufficient quantities of HIV particles to mount an immune response. Some tests measure the RNA or DNA of HIV itself. This test is used to screen blood supplies and the

⊕ Global Wellness

HIV/AIDS Covers the Globe

Since the worldwide HIV/AIDS pandemic began in the early 1980s, the prevalence of HIV/AIDS has increased dramatically such that, in 2007, 33.2 million people in the world are living with HIV (see accompanying figure); and 25 million people have died of AIDS. During the first quarter century of the pandemic, HIV/AIDS hit hardest in sub-Saharan Africa, where 75% of all people with HIV/AIDS lived. Since 2000, the number of HIV infections outside of Africa began a dramatic increase, particularly in Asia. In 2007, nearly 5 million people in Asia were living with HIV. India has nearly 2.5 million people with HIV, and China nearly 800,000. Without a vaccine and an all-out worldwide education/prevention effort to control it, it is estimated that by 2012 the number of people worldwide with HIV/AIDS will exceed 50 million.

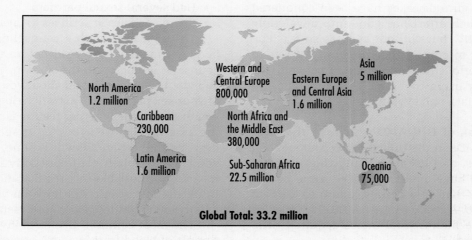

North America
1.2 million

Caribbean
230,000

Latin America
1.6 million

Western and
Central Europe
800,000

North Africa and
the Middle East
380,000

Sub-Saharan Africa
22.5 million

Eastern Europe
and Central Asia
1.6 million

Asia
5 million

Oceania
75,000

Global Total: 33.2 million

Source: Data from AIDS Epidemic Update, UNAIDS, 2007. Available: http://www.unaids.org.

Table 11.4

The Risk of HIV Infection from One Episode of Contact with an HIV-Positive Person

Type of contact	Risk (%)
Needle sharing	0.67
Occupational needlestick	0.30
Receptive anal intercourse	0.1–5.0
Receptive vaginal intercourse	0.1–0.2
Insertive vaginal intercourse	0.03–0.14
Insertive anal intercourse	0.06 or less
Receptive oral male intercourse	0.06 or less
Insertive oral male intercourse	Rare case reports
Female–female oral-genital contact	Rare case reports

Source: Modified from A. Harvey and R. H. Goldschmidt. (2005). HIV testing on demand. *American Family Physician, 71,* 1823–1825.

signs of AIDS are usually mononucleosis-like symptoms (e.g., swollen lymph glands, fever, night sweats) and possibly headaches and impaired mental functioning caused by HIV infection of the brain. As the disease progresses, individuals most often suffer weight loss, infections on the skin (shingles) or in the throat (thrush), one or more opportunistic infections, and cancer.

Because there is no way to rid the body of HIV and hence cure AIDS, treatment of the disease relies on (1) medically managing the opportunistic infections that result from immune suppression, and (2) attempting to suppress HIV infection within the affected

level of HIV in an infected individual (called the *viral load*).

An HIV-infected individual may not manifest symptoms of AIDS for as many as 15 or 20 years after the initial infection. During this latency period, the infected person is contagious and can spread the infection to others, even though she or he is symptomless. The first

TERMS

human immunodeficiency virus (HIV): the virus that causes AIDS; it causes a defect in the body's immune system by invading and then multiplying within certain white blood cells

pubic lice: small insects that live primarily in hair in the genital and rectal regions

scabies: infestation of the skin by microscopic mites (insects)

person's body. Treating HIV infection involves administering combinations of different drugs, but unfortunately, the combination therapies are not a cure and not all HIV-infected individuals respond. Also, because the drugs only suppress HIV, even those who do respond must take the drugs for life lest the virus begin multiplying again. Because HIV mutates rapidly, in many cases drug resistance develops. Finally, combination drug treatments cost about $10,000 per person per year, so they are unavailable for the economically disadvantaged, who make up 90% of the more than 45 million HIV-infected people in the world.

Because many viral diseases have been conquered by vaccination, much effort has gone into developing vaccines against HIV, but without success so far. The only effective way to control the spread of AIDS is to prevent the transfer of HIV from person to person. This is accomplished by using condoms, reducing exposure to infected individuals, and avoiding casual sex.

Reducing the Risk of HIV/AIDS Because the first reported cases of AIDS in the United States were among male homosexuals, and because many thousands of men in that group have died from AIDS, some people mistakenly believe that only homosexual men can get AIDS. This is not so. Anyone can get AIDS. The reasons that so many male homosexual males acquired AIDS include the following:

- Without knowledge of the infectious agent HIV, it was impossible to take precautions.
- In the late 1970s and early 1980s, sexual mores among young people, including male homosexuals, permitted multiple sexual partners, affording HIV rapid access to a large population.
- Anal intercourse provides HIV a highly efficient route of infection because microscopic tears in the rectum give the virus access to the recipient's blood. Microscopic tears in the penis also allow blood transmission, and blood in semen provides a further avenue of infection.

After it was determined that HIV caused AIDS, and once strategies were developed to stop its transmission, the frequency of new HIV infections among homosexual males declined dramatically. This decline demonstrated that educational efforts and motivation can prevent the transmission of HIV/AIDS and other STDs. Although AIDS is still a threat to male homosexuals, the majority of new cases of AIDS in the United States are among injection drug users who share their drug paraphernalia (needles and syringes) with others, and persons who engage in sexual intercourse with these individuals. Worldwide, most of the transmission of HIV/AIDS is through heterosexual intercourse. This being the case, researchers have found that adult males who undergo circumcision are much less likely to contract HIV/AIDS than are uncircumcised males (Cohen, 2005).

Testing for HIV Infection Health officials do not advocate that everyone be tested for HIV infection. But certainly those who suspect that they have been exposed to the virus are candidates for testing. These individuals include males who have had unprotected sex with other males and anyone who has

- Had unprotected sex with someone who is known or suspected to be infected with HIV
- Had a sexually transmitted disease
- Had unprotected sex with someone while drunk
- Had sex with someone whose AIDS-risky behaviors are unknown
- Had several sexual partners
- Shared needles or syringes to inject drugs of any kind

Testing begins with a counseling session. You will be given materials to read before the session with a counselor or doctor. In the session, you'll be asked why you want to be tested and about your behavior and that of your sex partner(s). This will help your counselor and you to determine whether testing is appropriate. If testing is appropriate, your counselor or doctor will describe the test and how it is done, provide basic AIDS education, explain confidentiality issues, discuss the meaning of possible test results and what impact you think the test result will have on you, and talk about whom you might tell about your result.

The most common HIV tests involve taking a small sample of blood from the arm or a drop of blood from a finger-stick. Less common are urine and oral-fluid tests. The blood, urine, or oral fluid is sent to a laboratory, where it is analyzed for antibodies to HIV. Commonly, the results are returned in a week or two. A rapid HIV test, which produces a result in 5 to 30 minutes, is also available. When your result is available, you will be asked to return to the counseling and testing center to receive the information. This is true for everyone tested regardless of the results.

Consumers should be wary of at-home HIV test kits. Most test kits advertised and sold over the Internet are faulty. The kits show a negative test result on samples that would test positive for HIV by standard methods. Using one of these kits could give a person the false impression that he or she is not infected. At-home *collection* kits are less error-prone. The sample is collected in private at home and sent to a lab that does the analysis and returns the results. Reliable at-home HIV testing kits are in development. Check the FDA Web site (http://www.fda.gov/oashi/aids/test.html) for up-to-date information on at-home test kits.

HIV tests can be obtained from physicians and a variety of health agencies. There are two kinds of HIV testing: anonymous and confidential. In the anonymous system, individuals are identified only by a self-selected number or alias, so the true identity is never recorded. In the confidential system, one's name is part of the medical record, which is supposed to be confidential. At-home HIV tests are also available. These require

Managing Stress

Why It Is Vital to Stay HIV Free

It's hard for me to remember the seemingly carefree life that I led in Los Angeles, San Francisco, and New York City before my AIDS diagnosis. It's been so long that I can barely remember what it felt like. I don't wish for anyone to have to lose that feeling. I take 37 pills every day: 14 drugs with breakfast, 9 vitamins and herbs with lunch (to help counteract and balance the drugs), and 14 more drugs with dinner. Doing this leads, of course, to the dreadful bouts of diarrhea, irritability, nausea, and fatigue that

accompany these medications and take place at times, it seems, without any rhyme or reason. Yet I take them religiously because they appear to enhance the quality of my life, but not without paying a price: the constant anxiety and doubt that goes along with swallowing toxic chemicals that no one really knows for sure what the long-term physical and mental effects may be. I don't wish this on anyone either.

Mark W. Baker
Provincetown Positive (newsletter)
Fall/Winter, 1997

---

individuals to collect a drop or two of blood from a finger-stick and mail the sample to a laboratory for analysis and follow-up telephone counseling.

Before HIV tests became available, thousands of people were inadvertently infected with HIV as a result of receiving HIV-tainted products derived from blood or blood transfusions (for example, tennis star Arthur Ashe). In the 1980s thousands of people with **hemophilia** (a hereditary blood disease) received clotting factor derived from pooled blood that was contaminated with HIV, and many have since been stricken with AIDS. In France, a national scandal erupted when it was learned that French health officials knowingly continued to allow hemophiliacs to receive contaminated blood products. All clotting factor products used today are manufactured by biotechnology companies and are free of viral contamination. In addition, all blood donations in the United States today are tested for HIV and other viral contamination. However, new strains of HIV continually arise, and tests are not available for all of them. For any elective surgery, patients often are advised to donate their own blood beforehand should a transfusion be required.

Reducing the STD Epidemic in the United States

STDs are an ongoing major health problem for both individuals and for all countries, including the United States. Recognizing this, the U.S. government made reducing the prevalence of STDs a major goal in Healthy People 2010. However, except for syphilis, that goal is not being met (**Table 11.5**).

The STDs of greatest concern are chlamydia and gonorrhea because they affect millions of Americans and are treatable with antibiotics. Current medical practice calls for treatment of people who seek treatment. These patients are instructed to tell their sexual partners about the infection and to encourage them to seek treatment also. This advice is rarely followed. So, for every person who is treated, many others go

untreated and continue to pass the infection to others (Erbelding & Zenilman, 2005).

An approach that appears to be more successful involves having the person undergoing treatment distribute antibiotics to known sexual partners so they can treat themselves anonymously. Public health officials hope this approach will reduce the rate of transmission of the more common, treatable STDs.

If the goal of reducing STDs in the United States is to be accomplished, all sexually active individuals need to practice safer sex and take all possible measures to avoid contracting an STD. Equally important is to avoid transmitting infections to others.

Preventing STDs

Preventing STDs requires that societies provide continuous, widespread public health programs and services for STD education and treatment. It is also crucial that infected individuals seek prompt treatment, take responsibility for not infecting other individuals, and practice safer sex to lower their risk of infection.

The stigma associated with STDs is a great hindrance to prevention efforts. Thinking about STDs in moral terms, that is, associating them with dirtiness and immorality, makes people reluctant to think and talk about them. It also makes society want to ignore STD epidemics. During World Wars I and II, American society supported massive gonorrhea and syphilis control programs; as a result, the incidence of these infections dropped tremendously. When the threat of a postwar STD epidemic seemed to wane, moralistic concerns thwarted the continuation of control efforts, and the

---

TERMS

hemophilia: a hereditary disease (primarily in men) caused by lack of an essential blood clotting factor; results in excessive bleeding in response to any scratch or injury

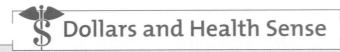

Dollars and Health Sense

Money Needed to Fight HIV/AIDS

More than 32 million people in the world have HIV/AIDS, and the number of cases is expected to climb to 50 million by 2012. Since the beginning of the worldwide epidemic nearly 40 years ago, more than 25 million people have died from AIDS.

About 95% of people with HIV/AIDS live in developing countries, where poverty is endemic and health care systems are inadequate. The World Health Organization states that HIV/AIDS will continue to be a serious international issue for the foreseeable future (UNAIDS, 2005).

In 2007, the world spent $10 billion for HIV/AIDS prevention and health care, principally anti-AIDs drugs; the United Nations estimated that $18 billion was needed. It is estimated that $50 billion will be needed by 2010. In 2008, the United States and Canada combined contributed more than

$6 billion for anti-HIV/AIDS programs in developing countries, and higher contributions have been pledged, not only for humanitarian reasons, but also for economic, security, and health ones.

The World Bank estimates per capita economic growth declines in poor countries hardest hit by HIV/AIDS. That's because when a poor country loses a large percentage of its young and middle-aged adult population to AIDS, there are not enough people to do the work of the country so it can advance economically. Also, when a poor country's meager financial resources are devoted to dealing with HIV/AIDS, insufficient money is available to build schools, roads, electricity generating plants, and other necessary infrastructure. So, all efforts to combat the spread of HIV/AIDS are important in helping to attain world peace and prosperity.

Table 11.5

Healthy People 2010 Sexually Transmitted Diseases Objective Status

HP 2010 objectives	Baseline year	Baseline	2000	2001	2002	2003	2004	2005	2006	HP 2010 target
Reduce the proportion of adolescents and young adults with *Chlamydia trachomatis* infections										
Females aged 15 to 24 years attending STD clinics	1997	12.2%	13.5%	13.3%	13.5%	14.1%	15.3%	15.4%	14.8%	3.0%
Males aged 15 to 24 years attending STD clinics	1997	15.7%	16.4%	17.0%	17.5%	19.3%	20.8%	20.5%	20.8%	3.0%
Reduce gonorrhea (cases per 100,000 population)	1997	123.0	128.7	126.8	122.0	116.2	112.4	114.6	120.9	19.0
Eliminate sustained domestic transmission of primary and secondary syphilis (cases per 100,000 population)	1997	3.2	2.1	2.1	2.4	2.5	NA	NA	NA	0.2
Reduce the proportion of adults aged 20 to 29 years with genital herpes infection	1988–94	17.0%	NA	NA	NA	NA	NA	NA	NA	14.0%
Reduce the proportion of females aged 15 to 44 years who have ever required treatment for pelvic inflammatory disease (PID)	1995	8.0%	NA	NA	NA	NA	NA	NA	NA	5.0%
Reduce the proportion of childless females with fertility problems who have had a sexually transmitted disease or who have required treatment for pelvic inflammatory disease (PID)	1995	27.0	NA	NA	NA	NA	NA	NA	NA	15.0%
Reduce congenital syphilis (cases per 100,000 live births)	1997	27.0	14.2	12.4	11.3	10.3	9.1	8.2	8.5	1.0

Source: U.S. Centers for Disease Control and Prevention, http://www.cdc.gov/std/stats01/2001AppHealthy2010.htm.

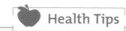 Health Tips

Condom Sense

Latex condoms are effective in preventing the transfer of organisms that cause HIV/AIDs and other STDs. Natural or skin condoms, which are somewhat effective as contraceptives, are too porous to block the transmission of infectious agents. The U.S. Food and Drug Administration tests both domestic and international condoms for cracks and other defects in the rubber, leaks, and resistance to breakage. Tested and approved European condoms carry the CE Mark; in the United Kingdom, approval is indicated with the Kitemark. Elsewhere in the world, condoms are also ISO approved.

Putting on a Male Condom

- Use a fresh condom to lessen the possibility of leakage or breakage. Condoms that have been in a wallet, purse, drawer, or auto glove compartment may have been weakened by the heat. Store condoms in a cool, dry place. Don't use a condom past its expiration date.
- Take the condom out of its package carefully so as not to damage it (no teeth, no fingernails). If there are holes or breaks, or if it's sticky or brittle, toss it out and use another.
- Put the condom on the erect penis before intercourse begins (see figure). Interrupting intercourse to put on a condom increases the chances of pregnancy and HIV transmission because the man might not be able to control ejaculation. Also, putting on the condom at the beginning offers the best protection against skin-to-skin transmission of STDs.
- Unroll the condom onto the erect penis (pull back the foreskin). Leave about one-half inch at the tip to catch semen. Some condoms have specially designed (reservoir) tips for semen collection. The tip of the condom should be pressed free of air to prevent breakage after ejaculation.
- Do not use Vaseline or mineral oil as a lubricant. They will destroy the latex. If a lubricant is desired, use a water-based lubricant such as K-Y Jelly or Astroglide.
- After ejaculation, withdraw the penis before it becomes soft. Otherwise, the condom might slip off. When removing the penis, hold the condom on the penis to be sure it does not slip off.

- Check the condom for holes or breaks. If any appear, spermicidal foam or jelly should be put into the vagina immediately, and possible emergency contraception ("the morning-after pill") should be sought.
- Condoms should be used only once and then discarded.

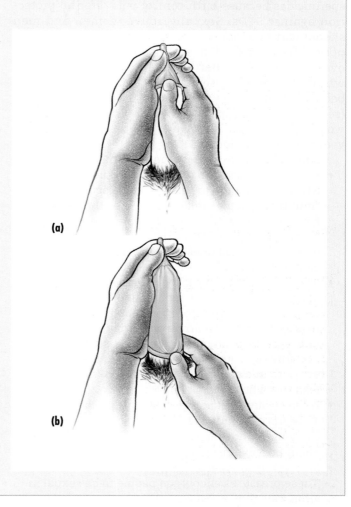

(a)

(b)

---

incidence of STDs increased. Public health officials realize that ongoing efforts are the only way to control STDs.

Judgmental attitudes also make talking about STDs difficult. To have to tell a partner that you have an STD, or even to say that you once had an infection and are now perfectly okay, can bring feelings of guilt and shame, which can lead to the avoidance of discussion altogether. Similarly, to ask about a partner's previous STDs may be interpreted as an accusation that the person is "loose" or immoral. To avoid feeling embarrassed or risk offending a sexual partner, people are likely to avoid the topic of STDs. Prevention would be enhanced if sexually active individuals developed an open atti-

tude about talking about STDs (and other aspects of sex) and acquired the necessary communication skills.

Practicing Safer Sex

The surest way to reduce the risk of acquiring a sexually transmitted disease is to abstain from sexual intercourse. This does not mean that one has to give up sexual interaction. There are many ways of giving and receiving sexual pleasure without engaging in sexual intercourse: touching, kissing, exchanging a massage, even sleeping together without intercourse.

Another way to reduce risk is to know a partner's sexual history, including all high-risk activities in which a partner may have engaged. Often this kind of information is difficult to gain early in a relationship because exchanging information about sexual histories requires a certain level of trust, which takes some time to develop.

Until you have this knowledge, it is essential to protect yourself by using condoms together with spermicides when having sex. Women and men who are sexually active should come to accept as standard practice with new partners the use of condoms together with spermicides because birth control pills offer no protection against STDs. Sexually active women and men should carry condoms and spermicides whenever the possibility of sex exists and use them. This requires overcoming the gender role stereotypes that women who admit to being sexual are "sluts" and men who behave the same way are "studs." The female condom (see Chapter 10), a polyurethane plastic sheath that a woman inserts into her vagina, has been shown to prevent the transmission of STDs.

Some barriers to safer sex include the following:

- *Denying that there is a risk.* Many people assume that STDs happen only to "dirty," "promiscuous," and "immoral" people, and because they themselves have sex only with people who are "clean" and "nice," getting an STD is impossible. Another form of denial is to tell oneself, "I eat right. I exercise. I can't get an STD."
- *Believing that the campus community is insulated from STDs.* The truth is that about half of college students are sexually active before they enter college. As a result, students can arrive on campus with an infection. Also, on many campuses, students in the same living groups and student organizations have sex with one another. One infected person could lead to a whole chain of infections.
- *Feeling guilty and uncomfortable about being sexual.* This prevents individuals from planning sex and carrying condoms and spermicides, and talking about possible risks with new partners.
- *Succumbing to social and peer pressure to be sexual.* These pressures encourage people to be sexual in situations that are potentially risky, such as one-night stands and brief relationships that are sexual virtually from the beginning. The risk of infection is lessened when individuals resist peer pressure to have sex with a relative stranger, and ask themselves instead, "Is this the right relationship?"

"Is this the right partner?" "Am I going to feel OK about this afterward?"

Effective Communication Skills

The pressure to be sexual early in a relationship, before the partners know each other well enough to talk about their past sexual experiences, may force partners to deny there may be a risk. A less risky strategy would be to postpone sexual interaction by saying, "I'd like to be close to you, but I'm not ready to have sex until we get to know each other better." "Not yet" and "maybe" are options when weighing an invitation to be sexual.

Even if a person is ready to talk about the sexual aspects of a new relationship, including birth control and possible exposure to STDs, it can be difficult because of fear of being rejected, offending the partner, or just spoiling the mood. Disclosing one's discomfort about talking about the subject is one way to relieve anxiety about it. A conversation could begin with one partner saying, "There's something I want us to talk about and I feel sort of uncomfortable about it, but I think it's important to both of us, so here goes."

After that introduction, the individual can offer information by saying something like, "We don't know each other very well; I'm concerned about sexual diseases. I want you to know this about me." That person should offer all of the information that he or she would like to be told. After hearing the disclosure, the other person is more likely to respond in kind. And if more information is desired, one could say something like, "Thanks for telling me all of that. I'd feel more comfortable if I knew a little more about . . . " whatever it is.

What if the other person gets offended or won't talk about this subject? Or what if the other person can't be trusted? If partners cannot discuss something as serious as STDs, it is prudent to postpone sexual interaction until the relationship has progressed to a greater level of trust. Potential sexual partners should remember that being under the influence of alcohol or other drugs can affect judgment in making decisions about what is and is not safe. Also, being drunk or stoned can impair using condoms effectively—or using them at all!

Safer sex does not mean no sex. It does not mean that sex is dangerous. It does not mean that sex cannot be fun. It does mean that sex is cooperative. It means that partners are making choices together.

Critical Thinking About Health

1. Research has consistently shown that a vast majority of college students know a lot about STDs and AIDS, and yet only 50% of students whose behavior puts them at risk for acquiring an STD or AIDS practice safer sex techniques. To many observers, such risk taking seems illogical, not to mention dangerous. One could postulate, however, that college students are behaving rationally (from their point of view) when they do not practice safer sex.
   a. Looking at your behavior and the attitudes of those of the people in your peer group, can you explain why some college students do not protect themselves from STDs and HIV?
   b. From your knowledge of your peer group's attitudes, how would you advise your college's administration to lessen the risk of STDs and HIV among its students?

2. From their first moments together it was obvious that Ilana and Jason were going to make a great couple. Every one of their friends said so. Yet Jason was troubled. Although they had agreed not to have sexual intercourse before marriage, as their intimacy deepened, Ilana felt obliged to tell him of the genital herpes infection she acquired when she was a wild 15-year-old. "I'm not that person anymore," she said, "and it's under control. Still, you never get rid of it."
   a. Do you think Jason should proceed in this relationship with Ilana?
   b. What factors should he consider in making his decision?

3. The monthly meeting of the Washington County School Board had never had so many attendees as the night of the vote on the new health curriculum for the county's middle schools. It seemed that everyone in the county had an opinion and was prepared to voice it to the seven board members. At issue was revising the module on sexual infections and HIV to include *how* such infections were actually transmitted. Some parents objected to including any discussion of STDs and HIV in the health curriculum, arguing that doing so only makes the students curious about sex and drugs and encourages experimentation. A second group of parents, while supporting a discussion of the diseases and the organisms that cause them, nevertheless objected to any discussion of behaviors involved in their transmission. They believed that the children ought to know about the biological aspects of the issue as a foundation for their own efforts at dissuading their children from any experimentation with unsafe sexual practices and experimentation with drugs. A third group of parents argued that the only way to ensure prevention was to discuss the behaviors involved. They claimed that the children would not take the discussion seriously unless all aspects of the issue were covered, and hence would be tempted either to disregard the information altogether or to become curious about what was not covered and put themselves at risk. If you were one of the school board members, how would you vote and how would you justify your vote to the parents in your district?

4. Because she had consistently voted to support research on HIV and AIDS, it shocked many people when Congresswoman Harmas refused to vote for the $7.8 billion appropriations bill to pay for protease inhibitor medicines for the medically indigent with AIDS in both the United States and around the world. "I have total compassion for these people," said Harmas, "but at $10,000 a year, we cannot afford to take care of everyone who is sick. Furthermore, in our country, most of the money will go to treating injection drug users, who ought to know better than to get the disease in the first place. And for all the poverty-stricken sick people, principally in Asia and Africa, all I can say is I'm sorry, complain to your own government. We're broke." Do you agree or disagree with the congresswoman's position?

Health in Review

- Sexually transmitted diseases are infections passed from person to person, most frequently by sexual contact.
- Millions of sexually transmitted infections occur each year in the United States.
- STDs are epidemic in the United States because people are uninformed about them, because they engage in high-risk behaviors, and because vaccines and cures (for several) are unavailable.
- The most common STDs in the United States are trichomoniasis, chlamydia, gonorrhea, syphilis, herpes, genital warts, pubic lice, and AIDS.
- Preventing STDs involves supporting public health efforts to inform the populace about STDs and their prevention and treatment. It also requires individuals to practice safer sex and to comply with treatment when they are infected.
- *Prevention* is the key!

Health and Wellness Online

The Web contains a wealth of information about health and wellness. By accessing the Internet using Web browser software, you can gain a new perspective on many topics presented in *Health and Wellness,* Tenth Edition. Access the Jones and Bartlett Publishers Web site at **health.jbpub.com/hwonline**.

References

American College Health Association. (2008). National College Health Assessment. Retrieved September 26, 2008, from http://www.acha-ncha.org/

Cohen, J. (2005). Male circumcision thwarts HIV infection. *Science, 309,* 860.

Drumright, L. N., Gorbach, P. M., & Holmes, K. K. (2004). Do people really know their sex partners? Concurrency, knowledge of partner behavior, and sexually transmitted infections within partnerships. *Sexually Transmitted Diseases, 31,* 437–442.

Dunne, E. F., et al. (2007). Prevalence of HPV infection among females in the United States. *Journal of the American Medical Association, 297,* 813–819.

Erbelding, E. J., & Zenilman, J. M. (2005). Toward better control of sexually transmitted diseases. *New England Journal of Medicine, 352,* 720–721.

UNAIDS. (2005). AIDS in Africa: Three scenarios to 2025. Retrieved October 2, 2005, from http://www.unaids.org/en/AIDS+in+Africa_Three+scenarios+to+2025.asp

Weinstock, H., Berman, S., & Cates, W., Jr. (2004). Sexually transmitted diseases among American youth. *Perspectives on Sexual and Reproductive Health, 36,* 6–9.

Suggested Readings

Centers for Disease Control and Prevention. Division of Sexually Transmitted Diseases. Statistics, health information, and treatment guidelines. Available: http://www.cdc.gov/std

Hayden, D. (2003). *Pox: Genius, madness, and the mysteries of syphilis.* New York: Basic Books. A discussion of the impact of syphilis on many of history's famous figures and the culture they created, including Oscar Wilde, Abraham Lincoln, and Hitler.

Holmes, K. K., et al. (2007). *Sexually transmitted diseases.* New York: McGraw-Hill. The most comprehensive medical text in the field.

Marr, L. (2007). *Sexually transmitted diseases: A physician tells you what you need to know.* Baltimore: Johns Hopkins Press. Detailed information on all STDs.

World Health Organization. Sexually transmitted infections. Available: http://www.who.int/topics/sexually_transmitted_infections/en/. A global view of activities, reports, news, and WHO programs.

Recommended Web Sites

Please visit **health.jbpub.com/hwonline** for links to these Web sites.

American Social Health Association
Dedicated to stopping sexually transmitted diseases and their harmful consequences to individuals, families, and communities.

HIVInsite
All about HIV/AIDS—medical issues, prevention, statistics, and policy analysis—from the University of California, San Francisco Medical Center.

Joint United Nations Programme on HIV/AIDS
International views of the AIDS epidemic.

National Center for HIV, STD, and TB Prevention
Public health surveillance, prevention research, and programs to prevent and control human immunodeficiency virus (HIV) infection and acquired immune deficiency syndrome (AIDS), other sexually transmitted diseases (STDs), and tuberculosis (TB).

U.S. Centers for Disease Control, Division of STDs
Up-to-date information on all aspects of STDs.

Part Four

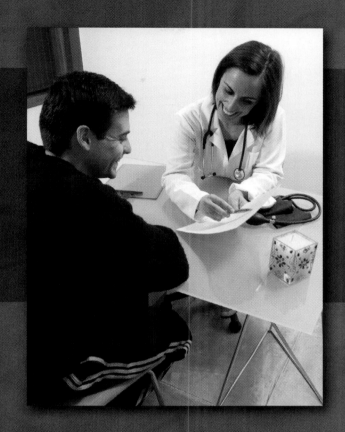

Understanding and Preventing Disease

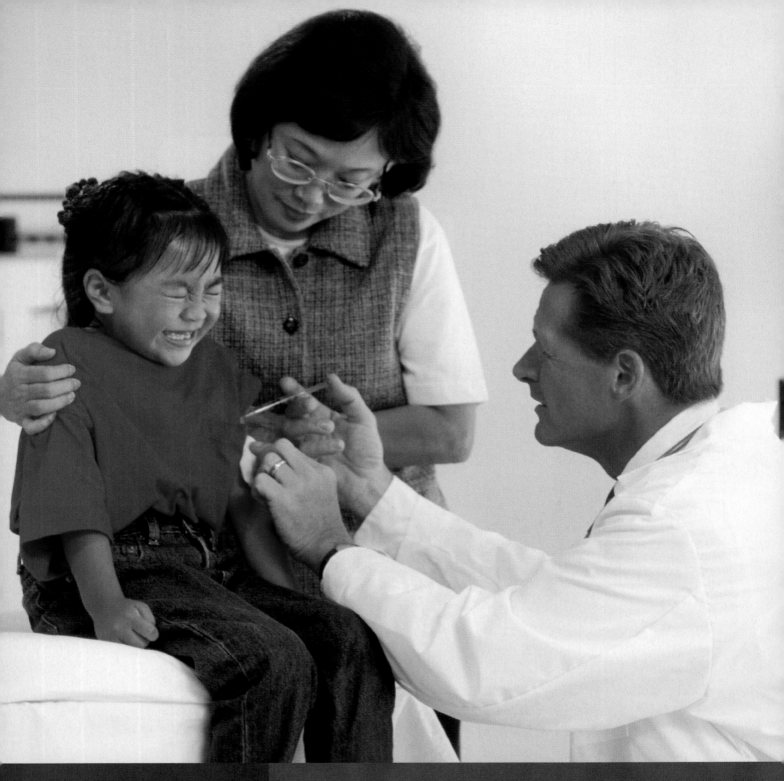

Health and Wellness online: **health.jbpub.com/hwonline**

Study Guide and Self-Assessment

12.1   My Vaccination Record

Chapter Twelve

Reducing Infections and Building Immunity: Knowledge Encourages Prevention

Learning Objectives

1. Define *pathogen, communicable disease, vector, immunizations, opportunistic infections, nosocomial disease, immune system, antibodies, antigens,* and *autoimmune diseases*.

2. Identify and explain how infectious diseases are prevented and treated.

3. Discuss the importance of antibiotics with regard to bacterial infections and the implications of antibiotic-resistant strains of bacteria.

4. Discuss how immunizations prevent infections.

5. Discuss the etiology, symptoms, and treatments for cold and flu, Lyme disease, mononucleosis, and ulcers.

6. Explain how antibodies battle infectious diseases.

7. Describe how unwanted activities of the immune system cause allergies.

8. Discuss organ transplants, blood transfusions, and the Rh factor.

9. Describe how HIV causes AIDS and ways to prevent HIV/AIDS infections.

In past centuries, hundreds of millions of people died from infectious diseases caused by bacteria, viruses, protozoa, and other microorganisms. Improvements in public sanitation, personal hygiene, nutrition, and immunizations have drastically reduced the amount of sickness and number of deaths from infectious diseases during the last one hundred years. However, infectious diseases such as malaria, tuberculosis, HIV/AIDS, and diarrhea from bacterial and viral infections still cause millions of deaths each year, primarily in poor, underdeveloped countries. Poverty and undernutrition create conditions that foster infectious diseases. Globally, infectious disease is still the single most common cause of death.

> Life is what happens when you're making other plans.
>
> *Tom Smothers*

After years of decline, some infectious diseases are again on the rise in the United States. Deaths from tuberculosis and pneumonia and from foodborne bacteria have increased in recent years. People living in urban or rural poverty and those who are addicted to drugs or alcohol are especially at risk for acquiring infectious diseases. New viruses and bacteria that cause serious disease and death in humans are emerging in communities in the United States and around the world. Bacterial contamination of beef, chicken, vegetables, and other foods has caused serious disease in the United States in recent years.

Even the healthiest person may contract an infectious disease. We all have occasional colds, flu, or stomach upsets that are caused by viruses. Usually these infections are self-limiting, and we become well in a few days or weeks. Other infectious diseases, such as pneumonia, tuberculosis, or "staph" infections, are caused by bacteria that can be destroyed with antibiotics. However, there is growing concern over the upsurge in disease-causing bacteria that are resistant to many antibiotics.

Understanding how infectious microorganisms cause disease and how your immune system battles infections is essential for maintaining wellness and for treating an infectious disease.

Infectious Microorganisms

Not all microorganisms are harmful when they are present in or on the body. In fact, bacteria perform many essential functions in many parts of the body, but there are also areas of the body that must remain sterile (**Table 12.1**). If normally sterile areas of the body become infected by microorganisms, an infectious disease results. Any microorganism that infects the body and causes disease is called a **pathogen**.

Bacteria in Health and Disease

The human body contains approximately 10 times as many bacteria as it has cells, and most of these trillions

---

Table 12.1

Bacteria in the Body

Some areas of the body harbor millions of bacteria, most of which are beneficial; other areas of the body are sterile (no bacteria).

Sterile body areas

Respiratory tract (below the vocal chords)

Sinuses and middle ear

Liver and gall bladder

Urinary tract above the urethra

Bones, joints, muscles, and blood

Cerebrospinal fluid (the brain and spinal column)

The linings around the lungs (pleura) and abdominal cavity (peritoneum)

Body areas that are colonized with bacteria

Skin: Contains thousands of bacteria per square centimeter and some fungi. The microorganisms are beneficial or harmless unless the skin is damaged or a person is already sick.

Nasopharynx and oropharynx: May contain billions of bacteria per milliliter of fluid, including pathogenic bacteria that can cause disease, but only in people whose immune systems are weak.

Esophagus and stomach: Thousands of bacteria are ingested with food. Most people have been infected with bacteria that cause ulcers (*Helicobacter pylori*) but do not have any symptoms of ulcers.

Small intestine: Low concentration of bacteria; species of *Lactobacillus* are common.

Large intestine: Billions of bacteria per milliliter of fluid are present; almost all are anaerobic species (bacteria that only grow in the absence of oxygen). All fecal matter contains billions of bacteria.

Vagina: Contains millions of bacteria, including species of *Lactobacillus* and *Escherichia coli* as well as other anaerobic bacteria.

---

of bacteria play some key role in keeping us healthy. Although it is true that preventing infections by disease-causing bacteria through sanitation, hygiene, and vaccinations and that treating bacterial infections with antibiotics have improved health enormously, we may have pushed the antibacteria war too far.

Widespread use of antibiotics in commercially raised animals such as cattle, hogs, and poultry has created strains of pathogenic bacteria that are not killed by antibiotic drugs (antibiotic resistance). The medical use of antibiotics to treat viral infections (viruses are not killed by antibiotics) also encourages the development of antibiotic-resistant strains of pathogenic bacteria, especially in hospitals. In addition, the growing use of antibacterial soaps, cosmetics, toothpaste, and other products may encourage the emergence of antibiotic resistance among bacteria and, in fact, may be counterproductive to promoting health. The development of immune system responses depends on early exposure to a wide range of environmental stimuli, including exposure to bacteria. When children play in the dirt, for example, they are getting valuable exposure to microorganisms that help their immune systems develop. Too much hygiene can be as detrimental to health as too little hygiene.

Proper functioning of the human intestinal system requires the concerted actions of trillions of bacterial cells from at least 500 different species (Silverman & Paquette, 2000). When we have digestive problems or diseases of the digestive system, it may be because the natural balance among the intestinal bacteria (called *flora*) has been disrupted. Also, it has been suggested that an imbalance of intestinal flora may contribute to obesity (Singer, 2007).

Probiotic therapy is the introduction of bacteria or other microorganisms into the body, usually by food or dietary supplements, to improve one or more bodily functions. For example, after taking antibiotics to cure an infection, bacterial flora in a person's gastrointestinal tract may be depleted or the balance of different bacterial species altered. Consuming active strains of the bacterium *Lactobacillus acidophilus* in yogurt or a supplement can restore the natural balance of bacteria in the intestines. Broad scientific support for the efficacy of probiotic therapy has yet to appear, but the National Center for Complementary and Alternative Medicine (NCCAM) reports that probiotic therapy may help in treating diarrhea due to viral infections, irritable bowel syndrome, and urinary tract and female genital tract infections (NCCAM, 2008). Although probiotic therapy seems promising for some conditions, consumers should be aware that the Food and Drug Administration (FDA) has yet to approve any probiotic medicine or product. Claims by manufacturers should be regarded with caution, as some people have been harmed by ingestion of presumed "helpful" bacteria (Raloff, 2008).

Recognizing Agents of Infectious Disease

A remarkable variety of microorganisms, including bacteria, viruses, protozoa, yeast, and small worms, can infect cells in the human body, causing disease, sickness, and death (**Figure 12.1**). Viruses are not alive in the same sense that a bacterium is; all microorganisms except viruses are cells that can grow and reproduce on their own. Viruses only grow and reproduce after they infect a cell and usurp the cellular machinery to make more viruses. Some common human diseases caused by viruses are colds, flu, polio, hepatitis, chicken pox, mumps, measles, herpes, and HIV/AIDS. Each of the viruses that cause these diseases is different and infects a specific tissue or organ in the body.

Other infectious diseases, such as pneumonia, tuberculosis, cholera, plague, typhoid fever, and gonorrhea, are caused by specific pathogenic bacteria. Often pathogenic bacteria and viruses cause disease only if the individual is already in a weakened state, particularly if the immune system is not functioning optimally.

If an infectious disease is shown to be caused by a specific microorganism, that cause is called its **etiology**. For example, tuberculosis usually is caused by a specific

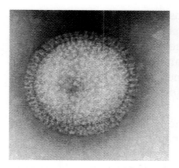

■ **Figure 12.1**

Infectious Organisms
Electron micrographs of *(upper)* an influenza virus that causes flu and *(lower)* *Salmonella* bacteria that cause food poisoning. Both the "flu" virus and the bacteria are easily passed from person to person and cause widespread epidemics.

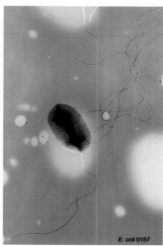

E. coli 0157

bacterium called *Mycobacterium tuberculosis,* infectious mononucleosis is caused by the Epstein-Barr virus, and giardiasis (an infection of the small intestine) is caused by the protozoan *Giardia lamblia.*

Infectious agents enter the body in a variety of ways. If the infectious organism is usually passed from person to person, the disease is called a **communicable disease.** Colds, measles, chicken pox, AIDS, and gonorrhea are all communicable diseases.

Infectious organisms also can be transferred to people from animals, especially insects. In these instances the animal or insect is said to be the **vector,** or carrier, of the disease-causing microorganism. For example, **malaria**

TERMS

communicable disease: an infectious disease that is usually transmitted from person to person

etiology: specific cause of disease

malaria: a disease of red blood cells that produces fever, anemia, and death

pathogen: a disease-causing organism

probiotic therapy: ingesting beneficial bacteria to help treat digestive disorders or other problems

vector: the carrier of infectious organisms from animals to people or from person to person

is usually caused by a microscopic protozoan called *Plasmodium falciparum*. When a person with malaria is bitten by a mosquito, blood (and the parasite) is taken up by the mosquito and injected into another person by a bite from the same mosquito. Thus, mosquitoes are the vectors for malaria. (Only a few species of mosquitoes carry the malarial parasite.)

Rabies is a disease of the nervous system caused by the rabies virus present in infected dogs, cats, bats, skunks, and other animals. The infected animals are the vectors for rabies, and the virus is transmitted in the saliva of the rabid animal.

Whether a person gets an infectious disease depends on a wide range of factors, including the competence of the immune system, nutritional status, stress, the presence of other diseases, and environmental conditions (**Figure 12.2**). For example, many people are exposed to bacteria that can cause pneumonia. However, pneumonia usually develops in older people whose immune systems are weak or in younger people who are susceptible to infections for the reasons stated earlier. Some people are more resistant to infectious organisms than others because of genes that they inherited.

Tuberculosis (TB) is not simply caused by infection with the bacterium *Mycobacterium tuberculosis*. Robert Koch, a famous nineteenth-century microbiologist, called TB the "disease of poverty" because it was associated with squalor, overcrowding, poor nutrition, and poor sanitation. Today, many people have small tubercular lesions in their lungs but have no symptoms of disease because they enjoy good nutrition, good living conditions, and are in good general health. However, in some urban areas where people live in squalor and poverty, TB is once again emerging as a problem.

In many areas of the globe, millions of people still die from infectious diseases (**Table 12.2**). Various kinds of worms (roundworm, pinworm, hookworm, and tapeworm) infect at least a billion people worldwide. Another 200 million people are debilitated by the waterborne parasite that causes the disease schistosomiasis.

Table 12.2

Estimated Annual Deaths Worldwide from Infectious Diseases

Acute respiratory infections	3,963,000
HIV/AIDS	2,777,000
Diarrheal diseases	1,798,000
Tuberculosis	1,566,000
Malaria	1,272,000
Measles*	611,000
Pertussis* (whooping cough)	294,000
Tetanus*	214,000
Meningitis, bacterial	173,000
Hepatitis B and C	157,000
Syphilis	157,000
Leishmaniasis	51,000
Trypanosomiasis	48,000
Dengue fever	19,000
Schistosomiasis	15,000

*Childhood diseases.

Source: World Health Organization, World Health Report, 2004.

Malarial parasites still infect as many as 300 million people each year and cause at least a million deaths annually around the globe. Surveys show that about a billion children in Asia, Africa, and Latin America contract severe diarrhea caused by infectious organisms, and over a million children die from diarrhea each year in these areas. Many countries lack the resources to ensure safe water supplies, public sanitation, safe waste disposal, and adequate health care—factors that can control the spread of most infectious diseases.

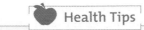 Health Tips

Wash Your Hands!

Several studies confirm that washing your hands is the best way to avoid picking up and transmitting viruses and bacteria that cause diseases such as colds, pneumonia, and diarrhea. Researchers provided bars of soap to hundreds of households with young children. In the families that were given soap, children had about half as many respiratory infections and bouts of diarrhea as did the children of control families that were not given soap. Another finding of the study was that antibacterial soap was no more effective at preventing infections than plain soap was. Between 1992 and 2000, the number of antibacterial household products increased from 26 to 700. These antibacterial products pollute the environment and contribute to the development of antibiotic-resistant strains of pathogenic bacteria (Levy, 2002).

At work and at home, *wash your hands* frequently with plain soap to prevent transmitting infectious microorganisms to yourself and to others.

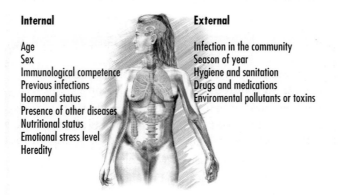

Internal	External
Age	Infection in the community
Sex	Season of year
Immunological competence	Hygiene and sanitation
Previous infections	Drugs and medications
Hormonal status	Enviromental pollutants or toxins
Presence of other diseases	
Nutritional status	
Emotional stress level	
Heredity	

■ **Figure 12.2**

Various internal and external factors determine whether disease will result from infections by viruses, bacteria, and other kinds of infectious agents.

🌐 Global Wellness

Travelers to Other Countries Should Obtain Health Information and Disease Outbreak Alerts

The U.S. Centers for Disease Control and Prevention (CDC) provide travelers to other countries with the latest information of disease outbreaks and health risks around the world. The CDC advisory system consists of four categories of warning.

The lowest category of risk is called "In the News." This describes outbreaks or health risks that are newsworthy but which present little or no health risk to travelers who take standard precautions such as drinking bottled water and not eating contaminated fresh fruits and vegetables.

The next lowest category, called "Outbreak Notice," also does not restrict travel but advises travelers of disease outbreaks in localized areas. Travelers are advised to make sure their vaccinations are up-to-date.

The third category is called "Travel Health Precaution." This category also does not restrict travel but usually advises travelers to avoid specific areas or to take additional health precautions. Outbreaks of infectious diseases occurring over a large geographic area usually fall into this category.

The category of highest risk is called "Travel Health Warning" and advises travelers not to travel to the area unless absolutely necessary. Vacationers should cancel their plans. The severe acute respiratory syndrome (SARS) epidemic in Asia a few years ago fell into this category.

Anyone traveling outside the United States should check the CDC travel advisory Web site at http://www.cdc.gov/travel or call (877) 394-8747 for the latest information on disease outbreaks and health information. If you want a list of English-speaking physicians in the area you are traveling to, contact the International Association for Medical Assistance to Travelers (http://www.iamat.org).

Fighting Infectious Diseases

Infectious diseases are fought in four ways: (1) sanitation, (2) treatment with antibiotics and other drugs, (3) vaccinations, and (4) healthful living. Stopping the spread of infectious organisms requires that they be destroyed both in infected people and in the environment. Thus, reducing the burden of infectious diseases is the responsibility both of individuals and of communities. Individuals need to practice good hygiene, avoid unsafe sex, and make sure required immunizations are up-to-date, especially for children. Communities have a responsibility to make sure water is safe to drink, the food supply is not contaminated, garbage and wastes do not pollute the environment, and that young people receive education and counseling on how to avoid sexually transmitted diseases.

Scientific understanding of the causes of infectious diseases first began in the late nineteenth century with the research of the French scientist Louis Pasteur, who established the germ theory of disease by showing that microscopic organisms could cause infections and disease. Pasteur discovered that these microorganisms could be rendered harmless by heat or by treatment with antiseptic chemicals. Like many radically new scientific ideas, Pasteur's admonitions were ignored at first.

The use of antiseptic (sterile) techniques to reduce the number of infections and deaths after surgery was adopted slowly in the United States, despite the fact that a famous American physician, Joseph Lister, had successfully implemented Pasteur's advice in his hospital. (The antiseptic mouthwash Listerine is named in his honor.) Before antiseptic techniques were introduced in hospitals, surgery or giving childbirth in a hospital often led to death from subsequent infection.

Sanitation, sterile techniques, and public health programs were not actively implemented in the United States until the beginning of the twentieth century. Only then did the incidence of many infectious diseases, such as tuberculosis, plague, pneumonia, and diphtheria, begin to decline dramatically. Many medical historians argue that sanitation is the most significant medical advance of all time because it contributed to preventing millions of cases of infectious disease caused by contaminated water and food.

Understanding Antibiotics

In the late 1940s another highly effective tool was discovered for combating infectious diseases caused by bacteria. The antibiotic **penicillin,** which is produced by a species of mold, was able to cure many kinds of bacterial infections. Today, hundreds of antibiotic drugs are available for treating infectious diseases caused by bacteria. Many other drugs are now available for treating diseases caused by viruses, protozoa, worms, and other microorganisms. These drugs either destroy the microorganisms or hold their numbers in check so the risk of disease is greatly reduced.

Antibiotics block essential biochemical reactions of microorganisms that infect the body, thereby preventing them from growing. The most useful antibiotics selectively interfere with the growth of bacteria without

TERMS

penicillin: an antibiotic produced by mold and capable of curing many bacterial infections

affecting the functions of body cells. Antibiotics kill both harmful and helpful bacteria in the body; however, once the harmful bacteria have been killed, the helpful bacteria quickly repopulate their normal sites.

Antibiotics do not prevent the growth of viruses because viruses are not living cells. Viruses infect and take over the cellular functions of body cells, thus ensuring their own growth and propagation. Finding a drug that will specifically kill a virus but not also kill body cells is very difficult.

When antibiotics were first discovered, they were greeted as wonder drugs capable of curing some of the most deadly bacterial infectious diseases, such as plague, tuberculosis, pneumonia, syphilis, and a slew of less serious diseases. Indeed, antibiotics have been exceptionally useful drugs over the past 50 years, but we are now witnessing a decline in their general effectiveness. One of the primary reasons is that many pathogenic bacteria have acquired new genes that make them resistant to one or several of the most common antibiotics.

Within a few years of the discovery of penicillin, penicillin-resistant bacteria began appearing in patients treated for bacterial infections. Bacteria also acquired resistance to other antibiotics, such as tetracycline, erythromycin, and chloramphenicol. Antibiotic resistance can be transferred among bacteria in nature in a small piece of **deoxyribonucleic acid (DNA)** that carries antibiotic-resistance genes. Harmless bacteria of one species can transfer antibiotic-resistance genes to many other species of bacteria, including ones that cause disease. In this way, bacteria that cause gonorrhea, pneumonia, tuberculosis, and "staph" infections have become resistant to many previously effective antibiotics.

For example, vancomycin is the only effective antibiotic for treating deadly bacterial infections of the circulatory system and surgical wounds. Since 1988, vancomycin-resistant bacteria have been increasing in patients with these infections; consequently, some patients die because the antibiotic is no longer effective. The antibiotics rifampin and isoniazid had been very effective in treating TB, but now these drugs are sometimes ineffective because the TB bacteria have acquired multiple antibiotic resistance.

Methicillin has been used for years as a very effective antibiotic in treating skin and soft tissue infections caused by the bacterium *Staphylococcus aureus*. Over the years, bacteria of this species have mutated until a very virulent strain, *methicillin-resistant Staphylococcus aureus (MRSA)* has emerged. These virulent "staph" infections were once found almost exclusively among patients in hospitals and nursing homes, where they frequently lead to death from blood infections. Now, however, MRSA infections are also occurring among nonhospitalized individuals. Annually, over 11 million people in the United States acquire MRSA infections, which are very

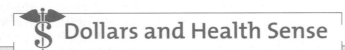

Dollars and Health Sense

Antimicrobial Products and "Superclean" Homes

Industries that market household cleaning products have discovered they can make a lot of money by preying on peoples' fears of germs and disease. More than 700 antibacterial household products are now sold (triclosan is a common antibacterial agent added to soaps and cleansers) to remove bacteria in the kitchen, bathroom, and elsewhere in the house (Aiello, Larson, & Levy, 2007). In addition, antibacterial agents are now added to food storage containers, towels, sheets, mattresses, pillows, and slippers. You can even buy antibacterial chopsticks. Where will it stop? Nowhere, if companies that sell this stuff have their way. To sell cleansers and other goods, companies fan public fear of microbial contamination and disease. In fact, living in a "superclean" home is actually counterproductive to a healthy environment and to healthy living. Exposure to common bacteria present in the home and outdoor environment is essential to immune system development in young children. All of us depend on the normal presence of beneficial bacteria on our skin, in our digestive system, and in other parts of the body. If the normal bacterial balance of the body is disturbed, it paves the way for colonization and infection by harmful bacteria.

Like the indiscriminate use of antibiotics in animal feed, widespread use of antimicrobial products in the home encourages the development of antibiotic-resistant strains of bacteria, thus rendering useless some of these products in hospitals and nursing homes, where they are essential for maintaining a hygienic environment so that sick patients do not become infected. Tons of antimicrobial household products are flushed and washed into the environment, where they foster development of antibiotic-resistant bacteria.

During the anthrax scare after the September 11 attacks, millions of homes stockpiled the antibiotic ciprofloxacin, in case it was needed for treating anthrax victims. The tons of "cipro" in bathroom cabinets invites its indiscriminate use whenever people feel sick. Also, unused cipro will probably wind up in the environment and further complicate the already serious problem of antibiotic-resistant bacteria.

The bottom line is that you do not need to use any antimicrobial products to clean your house or your body. A "superclean" home is unhealthy for you—and for the environment (Vastag, 2002). Do not contribute to the profits of companies jumping on the bandwagon of selling antimicrobial household products.

difficult to treat. In 2008, a quick test was approved for the detection of a MRSA infection. It is hoped that the availability of a test that gives a result in a couple of hours will improve treatment for MRSA infections and help prevent their spread.

The battle to abolish the use of antibiotics in animal feed has been going on for decades in the United States. In 2003, the World Health Organization (WHO) released a report concluding that the use of antibiotics endangered human health and was of little benefit to livestock. The European Union (EU) has ordered member countries to completely stop using antibiotics in feed for pigs and poultry. Even McDonalds', which buys more than a billion pounds of beef a year, has pledged to buy only antibiotic-free beef. The U.S. government has yet to ban the use of antibiotics in animal feed. This is another example in which profit and politics supercede scientific advice and human health.

In the 1990s, the FDA approved two drugs, Baytril and SaraFlox, that could be added routinely to poultry feed. These two drugs belong to a class of extremely effective antibiotics called fluoroquinolones; members of this family of drugs are used to treat the bacteria that cause anthrax and foodborne infections. Scientists and the American Medical Association warned that such use in animal feed would lead to the emergence of antibiotic-resistant strains. After several years of use, this is exactly what happened, and the FDA tried to ban the use of the drugs. Drug companies fought the FDA, and it was years before the drugs were finally withdrawn from the market. But it was too late; resistance had already occurred. Fluoroquinolone drugs are now much less effective in treating staph infections than they were before.

In 2007, the FDA again succumbed to drug company pressures and approved the use of a powerful antibiotic, cefquinome, for use in animal feed. Again the American Medical Association and many other health organizations warned that adding this drug to animal feed would, within a few years, lead to antibiotic-resistant strains of pathogenic bacteria and render this powerful class of drugs much less effective. Time after time over the last several decades, the FDA has bowed to industry pressures and has failed to perform its primary mission to protect the health of Americans.

How the Body Protects Itself

The best way to avoid infectious diseases caused by pathogenic microorganisms is to keep them out of the body. The skin and mucous membranes prevent the entry of most microorganisms into the body by functioning as physical barriers. That is why a wound often exposes the body to infection (**Figure 12.3**). The skin is mildly acidic and provides a poor habitat for most harmful microorganisms, although the skin is covered with beneficial bacteria.

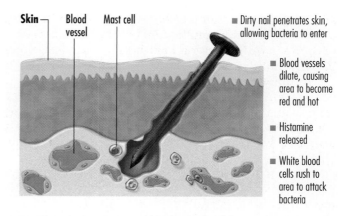

■ Figure 12.3

Inflammation Response
Penetration of the skin by any unsterile sharp object often produces an inflammation response, the normal response of the body to injury or infection.

The eyes, nose, throat, and breathing passages are protected by mucous membranes that continuously produce secretions that flush away harmful organisms and particles. Mucous membranes also secrete enzymes that can destroy toxic substances. The mouth, digestive system, and excretory organs also are protected by membranes that guard the internal organs.

Tears keep the surface of the eyes moist and serve to wash away foreign particles. Wax secreted from the ears protects the delicate hearing apparatus. The mucous coating of the respiratory tract is sticky and provides a trap for irritating particles and microorganisms in the air; microscopic hairs called **cilia** keep the mucus moving out of the bronchial tubes. Coughing and spitting are mechanisms that remove foreign material from the breathing passages. Sneezing and blowing the nose eliminate irritating particles that are inhaled.

Cells and enzymes in the blood quickly form clots that seal off any break in the skin, thereby preventing the entry of harmful substances and infectious organisms. If some bacteria do enter the wound before it is sealed off, other special cells that are part of the immune system attack and destroy the invaders.

If microorganisms or foreign particles penetrate the skin and enter the blood, they soon encounter specialized cells called **leukocytes**, the colorless white blood

TERMS

cilia: microscopic hairs in the lining of the bronchial tubes

deoxyribonucleic acid (DNA): a chemical substance that carries genetic information

leukocytes: white blood cells that fight infections

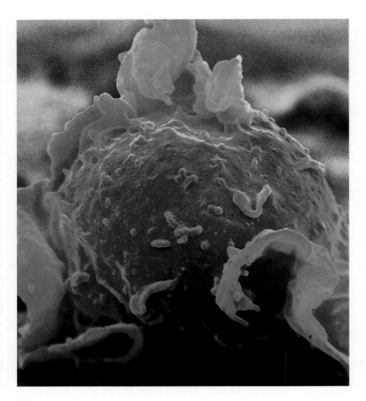

■ Figure 12.4

Macrophage
Photograph of a lung macrophage as visualized in an electron microscope.

cells that can be distinguished from the red blood cells that transport oxygen. Only about 1 in 700 cells in the blood is a leukocyte, but their number can increase dramatically if an acute infection occurs. That is why blood is tested for the number of white blood cells when an infection is suspected.

Specialized white blood cells called **macrophages** are associated with specific organs and are vital to the body's internal defense mechanisms. Macrophages are able to engulf and digest foreign cells and particles that invade the body. Organ-specific macrophages protect the lungs, stomach, and other organs from damage by foreign substances (**Figure 12.4**).

Common Infectious Diseases

Infectious diseases, depending on their cause and consequences, present special public health problems and personal concerns for many people. To better understand how to cope with infectious disease, we'll review colds and flu, Lyme disease, mononucleosis, hepatitis, and ulcers. AIDS is discussed later in this chapter and also in Chapter 11.

Colds and Flu

Most people, especially children, contract several colds and possibly flu every year. Both diseases are caused by viruses that infect cells of the respiratory tract. Colds are caused by more than 200 different viruses. A cold caused by one virus does not protect a person from catching a cold caused by a different strain, which explains why colds can occur one after another or several times a year.

Although cold symptoms may be quite discomforting, colds generally do not result in long-term illness or death. Billions of dollars are spent by Americans every year on medications that are supposed to alleviate cold symptoms, such as sore throat, cough, congestion, runny nose, and pain. Physicians joke that a cold will go away in about a week with rest and medications or in about seven days if nothing is done. It takes the immune system about a week to produce the specific proteins (antibodies) that inactivate the viruses and for tissues to heal.

High-tech modern medicine has nothing to offer that can prevent a cold, although enormous research efforts have been expended to find a drug that would reduce the risk of catching a cold. Although many of the "discoveries" of cold research were announced with great fanfare, none has worked.

Americans suffer an estimated 500 million colds a year. Missed work because of colds costs the U.S. economy about $20 billion a year. Anyone with a cold is caught between a rock and a hard place. Staying at home means lost income and possibly causing a major disruption at work. For example, if a physician with a cold stays away from work, all the appointments must be canceled or switched to other doctors whose schedules already are full. If a person decides to go to work despite being sick, sneezing, and coughing, other workers are likely to become infected and face the same problem of whether to stay at home or go to work. In the end, each sick person must decide how bad he or she feels. Is it worth going to work and infecting others? Are you really too sick to go to work? The choice is never easy.

Influenza, or flu, is caused by a different kind of virus than the ones that cause colds. Flu is a much more serious disease. The symptoms of flu are body aches, high fever, loss of appetite, and other complications. Infections of the respiratory system by a flu virus can so weaken people that they contract pneumonia, a bacterial infection, and die.

There are many different strains of flu virus, and new strains arise continually. Because flu is so debilitating and serious, vaccines are prepared each year that are supposed to be specific to the expected yearly epidemic. The problem is that scientists have to guess which flu strain will be the cause of the next epidemic, because it takes about a year to prepare and distribute the vaccine.

In some years, flu vaccine is quite effective, but in others, it is not effective at all because it was prepared with the wrong strains of the virus. People with respiratory problems such as asthma, people with immune system deficiencies, and the elderly, who are most sus-

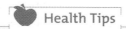 Health Tips

Stuffy Sinuses?

When your nose is stuffed up from a cold or allergies, instead of taking a decongestant pill or using a nasal spray, try soothing your swollen nasal passages with a dilute saline solution. Research shows that this method, called *nasal sinus irrigation*, really works (Harvey et al., 2007). Salt water irrigation washes the mucus, bacteria, allergens, and other debris from your nose, and it shrinks swollen membranes and improves the flow of air. Although you can buy prepared nasal solutions, it is easy to make your own using the following method.

1. Fill a clean 1-quart glass jar with tap or bottled water.
2. Add 2 to 3 heaping teaspoons of either pickling/canning or kosher salt. Do not use table salt, because it contains a large number of additives. If you prefer a weaker solution, use about half the amount of salt (best for kids).
3. Add 1 teaspoon baking soda (sodium bicarbonate).
4. Mix well and store at room temperature. Make fresh weekly.
5. Pour the amount of solution you plan to use into a clean bowl to avoid contaminating the entire jar. The solution can be warmed slightly in a microwave, but be sure the solution is just warm, not hot.
6. Fill an ear-cleaning rubber bulb or Water Pic with an irrigation tip with solution. Stand over the sink (or in the shower) and squirt liquid into each nostril, aiming the stream toward the back of your head, not the top. This will allow the solution to flow from your nose into your mouth so you can spit out the salty water. It does not matter if you swallow some of the liquid.
7. You can irrigate your nose two to three times a day. After a few days the stuffiness should disappear and you should breathe more freely.
8. Consult with a health professional before using this nasal irrigation procedure to be sure it is safe for your symptoms.

Source: University of Calgary School of Medicine. (2004). Instructions for nasal irrigation for nose and sinus patients. Available: http://www.headandneck.ucalgary.ca/nasal_irrig.htm.

ceptible to pneumonia, are advised to get a flu shot each year to help prevent infection.

Never catching a cold or flu is probably impossible in modern society. However, certain precautions can help reduce the risk. During seasons when colds and flu are present, try to stay away from crowds as much as possible. The viruses are easily transmitted in droplets from people who are coughing or sneezing. Being in a classroom, theater, bus, subway, or any crowded place increases the risk of being infected. The viruses also are easily transmitted by bodily contact, such as shaking hands with someone with a cold who has recently wiped his or her nose or mouth. So it's a good idea to wash your hands frequently during cold and flu season.

Structure of Influenza Viruses

Hundreds of different strains of the flu virus can be constructed by reassortment of its eight segments of genetic (RNA) information (**Figure 12.5**). Two proteins on the surface of the virus determine which cells it can attach to and its lethality to specific species. The hemagglutinin (H) protein binds to specific receptors on cells. Usually, the particular H protein restricts the infection to one or several species of animals. For example, avian flu viruses readily attach to receptors on bird cells but usually are unable to attach effectively to human cells. The neuraminidase (N) protein helps the viruses escape from infected cells so that they can infect other cells. There are 15 different H proteins and about 9 different N proteins; the combinations of the two proteins characterize the particular strain of flu.

Defining an Influenza Pandemic

The World Health Organization defines an influenza pandemic in six phases; in the final phase the virus has spread to many countries in at least two distinct regions of the world. During the last century there were three major influenza pandemics: one in 1918 and smaller ones in 1957 and 1968. The 1918 influenza pandemic was the worst in recorded history—estimates range up to 40 million deaths over a period of less than two years. The number of influenza deaths was greater than all the deaths in World War I or in the 25 years of the current AIDS pandemic.

On September 7, 1918, during World War I, a soldier at a training camp near Boston became very ill with a high fever. By September 16, several dozen new cases of influenza were admitted to the army hospital. By September 23, 12,604 cases of flu were reported among the 45,000 soldiers stationed in the camp (Taubenberger, 2005). By November, one-third of the U.S. population was infected (Holmes, 2004). These numbers show how swiftly a deadly strain of flu virus can spread in a population.

In a remarkable bit of scientific detective work, the strain that caused the 1918 flu pandemic has been reconstructed by recovering flu genetic material from victims

TERMS

macrophages: specialized cells that destroy and eliminate foreign particles and microorganisms from the body

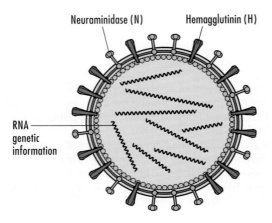

Neuraminidase (N)   Hemagglutinin (H)

RNA genetic information

■ **Figure 12.5**

Diagram of an Influenza Virus
The genetic information is contained in eight segments of ribonucleic acid (RNA). These can reassort and mutate to give rise to many different strains of viruses. Two proteins on the surface of each virus determine which species of animals it can infect. The hemagglutinin (H) protein recognizes specific cell receptors and allows the virus to infect those cells. The neuraminidase (N) protein helps new viruses to escape from infected cells.

who died and were buried in the arctic permafrost (Taubenberger, 2005). The 1918 virus was an H1N1 strain, the 1957 virus was an H2N2 strain, and the 1968 virus was an H3N2 strain. This last strain with slight variations is the strain that has been around since 1968.

The 2009 Influenza Pandemic

In April 2009, hundreds of cases of influenza were reported in Mexico. These infections were caused by a strain of virus that normally infects swine and so initially it was called "swine flu." Further analysis of the virus revealed that it contained genetic material from swine, bird, and human flu viruses. The virus was quickly identified as an H1N1 strain similar to the 1918 virus. This immediately raised fears of a serious worldwide flu pandemic.

Within a month, confirmed cases of H1N1 flu had spread from Mexico to 47 U.S. states and almost 40 countries around the world. Fortunately, the new H1N1 strain lacked the virulence gene that made the 1918 flu strain so deadly. Most cases of the H1N1 flu were relatively mild and infected people recovered quickly. Also, the new strain was susceptible to two antiviral drugs, oseltamivir phosphate (Tamiflu) and zanamivir (Relenza). These drugs interfere with the neuraminidase viral protein and prevent the release of new viruses from cells, thus slowing the spread of the infection in the body.

As of this writing, it is not known how long the 2009 flu pandemic will last or whether it will return at a later time in a more virulent form. Vaccines against the new virus are likely to be produced. One thing is clear from the 2009 flu pandemic: Health authorities in the United States and around the world must be ready to respond to influenza outbreaks that can arise at any time.

Avian Influenza

The strain of avian flu that is circulating among birds in Southeast Asia, Europe, and Africa is a strain called H5N1. Millions of domestic fowl have been killed in Thailand, Vietnam, Singapore, and elsewhere to try to stop the spread of the deadly strain of bird flu. However, because millions of wild birds also carry the virus, it is unlikely to be eradicated. Although the virus mainly infects and kills birds, about three hundred people have been infected by this H5N1 strain of bird flu. The mortality rate from human infections ranges from 44% to 79% (Writing Committee of the Second WHO Consultation on Clinical Aspects of Human Infection with Avian Influenza A (H5N1) Virus, 2008).

It is thought that almost all of the people who have been infected by the H5N1 avian flu strain acquired the infection from handling or eating birds that carried the virus. However, in a few cases, person-to-person transmission of the virus may have occurred. As of 2008, about 300 H5N1 infections in people had occurred worldwide, and about half of the people infected had died. Because of the enormous number of infected birds in the world, it is expected that the virus eventually will mutate and be capable of person-to-person transmission. The virulence of a new human virus derived from the avian virus cannot be predicted. Nor can scientists predict when such a virus will arise, although most expect it to happen sooner or later (Taubenberger, Morens, & Fauci, 2007).

Lyme Disease

Lyme disease was first recognized in 1975 when a number of children were diagnosed with an arthritis-like disease in Lyme, Connecticut. The disease was soon recognized as a distinct tickborne disease caused by pathogenic bacteria transmitted in a tick bite; the disease is called Lyme disease after the place where it was first discovered. In 1982, the first year of surveillance, 491 cases were reported. The number swelled to 17,029 in 2001 and increased to nearly 70,000 by 2005. About 95% of all cases of Lyme disease occur in Connecticut, Delaware, Rhode Island, Maine, Maryland, Massachusetts, Minnesota, New Jersey, New Hampshire, New York, Pennsylvania, and Wisconsin.

The most common place to get Lyme disease is in woods during warm months when ticks are abundant and are feeding on deer and small mammals, including household pets that can bring the ticks into the home. A specific bacterium called *Borrelia burgdorferi* is carried by a few species of tick (mainly, *Ixodes scapularis*). When this tick attaches to the skin and bites, the bacteria are injected into the blood.

If unrecognized and left untreated, Lyme disease progresses through three stages.

Stage 1: This stage begins a few days after the tick bite and lasts about a month. A red rash appears around the tick bite and gradually spreads out on

Table 12.3

Viruses That Remain in the Body for Life After Infection

Virus	Symptoms	Spread by	Remains in
Herpes simplex 1	Cold sores on lips or in mouth	Direct contact; most infectious when lesions are present	Nerve cells
Herpes simplex 2	Painful blisters on genital organs	Direct contact; oral–genital sex can transmit type 1 or 2 to mouth or genital area	Nerve cells
Cytomegalovirus (CMV)	No symptoms in most children and adults; CMV can cause stillbirth and mental retardation in fetuses	Body fluids: blood, urine, saliva	White blood cells
Varicella zoster virus	Chicken pox in children; shingles in adults	Person to person	Nerve cells
Epstein-Barr virus (EBV)	Mononucleosis	Saliva (kissing)	Lymph glands
Human immunodeficiency virus (HIV)	From none to full symptoms of AIDS	Sexual intercourse (homosexual or heterosexual), blood transfusions, contaminated needles of injection drug users, mother-to-child transmission before or after birth	T-cells of the immune system and other body cells

the skin. A person may not recognize the rash as stemming from a tick bite, but the rash is quite distinctive to an experienced physician's eye. The person may also feel tired, have headaches, and notice some joint pain.

Stage 2: After a month or two, about 15% of those persons bitten experience severe neurological symptoms such a meningitis and encephalitis. A few people will develop heart problems, and most will notice pain in the joints, muscles, tendons, and bones.

Stage 3: Within weeks and up to two years after the tick bite, about 60% of people develop arthritis characterized by pain and swelling of joints, especially the knees.

Because the symptoms of Lyme disease are similar to many other diseases, it is difficult to diagnose, especially if the patient does not report being bitten by a tick. Blood tests are helpful in making the diagnosis but are not completely reliable. Lyme disease is treated with antibiotics at all stages, and treatment is most effective if taken soon after the appearance of the characteristic rash.

In 1998, the FDA approved a vaccine that was 75% effective in protecting against Lyme disease. Three injections are needed, and protection lasts less than a year. The vaccine is effective only against Lyme disease and does not protect against other tickborne diseases or against strains found in Europe or other parts of the world. The cost is high and the vaccine is approved only for those 15 to 70 years of age, so children cannot be vaccinated. For all these reasons and because of low demand, the vaccine was withdrawn from the market in 2002. No vaccine for Lyme disease is currently available despite the rapid rise in the number of cases both in the United States and Europe (60,000 cases a year).

To avoid contracting Lyme disease, it is important to be completely covered with clothing—especially when hiking—in tick-infested areas. Pants should be tucked into boots. Proper dress alone can reduce the risk of contracting Lyme disease from a tick bite by at least 40% (Vazquez et al., 2008). Use light-colored clothing so that ticks can be seen more easily. If pets hike with you, examine them carefully afterward for ticks. Ticks embedded in the skin can be removed by pulling on them carefully with a tweezer, making sure that the head is removed.

If it is not treated soon after a person is bitten by a bacteria-infected tick, Lyme disease can become a chronic disease with ongoing medical problems. Some guidelines call for infected persons to be treated with antibiotics for 30 days; other authorities recommend longer treatment. Even if a person is apparently cured, symptoms related to the original infection can crop up years later.

Mononucleosis

Mononucleosis (commonly called "mono") is an infectious disease caused by the Epstein-Barr virus (EBV) that is ubiquitous in all human populations (Cohen, 2000). It is spread easily from person to person, especially in crowded conditions. It sometimes is called the "kissing disease" because the virus is present in saliva and readily

TERMS

Lyme disease: a serious, difficult-to-diagnose infectious disease caused by bacteria deposited by ticks when they bite

mononucleosis: an infectious disease caused by the Epstein-Barr virus, common among college-age adults

> There are two ways of being disappointed in life. One is to not get what you want and the other is to get it.
>
> *George Bernard Shaw*

transferred by mouth-to-mouth contact. About half of all children in the United States are infected by EBV by age 5, but in most children, the infection goes unnoticed because there are no symptoms. Once someone has been infected by EBV, he or she usually carries the virus for life without having symptoms or signs of disease. EBV and a number of other viruses can become permanently established in the body (**Table 12.3**).

If a teenager or young adult becomes infected by EBV, symptoms develop but usually clear up in several weeks without further illness. Symptoms of mononucleosis include swollen glands, sore throat, fever, chills, and, above all, complete exhaustion and loss of energy. About half of those infected develop an enlarged spleen, and a small percentage develop jaundice (yellow coloration of the skin and eyes). Fortunately, these symptoms resolve in two to four weeks in a healthy young adult.

There is no specific treatment for mononucleosis, but there are precautions that can facilitate recovery. The primary focus is rest and more rest. For the first two weeks, you may hardly be able to drag yourself out of bed. When you start to feel stronger, however, it is important to continue to rest. Trying to resume normal activities too soon can cause a relapse and extend the illness. Fluid intake is also important; drink as much water, juice, soup, or tea as you can. Some people find that taking herbs that act as immune system boosters (echinacea and astragalus) can speed recovery.

The primary reason to avoid strenuous activities, especially contact sports, for a month or more after a diagnosis of mononucleosis is to protect the spleen. If the spleen is enlarged, an injury could rupture it and create a serious medical problem that may necessitate surgery and removal of the spleen. Because mono affects young people who may be involved in competitive athletics, it is important that they understand why they must continue to be relatively inactive even when they no longer feel sick. Also, because EBV infection affects the liver, it is important not to drink alcohol or take other drugs that may further injure the liver.

The incubation time for EBV is quite long. Children may show symptoms in one to two weeks after infection; however, adults may not develop symptoms for one to two months. Thus, it is often difficult to know from whom you received the virus. Once you know that you have mononucleosis, it is important to try not to spread it among family and friends. Do not kiss anyone, and avoid sharing drinks or food. Try not to sneeze or cough when others are close by, and carry tissues to cover your mouth and nose. Even after all symptoms of mono have disappeared, active virus particles remain in the saliva for many months—up to six months in some

studies—so you still need to exert caution so as not to spread EBV to close associates and loved ones.

Ulcers

For most of the last century, it was thought that stomach **ulcers** (sores or holes in the lining of the stomach or duodenum, the first part of the small intestine) were caused by stress, anxiety, smoking, and alcohol consumption. However, in 1983, two medical researchers in Australia shocked the medical world by announcing that most stomach ulcers were caused by a bacterial infection in the lining of the stomach of susceptible persons. For several years this view was treated with skepticism, but now it has been established unequivocally that as many as 90% of ulcers are caused by particular stomach bacteria (*Helicobacter pylori*). Without the presence of these bacteria in the stomach, ulcers hardly ever occur.

Approximately 30% of the U.S. population is infected with *H. pylori*, and in developing nations the incidence of infections is estimated at 70% or higher. Most people become infected as children and do not experience any symptoms at the time. However, later in life some of those carrying the bacteria will develop ulcers. People get ulcers at any age, and men and women are affected equally. In addition to causing ulcers, *H. pylori* is associated with an increased risk of stomach cancer. About 1% to 3% of infected persons eventually will develop stomach cancer. That rate is six times greater than the rate for uninfected persons.

The most common ulcer symptom is a gnawing or burning pain in the abdomen between the breastbone and the belly button. The pain often occurs when the stomach is empty, between meals, and in the early morning hours, but it can occur at any other time. It may last from minutes to hours and may be relieved by eating food or taking antacids. Less common symptoms include nausea, vomiting, or loss of appetite. Sometimes ulcers bleed. If bleeding continues for a long time, it may lead to anemia with weakness and fatigue.

A physician can determine if an ulcer is caused by *H. pylori* infection by the following tests:

- *Blood:* A blood test can confirm if you have *H. pylori.*
- *Breath:* A breath test can determine if you are infected with *H. pylori.* In this test, you drink a harmless liquid and, in less than one hour, a sample of your breath is tested for *H. pylori.*
- *Endoscopy:* Your health care provider may decide to perform an endoscopy. This is a test in which a small tube containing a camera is inserted through the mouth and into the stomach to look for ulcers. During the endoscopy, small samples of the stomach lining can be obtained by biopsy and tested for *H. pylori.*

Antibiotics cure ulcers; therapy is one to two weeks of an antibiotic and a medicine that will reduce the acid in the stomach. This treatment is extremely effective in eliminating *H. pylori* with antibiotics and means that there is a greater than 90% chance that the ulcer can be cured for good.

Hepatitis

Serious liver disease is known as **hepatitis**. It can be caused by environmental agents such as excess alcohol consumption, exposure to pesticides, and drugs. Hepatitis also is caused by infection by any one of several different viruses that infect liver cells; the most common infections are caused by hepatitis A, hepatitis B, and hepatitis C viruses. The sources of infection and their severity vary for each of these viruses.

Hepatitis A This virus (HAV) causes liver disease in approximately 200,000 Americans each year but is fatal in less than 100 persons. At least one-third of Americans have been infected with hepatitis A at some time in their lives, and most suffer only mild symptoms and recover completely. The primary source of HAV infection is fecal–oral transmission; one can become infected from contaminated water or from eating food that has been handled by an infected person. Not washing hands after going to the toilet and subsequently handling food is the primary means of transmitting HAV. The symptoms of being infected include jaundice, fatigue, loss of appetite, abdominal pain, and intermittent diarrhea. The symptoms usually clear up within a few weeks, and there is no persistent liver infection. A very effective vaccine is available for those individuals who are at high risk of exposure to HAV or who travel to areas of the world where hepatitis A disease is widespread.

Hepatitis B Infection of the liver by hepatitis B virus (HBV) causes serious liver disease; it persists as a chronic infection and may eventually cause liver failure or liver cancer and death. Worldwide, as many as 350 million people are thought to have a chronic HBV infection; about 1.2 million HBV-infected people die each year from liver failure. Not all infections by HBV produce symptoms, but when they do the symptoms include jaundice, fatigue, abdominal pain, loss of appetite, nausea, and vomiting.

HBV is transmitted by blood; infection can result from blood transfusions, use of contaminated needles by injection drug users, sexual intercourse (heterosexual or homosexual) in which minute amounts of blood are exchanged, and by perinatal transmission, in which an infected pregnant woman passes the virus to her fetus. The incidence of hepatitis B disease has been decreasing as a result of the availability of a highly effective vaccine and prevention programs aimed at high-risk groups of people such as injection drug users and sexually active individuals. The blood used for transfusions now is screened routinely for the presence of HBV, and infection by this means is no longer a danger.

A vaccine against HBV is available, and it is recommended that all children be vaccinated for hepatitis B. In addition, all persons who are at high risk of exposure to hepatitis B—health care workers, hemodialysis patients, sexually active individuals, and injection drug users—are advised to obtain the HBV vaccination.

Hepatitis C Hepatitis C (HCV) is sometimes called the silent epidemic because until recently relatively little was known or publicized regarding this infection. However, HCV infection is now the most common reason for liver transplantation. It is estimated that 4 million people in the United States are chronically infected by HCV and that many eventually will develop serious liver disease. Among the 2 million persons in U.S. prisons, 20% to 60% are infected with HCV and receive no treatment.

Hepatitis C virus has been well characterized only since 1989; prior to that time millions of people became infected from contaminated blood without knowing it. HCV is not a single viral strain but consists of many related viruses. Like the flu virus, HCV can change its genetic information easily, which is one of the reasons that it is difficult to treat and why no vaccine has been developed. HCV is transmitted exclusively in blood and blood products; it is not transmitted by casual contact.

Americans who are infected with HCV generally were infected more than 20 years ago, before the virus was identified. Most do not even know they carry the virus until symptoms develop. A sensitive antibody test can detect if a person has been infected with HCV, and another test can detect the level of the viruses in the blood. Treatment involves administering two antiviral drugs, interferon and ribavarin, for six months; these drugs produce flulike symptoms, fatigue, and other side effects. The level of HCV is monitored at the end of treatment and six months later. A negative test for HCV indicates a probable cure, but only about 50% of patients so treated are cured (Lauer & Walker, 2001).

The risk of HCV infection in the United States today is quite low except for intravenous drug users who share needles, and health care workers who get an accidental needle puncture while treating a patient. The blood supply is screened for HCV, so transfusions are safe. However, HCV infections are still a risk in other parts of the world, especially from blood transfusions.

Hepatitis D This virus (HDV) is defective, is unable to grow by itself, and is only detected in the presence of HBV infection.

Hepatitis E This virus (HEV) is similar to HAV in that it is transmitted by a fecal–oral route in contaminated

---

TERMS

hepatitis: serious disease of the liver caused by hepatitis viruses A, B, C, D, or E; also caused by chemicals and alcohol

ulcers: open sores that occur in the stomach or small intestine from infection by the bacterium *H. pylori*

food and water. It causes the same symptoms as hepatitis A and does not result in chronic infection. Hepatitis E occurs primarily in underdeveloped countries where sanitation is poor. Travelers should avoid drinking unbottled water, using ice, or eating fresh fruits and vegetables that may be contaminated. No vaccine currently is available for hepatitis E.

Although viruses are the primary cause of hepatitis, remember the golfer in Ireland who suffered from non-viral hepatitis. It turned out that at each hole he licked his golf balls to clean them before teeing off. The herbicide residue on the balls eventually damaged his liver and caused hepatitis. The herbicide was used heavily on the golf course to control weeds, and the chemicals were picked up by the golf balls as they rolled in the grass.

Emerging Infectious Diseases

West Nile Virus

West Nile virus (WNV) is found throughout much of the world—Africa, the Middle East, India, Indonesia, and some areas of Europe. West Nile virus was first reported in the United States in 1999 when a large number of crows at the Bronx Zoo were found dead on the zoo grounds; this was followed by the death of a number of other birds in the zoo's collection. Soon afterward, several people in the New York area were hospitalized with symptoms of encephalitis. Blood samples were analyzed, and it was found that the RNA of the virus matched that of a West Nile virus strain previously isolated in Israel.

Mosquitoes that bite infected birds or other animals can transmit WNV to people. After about two weeks of incubation in a person, WNV may cross the blood–brain barrier (which restricts many infectious agents from reaching the brain) and infect the nervous system. In a few people, once the virus has infected the brain and nervous system, symptoms such as tremors, convulsions, paralysis, coma, and death may follow. The good news is that most people who are bitten by a WNV-infected mosquito will *not* develop serious symptoms and will recover completely without any lasting effects.

In 2007 WNV-related illness was reported in more than 3,600 persons in nearly all states (**Figure 12.6**). Many of these patients suffered from a serious neurological disease but eventually recovered. The spread of the disease and the number of reported cases are expected to continue to increase in the coming years. In addition to mosquito bites, people also can become infected with WNV through blood transfusions and organ transplants (Morse, 2003). People who have been infected by WNV do not show symptoms for some time or may even be without symptoms. Blood can be tested with an antibody test that can show whether a person has been infected by WNV. However, because it takes a week or

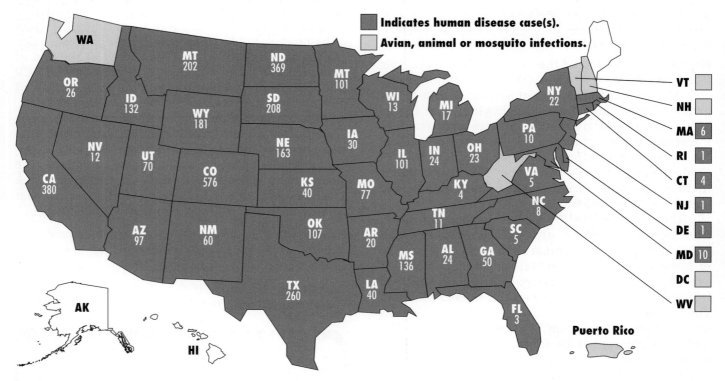

■ **Figure 12.6**

Number of Human West Nile Virus Infections Across the United States in 2007
Only five states (Maine, Vermont, Washington, Alaska, and Hawaii) had no reported cases.

Source: U.S. Centers for Disease Control and Prevention. (2008). West Nile virus: Statistics, surveillance, and control. Available: http://www.cdc.gov/ncidod/dvbid/westnile/Mapsactivity/surv&control08Maps.htm.

longer for antibodies to develop after an infection, an infected person may donate blood or an organ and the infection can go undetected.

Mosquito control is the major form of prevention: People are advised to avoid mosquito-infested areas where the West Nile virus is prevalent. Mosquito repellent may be of help in preventing infection.

Steps to prevent infection in areas where the virus is found include the following:

- Reduce outdoor activities in early evening when mosquitoes are active.
- Wear clothing that covers the arms and legs when going into mosquito-infested areas such as woods and wetlands.
- Spray clothing with insect repellent.
- Apply insect repellent sparingly to exposed areas of the body. (Read all precautions for using insect repellent.)
- If there are many mosquitoes in the house, put up mosquito nets around beds, especially those where children sleep.

SARS

In 2002–2003, a new disease called *severe acute respiratory syndrome* (SARS) emerged in Guangdong province in China and began to spread to other parts of China and to other countries around the world. The disease is caused by a new form of a family of viruses called *coronaviruses,* which are also the cause of many cases of the common cold. The new coronavirus, which apparently originated in an animal called the civet (a kind of cat whose meat is often sold in markets in parts of China), causes a severe respiratory disease with a fatality rate of about 15%. The disease rapidly spread around the world, carried by infected travelers. Ultimately, 8,000 cases of SARS were reported, causing 774 deaths in 26 countries (Peiris et al., 2003).

In a dramatic effort to halt the spread of the disease, early in 2003 the World Health Organization (WHO) issued its first-ever travel advisory. WHO recommended that nonessential travel to China, Hong Kong, Singapore, and other affected areas of the world be postponed. Public health officials in the United States and elsewhere hoped that by restricting travel from affected areas and by quarantining infected individuals, the spread of SARS could be halted. Fortunately, these worldwide efforts did succeed in ending the spread of SARS. By July 2003, travel bans were lifted and only a few cases of SARS were reported subsequently. No further cases of SARS have occurred to date. However, health officials will be vigilant for the foreseeable future.

As the world becomes a single global community in which people and other animals move rapidly from one part of the world to another, it is likely that more infectious diseases will appear. In fact, emerging infectious diseases have become one of the most serious global health problems.

The Immune System Battles Infections

The world teems with infectious viruses, bacteria, and other microorganisms that can cause disease if they invade the body. Most people stay well most of the time because the body contains a remarkable array of defense mechanisms that help keep disease-causing microorganisms out or that can destroy them if they invade the body. We only occasionally have an infectious disease because the **immune system** acts to protect the body from infectious organisms and foreign substances.

The immune system takes time to develop. At birth, a baby is protected from infectious diseases by antibodies that were present in the mother's blood and passed on to the newborn. **Antibodies** are proteins that recognize and inactivate viruses, bacteria, and harmful substances that can cause disease. Babies also receive antibodies in breast milk, which help to protect them while their own immune systems mature during the first year or so of life.

Many factors can adversely affect the development and functioning of the immune system. Perhaps the most important factor is poor nutrition, especially early in life. Without a healthy diet, a child is extremely susceptible to infections that a weak immune system cannot fight. Inadequate nutrition and infectious diseases are the principal reasons that children die in many undeveloped and impoverished countries of the world. Other factors that affect the development or functions of the immune system are hereditary disorders, viral infections, stress, and many drugs and chemicals, including alcohol and tobacco.

The Lymphatic System

The immune system, which is part of a larger and more complex system called the **lymphatic system,** has many organs and cells that must act in concert to protect people from infectious diseases (**Figure 12.7**). The lymphatic vessels contain fluid called lymph. At various intervals along the lymphatic vessels are nodules called **lymph nodes**.

TERMS

antibodies: proteins that recognize and inactivate viruses, bacteria, and other organisms and toxic substances that enter the body

immune system: an interacting system of organs and cells that protect the body from infectious organisms and harmful substances

lymph nodes: nodules spaced along the lymphatic vessels that trap infectious organisms or foreign particles

lymphatic system: a system of vessels in the body that trap foreign organisms and particles; the immune system is part of the lymphatic system

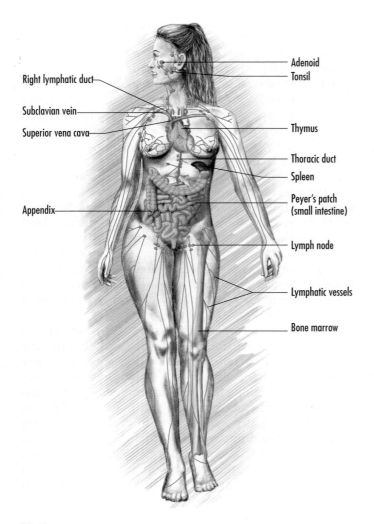

Right lymphatic duct

Subclavian vein

Superior vena cava

Appendix

Adenoid

Tonsil

Thymus

Thoracic duct

Spleen

Peyer's patch
(small intestine)

Lymph node

Lymphatic vessels

Bone marrow

■ **Figure 12.7**

The Lymphatic and Immune Systems
Bone marrow, lymph nodes, and other organs of the immune system are shown. The lymphatic system performs many functions in protecting the body from infectious diseases.

The "swollen glands" that people experience in the neck, under the arms, in the groin, or in other areas of the body are caused by enlarged lymph nodes that are engaged in filtering out infectious organisms or foreign particles capable of causing disease. Thus, swollen and sore lymph nodes are a sign that the body is fighting an infection.

Bone marrow, tonsils, adenoids, spleen, and thymus all produce cells that allow the body to mount an immune response against infectious microorganisms. When bacteria or viruses infect the body, the immune system produces diverse kinds of white blood cells that function in different ways to destroy them (**Table 12.4**).

The **T-cells** (also called T-lymphocytes) circulating in the blood are ready to attack infectious organisms immediately, because T-cells recognize the "foreign-ness" of specific proteins on the surface of bacteria, viruses, and other pathogens. The response of the T-cells

is called **cell-mediated immunity** because the T-cells attach directly to the infectious organisms and inacti-vate them. Once cells have been identified as foreign by the T-cells, the macrophages and other immune system cells complete the process of their destruction and elimination from the body.

The **B-cells** (also called B-lymphocytes) comprise the final and most effective immune system defense; the response of the B-cells is called **humoral immunity.** The B-cells function by producing antibodies, which recognize all proteins and other substances that are for-eign and potentially harmful to the human body.

All mammals have similar immune systems and manufacture antibodies; these immune systems evolved with the earliest animals on earth. Without a functional immune system, people and animals would quickly succumb to the countless infectious microor-ganisms in the environment. Because the immune sys-tems of all mammals are quite similar, researchers use rats, mice, and other small animals to study how cells of the immune system are synthesized and how they function.

The foreign proteins on viruses, bacteria, and other infectious organisms are called **antigens** (*antibody gen-erators*). Every person has a collection of B-cells circu-lating in the blood that can recognize any foreign pro-tein on any infectious organism in the world that may be encountered during a person's lifetime. How this col-lection of many millions of different B-cells develops in the human body is a fascinating but complex story, much of which is now well understood.

A particular B-cell can recognize a particular foreign antigen on a virus or bacterium and begin to make more B-cells just like itself. Eventually, these B-cells (at this stage called plasma cells) synthesize vast amounts of one specific kind of antibody that attaches to all of the specific pathogens in the body. Once the antibodies have recognized and inactivated them, other white blood cells finish the job of destruction. To produce the correct antibodies in large amounts takes about a week after an infection, which is why other quicker-acting immune system defense mechanisms are also needed.

The B-cells and T-cells interact among themselves in complex ways to produce a full-fledged immune response. Small molecules called **cytokines** coordinate the activities of the B-cells and T-cells. Many of the nat-ural cytokines, such as interferons and interleukins, that regulate functions of the immune system are now also manufactured by biotechnology companies. Some of these products are used in the treatment of cancer and other diseases in which the functions of the immune system are impaired.

T-cells are also divided into different classes according to their specific functions. Helper T-cells increase the proliferation of B-cells, killer T-cells destroy cancer cells and other pathogenic organisms, and suppressor T-cells retard the growth of other immune system cells. A special class of T-cells called

Table 12.4

Specialized White Blood Cells

All white blood cells originate in bone marrow and become specialized as they mature in different organs. Specialized cells carry out different functions of the immune system. The B-cells and T-cells recognize foreign proteins on infectious bacteria, viruses, and other organisms and substances. B-cells are converted to plasma cells that manufacture antibodies.

White Blood Cell Type	Description	Function	Life Span
Neutrophil	Spherical; with many-lobed nucleus, no hemoglobin, pink-purple **cytoplasmic granules**.	Cellular defense—phagocytosis of small microorganisms.	Hours to 3 days
Eosinophil	Spherical; two-lobed nucleus, no hemoglobin, orange-red staining **cytoplasmic granules**.	Cellular defense—phagocytosis of large microorganisms such as parasitic worms; releases anti-inflammatory substances in allergic reactions.	8 to 12 days
Basophil	Spherical; generally two-lobed nucleus, no hemoglobin, large purple-staining **cytoplasmic granules**.	Inflammatory response—contain granules that rupture and release chemicals enhancing inflammatory response.	Hours to 3 days
Monocyte	Spherical; **single nucleus** shaped like kidney bean, no cytoplasmic granules, cytoplasm often blue in color.	Converted to macrophages, which are large cells that entrap microorganisms and other foreign matter.	Days to months
B-lymphocyte	Spherical; round **singular nucleus**, no cytoplasmic granules.	Immune system response and regulation; antibody production sometimes causes allergic response.	Days to years
T-lymphocyte	Spherical; round **singular nucleus**, no cytoplasmic granules.	Immune system response and regulation; cellular immune response.	Days to years

CD4 cells are important indicators in the diagnosis and development of AIDS. When the level of CD4 cells in the blood falls, a person becomes extremely susceptible to infection by many different microorganisms, causing one of the more than two dozen infectious diseases that characterize AIDS.

Immunizations

One of the great achievements of modern medicine has been the development of **immunizations** (vaccinations) to prevent many serious infectious diseases caused by bacteria and, more important, by viruses. Viral diseases (whooping cough, measles, mumps, hepatitis, smallpox and polio) have been virtually eliminated or markedly reduced in the United States as a result of vaccinations.

TERMS

antigens: foreign proteins on infectious organisms that stimulate an antibody response

B-cells: cells of the immune system that produce antibodies

cell-mediated immunity: the response of T-cells to infections

cytokines: small molecules that coordinate the activities of B-cells and T-cells

humoral immunity: the response of B-cells to infections

immunizations: vaccinations to prevent a variety of serious diseases caused by both bacteria and viruses

T-cells: cells of the immune system that attack foreign organisms that infect the body

Vaccination is the administration, usually by injection (hence the name "shot"), of substances called **vaccines.** When you are vaccinated, inactivated viruses or bacteria (also toxins) are injected into the body. The body's immune system responds by producing antibodies (proteins) that can inactivate the infectious organisms. If you later encounter the active, disease-causing organisms, you are protected by "memory cells" that quickly produce the antibodies needed to destroy the infectious agents.

For example, the crippling disease poliomyelitis has been virtually eradicated in the United States as a result of the widespread use of the polio virus vaccine. The first polio vaccine was developed in 1954 by Jonas Salk, using chemically inactivated viruses. The polio vaccine now used is derived from a genetically inactivated virus developed in 1957 by Albert Sabin. Both methods of viral inactivation prevent the dead virus from causing disease and confer long-lasting immunity. However, a handful of polio cases occur each year as a result of the genetically inactivated polio vaccine now in use.

In general, vaccination is safe and effective in preventing a number of infectious diseases. Vaccinations are recommended for both children and adults, but vaccinations are crucial for young children and adolescents (**Figure 12.8**). Other vaccinations are recommended only for people at particular risk of exposure to a certain disease. For example, travelers to a country where cholera, typhoid fever, or hepatitis A is prevalent should be vaccinated for these diseases. Vaccination for influenza usually is recommended for people susceptible to lung infections, such as children and those who are elderly or have asthma.

In 2005, an improved vaccination for bacterial meningitis was approved in the United States. Each year about 3,000 Americans contract meningococcal disease, which infects the brain, spinal fluid, and blood. About 300 people die from this infection each year and others are seriously disabled. The new vaccine, called Menactra, is recommended for all adolescents aged 11 to 18, the group that is most at risk. The vaccine is not approved for children younger than 11.

Other New Vaccines

In 2006, a vaccine against several strains of human papillomavirus (HPV) was approved in order to protect women from developing cancer of the cervix. HPV is the most common sexually transmitted disease in the United States (see Chapter 11). About 10,000 American women are diagnosed with cervical cancer each year. For these reasons, the HPV vaccine (called Gardasil) is recommended for all females before they become sexually active. In 2007, a vaccine against herpes zoster was approved for use in adults older than 60 years. Herpes zoster viral infection causes chicken pox in children. In adults, it causes *shingles,* an extremely painful outbreak

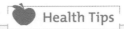 Health Tips

Boosting Immunity with Herbs

Several herbal remedies have been shown to safely and effectively stimulate the immune system. The herb echinacea, commonly known as coneflower, is an "immune booster"; that is, it stimulates certain cells of the body so that the immune system is better able to ward off disease and fight infection.

Laboratory studies of echinacea have shown that it stimulates phagocyte cells that help destroy cancer cells and infectious microorganisms. Echinacea also has been shown to stimulate the formation of interferon and tumor necrosis factor, substances in the body that fight infectious microorganisms and cancer cells. Other studies have shown that echinacea is about half as effective as steroid therapy in controlling the symptoms of arthritis.

Some people who use echinacea take it at the first sign of a cold and report that symptoms disappear within a day. Because some studies show that echinacea loses its ability to stimulate the immune system if taken on a daily basis, it is suggested that echinacea be taken for a few days, and then stopped for a few days, to maintain its stimulatory effects.

Another herb used to stimulate the immune system is *Astragalus membranaceus,* which has been used in China and other parts of Asia for thousands of years. The root is used in a dried form or boiled to make a broth or tea. Scientific studies of this herb show that it stimulates all functions of the immune system—in particular, the production of stem cells in bone marrow that are precursors to other immune system cells. Goldenseal is another herb purported to have immune-boosting properties.

of sores on the trunk of the body. A vaccine that will protect people from infection by hepatitis E virus (HEV) should soon become available. The lifetime risk of acquiring an HEV infection worldwide is 60%, and about 4% of HEV infections are fatal as a result of liver failure (Krawczynski, 2007). Like other hepatitis infections, there is no treatment for HEV, so a vaccine would be of great benefit to millions of people, particularly in Asia and Africa.

Vaccination Risks

Vaccination is widely regarded as one of the greatest public health achievements of all time and the principal cause of the dramatic global decrease in sickness and death from infectious diseases. Smallpox has been

TERMS

vaccines: inactivated bacteria or viruses that are injected or taken orally; the body responds by producing antibodies and cells that provide lasting immunity

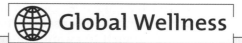 **Global Wellness**

The Long, Expensive Road to a New Vaccine

Severe diarrhea in children is a major cause of sickness and death around the world. Most cases of severe diarrhea are caused by rotaviruses. Approximately 2 million children die each year from rotavirus-induced diarrhea, primarily in Latin America and Africa. In the United States, about 50,000 people are infected by rotaviruses each year, and 20 to 40 die, usually children (King, 2005).

In 1998, the U.S. Food and Drug Administration (FDA) approved a vaccine that would prevent rotavirus-induced infections and diarrhea in children. Widespread immunization of millions of children around the world was expected to vanquish rotavirus deaths much as polio had been eliminated by the polio vaccine.

Wyeth, the drug company that developed the vaccine, had spent hundreds of million of dollars on large-scale clinical trials to prove the vaccine was safe and effective. However, an extremely rare, serious side effect was observed in about 1 in 10,000 children who received the shots. This did not prevent the FDA from giving its approval, however.

In 1999, after several children died from the rare side effect of the vaccination, the FDA halted sales of the drug in the United States. Meanwhile, another drug company, Glaxo Smith Kline (GSK), was also working on a rotavirus vaccine. Not wanting to risk the hundreds of millions of dollars that Wyeth lost, GSK decided to carry out its trials in poor countries first, thereby avoiding the need for FDA approval.

In Mexico, 1 in 50 children suffer from rotavirus infections, diarrhea, and possible death from dehydration. In July 2004, Mexico approved the use of the GSK vaccine. The vaccine proved to be 85% effective in preventing rotavirus infections and did not have the serious side effects of the previous vaccine. GSK has committed $550 million to construct a vaccine-manufacturing facility in Belgium. If the vaccine continues to be safe and effective in the poor countries that need it the most, GSK will probably seek FDA approval in a few years to market the vaccine in the United States.

Developing safe and effective vaccines is an incredibly costly and risky business. But the need for vaccines to protect against viruses that kill millions of people is too important a goal to give up.

Vaccine ▼ Age ▶	Birth	1 month	2 month	4 month	6 month	12 month	15 month	18 month	19–23 month	2–3 years	4–6 years
Hepatitis B[1]	HepB	HepB	HepB	see footnote[1]		HepB					
Rotavirus[2]			Rota	Rota	Rota						
Diphtheria, Tetanus, Pertussis[3]			DTaP	DTaP	DTaP	see footnote[3]	DTaP				DTaP
Haemophilus influenzae type b[4]			Hib	Hib	Hib[4]	Hib					
Pneumococcal[5]			PCV	PCV	PCV	PCV				PPSV	
Inactivated Poliovirus			IPV	IPV		IPV					IPV
Influenza[6]						Influenza (Yearly)					
Measles, Mumps, Rubella[7]						MMR					MMR
Varicella[8]						Varicella					Varicella
Hepatitis A[9]						HepA (2 doses)				HepA Series	
Meningococcal[10]										MCV4	

□ Range of recommended ages

■ Certain high-risk groups

■ **Figure 12.8**

Recommended Vaccination Schedule (2008) for Children Ages 0 to 6
In 2008, two new combination vaccines were approved that would reduce the number of shots a child receives. The first combines diphtheria, tetanus, pertussis, and polio in a single shot that can be given to preschool-aged children. The second combines five vaccines: diphtheria, tetanus, pertussis, polio, and *Haemophilus influenzae* type B (HiB). Four shots of this combination vaccine are required before age 2. Schedules are also available for those who missed shots or who need to catch up. Complete schedules are available at: http//www.cdc.gov/vaccines/.

eradicated from the world by vaccination, and polio is on the verge of being eradicated. Since 1912, the Centers for Disease Control and Prevention (CDC) has kept records of disease incidence before and after the introduction of a vaccine. In addition to the diseases just mentioned, there has been a 99% reduction in cases of measles, diphtheria, mumps, and rubella and a 97% reduction in whooping cough (pertussis) in the United States.

Vaccination is not 100% risk free. There are often mild reactions that generally disappear in a few days. Roughly speaking, about one per million vaccinations results in serious neurological damage or death. These cases are indeed tragic, but when counterbalanced by the millions of lives saved by being vaccinated, vaccination is probably as safe as taking a multivitamin. In recent years, however, a vocal minority has attacked vaccination as being unsafe and unnecessary despite firm scientific evidence to the contrary. Unsubstantiated claims about specific vaccines and adverse effects include the following:

Vaccine	Adverse Effect
Measles	Autism
Diphtheria, pertussis, and tetanus (DPT)	Sudden infant death syndrome
Haemophilus influenzae type B	Diabetes
Hepatitis B	Multiple sclerosis

Given the frequency and number of childhood vaccinations, it is not surprising that a condition surfaces by chance shortly after a child is vaccinated. It also is not surprising that distraught parents, looking for a cause, blame the vaccination. Despite rare problems, one medical expert advises, "Children everywhere deserve the protection that carefully developed, carefully monitored vaccines can provide against so much disease" (Campion, 2002).

The most controversy over vaccinations has arisen from the claim that a mercury-based preservative (thimerosal) in vaccines is the cause of the marked increase in autism among young children. The preservative has been used for years to prevent deterioration of the vaccines, particularly where refrigeration is not available. Because of parents' concerns, thimerosal was removed from all U.S. vaccines in 1999. A number of studies have concluded that there is no causal association between thimerosal-containing vaccines and childhood autism (Parker et al., 2004).

Despite scientific studies that support the overall safety of vaccinations, parents whose children acquired debilitating conditions after being vaccinated began to sue pharmaceutical companies that manufactured vaccines. Some of these suits were successful, and companies began to discontinue the manufacture of essential vaccines. To protect the nation's supply, the U.S. government passed the National Childhood Vaccine Injury Act in the late 1980s, which included establishment of a panel called the Vaccine Injury Compensation Program (VICP). This panel is empowered to award damages to parents who present evidence that their child's health was severely damaged by administration of a vaccine. In recent years the panel has been quite generous in making awards even though strong scientific evidence for the parents' case might be lacking (Offit, 2008). However, the existence of the VICP has provided the safeguards that encourage pharmaceutical companies to develop new and improved vaccines.

Vaccines for Unhealthy Lifestyles? Maybe Not Such a Good Idea

Diseases such as smallpox, polio, measles, mumps, diphtheria, typhoid fever, and others caused by viruses and bacteria have been eliminated or markedly reduced by vaccinations in the past century. The major threats to health in the present century derive from lifestyle behaviors such as smoking, drug addiction, and overweight. In the United States roughly 50 million people still smoke cigarettes, 6 million are addicted to drugs, and 60 million adults are characterized as obese. Now, researchers are trying to develop vaccines that will help people reduce their dependence on cigarettes, addictive drugs, and fattening foods.

The vaccines would work by binding to nicotine, methamphetamine, other drugs, or to an appetite-stimulating substance produced by the body called *ghrelin*. When bound to the vaccine, the drug or chemical cannot enter the brain to stimulate pleasure centers that are involved in addictive behaviors. Will this approach work? It's not yet proven, but early trials with a small number of subjects have demonstrated promising results.

Even if they work as hoped, the vaccinations are not a simple cure-all. Unlike vaccination for infectious diseases that provide long-term or lifetime immunity, lifestyle vaccinations are short lived and will probably have to be repeated every three months or so. Also, protection is not absolute; individuals still must modify their behaviors and stick to their decision to stop smoking, taking drugs, or eating to excess. The vaccinations facilitate the change in behavior but do not cure addictions. At some point the vaccinations must be stopped and persons must then rely on themselves not to return to unhealthy and destructive behaviors.

The use of behavior-modifying vaccines raises a number of ethical concerns, especially for children. Here are some ethical questions to consider.

- Should a judge sentence a robber who has stolen to obtain money to buy drugs to treatment by vaccination instead of a prison term?
- A parent wants his teenager vaccinated to prevent her from using nicotine and cocaine. The teenager

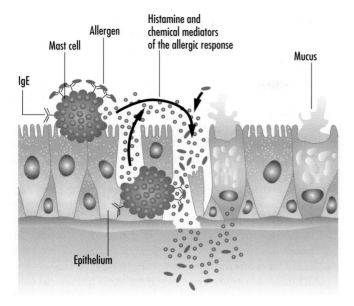

■ Figure 12.9

Chemistry of an Allergic Response

An allergen (a substance from a plant, insect, or other organism) binds to antibody proteins (IgE) on mast cells. This triggers the release of histamines and other inflammatory substances that characterize the allergic response. These reactions occur mainly in the nose, lungs, skin, and digestive tract.

objects but is underage. What is a physician to do in such a case?

- A pregnant woman is addicted to smoking and drugs. Can a judge force her to be vaccinated to protect the fetus from the effects of these substances?
- A parent wants her obese 8-year-old child vaccinated for the appetite protein to reduce his overeating behavior. If the child does not change his eating habits, the vaccinations might have to continue for years. No one knows the long-term effects of these vaccines on development. Should this child be vaccinated against the appetite-stimulating protein (ghrelin) to reduce his appetite?

Understanding Allergies

Allergies are the immune system's response to foreign substances called **allergens** that the body responds to as being harmful, but which usually are not. Pollens, molds, house dust, animal hair, foods, drugs, chemicals, and many other substances can act as allergens. The body responds by synthesizing a particular class of antibodies (immunoglobulin E, or IgE) that triggers the allergic reaction (**Figure 12.9**). No one knows why allergic responses evolved or what benefit they might have provided, but millions of people today can attest to the misery caused by allergic responses.

The allergic reaction is usually accompanied by the secretion of mucus and the release of **histamine,** an inflammatory chemical that is abundant in cells of the skin, respiratory passages, and digestive tract. That is why most allergic reactions are associated with the skin (eczema, hives, contact dermatitis), the respiratory passages (asthma, hay fever), and the digestive tract (swelling, vomiting, diarrhea).

Contact Dermatitis

Contact dermatitis affects millions of people because many of the things we touch or put on our skin can cause allergic reactions that manifest as rashes. Walking in the woods where poison ivy or poison oak grows can produce serious rashes in susceptible persons. Peeling a mango can cause people who are allergic to the skin of this fruit to break out in a rash; however, they usually can eat the flesh of the fruit without experiencing a reaction.

Contact dermatitis actually arises by two distinct mechanisms: *allergic contact dermatitis* involves reactions of the body's immune system cells with specific proteins that contact the skin, resulting in redness, itching, and inflammation. In contrast, *irritant contact dermatitis* does not involve an allergic response but rather is caused by cell damage and inflammation as a direct result of substances that contact the skin. Diaper rash is a common form of irritant dermatitis in babies. The hands also are frequently affected by irritant dermatitis arising from frequent contact with hard surface cleansers. Cosmetics also may cause irritant dermatitis, especially scented soaps and skin creams. When allergy tests are all negative and a skin condition persists, the condition is diagnosed as irritant dermatitis.

One increasingly common form of allergic contact dermatitis is latex allergy. It is estimated that latex allergies range from 1% to 6% in the general population, and among people who work in hospitals, such as nurses, the frequency is as high as 8%.

Latex is a form of sap extracted from rubber trees and is used in tires and rubber products of all kinds, especially protective gloves, which are used throughout the health care industry and other industries where materials must not be contaminated by touch. In the 1980s, the epidemics of AIDS and hepatitis B, both of

TERMS

allergens: foreign substances that trigger an allergic response by the immune system

contact dermatitis: an allergic reaction of the skin to something that is touched

histamine: a chemical released by cells in an allergic response; causes inflammation

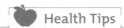 Health Tips

Getting Rid of Dust Mites May Help Allergies

Microscopic arachnids, dust mites, are a major contributor to peoples' allergies. Strictly speaking, it is not the mites but their feces that are highly allergenic. Mites live by the millions in bedding, clothing, carpets, drapes, wall coverings, and upholstered furniture. They are particularly abundant in mattresses, pillows, blankets, quilts, and fuzzy animals.

Getting rid of dust mites is difficult. Because they burrow deeply into objects and are so tiny, vacuum cleaners usually do not remove them. Removal of such items as carpets, plush furniture, drapes, and other cloth from rooms is recommended. Encasing mattresses and pillows with hypoallergenic covers may help. Frequent washing of pillows, bedding, and clothes is recommended. Soaking bedding and clothes in 1 part detergent to 3 parts eucalyptus oil for 30 minutes before washing removes 95% of mites and their debris. Try these steps if your allergies are severe.

which are caused by viruses transmitted in blood, created an unprecedented increase in the use of protective latex gloves. In 1987, the use of latex gloves in the United States jumped from 1 billion to 8 billion pairs, and it has been increasing ever since.

The milky latex sap extracted from rubber trees contains hundreds of different proteins; more than 50 have been purified and have been found to be allergenic. (Most allergies are caused by some kind of protein.) When these latex proteins interact with the skin, they can cause blisters and rashes. When they interact with sensitive mucous membranes in the vagina, rectum, or urethra from using condoms or other contraceptive devices, or during medical exams, the latex proteins can cause **anaphylactic shock** and death. Surgical instruments containing latex coverings or surgical gloves can cause severe reactions in sensitive patients.

The proteins in latex are similar to many proteins found in such fruits as banana, mango, papaya, cherry, peach, and avocado. Latex-related proteins also are found in milk, potatoes, and tomatoes. People who notice that they have become allergic to certain foods may, in fact, have become sensitive to latex. Physicians can test for latex allergies and can advise sensitive people on what foods to avoid.

Asthma

Asthma is a chronic disease involving inflammation and narrowing of the airways of the respiratory system, rendering breathing difficult and occasionally nearly impossible. The inflammation and narrowing are caused by the tightening of muscles that surround the airways, the swelling of cells that line the airways, and the production of mucus. Asthma is often a reaction to inhaling a respiratory irritant, such as cigarette smoke or cold air, or a substance to which someone is allergic. In susceptible individuals, exercise and stress also can trigger asthma. An intense asthmatic response is called an *asthma attack*. Asthma sufferers are counseled to avoid situations and substances that trigger attacks. They also can use inhalers that contain drugs that alleviate an asthma attack or drugs that help prevent attacks from occurring. Very severe asthma attacks may require emergency medical intervention. Asthma affects people of all ages, but it most often starts in childhood. In the United States, more than 22 million people suffer from asthma to some degree.

Although allergies are caused by both biological and environmental factors, they can also arise or be made worse by emotional upset and stress. Some asthmatic children often improve dramatically when separated from family situations that are stressful and emotionally upsetting. Adult asthmatics often notice that their attacks occur more frequently or become worse when they are upset or under stress that cannot be managed. Thus, asthmatics have an immunological makeup that makes them sensitive to allergens, but also respond physically to emotions and stress in ways that other people do not.

For example, an asthmatic person who gets into a violent argument with a husband, wife, or parent may begin to experience breathing difficulties, whereas an equally angry, nonasthmatic person would not. For these reasons asthma is classified as a psychosomatic disease, meaning that both the body and the mind contribute to the symptoms (see Chapter 2).

Since 1980, the prevalence of asthma and atopic dermatitis among children has doubled (Akinbami, 2006). Scientists are unsure of the reasons for this increase, but certain risk factors have been identified, including a family history of allergy, low socioeconomic status, non-Caucasian ethnicity, male gender, age greater than five years, and exposure to tobacco smoke, dust, or cockroaches (Higgins, Wakefield, & Cloutier, 2006). The roles of maternal diet, breastfeeding, the time of introduction of baby foods, and the use of formulas in developing allergies have also been examined (Greer et al., 2008). There is no evidence that maternal diet or breastfeeding affect the risk of asthma; however, in children with a family history of allergies, exclusive breastfeeding during the first four months may lessen the risk of atopic dermatitis and allergic reaction to cow's milk during the first two years of life.

Although the biological basis for allergies and asthma has been well documented by research, environmental factors also play a crucial role. African American children living in urban areas suffer from asthma much more frequently than other children, especially children living in the suburbs. Exposure to dust mites, cockroach feces, and other allergens may account for their higher rates of asthma.

Although the symptoms of asthma vary from mild to very severe, deaths resulting from asthma are rare, although increasing. People no longer need to suffer from asthma and endure the fear of not being able to breathe. A range of effective medicines is now available that can control symptoms, even the most serious. Short-acting bronchodilators that are inhaled at the onset of symptoms can provide immediate relief. For persistent asthma, short-term and long-term corticosteroid inhalers are available. With daily use, these can effectively suppress wheezing symptoms and breathing difficulties. Cromolyn inhalers also suppress symptoms in many people, and oral corticosteroids prevent asthma in the most severe cases.

Recently, a new class of drugs became available that blocks the actions of leukotrienes, chemicals produced in the body that cause muscles in the air passages to constrict. The goal of asthma treatment is to find the right medication at the lowest dose that leaves an asthmatic free of symptoms. And, of course, it is still important to eliminate as many allergens as possible from the home environment.

Many people with asthma receive allergy shots that are supposed to desensitize them to the substances (such as pollens or house dust) to which their bodies react. Some people do believe they benefit from the shots and that their asthma symptoms are reduced. However, scientific studies indicate that immunotherapy for asthma is of marginal benefit (Barnes, 1996). It is likely that getting a weekly shot acts as a powerful placebo in many asthmatics who believe in the efficacy of the injection.

Food Allergies

Food allergies, also called food intolerance, are allergic responses to a particular food. The reaction can be local (such as a stomach upset or swelling in the mouth) or it can involve the whole body. For example, an allergic reaction to a food or to an insect bite can cause hives to break out all over the body. Food allergies are most common in children but can occur in anyone at any age.

When people are tested for food allergies, six substances account for 90% of the allergic reactions—eggs, peanuts, milk, fish, soy, and wheat. Severe allergic reactions produce anaphylactic shock, a systemic reaction that can quickly cause death. Anaphylactic shock can be brought on by an immediate, strong allergic reaction to food, a bee sting, or a drug. Food allergies cause approximately 30,000 cases of anaphylactic reactions, 2,000 hospitalizations, and 200 deaths each year in the United States (Sampson, 2002).

Children are at particular risk of developing allergies to nuts, particularly peanuts. (Strictly speaking, the peanut is a legume, not a nut.) Children tend to outgrow most of their childhood allergies, but this is not true for nut allergies. In addition to peanuts, many persons are allergic to Brazil nuts, almonds, hazelnuts, and walnuts. Because the reactions in nut allergies can be quite serious, including anaphylactic shock, most people with nut allergies have to be extremely careful about what foods they eat because many manufactured products contain nuts.

Peanut allergies are especially common and dangerous—some people suffer to such a serious degree that even a minuscule amount of peanut protein can lead to anaphylactic shock and death. For years, people with peanut allergies had to learn how to live with them and avoid peanuts—something that is almost impossible to do all of the time. Now the health dangers of peanut allergies are widely recognized, and a number of steps have been taken to reduce potential exposure. Many airlines no longer serve peanuts, and many school lunch programs have eliminated peanuts or post warnings when they are served.

Eating in restaurants is always hazardous for those with peanut allergies, especially in Thai, Indonesian, or Vietnamese restaurants. If a pan has had peanut oil in it, enough remains to cause a reaction, even if it is cleaned before being used again. A 50-pound bag of dried molé from which the sauce is made has a handful of peanuts in it, more than enough to cause a reaction for someone eating in a Mexican restaurant.

A cutting board that has been used to cut peanuts a week ago still has enough peanut protein and oil on it to produce a reaction if it is used to cut something that goes into your dinner. A jelly jar also is very dangerous. If a spoon or knife that touched peanut butter is used to scoop out jelly, that jar is potentially harmful to someone with severe peanut allergies.

Shopping in a health food store is risky, although it is much better than it used to be when there were only a few scoops for all of the bins. Suppose someone uses a scoop to get some trail mix that has peanuts in it. That scoop is now contaminated. If it is used to scoop

TERMS

anaphylactic shock: a severe allergic reaction involving the whole body that can cause death

asthma: a chronic disease involving inflammation and narrowing of the airways that makes it difficult to breathe

food allergies: allergic responses to something that is eaten

food out of other bins, they all become contaminated with enough peanut protein to cause a reaction. Today, most health food stores have a separate scoop for each bin, and the scoop is wired down so it cannot be moved.

About 20% of people report food intolerance of one sort or another at some time in their lives, yet studies show that the actual number of people who are physiologically sensitive to foods actually is less (Rona et al., 2007). The discrepancy between what people report as an allergic reaction and what is demonstrated by allergy tests probably results from the power of suggestion. If someone reads or is told that many people are allergic to eggs, he or she may begin to experience a reaction when eggs are eaten. Also, vomiting after eating a particular food can produce a subsequent aversion or apparent allergic reaction to that food.

The power of suggestion in causing food allergies has been demonstrated by experiment (Jewett et al., 1990). In this study, patients who reported that they had a food allergy were given a series of injections to desensitize them to the food causing the allergy. One group was desensitized with a placebo (saline) injection; another group was desensitized with an injection of the allergen. Neither the patients nor the doctors knew which injections contained saline and which contained the allergen. Seven of 18 patients reported that their food allergies were prevented by the placebo shots. Others reported that their symptoms worsened when they received the saline placebo. Thus, placebo effects can cure food allergies or they can make them worse, as in this experiment. How we view food in our minds has a powerful effect on how it is received by the body (see Chapter 2).

The FDA now requires food manufacturers to list major food allergens on food product labels. Manufacturers are required to identify in plain English the presence of ingredients that contain protein derived from milk, eggs, fish, crustacean shellfish, tree nuts, peanuts, wheat, or soybeans.

Recognition of "Self"

The immune system is able to recognize and destroy virtually any foreign material, which is how it protects the body from infectious diseases. What prevents the immune system from recognizing and attacking the body's own cells and organs? By mechanisms that are not yet completely understood, the immune system can distinguish cells of the body that are recognized as "self" from all other cells (even those of another person) that are "nonself."

During fetal development, as the body's tissues are being formed, all of the antibody-producing cells that could attack the body's own cells are destroyed. It is not yet known how these particular antibody-producing

cells are selected out of the millions of different cells and destroyed, but such a mechanism is vital to protect the organs and tissues of the body from destruction.

Autoimmune Diseases

The immune system must function without mistakes to distinguish "self" from "nonself" because any mistake that caused antibodies to attack the body's own cells could result in serious disease or death. Unfortunately, mistakes in the functioning of the immune system do occur and produce **autoimmune diseases** (**Figure 12.10**). Some inherited disorders, fortunately quite rare, can result in the loss of the immune system's ability to distinguish "self" from "nonself." Environmental factors, such as viral infections, nutritional problems, and other unknown agents, may also cause the immune system to make mistakes that lead to autoimmune diseases.

Lupus erythematosus is an autoimmune disease that most frequently affects women between the ages of 18 and 35. In this disease, for reasons still unknown, antibodies are synthesized that attack the genetic information in cells (DNA), especially in cells of the blood vessels, skin, and kidneys. Many organs of the body are affected, and the symptoms—rashes, pain, and anemia—flare up and wane throughout life, which usually is shortened. In general, autoimmune diseases affect women more often than men.

Arthritis is one of the most common chronic diseases; approximately one in seven Americans has some form of arthritis. There are about 100 forms of arthritis and arthritis-related conditions, but the common denominator is pain and stiffness in joints throughout the body (**Figure 12.11**). The causes of arthritis vary widely, but many forms are the result of autoimmune disease in which the body's immune system mistakenly attacks cartilage and bone. Drugs can relieve many of the symptoms of arthritis, such as pain and inflammation, but the diseases themselves have no cure.

As with most chronic diseases of unknown etiology, the mind can exert a powerful role in controlling the symptoms of arthritis or in aggravating them. Relaxation and visualization exercises that emphasize mobility and comfort can be of great benefit in relieving the pain, stiffness, and inflammation associated with arthritis.

An autoimmune disease that affects the central nervous system is **multiple sclerosis (MS)**. Recent research suggests that MS may be initiated by a viral infection that somehow causes the immune system to produce antibodies that attack **myelin,** a substance that sheathes and insulates nerve fibers in the brain and spinal cord.

Although drugs can help reduce the symptoms of autoimmune diseases, these diseases are caused by complex malfunctions of the immune system. Because the mind also affects the functions of the immune system, many people who suffer from autoimmune dis-

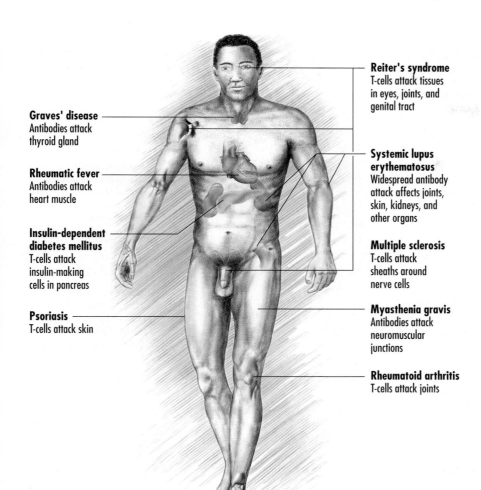

Graves' disease
Antibodies attack
thyroid gland

Rheumatic fever
Antibodies attack
heart muscle

**Insulin-dependent
diabetes mellitus**
T-cells attack
insulin-making
cells in pancreas

Psoriasis
T-cells attack skin

Reiter's syndrome
T-cells attack tissues
in eyes, joints, and
genital tract

**Systemic lupus
erythematosus**
Widespread antibody
attack affects joints,
skin, kidneys, and
other organs

Multiple sclerosis
T-cells attack
sheaths around
nerve cells

Myasthenia gravis
Antibodies attack
neuromuscular
junctions

Rheumatoid arthritis
T-cells attack joints

■ **Figure 12.10**

Autoimmune Diseases
These occur when the body's immune system goes
awry and cells of the immune system begin attacking
the body's own cells because they are mistakenly
recognized as foreign.

eases find relief in alternative therapies, mental relaxation techniques, and nutritional changes.

Organ Transplants

Like blood cells, all body cells have antigens on their surfaces that are different for everyone except identical twins. If tissue or organs from one person are grafted onto another, the immune system produces antibodies to the foreign cell antigens, causing destruction of the cells and rejection of the transplanted organ.

The more alike two persons are genetically, the more likely it is that the transplanted tissue will be accepted by the body. Identical twins are genetically identical; this is why tissue transplants between identical twins have the greatest chance of success. To minimize the rejection of transplanted organs, the **histocompatibility** (similarity of cell surface antigens) between the donor and recipient is determined by immunological tests. Just as red blood cells have particular groups of strongly antigenic proteins on their cell surfaces, so other cells in the body have antigenic proteins called **HLA (human leukocyte antigens)** that are

TERMS

arthritis: a variety of chronic diseases involving inflammation, stiffness, and pain in joints of the body

autoimmune diseases: mistakes in the functioning of the immune system that cause it to attack tissues in the body

histocompatibility: the degree to which the antigens on cells of different persons are similar

HLA (human leukocyte antigens): antigens that are measured to determine the suitability of an organ for transplantation from donor to recipient

lupus erythematosus: an autoimmune disease that mostly affects women

multiple sclerosis (MS): an autoimmune disease that affects the central nervous system

myelin: a substance that sheaths and insulates nerve fibers in the brain and spinal cord

■ **Figure 12.11**

Common Forms of Arthritis and Arthritis-Related Diseases and Their Symptoms

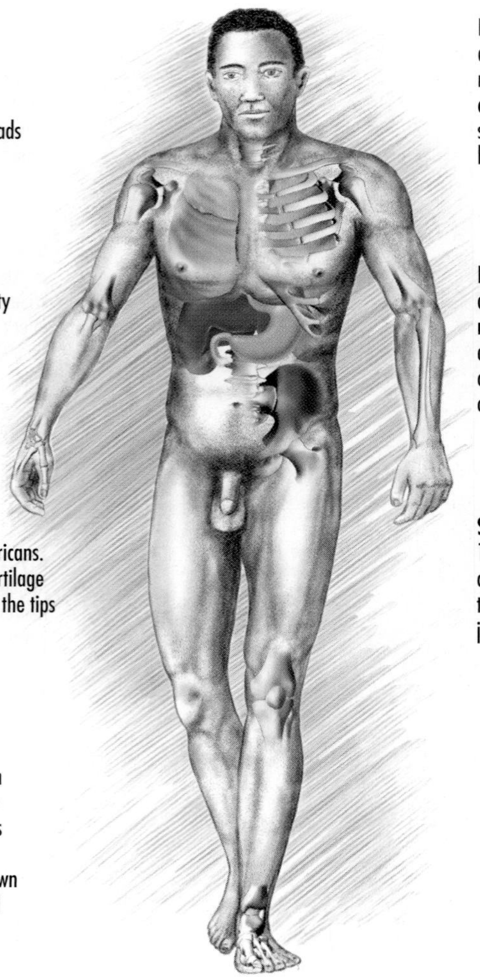

Ankylosing spondylitis affects about 300,000 Americans, usually younger men. It is caused by a spinal inflammation that spreads to other areas of the body.

Fibromyalgia affects about 4 million Americans, the majority of them women. The symptoms include fatigue, pain, insomnia, and stiffness but usually no inflammation of the joints.

Osteoarthritis affects an estimated 15 million older Americans. It is caused by the erosion of cartilage that acts as a shock absorber at the tips of bones.

Gout affects about 1 million Americans, the majority of them men. It is caused by the buildup of uric acid in the blood, crystals of which accumulate in joints, especially the big toe for unknown reasons. Overeating and alcohol are linked to the condition.

Polymyalgia rheumatica affects about 450,000 Americans, mostly older women. It is characterized by muscle pain and stiffness in the neck, shoulder, and hip.

Rheumatoid arthritis affects about 2 million Americans, the majority of them women. It strikes at any age and can eventually be crippling as a result of destruction of joints.

Scleroderma affects about 100,000 Americans. It is characterized by a thickening of the skin and inflammation of joints and internal organs.

crucial in determining whether a transplanted organ is accepted or rejected (**Figure 12.12**). The greater the similarity in HLA antigens between donor and recipient, the greater the chance that the tissue will be accepted and function normally in its new host. From the number of

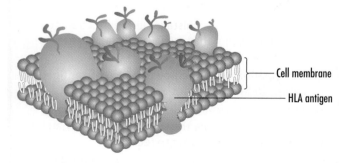

■ **Figure 12.12**

Antigens and the Immune System

A vast array of different HLA antigens is embedded in the outer membranes of cells, projecting beyond their surfaces. These antigens can be recognized by the body's immune cells and antibodies. Because every person's antigens are different, tissue transplanted from one person to another is usually rejected because the donor's HLA antigens are recognized as foreign and destroyed by the immune response of the recipient.

HLA antigens already determined, calculations show that there are so many different HLA combinations that each unrelated person is immunologically unique.

Today, the transplantation of hearts, kidneys, livers, and other organs has become a relatively common procedure in many hospitals. However, organ transplants are extremely costly, complicated procedures and are not always successful. Many more people are waiting for suitable organs than can be supplied from living donors or accident victims. Patients whose survival depends on the availability of a suitably matched organ often wait months to receive one, and often no organ becomes available before the patient dies (see Chapter 19).

The organ transplanted most often is the kidney. Because people have two kidneys, relatives sometimes donate one of their healthy kidneys to another close relative if their HLA genes are well matched. If the match is perfect for HLA antigens and ABO blood type, the success rate is 90% survival at one year. Brothers and sisters have one chance in four of inheriting the same HLA genes from their parents, which is why close relatives are examined first as possible donors. Bone marrow transplants also are used as a last resort in cases of aplastic anemia, acute leukemia, and radiation sickness.

Table 12.5

Permissible Transfusions Determined by ABO Blood Group

Blood group	Genotype	Antigens on red blood cells	Transfusions cannot be accepted from	Transfusions are accepted from
O (universal donor)	OO	None	A, B, AB	O
A	AA, AO	A	B, AB	A, O
B	BB, BO	B	A, AB	B, O
AB (universal recipient)	AB	A, B	None	A, B, AB, O

The rejection of transplanted organs can be controlled to some degree with **immunosuppressive drugs** (corticosteroids, cyclosporine); however, treatment with these drugs lessens resistance to infections and sometimes enhances development of other diseases. Long-term immunosuppressive drug therapy itself results in increased susceptibility to cancer. It makes more sense to seek ways to prevent kidney and heart diseases so that surgical transplants are not necessary.

Blood Transfusions: ABO and Rh Factors

In the early part of the twentieth century, a blood transfusion often led to the patient's death. Because the patient's immune system recognized the donor's blood cells as being "foreign," it attacked them with both T-cells and antibodies. The antibodies caused clumps of blood cells to form in the veins and arteries, impeding the flow of blood and oxygen and causing death.

The two most important human red blood cell surface antigens are the ABO and Rh-positive/Rh-negative proteins. There are actually many other groups of antigens on red blood cells, but these two are by far the most important ones in evoking an immune response that can endanger health. **Table 12.5** shows the pattern of donor–recipient ABO blood types that must be matched for a successful transfusion.

People with type O blood have neither A nor B antigens on their red blood cells and are **universal donors;** their blood cells will not stimulate an antibody response in the recipient, no matter what the blood type. People with type AB blood have both antigens present on their red blood cells and do not synthesize A or B antibodies because these antigens are recognized as "self" and those antibody-producing cells are destroyed. People with type AB blood are **universal recipients** and can accept blood from any of the four groups.

The Rh-positive antigen and the antibody that reacts against it cause problems primarily in pregnancy. A woman is Rh-negative if her red blood cells do not contain any of this antigen. If the red blood cells of a developing fetus have the Rh-positive antigen (inherited from the father) and if some of the fetus's red blood cells enter the mother's blood supply, production of anti-Rh antibodies can be stimulated by her immune system, which recognizes the fetal cells as foreign. This usually does not cause any difficulty during the first

pregnancy and might even go unnoticed until the woman becomes pregnant again.

Now, if the second fetus is also Rh-positive, the Rh-positive antibodies (synthesized during the first pregnancy) in the mother's blood attack the developing infant's red blood cells, resulting in anemia, brain damage, or even death. Fortunately, doctors can manage this problem safely and effectively. At the time the first child is delivered, the mother is given an injection of anti-Rh antibodies that destroys any Rh-positive antibodies in her blood. In this way, any danger to the fetus during a subsequent pregnancy is avoided.

AIDS and HIV

AIDS (acquired immune deficiency syndrome) was first recognized as a distinct disease in the early 1980s in the United States. It has progressively spread worldwide and now is a major threat to global health (see Chapter 11). More than half of the world's AIDS victims live in Africa, and most have no access to drugs that can retard the spread of **HIV (human immunodeficiency virus)** in the body. Left untreated, AIDS will eventually develop.

Although diseases, such as smallpox and polio can be traced back in human history for thousands of years, it is thought that AIDS is a disease of very recent origin. Considerable evidence now indicates that the virus

---

TERMS

AIDS (acquired immune deficiency syndrome): a syndrome of more than two dozen diseases caused by HIV

HIV (human immunodeficiency virus): the virus defined as the cause of AIDS

immunosuppressive drugs: drugs to suppress the functions of the immune system (e.g., after organ transplants)

universal donors: people whose blood is accepted by everyone during transfusion

universal recipients: people whose blood type is compatible with anyone else's blood

originally infected chimpanzees and probably infected humans who ate chimpanzee meat or who received bites or scratches while handling infected chimpanzees. After infecting people, the virus gradually changed its genetic makeup, evolving into a virus that could infect human immune system cells and destroy them. At least two distinct strains of HIV have been isolated from patients with AIDS, and it is likely that other strains will emerge as the virus spreads around the world.

AIDS is called a syndrome because it is defined by the appearance of any one of several different infectious diseases. It also is characterized by a very low level of a particular immune system cell called the CD4 T-cell. In an uninfected person the CD4 T-cell level is 800 to 1,200 cells/milliliter; in an AIDS patient the level can be 100 cells/milliliter or less. Once HIV infects CD4 T-cells, it replicates and releases viruses that infect additional cells.

HIV is a very small virus with little genetic information; however, it is very effective at infecting cells. One reason for the efficiency is HIV's ability to take control of an infected cell's normal biochemical activities and utilize them during infection. The elements of a cell that HIV takes over are called *dependency factors*. More than 275 cellular HIV dependency factors have been identified that play some role in the ongoing infection and continued virus production. The importance of identifying these HIV dependency factors is that some are potential targets for drugs that could prevent growth of HIV in cells. One such drug that blocks HIV dependency factor CCR5 has already been approved for use.

AIDS and the Immune System

Infection with HIV gradually weakens the body's immune system, exposing it to **opportunistic infections** caused by any of a wide variety of microorganisms. AIDS patients become progressively weaker with each infection and eventually die. The course of HIV infection is unpredictable; some individuals progress to full-blown AIDS and die within months. Others have no symptoms even after 10 years or more of HIV infection (**Figure 12.13**).

The mystery of long-term survival of untreated HIV-infected individuals has now been partially solved. Modern gene-scanning techniques have discovered three human genes that are unique to the long-term HIV-infected survivors; the products of these genes apparently keep the HIV level low enough to maintain immune function and prevent development of AIDS.

For the majority of HIV-infected patients, powerful drugs must be taken to keep HIV in check and prevent progression to AIDS. More than 30 anti-HIV drugs are currently available for treating AIDS. These drugs fall into several different classes: nucleoside reverse transcriptase inhibitors (NRTIs), non-nucleoside reverse transcriptase inhibitors (NNRTIs), protease inhibitors (PIs), fusion inhibitors, entry inhibitors, and HIV integrase and transfer inhibitors. Drugs usually are given in combinations to maximize effectiveness and reduce the chance that the patient will develop a drug-resistant strain of HIV. Drugs must be taken daily to prevent HIV proliferation. Because all of these drugs are toxic, there is a time limit as to how long they can be taken. Also, because of cost and other considera-

■ **Figure 12.13**

HIV and the Immune System
After infection, the virus level rises sharply in the blood, but within three months is undetectable. However, the virus is usually multiplying slowly in lymph nodes. The infected CD4 T-cells gradually decrease in number over many years. At some point, the immune system is weakened so that the person becomes susceptible to opportunistic diseases. Although this figure shows a disease latency of 8 years, some HIV-positive individuals have had no symptoms for as long as 15 years.

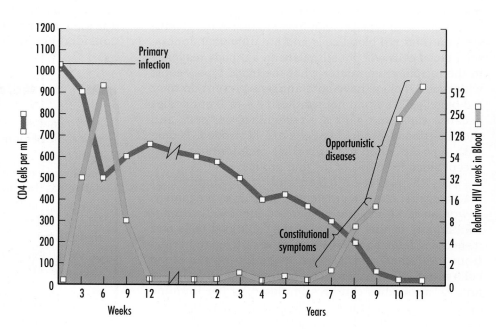

tions, not all AIDS patients receive the most effective drug regimens.

Although treating HIV infections is effective, a cure for HIV/AIDS is still a remote hope. Eventually, scientists hope to develop a vaccine for HIV infection; although many potential vaccines have been tested, none has proved effective. In Asia and Africa, millions of people are still becoming infected with HIV annually; however, they have little hope of receiving the expensive and complicated treatments used in the United States and other Western countries. In some countries in Africa, HIV infection rates exceed 20%. In South Africa and Zimbabwe, as many as one-half of the population is infected. Average life expectancy in these countries is falling rapidly.

The AIDS Antibody Test

Upon infecting a person, HIV acts like all other viral infections by stimulating synthesis of antibodies capable of inactivating the virus. Detection of these antibodies is the basis of the **AIDS antibody test.** In reality, the test is an indirect measure of HIV infection; it does not measure whether a person has AIDS or will get AIDS.

The test is positive only after antibodies have reached a detectable level, which can take several weeks or even months after infection. In the interim, a person is highly infectious but will show negative results on the AIDS anti-

body test. Thus, even a recent negative AIDS antibody test may not mean that a person is uninfected if the person has been sexually active or uses injected drugs.

Another problem with AIDS antibody tests is false-positive results that create unnecessary anxiety. A false positive means that the test shows that the person has antibodies in his or her blood that resemble ones produced in response to HIV. In reality, the person is not infected and the test is in error. Infection by other viruses or bacteria whose antigens resemble those of HIV can lead to a false-positive result on the HIV antibody test. Any positive AIDS test result should be rechecked. The most accurate test for HIV infection is the **Western blot,** which tests for the presence of specific HIV proteins.

Preventing HIV Infection

Compared with other viral infections, such as ones that cause colds, flu, or hepatitis, HIV is not very infectious. The virus is *never* transmitted by casual contact between an infected person and uninfected persons. "Never," in this context, means that no well-documented cases of HIV infection have been reported except as a result of sexual intercourse or the receipt of HIV-contaminated blood (see Chapter 11 for a discussion of the sexual transmission of HIV). HIV is not transmitted in saliva, spit, sweat, air, water, or by objects that have been used by an HIV-infected person.

Preventing Infections

Infections to some degree are unavoidable. However, the elements of healthy living that we have been emphasizing can both reduce the risk of contracting an infectious disease and also hasten recovery. Foremost is maintaining health by proper nutrition and a reasonable amount of exercise. These factors, as well as sufficient rest and sleep, increase the ability of the immune system to fight infectious organisms.

Vaccinations against certain infections can provide almost complete protection. Check your record of immunizations with your family physician and update

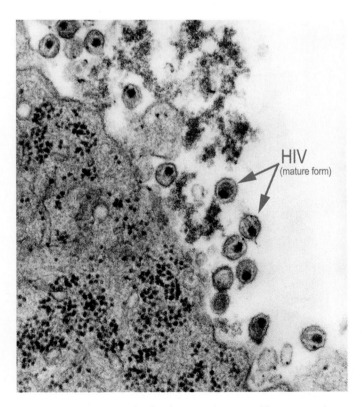

HIV
(mature form)

The AIDS virus as seen under the electron microscope. The arrows point to human immunodeficiency viruses being released from infected cells.

| TERMS |

AIDS antibody test: detects antibodies in blood that are produced in response to infection by HIV

opportunistic infection: any infectious disease in a patient with a weakened immune system; often occurs in AIDS patients

Western blot: a test to determine the presence of specific HIV proteins; very accurate

any that have not been received on schedule or that you are not sure that you received as a child. Many infections, such as mumps or measles, that are usually mild in childhood can be serious if acquired as an adult.

Never forget that the mind interacts with the immune system and also contributes to the body's propensity to ward off or to succumb to infections. Stressful situations and emotional upsets lower the body's defenses and make it more vulnerable to infectious microorganisms. Finally, use common sense and stay away from people and situations that are known to carry a high risk of infection. For example, do not travel to an area that is having a cholera epidemic. Do not expose yourself unnecessarily to people with colds, flu, chicken pox, or other highly contagious diseases. With reasonable precautions many infectious diseases are preventable. And by maintaining good health, the body will quickly and completely recover from most infections when they do occur.

Critical Thinking About Health

1. Describe one infectious disease you have had in the past few years (other than a cold). Discuss the following: (a) how you think you caught the disease, (b) what kind of microorganism caused it, (c) what the symptoms were, (d) how the disease was treated, and (e) any advice you were given on how to avoid contracting the disease in the future. Have you made any changes in your lifestyle to reduce the risk of contracting an infectious disease as a result of this experience?

2. What kind of infectious disease worries you the most: Lyme disease, AIDS, hepatitis, tuberculosis, sexually transmitted diseases in general, or others? Explain your concerns over contracting this disease, including any circumstances in your life that might have given rise to your concerns. Describe all that you know about this particular disease and how your concerns have altered your lifestyle or behaviors.

3. Find out all that you can on foodborne infectious diseases. Describe the kinds of microorganisms in foods that cause disease and ways that people can protect themselves from becoming infected. Do you have any concerns about the foods that you eat? Can you reduce or eliminate these concerns by making changes in your diet?

4. A variety of mind–body exercises is effective in controlling the symptoms of allergies, asthma, arthritis, and other immune system diseases. Learn as much as you can about how the immune system works. Discuss how you think the mind affects the immune system and how it can affect symptoms of the diseases just mentioned. Have you had any personal experience in using your mind to change the symptoms of a disease that has its roots in some form of immune system malfunction?

Health in Review

- Infectious diseases are caused by a myriad of pathogenic organisms: viruses, bacteria, fungi, protozoa, and worms. Growth of certain microorganisms in the body can cause a wide range of diseases and sickness; some produce only mild symptoms, but others produce serious disease and death.
- Some pathogenic microorganisms are easily passed from one person to another and cause communicable diseases.
- Some infectious diseases are caused by a vector, such as an insect or other animal, that transmits the pathogenic microorganism to an uninfected person.
- Hepatitis B and C infections are transmitted in blood and affect millions of people worldwide.
- In the United States, emerging infectious diseases are of concern: West Nile virus that causes encephalitis is one. Concerns over possible SARS and avian flu epidemics are also high.
- Many pathogenic bacteria are becoming resistant to antibiotics, making treatment of serious infectious diseases difficult.
- Antibiotics kill microorganisms but do not kill viruses, which are not alive in the sense that cells are.
- Infectious disease is fought in four ways: sanitation, antibiotics, vaccination, and healthful living.
- Vaccinations are vital to preventing serious infections. Approved vaccines are safe except in rare cases of adverse reactions.

- The skin and mucous membranes keep harmful substances from entering the body.
- Specialized white blood cells circulate in the body, attacking and destroying invading foreign organisms.
- The immune system produces cells that make antibodies, which are proteins that recognize any foreign substance or organism.
- Malfunctioning of the immune system causes autoimmune diseases and allergies.
- Each person carries a unique set of antigens on cells of the body that makes tissues and organs unique to each individual.
- Transplantation of organs or blood requires that the donor and recipient be matched with respect to histocompatibility, which is the matching of HLA or ABO antigens.
- AIDS results from infection by HIV, which destroys CD4 cells of the immune system. Immunodeficiency leads to opportunistic infections that eventually cause death.
- Long-term survivors of HIV infection have genes that make them resistant to infection by HIV and to development of AIDS.
- Many drugs help to keep HIV in check in persons infected with AIDS.

Health and Wellness Online

The Web contains a wealth of information about health and wellness. By accessing the Internet using Web browser software, you can gain a new perspective on many topics presented in *Health and Wellness*, Tenth Edition. Access the Jones and Bartlett Publishers Web site at **health.jbpub.com/hwonline**.

References

Aiello, A. I., Larson, E. L., & Levy, S. B. (2007). Consumer antibacterial soaps: Effective or risky? *Clinical Infectious Diseases, 45,* Supplement 2, 137–147.

Akinbami, L. J. (2006). The state of childhood asthma, United States, 1980–2005. Advance data from Vital and Health Statistics no. 381. Hyattsville, MD: National Center for Health Statistics. Retrieved October 14, 2008, from www.cdc.gov/nchs/data/ad/ad381.pdf

Barnes, P.J. (1996). Is immunotherapy for asthma worthwhile? *New England Journal of Medicine, 334,* 530–531.

Campion, E. W. (2002). Suspicions about the safety of vaccines. *New England Journal of Medicine, 347,* 1474–1475.

Cohen, J.I. (2000). Epstein-Barr virus infection. *New England Journal of Medicine, 343,* 481–490.

Greer, F. R., et al. (2008). Effects of early nutritional interventions on the development of atopic disease in infants and children: The role of maternal dietary restriction, breastfeeding, timing of introduction of complementary foods, and hydrolyzed formulas. *Pediatrics, 121,* 183–191.

Harvey, R., et al. (2007). Nasal saline irrigations for the symptoms of chronic rhinosinusitis. *Cochrane Database of Systematic Reviews.* Retrieved August 7, 2007, from http://www.cochrane.org/reviews/en/ab006394.html

Higgins, P. S., Wakefield, D., & Cloutier, M. M. (2006). Risk factors for asthma and asthma severity in nonurban children in Connecticut. *Chest, 128,* 3846–3853.

Holmes, E. C. (2004). 1918 and all that. *Science, 303,* 1787–1788.

Jewett, D. L., et al. (1990). A double-blind study of symptom provocation to determine food sensitivity. *New England Journal of Medicine, 323,* 429–433.

King, J. (2005, June). The vaccine that almost wasn't. *Technology Review,* 36–38.

Krawczynski, K. (2007). Hepatitis E vaccine: Ready for prime time. *New England Journal of Medicine, 356,* 949–950.

Lauer, G.M., & Walker, B.D. (2001). Hepatitis C virus infection. *New England Journal of Medicine, 345,* 41–52.

Morse, D.L. (2003). West Nile virus—not a passing phenomenon. *New England Journal of Medicine, 348,* 2173–2174.

National Center for Complementary and Alternative Medicine. (2008). An introduction to probiotics. Retrieved February 20, 2009, from http://nccam.nih.gov/health/probiotics

Offit, P. A. (2008). Vaccines and autism revisited: The Hannah Poling case. *New England Journal of Medicine, 358,* 2089–2091.

Parker. S. J., et al. (2004). Thimerosal-containing vaccines and autistic spectrum disorder: A critical review of published original data. *Pediatrics, 114,* 793–804.

Peiris, J. S. M., et al. (2003). The severe acute respiratory syndrome. *New England Journal of Medicine, 349,* 2431–2440.

Raloff, J. (2008). Nurturing our microbes. *Science News, 173,* 138–140.

Rona, R. J., et al. (2007). The prevalence of food allergy: A meta-analysis. *Journal of Allergy and Clinical Immunology, 120,* 638–646.

Sampson, H. A. (2002). Peanut allergy. *New England Journal of Medicine, 346,* 294–298.

Silverman, N., & Paquette, N. (2008). The right resident bugs. *Science, 319,* 734–735.

Singer, E. (2007, July/August). Our microbial menagerie. *Technology Review,* 58–61.

Taubenberger, J.K. (2005, January). Capturing a killer flu virus. *Scientific American,* 63–71.

Taubenberger, J. K., Morens, D. M. & Fauci, A. S. (2007). The next influenza pandemic: Can it be predicted? *Journal of the American Medical Association, 297,* 2025–2027.

Vastag, B. (2002). "Cipromania" and "superclean" homes are now increasing antibiotic resistance. *Journal of the American Medical Association, 288,* 947–948.

Vazquez, M., et al. (2008). Effectiveness of personal proactive measures to prevent Lyme disease. *Emerging Infectious Diseases, 142,* 210–216.

Writing Committee of the Second WHO Consultation on Clinical Aspects of Human Infection with Avian Influenza A (H5N1) Virus. (2008). Update on avian influenza A (H5N1) virus infection in humans. *New England Journal of Medicine, 358,* 261–272.

Suggested Readings

Bakalar, N. (2003). *Where the germs are: A scientific safari.* New York: Wiley. If you are curious about germs, both healthy and unhealthy, this is a fun book for information.

Cowley, G. (2002, April 22). Hepatitis—the insidious spread of a killer virus. *Newsweek,* 47–53. Covers the epidemic of hepatitis C infections and the expected surge in the number of people with serious liver disease.

Finkel, M. (2007, July). Bedlam in the blood: Malaria. *National Geographic,* 32–67. Describes in depth the efforts that are being made worldwide to eradicate malaria, a disease that is acquired by 500 million people each year.

Harder, B. (2004, November 27). Asthma counterattack. *Science News,* 344–345. Describes studies that show how cleaning up the home environment can reduce asthma attacks in children.

Mitman, G. (2007). *Breathing space: How allergies shape our lives and landscapes.* New Haven, CT: Yale University Press. An excellent discussion of all aspects of allergies, including their history, treatment, desensitization, and ways to avoid allergens.

National Center for Infectious Diseases. (2003). Health information for international travel, 2003–2004. Available: http:/bookstore.phf.org. Contains a wealth of information on specific countries, diseases likely to be encountered, and drugs and vaccinations recommended.

Specter, M. (2003, February 3). The vaccine. *The New Yorker,* 54–65. A devastating account of the AIDS epidemic and the efforts scientists are making to find a vaccine to prevent HIV infection.

Specter, M. (2005, February 28). Nature's bioterrorist. *The New Yorker,* 50–61. An excellent article that explains why the current bird flu epidemic in Asia poses such a grave threat of a human flu pandemic.

Spector, M. (2007, December 3). Darwin's surprise. *The New Yorker,* 64–73. Explains how human health and evolution actually depend on viruses and bacteria within us. If you read no other science article, read this one.

Taubenberger, J. K. (2005, January). Capturing a killer flu virus. *Scientific American,* 63–71. An exciting account of how the genetic information of the deadly 1918 flu virus was reconstructed from frozen remains of victims.

Recommended Web Sites

Please visit **health.jbpub.com/hwonline** for links to these Web sites.

Allergy Newswire
A good site for current information and advice on allergic conditions.

Emerging Infectious Diseases
An online journal from the U.S. Centers for Disease Control and Prevention (CDC).

Food Allergy Network
Information and education on food allergies.

MedlinePlus on Infectious Diseases
From the U.S. National Library of Medicine.

U.S. Centers for Disease Control and Prevention
The CDC is the research and education division of the U.S. Public Health Service.

World Health Organization Report on Infectious Diseases
Updates on outbreaks of infectious diseases around the world.

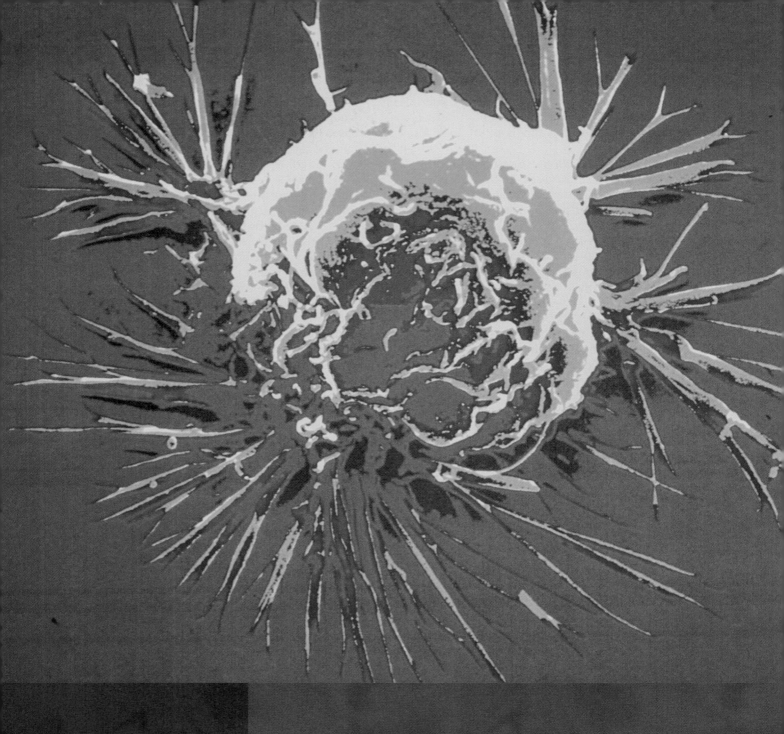

Health and Wellness Online: **health.jbpub.com/hwonline**

Study Guide and Self-Assessment

Chapter Thirteen

Cancer: Understanding Risks and Means of Prevention

Learning Objectives

1. Identify and describe the most important ways to prevent cancer.

2. Briefly discuss the incidence of cancer today and why mortality has not fallen.

3. Define the following terms: *cancer, tumor, benign tumor, malignant tumor, metastasis,* and *xenoestrogen*.

4. Explain the difference between inherited diseases and genetic diseases.

5. Describe the kinds of environmental agents that cause cancer.

6. Explain ways to prevent skin cancer.

7. Discuss some risk factors associated with breast cancer.

8. Describe how to do a breast self-exam (BSE).

9. Discuss how cigarette smoke contributes to cancer.

10. Discuss the association between diet and cancer.

11. Briefly describe the three medical treatments for cancer.

12. Describe several coping mechanisms for someone with cancer.

13. Explain the risks and benefits of being tested for a cancer susceptibility gene.

On the basis of recent statistics, one of two men and one of three women in the United States will develop some type of cancer during their lifetime; in 2008, it was estimated that approximately 565,650 Americans would die from cancer. Despite the dismal statistics, the news about cancer is not all bad. Most cancers *are* preventable if people adopt healthy lifestyles. Avoiding cigarette smoke and tobacco in *any* form is the most important action anyone can take to prevent cancer, especially lung and pancreatic cancers, which are most often incurable. Cigarette smoke is estimated to be the primary cause in the development of at least 30% of all cancers (see Chapter 17). Overweight and obesity, low levels of physical activity, and poor nutrition also increase the risk of cancer.

> Pain has an element of blank:
> it cannot recollect
> when it began, or if there were
> a day when it was not.
>
> *Emily Dickinson*

A healthy diet that includes low levels of beef and high levels of fresh fruits, vegetables, and fiber will also markedly reduce the risk of cancer. Avoiding excess exposure to ultraviolet (UV) radiation in sunshine and tanning booths is essential to lessen the risk of skin cancer later in life. Finally, knowing what chemicals in the environment are cancer-causing can help you avoid dangerous substances. Overall, if everything known about cancer prevention were practiced by everyone, up to two-thirds of *all* cancers could be prevented.

Another positive note is that about half of all cancer patients can be cured if their cancer is detected at an early stage before cancer cells have spread. Being "cured" of cancer means that a person's life expectancy is the same as for a person who never had cancer. It is important to have cancer screening tests as indicated for your age and risk group (**Table 13.1**). You should also watch for early warning signs in functions of the body that may indicate that a cancer is developing.

Understanding Cancer

Incidence of Various Cancers

The annual number of new cases of cancer at various body sites is shown in (**Figure 13.1**). Although the incidence of some cancers has decreased somewhat since 2000, the incidence of other cancers, such as non-Hodgkin's lymphoma and melanoma, has increased. Thus overall, cancer rates have not changed much since the 1980s, despite th introduction of sophisticated medical screening methods. That the incidence of cancer has not changed suggests that medical science and society at large must turn more attention to prevention if cancer rates are to decline.

What Is Cancer?

The term *cancer* comes from the Latin word meaning "crab." Cancer was characterized as a crablike disease by the Greek physician Hippocrates, who observed that cancers spread throughout the body, eventually cutting off life. Now **cancer** generally is defined as the unregulated multiplication of specific cells in the body. The word *cancer* actually refers to more than 200 different

---

Table 13.1

Recommended Screening Tests for Cancer Detection and Prevention

Test	Sex	Age	Frequency of testing
Colonoscopy[1]	M & F	50 and over	Every 10 years
Flexible sigmoidoscopy[1]	M & F	50 and over	Every 5 years
Double-contrast barium enema[1]	M & F	50 and over	Every 5 years
Fecal occult blood test (FOBT)[1]	M & F	50 and over	Every year
Digital (finger) rectal examination[2]	M	50 and over	Every year
Prostate specific antigen[2]	M	50 and over	Every year
Pap test[3]	F	18 and over	Women should begin getting a Pap test with the start of sexual activity, but no later than at 21 years of age, and repeat the test at least every 3 years
Breast self-examination[4]	F	20 and over	Every month
Breast clinical examination[4]	F	20–40	Every 3 years
		40 and over	Every year
Mammography[3]	F	40 and over	Every 1–2 years

[1]Colorectal cancer screening fact sheet. CDC Publication No. 99-6949. CMS Publication No. 11011 Revised August 2008.

[2]Prostate cancer screening: A decision guide. U.S. Department of Health and Human Services, Centers for Disease Control and Prevention (CDC), September 2006.

[3]Department of Health and Human Services, Centers for Disease Control and Prevention, Fact sheet: Breast and Cervical Cancer Detection Program, 2008.

[4]Breast Cancer Screening, Centers for Disease Control and Prevention, 2008.

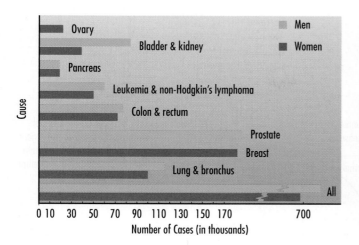

Figure 13.1

Estimated Number of New Cancer Cases, United States, 2008

Source: Data from U.S. National Cancer Institute.

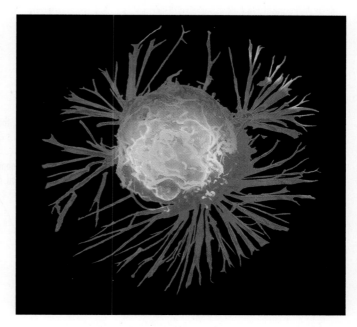

Electron micrograph of a breast cancer cell.

diseases, but in all cases, certain body cells multiply in an abnormal, unregulated manner.

Normally, the growth and reproduction of every cell in the body are regulated; this regulation, in turn, determines the size and functions of tissues and organs. If a normal body cell begins to grow abnormally and reproduces too rapidly, a mass of abnormal cells eventually develops that is called a **tumor**. A tumor generally contains millions of genetically identical abnormal cells before it can be detected or diagnosed.

If the cells of the tumor remain localized at the site of origin in the body and if they multiply relatively slowly, the tumor is said to be benign. **Benign tumors,** such as cysts, warts, moles, and polyps, do not spread to other parts of the body. Benign tumors usually can be removed surgically and generally are not a threat to life; in fact, a benign tumor weighing several hundred pounds was surgically removed from a woman who recovered fully. Benign tumors cannot regrow if all of the abnormal cells are removed by surgical excision of the tumor.

Malignant tumors are composed of cells that multiply rapidly, have other abnormal properties that distinguish them from normal cells, and invade other normal tissues. In particular, malignant cells may have altered shapes and cell-surface characteristics that contribute to their rapid proliferation. Many malignant cells also have abnormal chromosomes or altered genes, and they manufacture abnormal proteins. The numerous altered properties of malignant cells enable a **pathologist,** a physician who specializes in the causes of diseases, to determine whether the cells removed from a tumor are malignant and to what degree, a process called "staging" the tumor.

The cells of most malignant tumors also undergo **metastasis,** a process in which cells detach from the original tumor, enter the lymphatic system and bloodstream, and are carried to other organs. Once the malig-

nant cells spread to other organs, they develop into new tumors that often grow more rapidly than cells in the original tumor. Metastases and the growth of new tumors in many organs of the body eventually disrupt a vital body function, which is the cause of death.

Cancers are medically classified according to the organ or kind of tissue in which the tumor originates. The four major categories of cancers are *carcinomas, sarcomas, leukemias,* and *lymphomas* (**Figure 13.2**). Within these major categories are numerous subgroups that generally describe the organ in which the cancer originates, such as adenocarcinoma of the stomach or small cell carcinoma of the lung. About half of all human cancers originate in one of four organs: the lung, breast, prostate, or colon, which is why so much research is devoted to these particular forms.

TERMS

benign tumor: a tumor whose cells do not spread to other parts of the body

cancer: unregulated multiplication of cells in the body

malignant tumor: a tumor whose cells spread throughout the body

metastasis: the process by which cancer cells spread throughout the body

pathologist: a physician who specializes in the causes of diseases

tumor: a mass of abnormal cells

■ **Figure 13.2**

Four Major Categories of Cancers and
Approximate Frequencies of Occurrence

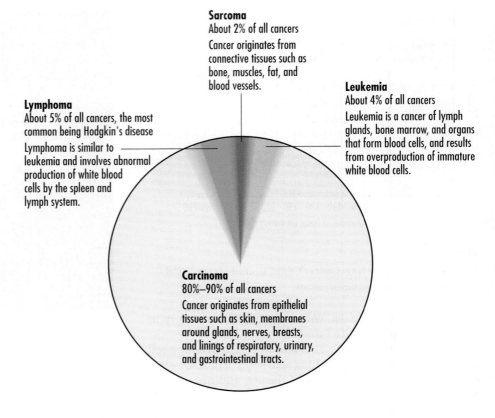

Sarcoma
About 2% of all cancers
Cancer originates from
connective tissues such as
bone, muscles, fat, and
blood vessels.

Lymphoma
About 5% of all cancers, the most
common being Hodgkin's disease
Lymphoma is similar to
leukemia and involves abnormal
production of white blood
cells by the spleen and
lymph system.

Leukemia
About 4% of all cancers
Leukemia is a cancer of lymph
glands, bone marrow, and organs
that form blood cells, and results
from overproduction of immature
white blood cells.

Carcinoma
80%–90% of all cancers
Cancer originates from epithelial
tissues such as skin, membranes
around glands, nerves, breasts,
and linings of respiratory, urinary,
and gastrointestinal tracts.

Cancer does not develop all at once in a cell. Several changes must occur in the genetic information (i.e., DNA) carried in a single cell before it can become a cancer cell and multiply into a tumor. Cells change their abnormal growth properties one step at a time; each genetic change pushes the cell further along the spectrum of abnormal growth. Not all cells acquire the same genetic changes, nor can anyone predict when the changes will occur. That explains why some cancers develop and grow rapidly and cause death in months, whereas other cancers grow so slowly that the person eventually dies from a cause other than cancer.

Once a tumor has been detected, cells can be removed from it in a procedure called a **biopsy;** the cells are then examined under the microscope by a pathologist. In stage I, cancer cells can be distinguished from normal cells. The cancer cells are still localized (usually referred to as cancer *in situ*) and surgical removal of the tumor usually results in a cure. In stage II, the cancer cells have begun to metastasize and may have migrated to nearby lymph nodes. That is why lymph nodes near the tumor are removed and examined during surgery to determine if cancer cells have spread. By stage III, the cancer cells have spread throughout the body, and tumors may have begun to grow in other organs. In stage IV, often a terminal stage, tumors are found throughout the body and usually are resistant to treatment.

The numbers of deaths from cancer by organ and by sex are shown in **Figure 13.3**. Lung cancer is now the leading cause of death in both women and men. Cancer of the colon and rectum, the third leading cause of death for both men and women, is believed to be strongly associated with fat-rich diets, low fiber, and overweight and obesity.

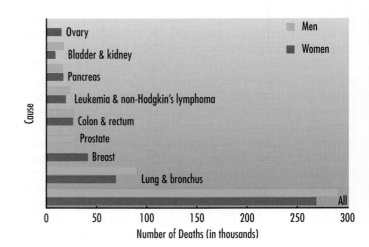

■ **Figure 13.3**

Deaths from Common Cancers, United States, 2005

Source: Data from Centers for Disease Control and Prevention, *National Vital Statistics Reports, 56,* 2008.

Causes of Cancer

Most Cancers Are Not Inherited

Many people live in fear of cancer, often because one or more closely related family members have died from some type of cancer. They may believe that cancer is passed on in the genes or that, at least, the susceptibility to cancer is inherited. Neither of these beliefs is correct for the vast majority of cancers. However, a persistent fear of developing cancer can generate stress that may weaken the immune system and contribute to the development of disease, including cancer.

Scientific studies indicate that 90% to 95% of *all* cancers, including breast, lung, stomach, colon, skin, or prostate, are *not* inherited from parents except in a few rare families in which members do inherit one or more cancer susceptibility genes (Lichtenstein, et al., 2000).

Confusion about genes often stems from misunderstanding the meanings of the words "genetic" and "inherited." The two are not synonymous. All of your cells (except for red blood cells) contain exact copies of the chromosomes and genes that were in the fertilized egg from which you developed. The genes in the chromosomes of any cell of your body, such as skin, lung, or stomach cells, can be chemically changed by environmental agents such as chemicals and radiation. These genetic changes in skin, lung, or stomach cells may transform them into cancer cells. Thus, cancer is a genetic disease in that genes are changed in a person's body cells; however, it is *not* an inherited disease because defective genes were not usually passed on from parents. Thus, a parent who acquires cancer cannot pass it on to his or her child.

Even if several close family members have died of cancer, it does not mean that cancer "runs in the family" and is an inherited disease. Currently, about one of every four deaths each year in the United States is due to cancer. If your grandparents and eight aunts or uncles have died, probably two or three of them died of cancer simply by chance. If they all smoked cigarettes, it would not be surprising if more than three of ten close relatives died of cancer.

One of the best pieces of evidence showing that most cancers are *not* inherited comes from a study of World War II veterans. The health of 15,000 pairs of identical or nonidentical (fraternal) twin brothers was followed for many years after World War II. No difference was observed in the different twin pairs in the development of cancer. That is, if one identical twin contracted cancer, the other identical twin was no more likely to get cancer than the average person.

Because identical twins share identical genes (i.e., they are natural clones that developed from the same fertilized egg that split into separate embryos), they should carry identical cancer-causing genes. The fact that identical twins do not *both* have cancer at significantly higher rates than the average person means that most cancers are *not* caused by inherited genes. For most people, lifestyle (e.g., diet, weight, smoking, drinking alcohol) plays a far greater role in causing cancer than any genes that are passed on from parents.

Cancer Susceptibility Genes

Although only a small fraction (estimates range between 5% and 10%) of all cancers are strongly influenced by heredity, some families do transmit cancer susceptibility genes to children. A **cancer susceptibility gene** does not cause cancer directly; however, it makes a person carrying such a gene more vulnerable to environmental factors that contribute to the risk of developing cancer.

In 2006, the U.S. National Institutes of Health launched a search for cancer susceptibility genes. Prior to this project, a few cancer susceptibility genes had been identified that increased the risk of cancer in specific organs, sometimes to a considerable degree (**Table 13.2**). By 2008, almost 100 tentative or "candidate" cancer susceptibility genes had been identified (Dong et al., 2008), the significance of which remains to be determined by further research. BRCA1 and BRCA2 genes are susceptibility genes for breast or ovarian cancer; APC, MSH2, and MLH1, for colon cancer. People who carry mutant (abnormal) copies of these genes are at higher risk for certain cancers than are people who carry normal genes.

Many genes that increase the risk of colon cancer have been identified, and some of their biological functions in cells also are understood (**Figure 13.4**). If a person inherits an abnormal form of any one of three genes, APC, MSH2, or MLH1, the risk of colon cancer is increased. However, fewer than 5% of all colon cancer patients inherit any of these colon cancer susceptibility genes.

During a person's lifetime, mutations continue to arise and accumulate in cells lining the colon. For example, suppose a person inherited an MSH2 mutation and 20 years later a colon cell acquired an APC mutation. Those two mutations make that colon cell begin to reproduce itself at a faster rate; at some point, one cell among the faster-growing ones acquires a third mutation in either a K-*ras*, DDC, or p53 gene. That cell now has three mutations and may develop into cancer of the colon. Along the way to tumor formation, other mutations also

---

TERMS

biopsy: removal of cells from a tumor for examination under a microscope

cancer susceptibility gene: gene responsible for familial breast cancer and genes that cause susceptibility to colon cancer; increases the risk of a person developing cancer in his or her lifetime

Table 13.2

Cancer Susceptibility Genes

Abnormalities (mutations) in these genes can be inherited. Each abnormal gene contributes to the development of cancer in a specific organ.

Gene	Organ affected
Breast cancer	
BRCA1	Breast, ovary
BRCA2	Breast
p53	Breast, brain
Colon cancer	
MSH2	Colon, uterus
MLH1	Colon, uterus
PMS1, PMS2	Colon, other
APC	Colon
Melanoma	
MTS1 (CDKN2)	Skin, pancreas
CDK4	Skin
Prostate cancer	
HPC1	Prostate
MSR1	Prostate
AR	Prostate
CYP1	Prostate
SRD5A2	Prostate

may occur. On average, when colon cancer cells are examined, they have at least three of the mutations described in Figure 13.4. Now you can understand why chance genetic changes and exposure to environmental agents that cause mutations play such important roles in the development of cancer.

A word of caution is in order. Several companies offer tests for a wide variety of purported cancer susceptibility genes. The tests cost a lot of money. Being identified as a carrier of a cancer susceptibility gene whose significance or function is unknown provides you with nothing except a large dose of worry. For the vast majority of people, cancer susceptibility genes are of no consequence and should be of no concern. The most important thing in cancer prevention, as discussed next, is avoiding or mitigating the environmental factors that actually cause normal cells to become cancer cells.

Environmental Factors That Cause Cancer

The causes of cancer or, more correctly, the risk factors associated with the development of cancer are numerous and complex. It often is difficult to point to a single cause of a cancer, but certain environmental factors are strongly correlated with the occurrence of particular cancers. Two examples are the strong correlation between cigarette smoking and lung cancer and exposure to ultraviolet light and skin cancer. Even in these examples, not everyone who smokes heavily or stays in the sun day after day will get lung or skin cancer.

Epidemiology is the branch of science that investigates the causes and frequencies of diseases in human populations. Many epidemiological studies show that as many as 80% to 90% of cancers are caused by exposure to environmental factors that are known to increase the risk of cancer (**Table 13.3**). For example, smoking cigarettes while young puts a person at 10 to 20 times higher risk of developing cancer later in life than persons who

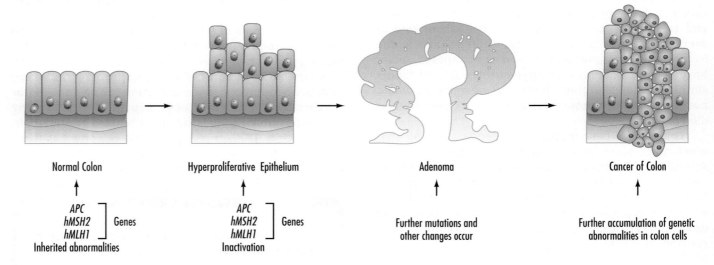

■ **Figure 13.4**

Mutant Genes Contribute to Development of Cancer Cells

Changes in several genes can lead to increased risk of colon cancer. Abnormalities in APC, MSH2, or MLH1 genes can be inherited from parents. Other changes may occur in genes of colon cells during the course of a person's life before development of a cancer. Examination of colon cancer cells indicates that most of them have accumulated several genetic changes, either inherited or acquired.

Table 13.3

Environmental and Lifestyle Risk Factors That Contribute to Cancer

Factor	Amount of risk	Types of cancer
Nutrition	About *half* of cancer deaths are caused by nutritional problems: Excess calories Excess fat consumption Obesity Nutritional deficiencies, especially fiber and vitamin A	Cancers of the colon, rectum, stomach, breast, and ovaries
Cigarettes and alcohol	About *one-third* of cancer deaths are caused by smoking cigarettes and excessive alcohol consumption	Cancers of the lung, pancreas, mouth, larynx, liver, esophagus, and bladder
Occupation	About 5% of cancer deaths are caused by substances in the workplace, such as asbestos, benzene, and vinyl chloride	Cancers of the bladder, lung, stomach, blood, liver, bones, and skin
Radiation	About 3% of cancer deaths are caused by ionizing radiation, such as x-rays and ultraviolet light	Blood, skin
Other	Other cancer deaths result from heredity, chronic disease, drugs, and infections	Various cancers

■ **Figure 13.5**

Environmental factors change both genes and the growth properties of cells that may lead to the development of cancer.

Factors that change genes in cells

Ionizing radiation

Infectious microorganisms (viruses and bacteria)

Carcinogenic chemicals

Tumor

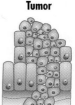

Factors that promote growth of genetically abnormal cells

Hormones
Nutritional deficiencies
Reduced immune system
Aging
Immunosuppressive drugs

do not smoke. Eating fat-laden fast food frequently may be convenient, but it is ultimately unhealthy and may contribute to the development of certain cancers. Because each of us can change our diets, stop smoking, and avoid other cancer-causing risks in the environment, preventing cancer is a realistic and attainable goal for most people.

Three classes of environmental agents—ionizing radiation, infectious microorganisms (viruses and bacteria), and cancer-causing chemicals (carcinogens)—have been shown to increase the risk of cancer in both laboratory animals and people. Each of these agents increases the risk of cancer by producing chemical changes (**mutations**) in genes in any cell in the body and cause it to multiply abnormally (Croce, 2008). If a cell undergoes one or more mutations in genes that regulate its growth, it may begin to multiply rapidly and develop into a tumor. Environmental factors cause mutations and also affect the rate of abnormal cell growth (**Figure 13.5**).

Ionizing Radiation

Ionizing radiation consists of x-rays, ultraviolet (UV) light, and radioactivity whose energy can damage cells and chromosomes. The high rate of leukemia among survivors of the Hiroshima and Nagasaki atomic bomb

blasts in 1945 leaves no doubt that radioactivity increases the risk of cancer.

In the United States, among children born in southern Utah in the 1950s who were exposed to radioactive fallout from nearby atomic tests, leukemia deaths were two to three times greater than among children born in southern Utah before and after the atomic tests. In a landmark legal decision in 1984, a federal court ruled that the U.S. government was negligent in conducting atomic bomb tests in southern Utah in the 1950s because the tests released radioactive material into the

TERMS

epidemiology: a branch of science that studies the causes and frequencies of diseases in human populations

ionizing radiation: radiation, such as x-rays, that can damage cells and cause cancer; also used to treat cancer

mutations: permanent changes in the genetic information in a cell; only mutations in sperm and eggs are inherited

atmosphere. The court ruled that the families who were exposed to radioactivity as a result of these tests, and whose members died as a result of exposure to the radioactivity, were entitled to compensation.

The nuclear reactor accident at Chernobyl in Ukraine in 1986 also released large amounts of radioactivity, particularly radioactive iodine, strontium, and cesium, into the atmosphere. Not only was the region around the reactor affected, but radioactive fallout occurred over much of Europe. In some countries, milk and crops were so contaminated that they had to be destroyed. Some of the radioactivity was detected in countries as distant as the United States and Japan.

The toll in human sickness and deaths from this nuclear accident continues to mount even today. Approximately 32,000 persons died directly or indirectly as a result of the reactor explosion; another 30,000 suffered some degree of radiation sickness. Children are especially at risk from radioactive iodine, which causes thyroid cancer; in Ukraine, thyroid cancer among children increased by a factor of 10 over what it was before the accident occurred.

Because any amount of ionizing radiation, however small, has the potential for causing damage to chromosomes and genes, one should minimize exposure to x-rays. For example, if you are healthy, periodic chest x-rays are unnecessary. CAT scans also expose the body to significant amounts of radiation. Some homes release radon, a radioactive gas present in some building materials. Long-term exposure to the invisible radon gas contributes to the risk of cancer (see Chapter 24).

The most common source of ionizing radiation in nature is UV radiation in sunlight. Because children and young people spend long hours in the sun, people acquire as much as 80% of their lifetime UV exposure by age 20.

Ultraviolet radiation in sunlight is characterized by two different wavelengths, called UVA and UVB. Until recently, it was thought that only UVB was dangerous, but now it appears that both forms of UV radiation are harmful. Reducing the time of exposure to intense sunlight and using sunscreen creams to protect exposed areas of the body reduce the risk of skin cancer.

Infectious Microorganisms

In 1911, Peyton Rous, a scientist working at the Rockefeller Institute in New York, showed that cancer could be produced in chickens by injecting them with a virus isolated from chicken tumors. Since then, other viruses, called **tumor viruses,** have been found in animals such as mice, cats, and monkeys.

Finding tumor viruses that infect people has been generally unsuccessful despite considerable research. Only four viruses have been associated with specific human cancers; in the vast majority of people, infection by these viruses will not cause cancer, although it will increase its risk. Increased cancer risk is associated with infection by hepatitis B and C viruses (liver cancer), papillomavirus (genital and cervical cancer), human T-cell leukemia-lymphoma virus (leukemia and lymphoma), and Epstein-Barr virus (cancer of the nose or pharynx). Infection by HIV, the virus that causes AIDS, is associated with the development of a particular cancer called Kaposi's sarcoma. And a bacterium that is found in the stomach and causes ulcers (*H. pylori*) is associated with an increased risk of gastric cancer, one form of lymphoma, and possibly pancreatic cancer.

Chemical Carcinogens

A **chemical carcinogen** is an environmental substance that can interact with cells to initiate cancer, usually by chemically altering the chromosomes or genes in cells. Genes are responsible for manufacturing the enzymes and other proteins a cell needs to function properly. An altered gene usually makes an abnormal protein that may change the growth properties of a cell and cause it to become a cancer cell.

Many chemicals that are developed are now tested to determine their cancer-causing potential. Unfortunately, many thousands of chemical substances already in use have not been adequately tested. Of the thousands of chemical substances that have been tested, many have been found to be carcinogenic and should be avoided if at all possible. Carcinogens include cigarette smoke, pesticides, asbestos, heavy metals (lead, mercury, cadmium), benzene, and nitrosamines.

Despite the long list of carcinogenic substances, some scientists and public health officials argue that tobacco is the only substance of consequence with respect to the numbers of cancers caused. Although the argument has some basis, it is of small consolation to persons who acquire cancer from exposure, often without their knowledge, to carcinogenic substances in the environment or workplace (**Table 13.4**).

In some industries, workers have cancers that almost never arise in the general population. For example, **mesothelioma** is a rare form of lung cancer that only occurs among persons exposed to asbestos fibers. Long-term exposure to the heavy metals beryllium and cadmium increases workers' risk of prostate cancer. Workers exposed to vinyl chloride, the starting material for polyvinyl chloride (PVC) pipes and other products, develop a rare form of liver cancer not found in the general population. Fortunately, with current occupational and safety regulations, these types of occupational cancers occur infrequently.

The total number of cancers attributable to industrial chemicals is small compared with those caused by tobacco and diet; however, cancers caused by industrial chemicals are preventable or avoidable. Before you accept a job it might be wise to determine what chemicals you will be exposed to for long periods.

Table 13.4

Examples of Occupational Cancers

Chemical/physical agent	Cancer type	Exposure of general population	Examples of workers frequently exposed or exposure sources
Arsenic	Lung, skin	Rare	Insecticide and herbicide sprayers; tanners; oil refinery workers
Asbestos	Mesothelioma, lung	Uncommon	Brake-lining, shipyard, insulation, and demolition workers
Benzene	Myelogenous leukemia	Common	Painters; distillers and petrochemical workers; dye users; furniture finishers; rubber workers
Diesel exhaust	Lung	Common	Railroad and bus-garage workers; truck operators; miners
Formaldehyde	Nose, nasopharynx	Rare	Hospital and laboratory workers; manufacture of wood products, paper, textiles, garments, and metal products
Hair dyes	Bladder	Uncommon	Hairdressers and barbers (inadequate evidence for customers)
Ionizing radiation	Bone marrow, several others	Common	Nuclear materials; medicinal products and procedures
Mineral oils	Skin	Common	Metal machining
Nonarsenical pesticides	Lung	Common	Sprayers; agricultural workers
Painting materials	Lung	Uncommon	Professional painters
Polychlorinated biphenyls	Liver, skin	Uncommon	Heat-transfer and hydraulic fluids and lubricants; inks; adhesives; insecticides
Radon (alpha particles)	Lung	Uncommon	Mines; underground structures; homes
Soot	Skin	Uncommon	Chimney sweeps and cleaners; bricklayers; insulators; firefighters; heating-unit service workers
Synthetic mineral fibers	Lung	Uncommon	Wall and pipe insulation; duct wrapping

Do Xenoestrogens Cause Cancer?

Estrogens are hormones that regulate a variety of biological functions in women, including the growth and development of breast tissue. Many chemicals that we are exposed to in the environment mimic the action of normal estrogen to some degree; such chemicals are called **xenoestrogens** (literally, foreign estrogens).

Substances that contain xenoestrogens include the pesticides DDT (banned in the United States, but still used elsewhere), methoxyclor, kepone, chlordane, atrazine, and endosulfan. Polychlorinated biphenyls (PCBs), which were used in electrical transformers for many years, also are xenoestrogens. Bisphenol-A, a component of polycarbonate plastics that are widely used in water bottles, baby bottles, food cans, and many other plastics, also is a xenoestrogen (see Chapter 24).

A variety of evidence points to environmental xenoestrogens as agents in the development of some cancers, particularly breast cancer (see Chapter 24). Clues came from wildlife that suffered reproductive abnormalities after being exposed to xenoestrogens. Male fish collected near the outflow from sewers showed production of vitellogin, a female protein. Alligators hatched in a lake in Florida contaminated with a pesticide grew abnormally small penises and had altered hormone levels. And military dogs that served in Vietnam (where Agent Orange, a xenoestrogen, was widely dispersed) had twice the rate of testicular cancer and reproductive defects compared with dogs that did not serve in Vietnam. So xenoestrogens may not only be involved in breast cancer, but may also play a role in reproductive problems and testicular cancer.

The effects of xenoestrogens can be tested on human cells grown in the laboratory. Normal estrogen binds to many cells and affects their growth. Xenoestrogens bind to the same cellular receptors as normal estrogen and exert some of the same effects on the growth of cells. The evidence that xenoestrogens can affect cell proliferation and reproductive organs is now well established.

In the 1960s and 1970s, Israel had one of the highest incidences of breast cancer in the world. In 1976, Israel banned all chlorinated pesticides and made it illegal for milk products to have any detectable pesticide residues. In the years following the pesticide ban, rates of breast cancer declined dramatically. These findings support the theory that pesticides acting as xenoestrogens are a major contributor to breast cancer.

TERMS

chemical carcinogen: a chemical that damages cells and causes cancer

mesothelioma: a form of lung cancer caused by asbestos

tumor viruses: viruses that infect cells, change their growth properties, and cause cancer

xenoestrogens: environmental chemicals that mimic the effects of natural estrogen; may cause cancer

It is impossible to avoid all exposure to xenoestrogens because they are everywhere in the environment. Eating broccoli, cabbage, and soy products may help counteract the effects of xenoestrogens. This advice comes from the observation that Asian women have much lower rates of breast cancer in comparison with white or black American women. Asian diets are richer in these vegetables, which may contain chemicals that block the biological activities of the xenoestrogens.

Facts About Common Cancers

Lung Cancer

Lung cancer is the deadliest of all cancers worldwide. In the United States, lung cancer is the number one cause of cancer deaths for both men and women. In 2008, it was estimated that 215,000 lung and bronchus cancers would be diagnosed in the United States, which accounts for about 15% of all cancers. Since 1987, more women have died each year from lung cancer than from breast cancer. Smoking cigarettes is the primary cause of 80% to 90% of all lung cancers (see Chapter 17).

The survival rate of lung cancer patients is dismal; among all patients receiving a diagnosis of lung cancer, only 14% live another five years. Even if diagnosed and treated at the earliest stage, survival for five years is only 67%. Medical costs of treating lung cancer are about $10 billion annually, making it the costliest of all cancers.

The risk of lung cancer varies significantly among ethnic and racial groups (Haiman et al., 2006). African Americans and native Hawaiians are at highest risk, especially at lower levels of cigarette smoking (less than a pack a day). White Americans, Japanese Americans, and Latinos are about half as likely to get lung cancer as the other two groups at comparable levels of smoking. The reasons for racial and ethnic differences are not clear but may have to do with inherited lung cancer susceptibility genes that vary among groups of people.

The rate of lung cancer in other nations is rising rapidly as more and more people take up cigarette smoking. Women in developing countries begin to smoke at early ages to appear sophisticated and because of peer pressure. International efforts are under way to reduce smoking around the world among young people, especially among young girls (see Chapter 17). China and other developing nations will have to cope with epidemics of lung cancer soon. The concerted effort in the United States to get people to stop smoking and to prevent access of young people to cigarettes is an attempt to reverse the epidemic of lung cancer in this country.

Breast Cancer

Both men and women can develop breast cancer, but it occurs very rarely among men. Although more women die from lung cancer than breast cancer, more than twice as many women contract breast cancer. Since

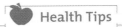

Health Tips

Abortion Does Not Increase Risk of Breast Cancer

In 2002, the National Cancer Institute (NCI) Web site announced that scientists had found no association between abortion and subsequent risk of breast cancer. Some members of Congress raised a hue and cry, and the information was removed from the NCI Web site.

NCI then assembled more than a hundred scientific experts from various fields to review the data. Only one member disagreed with the otherwise unanimous conclusion: "There is no association between abortion and the risk of breast cancer" (Couzin, 2003).

1940, the incidence of breast cancer among American women has more than doubled.

Increased weight, lack of exercise, and high levels of dietary fat have all been proposed as factors contributing to an increased risk of breast cancer. However, recent research does not support the view that the amount of fat in the diet increases the risk of breast cancer. Other factors that increase the risk of breast cancer among women to varying degrees are the following:

- Mother who had breast cancer before age 60
- Onset of menarche before age 14
- First child born after age 30
- No biological children
- Menopause after age 55
- Benign breast disease
- Estrogen replacement therapy after age 55
- Consuming more than 3 ounces of alcohol a day
- Inheritance of BRCA1, BRCA2, and other susceptibility genes
- Exposure to xenoestrogens

Does Routine Mammography Help Prevent Breast Cancer?
In 1997, a blue ribbon panel of experts at the National Institutes of Health created a furor when it recommended that routine mammogram screening for breast cancer not begin until women reached age 50; the panel concluded that women in their 40s would not benefit from **mammograms.** The controversy intensified significantly in 2000, when a meta-analysis of all breast cancer outcomes and mammography concluded that mammograms did not prolong life in women who had breast cancer (Horton, 2001). One expert summed up the controversy with this observation: "Everyone agrees that mammograms detect early tumors, smaller tumors, and give women more treatment options. The question is whether it saves more lives in the long run" (Christensen, 2002). Despite all the arguments, mammograms are still recommended for all women by the World Health Organization. The American Cancer Society recommends women get mammograms every one to two years beginning in their 40s.

🌓 Wellness Guide

Breast Awareness and Breast Self-Exam

Women should know how their breasts normally look and feel so they will be aware of any changes that might signal a problem. Doing breast self-exam (BSE) monthly is a good way to do this. When breast cancer is found early, treatment and recovery are more likely to be successful. Even though breast cancer tends to occur late in life, young women are encouraged to learn and do BSE so they will know what is normal for them.

Abnormal signs (see accompanying figures) that signal the need to consult a health professional are as follows:

- A hard lump or knot in or near the breast or underarm
- Dimpling, puckering, or ridges of the skin on the breast
- A nipple that is pushed inward rather than sticking out

- Redness, warmth, swelling, or pain
- Itchy, scaly sore or rash on the nipple
- Nipple discharge other than breast milk
- Change in color, shape, size, or texture of a breast

Breast self-exams should not replace regular screening mammograms or clinical breast exams performed by a health professional. Women aged 20 to 39 should have a clinical breast exam at least once every three years. Women older than 40 should have a clinical breast exam each year and a screening mammogram every one to two years. The American Cancer Society offers a guide for doing BSE properly; this information can be found online by searching on "ACS BSE."

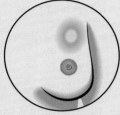
Lump

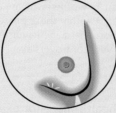
Skin dimpling

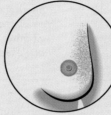
Change in skin color or texture.

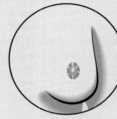
Change in how the nipple looks, like pulling in of the nipple.

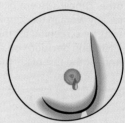
Clear or bloody fluid that leaks out of the nipple

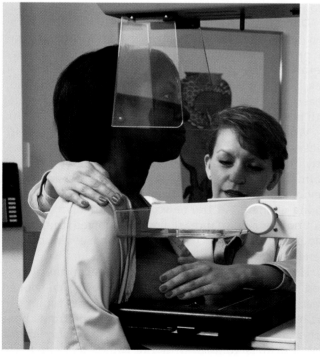

Mammograms can detect breast cancer at an early stage and improve chances for successful treatment.

Lifestyle Changes Help Prevent Breast Cancer Among Western women, the lifetime risk of developing breast cancer is about 10%, and breast cancer remains a leading cause of death among women in developed countries. In the United States, breast cancer is diagnosed in about 182,000 women each year; about 40,000 women die annually. The incidence of breast cancer among African American women is significantly higher than for white American women. Also, breast cancer in African American women is much more deadly for reasons that are unknown. The five-year rate of survival of white women after a diagnosis of breast cancer is 90%; the five-year survival rate of African American women after a diagnosis of breast cancer is only 77% (Couzin, 2007). For women with BRCA1 or BRCA2 mutations, the lifetime risk is considerably higher—some estimates put it as high as 80% to 90%.

> TERMS
>
> mammogram: x-ray picture used to detect tumors in the breast

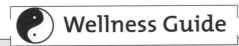

Wellness Guide

Inherited Genes for Breast Cancer and Breast Removal: What to Do?

The genes BRCA1 and BRCA2 confer an inherited predisposition to development of breast and ovarian cancer. About 5% to 10% of all breast cancer cases are thought to be influenced by inheritance of these cancer susceptibility genes. These genes do not cause breast cancer, but they increase a woman's lifetime risk. However, any estimated risks are really only educated guesses from studies of a few families whose female members have an exceptionally high rate of breast or ovarian cancer. Whether the risks calculated for these families can be extrapolated to other families is speculative. The increased risk, however great, is vitally important to each woman who has to make crucial health decisions.

Knowing that one is carrying a BRCA1 or BRCA2 gene (or other cancer susceptibility genes) creates stress and problems for any woman (or couple) who chooses to use the available tests for screening for these genes. Personal relations (including decisions on childbearing) are bound to be affected. And for the rest of her life, a woman will worry about the appearance of breast or some other cancer; such ongoing stress is bound to have a negative effect on health and on relationships.

Until 2008, people who used genetic tests also had to worry about loss of health and life insurance, loss of a job, and other forms of genetic discrimination if the results of genetic tests were shared with insurers and employers. In 2008, the U.S. Congress passed the Genetic Information Nondiscrimination Act (GINA), which makes it illegal for a company to deny insurance, benefits, or employment to any person based on genetic testing results that indicate that they are susceptible to a disease in the future (see Chapter 15).

For some women, knowing that they are at very high risk of developing breast cancer is sufficient cause for them to opt for prophylactic mastectomy; that is, they have their breasts removed while young to avoid the chance of breast cancer later in life. Prophylactic oophorectomy (removal of ovaries) is another option for women who are at high risk for breast and ovarian cancer. Whether these procedures prolong life or whether the potential benefits offset the damage to the quality of life are still very controversial.

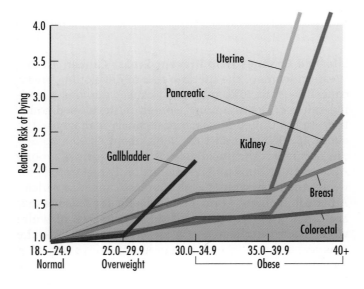

■ **Figure 13.6**

Estimated Extra Cancer Risk for Women Who Are Overweight or Obese

As a woman's body mass index (BMI) increases, so does the risk of various cancers. The greatest risk is for uterine and kidney cancers. Just being somewhat overweight may double the risk of gallbladder and uterine cancers. Breast and uterine cancer risk increases significantly with obesity.

Copyright September 2007. Reprinted with permission from Nutrition Action Healthletter, a publication of the nonprofit Center for Science in the Public Interest. www.cspinet.org.

Living healthfully—for example, maintaining a normal body weight—is effective in reducing women's risk of breast and other cancers (**Figure 13.6**). Other ways that help prevent breast cancer include maintaining a low-fat diet, consuming adequate amounts of fresh fruits and vegetables, engaging in physical activity, and limiting alcohol consumption.

One bit of encouraging news is that women who have first-degree female relatives who had breast cancer are only at slightly greater risk for breast cancer than average (Collaborative Group on Hormonal Factors in Breast Cancer, 2001). Eight of nine women who develop breast cancer do *not* have a mother, sister, or daughter with breast cancer.

Women with a diagnosis of breast cancer can increase their chances of survival by engaging in physical activities such as walking briskly for 3 to 5 hours a week (Holmes et al., 2005). Physical activity had been shown previously to reduce the incidence of breast cancer among women, but the new research involving almost 3,000 women with breast cancer showed that those who exercised survived longer than those who did not exercise.

How aggressively to treat breast cancer has always been a problem for physicians. A newly developed genetic test of the DNA in a particular breast tumor can distinguish patients with a good prognosis from those with a poor prognosis (**Figure 13.7**). The prediction of the genetic test is valid even if the tumor has spread to lymph nodes, which usually is considered a poor prognostic sign by physicians.

☯ Wellness Guide

Testicular Cancer—Self-Exam

The testicles (also called testes or gonads) are located behind the penis in a pouch of skin called the scrotum. The testicles produce and store sperm, and they are also the body's main source of male hormones. These hormones control the development of the reproductive organs and other male characteristics, such as body and facial hair, low voice, and wide shoulders.

Testicular cancer is rare. It accounts for only about 1% of all cancers in American men. However, cancer of the testicle is the most common cancer in men 15 to 35 years old. Men who have an undescended testicle (a testicle that has never moved down into the scrotum) are at higher risk of developing cancer of the testicle than other men whose testicles have moved down into the scrotum. This is true even if surgery has been done to place the testicle in the appropriate place in the scrotum. The symptoms of testicular cancer include the following:

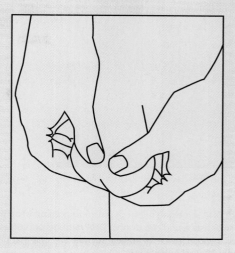

- A lump in either testicle
- Any enlargement of a testicle
- A feeling of heaviness in the scrotum
- A dull ache in the lower abdomen or the groin
- A sudden collection of fluid in the scrotum
- Pain or discomfort in a testicle or in the scrotum
- Enlargement or tenderness of the breasts

These symptoms are not sure signs of cancer. They can also be caused by other conditions. However, it is important to see a doctor if any of these symptoms lasts as long as two weeks. Any illness should be diagnosed and treated as soon as possible. Early diagnosis of testicular cancer is especially important because the sooner testicular cancer is found and treated, the better a man's chance for complete recovery.

Most testicular cancers are found by men themselves, by accident or when doing testicular self-examination (TSE). The testicles are smooth, oval-shaped, and rather firm. Men who examine themselves regularly become familiar with the way their testicles normally feel. Any changes in the way they feel

from month to month should be reported to a doctor. Men can improve their chance of finding a tumor by performing a testicular self-examination once a month (see the accompanying figure). TSE should be performed after a warm bath or shower. The heat relaxes the scrotum, making it easier to find anything unusual. To perform a self-exam follow these suggestions:

- Stand in front of the mirror. Look for any swelling on the skin of the scrotum.
- Examine each testicle with both hands. The index and middle fingers should be placed under the testicle while the thumbs are placed on the top.
- Gently roll the testicle between the thumbs and fingers. It's normal for one testicle to be larger than the other.
- Find the epididymis (the soft, tubelike structure at the back of the testicle that collects and carries the sperm). Do not mistake the epididymis for an abnormal lump.
- If you find a lump, contact your doctor right away. Most lumps are found on the sides of the testicle, but some appear on the front. Remember that testicular cancer is highly curable, especially when treated promptly.

Several drugs are now available that significantly reduce the risk of breast cancer reoccurring in women who have been treated successfully for breast cancer. Tamoxifen has been used for years to prevent the reoccurrence of breast cancer. Other drugs called *aromatase inhibitors* also are effective in preventing a reoccurrence of breast cancer.

Testicular Cancer

The rate of testicular cancer among young men has been increasing but, as with breast cancer, the causes for the increase are unknown. It may be that exposure to xenoestrogens plays a role, but that has not been confirmed. Testicular cancer is still quite rare but usually can be cured if detected early. That is why it is recom-

mended that young men perform a testicular self-exam regularly. The most publicized example of a testicular cancer cure is that of bicyclist Lance Armstrong, who won the grueling Tour de France six years in a row after recovering from testicular cancer.

Prostate Cancer

Prostate cancer occurs primarily in men over age 65, although abnormal prostate cells can be detected at autopsy in young men who die from other causes. Generally, prostate cancers are very slow-growing and, in many cases, may never become life-threatening.

Early diagnosis of prostate cancer is facilitated by two tests. One is the finger rectal exam, in which a trained person can detect if the prostate is enlarged or otherwise

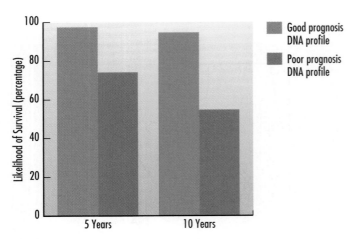

■ Figure 13.7

Using modern DNA screening methods (*microarray analysis*) on breast cancer cells, scientists found two distinct DNA patterns or profiles—one that predicted a good chance for 10-year survival and one that predicted a poor chance for 10-year survival.

Source: Data from M. J. van de Vijver. (2002). A gene-expression signature as a predictor of survival in breast cancer. *New England Journal of Medicine, 347,* 1999–2009.

feels abnormal. The **prostate-specific antigen (PSA) test** detects a protein in blood that is associated with abnormal growth of the prostate gland. A high PSA level may indicate prostate cancer, but also occurs with many other noncancerous conditions. Only additional tests can confirm the meaning of a high PSA level in blood.

The primary risk factor for prostate cancer is being elderly; about 80% of cases and 90% of deaths occur in men over age 65. An estimated 25 million American men over age 50 have some detectable abnormal prostate cells; however, the vast majority never develop prostate cancer because most prostate cancers grow extremely slowly. Even among those who do, most eventually die from causes other than prostate cancer. Thus, the first question is whether it is worth screening for prostate cancer, and second, whether slow-growing prostate cancers should even be treated. The U.S. Preventive Services Task Force recommends *against* any routine screening for prostate cancer, including the digital exam, the PSA test, and ultrasound scan.

One form of treatment for prostate cancer, radical prostatectomy, often causes urinary, sexual, or bowel dysfunction and makes life generally miserable. In the last 20 years the number of radical prostatectomies has increased dramatically. The number of deaths from prostate cancer fell from about 40,000 in 1995 to about 28,000 in 2008. Whether early detection and surgery accounted for the decline is difficult to determine. Presently, there are a number of treatment options for prostate cancer, including "watchful waiting."

As with breast cancer and colon cancer, several susceptibility genes for prostate cancer have been identified. About 40% of prostate cancers are caused by inherited susceptability genes (Gelmann, 2008). When screening tests become available, men will have to decide whether or not they want to know if they carry a gene that puts them at higher-than-average risk for prostate cancer.

Skin Cancer

Skin cancers are on the rise everywhere, but they are especially prevalent in regions of the world exposed to intense sunlight. **Melanoma,** a malignant form of skin cancer, has increased almost 20-fold since 1930. Melanoma is now the most common cancer in women aged 25 to 29 and the second most common in women aged 30 to 34. Worldwide, melanoma is diagnosed in about 132,000 persons each year. Dark-skinned individuals are at least 500 times less likely to get melanoma than are fair-skinned individuals (Marx, 2007). As with other cancers, a number of susceptibility genes for melanoma have been identified.

The skin (epidermis) consists of several layers and kinds of cells. The upper layer consists of flat squamous cells, and the bottom layer contains basal cells. Interspersed among the squamous and basal cells are melanocytes, cells that give skin its characteristic pigmentation. People with more melanocytes are less susceptible to skin cancer than are light-skinned people.

Exposure to sunlight is the primary cause of all forms of skin cancer. The exposure to sunlight that most of us receive as children largely determines the risk of skin cancer later in life. Two factors contribute to the dramatic rise in the rate of skin cancers. First, in the last generation or two we have become a nation of sun bathers and sun worshippers. Tans are associated with health, vigor, and beauty. Second, the continuing depletion of the ozone layer (see Chapter 24) has resulted in more UV radiation reaching the earth's surface; it is the UV radiation in sunlight that causes mutations in skin cells that may lead to cancer. To reduce the risk of skin cancer, you must reduce your exposure to sunlight.

About a million cases of skin cancer are diagnosed every year in the United States. **Basal cell carcinoma** and **squamous cell carcinoma** are usually not life-threatening, and the abnormal cells can be removed surgically or by scraping, freezing, or burning. Even melanomas, if discovered and removed while the tumor is less than 1 millimeter thick, can be treated successfully. However, melanomas grow rapidly, and once the cells have metastasized, malignant melanoma often leads to death.

To protect yourself from melanoma, remember these "ABCD" rules when examining moles on your body for any changes. If you suspect anything, consult a physician immediately.

- **A**symmetry—one half of a mole looks different from the other half.
- **B**order irregular—the edges of a mole are ragged or indistinct.
- **C**olor—the pigmentation in the mole is uneven.

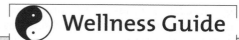
Wellness Guide

health.jbpub.com/hwonline

Ways to Prevent Skin Cancer

The number of people in the United States with various types of skin cancer, especially melanoma, has been increasing yearly. This need not be so because skin cancers are among the most preventable of all cancers. The primary cause of most skin cancers is overexposure to sunlight. Use of indoor tanning lamps also poses a hazard. The best way to prevent skin cancer is to follow the **WAR** rule:

- **W**ear protective clothing.
- **A**void the sun between 10 A.M. and 3 P.M.
- **R**egularly apply sunscreen with an SPF greater than 15 when outdoors, even on cloudy days. Sunscreen should be reapplied every two hours, and more often to replace what is washed from the body if swimming or exercising.

Protecting children from sunburn and overexposure is especially important because it is the lifetime exposure to UV that is associated with skin cancers in later life. By age 65, about one American in two has had some form of skin cancer. The ozone layer in earth's upper atmosphere filters out much of the sun's UV light; thinning of the ozone layer in recent years markedly increases the danger of overexposure to sunlight. Unless more people follow the WAR rule, the incidence of skin cancers is expected to continue to rise in the years ahead.

Wearing sunglasses that block at least 99% of all UV light is important for protecting eyes. Polarized lenses block glare

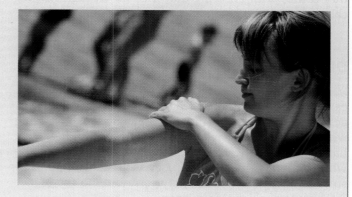

but do not necessarily block UV unless the label says so. "Photochromic" lenses that darken in bright light also may not block UV light; always read the label. Over time, eye exposure to UV can cause cataracts.

The Environmental Protection Agency and the National Weather Service offer a daily e-mail advisory to anyone wanting to know the UV levels in their area. UV intensity is rated on a point scale of 1 to 11; 6 or higher means that the UV intensity is high for the area and that exposure should be limited. The UV advisory can be accessed at http://epa.gov/sunwise/uvindex.html.

- **D**iameter—any mole that is larger than the diameter of a pencil or that has increased in size.

Colon Cancer

Mortality from colon cancer is exceeded in the United States only by that from lung cancer, prostate cancer, and breast cancer. Colon cancer affects men and women equally and causes about 50,000 total deaths annually in the United States. As with many cancers, if discovered in the earliest stages, many cases of colon cancer can be cured surgically.

Colon cancer is rarely diagnosed in persons under age 40 but begins to appear more frequently in persons over age 50. The primary screening tests for colon cancer are occult blood tests and flexible sigmoidoscopy and colonoscopy. In the occult blood test, stool samples are analyzed for the presence of blood, which may be a sign of colon cancer. In sigmoidoscopy, a flexible instrument is inserted via the rectum into the lower part of the colon to allow the health provider to visually examine the lining of the colon. If any abnormal tissue is observed, a complete examination of the colon (colonoscopy) is recommended.

Occult blood tests for colon cancer are not very accurate, and some risk is involved with sigmoidoscopy because it is invasive. A positive sign from an occult blood test in a stool is usually cause for additional tests for colon cancer.

In a colonoscopy, death occurs in approximately 1 of 10,000 procedures. However, the rate of death from colon cancer in persons aged 50 to 54 is only about 1.8 per 10,000, so deciding to have a colonoscopy is not a simple decision. Each person needs to weigh the risks and benefits for his or her particular situation.

Certain inherited genes (see Table 13.2 and Figure 13.4) are known to increase a person's risk for colon cancer. Persons from families known to be at high risk can be genetically tested to see if they have inherited a colon cancer susceptibility gene. They may benefit from the genetic

---

TERMS

basal cell carcinoma: a form of skin cancer that usually can be removed surgically

melanoma: a particularly dangerous form of skin cancer

prostate-specific antigen (PSA) test: a blood test that detects a protein associated with abnormal growth of the prostate gland

squamous cell carcinoma: cancer of the top layer of skin; most are curable if removed early

information by more frequent examination of their colon, but they also must be willing to accept the lifelong stress that comes with knowing that they are at high risk for colon cancer.

Diet and Cancer Risk

Many epidemiological studies show that the risk of certain cancers is strongly influenced by diet. For example, stomach cancer is common in Japan but uncommon among white Americans in Hawaii. Japanese Americans in Hawaii have stomach cancer rates that are almost as low as the white American population. Excessive consumption of smoked and pickled foods may contribute to the higher rates of stomach cancer in Japan.

Despite the scientific uncertainty over what specific foods increase the risk of cancer, certain dietary choices may help in preventing cancer (**Table 13.5**). Most of these dietary recommendations also help boost the immune system, which is the body's main defense against foreign cells (see Chapter 12). B vitamins, vitamin C, and folic acid have been shown to boost the immune system and, as a consequence, may also help destroy cancer cells. These substances can be taken as supplements, but also are readily available in fresh fruits and vegetables.

Scientists continue to speculate over why certain kinds of cancer are so dependent on diet. One possibility is that we are asking the body to do things chemically for which it is unprepared by the course of human evolution. That is, cancer may be thought of as a disease of maladaptation.

Our ancestors foraged for their food. They collected and ate seeds, roots, fruits, and vegetables and rarely ate meat. Thus, the diet we consume today, filled with excess sugar, salt, fat, and meat, may be incompatible with the body chemistry we have inherited from our ancestors. The modern diet, heavy with processed foods, may result in the accumulation of toxic chemicals or an insufficient amount of some essential nutrients found in fresh fruits and vegetables, nuts, and grains.

Cancer Treatments

The three medical treatments for cancer are surgery, **radiation therapy**, and **chemotherapy**. Surgical removal of all or as much of a tumor as possible is considered the best treatment for cancer, particularly if the tumor is small and cells have not spread throughout the body. If even a few cancer cells remain, however, they may grow into new tumors, which is the reason that surgery, such as mastectomy, often removes a great deal of tissue in addition to the tumor.

If there is evidence that tumor cells have spread, or if some of the tumor could not be removed surgically, then radiation or chemotherapy, or both, are used to kill the remaining cancer cells. X-rays or other forms of high-energy radiation can destroy cancer cells, as can the powerful drugs used in chemotherapy. Because radiation therapy and chemotherapy destroy normal cells as well as cancer cells, only limited amounts of each treatment can be administered.

Despite improvements in surgical techniques and development of new chemotherapeutic drugs, cancer treatments today are not noticeably more successful than they were in the past, a fact that is reflected in the more or less unchanged death rates for most cancers. However, a few specific cancers can be treated successfully.

An analysis of cancer mortality over the past 40 years in the United States led to the following conclusion:

> The best of modern medicine has much to offer to virtually every patient with cancer, for palliation if not always for cure, and every patient should have access

Table 13.5

Dietary Recommendations to Help Prevent Cancer

About 50% of all cancers are thought to derive from nutritional deficiencies.

Substance or food	Effect on cancer risk	Advice
Fiber	Helps decrease colon and rectal cancer	Obtain fiber from vegetables, fruits, whole grains
Cruciferous vegetables (broccoli, cauliflower, brussels sprouts)	Phytochemicals in these vegetables may detoxify cancer-causing chemicals	Eat more; raw or undercooked is best
Allium vegetables (onion, garlic, chives)	Sulfur-containing chemicals in allium vegetables may help prevent cancer	Eat more
Beta-carotene (15 mg), vitamin E (400 IU), and selenium (50 µg)	A daily supplement reduced cancer (mainly stomach and esophagus) in a large Chinese population	Use supplements in moderation; selenium in high doses is toxic
Folic acid	Deficiency in this vitamin increases genetic damage that may contribute to cancer	Supplement if diet is deficient
Green tea	Reduced esophageal cancer in Chinese population	Most tea drunk in United States is black tea; try green tea
Shiitake mushrooms	Extracts of shiitake mushrooms reduced tumors in laboratory animals; also reduces blood cholesterol	Add to diet

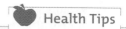 Health Tips

Don't Be Fooled by "Miraculous" Cancer Cures

Most people who are diagnosed with cancer become depressed or angry, especially if their doctor is pessimistic about the outcome or cannot offer hope of a cure. People who cannot be helped by conventional medicine (and many who can) often turn to an alternative medicine that offers hope of cures for untreatable, advanced cancer. Alternative medicines run the gamut from nutritional therapies, immune therapies, and light therapies to spiritual cures.

Most of the alternative cancer therapies are designed to take money from desperate patients. If you would like information on any alternative therapy you or a loved one is contemplating using, a good place to look for information is at quackwatch.com. This site has links to many other sources of reliable information. If it is too good to be true, it usually is not true.

Table 13.6

Unproven Cancer Therapies

Many cancer patients who are desperate or who have exhausted all medical treatments turn to unconventional therapies for which benefits are scientifically unproven.

Therapy	Rationale
Metabolic therapy	Toxins and wastes in the body cause cancer. Treatments remove cellular poisons and detoxify the body.
Herbal remedies	Herbs have natural, sacred, curative properties not known to science.
Megavitamins	High doses of vitamins kill cancer cells and rejuvenate the body.
Diet therapy	Special diets (grape, macrobiotic, shark cartilage) restore balance to the body and cure the cancer.
Electronic devices	Electrical or magnetic energy harmonizes the life forces and kills the cancer cells.
Immunotherapy	Treatments stimulate or restore immune system functions, which will then be able to destroy cancer cells. (Immunotherapies are being tested by scientists but are a long way from clinical use.)

to the earliest possible diagnosis and the best possible treatment. The problem is the lack of substantial improvement over what treatment could already accomplish some decades ago. A national commitment to the prevention of cancer, largely replacing reliance on hopes for universal cures, is now the way to go. (Bailar & Gornik, 1997)

As might be expected from such a radical suggestion, the restructuring of the nation's priorities toward cancer prevention rather than cures of advanced cancers was vigorously opposed by the head of the National Cancer Institute and other medical researchers (Kramer & Klausner, 1997). Scientists seeking cancer cures will continue to do battle with scientists hoping to prevent cancer.

There are hundreds of cancer drugs on the market, many of them quite effective for treating a specific cancer. However, many of the chemotherapeutic drugs that have been created by innovative technologies are extremely expensive. Many cancer drugs cost thousands of dollars annually, and cancer treatments can end up costing hundreds of thousands of dollars, far more than most cancer patients can afford without comprehensive health insurance. Doctors who treat cancer patients now spend time explaining the different drug options and their costs to cancer patients.

Cancer patients often become desperate and depressed about their condition, the pain of treatments, and the prospect of death. In this state, some patients turn to unconventional therapies and promises of "miracle" cures (**Table 13.6**). Many cancer patients turn to alternative therapies in hope of a cure when conventional medicine has nothing to offer. Although unconventional therapies may be helpful or at least produce more peace of mind, patients and their families need to

be wary of practitioners who make unfounded claims for unlicensed drugs and unproven therapies.

Curing Childhood Cancers

Each year in the United States, about 20,000 children younger than 21 years receive a diagnosis of cancer. Because of advancements in treating these childhood cancers, about 80% of these children are cured and enter adulthood with no signs of cancer. Curing many forms of childhood cancer has been hailed as a great success story in the fight against cancer. However, studies of thousands of childhood cancer survivors have revealed a dark side to the cures (Oeffinger & Robison, 2007).

Childhood cancers are cured by aggressive treatment with a battery of toxic chemotherapeutic chemicals and radiation that destroy cancer cells. The Childhood Cancer Survivor Study (CCSS) was established in 1994 to study the health of persons who were cured of cancer as children. These people were treated between 1970 and 1986 when most of the successful treatments were introduced. Twenty-five pediatric cancer treatment centers from around the country pooled their survivor

TERMS

chemotherapy: use of toxic chemicals to kill cancer cells and treat some forms of cancer

radiation therapy: use of high-energy radiation, such as x-rays, to kill cancer cells and treat some forms of cancer

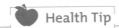 Health Tip

Video Game Helps Kids Battle Cancer

A nine-year-old and a software engineer teamed up to design a video game that would help kids with cancer battle the "bad" cells and accept the "good" chemical in chemotherapy. The game can be downloaded at www.makewish.org/ben.

data. The findings of this large, long-term study show that a majority of the survivors had serious chronic health problems and were likely to die prematurely. They suffered from other cancers, heart disease, musculoskeletal disorders, and other serious conditions. The study emphasizes that survivors of childhood cancers must receive ongoing medical attention throughout their lives to detect and treat new health problems.

For cancer survivors of any age, a healthy lifestyle is crucial to help reduce the damaging effects of the toxic treatments used to cure their cancer. Childhood cancer survivors should concentrate on eating the healthiest diet possible. They should avoid smoking and try to live in areas where the environment, especially the air, is not polluted. They should exercise regularly and avoid excess weight gain. Finally, they should regularly consult a physician who is knowledgeable about the subsequent health problems of childhood cancer survivors.

Experimental Cancer Therapies

When abnormal cells arise in the body, in most instances they are recognized and destroyed by the body's immune system. Only when abnormal cells fail to be eliminated and continue to grow and reproduce does a cancer develop. Medical researchers are currently looking for ways to develop cancer vaccines and ways to boost the body's immune system so that it is better able to fend off cancer.

> More harm is done by fools through foolishness than is done by evildoers through wickedness.
>
> *Sufi proverb*

In 2006, a cancer vaccine was approved that, if widely used, would almost eliminate cervical cancer in women. This vaccine is safe and 100% effective in blocking infection by the strains of human papillomavirus (HPV) that cause cervical cancer (Gostin & DeAngelis, 2007). Globally, an estimated 493,000 cases of cervical cancer are diagnosed each year, with about 274,000 deaths.

These new cases of cervical cancer are now preventable. It is recommended that all girls over age 11 receive a series of three shots; older girls and women should get a "catch-up" vaccination. Despite its enormous potential for preventing cervical cancer, some people object to the vaccination because they believe it will increase sexual activity among teenage girls.

For a tumor to grow rapidly, it must be well supplied with nutrients. To accomplish this, the tumor develops a network of new blood vessels that can supply the necessary nutrients, a process called angiogenesis. More than 30 years ago, physician Judah Folkman proposed that finding ways to destroy the new blood vessels in tumors might be a powerful way to arrest cancer growth and destroy tumors. Today, drugs that inhibit angiogenesis in tumors are being developed.

Coping with a Diagnosis of Cancer

A diagnosis of cancer raises serious problems for the patient and for family and friends. Often the patient enters a state of disbelief or shock. The family has to cope with new problems. The patient must face surgery or other treatment. Along with treatment, the patient usually must deal with fear of death, anger at the disease, loss of income, changes in living habits, and, above all, the uncertainty of the outcome, which may last for months or years. These are some of the reasons why coping with cancer can be difficult. Stress and emotional upset can depress the normal functions of the immune system. There also is evidence that hostile feelings, resentment, deeply felt personal loss, and feelings of hopelessness may be important factors in cancer development and lowering of disease resistance.

Pain also contributes to a cancer patient's stress and depression. Some cancers cause intense, unremitting pain that can be relieved only by opioid therapy. Yet many physicians still are reluctant to prescribe adequate doses of appropriate drugs to alleviate the pain of cancer patients, even among those who clearly are dying. Some physicians worry more about creating addiction in their patients than about relieving their pain and suffering. They also worry about prosecution for drug offenses by overzealous drug enforcement authorities. Attitudes are changing slowly, but many—probably a majority—of cancer patients undergoing therapy do not receive adequate relief for their pain. In June 2001, a physician in Berkeley, California, was sued for not providing adequate pain relief to a patient dying from cancer. The family of the deceased sued the physician; a jury agreed and awarded significant monetary damages.

The coping strategies for dealing with the emotional distress resulting from cancer, AIDS, and other serious diseases are similar. They all depend on using the mind in positive ways. The effectiveness of any therapy and the ability to cope with a life-threatening illness depend on focusing the mind on ways to enhance the healing process. Meditation and relaxation techniques are important in reducing stress. Learning how to use visual imagery can help with the effectiveness of treatments. Along with mental relaxation techniques, the mind can focus on images and suggestions that may help the immune system fight and destroy cancer cells.

🧘 Managing Stress

The Art of Visualization

As director of Biofeedback Research at the Menninger Clinic in Topeka, Kansas, Dr. Patricia Norris has documented several cases where mental imagery and visualization were used successfully to complement traditional medical treatment. Dr. Norris cites eight specific characteristics that help to make mental imagery and visualization effective as a healing tool, specifically with regard to cancer:

1. **Make the visualization personal.** The images must be self-generated. Images that are created by the practitioner and not the patient appear to be ineffective.

2. **Make the imagery "egosyntonic."** Egosyntonic means that the image must fit the values and ideals of that person. If, for example, the individual is pacifistic, then combative or warlike imagery will undermine the effectiveness of this type of treatment.

3. **Make the imagery positive.** Negative imagery reinforces negative thoughts, which are not conducive to healing. As an example, Norris notes that sharks, as a healing image, are not a good idea.

4. **Take an active role in the imagery.** Rather than imagining watching the imagery on a movie screen, you must feel the sensations of your images in the first person. You must have a sense that what you are seeing is happening inside your body, not "out there somewhere."

5. **Make the image anatomically correct and accurate.** Knowing exactly what body region and physiological system is in a disease state will dictate the type of imagery used. Consequently, you need to know whether to access the central nervous system or the immune system. Norris states that more than one image can be used in the healing process.

6. **Be constant, use dialogue.** Constancy means to be regular in generating your imagery. Norris suggests three 15-minute sessions per day, with intermittent shorter sessions throughout the day. When you feel pain, your body is communicating to you. She suggests making pain your friend. In the dialogue style of self-talk, she suggests thanking the pain for making you aware of the problem so that you may be able to fix it. Finally, she suggests "destroying" a tumor with its permission. Respond with love. Make peace with your body.

7. **Create a blueprint.** The concept of the blueprint is a strategy. A blueprint visualization is like time-lapse photography where a flower (symbolizing a tumor) is shown to bloom within seconds, and then closes up again and fades away. An example would be to see the construction of a building, starting from the hole in the earth to opening day, where you are cutting the ribbon at the front entrance.

8. **Include the treatment in the imagery.** Norris has found that patients who use mental imagery with chemotherapy treatment and radiation do better than those who "fight" these medical procedures. She notes that it helps to have benevolent feelings versus ambivalent feelings toward the treatment. She suggests one mentally "welcome the treatment into the body." Consider the treatment as a guest in your house. Based on her patient research, she offers these examples:

(a) *Chemotherapy*—a gold-colored fluid that healthy cells, acting as a bucket brigade, pass along to the cancer cells, who in turn drink up the chemotherapy

(b) *Radiation treatment*—a stream of silver energy aimed at the cancerous tumor(s). Ask the white blood cells to move away or to shield themselves and act like mirrors to reflect the radiation toward the cancer cells, then watch the cancer cells die.

A dramatic illustration of the power of belief in altering the course of cancer is the case of Mr. Wright, a patient in the 1950s. At that time, a drug called krebiozen was touted by some as a "miracle drug" that could cure cancer. Mr. Wright, who had terminal lymphosarcoma, was given a life expectancy of two weeks by his physician. However, Mr. Wright had enormous faith in the miracle drug and insisted that he be treated with it. After a single injection, his doctor noted that "the tumor masses had melted like snowballs on a hot stove, and in only these few days, they were half their original size" (Klopfer, 1957).

Mr. Wright was symptom free for two months until he read in the newspaper that krebiozen was worthless in treating cancer, whereupon he relapsed and was readmitted to the hospital. With nothing to lose, his doctor assured him that a fresh, double-strength injection of krebiozen would cure him. In actuality, Mr. Wright received an injection of salt water. Once again he was symptom free for two months. Then headlines again proclaimed "nationwide tests show krebiozen to be a worthless drug in treatment of cancer." Mr. Wright relapsed and died in two days.

Coping with cancer requires courage and conviction. A cancer patient must not give up hope, despite what the statistics predict or what physicians say about the prognosis. The patient must believe that a cure is possible and work toward that end. For many people, coping with cancer is a transforming experience and gives renewed meaning to life.

The most important thing to remember about cancer is that most cancers *are* preventable. Abstain from smoking or using tobacco and follow a diet rich in fresh fruits and vegetables. Also avoid excess exposure to sunlight and to chemicals that are known to be carcinogenic.

Critical Thinking About Health

1. Consider this hypothetical case of a female college student. Several women in her family, including her grandmother and an aunt, died of breast cancer before they reached 65 years of age. She is only 21 years old but is very concerned about her own risk of developing breast cancer. She decides to be tested for the breast cancer susceptibility genes BRCA1 and BRCA2, even though her physician explains that no medical treatment short of prophylactic mastectomy is available. The genetic test is positive for gene BRCA1, and her risk of breast cancer is significantly higher than for other women who do not have this gene. Discuss, from your own perspective, what this woman should now do to preserve her health. Gather as many facts as you can on breast cancer and the effects of these susceptibility genes.

2. Make a list of all the factors you can think of that increase the risk of developing cancer. Order the items in your list from highest risk to lowest in your judgment. Are any of the risk factors relevant to your life? If so, describe how you could modify your lifestyle or behaviors to reduce the risk of developing cancer.

3. A number of strategies are presented in this chapter that can help prevent cancers of various types. List and discuss ways to help prevent lung cancer, skin cancer, breast cancer, and colon cancer.

4. The "war against cancer" is fought by physicians and scientists in two fundamentally different ways. On the one hand, medical research tries to discover better treatments for all forms of cancer. On the other hand, epidemiologists and other researchers believe that we need to shift the scientific emphasis from seeking cures to prevention because we understand many of the environmental factors that cause cancer. Reducing exposure to risk factors could prevent as many as half of all human cancers. In your judgment, which of these positions is correct? Or do you believe both positions are equally valid? Develop facts and arguments that substantiate your views and write a report of your conclusions.

Health in Review

- *Cancer* refers to a number of different diseases, all of which share the common property of abnormal, unregulated cell growth in the body.
- Dietary factors and environmental agents, such as smoking and sunlight, act on the genetic material in cells to cause chemical changes that may initiate a tumor, which is a mass of abnormal cells.
- Cigarette smoking is responsible for about one-third of all cancers, especially lung cancer.
- The principal environmental agents that cause cancer are ionizing radiation, tumor viruses, carcinogenic chemicals, and, possibly, xenoestrogens.
- If everything known about cancer prevention were practiced, up to one-half of cancers would not occur; thus, cancer is largely a preventable disease.
- Only 5% to 10% of cancers are caused by genes that have been inherited. The genetic changes in body cells that result in cancer are not passed on to children because these genetic changes have not occurred in sperm or eggs.

- The treatments for cancer include surgery, radiation, and chemotherapy. The goal of all three cancer treatments is the removal or destruction of as many cancer cells as possible.
- Recovery from cancer depends on good nutrition, positive attitudes, healing mental images, and medical treatment appropriate for the particular cancer. A healthy, active immune system also is an essential component in cancer prevention and recovery.
- Both breast and testicular self-examinations are positive means of early cancer detection.
- Dietary deficiencies or excesses are responsible for about one-half of all cancers.
- Overexposure to sunlight causes skin cancer, which is on the increase.
- Significantly reducing cancer requires major changes in people's lifestyles, including more attention to a healthy diet, elimination of tobacco use, limiting alcohol consumption, and reducing exposure to intense sunlight and chemical carcinogens.

Health and Wellness Online

The Web contains a wealth of information about health and wellness. By accessing the Internet using Web browser software, you can gain a new perspective on many topics presented in *Health and Wellness,* Tenth Edition. Access the Jones and Bartlett Publishers Web site at **health.jbpub.com/hwonline.**

References

American Cancer Society. (2008). *Cancer facts and figures, 2008.*

Bailar, J.C., & Gornik, H.L. (1997). Cancer undefeated. *New England Journal of Medicine, 336,* 1569–1574.

Christensen, D. (2002). Mammograms on trial. *Science News, 161,* 254–266.

Collaborative Group on Hormonal Factors in Breast Cancer. (2001). Familial breast cancer: Collaborative reanalysis of individual data from 52 epidemiological studies including 58,209 women with breast cancer and 191,986 women without the disease. *Lancet, 358,* 1389–1398.

Couzin, J. (2003). Review rules out abortion cancer link. *Science, 299,* 1498.

Couzin, J. (2007). Probing the roots of race and cancer. *Science, 315,* 592–595.

Croce, C. M. (2008). Oncogenes and cancer. *New England Journal of Medicine, 358,* 502–527.

Dong, L. M., et al. (2008). Genetic susceptibility to cancer. *Journal of the American Medical Association, 299,* 2423–2436.

Gelmann, E. P. (2008). Complexities of prostate-cancer risk. *New England Journal of Medicine, 358,* 961–962.

Gostin, L. O. & DeAngelis, C. D. (2007). Mandatory HPV vaccination. *Journal of the American Medical Association, 297,* 1921–1923.

Haiman, C. A., et al. (2006). Ethnic and racial differences in smoking-related risk of lung cancer. *New England Journal of Medicine, 354,* 333–342.

Holmes, M. D., et al. (2005). Physical activity and survival after breast cancer diagnosis. *Journal of the American Medical Association, 293,* 2479–2486.

Horton, R. (2001). Screening mammography—An overview revisited. *Lancet, 358,* 1284–1285.

Klopfer, B. (1957). Psychological variables in human cancer. *Journal of Prospective Techniques, 21,* 331–340.

Kramer, B.S., & Klausner, R.D. (1997). Grappling with cancer—Defeatism versus the reality of progress. *New England Journal of Medicine, 337,* 931–934.

Lichtenstein, P., et al. (2000). Environmental and heritable factors in the causation of cancer. *New England Journal of Medicine, 343,* 78–86.

Marx, J. (2007). A healthy tan? *Science, 315,* 1214–1216.

Oeffinger, K. C., & Robison, L. L. (2007). Childhood cancer survivors, late effects, and a new model for understanding survivorship. *Journal of the American Medical Association, 297,* 2762–2764.

Suggested Readings

Christensen, D. (2002). Mammograms on trial. *Science News, 161,* 254–266. A good overview of the controversy regarding whether women should get mammograms.

Collins, F. S., & Barker, A. D. (2007, March). Mapping the cancer genome. *Scientific American,* 50–57. Describes the project to map all of the variant human genes that may contribute to the development of cancer.

Esteva, F. J., & Hortobagyi, G. N. (2008, June). Gaining ground on breast cancer. *Scientific American,* 58–65. An update on the new treatments for breast cancer.

Gibbs, W. W. (2003, July). Untangling the roots of cancer. *Scientific American,* 57–65. Discusses the many ways cancers can develop in people and possible new therapies.

Nathan, D. G. (2007). *The cancer treatment revolution.* Hoboken, NJ: John Wiley & Sons. A valuable resource for someone who has been diagnosed with cancer and wants to understand treatment options.

Rados, C. (2005, March/April). Teen tanning hazards. *FDA Consumer,* 8–9. Explains why using indoor tanning lamps increases skin cancer risks. Young people are the biggest users of indoor tanning lamps.

Spector, M. (2006, March 13). Political science. *The New Yorker,* 58–69. Describes how the political weight of the U.S. government was used to delay the approval of a vaccine that prevents cervical cancer in women based on the beliefs of some politicians that such a vaccine would encourage premarital sex.

Welch, H. G. (2004). *Should I be tested for cancer? Maybe not—and here's why.* Berkeley: University of California Press. Many tests for various cancers exist, but they often are not helpful. This book explains why.

Recommended Web Sites

Please visit **health.jbpub.com/hwonline** for links to these Web sites.

American Cancer Society
Information on types of cancer, prevention, treatment options, and medical issues.

CancerNet
The U.S. National Cancer Institute's database of cancer information.

National Alliance of Breast Cancer Organizations
Information and educational resources.

National Toxicology Program, Department of Health and Human Services
This Web site contains a list of all carcinogenic substances that have been tested by the government. The list is updated every two years.

Oncolink
Comprehensive cancer information from the University of Pennsylvania School of Medicine.

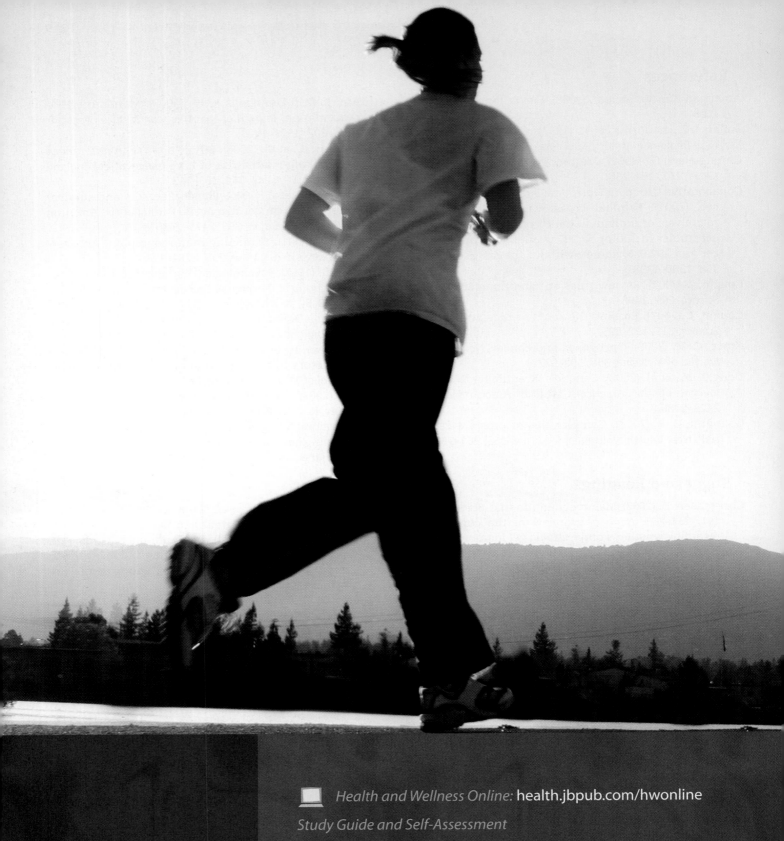

Chapter Fourteen

Cardiovascular Diseases: Understanding Risks and Measures of Prevention

Learning Objectives

1. Describe how the heart functions.

2. Define *cardiovascular disease, infarction, coronary heart disease, stroke,* and *heart attack.*

3. Explain the role atherosclerosis plays in heart disease.

4. Identify and explain types of heart surgeries used to repair blocked arteries.

5. Identify the major risk factors of heart disease that cannot be changed, major risk factors that can be changed, and other contributing factors.

6. Explain the role of homocysteine in heart disease.

7. Discuss various ways to reduce cholesterol levels.

8. Explain how stress contributes to hypertension.

9. List dietary supplements and foods that help maintain a healthy cardiovascular system.

The human heart has long been a symbol of human love as it is expressed in poetry, stories, and everyday customs. Our language still reflects the idea that love and feelings reside in the heart. The word "heartfelt" implies deep feelings of caring and sincerity; "heartless," however, implies being cold and uncaring. When love relationships collapse, people refer to their "broken hearts" or the "heartlessness" of the former lover. People are described by the nature of their hearts—cruel, kind, warm, or cold; some are even referred to as having a heart of stone. When people refer to distressing experiences in life, they talk of "heartache," and when they are happy, their hearts may "leap with joy."

> Have a heart that never hardens
> A temper that never tires
> A touch that never hurts.
>
> *Charles Dickens*

Today we know that emotions, thoughts, and feelings of every kind originate in the brain, not the heart. The heart's only function is to pump blood and circulate it throughout the body. The heart is an extraordinarily effective pump; it pumps slightly more than a gallon of blood per minute through approximately 60,000 miles of blood vessels in the body. In this gallon of blood are about 25 trillion red blood cells that carry oxygen from the lungs to all the body's cells and remove the carbon dioxide that is exhaled as waste. Each day about 200 billion new red blood cells are synthesized in bone marrow (the soft material at the center of large bones) and released into the circulation. Each day the heart expands and contracts (beats) 100,000 times and pumps about 2,000 gallons of blood. A healthy heart and blood vessels are essential for survival.

Understanding Cardiovascular Diseases

Cardiovascular disease refers to any of a number of conditions that damage the heart or the arteries that carry blood to and from the heart (**Table 14.1**). If the **coronary arteries** (the blood vessels that carry blood to the heart) become diseased or blocked, a **heart attack** may result. If the cells of the heart do not receive a continual supply of blood and oxygen, the cells die, a condition known as an **infarction**. If the blood supply to the heart is only partially blocked, the process is known as **ischemia**.

According to current estimates, more than 70 million Americans (34% of the population) have some form of cardiovascular disease (American Heart Association, 2008). About one-third of all deaths each year in the United States result from cardiovascular diseases that lead to heart attacks and strokes. A **stroke** occurs when an insufficient supply of blood to brain cells causes them to die. Although cardiovascular diseases tend to occur in the elderly, heart attacks can occur at any age, often without warning.

Table 14.1

Categories of Cardiovascular Disease

Disease	Description
Atherosclerosis	Partial or complete blockage of one or more coronary arteries; the leading cause of heart attack and stroke
Arrhythmia	Heart rhythm disorders; includes atrial fibrillation and flutter
Cardiomyopathy	Inflammation and reduced function of the heart muscle
Endocarditis	Bacterial infection of the heart lining or valves
Congenital heart defects	Heart defects present at birth; about 30,000 babies are born each year with any one of three dozen different defects
Congestive heart failure	Occurs when the heart is unable to pump all the blood that is returned to it
Rheumatic heart disease	Damage to the heart caused by the immune system in response to certain bacterial infections occurring during childhood
Valvular heart disease	Results from defective heart valves, usually the aortic or mitral valves

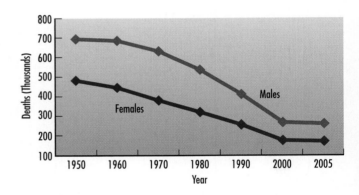

■ Figure 14.1

Mortality from Cardiovascular Disease in the United States (1950–2005)

Source: Data from U.S. Centers for Disease Control and Prevention.

The rate of death from cardiovascular diseases among men has been declining steadily in the United States but has increased somewhat in the last decade for women (**Figure 14.1**). Certainly, public awareness of the risk factors in cardiovascular disease has been a major contributor to the overall decline in mortality. Overall, deaths from heart disease have declined in the United States from 336 per hundred thousand in 1980 to 236 per hundred thousand in 2004. Much of this decline in deaths is thought to be due to more effective treatment of heart disease and heart attacks. Less fat and cholesterol in the diet, less cigarette smoking, and more exercising have also contributed to reducing deaths from cardiovascular dis-

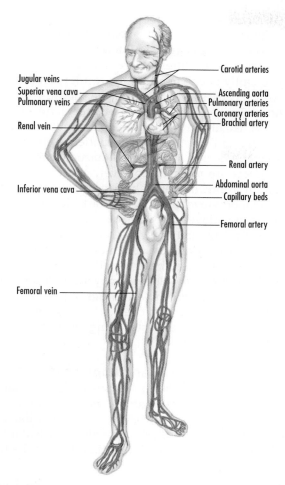

Jugular veins
Superior vena cava
Pulmonary veins
Renal vein
Inferior vena cava
Femoral vein

Carotid arteries
Ascending aorta
Pulmonary arteries
Coronary arteries
Brachial artery
Renal artery
Abdominal aorta
Capillary beds
Femoral artery

■ Figure 14.2

Cardiovascular System
Includes the heart, arteries, and veins. The heart receives oxygenated blood from the lungs and pumps it to all tissues in the body.

ease. Like cancer, most heart disease is preventable and is caused primarily by unhealthy lifestyles, poor diet, high blood pressure, and cigarette smoking.

The Heart and Blood Vessels

The human cardiovascular system consists of the heart (the pump) and the various blood vessels (**Figure 14.2**). **Arteries** carry oxygenated blood from the heart to all organs and tissues in the body. **Veins** return blood to the heart after oxygen and nutrients have been exchanged for carbon dioxide and waste products. **Capillaries** are tiny blood vessels that branch out from arteries and veins and circulate blood to all of the cells in the body. Blood vessels can be damaged by injury or by disease; this damage may obstruct the flow of blood carrying oxygen and nutrients.

The organ that keeps the blood circulating throughout the body is the heart, a highly specialized muscle about the size of an adult fist that pumps blood (**Figure 14.3**). The muscular wall of the heart is called the

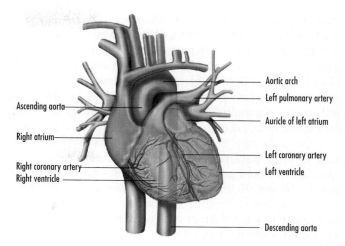

Ascending aorta
Right atrium
Right coronary artery
Right ventricle

Aortic arch
Left pulmonary artery
Auricle of left atrium
Left coronary artery
Left ventricle
Descending aorta

■ Figure 14.3

Heart and Major Arteries
Oxygenated blood is pumped through the arteries (red), and oxygen-depleted blood is returned to the heart via the veins (blue).

myocardium. If the blood supply to heart cells is blocked, cells begin to die and a heart attack results.

The heart consists of four separate chambers: The upper two chambers are called the left atrium and the right atrium; the lower two chambers are the right ventricle and the left ventricle. Blood that is depleted of oxygen returns to the heart via the right atrium and then flows to the right ventricle. From there blood is pumped to the lungs, where it is reoxygenated and returned via the pulmonary veins to the left atrium. Finally, the fresh blood is

TERMS

arteries: any of a series of blood vessels that carry blood from the heart to all parts of the body

capillaries: extremely small blood vessels that carry oxygenated blood to tissues

cardiovascular disease: any disease that causes damage to the heart or to major arteries leading from the heart

coronary arteries: two arteries arising from the aorta that supply blood to the heart muscle

heart attack: death of, or damage to, part of the heart muscle caused by an insufficient blood supply

infarction: death of heart cells resulting from a blocked blood supply

ischemia: an insufficient supply of blood to the heart

myocardium: muscular wall of the heart that contracts and relaxes

stroke: an insufficient supply of blood to the brain, resulting in loss of muscle function, loss of speech, or other symptoms

veins: blood vessels that return blood from tissues to the heart

pumped throughout the body's tissues from the left ventricle through the large artery called the **aorta.**

The heart contracts from 60 to 100 times a minute, depending on the body's activity. The entire volume of blood in the body is recirculated almost once every minute. During an average lifetime of 70 years, the heart will pump between 30 and 40 million gallons of blood, and it will beat 2.5 billion times!

The beat of a healthy heart is characterized by its rate and its pattern, or *rhythm*. The heart rate is the number of times per minute the lower chambers of the heart (the ventricles) contract to move blood out of the heart. The heart rhythm is a sequence of coordinated biological events that create ventricular contractions strong enough to move blood. The heart rate is controlled by a region in the right atrium called the **sino-atrial node**. This region sends electrical signals across the surface of the heart, which causes heart muscle fibers to contract. The heart rate is also influenced by electrical signals from the brain, which explains how emotions, excitement, fear, and stress can suddenly change the heart rate.

A biological anomaly, injury, or disease can cause the heartbeat to lose its normal rhythmic pattern. An irregular heartbeat is called an *arrhythmia*. Symptoms of arrhythmias include a fast or slow heartbeat, skipping beats, shortness of breath, chest pain, lightheadedness, dizziness, and sweating. Types of arrhythmias are presented in **Table 14.2**.

The heartbeat also can be affected by nerve impulses that originate in areas of the heart other than the sino-atrial node. If these signals interfere with the normal heartbeat, causing different areas of the heart to beat independently of one another, the result is **atrial fibrillation,** which causes a change in the heartbeat.

Atrial fibrillation involves the upper chambers of the heart and usually develops as people age; it is estimated that about 2 million Americans experience atrial fibrillation to some degree. Usually the episodes are brief and no ill effects are noticed. However, persons with atrial fibrillation are at higher risk of stroke. Because of the reduced blood movement in the heart, clots can form in the heart and travel through the arteries to the brain, where a blockage may result. Atrial fibrillation can be managed with various drugs, and anyone who experiences an irregular heartbeat (usually noticed as a palpitation in the chest) should see a physician. If the fibrillation cannot be controlled with drugs, a **pacemaker** can be implanted in a person's chest. This is a small electrical device that supplies a steadying electrical signal to the heart.

Defibrillators: External and Implanted

Each year, about 460,000 Americans experience sudden cardiac arrest, and about half die within an hour of the onset of symptoms. About 60,000 cases of cardiac arrest are associated with fibrillation, usually ventricular fibrillation, which occurs in the lower chambers of the heart.

Table 14.2

Types of Irregular Heart Rhythms

Type	Description
Premature (extra) beats	A sensation of fluttering in the chest or a skipped beat. Very common; most of the time requires no treatment, especially in healthy people. Premature beats in the atria are called premature atrial contractions, or PACs. Premature beats in the ventricles are called premature ventricular contractions, or PVCs.
Atrial fibrillation (AF)	A rapid, irregular contraction of the atria resulting from abnormal electrical signals coursing in a disorganized way through the heart tissue. This causes the walls of the atria to quiver (*fibrillate*) to be able to pump blood in the normal way. Stroke and heart failure are serious complications of ongoing, untreated AF.
Atrial flutter	Similar to atrial fibrillation; the spread of electrical signals through the atria is too fast and regular (as opposed to irregular). Similar symptoms and complications as atrial fibrillation.
Paroxysmal supraventricular tachycardia (PSVT)	A very fast heart rate that begins and ends suddenly. It occurs due to problems with the electrical connection between the atria and the ventricles. Not usually dangerous, and tends to occur in young people. It can happen during vigorous exercise.
Ventricular tachycardia	A fast, regular beating of the ventricles. A few beats of ventricular tachycardia often do not cause problems, but episodes lasting for more than a few seconds can be dangerous.
Ventricular fibrillation	Disorganized electrical signals make the ventricles quiver instead of pump normally. When ventricles do not pump blood out of the heart, a person will lose consciousness within seconds and may die. To prevent death, the condition must be treated immediately with defibrillation, an electric shock to the heart.
Bradyarrhythmias	The heart rate is much slower than normal. A very slow heart rate may result in not enough blood reaching the brain.

In these cases, the heartbeat is very erratic and death ensues unless a regular heartbeat can be restored quickly. A **defibrillator** is an electrical device that can restore normal heart rhythm by delivering electrical shocks through the chest to the heart. For a heart attack victim to survive, defibrillation should be initiated within a short period (a few minutes) after the beginning of the heart attack. By the time a patient reaches an emergency room, it is often too late for defibrillation.

For these reasons, automated external defibrillators (AEDs) have been developed and are now placed in many public areas where people congregate, such as shopping malls, sports arenas, stadiums, and airplanes. AEDs also can be purchased by individuals and kept in the home, where most heart attacks occur.

Because about 80% of sudden heart attacks occur at home, the usefulness of publicly placed AEDs is questionable (Callans, 2008). On the other hand, if one waits for paramedics to arrive to administer an electrical shock to the heart, statistics show that only about 6% of those patients survive to be discharged from a hospital. Controversy still surrounds the placement and use of AEDs in public places, especially by untrained personnel.

People who suffer from frequent abnormal heart rhythms (cardiac arrhythmias) may be candidates for an implantable cardioverter defibrillator (ICD). A small unit is implanted in the chest with wires attached to the heart. If the heart begins to beat irregularly, the defibrillator will deliver a pulse of electricity to the heart to restore normal heartbeats. Each year in the United States, about 200,000 patients receive an ICD at a cost of up to $50,000 per patient (Harder, 2006). The batteries last about five years; then, the surgery must be repeated. Most patients with ICDs will not experience an arrhythmia severe enough to trigger an electrical shock. But doctors still cannot distinguish with certainty those patients who definitely need an ICD from those who probably do not need one.

Regulating Blood Flow

To maintain uniform blood flow in the correct direction through arteries and veins, the cardiovascular system is equipped with one-way valves both in the chambers of the heart and in blood vessels (**Figure 14.4**). With every heartbeat, the valves in the heart open and close to allow blood to circulate in one direction. In rare cases, one or more of the heart valves may be defective at birth because of developmental abnormalities. With modern techniques of open-heart surgery, defective heart valves can be repaired or replaced with artificial valves that allow the heart to function normally.

Heart valves can also be damaged by childhood throat infections caused by *Streptococcus* bacteria. Repeated streptococcal infections can cause rheumatic heart disease (formerly called rheumatic fever), a serious inflammatory disease of the heart valves. In susceptible people, the immune system overreacts to the presence of

the bacteria. Some proteins on the heart cells are similar in structure to proteins on the bacteria, so the immune system attacks heart valve cells as well as the infectious bacteria.

The mitral and aortic valves are particularly susceptible to damage by infections. Scar tissue forms and prevents the valves from opening and closing correctly. By listening to the heartbeat, a **cardiologist,** a physician who specializes in heart diseases, can detect abnormalities in the heart's valves. Because of potential heart problems, it is important that all "strep throat" in

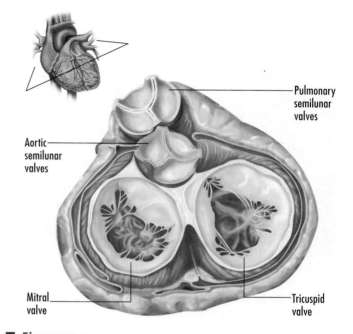

■ Figure 14.4

Heart Valves
The heart's valves keep the blood flowing in one direction into and out of the chambers of the heart.

TERMS

aorta: the large artery that transports blood from the heart to the body

atrial fibrillation: rapid, erratic contraction of the upper chambers of the heart

cardiologist: a physician who specializes in diseases of the heart

defibrillator: an electrical device that can restart a heart that has stopped beating by delivering electrical shocks to it

pacemaker: an electrical device implanted in the chest to control irregular heartbeats

sinoatrial node: the region of the heart that produces an electrical signal that causes the heart to contract

children be treated with antibiotics to reduce the risk of developing rheumatic heart disease.

Another common, but less serious, defect of the circulation is in valves in the veins that cause **varicose veins.** These appear as unsightly, bluish bulges in veins, usually in the legs. Blood returning to the heart from the legs has to flow against the pull of gravity, and one-way valves in the veins normally prevent the blood from draining downward. If the valves in the veins of the legs become weakened, blood tends to accumulate, distending the veins and producing visible varicose veins. The valve failures in the veins are not life-threatening and often can be corrected by surgical removal of the damaged areas.

Atherosclerosis

Arteriosclerosis, which literally means hardening of the arteries, includes all kinds of diseases that damage the arteries and eventually lead to coronary artery disease (CAD). However, the one form of arteriosclerosis that is of primary concern is **atherosclerosis.** This arterial disease begins with damage to cells of the heart's arteries and leads to the formation of a fibrous, fatty deposit called **plaque.** The arterial plaque slowly increases in size until eventually the amount of blood flowing through the artery is greatly reduced or completely blocked (**Figure 14.5**).

Obstruction of blood flow in an artery is very serious because heart cells are deprived of oxygenated blood and die. Oxygen is supplied to the heart by the coronary arteries, which are the first to branch from the aorta. Despite its relatively small size, the heart uses about 20% of the total oxygenated blood circulated through the body.

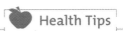
Health Tips

Infected Gums Contribute to Heart Disease

We all know that cleaning your teeth and gums prevents dental caries. Here is another strong reason for oral cleanliness. Some research has shown an association between infected gums and risk of heart disease. Bacteria found in the mouth have also been detected in the plaques that block arteries.

About one-half of all Americans over age 30 have *gingivitis,* a mild inflammation of the gums caused by oral bacteria; about one-third over age 30 have *periodontitis,* acute gum inflammation and gum disease. (Smoking is a primary cause of this condition.) If your gums bleed when you brush or floss, see your dentist for treatment for gum disease. Maintaining oral health when you are young may also prevent heart disease later in life.

If the coronary arteries become partially blocked and the heart cells do not get enough oxygen, chest pain called **angina pectoris** results. The drug nitroglycerin dilates blood vessels and is used to relieve the pain of angina. If a plaque ruptures and a coronary artery becomes completely blocked, the person may have a fatal heart attack.

Diagnosis of a Heart Attack

Each year in the United States about a million people are admitted to hospitals because of possible heart attacks. Tests eventually rule out a heart attack in about 50% of those admitted. Chest pains that mimic those of a heart attack can be brought on by severe indigestion (heartburn), panic, and stress.

Distinguishing between a heart attack and less serious causes of chest pain is crucial if appropriate treat-

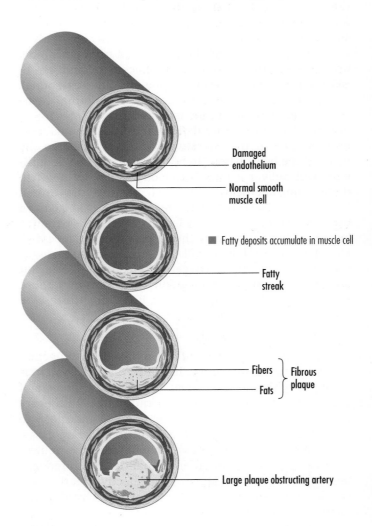

Damaged endothelium

Normal smooth muscle cell

■ Fatty deposits accumulate in muscle cell

Fatty streak

Fibers ⎫ Fibrous
Fats ⎬ plaque

Large plaque obstructing artery

■ **Figure 14.5**

Development of an Atherosclerotic Lesion (Plaque) Inside an Artery
Plaque can eventually block blood flow, causing a heart attack or stroke. Many factors are involved in the formation of a plaque, including cholesterol and lipid levels, immune system cells, and inflammation.

ment is to be started. At present, diagnosing a heart attack involves a number of different laboratory tests.

If a heart attack has occurred, the levels of certain proteins in the blood, such as creatine kinase, troponin, myoglobin, and myosin, begin to change. Measuring the levels of these proteins allows physicians in emergency rooms (ERs) to determine quickly whether a heart attack has occurred and to initiate appropriate treatment.

Even after extensive tests show that the heart and arteries are functioning normally, 15% to 30% of patients with severe chest pains continue to experience pain and symptoms of cardiovascular disease. In most of these patients, the angina pain can be controlled with medications, and they are not at any greater risk of a heart attack than persons without angina.

Repairing Blocked Arteries

When medical tests show that one or more coronary arteries are blocked, surgery is usually recommended to remove the blockage.

A precise image of the flow of blood through the coronary arteries that supply blood to the heart is obtained by an invasive procedure called **cardiac catheterization**. A thin tube is threaded from an artery in a leg or arm up into the coronary arteries. A dye is injected, and high-speed x-ray film records the flow of the dye in the arteries. More than a million cardiac catheterizations are performed each year in the United States on patients with suspected partial blockage of their coronary arteries.

In **coronary artery bypass surgery,** the diseased segment of an artery is cut out and a segment of a healthy vein or artery is grafted onto the damaged artery to restore normal flow of blood to the heart. If one graft is made into a blocked artery, the surgery is called a single coronary bypass; if four grafts are made, it is called a quadruple bypass.

Coronary artery bypass surgery is a form of **open-heart surgery** and usually requires several months of recuperation. In open-heart surgery, while the heart is exposed and being repaired, the bloodstream is diverted through a heart–lung machine. More than half a million bypass surgeries are performed every year in the United States, at an average cost of approximately $60,000 each. Although bypass surgeries are successful and save many lives, as many as half of bypass patients experience another arterial blockage within five years, especially if they do not modify their lifestyle to reduce the risk factors contributing to heart disease.

TERMS

angina pectoris: medical term for chest pain caused by coronary heart disease; a condition in which the heart muscle doesn't receive enough blood, resulting in chest pain

arteriosclerosis: hardening of the arteries

atherosclerosis: a disease process in which fatty deposits (plaques) build up in the arteries and block the flow of blood

cardiac catheterization: visualization of blocked coronary arteries by using a catheter and monitoring blood flow in coronary arteries; a dye is injected through the catheter

coronary artery bypass surgery: surgery to improve blood supply to the heart muscle by replacing the damaged portion of the artery with a graft

open-heart surgery: surgery performed on the opened heart while the blood supply is diverted through a heart–lung machine

plaque: deposit of fatty substances in the inner lining of arteries

varicose veins: swelling of veins (usually in the legs) resulting from defective valves

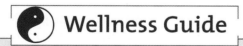 Wellness Guide

Concussion to the Heart

Most everyone knows what a brain concussion is—a blow to the head that may cause unconsciousness, problems in mental functioning, and headaches for weeks or months after the concussion. Concussions are frequent in contact sports such as football, and NFL quarterbacks Troy Aikman and Steve Young were forced to retire after each suffered a series of concussions.

A blow to the left side of the chest caused by a punch, thrown baseball, hockey puck, or other object may cause a concussion to the heart that is medically known as *commotio cordis.* Such a blow, even a light blow, if delivered at a very precise moment during the rhythmic beating of the heart, can induce instant fibrillation (irregular heartbeat) and sudden death. Cases of commotio cordis are rare. Only about 130 cases have been reported in the United States (Maron et al., 2005), but sports medicine experts suspect that many more go unreported. Unfortunately, only about 15% of affected persons—most of whom are children—survive. The sports carrying the highest risk of sudden death from commotio cordis are baseball, softball, and hockey.

Use of chest protectors and softer balls can reduce the risk of commotio cordis in some sports, especially among children and young athletes. Also, never punch or poke anyone in the chest.

$ Dollars and Health Sense

Coronary Artery Bypass Surgery and Angina

High-tech surgical procedures, such as coronary artery bypass, angioplasty, and pacemaker implantation, have revolutionized the treatment of coronary heart disease (CHD). Although these surgeries prevent some heart attacks and save lives, in many instances they are performed for heart conditions such as angina (chest pain) that can be controlled with medications.

In the 1950s, angina from partially blocked coronary arteries was relieved by an operation in which a chest artery was tied off in the hope that more blood would be supplied to the patient's heart. About 40% of the patients had reduced pain following this operation. To determine whether

Block in left coronary artery
■ Once bypass is performed, this blocked section is removed

Saphenous vein graft to right coronary artery

Aorta
Pulmonary artery
Saphenous vein graft to left coronary artery

Diagram of the coronary arteries showing where grafts are made to correct blockages.

the relief of angina pain was a placebo effect or actually resulted from the surgery, a number of mock operations were performed. (In the 1950s, informed consent was not mandatory in most hospitals.) Patients were given anesthesia, the chest was cut open, but nothing else was done to correct blood flow to the heart. Patients who underwent mock surgeries had just as much relief from angina as patients who had the chest artery tied off (Frank, 1973). As a result, this operation was abandoned.

In a similar fashion, coronary artery bypass operations may relieve angina as a result of the long period of rest and recuperation that patients undergo; lifestyle changes that people make also may contribute to their relief. A large part of the success of bypass surgery may be a result of a placebo effect (see Chapter 2).

Although effective in restoring normal blood flow to the heart, coronary artery bypass surgery carries the risk of neuralgic damage and cognitive loss. Stroke is the most serious complication, occurring in 1% to 6% of patients undergoing bypass surgery. Many patients also notice some loss of both short- and long-term memory. Some patients show a cognitive decline even five years after bypass surgery. The death rate during bypass surgery is approximately 2.2%, a relatively high risk.

An alternative surgical approach to opening a blocked artery is **percutaneous transluminal coronary angioplasty (PTCA),** or simply angioplasty). In this procedure, a thin wire is threaded from the femoral artery in the thigh up to the point of blockage in a coronary artery. Another thin tube containing a deflated balloon is then slipped over the wire and threaded up to the area of the arterial plaque. The balloon is inflated and pushes the plaque back into the wall of the artery, thereby opening it up. Angioplasty costs about half as much as a bypass operation, but the frequency with which the blockage recurs is quite high, making a repeat procedure necessary.

An alternative to bypass surgery for clogged arteries is a procedure called *stenting*. This procedure also involves inserting a catheter into an arm or leg and threading it up to the point of blockage in either a coronary artery or the carotid artery in the neck. If a blockage is found, an object called a stent is inserted that props the artery open.

Stenting has become widely used because it is a simpler, cheaper, and safer procedure than bypass surgery. However, there are still questions as to whether bypass surgery or stenting is better for long-term survival. The original stents inserted into arteries consisted of bare metal. In a large number of patients, the stents and arteries often became blocked again within months or years, and the procedure had to be repeated. A few years ago, drug-eluting stents were introduced. These stents slowly release a drug that helps prevent the artery from becoming blocked again. Despite the initial enthusiasm for drug-eluting stents, it soon became apparent that there were problems with them (Vastag, 2007). Life-threatening blood clots developed in some patients who had drug-eluting stents implanted in one or more arteries. Other large-scale studies indicated that for partial arterial blockage, drugs were safer and more effective than surgical insertion of drug-eluting stents. How to treat patients with one or more blocked arteries is still questionable. However, most cardiologists agree that if at least three arteries are blocked, bypass surgery is the best option.

All forms of cardiovascular operations and procedures have been increasing rapidly in recent years (**Figure 14.6**). Overall, almost 7 million coronary and carotid procedures are performed annually in the United States to repair clogged arteries and prevent heart attacks and strokes. More effort is need by public health officials and the public to help people adopt lifestyles that will reduce

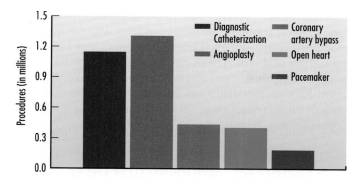

■ **Figure 14.6**

Number of Cardiovascular Surgeries and Procedures Performed in the United States in 2006
Data are for inpatient (hospital) procedures only. Diagnostic catheterization is for assessing the amount of blockage in the coronary arteries. Angioplasty (also called percutaneous transluminal coronary angioplasty [PTCA], or percutaneous transluminal intervention [PCI]) is opening a clogged artery by inflatable balloon or stent. A pacemaker is a device that regulates the heartbeat. Open heart procedures include heart valve replacements and implanting defibrillators.

Source: C. J. DeFrances. (2008, July 30). 2006 National Hospital Discharge Survey. National Health Statistics Reports, No. 5, 1–20.

the need for invasive medical procedures to repair clogged arteries.

Some physicians question whether all the coronary artery bypass and other surgeries really are always necessary. In Canada and Great Britain, where far fewer of these surgeries are performed, patients with cardiovascular disease live just as long. Like other aspects of American culture, coronary artery bypass surgery has become a "celebrity procedure." (David Letterman displayed his quadruple bypass on his TV show, direct from the hospital the day after surgery.) It also is extremely profitable for hospitals and surgeons. However, despite the glamour and profit, there is growing evidence that lifestyle changes and appropriate medicines are as effective, safer, and less costly than surgery is in treating cardiovascular disease.

Until recently, it was medical dogma that atherosclerosis was a progressive and irreversible disease. However, clinical studies involving patients with partially blocked arteries have consistently shown that the blockages can be improved through lifestyle changes and that this entrenched medical view is incorrect (Ornish et al., 1998). Patients who are motivated and who change their lifestyle dramatically can improve the health of their arteries and avoid surgery. However, most patients with blocked arteries still opt for the quick fix of surgery, even though, for many, it is only a temporary solution to their cardiovascular problems. (Arteries often become blocked again within a few years after surgery.) Many physicians still feel obligated to perform bypass surgery or stenting for fear of being sued for not recommending the standard and accepted medical treatment. Thus, heart and artery surgeries probably will

continue to be performed excessively in our society until views change.

Cardiopulmonary Resuscitation

Cardiopulmonary resuscitation (CPR) is an emergency procedure administered to a person who has stopped breathing, which usually results from a heart attack, electrocution, or near drowning. CPR involves two actions by the person administering it: (1) mouth-to-mouth breathing, and (2) repeated compression of the chest. In 2005, the rules for administering CPR were changed; the new rules reduce the importance of mouth-to-mouth breathing and emphasize repeated, rapid, and vigorous compressions of the chest.

The new rules make it easier for someone to learn CPR because the same rules now apply to both adults and children. The new rules also make it unnecessary to stop compressing the chest to periodically check the victim's breathing. The new rules call for 30 rapid, forceful compressions of the chest followed by two mouth-to-mouth breaths. The chest compressions force the blood to circulate, which is critical to supplying vital organs and the brain with the oxygen remaining in the blood. The new rules also call for giving only one shock to the victim's heart with a defibrillator before beginning CPR. In the past, several shocks were recommended. Studies have shown that people who take a CPR training course can learn how to use a defibrillator in about 5 minutes and CPR in about 20 minutes. The four steps in CPR are as follows:

Step 1: Place the person carefully on his or her back. Tilt the head back and lift the chin until the teeth almost touch. Look for signs of breathing.
Step 2: If the person is not breathing, pinch the nose and give the person two full breaths about two seconds long to produce a visible chest rise.
Step 3: Place your hands in the center of the person's chest between the nipples. Place one hand on top of the other and with elbows locked press the heel of your hand into the chest.
Step 4: Give 30 rapid compressions for every two full breaths; repeat until medical help arrives or until the person starts breathing.

Immediate administration of CPR can double the chance of a person surviving sudden cardiac arrest. By making CPR rules simpler and easier to learn, it is hoped that more people will become proficient in the technique. For more information about the new CPR

TERMS

cardiopulmonary resuscitation (CPR): an emergency lifesaving procedure used to revive someone who has stopped breathing or suffered cardiac arrest

percutaneous transluminal coronary angioplasty (PTCA): a procedure to open blocked arteries

rules or to enroll in a CPR course, contact the American Heart Association at www.americanheart.org.

Stroke

Stroke, also called brain attack, is the third leading cause of death in the United States, after heart disease and cancer. As with the latter two diseases, stroke is, in most cases, a preventable disease. High blood pressure is the most important risk factor and plays a role in at least 70% of all strokes.

Stroke is a form of cardiovascular disease that affects arteries supplying blood to the brain. If a brain artery becomes blocked or ruptures, brain cells die within minutes from lack of oxygen. Parts of the body whose functions depend on these damaged areas in the brain also are affected. Thus, a person who has a stroke can lose the ability to speak or to see, become paralyzed in an arm or leg, or lose the use of one whole side of the body. Strokes can result from injuries to the head or from weak spots in the arteries called **aneurysms** that balloon out and rupture. Strokes also can result when the heartbeat is weak and the heart does not pump enough blood through the arteries to the brain. The effects of strokes vary greatly, ranging from mild or unnoticed symptoms to sudden death.

Two main classes of stroke or brain attack are defined medically. *Ischemic stroke* results when one or more blood vessels in the brain become blocked due to a clot in an artery in the brain or in one leading to the brain. Brain cells that are deprived of oxygen supplied in arterial blood begin to die almost immediately. *Hemorrhagic stroke* results when a blood vessel in the brain ruptures, which also deprives brain cells of oxygen.

The warning signs of a stroke are any of the following conditions that occur suddenly. Immediate medical attention is needed if any of these symptoms of stroke occur:

- Sudden weakness or numbness of the face, arm, or leg on one side of the body
- Sudden dimness or loss of vision, especially in one eye
- Loss of speech, difficulty understanding speech, or trouble talking
- Sudden, severe headaches with no known cause
- Unexplained unsteadiness, dizziness, or sudden falls, especially with one of the other symptoms

Some patients at risk for strokes may benefit from a surgical procedure called **carotid endarterectomy** that removes fatty deposits by inserting a stent in the clogged artery in the neck. These arteries supply blood to the brain and, if they become blocked, may cause a stroke. Blocked neck arteries can be detected by listening to the blood flow with a stethoscope and can be confirmed by an ultrasound scan. The principal danger of the surgery is that it may precipitate a stroke—the very thing that it is designed to prevent.

The best way to prevent a stroke is to reduce the risk factors. There are five controllable risk factors for a stroke:

(1) high blood pressure; (2) heart disease; (3) cigarette smoking; (4) transient ischemic attacks; and (5) high red blood cell count, which thickens the blood and facilitates formation of a clot. These risk factors can, for the most part, be controlled by lifestyle changes or medications or both. Risk factors for a stroke that cannot be changed include (1) increasing age, (2) being male, (3) race, (4) diabetes mellitus, (5) prior stroke, and (6) heredity.

Risk Factors for Cardiovascular Disease

What starts the development of plaque in arteries and leads to cardiovascular disease, heart attacks, and brain attacks? No one knows for certain. Arterial plaques are found in the hearts of healthy young people who die accidentally, suggesting that the disease process begins early in life in some individuals. Atherosclerosis is primarily a disease of modern, industrialized societies. Tribal people in New Guinea, Kung tribes in Africa, and Inuit in Greenland have a low incidence of cardiovascular disease. Tarahumara Indians in Mexico have virtually no heart disease or high blood pressure as long as they consume their native diet. However, when researchers switched a group of Tarahumara Indian volunteers to a typical American diet, they gained weight and had dramatic increases in lipid and cholesterol levels in their blood (McMurry et al., 1991).

Although specific causes of cardiovascular disease are still not completely understood, there is general agreement that four factors contribute to its risk: (1) smoking, (2) overweight and diabetes mellitus, (3) hypertension, and (4) hypercholesterolemia. Other factors that play a role but whose precise contribution is uncertain are stress, inflammation, age, sex, and heredity.

The epidemic of overweight and obesity among young people (see Chapter 6) is expected to produce a large increase in heart disease, heart attacks, strokes, and

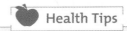 Health Tips

Naps Reduce Risk of Dying from a Heart Attack

Southern Europeans love a big lunch and a siesta, especially the Greeks. A survey of thousands of Greek workers found that those who took a 30-minute nap at least three times a week in the afternoon were 64% less likely to die from a heart attack compared with workers who did not take a nap. Even a 5-minute nap a couple of times a week showed a 12% reduction in heart attack deaths. Although the results are impressive, critics point out that the Greek workers who napped may already have had very low stress levels or some other behavior that benefited their hearts. Although the work situation in the United States is very different from that in Greece, it might be worth a try if you are one of the lucky ones who can slip away for an afternoon "power" nap.

deaths as these individuals enter middle age. The burden on the U.S. health care system and the increased costs are expected to be staggering. Overweight now rivals cigarette smoking as the leading preventable risk factor for heart disease. Overweight smokers are expected to develop heart disease at relatively young ages.

The more risk factors a person has, the greater is the likelihood for developing cardiovascular disease (**Figure 14.7**). Fortunately, each of these major risk factors can be markedly reduced by lifestyle changes and/or medications.

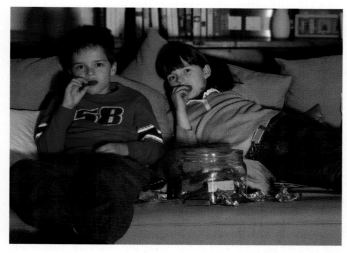

Risk factors for cardiovascular disease include cigarette smoking, high blood pressure, high blood cholesterol, sedentary lifestyle, overweight, and excessive alcohol consumption.

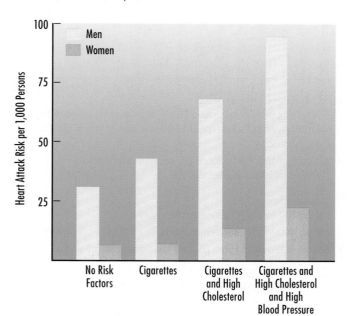

■ Figure 14.7

How Risk of Heart Attack Increases
The graph shows how risk increases for a male or female, age 55, with the following risk factors: smoking 20 cigarettes per day, having a blood cholesterol level greater than 260 mg/dl, and having a systolic blood pressure higher than 150 mm Hg.

Cholesterol

Cholesterol is an essential component of body cells and is synthesized in the body as well as being obtained from food (**Table 14.3**). Cholesterol circulates in the blood mostly in the form of particles consisting of proteins, triglycerides (fats), and cholesterol. These particles are divided into two kinds: **high-density lipoproteins (HDL)** and **low-density lipoproteins (LDL)**. These have different functions that, in some sense, are opposite to one another. Other kinds of cholesterol-carrying particles also are found in the blood, but these are ultimately converted into LDL particles.

The cholesterol that gets deposited in plaques and blocks the arteries comes mainly from LDL particles. As LDL particles circulate in the blood, cholesterol is used by tissues to build new cells. Any excess cholesterol is processed in the liver, and the cholesterol level in the blood is maintained by regulatory mechanisms in the

Table 14.3

Amount of Cholesterol in Various Foods

Food	Cholesterol
Lard, 1 tablespoon	12 mg
Cream, 1 oz.	20 mg
Cottage cheese, 1/2 cup	24 mg
Ice cream, 1/2 cup	27 mg
Cheddar cheese, 1 oz.	28 mg
Whole milk, 1 cup	34 mg
Butter, 1 tablespoon	35 mg
Oysters, salmon, 3 oz.	40 mg
Clams, tuna, 3 oz.	55 mg
Beef, pork, lobster, chicken, turkey, 3 oz.	75 mg
Lamb, veal, crab, 3 oz.	85 mg
Shrimp, 3 oz.	130 mg
Beef heart, 3 oz.	230 mg
Egg, one yolk	250 mg
Liver, 3 oz.	370 mg
Kidney, 3 oz.	680 mg
Brains, 3 oz.	1,700 mg

The most common source of cholesterol in the diet is egg yolk. Only about half of the consumed cholesterol is absorbed. Additionally, the human liver itself synthesizes 1,000 to 1,500 mg of cholesterol a day.

TERMS

aneurysm: a ballooning out of a vein or artery

carotid endarterectomy: removal of fatty deposits in arteries in the neck to prevent a stroke

high-density lipoprotein (HDL): the carrier of cholesterol from tissues to the liver for removal from the circulation; carrier of "good" cholesterol

low-density lipoprotein (LDL): the carrier of "bad" cholesterol in blood

liver. Receptor proteins on the surface of liver cells bind LDL particles and remove excess cholesterol. If the liver is overwhelmed with LDL particles, it may not be able to process all of them. When that occurs, too much cholesterol circulates in the blood and may be deposited in the walls of the arteries.

HDL particles are produced in the liver and intestines and are released into the bloodstream. As HDL particles circulate through the body, they pick up cholesterol and return it to the liver for removal. Thus, HDL particles scavenge excess cholesterol from the blood and arteries, thereby reducing the buildup of plaques.

People differ markedly in their ability to process excess cholesterol, just as they differ in other traits. The most dramatic example of cholesterol metabolism is that of an 88-year-old man who had eaten 25 eggs a day for more than 15 years and yet had completely normal blood cholesterol levels (Kern, 1991).

At the other extreme of the body's ability to process cholesterol are persons with an inherited disease called **familial hyperlipidemia (FH),** which results in markedly elevated levels of cholesterol in the blood. People with this disease have two defective genes, one inherited from each unaffected parent. The normal forms of these genes are responsible for synthesizing LDL receptor proteins on liver cells that bind LDL particles and remove cholesterol from the blood. As a result of their defective genes, people with FH cannot synthesize these essential LDL receptor proteins. Cholesterol cannot be removed and processed in the liver, and it accumulates to exceptionally high levels in the blood. People with this disease usually have heart attacks at an early age. In a few cases, transplant of a nor-

mal liver has successfully reversed the effects of FH to a significant degree.

Measuring Cholesterol Levels Cholesterol and lipid levels in the blood are measured in various ways. Total cholesterol levels are measured in milligrams per deciliter (mg/dl) of blood. Generally, a cholesterol level below 200 mg/dl indicates a relatively low risk of coronary heart disease (CHD); 240 mg/dl or higher doubles the risk of CHD. Blood cholesterol values between 200 and 239 mg/dl indicate moderate and increasing risk of CHD. However, the total cholesterol level may not be a reliable indicator of cardiovascular disease risk because the level of HDL in the blood is also important and can modify the risk inherent in high cholesterol levels.

For example, a cholesterol level of 240 might not be considered dangerous if your HDL level also was high. Generally, if the ratio of the total cholesterol divided by the HDL level is about 4.5, the risk is said to be average. A ratio above 4.5 increases the risk of heart disease; a ratio below 4.5 reduces it. The various numbers used to establish the risk of heart disease are quite confusing, but the general rules are explained in the Wellness Guide feature on interpreting blood cholesterol and lipid measurements.

Extensive research has shown a strong association between blood cholesterol levels and coronary heart disease: The higher the blood cholesterol level, the greater the risk of all forms of cardiovascular disease. However, many epidemiological studies show that diet is not always a good predictor of heart disease.

For example, the French enjoy a diet laden with eggs, meats, and fats. They have cholesterol levels that,

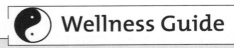

Wellness Guide

How to Interpret Blood Cholesterol and Lipid Measurements

In evaluating your risk of heart and artery disease, the level of four different "fat" molecules are measured: cholesterol, high-density lipoprotein (HDL), triglycerides, and low-density lipoprotein (LDL). The range of values for each is indicated below.

Cholesterol
- Below 200 mg/dl: Safe, unless the HDL level is below 35 mg/dl.
- 200 to 239 mg/dl: Borderline high. If you have other risk factors for heart disease, such as high blood pressure or an HDL level below 35 mg/dl, then you are at risk and some corrective action is needed.
- Above 240 mg/dl: High. Further tests are needed; dietary changes, as well as drugs to lower the level, may be recommended.

High-Density Lipoprotein
- 35 mg/dl: Low. Exercise and other steps may be needed to raise the level. Women generally have higher levels of HDL than men do.
- 35 to 60 mg/dl: Considered protective, especially if cholesterol levels are below 240.

Triglycerides
- Below 200 mg/dl: Considered normal range.
- 200 to 400 mg/dl: Borderline high.
- Above 400 mg/dl: High. Dietary changes recommended.

Low-Density Lipoprotein
LDL is not measured directly, but levels are calculated according to the following formula:

$$LDL = \text{Total cholesterol} - HDL - (\text{Triglycerides}/5)$$

Using this formula, an LDL value below 130 is considered safe; a value above 160 is considered high, and lipid-lowering drugs may be prescribed. However, even this formula does not satisfy all the experts, some of whom believe that the ratio of LDL to HDL is the really significant measure of risk for heart disease.

on average, are much higher than those of Americans. Yet the French die of heart disease at less than half the rate observed in the United States (sometimes called the "French paradox"). There is no satisfactory explanation for the discrepancy; some heart experts attribute it to drinking wine with meals (which may reduce stress) and eating more vegetables (which may be protective in some way).

Other epidemiological studies show that populations vary greatly in the level of cholesterol that constitutes a risk for CHD. People with a blood cholesterol level of 200 in the United States are five times as likely to die of CHD as people in Japan with the same cholesterol levels. People in southern Europe are also at a relatively low risk for a heart attack, even when their cholesterol level is above 250 mg/dl. Another unexplained piece of the elevated cholesterol–heart attack puzzle is the following fact: 50% of Americans who die of a heart attack have normal levels of blood cholesterol (Mandelbaum-Schmid, 2004).

Although there is no disagreement that high cholesterol levels are a major risk factor for cardiovascular disease, the level at which the risk begins to be significant is controversial. In general, physicians in this country view cholesterol levels above 200 mg/dl as cause for intervention with dietary measures, drugs, or both.

Cholesterol, Statins, and Inflammation Statins are a class of drugs that reduce the level of blood cholesterol dramatically. Statins are among the top-selling prescription drugs in the United States. Statins act by inhibiting an enzyme (HMG-CoA reductase) in liver cells that manufactures cholesterol, so production of cholesterol by the body is markedly reduced. Another benefit of statins is that, by blocking the production of cholesterol, they force the liver to increase production of the receptors on liver cells that bind LDL cholesterol. This also aids in the removal of excess cholesterol from the circulation.

People with high cholesterol levels (hypercholesterolemia) invariably respond to treatment with statins by a marked reduction in their blood cholesterol levels. The two significant side effects of statins are liver problems, which occur in about 1% of patients, and muscle weakness (myopathy), which occurs in about 0.1% of people taking statins. Switching from one statin to another often resolves the side effects for those who are affected.

Although no one really knows what causes plaques in arteries, inflammation is now thought to be a significant factor (Hansson, 2005). Recent studies show that inflammation plays an important role in the development of coronary artery disease (CAD) just as it does in other diseases such as asthma and arthritis. A particular protein in blood (**C-reactive protein, CRP**) rises when inflammation is present. Some studies show that people with more advanced coronary artery disease have higher levels of CRP, so it was hoped that measurement of CRP would provide a useful indicator of peoples' risk of heart disease or heart attack. However, so many factors affect the level of CRP in the circulation (e.g., smoking, infections, inflammatory diseases) that it is not a useful biomarker for the risk of heart disease or a heart attack (Braunwald, 2008).

Statins also reduce inflammation in arteries by blocking actions of certain immune system cells that cause inflammation. And statins reduce the level of C-reactive protein in the blood, another indication of their activity as anti-inflammatory drugs.

High Blood Pressure

Medical surveys indicate that about one in three older Americans suffers from high blood pressure (**hypertension**). At 42% for older men and 44% for older women, the prevalence of high blood pressure among African Americans is among the highest in the world. About a third of individuals with high blood pressure are unaware that their blood pressure is high. Consequently, they also are unaware that they are at risk for heart disease, kidney disease, and stroke. The cause of high blood pressure in 90% to 95% of cases is unknown; the medical term for this is **essential (primary) hypertension**.

The remaining cases of high blood pressure are symptoms of a recognizable problem, such as a kidney abnormality, congenital defect of the aorta, or adrenal gland tumor. This type of high blood pressure is called **secondary hypertension**. Generally, when the cause of secondary hypertension is determined and corrected, blood pressure returns to normal.

High blood pressure may be caused by psychosocial factors, although the mechanisms by which these factors could cause it are not understood. For example, people with low income and poor education are at higher risk for high blood pressure. Being poor or jobless may generate stress and raise blood pressure. African and Hispanic Americans have a higher prevalence of high blood pressure than white Americans. The stress of being a member of a minority group may also increase

---

TERMS

C-reactive protein (CRP): a protein in blood that is a measure of chronic inflammation and risk of a heart attack

essential (primary) hypertension: high blood pressure that is not caused by any observable disease

familial hyperlipidemia (FH): an inherited disease causing extremely high levels of cholesterol in the blood

hypertension: high blood pressure

secondary hypertension: high blood pressure caused by a recognizable disease

statins: a class of drugs that block synthesis of cholesterol in the liver and reduce the amount of cholesterol in the blood.

the risk of high blood pressure and heart disease. Hypertension is a disease of modern societies; even today remote tribes in New Guinea or in the forests of Brazil do not develop hypertension.

High blood pressure is a major risk factor for heart attacks and stroke because blood vessels in the heart or brain are more likely to rupture under increased pressure. Hypertension is often called the "silent killer" because it is a disease without symptoms until something serious occurs. About 20% of the world's population has hypertension. The vast majority do not know it and are untreated.

Each time the heart contracts, blood is pumped through the arteries and exerts pressure on the arterial walls (**Figure 14.8**). In fact, there are two pressures that are measured. The maximum pressure in the arteries occurs when the heart contracts (**systole**), pumping blood from the heart to the lungs and body. Between contractions, the pressure falls (**diastole**) as blood flows from one chamber of the heart to another. Normal blood pressure is defined as a value less than 120/80 mm Hg (systole/diastole). In addition to what has been defined as "normal" blood pressure, a new, "prehypertensive" category has also been added. People with a systolic pressure of 120–139 or a diastolic pressure of 80–89 are said to be prehypertensive. Most of these individuals will have further increases in their blood pressure until they eventually will need to be treated for high blood pressure also.

High blood pressure can be lowered by making certain changes in lifestyle. Overweight and overeating are major risk factors that can be changed; increasing physical exercise also is required to reduce hypertension. Moderating salt and alcohol consumption also is benefi-cial. And ensuring that you are obtaining an adequate amount of potassium (eat more bananas) will also reduce blood pressure.

Blood pressure is the result of two forces. The first is created by the heart as it pumps blood into the arteries; the second is created by the arterial blood vessels as they resist blood flow from the heart. Tiny receptors in the walls of the arteries respond to changes in blood pressure. If blood pressure rises, these receptors send signals to the nerves to relax the arteries and to slow down the heartbeat, thus returning blood pressure to normal levels. However, these regulatory mechanisms can be overcome by signals from the brain. Arteries can be constricted and blood pressure raised by thoughts and emotions. Fear, tension, anger, and anxiety activate the sympathetic nervous system, which sends signals to the arteries, causing them to constrict. If one's life is overly stressful or full of anger and frustration, arteries may stay constricted and blood pressure remains elevated.

Although drugs are the most effective means of controlling hypertension, mental relaxation techniques are also effective. By using biofeedback equipment that displayed blood pressure values, some people learned how to develop mental relaxation states that lowered their blood pressure. In fact, many studies demonstrate that a variety of relaxation techniques is effective in lowering blood pressure in hypertensive patients.

The Antihypertensive and Lipid-Lowering Treatment to Prevent Heart Attack Trial (ALLHAT) is the most comprehensive clinical trial yet to determine optimal treatments for high blood pressure and high cholesterol (Appel, 2002). The study concluded that drugs called thiazide diuretics, which increase urine output and remove

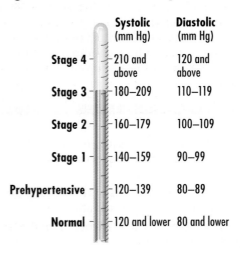

	Systolic (mm Hg)	Diastolic (mm Hg)
Stage 4	210 and above	120 and above
Stage 3	180–209	110–119
Stage 2	160–179	100–109
Stage 1	140–159	90–99
Prehypertensive	120–139	80–89
Normal	120 and lower	80 and lower

■ **Figure 14.8**

Stages of High Blood Pressure
According to current guidelines, normal blood pressure is less than 120/80 (systole/diastole). High blood pressure (hypertension) is defined in four stages, the risk of heart disease being greater the higher the blood pressure. Weight loss, exercise, not smoking, and stress reduction are recommended ways to control hypertension at earlier stages; drugs may also be necessary at later stages.

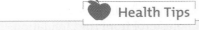

🍎 Health Tips

Breathing Exercise to Reduce Hypertension

Breathing exercises are often the most efficient way to reduce stress and lower blood pressure. There are many forms of breathing exercises, ranging from simple to complicated. The following breathing exercise is a simple and effective way to reduce stress and lower blood pressure.

1. Sit comfortably upright in a chair.
2. Exhale through your mouth as completely as possible.
3. Close your mouth and breathe in through your nose slowly to a count of four. Use abdominal breathing.
4. Hold your breath for a count of seven or as long as you can.
5. Exhale slowly through your mouth to a count of eight.
6. Repeat this cycle three more times, then stop and breathe normally.

Practice at least twice a day every day. The cycle can be increased slightly as the exercise becomes easier over time.

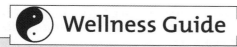

Wellness Guide

Home Blood Pressure Monitors and Internet Consultations to Help Patients Reduce Hypertension

High blood pressure is the leading reversible risk factor for heart attacks and brain attacks. For people with high blood pressure, a 10-mm reduction in systolic blood pressure means a 30% to 40% reduced risk of dying from a heart attack or brain attack (Jones & Peterson, 2008). Despite effective therapies for reducing high blood pressure, efforts to do so are largely unsuccessful. Physicians who diagnose high blood pressure in patients usually recommend lifestyle changes if people smoke, are overweight, or do not exercise. Medications are also prescribed that are very effective in lowering blood pressure to

more acceptable levels. Yet, fewer than a third of patients with high blood pressure achieve goals for lower blood pressure. A new strategy is to supply patients with a home blood pressure monitor with which to take frequent measurements. They also are supplied with an Internet site where their progress is monitored and questions answered by a health professional. It is hoped that increased patient involvement with controlling their high blood pressure will increase the number of patients who successfully lower their blood pressure and thus their risk of cardiovascular disease.

salt, are the preferred initial treatment. Other drugs should be used only if diuretics do not lower blood pressure sufficiently.

A large study funded by the National Institutes of Health showed that high blood pressure could be lowered significantly by dietary changes. The clinical trial was called Dietary Approaches to Stop Hypertension (DASH). The DASH diet emphasizes consuming several daily servings of fruits and vegetables; a greater intake of potassium, magnesium, and calcium; and less consumption of meat, fat, and sweets. Adopting the DASH or a DASH-like diet is the best way to lower blood pressure without drugs and to help maintain a healthy heart (see Chapter 5).

Cigarettes and Cardiovascular Disease

Smoking cigarettes is another major risk factor for the development of cardiovascular disease, heart attacks, and strokes. Smokers are at two to four times greater risk of dying from a heart attack than are nonsmokers. The risk of heart disease from tobacco smoke extends to those who breathe secondhand smoke at work or at home. The more tobacco smoke a person is exposed to, the greater the risk of cardiovascular disease and a heart attack (**Figure 14.9**).

Stopping smoking at any time can reverse many of the harmful physiological effects of tobacco on the cardiovascular system. After several years of not smoking, ex-smokers have about the same risk of cardiovascular disease as nonsmokers. One key to protecting your heart is not smoking and not living or working in a smoke-filled environment.

The Metabolic Syndrome

A model that pulls together many of the factors that are shared by people at risk for diabetes, cardiovascular disease, and heart attacks is called the **metabolic syndrome**. A person with three or more of the following risk factors is defined as having metabolic syndrome:

- Waist circumference greater than 40 inches for men and 35 inches for women
- Elevated triglyceride level of 150 mg/dl or greater
- High-density lipoprotein (HDL) level of 40 mg/dl or lower for men and 50 mg/dl or lower for women
- Fasting blood glucose level of 100 mg/dl or higher (hyperglycemia)
- High blood pressure (130/85 or higher)

A national survey indicated that 6.7% of participants between the ages of 20 and 29 met the criteria for metabolic syndrome. The prevalence increased to 43.5% for participants aged 60 to 69 years (Holvoet, 2008). Because of the enormous number of people with metabolic syndrome in the United States who are at high risk of diabetes, cardiovascular disease, and premature death, metabolic syndrome is regarded as a pressing public health problem. Despite the fancy name, metabolic syndrome is really the result of poor lifestyles—smoking, overeating and overweight, lack of exercise, and poor diet.

TERMS

diastole: the pressure in the arteries when the heart relaxes (the lower number)

metabolic syndrome: a model embracing five risk factors that puts people who have at least three risk factors at risk for cardiovascular disease, diabetes, and premature death

systole: the pressure in the arteries when the heart contracts (the higher number)

A
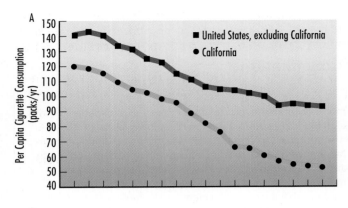

B
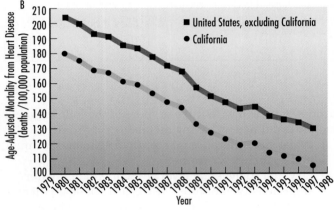

■ **Figure 14.9**

Relation Between Cigarette Consumption and Death from Heart Disease

An aggressive antismoking campaign in California from 1989 to 1992 resulted in a significant decrease in cigarette consumption in the state as compared with the rest of the United States. Deaths from heart disease also were much lower in California than in the rest of the country in this period. These graphs show that the amount of cigarette smoking is directly related to deaths from heart disease.

Stress

In the 1960s, two physicians, Meyer Friedman and Ray Rosenman, created a furor by suggesting that almost all heart disease is of behavioral origin. They claimed that in the absence of a pattern they called **type A behavior**, all the other risk factors would not cause cardiovascular disease. They argued that these other factors—smoking, lack of exercise, high cholesterol, hypertension—contribute to the development of heart disease, but that the main risk factor was stress caused by how people live and act.

Type A behavior is characterized by the following traits:

• Time urgency, impatience
• Hostility
• Achievement striving

The association between type A behavior and heart attacks has been difficult to prove because of the difficulty in measuring the subjective behaviors. At least five large studies subsequently failed to find any connection

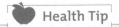
Health Tip

Laughter Helps Heart Stay Healthier

In 1979, a well-known magazine editor, Norman Cousins, published a memoir called *Anatomy of an Illness*. In this book he described how he cured himself of a rare, untreatable disease called ankylosing spondylitis by watching humorous movies over an extended period of time. He became famous for advocating laughter as a cure for most serious diseases, including cancer and heart disease. Since his original account, scientists have been pursuing evidence that laughter heals. One of the best demonstrations that laughter is good for the heart comes from experiments in which volunteers were asked to watch "happy" or "sad" movies (Miller et al., 2006). After watching a happy, humorous movie, blood flow to the heart increased in 19 of 20 subjects. Conversely, after watching a sad, depressing move, blood flow to the heart decreased in 14 of the 20 subjects. Overall, blood flow levels to the heart changed by as much as 50 percent. Anyone at risk for heart disease should probably watch more comedies than war movies.

between type A behavior and cardiovascular disease; however, a few studies did find an association. Using more sophisticated interviewing procedures, researchers found that anger and hostility are key psychological factors associated with an increased risk of cardiovascular disease. Time urgency/impatience also contributes to increased risk. Psychosocial factors such as stress, anger, hostility, depression, work overload, and anxiety all contribute to cardiovascular disease risk and heart attacks (see Chapter 3). Stress at work also is a risk factor for a heart attack. Work stress derives mainly from psychological demands and low decision-making latitude (Aboa-Eboule, 2007). Job stress contributes to both a first heart attack and also reoccurrences.

Salt

One of the most controversial risk factors for cardiovascular disease and a stroke is dietary salt (Frohlich, 2007). For decades, Americans have been urged to reduce their consumption of salt—from an average of 10 grams per person per day to 6 grams or less. Many people find it difficult to reduce their salt intake because 80% of the salt consumed comes from processed foods. Because the taste of foods is determined by salt (and fat), food manufacturers are reluctant to reduce the amount of salt in their products.

Some of the problems in resolving the salt controversy include conflicting scientific studies, marginal effects one way or the other, and disagreement over the interpretation of the scientific results between health agencies and their critics. The primary reason for recommending reduced salt intake is salt's presumed effect in raising blood pressure. However, there is no compelling scientific evidence that reducing salt intake lowers blood pressure.

Diet and Cardiovascular Disease

As already mentioned, diet plays a major role in heart disease, especially as it contributes to being overweight and overfat and to elevated levels of cholesterol. However, certain foods and vitamins in the diet seem to provide some protection from cardiovascular disease.

Vitamin E, Vitamin C, and Beta-Carotene

Although the oxygen gas that we breathe is essential to life, uncombined oxygen atoms in cells can react with many substances and cause damage. For example, consider what happens to iron that is exposed to the oxygen in air under moist conditions: It quickly rusts and disintegrates. Body tissues also can be destroyed by oxygen atoms. The body has many mechanisms for protecting cellular constituents from oxidation, among them the antioxidant action of vitamin E and vitamin C.

Vitamin E acts as an **antioxidant** in blood and reduces the amount of oxidized LDL that is formed. When volunteers took vitamin E supplements (800 IU), their LDL particles were more resistant to oxidation. Like vitamin E, vitamin C is an antioxidant and can neutralize destructive oxygen atoms and other oxidizing substances called **free radicals.** Free radical compounds in the blood may damage the elastic tissues in arteries that allow blood vessels to expand and contract. If a blood vessel is damaged and cannot relax, blood pressure rises. Vitamin C is thought to prevent such damage from occurring by eliminating the free radical compounds in blood. Taking up to a gram of vitamin C supplement a day is safe; any that is not used is excreted in urine. However, taking megadoses of vitamin C (10 grams a day) can cause serious side effects, such as stomach irritation and kidney stones.

Beta-carotene is another vitamin with antioxidant properties. Vitamin E, vitamin C, and beta-carotene together have been regarded as essential dietary nutrients that help reduce the risk of cardiovascular disease and cancer.

> A man's worst enemies can't wish on him what he can think up himself.
> *Yiddish Proverb*

Current thinking is that antioxidant vitamin supplements are of little proven benefit in reducing the risk of cardiovascular disease or cancer; in fact, vitamin E supplements seemed to increase risks slightly.

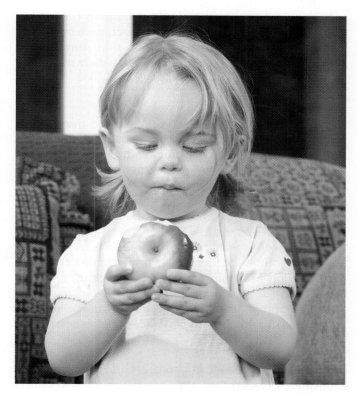

It's important to encourage children to eat heart-healthy snacks, so they won't have to break bad eating habits later in life.

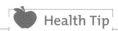 Health Tip

Air Pollution Around the Home Increases the Risk of Heart Disease

Probably the last thing you think about when you buy a home or rent an apartment is the air quality in the neighborhood. But maybe you should. Recent research shows quite convincingly that air pollution in the form of tiny dust particles (not smog) causes, over time, thickening of the arteries and atherosclerosis.

The air pollution level around homes of about 800 people in Los Angeles was measured at various intervals. Increased thickening of the walls of arteries was observed in people who were exposed to higher levels of air pollution. The Environmental Protection Agency (EPA) is now financing a larger, 10-year study to confirm the results. However, it may be difficult finding a home 10 years from now in an urban area that does not have significant air pollution.

TERMS

antioxidant: substance that in small amounts inhibits the oxidation of other compounds

free radicals: oxidizing substances in the body that can damage blood vessels and tissues

type A behavior: behaviors characterized by traits, such as time urgency or hostility, that contribute to the risk of heart disease

Nutritional guidelines often fluctuate as often as clothing fashions. Taking a one-a-day vitamin supplement still seems safe and prudent to maintain optimal health. However, vitamin supplements are no substitute for a nourishing diet consisting of plenty of fresh fruits and vegetables.

B Vitamins

Other vitamins that protect against heart disease are three B vitamins: B_6, B_{12}, and folic acid (folate). As described previously, high levels of the amino acid homocysteine are associated with atherosclerosis and heart disease. People with high levels of homocysteine in their blood also had low levels of the three B vitamins. On the other hand, people with low homocysteine levels had high levels of the B vitamins and were less likely to develop heart disease.

The key B vitamins can be obtained from food; however, many people do not obtain enough in their diets. The evidence that B vitamins do, in fact, protect against heart disease is now strong enough that some health authorities recommend taking them in a daily multivitamin supplement.

Calcium

Food profile studies indicate that half or more of all Americans of both sexes consume amounts of calcium that are less than the recommended amounts for bone development and health. Populations that are especially at risk are African Americans, pregnant women, obese persons, and the elderly. Unless you consume foods that are high in calcium, such as milk and cheese, your daily calcium intake may be low.

Calcium deficiency is not only a risk factor for osteoporosis in women, but also is a significant risk factor for hypertension in persons of all ages. Calcium is readily obtained in the diet, but levels can also be increased by taking calcium supplements, which cost much less and are much safer than antihypertensive medications.

Soy Products

Soybeans have been cultivated around the world for thousands of years; the Chinese name for soybean is *tatou*, which means "greater bean." Soy seems to boost the activity of LDL receptors in the liver, and thereby helps to remove cholesterol from the blood. Soy also seems to block oxidation of the LDL particles, which prevents them from sticking to the walls of arteries.

Studies in which people ate 1 to 2 ounces of soy daily showed that both cholesterol and LDL levels dropped about 10%. Other studies indicate that soy is especially effective among people with cholesterol levels above 240 mg/dl. Soy is available in a multitude of products, such as soy milk, soft and firm tofu, and tofu burgers.

Fish Oils

Populations that consume large amounts of fish in their diets—Greenland Inuit and Japanese islanders—have lower rates of CHD than others. Americans who consume fish regularly in their diets also have healthier hearts. The protective effects of dietary fish have been ascribed to fish oils, in particular to omega-3-polyunsaturated oils. In some studies, supplements of fish oil have reduced levels of cholesterol and blood pressure. Not all fish are safe to eat because of high levels of mercury (see Chapter 24).

One of the best studies demonstrating the beneficial effect of fish was carried out in Tanzania among Bantu villagers. One group of Bantu lived on the shores of a lake, and people consumed about a pound of fish a day. The other Bantu population lived in nearby hills and had a diet that consisted primarily of vegetables. The Bantu people who ate fish had high levels of n-3-polyunsaturated oils in their blood. They also had lower levels of cholesterol and lipoproteins (Pauletto et al., 1996). Sardines, salmon, and mackerel have high levels of omega-3-polyunsaturated oils, but all fish have some.

Trans Fats

When food manufacturers convert liquid oils to solid fats such as margarine, they create trans fats by adding hydrogen atoms (hydrogenation) to molecules of liquid fat. High levels of trans fat are found in margarine and in fast foods such as french fries, doughnuts, cakes, and cookies. Like saturated fat and cholesterol, trans fat increases the risk of cardiovascular disease (Mozaffarian et al., 2006).

Since 1993, nutrition labels on manufactured foods have listed the amount of cholesterol and saturated fat in the product. As of January 1, 2006, the nutrition fact labels on foods also listed the amount of trans fat in the product. Health professionals recommend that people reduce the amount of trans fat they consume.

New York City has ordered all restaurants and food suppliers to stop using and cooking with oils that contain trans fats. In 2008, California enacted a statewide ban on the use of trans fats in all foods served in restaurants and sold in stores. Countries such as Denmark and Canada also are considering banning the use of trans fats in foods completely.

Tea

Both green and black tea contain antioxidant chemicals that help block oxidation of LDL particles in the blood; herb teas do not contain antioxidants. Consuming green or black tea helps protect the coronary arteries in a manner similar to that of the C and E antioxidant vitamins. Asian people drink green tea daily, which may contribute to their reduced risk of CHD.

Aspirin

A commonly used drug can significantly reduce the risk of CHD and heart attacks. Aspirin helps to "thin" blood and also acts to combat inflammation. Studies have been carried out in which aspirin was given to both healthy people and to people who had had a heart attack or stroke. In all studies, small amounts of aspirin reduced the risk of a heart attack. The recommended dose of aspirin to reduce heart attack risk is 81 mg per day, the amount in a baby aspirin.

It is now recommended that if you think you might be having a heart attack, first call 911 and then take a couple of aspirin, which will help prevent clotting. Whether healthy people who are at low risk of a heart attack should take aspirin on a regular basis is still an open question. As with vitamin supplements or drinking alcohol, each person must decide what is best for his or her health.

Alcohol

A large study of 275,000 middle-aged American men showed that one or two drinks a day over 12 years reduced their risk of dying from a heart attack by about 20% in comparison with men who did not drink alcohol. Other studies show that moderate alcohol consumption also reduces the risks of stroke. However, more than two drinks a day *increases* the risk of both heart attack and stroke significantly.

A larger study looked at the drinking habits of 80,000 Japanese men and women over a 14-year period and their risk of death from heart or brain attacks. This study found that men and women differ considerably in the health effects of drinking. Men who drank up to four drinks a day had a slightly reduced risk of death from a heart attack but a slightly higher risk of death from a brain attack as compared with nondrinkers. On the other hand, women who drank about four drinks a day

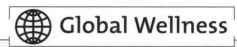
Global Wellness

Deaths from Cardiovascular Disease Are Increasing Worldwide

Despite the death toll from HIV/AIDS and other infectious diseases in poor, underdeveloped countries, cardiovascular disease is still the leading cause of death in most of these countries. In 2005, it was estimated that about 14 million people in developing countries died from cardiovascular diseases; by 2015 that number is expected to rise to 16 million (WHO, 2009). Already, 80% of all deaths from cardiovascular disease occur in low- and middle-income countries (see the accompanying figure). Moreover, most of the cardiovascular deaths in these underdeveloped countries occur among people who are, on average, 10 to 20 years younger than in industrialized Western countries.

China has recorded a doubling of cardiovascular disease deaths over the past 20 years, and the majority of these deaths have occurred in the 35- to 54-year-old age group. Also, stroke is a major killer in China, Southeast Asia, and sub-Saharan Africa; heart attack is the primary killer in urban India, Latin America, and the Middle East. The worldwide epidemic of cardiovascular disease is largely caused by changes in lifestyle brought about by globalization and change in peoples' lifestyles and diets. As a companion to greater wealth, diets become more westernized, physical activity decreases, and tobacco use increases, as do pollution and stress. Thus, along with the new car, cell phone, and computer come cardiovascular disease, diabetes, obesity, stroke, and heart attacks.

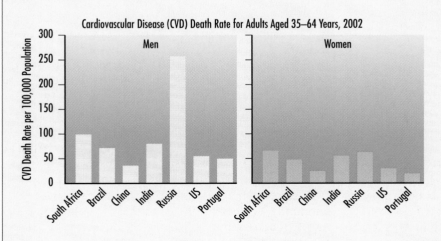

Cardiovascular Disease (CVD) Death Rate for Adults Aged 35–64 Years, 2002

Men — Women

CVD Death Rate per 100,000 Population

South Africa, Brazil, China, India, Russia, US, Portugal

Death Rates from Cardiovascular Disease in Various Countries

Source: Data from the World Health Organization.

quadrupled their risk of death from a heart attack and doubled their risk of a brain attack. However, if the women had two drinks or less per day, they also had a slightly reduced risk of death from a heart attack. The basic conclusion from this large study is that heavy drinking is far more dangerous for women than for men.

Although moderate alcohol drinking does have some health benefits, the issue of drinking is so controversial (and alcohol is potentially harmful) that no recommendation can be made to drink because it may protect you from a heart attack (Goldberg, 2003). Many dietary and lifestyle changes are much more beneficial to your heart than drinking alcohol. On the other hand, persons who enjoy a drink occasionally need not feel guilty that they are damaging their health.

Coffee, Tea, and Cocoa

The caffeine in coffee has sometimes been associated with an increased risk of high blood pressure, although studies have differed in that conclusion. Recent evidence suggests that drinking moderate amounts of coffee does not increase the risk of high blood pressure, although drinking cola sodas does increase the risk somewhat. There is no explanation for why the caffeine in coffee does not raise blood pressure whereas cola sodas seem to.

Most studies point to the fact that regular drinkers of green tea have less cardiovascular disease than people who do not drink green tea. All tea comes from the same leaves; differences in processing produce white, green, or black tea. Chemicals called *polyphenols* in tea seem to provide the cardiovascular protective effects.

Cocoa also has been implicated in reducing high blood pressure. The Kuna are a native people who live on sparsely inhabited islands in the Caribbean. Researchers observed that these island people have a very low incidence of high blood pressure, which seems to be associated with drinking several cups of relatively unprocessed cocoa a day. Kuna who move away from the islands usually stop drinking cocoa and also develop high blood pressure. Chemicals called *flavonoids* that are present in cocoa seem to increase blood flow and reduce the development of high blood pressure. Unfortunately, most of the cocoa sold in the United States is highly processed and sweetened to make it palatable. The cocoa the Kuna drink is unprocessed and quite bitter.

Preventing Cardiovascular Disease

With the increased attention given to risk factors that cause cardiovascular disease, people are now armed with knowledge that can reduce their chances of heart attacks and brain attacks. People should maintain normal weight and avoid consumption of foods containing large amounts of saturated fats, trans fats and cholesterol. A diet rich in fresh fruits and vegetables helps protect your heart and arteries. Understanding the adverse consequences of cigarette smoking should encourage smokers to quit. Also, taking supplements of B vitamins and calcium might be helpful, as might green tea and glass of wine with dinner. However, nothing is better for the heart than a healthy diet and plenty of exercise.

Critical Thinking About Health

1. African Americans as a group have higher blood pressure, on average, than white Americans. Various hypotheses have been advanced to explain the differences in blood pressure between the races, including genetic differences, social factors, economic factors, diet, and behavioral differences. Find out all that you can on racial differences in blood pressure (your local branch of the American Heart Association is a good place to start looking for information). Then write a report giving your views as to why the blood pressure discrepancy exists among races and ethnic groups in our society.

2. Use a printed cholesterol counting guide from the U.S. Department of Agriculture's Nutrient Data Laboratory Web site to determine approximately how much cholesterol you consume in an average week. Then try to construct a diet for yourself, either by reducing amounts of certain foods or by eliminating them altogether, that will reduce your average weekly cholesterol intake by at least 20%. Can you construct a diet that satisfies you and that contains 50% less cholesterol? Write up your findings in a report.

3. Make a list of all the factors discussed in this chapter that increase the risk of cardiovascular disease, heart attacks, and stroke. How many of the risk factors do you have? Among the risk factors that can be changed, discuss how you would go about reducing them in your life to improve your cardiovascular health now and for the future.

4. People in Japan or southern European countries have one-half to one-third the risk of dying from heart disease in comparison with people from the United States or northern Europe, even when their cholesterol levels, on average, are the same. A person with a cholesterol level of 250 mg/dl in Denmark has a two to three times greater risk of a fatal heart attack compared with an Italian with the same cholesterol level. Develop arguments to explain this difference that seem reasonable to you and organize your facts and ideas in the form of a hypothesis.

Health in Review

- The heart is a pump that maintains blood circulation in the arteries and veins. The arteries carry oxygen and nutrients to cells, and the veins carry carbon dioxide back to the lungs.
- Damage to the heart or arteries is called cardiovascular disease, which is the leading cause of death in the United States.
- Major risk factors of heart disease that cannot be changed are heredity, gender, and age.
- Major risk factors for cardiovascular disease that can be changed are cigarette or tobacco use, high blood cholesterol, high blood pressure, physical inactivity, and poor diet.
- Other factors that contribute to heart disease are diabetes, obesity, and stress.

- Various surgeries are performed to repair clogged arteries: coronary artery bypass surgery, angioplasty (stenting), and endarterectomy.
- One baby (81 mg) aspirin each day may reduce the risk of a heart attack for someone at risk.
- Calcium, soy products, fish oils, cocoa, and green tea all help keep the heart healthy.
- Heart disease is caused by modern lifestyles and can be prevented. Making changes in your diet, not smoking, and increasing exercise while you are young can help keep the heart, arteries, and brain healthy throughout life.

Health and Wellness Online

The Web contains a wealth of information about health and wellness. By accessing the Internet using Web browser software, you can gain a new perspective on many topics presented in *Health and Wellness,* Tenth Edition. Access the Jones and Bartlett Publishers Web site at **health.jbpub.com/hwonline.**

References

Aboa-Eboule, C., et al. (2007). Job strain and risk of acute recurrent coronary heart disease events. *Journal of the American Medical Association, 298,* 1652–1660.

American Heart Association. (2008). *Heart disease and stroke statistics—2008 update.* Dallas, TX: Author.

Appel, L. (2002). The verdict from ALLHAT—Thiazide diuretics are the preferred initial therapy for hypertension. *Journal of the American Medical Association, 288,* 3039–3041.

Braunwald, E. (2008). Biomarkers in heart failure. *New England Journal of Medicine, 358,* 2148–2159.

Callans, D. J. (2008). Can home AEDs improve survival? *New England Journal of Medicine, 358,* 185–186.

Frank, J. D. (1973). *Persuasion and healing.* Baltimore, MD: Johns Hopkins University Press.

Frohlich, E. D. (2007). The salt conundrum. *Hypertension, 50,* 161–163.

Goldberg, I. J. (2003). To drink or not to drink? *New England Journal of Medicine, 348,* 163–164.

Hansson, G. K. (2005). Inflammation, atherosclerosis, and coronary artery disease. *New England Journal of Medicine, 352,* 1685–1694.

Harder, B. (2006, September 23). Calling death's bluff. *Science News,* 202–204.

Holvoet, P., et al. (2008). Association between circulating oxidized low-density lipoprotein and incidence of the metabolic syndrome. *Journal of the American Medical Association, 299,* 2287–2293.

Jones, D. W., & Peterson, E. D. (2008). Improving hypertension control rates: Technology, people or systems? *Journal of the American Medical Association, 299,* 2896–2898.

Kern, F. (1991). Normal plasma cholesterol in an 88-year-old man who eats 25 eggs per day. *New England Journal of Medicine, 324,* 13.

Mandelbaum-Schmid, J. (2004, July/August). Beyond cholesterol. *Body and Soul,* 72–99.

Maron, B. J., et al. (2005). Task Force II: commotio cordis. *Journal of the American College of Cardiology, 45,* 1371–1373.

McMurry, M. P., et al. (1991). Changes in lipid and lipoprotein levels and body weight in Tarahumara Indians after consumption of an affluent diet. *New England Journal of Medicine, 325,* 1704–1708.

Miller, M., et al. (2006). Impact of cinematic viewing on endothelial function. *Heart, 92,* 262–263.

Mozaffarian, D., et al. (2006). Trans fatty acids and cardiovascular disease. *New England Journal of Medicine, 354,* 1601–1613.

Ornish, D., et al. (1998). Intensive lifestyle changes for reversal of coronary heart disease. *Journal of the American Medical Association, 280,* 2001–2007.

Pauletto, P., et al. (1996). Blood pressure and atherogenic lipoprotein profiles of fish-diet and vegetarian villagers in Tanzania: The Lugalawa study. *Lancet, 348,* 784–788.

Vastag, B. (2007, June 23). Stents stumble. *Science News,* 394–395.

World Health Organization. (2009). Cardiovascular diseases. Retrieved May 15, 2009, from http://www.who.int/mediacentre/factsheets/fs317/en/index.html

Suggested Readings

Cooper, R. S., Rotimi, C. N., & Ward, R. (1999, February). The puzzle of hypertension in African-Americans. *Scientific American*, 56–63. Discusses both the genetic and environmental factors that have been investigated to explain why African Americans have a much higher prevalence of hypertension than white Americans.

How to keep your heart healthy. (2003, November/December). *FDA Consumer*, 18–25. Suggestions on how to make dietary and other lifestyle changes that will help keep your heart healthy.

Hu, F. B., & Willett, W. C. (2002). Optimal diets for prevention of coronary heart disease. *Journal of the American Medical Association, 288*, 2569–2575. Discusses what to eat and what to do to lower risk of heart disease.

Mozaffarian, D., et al. (2006). Trans fatty acids and cardiovascular disease. *New England Journal of Medicine, 354*, 1601–1613. Explains what fatty acids are and how they affect health in many ways.

Ornish, D., et al. (1998). Intensive lifestyle changes for reversal of coronary heart disease. *Journal of the American Medical Association, 280*, 2001–2007. A report documenting that the blockages in arteries can be reversed by changes in lifestyle and that the beneficial changes persist for years.

Underwood, A. (2005, October 3). The good heart. *Newsweek*, 49–84. Evidence is accumulating that a person's psychological state is just as important as diet and exercise in maintaining a healthy heart.

Recommended Web Sites

Please visit **health.jbpub.com/hwonline** for links to these Web sites.

American Heart Association
Information and education on all aspects of cardiovascular disease.

MedlinePlus on Heart Disease
From the U.S. National Library of Medicine. General information.

National Heart, Lung and Blood Institute
Information on heart disease and high blood pressure.

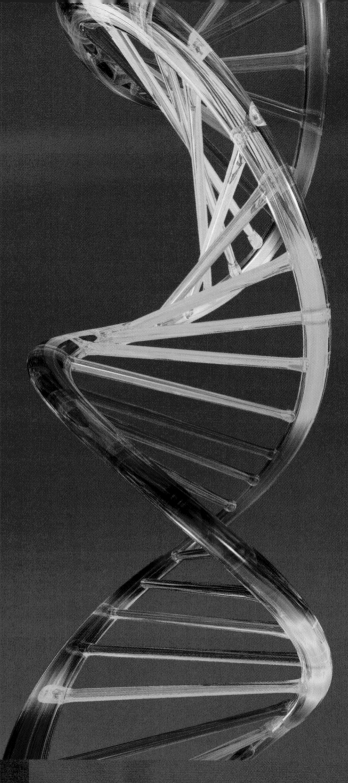

Chapter Fifteen

Heredity and Disease

Learning Objectives

1. Describe the functions of DNA, genes, and chromosomes.

2. Describe several inherited diseases caused by chromosomal abnormalities.

3. List several chemicals that cause birth defects and what they were used for.

4. Explain how a familial pattern of disease differs from a hereditary (genetic) disease.

5. Describe the symptoms of fetal alcohol syndrome and how it can be prevented.

6. Explain the role of genetic counseling in preventing hereditary diseases.

7. Explain the procedure of amniocentesis.

8. Define *genetic discrimination* and its consequences for people.

9. Discuss how gene therapy and embryonic stem cells may be used to treat and cure disease.

10. Define *cloning* and list some animals that have been cloned.

When the sperm from your father joined with the egg from your mother, you were conceived. You inherited from each parent about 25,000 to 30,000 genes. Beginning with conception and continuing throughout life, those genes direct and control the development and repair of your body's tissues and organs. The genes control the chemistry that keeps you alive, your particular disease susceptibilities, and, to a large extent, your overall health and life expectancy.

> People through finding something beautiful, think something else unbeautiful. Through finding one man fit, judge another unfit.
>
> *Lao Tzu,* The Way of Life

Genes are arranged in a linear array along threadlike structures called **chromosomes,** which are present in almost all cells of the body. Each person carries 23 pairs of chromosomes (a total of 46) in virtually every cell of the body. (The only major exception is red blood cells, which lose their chromosomes before they enter the blood circulation.) Males and females differ only in one pair of chromosomes, called the sex chromosomes. Men have an XY pair and women have an XX pair. The original parental chromosomes present in the fertilized egg are replicated into every cell of the fetus during development; skin, liver, heart, lung, and brain cells all contain identical sets of chromosomes. Only half of each parent's set of chromosomes is passed on in the fertilized egg, thus keeping

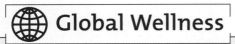 Global Wellness

Lactose Intolerance: A Mutation That Influenced Human Evolution

The sugar *lactose* is present in mother's milk and is the primary source of energy for all babies when breastfed. Digestion of the sugar lactose is accomplished by an enzyme—called *lactase*—that is present in the digestive system of all newborns. The gene for producing the enzyme that digests lactose is situated on chromosome 2, and almost all babies are born with this gene activated so that they can digest breast milk or cow's milk. Very infrequently, a baby is born with an inactive gene that causes a condition known as *alactasia* These infants cannot digest lactose in breast milk or in any milk product. If they are breast fed or given cow's milk, these infants have watery diarrhea, which can be life-threatening due to dehydration and nutrient depletion.

A much more common condition involving inability to digest the sugar lactose occurs later in life and is called *lactose intolerance.* The extent of lactose intolerance varies widely among the world's adult population (see accompanying figure).

Lactose intolerance occurs in the following way. As mentioned previously, the gene that allows babies to digest lactose is switched on in all newborns so that they can thrive on breast milk. In a majority of the world's children, the gene is switched off sometime between two and five years of age. This corresponds to the normal time of weaning in most cultures. The explanation for this switching off of the gene is that, until quite recently in human evolution, people did not consume milk after weaning. The body could conserve energy for other uses by not producing an unnecessary enzyme.

About 10,000 years ago, people in northern Europe and a few tribes in Africa began to raise cows, goats, sheep, and other animals for their milk, which became an important part of the diet. Mutations in the lactase genes arose among these milk drinkers that permitted continued lactase enzyme production for life, and this genetic change was passed on from one generation to the next.

Modern genetic research has now shown that two mutations account for all the lactose-tolerant people in the

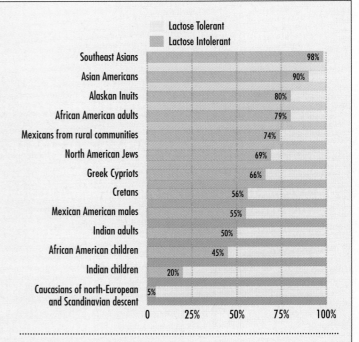

Source: World Health Organization.

world (Enattah, 2002; Gibbons, 2006). All of the adults who can drink milk without any ill effects have one or the other of these two mutations. Today, populations around the world vary from being almost completely lactose intolerant (Southeast Asians) to being almost completely lactose tolerant (Scandinavians). In the thousands of years since these mutations arose, people have carried the lactose-tolerance genes to all parts of the world.

Until recently, it has been difficult to diagnose lactose intolerance. Generally, the diagnosis is made by stopping the ingestion of milk products to see if the symptoms disappear. Now, however, a genetic test is available to determine if a person with symptoms actually lacks the genes to produce lactase. (*Note:* Lactose intolerance is not true milk allergy; milk allergy is an immune response to milk proteins; see Chapter 12.)

the chromosome number the same from generation to generation.

Cells and organs differ in the body because of the particular genes that are expressed in different tissues. The orchestrated turning on and turning off of genes in cells is the key to development and correct functioning of the body throughout life. The flow of information from DNA in chromosomes to functional proteins in cells is the same in all living organisms, attesting to a common cellular evolutionary history (**Figure 15.1**).

Human chromosomes have a characteristic shape, size, and banding pattern that can be seen when they are stained with dyes and examined under the light microscope. Each of the 23 different human chromosome pairs can be distinguished and identified. Human chromosomes are viewed under the microscope and then photographed and arranged in pairs in a standard display called a **karyotype.**

The information carried in genes along the chromosomes is contained in a chemical substance called **DNA (deoxyribonucleic acid).** Each chromosome, depend-

ing on its size, contains thousands of different genes whose information is encoded in the chemistry of the DNA. Together, these genes determine the uniqueness of each human being. (Identical twins share identical sets of genes but differ in their traits to some extent because of environmental effects on the expression of their genes.) Because chromosomes occur in pairs, each person carries

TERMS

chromosomes: threadlike structures in the nuclei of cells that carry an individual's genetic information

DNA (deoxyribonucleic acid): the chemical substance that carries all of a person's genetic information in chromosomes in cells

karyotype: visual display of all of a person's chromosomes that can detect chromosomal abnormalities characteristic of inherited diseases

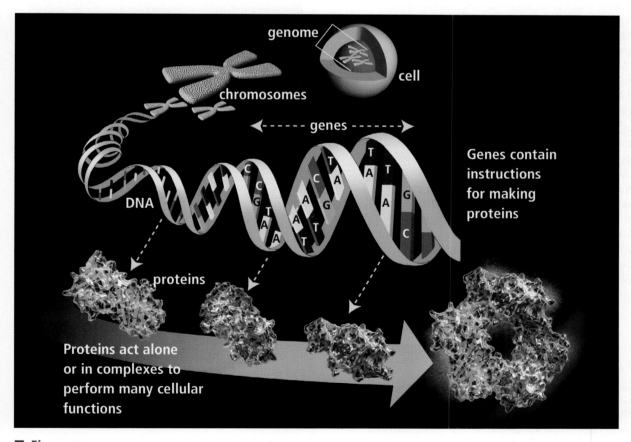

■ Figure 15.1

DNA—The Molecule of Life

The diagram shows the relation among DNA, genes, chromosomes, and proteins in all cells of the body. Chromosomes contain the hereditary chemical DNA. Specific short segments of DNA contain genes, most of which carry information for the synthesis of specific proteins. The information in each gene is copied into a molecule of RNA (ribonucleic acid), which is then translated into a specific protein that the cell needs.

Source: U.S. Department of Energy.

two copies of each gene; these may be identical in information or differ slightly from one another.

Most American babies are born healthy. However, about 3% to 4% of newborns have an observable **congenital (birth) defect**—an anomaly in some aspect of the body's structure or functioning that occurred during development in the mother's uterus. Congenital defects are caused by one or more of the following factors:

- Presence of an abnormal chromosome or abnormal number of chromosomes
- A chemical error in one or more genes inherited from parents; the defective gene alters body structure or functions
- The effect of toxins, drugs, or other environmental factors on normal fetal development

In this chapter, we discuss the origin, prevention, and treatment of common birth defects and inherited diseases.

Chromosomal Abnormalities

Errors may occur when chromosomes are distributed to sperm or egg. The distribution may result in too few or too many chromosomes being transmitted (other forms of physical chromosomal abnormalities also occur). These chromosomal abnormalities result in hereditary diseases (**Table 15.1**). About 20% of all human conceptions have a chromosomal abnormality of some kind. The majority of fetuses with chromosomal abnormalities abort spontaneously, ending the pregnancy (Sluder & McCollum, 2000).

Viewing cells removed from a fetus, child, or adult can identify chromosomal abnormalities, such as the extra chromosome 21 that causes *Down syndrome* (**Figure 15.2**).

This serious inherited birth defect occurs in about 1 in every 700 babies born in the United States. However, the rate begins to increase in women around age 35 and increases dramatically after age 40. Because of the increase in Down syndrome with increased maternal age, all pregnant women over age 35 are advised to undergo genetic tests of fetal cells (see section on prenatal testing) to determine if they are carrying a fetus with Down

syndrome. If the tests are positive, women can elect to have an abortion or continue the pregnancy, knowing that they will deliver a child with Down syndrome.

The extra chromosome 21 carried in all cells of individuals with Down syndrome causes heart defects,

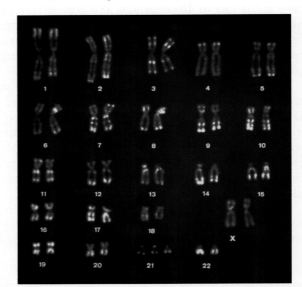

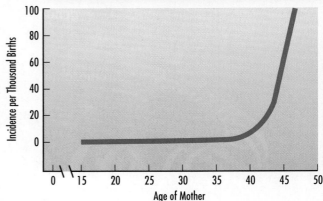

■ **Figure 15.2**

Karyotype of Individual with Down Syndrome
Note three copies of chromosome 21. Frequencies of children born with Down syndrome are shown in relation to the age of the mother. At age 35 the risk of this particular chromosomal defect begins to rise sharply.

Table 15.1

Chromosomal Abnormalities

Some genetic diseases are associated with an extra or missing chromosome. Most abnormalities in chromosome number (more or less than the normal 46) are incompatible with survival; in most cases, affected babies die before birth. However, abnormalities in chromosomes 21, X, or Y are compatible with survival but usually produce physical and mental abnormalities.

Genetic disease/disorder	Chromosomal defect	Incidence per live births	Symptoms
Turner's syndrome (female)	Missing X	1/1,000	Absence of ovaries, short stature, underdeveloped breasts
Klinefelter's syndrome (male)	Extra X	1/1,000	Small, undeveloped testes, sterility, mental retardation
Down syndrome (male or female)	Extra chromosome 21	1/700	Physical abnormalities, mental retardation, heart defects
XXX syndrome (female)	Extra X	Uncertain (1/1,000)	No clinical abnormalities, height above average, possible mental retardation
XYY (male)	Extra Y	Uncertain (1/1,000)	No clinical abnormalities, height above average, controversy over "criminal" tendency

altered facial features, and mental retardation. With modern medical care, the life expectancy of a person with Down syndrome is 40 to 50 years. However, caring for a Down syndrome person beyond childhood is taxing on families both emotionally and financially. Eventually, most individuals with Down syndrome are placed in special living situations with trained caregivers.

Hereditary Diseases

A **hereditary (genetic) disease** results from the following sequence of events. An abnormal gene (one whose chemistry has been altered) is passed on to a child from one or both parents. As a result of inheriting the defective gene (or genes), a protein is produced that is abnormal or even missing completely. For example, if an essential muscle protein is defective or missing during fetal development, muscle tissues develop abnormally. Several forms of *muscular dystrophy* are inherited in this way. If a protein necessary for bone formation is defective, short stature, or *dwarfism*, results.

> Life is not a matter of holding good cards, but of playing a poor hand well.
>
> *Robert Louis Stevenson*

If the defective protein is an enzyme, an essential chemical reaction in the body will be affected and some aspect of metabolism will be abnormal. For example, in *hemophilia*, a chemical called factor VIII, required for normal blood clotting, is defective as a result of an altered gene on an X chromosome. *Phenylketonuria* (PKU) is an inherited disease caused by a defect in an enzyme that is needed to digest the amino acid phenylalanine, which is present in food. If excess phenylalanine in the blood is not broken down, it accumulates in tissues and causes abnormal brain development and mental retardation.

Sickle cell disease is caused by a defect in hemoglobin proteins present in all red blood cells. Hemoglobin molecules pick up oxygen as blood circulates through the lungs. In sickle cell disease, the defective hemoglobin proteins change the shape of red blood cells so that they

TERMS

congenital (birth) defect: any abnormality observed in a newborn that occurred during development

hereditary (genetic) disease: any disease resulting from the inheritance of defective genes or chromosomes from one or both parents

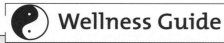 Wellness Guide

Is There a Gay Gene?

In modern society, the word *gay* is used to refer to a homosexual male. Historically, the word meant "mirthful, high spirited"; later, it began to be associated with sexual conduct as in "gay blade." But how the term *gay* came to be associated with male homosexuals is still uncertain.

In 1993, a scientific research team claimed to have discovered the biological basis of male homosexuality by identifying a "gay gene." However, their methods involved statistical associations, and no actual gene was ever identified. Furthermore, genetic studies by other researchers failed to confirm the original observations or analysis. Although researchers presume that homosexuality has a basis in biology and genes, there is still no convincing evidence to support this presumption. Perhaps the best evidence is that many gay persons report that they were aware at a very early age of their attraction to other males. But this is not scientific evidence for a gay gene.

Should future research uncover specific genetic influences on sexual orientation, and given its complex nature, it seems highly unlikely that a single gene (or even a few genes) can account for homosexuality. Sexual orientation is most likely determined by hundreds of genes and numerous environmental factors that affect brain development *in utero* as well as after birth. The factors underlying sexual orientation are probably at least as complex as the ones that affect intelligence.

Research on the genetic basis of homosexuality is extremely controversial for many reasons. In the past, and even now,

most homosexual men would have chosen to hide their sexual orientation because of the dire consequences of "coming out." In the United States, prior to the 1970s, homosexuality was medically classified as a disease and homosexual men were often forced to undergo painful psychological or physical treatments to "cure" their homosexuality. Until recently, in China, shock therapy was used to "treat" homosexuals. Although gay men are well integrated in most aspects of American society today, strong prejudice still exists in many areas of the United States and in other countries around the world (read the story "Brokeback Mountain" by Annie Proulx or watch the movie based on it). Extreme prejudice or hatred of homosexuals is called *homophobia* and is still a problem in the United States and elsewhere in the world.

Anthropological evidence indicates that homosexuality has existed in all human cultures past and present and that, in general, male homosexuals constitute between 2% to 4% of any human population. Thus, homosexuality is a typical variation among people, just like genetic variation in height or intelligence. For example, only a few percentage of people are over seven feet tall or have the mind of a genius, but they are not stigmatized. If one or several genes are eventually found that make an individual more likely to have a same-sex orientation, it is not hard to imagine many people wanting to undergo genetic testing for such genes. A positive test for homosexuality susceptibility genes could be used to determine the suitability of a marriage partner or to abort a fetus. The hypothetical possibility of a genetic test for homosexuality is disturbing and could create significant social problems (see the section "Genetic Testing" later in this chapter).

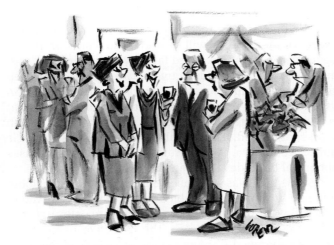

"Everybody thinks we're sisters, but we're actually mother and son."

© The New Yorker Collection 2008 Lee Lorenz from cartoonbank.com.
All rights reserved.

Table 15.2

Increased Risk of Certain Diseases and Disorders Among Children When One Parent Is Affected

Although genes probably are involved to some degree, the number of genes conferring risk, or the extent of the genetic contribution, is basically unknown. In all cases, environmental factors also are involved.

	Lifetime risk (%)	
	General population	One parent affected
Alcoholism (men)	10	40
Alcoholism (women)	3–5	12–20
Alzheimer's	5–10	10–20
Colon cancer	6	12–18
Diabetes, type 2	3–7	10–15
Depression, bipolar	1–3	9–27
Dyslexia	5–10	30–60
Psoriasis	1–2	25
Rheumatoid arthritis	1	5
Schizophrenia	1	10

tend to clog small blood vessels. As a result, essential oxygen cannot reach tissues and organs.

Familial Diseases Hereditary diseases are *always* caused by defective chromosomes or genes that change body structure or chemistry in some way. However, determining if a disease or physical abnormality is inherited is not a simple matter. Many birth defects are caused by infections, teratogens, or other environmental factors, as well as by defective genes.

Sometimes a disease is said to "run in the family," which means that several members of a family have the same disease. Children of parents who suffer from certain diseases are at higher risk of developing these diseases compared with the average risk in the general population (**Table 15.2**). Allergies, obesity, or alcoholism may run in the family, but this does not mean that these diseases are inherited or are caused by defective genes. Families share many environmental factors as well as genes. For example, families share the same water, food, and air, any one of which may contain harmful or toxic substances. When parents have a poor diet, children usually do also. To appreciate the difference between an inherited disease and one that "runs in the family," consider these examples. Being a Muslim or a Catholic runs in families, as does being a Republican or a Democrat, but these traits clearly are not determined by any genes that have been inherited. Only a physician or scientist trained in medical genetics can determine whether a disease or defect is a result of inherited genes, environmental factors, or a combination of both.

Congenital Defects

Each newborn is examined immediately after birth for any observable physical abnormalities, which are called congenital defects. Such defects are not necessarily inherited,

although defective genes passed on from parents may play some role. Most congenital defects are caused by a complex interaction of genes and environmental factors. Examples of congenital defects are cleft lip, cleft palate, and spina bifida (cleft spine), which result from developmental abnormalities in the formation of the oral cavity and the spine, respectively (**Figure 15.3**).

Cleft lip has been known to occur in only one of a pair of identical twins, so environmental factors other than genes must contribute to this abnormality. The importance of environmental factors during fetal development also is borne out by the observation that even though identical twins share identical genes, they usually are born with different birth weights. This shows that identical twins are affected differently by environmental factors even during development in the same uterus.

Spina bifida is a congenital defect that affects 1 of every 1,000 newborns. It occurs when one or more spinal vertebrae fail to close and the spinal cord and nerves bulge through the cleft, forming an easily damaged, fluid-filled sac. The protruding spinal nerves are vulnerable to paralysis-causing damage and also to life-threatening infections. The most serious congenital defect of the nervous system is *anencephaly*, which refers to very abnormal brain development; affected babies are either stillborn or die soon after birth. Surgery can repair some of the damage resulting from spina bifida; however, nothing can be done for anencephaly.

Supplementing the diet of pregnant women with the vitamins folic acid and B_{12} dramatically reduces the risk of spina bifida and other birth defects. Folic acid is the most effective in preventing birth defects and should be taken before pregnancy occurs. Women who plan on becoming pregnant should take folic acid (400 micrograms per day) before and after becoming pregnant. Flour and cereals have been supplemented with folic acid for

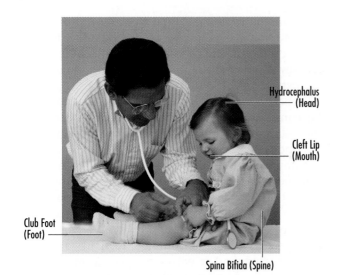

Hydrocephalus (Head)

Cleft Lip (Mouth)

Club Foot (Foot)

Spina Bifida (Spine)

■ **Figure 15.3**

Congenital defects arise during fetal development and are detected at birth.

the past decade. As a result, the incidence of spina bifida birth defects has decreased significantly.

However, in recent years the number of birth defects has been increasing as fewer women supplement their diets with folate before becoming pregnant. They also are not consuming enough folate-supplemented grains, perhaps because of the fad for "low-carb" diets. The folate solution to reducing birth defects also has come under attack by researchers who claim that excess folate in the diet may be harmful to the elderly. The bottom line: If you are female and think you may become pregnant, take a folate supplement. It can reduce the risk of having a child with a birth defect by as much as 70%.

Any environmental agent that causes a defect in a developing fetus is called a **teratogen** (Table 15.3). Many environmental agents, such as prescription and illegal drugs, viral and bacterial infections, alcohol consumption, and cigarette smoke, act as teratogens (from the Greek, "to produce a monster") during pregnancy and may cause abnormal development in a fetus. With a little care, many teratogens can be avoided, thereby increasing the likelihood of a healthy baby. In particular, smoking cigarettes and drinking alcohol should be avoided by any woman who is pregnant or attempting to become pregnant. Alcohol is concentrated when crossing the placenta, so that even one or two drinks can lead to high alcohol levels in the fetus and affect its development.

Thalidomide

Thalidomide was developed by a Swiss pharmaceutical company in 1953. Originally tested as a drug for epilepsy, it was subsequently found to be an effective tranquilizer and sedative. In 1957, thalidomide was marketed in Europe and other countries around the world as the drug of choice for pregnant women experiencing "morning sickness." The drug was thought to be extremely safe and had been tested in pregnant animals, where it did not act as a teratogen.

Table 15.3

Teratogens

Environmental agents (e.g., infectious viruses and other microorganisms, chemicals, medicines) can act as teratogens and cause birth defects. Many agents in addition to those listed below are suspected of causing abnormal development of the fetus.

Environmental agent	Effects
Accutane (acne drug)	Spontaneous abortion, stillbirth, malformation of the brain and heart
Alcohol	Growth deficiencies, mental retardation
Antithyroid drugs	Thyroid defects
Carbamazepine	Neural tube defects
Cocaine	Fetal death, nervous system and genital abnormalities
Cytomegalovirus, herpes simplex virus, varicella zoster virus	Growth deficiencies, mental retardation
Diethylstilbestrol (DES)	Masculinization of female, abnormalities of vagina and cervix, risk of vaginal cancer
Ionizing radiation	Growth deficiencies, mental retardation, organ malformation (depending on dose)
Lithium carbonate	Heart and blood vessel defects
Methotrexate and etretinate	Prescription drugs that cause severe birth defects
Nonsteroidal anti-inflammatory drugs	Circulation defects
Phenytoin	Central nervous system defects
Polychlorinated biphenyls	Growth deficiencies, pigment abnormalities
Poor nutrition during fetal development	Growth deficiency, mental retardation
Rubella virus (German measles)	Heart and eye abnormalities, mental retardation
Tetracycline (antibiotic)	Teeth and bone abnormalities
Thalidomide	Limb malformation
Tobacco smoke	Growth deficiencies, increased risk of sickness and death soon after birth
Warfarin	Central nervous system defects

However, thalidomide is *not* safe for any woman who is pregnant. Thalidomide interferes with normal development of the bones of the arms and legs of a fetus and causes other developmental abnormalities. Between 1956 and 1961, when the teratogenic effects of the drug were finally recognized, thousands of babies in Europe and elsewhere in the world had been born with severe deformities of the arms and legs. Many thousands more were stillborn, but no one knows for sure how many

TERMS

teratogen: any environmental agent that causes abnormal development of a fetus

pregnant women lost their fetuses or gave birth to deformed babies. The drug was never approved for sale in the United States largely because of Francis Kelsey, a physician at the Food and Drug Administration (FDA) who was responsible for new drug applications. She was concerned about the drug's side effects and delayed its approval until the devastating effects of the drug were discovered in other countries. Most countries had banned the use of thalidomide by 1961.

However, interest in the therapeutic potential of thalidomide and related drugs has not subsided. Research has continued and, in an ironic twist of fate, thalidomide (trade name, Thalomid) was approved by the FDA in 1998 for use in treating skin lesions associated with leprosy. The drug now comes with a strong warning advising doctors not to prescribe the drug for any condition for which it is not approved or for women who might become pregnant. The lesson from thalidomide is that women who may become pregnant should not take any drug—prescription, over-the-counter, or illegal—in order to protect a fetus should they become pregnant.

DES

In the 1950s and 1960s, the synthetic hormone DES (diethylstilbestrol) was prescribed to help prevent miscarriage. DES was not identified as a teratogen until the 1970s. Many daughters of women who took DES before or during pregnancy discovered that they had abnormalities in their reproductive organs when they tried to become pregnant. These daughters also have a higher risk of developing vaginal cancer. Although the drug did not cause abnormalities in all children of DES mothers, the risk is sufficiently great that most DES women carry the psychological burden of their potential for reproductive problems and cancer.

Accutane

Isotretinoin is an analogue of vitamin A and is sold as a drug called Accutane that is used to treat severe acne and other skin disorders. Accutane was tested in laboratory animals and labeled a teratogen because it caused birth defects when administered to pregnant mice and rats. The drug was finally released with the warning that it should not be used during pregnancy. However, during the 1980s, hundreds of babies with congenital defects were born to women who became pregnant while taking Accutane for skin problems. In some cases, the women may have become pregnant by accident while taking the drug; in others, the desire to improve their skin condition may have caused them to disregard the warning. This points out a dilemma faced by the FDA, the government agency that regulates drugs. Should an effective drug that is known to be a teratogen be released with a warning or should it be banned entirely?

Fetal Alcohol Syndrome

Consumption of alcohol in any amount during pregnancy increases the risk of a *fetal alcohol spectrum disorder,* the most common form being **fetal alcohol syndrome** (FAS). This condition is diagnosed if an infant has certain characteristic abnormal facial features, growth reduction, and neurodevelopmental abnormalities (Sokol, Delaney-Black, & Nordstrom, 2003).

Although most babies with FAS are born to women who consume large amounts of alcohol during pregnancy, studies show that even moderate drinking during pregnancy may increase risk.

Many women think that an occasional drink during pregnancy cannot cause any harm. They may be right, but it still is a gamble even if the risk is low. Nine months is a long time between drinks for someone who is used to drinking, even occasionally. Women who are light drinkers before becoming pregnant (about one drink per day) find it easier to give up alcohol than women who are heavy drinkers (three or more drinks per day). Despite warnings on alcoholic beverage containers, the incidence of FAS and other alcohol-related disorders in developing fetuses has remained quite high—as many as 1 in 10 newborns have been exposed to alcohol during pregnancy.

The drinking of alcohol by pregnant women who give birth to a handicapped child raises questions about individual rights. Does a mother have a right to do with her body as she sees fit even if it means harming the baby? Does society have the right to regulate the consumption of alcohol and other harmful substances by a pregnant woman? Some people argue that a pregnant woman who irresponsibly uses alcohol or drugs during pregnancy should be imprisoned while pregnant so that her use of dangerous substances can be controlled. The ethical and legal questions surrounding pregnancy, alcohol, and drugs are unresolved.

Preventing Hereditary Diseases

Prenatal Testing

An important goal of modern medicine is preventing inherited diseases caused by abnormal genes or chromosomes. Genetic counseling of couples who are at risk for having a child with a hereditary disorder can help prevent them from having a handicapped child by counseling them before and during pregnancy. Genetic counseling can provide useful information, but, in the end, the parents must make the decisions. Prenatal testing is not advised or necessary for all pregnant women or couples planning to have a child. Only those who are at higher-than-average risk for bearing a child with a hereditary defect are advised to undergo prenatal testing and genetic counseling.

Hundreds of single-gene defects that cause hereditary diseases now can be detected *in utero* with a prenatal procedure called **amniocentesis** (**Figure 15.4**). In this procedure, fetal cells are obtained by removing a sample of amniotic fluid from the womb around the fifteenth week of pregnancy. Although amniocentesis is very safe, there is still a small risk of harming the fetus or inducing a miscarriage. The physician should discuss the risks and benefits of the procedure as part of the genetic counseling. Amniocentesis is performed so that prospective parents can decide whether to continue the pregnancy or abort the fetus. The decision is generally made after discussion with their physician and a counselor.

The fetal cells obtained by amniocentesis are grown in the laboratory and tested for biochemical and genetic abnormalities. Examination of the chromosomes in the karyotype analysis also identifies the sex of the fetus, but this information is provided only if the pregnant woman specifically requests it. (Although most people in American society are joyful at the birth of either a boy or a girl, in other countries, male children are still considered more desirable. In fact, determination of a female fetus by amniocentesis and karyotype analysis is the most common cause of elective abortion in many countries.)

Another prenatal procedure, called **chorionic villus sampling (CVS)**, can be performed as early as eight weeks after conception. This earlier test provides infor-

mation regarding the health of the fetus, allowing the parent(s) to make an earlier decision with respect to terminating the pregnancy.

A noninvasive form of prenatal testing is **ultrasound scanning,** which is used to visualize the developing fetus (**Figure 15.5**). Ultrasound scans use high-frequency sound waves that bounce back from the various tissues in the fetus with different intensities. The sound waves reflected from the fetus are displayed on a screen, and the image is interpreted by a physician trained in the use of this technique.

Ultrasound scans are used to detect multiple fetuses and to determine the location of the placenta, which is important if amniocentesis is to be performed. The scans can gauge the fetus's head size, thereby providing determination of the age of the fetus. Abnormal brain development and neural tube defects also can be diagnosed with an ultrasound scan. Despite the safety of these tests, pregnant women are advised not to have an ultrasound scan unless their health or that of the fetus requires one.

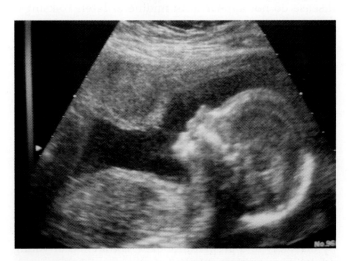

Amniocentesis

Amniotic cavity

Centrifuge

- Amniotic fluid withdrawn from cavity

Cells from amniotic fluid

Cell culture

- Analyzed for biochemical or chromosomal defects

■ **Figure 15.4**

Amniocentesis

In the diagnostic procedure called amniocentesis, a sample of the fluid that surrounds the developing fetus is collected. Both the fluid and the fetal cells it contains are then analyzed for biochemical or chromosomal defects.

■ **Figure 15.5**

Ultrasound Scanning

Image of a fetus obtained by ultrasound scanning. Such ultrasound scans reveal the position of the fetus and may also indicate certain physical abnormalities.

> ┃ T E R M S ┃
>
> amniocentesis: a procedure in which amniotic fluid is removed from the uterus and tested to determine whether genetic or anatomical defects exist in the fetus
>
> chorionic villus sampling: a prenatal procedure used to determine whether genetic or anatomical defects exist in a fetus; an alternative to amniocentesis
>
> fetal alcohol syndrome: birth defects and mental disabilities caused by ingestion of alcohol by the mother during pregnancy
>
> ultrasound scanning: use of sound waves to visualize the fetus in the womb

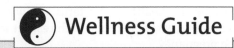

Wellness Guide

Determining If You Are at Risk for Bearing a Genetically Handicapped Child

Prenatal testing and genetic counseling are advised if a person falls into any one of the following risk categories:
- Maternal age over 35 years (risk of Down syndrome)
- High or low levels of alphafetoprotein during pregnancy (risk of neural tube defect)
- Woman had a previous child with a chromosomal abnormality or neural tube defect
- Woman had a previous stillbirth or neonatal death
- Woman or mate carries a previously diagnosed chromosomal or genetic abnormality
- Woman carries a previously diagnosed defective gene
- Woman and mate carry the same previously diagnosed defective gene
- Close relatives have a child with an inherited disorder
- Woman has been exposed to a teratogenic agent during pregnancy
- Woman has recently been infected by rubella (measles) virus or cytomegalovirus

Genetic Counseling

Genetic counseling is necessary both before and after a pregnancy occurs to help high-risk individuals have a healthy baby. Genetic counseling begins with objective calculations of genetic risks to a fetus, which, in some cases, guarantee that an abnormal fetus is being carried. However, after risks have been evaluated, subjective values inevitably enter into the decisions. For example, religious convictions may preclude an abortion and lead some women to continue a pregnancy even though a child with Down syndrome will be born.

Although genetic counselors strive to be objective, the counseling process is subtle and counselors may inadvertently interject personal opinions. For example, prospective parents who each carry a defective gene may be told that they have one chance in four of having a genetically handicapped child. Or they can be told that the odds are three to one that they will have a normal child. Both statements express the same truth about the probabilities, but the prospective parents may well interpret the two statements quite differently. One statement emphasizes a negative outcome; the other a more positive outcome.

Giving advice or making recommendations that affect the life of another person invariably involves difficult moral decisions and many conflicting views. Ideally, the personal views of a genetic counselor should not influence the decision-making process of the couples or families involved. Clients should arrive at their own informed decisions after careful consideration of all of the medical facts and risks that have been explained to them.

Genetic Testing

One of the major goals of genetic testing is to alert people to their own risk of developing a disease or to their risk of passing on a defective gene to a child. Sometimes a defective gene passed on from one parent is sufficient to cause an inherited disease; in other cases a defective gene must be inherited from each parent. Once the underlying genetic cause of a disorder or disease has been identified and the DNA in the gene analyzed, it is possible to devise a genetic test that can quickly determine whether a person carries a "normal" gene or one that is defective and that may cause an inherited disease if passed on to progeny. Depending on the individual and the disease, genetic testing can be helpful or harmful.

Genetic tests are most useful when they can be used to prevent passing on genes that cause serious inherited disorders. Some common inherited disorders for which genetic tests are available include cystic fibrosis, sickle cell anemia, hemophilia A, Duchenne muscular dystrophy, Huntington's disease, Fragile X syndrome, and many others. People who are concerned whether they or other family members carry a defective gene should consult with a physician trained in genetic testing and counseling. Despite the explosion of genetic knowledge and development of genetic tests in recent years, not all medical experts are convinced that they are necessarily beneficial or should be incorporated into general medical practice.

Two examples serve to illustrate the complex issues surrounding genetic testing. Symptoms of Huntington's disease do not appear until midlife or later. Folksinger Woody Guthrie died of Huntington's disease, and his son, Arlo Guthrie, did not know whether he had inherited the abnormal gene from his father. (Arlo had a 50-50 chance of having inherited the gene. The genetic test for Huntington's disease had not yet been developed.) Arlo took the chance and had his children before he reached the age when symptoms appear. Luckily, Arlo did not inherit the gene from his father, so his children will not get Huntington's disease either.

If a parent has died of Huntington's disease, the children of that parent can be tested for the presence or absence of the gene. Suppose a child finds out at age 15 that the Huntington gene has been passed on and that symptoms likely will begin to appear in midlife followed by disability and premature death. For a child or young adult to cope with that knowledge may well be too much of a psychological burden. Some people whose families have a history of members with Huntington's disease choose not to know or to be tested; others want to know their status. Either choice is difficult and may result in

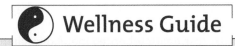

Wellness Guide

Biomarkers for Disease Susceptibility

An outcome from knowing the complete DNA sequence of human chromosomes is the ability to pinpoint differences that make one individual more susceptible to a disease than someone else. For example, a single chemical change in a chromosome might make a person prone to developing diabetes, heart disease, prostate cancer, or depression.

Technologies developed in the past few years allow scientists to rapidly screen a person's DNA for *biomarkers* that signal an increased susceptibility to dozens of diseases, mental disorders, and unhealthy behaviors. This process, called *whole genome scanning*, utilizes methods that can compare virtually all of a person's genes with a standard set to uncover differences that are associated with increased disease risk. The risks may be small or very large: a 10% to 20% increased risk is regarded as small; a 5- to 10-fold increased risk is quite large.

In 2005, a gene was discovered that increases the risk of developing macular degeneration (a condition that causes blindness in older adults; see Chapter 22) four- to six-fold. In 2007, gene variants were discovered that increase the risk of diabetes (80%), obesity (67%), and heart disease (20–40%) (Couzin & Kaiser, 2007). The pace of discovery of disease susceptibility genes is expected to increase in the coming years. Soon it may be possible for a primary care physician to take a drop of blood, insert it into a gene-scanning machine, and give a patient a printout listing dozens of diseases that she or he is susceptible to, along with a calculated risk.

What is a patient or a doctor to do with such information? The answer is really "nothing" for the foreseeable future. There are no treatments or drugs that can reduce or change a person's genetic susceptibility. A healthy lifestyle is helpful but no guarantee that a disease can be prevented. So, is testing for all the known (and soon to be known) variant genes worthwhile? One thing is certain: The companies that develop these testing methods will want to market them aggressively.

---

serious psychological stress whether the result is positive or negative. (A negative result may produce overwhelming feelings of guilt if a sibling's result is positive.)

Another dilemma arises with breast cancer. The risk of developing breast cancer in women is strongly influenced by inheriting one or both cancer susceptibility genes called BRCA1 and BRCA2 (see Chapter 13). Inheriting both susceptibility genes means a woman has an 80% to 90% probability of developing breast cancer at some time in her life, usually while quite young. In families whose female members have a high incidence of breast cancer, young women can be tested for the presence of these susceptibility genes. If both genes are found to be present, a young woman is faced with two demoralizing choices. She can worry and wait for signs of breast cancer. Or she can elect to have prophylactic mastectomy in which both breasts are surgically removed while she is young to avoid the development of breast cancer later in life.

In Great Britain, women who carry breast cancer susceptibility genes can choose to have a child using *in vitro* fertilization (see Chapter 9). A single cell from the embryo can be tested to make sure it does not carry BRCA1 or BRCA2 genes before it is implanted. In this way, parents can be sure the harmful genes will not be passed on to their child. However, preimplantation genetic screening of embryos and subsequent procedures also can have unfortunate outcomes, such as multiple pregnancies (Collins, 2007).

Genetic tests for serious diseases are a great medical advance but also create serious problems. Any person thinking about getting a genetic test should consult a genetic counselor before proceeding with such tests. Knowing what your disease risks are can change your life

forever. And if others obtain the results of your genetic tests, it could lead to insurance or employment problems.

Genetic Discrimination

One of the potential harmful consequences of genetic testing is the possibility of discrimination against a person because he or she carries a particular gene that predisposes the person toward a disease. We all understand what discrimination based on sex or race means, and laws have been passed to prevent racial or sexual discrimination in employment, housing, the armed services, and in other public settings. Although rarely described in genetic terms, racial and sexual discrimination are actually a form of genetic discrimination because sex and skin color are determined by the genes that were inherited from parents.

Employers and insurance companies are the organizations most interested in knowing what defective genes a person may have inherited. Companies would obviously prefer not to hire someone who was likely to have a serious health problem after working a few years. Such a person is costly to a company because of wasted training, lost work, and costs of health benefits. A company's health insurance plan might even be canceled if the benefits paid became too high.

Health insurance and life insurance companies also would like to have information about a person's genetic profile so that they could select members who are "good"

TERMS

genetic counseling: information to help prospective parents evaluate the risks of having or delivering a genetically handicapped child

risks and reject those who are "poor" risks. Insurance companies are profit driven like all companies and usually can obtain information about genetic tests from a person's medical record. Thus, everyone needs to be very cautious in allowing others to have access to their medical records.

After more than 10 years of intense effort to deal with the problems of genetic discrimination, the Genetic Information Nondiscrimination Act (GINA) was finally passed by Congress and signed into law in 2008. The law forbids:

- An employer from firing or not hiring a person based on information obtained from genetic testing
- Insurance companies from denying health or life insurance to persons based on information obtained from genetic tests
- Companies from charging higher premiums for persons with disease susceptibility genes

It is hoped that the federal law will make people feel safer if they choose to undergo the increasing number of genetic tests that are available and will not fear reprisal from employers or insurers.

Treating Hereditary Diseases

Very few of the thousands of known hereditary diseases can be treated effectively. Phenylketonuria (PKU) is an exception; it can be managed if the affected newborn is diagnosed at birth. Because PKU is treatable and because the test is accurate and inexpensive, all newborns in the United States are tested for PKU. The amino acid phenylalanine is present in any normal diet and, if it is eaten by a child with PKU, it accumulates in the blood, affecting brain development and causing mental retardation. A person with PKU lacks an enzyme that is essential for the chemical breakdown of the phenylalanine present in most proteins, including proteins in milk. Thus, any baby with PKU is immediately put

> In nature there is no blemish but the mind.
> None can be called deformed but the unkind.
>
> *William Shakespeare,*
> Twelfth Night

on a phenylalanine-free diet, which must be maintained at least until, and often beyond, puberty.

Mandatory testing for inherited metabolic (chemical) disorders in newborns varies from state to state; some states test for as few as 3 disorders, whereas others test for almost 30. With modern technology, a single drop of blood taken from the heel of a newborn can be tested for at least 40 different inherited metabolic disorders. One problem with the tests is that for every infant who actually has an inherited disorder, up to 60 false positives also result. These false-positive results must be ruled out by further tests, during which time parents will continue to worry. Each metabolic disorder creates its own set of medical problems, some of which may be treatable and others not.

Gene Therapy

Thousands of human disorders are caused by the inheritance of a gene that is abnormal. Because genes contain the information for making proteins, inheriting an abnormal gene means that a defective protein is synthesized; the result is some abnormality in body chemistry that is manifested as a disease. People with sickle cell anemia inherit abnormal genes for hemoglobin synthesis. In cystic fibrosis, the defective protein is in cell membranes that determine how chemicals enter and exit cells. And in muscular dystrophy, proteins that are used to build muscle are defective. The problem for medical science is how to cure these inherited diseases.

Occasionally the defective protein can be manufactured and injected into patients to replace the missing one, as in the treatment for hemophilia. In other cases, drugs are used to lessen the severity of symptoms, as in cystic fibrosis and sickle cell anemia. However, because a fundamental gene is defective in all of the cells in a person's body, these kinds of treatments do not permanently cure the patient. That is the goal of **gene therapy**.

As more and more human genes are isolated and cataloged by laboratories around the world, the normal genes corresponding to the defective ones become avail-

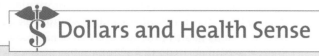

$ Dollars and Health Sense

The Stem Cell Business

Whereas stem cell research in the West is proceeding by fits and starts, China already has a booming business in treating "medical tourists" with fetal and embryonic cells of all kinds. Most of the patients have neurological disorders such as Parkinson's disease or spinal injuries that have left them paralyzed. Others have a condition called macular degeneration that leads to blindness (see Chapter 22). For $20,000 plus the cost of the trip, patients can receive injections of fetal or embryonic cells that are supposed to restore some degree of normal function. Some patients claim that they have been helped by the treatments, but objective tests performed

in the United States do not substantiate the benefits. Some patients who have received injections of cells directly into the brain have had subsequent infections.

People who are desperate for some kind of treatment even when none is available in the United States will seek it elsewhere if they can afford it. In the 1960s, desperately ill people went to "psychic surgeons" in the Philippines who purportedly removed tumors from deep in the body with their bare hands, and some people returned claiming that they were cured. Faith and belief are powerful healers (see Chapter 2). If a cure for something that is incurable sounds "too good to be true," however, then it probably is.

able for gene therapy. Once a normal human gene has been purified, it can be inserted into affected patients by a variety of medical techniques. The hope is that the normal gene will function once it is in the cells, and that the protein will be produced in sufficient quantity to cure the inherited disease permanently.

The logic of gene therapy is sound; however, in practice it has proved exceptionally difficult to overcome the technical and biological obstacles. In 2000, it appeared that gene therapy had its first major success. Several children in France suffering from a severe inherited immune system disease were given healthy genes, and their immune systems began functioning normally. The normal genes were transferred to their cells using what was thought to be a harmless virus as a vector to carry the genes into cells. Scientists hailed the results. By the end of 2002, however, two of the children had contracted leukemia, presumably from the virus that had been used in the gene therapy experiment.

The use of this method of gene therapy was suspended, and scientists are searching for other means of transferring genes to cells. Most of the gene therapy experiments currently in progress involve attempts to cure cancer in advanced stages. If safe and effective gene therapy techniques can be developed, incurable inherited diseases may be cured.

In 2007, gene therapy technology experienced a major setback with the death of a patient who had been undergoing gene therapy to cure rheumatoid arthritis. Because of this death, all gene therapy trials in the United States were suspended until additional safety procedures could be implemented. Although gene therapy may eventually succeed in curing some inherited diseases, the ultimate solution to eliminating inherited disorders may be the detection of defective genes in prospective parents and prevention of their transmission to offspring.

Embryonic Stem Cells

A generation ago there was great consternation and public debate over the ethical and social issues associated with *in vitro* fertilization (IVF). Today, the benefits and risks of IVF are widely accepted, and millions of children, many of whom have reached reproductive age themselves, have been conceived using assisted reproductive technologies (see Chapter 9). However, the ability to create human embryos in the laboratory has led to research with unused laboratory-derived embryos to generate **embryonic stem cells.** Such cells hold great promise for treating presently incurable diseases such as Parkinson's disease, amyotrophic lateral sclerosis (ALS), spinal injuries, and type 1 diabetes.

A human being begins with a fertilized egg that develops over a span of nine months in the uterus into a fully developed infant. When a human embryo develops to the point where it contains several hundred cells, it is called a blastocyst (**Figure 15.6**). The internal cells in the blastocyst are embryonic stem cells because they

possess the capability of developing into specific tissues such as lung, heart, liver, brain, and so forth when they are exposed to specific environmental factors that cause them to differentiate (become specialized). In the laboratory, cells can be removed from early-stage embryos and grown in large numbers in laboratory dishes, where some develop into stable embryonic stem

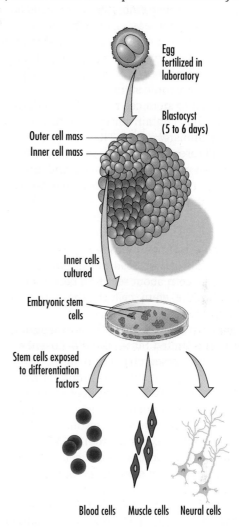

■ **Figure 15.6**

Isolation of Embryonic Stem Cells
A fertilized egg is allowed to develop in the laboratory until it contains several hundred cells. Some of these cells are spread on laboratory dishes where they grow into colonies of embryonic stem cells. These cells can be grown almost indefinitely; when they are exposed to certain environments, they differentiate into cells characteristic of specific tissues and organs.

TERMS

embryonic stem cells: cells derived from human fertilized eggs and grown in laboratory dishes; stem cells have the capacity to differentiate into many different tissues and organs

gene therapy: a technique for replacing defective genes with normal ones in certain tissues of a person affected with a hereditary disease

cell lines that can be stored or grown under special conditions during which they develop into specialized cells and tissues. Stem cell lines retain the potential for developing into specific tissues almost indefinitely. When injected into organs in the body, stem cells can replace tissues that may have been damaged or destroyed by disease.

For example, mouse embryonic stem cells have been injected into the pancreas of diabetic mice where the cells developed into pancreatic cells capable of producing insulin. The research with mice suggests that some forms of human diabetes (type 1) might be helped by the use of human embryonic stem cells.

A major goal of stem cell research is to develop lines of stem cells that contain an individual's own genetic information (Phimister, 2005). This can be accomplished as follows. Cells are removed from a patient with a serious disease. Several nuclei are removed and injected into human eggs from which the nuclei have been carefully removed (enucleated eggs). Each egg with the patient's cell's nucleus will develop into a blastocyst in a laboratory dish. Then single cells are removed and grown into stable embryonic stem cell lines. If this is successful, the individualized stem cells can be used to treat the patient's disease without concern about rejection because the genetic information in the stem cells is the same as in the patient's own cells.

Embryonic stem cell research is exceptionally controversial in the United States (Kalb & Rosenberg, 2004). Supporters of such research point to its enormous potential for relieving human suffering and treating incurable diseases. Opponents believe that every human embryo, regardless of how it was created, is a potential "person" and that the "soul" enters when fertilization takes place or when an embryo exists (Sandel, 2004). Other opponents argue that embryonic stem cell research is the beginning of a "slippery slope" that will lead to cloning babies, manufacture of organs for sale, and other deplorable uses of human cells derived from embryos.

In 2008, several groups of researchers showed that cells with properties similar to embryonic stem cells could be derived from adult cells. By adding a number of genes to adult cells, the scientists were able to reprogram the cells so that some of them gained the capacity to develop into all kinds of cells and tissues just as embryonic stem cells do. However, it is not clear yet whether these adult-derived stem cells have the same therapeutic potential as embryonic stem cells or whether they are safe to inject into people (Higgs, 2008).

Cloning

Cloning refers to the production of genetically identical plants or animals. Cloning is quite easy with plants; anytime you take a cutting from a plant and start a new one, you have created a clone. However, cloning an animal is considerably more difficult. A nucleus must be removed from a cell in the adult animal that is to be cloned. Then

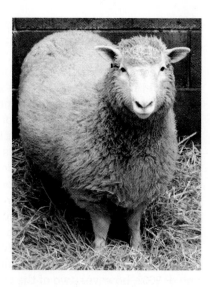

Dolly, a sheep, was in 1997 the first large animal to be cloned. Since then cows, pigs, horses, mules, cats, dogs, and other animals have been cloned.

this nucleus must be gently inserted into an egg of the same species in which the nucleus has been destroyed or removed. All these manipulations are done by a skilled researcher peering into a microscope. The egg is then implanted into the uterus of a female animal who has been hormonally prepared for pregnancy.

In 1997, Dolly, a sheep in Scotland, was the first animal to be cloned. Since then, more than 15 other animal species have been cloned in laboratories around the world; these include wolf, African wild cat, dog mule, domestic cat, buffalo, mouse, goat, rabbit, horse, cow, pig, rat, and ferret. Despite these accomplishments, success in cloning is quite rare. Most implanted embryos do not develop normally, and usually the fetus is aborted or born so defective that it does not survive. Among those that do survive, many become sick and die prematurely.

However, some of the cloned animals do appear normal and are being studied as they age to see what diseases or problems occur as they get older. Perhaps the most remarkable thing about cloning mammals is that it works at all, even if only rarely, given the complexity of fetal development and the precision with which thousands of genes must be activated and deactivated during development (Cibelli, 2007).

Should we clone humans? "Unthinkable," say most scientists for scientific, ethical, and social reasons. Even though cloning of people is universally forbidden, the cloning of animals for purposes such as to improve the quality of meat, to produce drugs secreted in the animal's milk, and to satisfy pet owners will continue to increase in the years ahead.

TERMS

cloning: the process of making genetically identical plants or animals

Critical Thinking About Health

1. A woman friend who is about 25 years old has just learned that she is pregnant. The woman smokes cigarettes and likes to party on weekends. Based on what you have learned about the causes of congenital defects in this chapter, make a list of all the behavioral, dietary, and lifestyle changes you would recommend to your friend to help ensure that she gives birth to a healthy child. Discuss the rationale for each of your recommendations.

2. Abortion is one of the most controversial issues in American society. At one end of the spectrum of views are people who think that all abortions should be prohibited for any reason whatsoever, even if the life of the pregnant woman is in jeopardy. At the other extreme are people who believe that each pregnant woman should have complete freedom to do whatsoever she chooses with respect to her pregnancy because it is her body. Evaluate these two views of abortion and present your own views in as much detail as possible. Substantiate each of your views.

3. You and your spouse decide now is the time to begin a family. Your spouse has a younger brother who is mentally handicapped and you have an older sister who was born with a cleft palate that was corrected by surgery. Do you believe that your risks of having a child with a congenital defect or inherited disorder are higher than average? Based on what you have learned in this chapter, are there any precautions that you should take or any genetic tests that you think would be appropriate to reduce any anxiety about becoming pregnant? Make a list of questions that you both would like to discuss with your physician regarding things that you should know or tests that you should take to help ensure giving birth to a healthy child.

4. A few years ago, the U.S. military ordered all service personnel to have a blood sample taken so that the DNA of each individual's cells could be analyzed and the pattern placed on file, much as the FBI keeps files of fingerprints of criminals and others. The reason the military wants each person's DNA analyzed is so that remains can be positively identified in case that person dies in a future conflict. One soldier refused to give a blood sample in violation of a direct order and was ordered to stand before a court martial. The soldier argued that he had no assurance that his DNA information would be kept private and would not be used for purposes of discrimination or to his detriment in other ways.

   a. Do you think the military is justified in wanting each person's DNA on file?

   b. In what ways might the DNA information be used to the detriment of the soldier either in the military or after his release from military service?

   c. Discuss the pros and cons of having the DNA profile of every person in the United States on file in a federal agency so that any person could be positively identified by law enforcement authorities, government agencies, or other organizations, should the need arise.

Health in Review

- Every newborn inherits 23 chromosomes and about 20,000 genes from each parent. Inheriting abnormal chromosomes or abnormal genes can result in an inherited disease.
- Genetic information is carried in DNA.
- Congenital birth defects are observed at birth in about 1 of 50 newborn babies in the United States. Abnormal development of the fetus during pregnancy can be caused by environmental factors, abnormal genes that were passed on from one or both parents, or a combination of both.
- Ultrasound, amniocentesis, and chorionic villus sampling are prenatal diagnostic procedures that can determine whether fetal development is normal or whether there is a physical or biological defect.
- Taking prescription or illegal drugs, drinking alcohol, or becoming infected by viruses during pregnancy also can harm the fetus. If drugs or alcohol are used by a pregnant woman, especially in early pregnancy, the fetus may abort spontaneously or the newborn may suffer growth deficiencies, mental retardation, or other problems.

- Couples who are at higher-than-average risk for having a genetically handicapped child should undergo genetic counseling before and after pregnancy is established.
- Modern genetic diagnostic tests can detect genes responsible for hundreds of hereditary diseases; however, only a few can be treated successfully.
- Genetic discrimination may occur when people find out that they or others carry genes that predispose them to diseases and disorders. A federal law prohibits genetic discrimination.
- Gene therapy is a promising new method of treating genetic diseases.
- Embryonic stem cells are derived from early-stage embryos produced in the laboratory. Such cells have the potential to differentiate into any desired tissues. Such cells may help cure serious diseases.
- Cloning human beings is unjustified for scientific, ethical, and social reasons; cloning other animals is relatively common but still unreliable.

Health and Wellness Online

The Web contains a wealth of information about health and wellness. By accessing the Internet using Web browser software, you can gain a new perspective on many topics presented in *Health and Wellness*, Tenth Edition. Access the Jones and Bartlett Publishers Web site at **health.jbpub.com/hwonline**.

References

Cibelli, J. (2007). A decade of cloning mystique. *Science, 316*, 990–992.

Collins, J. A. (2007). Preimplantation genetic screening in older mothers. *New England Journal of Medicine, 357*, 61–62.

Couzin, J., & Kaiser, J. (2007). Closing the net on common disease genes. *Science, 316*, 820–822.

Enattah, N. S., et al. (2002). Identification of a variant associated with adult-type hypolactasia. *Nature Genetics, 30*, 233–237.

Gibbons, A. (2006). There's more than one way to have your milk and drink it, too. *Science, 314*, 1672.

Higgs, D. R. (2008). A new dawn for stem-cell therapy. *New England Journal of Medicine, 358*, 964–966.

Kalb, C., & Rosenberg, D. (2004, October 25). Stem cell division. *Newsweek,* 43–50.

Phimister, E. G. (2005). A tetraploid twist on the embryonic stem cell. *New England Journal of Medicine, 353*, 1046–1054.

Sandel, M. J. (2004). Embryo ethics—The moral logic of stem cell research. *New England Journal of Medicine, 351*, 207–212.

Sluder, G., & McCollum, D. (2000). The mad way of meiosis. *Science, 289*, 254–255.

Sokol, R. J., Delaney-Black, V., & Nordstrom, B. (2003). Fetal alcohol spectrum disorder. *Journal of the American Medical Association, 290*, 2996–2999.

Suggested Readings

Brownlee, C. (2005, April 9). Code of many colors. *Science News,* 232–234. Evaluates the never-ending controversy about biology and race.

Collins, F. S., & McKusick, V. A. (2001). Implications of the Human Genome Project for medical science. *Journal of the American Medical Association,* 540–545. Discusses what the Human Genome Project means for medicine and treatments in the twenty-first century.

The future of stem cells. (2005, July). *Scientific American,* A3–A35. A collection of articles discussing all aspects of stem cell research and future prospects for treating incurable diseases.

Gawande, A. (2004, December 6). The bell curve. *The New Yorker,* 82–91. A doctor describes the complexities of getting treatment for a common inherited disease, cystic fibrosis.

Hall, M., & Olopode, O. I. (2005). Confronting genetic testing disparities. *Journal of the American Medical Association, 293*, 1783–1785. Explains the many problems associated with genetic testing.

Nuzzo, R. (2008, June 2). Nabbing suspicious SNPs. *Science News,* 20–24. An excellent short article describing how the hundreds of disease susceptibility genes are being discovered.

Venter, C. (2007). *A life decoded: My genome, my life.* New York: Viking. The personal story of the man who beat everyone in the race to sequence the human genome.

Recommended Web Sites

Please visit **health.jbpub.com/hwonline** for links to these Web sites.

GeneWatch

The Council for Responsible Genetics (CRG) publishes a monthly magazine called *GeneWatch*. CRG is an activist organization that focuses public attention on the moral and ethical issues of the genetic advances in medicine, food, and technology.

The Human Genome Project

Information on the scientific, medical, ethical, legal, and social aspects of medical genetics.

U.S. National Center for Birth Defects and Developmental Disabilities

Information on causes and prevention of birth defects.

Part Five

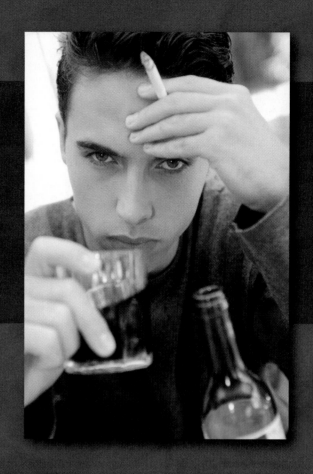

Explaining Drug Use and Abuse

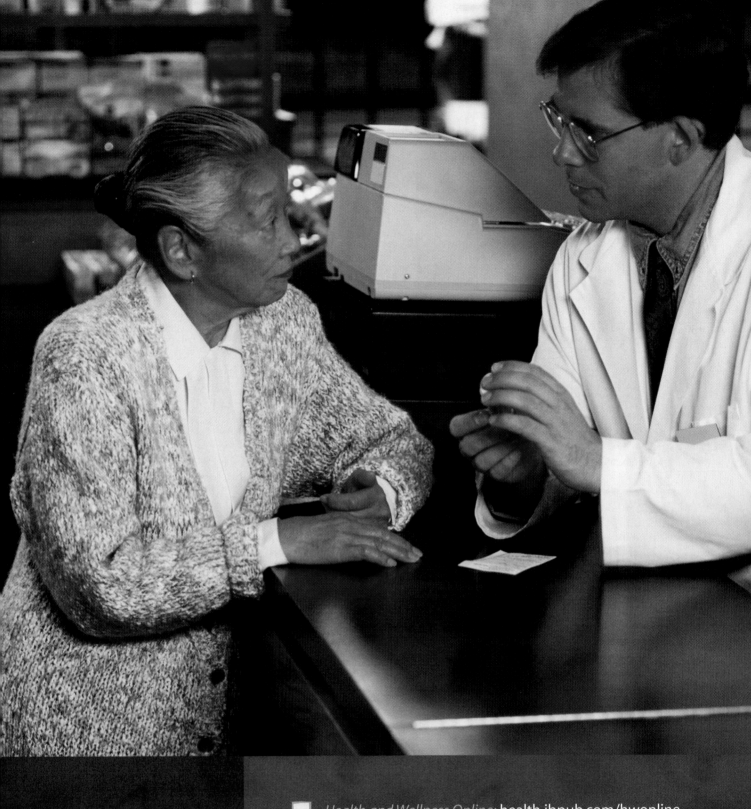

Chapter Sixteen

Using Drugs Responsibly

Learning Objectives

1. Explain the difference between a drug and a medicine.

2. Explain the concept of a drug receptor and its relation to drug side effects.

3. Describe the logic of a double-blind drug effectiveness study.

4. Define *lifestyle drugs*.

5. Give examples of the overuse of legal drugs in American society and the influences of drug advertising on drug use.

6. Explain the FDA's drug approval process.

7. Define *addiction*, *physical dependence*, *habituation*, *tolerance*, and *withdrawal*.

8. Describe the different effects of the major classes of psychoactive drugs: stimulants, depressants, marijuana, hallucinogens, PCP, and inhalants.

9. Describe the health hazards of using anabolic steroids.

For thousands of years, people have been ingesting substances to heal themselves, change consciousness, produce sleep, drive out evil spirits, and promote tribal and family harmony. For most of that time, such substances were obtained by chewing the leaves of a particular plant, brewing a tea from a plant's bark or roots, or mixing a potion made up of plant and animal materials, as the three witches in Shakespeare's *Macbeth* did when they concocted "eye of newt and toe of frog, wool of bat and tongue of dog." Today, some substances used for healing or nonmedicinal purposes are still obtained by ingesting plant and animal tissues or their extracts directly, whereas others are chemically pure substances that are manufactured by modern chemical and biological technologies.

No matter how they are obtained, many substances are of enormous value in relieving pain, preventing disease, and facilitating healing. However, indiscriminate or inappropriate use and overuse of drugs also are major problems in our society. For example, overuse of antibiotics has led to the creation of antibiotic-resistant bacteria, against which many antibiotic drugs are no longer effective (see Chapter 12). Many people use medicines, such as pain relievers and stimulants, for reasons other than approved medical ones. Alcohol use is responsible for thousands of deaths and incalculable personal and family trauma. Each year in the United States, about 2 million people suffer an adverse drug reaction from a medically prescribed drug, and about 100,000 die from taking the drug (Nakamura, 2008). And everyone has heard of the "war on drugs," which is concerned with the social and legal problems associated with the use of amphetamines, cocaine, heroin, and other illegal substances.

> Too much of a good thing is wonderful.
> *Mae West*

The use of drugs in our society has become so commonplace and accepted that many people automatically turn to drugs to solve their physical, mental, and emotional problems, failing to appreciate the values of nondrug alternatives and to understand the associated dangers and health hazards. When they are stressed, anxious, depressed, or tired, or if they have a headache or gastrointestinal upset, many people believe that taking drugs is the *only* source of relief. Although many medicines are extremely valuable, reliance on drugs to solve life's problems is much more likely to mask than to solve them, and may also open the way for chemical dependency.

What Is a Drug?

A **drug** is a single chemical substance in a medicine that alters the structure or function of some of the body's biological processes. The alteration can start, stop, speed up, or slow down a process, depending on the specific drug and its effect. A **medicine** is a drug (or combination of drugs) that is intended to (1) prevent illness, as vaccines do; (2) cure disease, as antibiotics do; (3) aid healing, as heartburn medications do; or (4) suppress symptoms, as pain relievers do. Not all drugs—for example, alcohol and nicotine—are medicines.

Drugs are usually classified according to the particular biological process they affect rather than by their chemical properties. For example, all substances that increase urine production, regardless of their chemical structure, are called *diuretics,* those that reduce pain are *analgesics,* and those that produce nervous system excitation are *stimulants.*

Drug Laws

American society regulates chemicals that change physiology (the definition of a drug) by placing them into one of five groups:

1. Chemicals that are presumably so potent that only a doctor can permit their use so as to limit any harm that might arise from their use (so-called prescription drugs)
2. Chemicals that are not so potent or dangerous that consumers can obtain them directly from stores or other sellers (so-called nonprescription or over-the-counter drugs)
3. Chemicals, plant extracts, and vitamins that are called "dietary supplements" rather than drugs, even though biologically they act as drugs, which consumers can obtain directly from stores or other sellers
4. Tobacco and alcohol, which are addictive drugs with no therapeutic value and are used by choice for a variety of reasons
5. Chemicals that are considered so dangerous to users and society that they are outlawed (so-called illegal or illicit drugs)

It is important to realize that regardless of its legal category, no drug is entirely safe. Any substance that can alter physiology has the potential to be harmful. The federal government screens only prescription drugs for potential harm. For chemicals in the other four categories in the preceding list, consumers are pretty much on their own with respect to risks and benefits.

The United States spends billions of dollars each year on the "war on drugs." It is important to see that this expenditure is about enforcement of laws and not necessarily about protecting health. The number of people whose health is affected by all illegal drug use combined is far less than those harmed by alcohol and tobacco (**Figure 16.1**). And it is estimated that each year millions of Americans are made sick and many thousands die from taking too much of—or the wrong—prescription medicines. This is not to say that there should not be laws regarding drug use. For health reasons, however, it is wise not to think of legal drugs as safe and good and of illegal drugs as harmful and bad.

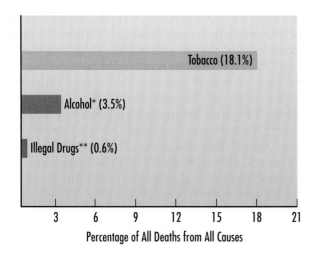

Tobacco (18.1%)

Alcohol* (3.5%)

Illegal Drugs** (0.6%)

3   6   9   12   15   18   21

Percentage of All Deaths from All Causes

■ **Figure 16.1**

Percentage of All-Cause Annual Deaths from Drug Use, United States

*Includes deaths from alcohol-related car crashes.

**Deaths associated with suicide, homicide, motor vehicle injury, HIV infection, pneumonia, violence, mental illness, and hepatitis.

Source: Data from A. H. Mokdad, et al. (2004). Actual causes of death in the United States, 2000. *Journal of the American Medical Association, 291,* 1242.

The situation is much more complex than that. This is why the healthiest course of action is to be a cautious, knowledgeable consumer of drugs of any kind.

How Drugs Work

Many drugs act by binding to **receptors** on the surface of, or within, specific cells in the body. A drug–receptor interaction is akin to a key (the drug) fitting into a lock (the receptor) (**Figure 16.2**). When a drug binds to a cell's receptor, it alters one or more biological processes of the cell. Frequently, a drug may chemically resemble a natural body component, such as a hormone or a neurotransmitter, which interacts with the receptor as part of normal functioning. The drug binds to the receptor in place of the natural substance and thereby alters physiology.

For example, the receptors for many antibiotics are on structures within bacteria that are responsible for manufacturing vital bacterial proteins. When an antibiotic binds to its receptor in a bacterium, it blocks the manufacture of bacterial proteins, the bacteria do not reproduce, and the infection stops. The receptors for many antidepressant drugs are located in the brain on cells that utilize the neurotransmitter serotonin. When an antidepressant binds to its receptor, serotonin transport into those cells is blocked, and depression is relieved.

Pharmacogenetics

A major assumption in the prescribing of drugs is that everyone's body uses a drug in the same way. This is the reason that drugs have "standard" dosages and expected side effects, and that adverse effects occur in only a small number of people. However, doctors and scientists know that individuals respond to drugs differently,

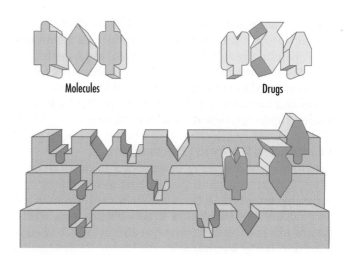

Molecules   Drugs

■ **Figure 16.2**

Bindings of Drugs to Cellular Receptor Sites
The molecular structures of many drugs are similar to molecules normally produced in the body. The drugs attach to receptor sites on cells and alter the physiological functioning of organs and tissues.

sometimes quite dramatically. The degree to which a person responds to a drug can depend on that person's genetic makeup. As discussed in Chapter 15, genes control nearly all the body's chemical reactions. Just as variations in genes produce different eye color pigments, genetic variations determine how the body responds to a particular drug and how it is eliminated from the body. This is why one person may tolerate and respond positively to a particular dose of a drug while another person may have an adverse reaction or even die. In some instances, scientists can now determine which of a person's genes may affect her or his response to a particular drug. This is the science of **pharmacogenetics** (Shurin & Nabel, 2008).

For example, the drug *warfarin* is used to prevent the formation of potentially fatal blood clots. To be effective and safe, the amount of warfarin in a person's blood must be maintained within narrow limits; too little may allow a clot to form, and too much may cause internal bleeding. It's been determined that individuals differ genetically with regard to how they utilize and excrete

---

TERMS

drug: a single chemical substance in a medicine that alters one or more of the body's biological functions

medicine: drugs used to prevent, treat, or cure illness; aid healing; or suppress symptoms

pharmacogenetics: tailoring drugs to a particular individual to match her or his biology

receptor: protein on the surface or inside of a cell to which a drug or natural substance can bind and thereby affect cell function

warfarin. Genetic tests are now available so doctors can match the appropriate dose of warfarin with a patient's corresponding genetic profile. The goal of pharmacogenetics is to identify many of the genes that affect drug responses and adverse effects. The hope is that one day drugs can be tailored to a patient's specific biology to produce optimum benefit with minimal risk.

Unintended Harmful Effects of Drugs

Even though a drug may be intended to have a single effect, it often has more than one because it binds to a variety of receptors in or on different cells. Unintended drug actions are called **side effects** (**Figure 16.3**), which may be minor or severe. Some side effects include allergic reactions (**drug hypersensitivity**); harm to developing embryos and fetuses (**teratogen**); or physical dependence.

Drug side effects can be quite dangerous. One study estimated that, each year in the United States, drug side effects are responsible for injury and illness in more than 2 million hospitalized patients (Classen, 2003). Furthermore, drug side effects are responsible for the deaths of 100,000 hospitalized patients per year, making them the sixth leading cause of death in the United States. These adverse drug reactions are caused by the unintended effects of the drugs and not to errors in prescribing or dosing, drug abuse, or accidental poisoning. This means that in the present climate of heavy drug advertising, it is necessary for good health for you to remember and respect that drugs are potent biological agents with both benefits and potentially fatal drawbacks.

In addition to side effects, a drug also may be harmful if the drug taker has a condition that is aggravated by that drug. A medical reason for not taking a drug is called a **contraindication.** For example, a history of blood vessel disease is a contraindication for taking birth control pills. The need to screen for contraindications is one reason that many medicines are available only by prescription.

Medical practitioners should be knowledgeable about the side effects and contraindications of drugs, but sometimes these are overlooked. About one-third of hospital stays are needlessly extended because inappropriate medications are administered or medications are managed improperly by medical staff. The United States Institute of Medicine estimates that 7,000 Americans die each year from medication errors. Consumers of medications should learn as much as they can about the intended use and side effects of their drugs, and they should ask their medical providers to explain the rationale for the medications prescribed (**Table 16.1**).

Routes of Drug Administration

Drugs can be taken by mouth, inhalation, or injection into the muscles, under the skin (from which they diffuse into surrounding tissues and blood), or directly into the bloodstream (intravenous or IV). Drugs also can be absorbed through the skin and the mucous membranes of the nose, eyes, vagina, and anus. Regardless of the route of entry, most drugs remain active in the body for several hours.

Once in the body, drugs are degraded or destroyed by the liver and the lungs. Drugs are also filtered by the kidneys and eliminated from the body in urine. Drugs such as inhalatory anesthetics or nitrous oxide are eliminated in expired air.

Effectiveness of Drugs

The **dose** of a drug is the amount that is administered or taken. The effectiveness of a particular dose of a drug is influenced by a person's body size, how rapidly the drug breaks down and is eliminated, and sometimes by the presence of other drugs and foods recently consumed (**Table 16.2**). A drug's effectiveness also depends on the person's expectations of the drug's efficacy (placebo effect) and the person's mental state. For example, when stressed or anxious, many people require higher doses

■ **Figure 16.3**

Common Side Effects of Drugs of Abuse

The functions of almost every organ or system in the body can be unintentionally altered by the effects of a drug.

Source: G. Hanson, P. J. Venturelli, & A. Fleckenstein. (2009). *Drugs and society* (10th ed.). Sudbury, MA: Jones and Bartlett Publishers.

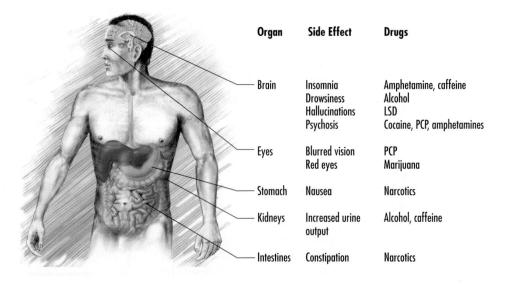

Organ	Side Effect	Drugs
Brain	Insomnia	Amphetamine, caffeine
	Drowsiness	Alcohol
	Hallucinations	LSD
	Psychosis	Cocaine, PCP, amphetamines
Eyes	Blurred vision	PCP
	Red eyes	Marijuana
Stomach	Nausea	Narcotics
Kidneys	Increased urine output	Alcohol, caffeine
Intestines	Constipation	Narcotics

Table 16.1

Latin Terms Commonly Used in Prescriptions

Latin	Abbreviation	Meaning
ante cibum	ac	before meals
bis in die	bid	twice a day
gutta	gt	drop
hora somni	hs	at bedtime
oculus dexter	od	right eye
oculus sinister	os	left eye
per os	po	by mouth
post cibum	pc	after meals
pro re nata	prn	as needed
quaque 3 hora	q 3 h	every 3 hours
quaque die	qd	every day
quater in die	qid	four times a day
ter in die	tid	three times a day
†, ††, or †††		1, 2, or 3 (of the dosage form, such as tablets)

very close to giving the same relief as do the drugs (see Chapter 2).

In 1984, ibuprofen was introduced into the over-the-counter market. Because aspirin and acetaminophen compounds commanded over 90% of the pain-reliever market, manufacturers of ibuprofen advertised heavily in medical journals to get physicians to recommend or prescribe the new drug. One advertisement showed that after four hours, Nuprin, the trade name for one ibuprofen drug, relieved headaches about 8% more effectively than acetaminophen (**Figure 16.4**). From a holistic health perspective, however, the more significant result is that almost 40% of headache sufferers got the same relief with a placebo. Thus, 4 of 10 headache sufferers found relief simply by believing that they had taken a pain-relief medicine.

An even more remarkable placebo effect is shown by the ability of balding men to stimulate hair growth simply by believing that they are using a hair-stimulating drug called Rogaine. The Pfizer Company, manufacturer of Rogaine, advertises extensively in the most prestigious

of analgesics to relieve pain than when they are relaxed. Most drugs have a narrow range of effectiveness, that is, doses that produce intended results. In excess, many drugs are toxic and some are lethal. If the dose is too low, insufficient therapeutic effect may result.

The effects of a drug or medicine are often determined scientifically by performing double-blind clinical trials, which involve administering the drug and a look-and-taste-alike placebo to matched groups of patients. Neither the people administering the drug nor the patients know who is receiving the drug and who is receiving the placebo (thus the expression **double-blind**). Only after the trial is the code revealed that tells which patients received the drug. What is most remarkable about many of these drug trials is not that drugs show a therapeutic effect, but that placebos often come

TERMS

contraindication: any medical reason for not taking a particular drug

dose: amount of drug that is administered

double-blind: when neither the person receiving the drug nor the person administering the drug knows whether it is a placebo or the real drug

drug hypersensitivity: an allergic reaction to a drug

side effects: unintended and often harmful actions of a drug

teratogen: any environmental agent or drug that alters development of a fetus

Table 16.2

Drug and Food Interactions That Should Be Avoided

If you take	Avoid	Because
Erythromycin or penicillin-type antibiotics	Acidic foods: pickles, tomatoes, vinegar, colas	These antibiotics are destroyed by stomach acids.
Tetracycline-type antibiotics	Calcium-rich foods: milk, cheese, yogurt, pizza, almonds	Calcium blocks the action of tetracycline.
Antihypertensives (to lower blood pressure)	Natural licorice (artificial is OK)	A chemical in natural licorice causes salt and water retention.
Anticoagulants (to thin blood)	Vitamin K: green leafy vegetables, beef liver, vegetable oils	Vitamin K promotes blood clotting.
Antidepressants (monoamine oxidase inhibitors)	Tyramine-rich foods: colas, chocolate, cheese, coffee, wine, avocados	Tyramine elevates blood pressure.
Diuretics	Monosodium glutamate (MSG)	MSG and diuretics both increase water elimination.
Thyroid drugs	Cabbage, brussels sprouts, soybeans, cauliflower	Chemicals in these vegetables depress thyroid hormone production.

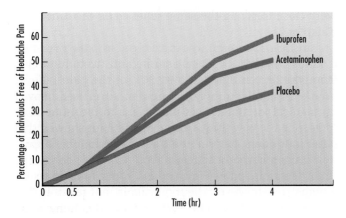

■ Figure 16.4

A Study of the Effectiveness of Ibuprofen Versus Acetaminophen in Relieving Headaches
Note that almost 40% of headache sufferers get relief with no drug at all.

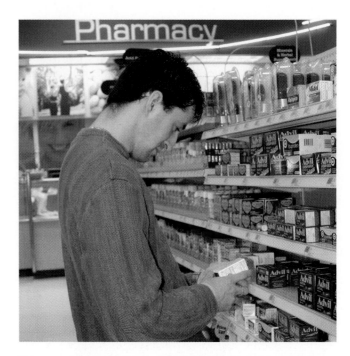

More over-the-counter drugs are available in the United States than anywhere else in the world.

medical journals and on TV. In these ads, the company emphasizes the effectiveness of Rogaine compared with a placebo solution applied to the scalp. Rogaine produces minimal to moderate growth of new hair in 33% of patients receiving the drug. However, a placebo containing no active ingredient produces minimal to moderate hair growth in 20% of patients. Although this fact is ignored by the advertising, it means that one of five men who have pattern baldness (an inherited trait) can stimulate new hair growth simply because they believe they are using a drug. How the mind changes physiology to accomplish this is unknown. The point, however, is never to underestimate the power of your mind to act like a drug and help you to heal an injury or illness.

The Overmedicating of Americans

Americans consume an enormous quantity of drugs. In the United States, about 3.5 billion drug prescriptions are filled each year at an annual cost of nearly $200 billion (**Table 16.3**). In addition, there are about 100,000 different kinds of nonprescription drugs, or **over-the-counter (OTC) drugs,** purchased, for which Americans pay nearly $20 billion a year. Millions of people ingest herbal extracts and teas for their purported medicinal value, and millions more take vitamins, not as nutritional supplements, but as medicine. Indeed, when Americans are sick, four out of five times they self-treat with OTC drugs and so-called alternative medicines (see Chapter 20).

More than one-fourth of the legal drugs sold in the United States are **psychoactive,** that is, they alter thoughts, feelings, and sensations. Psychoactive drugs include tranquilizers, sleeping pills, and mood modifiers. About 100 million Americans use alcohol regularly, another 45 million smoke cigarettes or chew tobacco for the stimulant effects of nicotine, and more than one-third of adult Americans ingest caffeine daily for its

stimulatory effects. In addition, about 12 million Americans regularly use illegal drugs (e.g., marijuana, cocaine, LSD, heroin).[1]

As a group, older persons tend to take the most drugs, usually because they have chronic medical conditions. It is not uncommon for some older people to take 10 or more different medications daily, which may have been prescribed by different physicians at different times. Occasionally, these drugs interact with each other to cause additional problems. That's why it is important for older people and their families and caretakers to keep a list of all medications and their doses and to inquire of health providers about possible harmful drug interactions.

In American society, the belief that drugs are legitimate and desirable solutions to life problems is pervasive. Consider this ad that appeared in a medical journal: A middle-aged man sits at a table in a restaurant on which there's a bowl of chili, a plate of fried food, and a bottle of hot sauce. The man's face signals discomfort and his right hand is placed on his obviously upset stomach. The headline in the ad says "Oh, my GERD," referring to the man's recurring problem with severe heartburn (called "gastroesophageal reflux disease," or GERD, in medical language). The ad, of course, is for a drug that relieves the symptoms of heartburn. No mention is made of the possibility that avoiding foods that cause this man to be so miserable (the ones on the table before him) is another way for him to feel better.

_____

[1] These data pertain to Americans over the age of 18.

About half of all doctor visits are for nonmedical or mental health problems that manifest as fatigue, lethargy, gastrointestinal upset, aches and pains, and sleeplessness. Often patients expect health care providers to prescribe a medicine, and just as often, health care providers feel obligated to offer some remedy, even if a medically legitimate one does not exist. The answer to this dilemma is provided by pharmaceutical companies that manufacture and advertise drugs for just about any patient complaint (Table 16.3).

Sometimes people become so depressed or upset over a life situation that they cannot muster the clear thinking and action necessary to deal with the problem. In such instances, a sleeping pill, tranquilizer, or antidepressant may help temporarily. Unfortunately, too many people mistakenly assume that the drug itself will solve the problem, whereas it may instead substitute for proper help and treatment.

Many physicians recognize this problem. They would prefer to deal only with physically ill people—the patients whose problems they were educated to treat. But many patients resist the suggestion that they do not have a disease for which there is a diagnosis and insist that they receive a drug. As people become more informed and aware of the undesirable consequences of unnecessarily taking drugs, hopefully they will elect to cope with stress and anxiety in ways that do not involve drugs.

Being healthy means, among other things, being responsible for the drugs you use. You do not have to resort to "chemical coping" for emotional problems. You can resist being pushed into pill popping by drug company advertising. Seeking alternatives to prescription or OTC drug use may be the most healthful action you can take (see Chapter 20).

Lifestyle Drugs

Many Americans have come to accept pharmaceutical solutions (called **lifestyle drugs**) for symptoms, behaviors, and moods that are caused by unhealthy behaviors (smoking, drinking alcohol, overeating, lack of exercise) or from the stress and anxiety of daily living. Instead of changing unhealthy behaviors or seeking nonchemical ways to reduce excessive stress and anxiety, many people prefer to pop a pill. They are encouraged to do so by an unrelenting barrage of drug company advertising (see next section) urging them to use drugs as the best way to solve life's problems. As one health professional has pointed out, "Americans have long craved chemical solutions to their problems of living. The many names that psychiatrists have given to the various manifestations of 'the problem that has no name' will change, and the newest blockbuster drugs to treat them will come and go. The angst that drives the voracious and profitable consumption of psychotropic drugs is, however, unlikely to subside" (Horvitz, 2009).

Psychotropic drugs (major tranquilizers, benzodiazepines, and selective serotonin reuptake inhibitors [SSRIs]) are useful in treating specific diseases such as severe depression, schizophrenia, or obsessive-compulsive disorder. However, they are not intended to be used to mask the problems caused by stress and to relieve, temporarily at least, the anxieties of daily living. Instead of seeking healthy ways of coping, people turn to doping. In fact, modern psychotropic drugs generally have replaced opium, marijuana, and morphine, which were widely used in the nineteenth century to alleviate lifestyle problems and symptoms deriving from overwork, poverty, unhealthy living conditions, and stress.

Prozac, an SSRI, is arguably the most successful of the modern drugs that elevate and alter mood and decrease feelings of depression. No doubt that there are many legitimate medical uses for Prozac and other psychotropic drugs, but the extent to which their use is

Table 16.3

Most-Prescribed Drugs in the United States

Drug	Purpose	Number of prescriptions (in millions)
Lipitor	Lower cholesterol	55.1
Singulair	Relieve asthma	27.2
Lexapro	Antidepressant	27.0
Nexium	Reduce heartburn	26.4
Synthroid	Treat thyroid disease	25.5
Plavix	Anticlotting	22.3
Toprol XL	Lower blood pressure	21.0
Prevacid	Treat dudenal ulcer	20.4
Vytorin*	Lower cholesterol	19.4
Advair Diskus	Treat asthma	18.1
Zyrtec	Relieve allergy symptoms	17.9
Effexor XR	Antidepressant	17.2
Protonix	Reduce heartburn	16.0
Diovan	Lower blood pressure	15.2
Fosamax	Prevent osteoporosis	15.0

*Removed from the market in 2007
Source: Data from Top 200 drugs, 2007.
Available: http://www.rxlist.com/script/main/hp.asp

TERMS

lifestyle drugs: drugs prescribed for conditions that arise from certain living habits or from the natural process of aging

over-the-counter (OTC) drugs: drugs that do not require a prescription

psychoactive: any substance that primarily alters mood, perception, and other brain functions

encouraged by drug manufacturers, prescribed by physicians, and accepted by patients as solutions to lifestyle problems is, to say the least, a significant problem in American society. Lifestyle problems should first be addressed conservatively with lifestyle changes, not lifestyle drugs.

Other targets of lifestyle drugs are the normal changes that occur with aging (hair loss, reduced sexual drive, and sagging or wrinkled skin). If you believe all the advertisements you see, you should aspire to be eternally youthful, attractive, and sexually active. Skin should not be allowed to wrinkle or sag. Loss of hair is not to be accepted and requires medical intervention. Flagging sexual desire is to be avoided at any cost; actually at whatever cost the drug companies can exact from worried consumers. Rogaine is a highly profitable drug for restoring thinning hair in men even if it is only marginally successful in actually restoring hair. Viagra has been an enormously successful drug for those seeking to enhance their sexual performance or satisfaction. Originally marketed to men who experienced difficulty in achieving and maintaining an erection, it soon was advertised to men and women as a panacea for any and all sexual difficulties and dissatisfactions.

And, of course, there are weight-loss and appetite-suppressant drugs that prevent people from adopting sensible eating and exercise habits that could actually improve their health and self-esteem. Many athletes take the arduous path to success by rigorous training and healthy eating. Others seek advantage with steroids and other drugs that may give them an edge in strength and endurance.

Lifestyle drugs are not about to disappear from American culture, especially not if drug companies continue to have a strong influence. But as a consumer and as a person who desires to be as physically and emotionally healthy as possible, aim for a lifestyle that will help you to achieve your goals without lifestyle drugs.

Drug Company Advertising

Because the greatest drug company profits come from prescription medications, most drug company advertising is directed toward physicians. Drug companies spend billions of dollars per year—about $10,000 per year per physician—trying to persuade doctors to prescribe drugs that the companies manufacture. Drug companies send sales representatives to doctors' offices, hospitals, and health maintenance organizations to inform them of their products and to leave free samples. Drug companies sponsor seminars and courses often accompanied by free meals or vacations to update physicians on the diagnosis and treatment of particular diseases (for which the company offers a drug). And drug company advertising supports the publication of almost all professional medical magazines. Doctors often say that their medical judgment is not influenced

by these obvious attempts at persuasion, but research shows otherwise (Steinman et al., 2007). Moreover, drug companies would not spend so much money promoting their products to physicians if it were not profitable. Recognizing that attempts to influence physicians' prescribing behavior may not be in the best interests of patients, several doctors' organizations and medical schools have developed guidelines and policies to curtail such influence, and some state legislatures and the U.S. Congress are considering legislation to do likewise (Steinbrook, 2008).

In addition to physicians and other health care professionals, consumers also are targets of prescription drug advertising, especially in magazines and on TV. In 1997, the Food and Drug Administration (FDA) relaxed its regulations regarding the advertising of prescription drugs directly to consumers (the United States and New Zealand are the only industrialized nations that permit this), and pharmaceutical companies quickly found that **direct-to-consumer advertising (DTCA)** is very profitable. In 1999–2000, sales of the 50 most heavily advertised drugs to consumers rose 32%, but sales for nonadvertised drugs rose only 13%. In 2005, about $4.2 billion was spent on DTCA, up from $2.5 billion in 2002.

Direct-to-consumer advertising is designed to encourage consumers to demand advertised drugs from their doctors in the belief that the drugs they see advertised are superior, whereas unadvertised, lesser known drugs are inferior. This creates pressure on doctors to prescribe advertised drugs even if other, equally effective (and sometimes more effective!) medications are available, and even if no drug is medically warranted (Kravitz et al., 2005). Many doctors are "rated" by the HMOs that pay them, so they do not want to make patients angry.

Since the inception of DTCA, the FDA and medical organizations have frequently chastised pharmaceutical companies for making misleading claims in their advertising. In general, DTCA overstates or overemphasizes the benefits of a drug while not making clear the measured efficacy of the drug or the known risks of taking it (Boden & Diamond, 2008).

The Internet plays a role in DTCA, too. Many Web sites carry ads for drugs. And many that purport to offer information about a particular medical condition are merely fronts for the advertising and sale of particular drugs. To get more information about a medical condition, a visitor to these Web sites may fill out a form or leave an e-mail address, only to become the recipient of a discount coupon for a medication.

Proponents of DTCA say it benefits consumers by making them more aware of both illnesses and medications and encourages them to seek medical advice and attention when they otherwise might not. Opponents of DTCA argue that it often makes it difficult for doctors to prescribe appropriate medications and that it creates a demand for drugs *in lieu* of nondrug treatments and disease prevention. Moreover, DTCA reinforces the general message that a drug is the first-line response to any health or medical problem.

Only one in 10,000 drugs that initially show promise in the laboratory is ever tested in people. Of that group of chemicals, only one in five ever passes all three pre-market tests and gets approved. Because the pharmaceutical company developing the drug pays for all the testing—at a cost of many millions of dollars per new drug—any drug that is approved needs to sell well to make up for the costs of drugs that never make it to market. The drugs Celebrex and Bextra were approved in the late 1990s to reduce arthritis pain. They were advertised heavily in magazines and on TV, and within a few years they were generating enormous profits. However, in 2005, the FDA halted the advertising of Celebrex and Bextra, citing that the ads were misleading about the risks of heart disease and stroke associated with taking those drugs. When it comes to heavily advertised prescription drugs, consumers are best served by caution.

The FDA and You

In 1906, the U.S. Congress passed the Federal Food and Drugs Act, which ultimately gave rise to the Food and Drug Administration, to ensure the safety of products sold as foods or medicines. The original 1906 law was revised and strengthened in 1938 as the Federal Food, Drug, and Cosmetic (FDC) Act. Prior to passage of the law, anyone could put anything in a package or bottle and sell it as a food or medicine. You can imagine how many people either wasted their money, or worse, got sick or died from chemicals they ingested. Now, the FDA regulates the safety of nearly all foods (the USDA oversees meat and poultry), all prescription and over-the-counter drugs (but not dietary supplements) and medical devices, cosmetics, and animal feed.

A major function of the FDA is the approval of new prescription drugs, a process that usually proceeds in the following way:

Step 1: Someone discovers or invents a chemical that in laboratory animals shows promise as a medicine. Often this is a scientist at a research university or a medical school. Financial support for the research comes from tax dollars in the form of grants administered by the U.S. government's National Institutes of Health or the National Science Foundation. Occasionally, the initial research is carried out by drug-company researchers or academic scientists who receive financial support from a drug company to carry out specific research.
Step 2: Based on laboratory studies, a drug company decides that a chemical has promise as a human

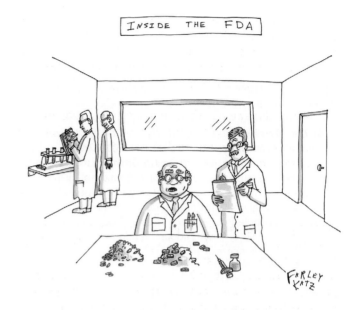

"These medicines all taste pretty good—let's approve them."

© The New Yorker Collection 2008 Farley Katz from cartoonbank.com. All rights reserved.

medicine and applies for FDA approval to conduct tests on people. These tests cost many millions of dollars, which the pharmaceutical company pays for. There are three kinds of tests, or trials, each carried out on a different group of people:

Phase 1 trial: The test drug is given to 50 to 100 healthy volunteers to determine how the healthy human body responds to different doses of the drug.
Phase 2 trial: The test drug is given to several hundred people with the disease or condition the drug is intended to treat to determine whether it is safe and possibly effective.
Phase 3 trial: The test drug is given to as many as 3,000 to 5,000 people with the disease or condition for which the drug is intended to determine its safety and efficacy.
Step 3: If the test drug passes all three trials, the pharmaceutical company applies to the FDA for approval to manufacture and market the drug. A public meeting is convened in Washington, D.C., at which interested parties testify before a panel of FDA-appointed scientists on whether the new drug meets criteria for approval, that is, safety,

TERMS

direct-to-consumer advertising (DTCA): the marketing of prescription drugs to consumers to stimulate demand for a drug

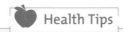

Use the Five-Year Rule for New Drugs

The Food and Drug Administration requires that every new prescription drug be tested for safety and efficacy before it can be distributed. About 10% of the time, however, the dangers of a new drug are not uncovered until it has been in use in the general population (Lasser et al., 2002). Then, a dangerous drug must begin to carry a warning on its label, or, in the most serious cases, it is withdrawn from the market.

Because serious health problems caused by a new drug may not appear until the drug has been prescribed for millions of people, Public Citizen's Health Research Group suggests that all consumers adopt this rule: *Do not use any new drug that has been on the market for less than five years if any older, effective drug is available.*

For most medical conditions, safe, effective drugs that have been on the market for decades are the ones to use. Follow the five-year rule unless you have a serious medical problem that can only be treated with a newer drug.

effectiveness, and need. At the end of a day or two of testimony, the scientific panel votes whether or not to approve. Word-for-word transcripts of approval hearings for new drugs are on the FDA's Web site (www.fda.gov).

Step 4: After a drug is approved and on the market, its safety and efficacy are monitored (so-called postmarket evaluation). That's because unknown problems with a drug can arise once it's in widespread use. Preapproval testing by a drug company takes place on only a few thousand people. That's enough to uncover obvious problems with a new drug. However, some drugs cause problems only in a small percentage of people, and these problems don't show up until many thousands or millions of people take the drug. After a drug is approved, doctors are supposed to be on the lookout for problems and they are supposed to report them to the FDA through a system called MedWatch (www.fda.gov/medwatch). If postapproval experience shows that a drug is dangerous, the FDA can revoke approval and the drug can no longer be sold.

The standard procedure for testing a new drug can take two years or more. However, if, while in testing, a new drug for a life-threatening condition shows promise and there are no alternative drugs, the FDA can grant a drug company accelerated, conditional approval ("fast-track approval") to market the drug. The condition is the drug company's promise that it will continue testing the drug in the postapproval period and be prepared to withdraw the drug from distribution if unknown problems are uncovered. Fast-track drugs can be sold without warnings or special restrictions, and patients may not be aware that a drug is still under study. Each year, the FDA must report to Congress whether required tests of fast-track drugs are

proceeding on schedule or whether they have been completed by the drug companies promising to do them. As of September 30, 2007, 1,682 products had been ordered to undergo postmarketing studies. Over 80% had been on the market for more than two years without their evaluations being begun. Required progress reports on over 40% of the ongoing studies were over 60 days late.

In 2004, a very popular anti-inflammatory drug called Vioxx was withdrawn from the market for increasing the risk of heart disease and stroke. Prior to approval, the drug had been tested for its ability to reduce arthritis symptoms while causing less stomach irritation and damage than other pain medicines. During the initial testing phases, the increased risk of heart attack and stroke from taking Vioxx was suspected from clinical observations and on biological grounds. Nevertheless, neither the pharmaceutical company (Merck) nor the FDA warned doctors and consumers of the potential life-threatening risks. A scientifically sound approval process depends on unbiased research on the safety and efficacy of the drugs being tested. Because testing is paid for by drug companies, however, the results of *all* tests of Vioxx were not always reported; positive results were reported in the form of articles in medical journals, and negative results were relegated to a secret filing cabinet. Congress and the FDA are now requiring that all tests be reported to the approval committee, not just the ones chosen by the sponsoring drug companies. The Health Tip suggests that people not take a new drug within five years of its approval if other, known-to-be-safe drugs are available.

Like any government agency, the FDA can be pulled this way and that by political winds and the efforts of lobbyists. On occasion (we don't know how rarely), approval of a new drug is influenced by the pharmaceutical company making application for approval. Pharmaceutical companies pay the FDA hundreds of thousands of dollars to cover the FDA's costs in the approval process. (Remember, the drug company also pays for the actual drug testing.) These fees are part of the FDA's budget. Some critics of the approval system argue that these big fees provide pharmaceutical companies access to FDA regulators, which may influence the regulators' vote on approval of a new drug. Not long ago such influence was uncovered in the approval of a drug for type 2 diabetes called Rezulin, which caused liver damage and death in several people and which had already not been approved in Europe and Japan. The drug was pulled from the market about two years after its approval.

Prompted by the withdrawal of Vioxx from the market and disclosures that the FDA failed to protect children from known dangers of certain antidepressants, in 2006 the Institute of Medicine, a division of the National Academy of Sciences, issued a report with suggestions to improve the FDA's systems for determining the safety of new drugs (Hennessey & Strom, 2007). Among the report's suggestions were to increase the agency's funding substantially so that it is less dependent on user fees from drug companies and to improve greatly the methods for postmarket monitoring of drug safety. In 2007, Congress passed a law (the Prescription Drug User Fee Act) incorporating many of the Institute of Medicine's suggestions, including the following provisions:

- The FDA will have more authority over post-marketing surveillance and approval of new drugs.
- Drug advertisements will have a toll-free phone number and Web address to assist patients in reporting adverse effects with new drugs.
- There will be greater penalties for advertisements that overstate a drug's efficacy and understate its adverse effects.
- The results of all tests of all new drugs must be put in a public (Web-based) database.

Despite the 2007 law bolstering its systems for drug testing and safety monitoring, more improvement at the FDA is required to restore confidence in the agency (Schweitzer, 2008).

Drug Misuse, Abuse, and Addiction

A large number of Americans regularly use drugs that are not intended as medicines:

- 126 million Americans, or 51% of the population, drink alcohol.
- 44 million Americans, or 20% of the population, use tobacco products, principally cigarettes.
- 19.8 million Americans, or 8% of the population, use an illegal drug (principally marijuana).[2]

Moreover, many Americans misuse prescription-only or over-the-counter drugs by taking them for purposes other than intended by the manufacturer or a doctor (for example, to get "high") or in quantities not intended by the manufacturer or a doctor. For example, in 2004, millions of Americans regularly used psychotherapeutic drugs for nonmedical reasons. These included 4.4 million who used pain relievers (principally opiates), 1.6 million who used tranquilizers, 1.2 million who used stimulants, and 0.3 million who used sedatives.

The human body is capable of tolerating and eliminating small quantities of virtually any substance or drug with no permanent harmful effects. However, it may be harmful to ingest large doses or to use a drug often even in small quantities. Generally, using any drug to the point where health is adversely affected or the ability to function in society is impaired can be defined as **drug abuse**. Characteristics of drug abuse include the following:

- Failure to fulfill major obligations at work, school, or home (e.g., repeated absences or poor work performance; absences, suspensions, or expulsions from school; neglect of children or household)

- Recurrent substance use in situations in which it is physically hazardous (e.g., driving an automobile or operating a machine)
- Recurrent substance-related legal problems (e.g., DUIs, arrests for substance-related disorderly conduct)
- Continued substance use despite having persistent or recurrent social or interpersonal problems caused or exacerbated by the effects of the substance (e.g., arguments with spouse, physical fights)

Drug abuse refers not to the type or amount of a drug taken but to whether or not the person taking the drug is personally or socially impaired. If a drug is used to mask anxiety or facilitate undesirable behaviors, it is being abused. If a drug is used continually to combat the effects of stress, it is being abused. If pleasure is experienced only when a drug is taken, the drug is being abused. If a person cannot control the use of a drug, it is being abused.

Most of the commonly abused drugs are psychoactive substances that affect thoughts, perceptions, feelings, and moods; in other words, they change consciousness (**Table 16.4**). Consciousness is the state of being aware of one's mental processes. Each of us has a "normal" state of consciousness, although many people would have difficulty describing what they mean by "normal." However, everyone knows when his or her state of consciousness deviates from normal—for example, when drunk, extremely angry, sad, or depressed. A high fever can alter consciousness even to the point of hallucinations.

There are numerous activities not generally regarded as consciousness-altering that produce changes in consciousness comparable in many respects to those produced by psychoactive drugs. Long-distance runners may experience a change of consciousness that is described as a "runners' high"; dancing can produce psychic "highs" and even ecstatic states of consciousness, which is the goal of the whirling dervishes who practice particular forms of Sufi dancing. Fasting can produce profound changes in consciousness, which is why prolonged fasts are often part of religious training. Many "thrill" activities, such as riding on roller coasters, shooting the rapids on river rafts, or bungee-jumping, change consciousness and presumably are enjoyed for that reason. Put into this perspective, ingesting psy-

> Freedom's just another word for nothing left to lose.
> *Janis Joplin*

TERMS

drug abuse: persistent or excessive use of a drug without medical or health reasons

---

[2] These data pertain to Americans over the age of 12.

Table 16.4

Classifications of Drugs That Affect the Central Nervous System

Drug classification	Common or trade name	Medical uses	Effects of average dose	Physical dependence	Tolerance develops
Opiates	Codeine	Analgesic (pain relief)	Blocks or eases pain; may cause drowsiness and euphoria; some users experience nausea or itching sensations	Marked	Yes
	Darvon				
	Demerol				
	Fentanyl				
	Heroin				
	Methadone				
	Morphine				
	Opium				
	Oxycontin				
	Percodan				
	Vicodin				
	Dextromethorphan	Cough suppressant			
Sedatives	Amytal	Sedation, tension relief	Relaxation, sleep; decreases alertness and muscle coordination	Marked	Yes
	Nembutal				
	Phenobarbital				
	Seconal				
	Doriden				
	Quaalude				
	Halcion				
Minor tranquilizers	Dalmane	Anxiety relief, muscle tension	Mild sedation; increased sense of well-being; may cause drowsiness and dizziness	Marked	No
	Equanil/Miltown				
	Librium				
	Valium				
	Xanax				
Major tranquilizers (phenothiazines)	Mellaril	Control psychosis	Heavy sedation, anxiety relief; may cause confusion, muscle rigidity, convulsions	None	No
	Thorazine				
	Prolixin				
Alcohol	Beer	None	Relaxation; loss of inhibition; mood swings; decreased alertness and coordination	Marked	Yes
	Wine				
	Liquor				
Inhalants	Amyl nitrite	Muscle relaxant, anesthetic	Relaxation, euphoria; causes dizziness, headache, drowsiness	None	?
	Butyl nitrite				
	Nitrous oxide				
Stimulants	Benzedrine	Weight control; narcolepsy; fatigue and hyperactivity in children	Increased alertness and mood elevation; less fatigue and increased concentration; may cause insomnia, anxiety, headache, chills, and rise in blood pressure; organic brain damage after prolonged use	Mild to none	Yes
	Biphetamine				
	Desoxyn				
	Dexedrine				
	Methedrine				
	Preludin				
	Ritalin				
Cocaine	Cocaine hydrochloride	Local anesthetic, pain relief	Effects similar to stimulants	Marked	No
Cannabis	Marijuana	Relief of glaucoma, asthma, nausea accompanying chemotherapy	Relaxation, euphoria, altered perception; may cause confusion, panic, hallucinations	None	No
	Hashish				
Hallucinogens	LSD	None	Altered perceptions, visual and sensory distortion; mood swings	None	Yes
	PCP				
	Mescaline				
	Peyote				
	Psilocybin				
Nicotine	(In tobacco)	None	Altered heart rate; tremors; excitation	Yes	Yes

choactive drugs is only one of many ways people change their consciousness.

Taking psychoactive drugs to alter consciousness is particularly dangerous because the cognitive, emotional, and behavioral processes that the drugs alter are required for harmonious adaptation to one's environment. Drugs that induce pleasant emotions can give a false sense of benefit. Drugs that block uncomfortable emotions (e.g., sadness, fear, pain) can impair useful defenses. Furthermore, regular use of psychoactive drugs can alter the biology of the brain to the point that drug using becomes a goal in itself, irrespective of any desire to alter thoughts and emotions (**Figure 16.5**).

Addiction

One of the many dangers of drug abuse is **addiction**, which is a progressive, chronic condition that is characterized by the following:

- *Compulsion:* An overwhelming preoccupation, desire, or drive to use a psychoactive drug, which can include obsessive thinking about a drug and drug-seeking and drug-hoarding behavior
- *Loss of control:* The inability to control use of a drug or loss of control over one's behavior because of taking a drug (e.g., impulsive actions, verbal or physical violence, impulsive sexual behavior)
- *Continued drug use despite adverse consequences:* The tendency not to stop drug use in the face of arrest, job loss, family breakdown, and health problems
- *Distortions in normal thinking:* Not admitting that problems are the result of drug taking (denial)

About 8% of Americans have abused drugs and 2.6% have been addicted at some point in their lives (Compton et al., 2007). Adults between the ages of 18 and 44 are the most likely to have drug abuse and addiction problems. Many people who are addicted to drugs have coexistent mental health issues, such as bipolar disorder, panic disorder, generalized anxiety disorder, and antisocial and dependent personality.

Addiction is chronic and progressive: It tends to get worse over time. Family members who wait for an addicted family member to "get better" generally are severely disappointed.

Physical Dependence

Addiction is often associated with **physical dependence** (also called tissue dependence), which is biological adaptation to long-term exposure to a drug. First-time or infrequent use of a psychoactive drug causes intoxication because the drug upsets the biological balance in the brain. With continued use of a psychoactive drug, actual physical changes take place in brain tissues to adapt to the continual presence of the drug.

Both legal and illegal drugs can cause physical dependence. The legality of a drug is more a function of social, political, and economic considerations than the drug's toxicity or pharmacology. From a personal and

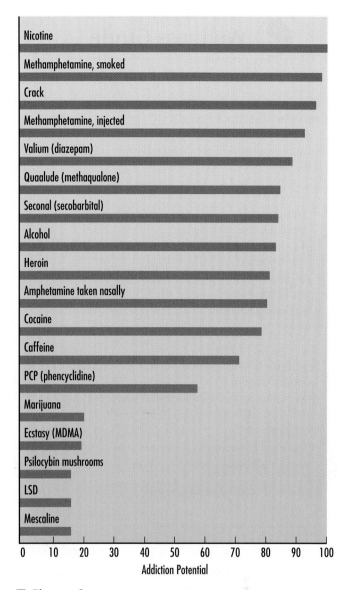

■ **Figure 16.5**

Health experts' ratings of how easy it is to become addicted and how difficult it is to stop using various drugs, with 100 being the highest addiction potential. Note that both legal and illegal drugs can be highly addictive.

Source: G., Hanson & P. J. Venturelli. (2001). *Drugs and society* (6th ed.). Boston: Jones and Bartlett Publishers, p. 95.

TERMS

addiction: physical and psychological dependence on a drug, substance, or behavior

physical dependence: a physiological state that depends on the continuous presence of a drug; absence of the drug may cause discomfort, nervousness, headaches, and sweating (withdrawal symptoms) and sometimes death

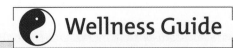

Wellness Guide

Risk Factors for Addiction

Biologically based risk factors (e.g., genetic, neurological, biochemical)	**Leading to this effect**
• A less subjective feeling of intoxication	• More use to achieve intoxication (warning signs of abuse absent)
• Easier development of tolerance; liver enzymes adapt to increased use	• Easier to reach the addictive level
• Lack of resilience or fragility of higher (cerebral) brain functions	• Easy deterioration of cerebral functioning, impaired judgment, and social deterioration
• Difficulty in screening out unwanted or bothersome outside stimuli (low stimulus barrier)	• Feeling overwhelmed or stressed
• Tendency to amplify outside or internal stimuli (stimulus augmentation)	• Feeling attacked or panicked; need to avoid emotion
• Attention deficit hyperactivity disorder and other learning disabilities	• Failure, low self-esteem, or isolation
• Biologically based mood disorders (depression and bipolar disorders)	• Need to self-medicate against loss of control or the pain of depression; inability to calm down when manic or to sleep when agitated
Psychosocial and developmental "personality" factors	
• Low self-esteem	• Need to blot out pain, gravitate to outsider groups
• Depression rooted in learned helplessness and passivity	• Need to blot out pain; use of a stimulant as an antidepressant
• Conflicts	• Anxiety and guilt
• Repressed and unresolved grief and rage	• Chronic depression, anxiety, or pain
• Posttraumatic stress disorder (as in veterans and abuse victims)	• Nightmares or panic attacks
Social and cultural environment	
• Availability of drugs	• Easy, frequent use
• Chemical-abusing parental model	• Sanction; no conflict over use
• Abusive, neglectful parents; other dysfunctional family patterns	• Pervasive sense of abandonment, distrust, and pain; difficulty in maintaining attachments
• Group norms favoring heavy use and abuse	• Reinforced, hidden abusive behavior that can progress without interference
• Misperception of peer norms	• Belief that most people use or favor use or think it's "cool" to use
• Severe or chronic stressors, as from noise, poverty, racism, or occupational stress	• Need to alleviate or escape from stress via chemical means
• "Alienation" factors: isolation, emptiness	• Painful sense of aloneness, normlessness, rootlessness, boredom, monotony, or hopelessness
• Difficult migration or acculturation with social disorganization, gender or generation gaps, or loss of role	• Stress without buffering support system

Source: G., Hanson, P. J., Venturelli, & A. Fleckenstein, (2006). *Drugs and society,* (9th ed.). Boston: Jones and Bartlett Publishers, p. 60.

community health standpoint, alcohol causes far more harm than all other drugs combined, yet it is legal.

The legal status of drugs changes with social customs and people's beliefs. In the 1920s and 1930s, alcohol was illegal in the United States but marijuana was legal. During the early twentieth century, opium, morphine, and cocaine were openly advertised and sold in the form of tonics and cough syrups. Coca-Cola, concocted by a Georgia pharmacist in 1886, was sold as both a remedy and an enjoyable drink. "Coke" contained cocaine until 1906, when the cocaine was replaced by caffeine.

Tolerance

Tolerance is an adaptation of the body to a drug so that larger doses are needed to produce the same effect. Thus, the longer one uses a drug, the more of that drug must be consumed to produce the desired effect. Because not all parts of the body become tolerant to a drug to the same degree, these higher doses may be dangerous. For example, a heroin or barbiturate user can become tolerant to the psychological effects of the drug, but the user's respiratory center in the brain, which controls breathing, does not. If the person takes a high dose of heroin or barbiturate to overcome the tolerance to the drug's psychological effects, the brain's respiratory center may cease to function as a result of the overdose, and the person may stop breathing.

Withdrawal

A consequence of physical dependence is the experience of withdrawal (or abstinence syndrome), which occurs when the body adapts to the absence of a drug on which it has become physically dependent. Withdrawal is often uncomfortable, and it may be fatal. For example, someone physically dependent on heroin may experience anxiety, pain, sweating, muscle cramps, frightening hallucinations, and fatal seizures when deprived of the drug. Indeed, for those who have experienced withdrawal, the fear of experiencing it again may become a greater motivator to continue drug use than the effects of the drug itself.

With many drugs, **withdrawal symptoms** are the opposite of the drug's primary effects. In general, withdrawal from central nervous system depressants, such as alcohol, opiates, tranquilizers, and sedatives, leads to symptoms such as hyperexcitedness, anxiousness, irritability, and susceptibility to seizures. Withdrawal from stimulants, such as cocaine, amphetamines, and caffeine, on the other hand, can produce sleepiness, depression, and loss of consciousness.

Psychological Dependence

Besides physical dependence, drugs can create **habituation** or **psychological dependence**, which is manifested as an intense craving for the drug. Habituation becomes injurious when a person becomes so consumed by the need for the desired drugged state that all of that person's energy is siphoned into compulsive drug-seeking behavior. Physically addicting drugs such as heroin, alcohol, and nicotine often produce habituation. As a consequence of compulsive drug-seeking behavior, relationships, jobs, and families may be destroyed.

Stimulants

Stimulants are substances that increase the activity of the central nervous system. These drugs include cocaine, amphetamine, amphetamine-like drugs, and caffeine. Their main effects are an increase in mental arousal and physical energy and production of a state of euphoria, which is why they are referred to as "uppers." Stimulants also can cause restlessness, talkativeness, and difficulty sleeping. Long-term use of stimulants tends to produce physical and psychological dependence.

Cocaine

Cocaine is obtained from the leaves of the coca shrub, *Erythroxylum coca,* a plant indigenous to the Andes. For thousands of years, inhabitants of Peru, Bolivia, and Colombia have chewed coca leaves to obtain a moderate stimulant effect intended to overcome fatigue. After the Spanish conquest of the Inca empire in the sixteenth century, coca leaves were introduced to Europe and later to North America. In the late nineteenth century, Angelo Mariani, a Corsican, received a medal from the pope for manufacturing an extract of coca leaves that "freed the body of fatigue, lifted the spirits, and induced a sense of well-being." In the United States in the 1880s, Atlanta pharmacist J. C. Pemberton mixed extracts of coca leaves and kola nuts to produce Coca-Cola, claimed at the time to be not only refreshing but also "exhilarating, invigorating, and a cure for all nervous afflictions." Today, of course, Coke no longer contains cocaine, although cocaine-free extracts of coca leaves are still used for flavoring. Sigmund Freud extolled the use of cocaine as a

---

▌TERMS▐

cocaine: a stimulant drug, obtained from the leaves of the coca shrub, that causes feelings of exhilaration, euphoria, and physical vigor

habituation: psychological dependence arising from repeated use of a drug

psychological dependence: dependence that results because a drug produces pleasant mental effects

stimulants: substances that increase the activity of the central nervous system

tolerance: a condition in which increased amounts of a drug or increased exposure to an addictive behavior are required to produce desired effects

withdrawal symptoms: uncomfortable and sometimes dangerous reactions that occur after a person stops taking a physically addicting drug

Global Wellness

Tracking Cocaine Use

European countries know that cocaine is widely used, but until recently the actual amounts and locations of use were unknown. Now sophisticated analytical techniques can monitor the use of cocaine by testing a country's currency (Bohannon, 2007). Euros that have been in circulation for only a few months are likely to have been rolled up and used to snort cocaine. The chemical structure of cocaine is such that it binds tightly to fibers in the euro bill. Because each country in Europe has its own distinct euro, the amount of cocaine in a country's currency is a measure of cocaine use. Typically, about 1 in 20 euros is contaminated with cocaine, and the amount can be as high as 10 micrograms. (A line of cocaine powder contains about 100 milligrams.) Some of the most cocaine-contaminated euros are found in Dublin, Ireland, where all of the bills in some samples showed traces of the drug. Spain, Italy, and Ireland have the highest use of cocaine,

Testing wastewater for a chemical by-product of cocaine can also determine the amount of cocaine being used. Surveys of 29 locations in Germany led to the estimate that Germans consume about 20 tons of cocaine each year. Tests of wastewater in London suggest that about 4% of Londoners between the ages of 15 and 30 use cocaine, an estimate close to the number arrived at by more traditional methods. A U.S. researcher planned to do a similar study for the city of San Diego, but the city refused to supply wastewater samples. Sewer epidemiology is a fast-growing science that not only can test for cocaine but also for many other drugs (legal and illegal) as well.

mood elevator, a possible antidote to depression, and a treatment for morphine addiction. However, witnessing a friend's severe and terrifying psychotic reaction to cocaine tempered Freud's enthusiasm for the drug.

As an illegal recreational drug, cocaine is most commonly taken into the body by sniffing ("snorting") it as a white powder, injecting it directly into the bloodstream (an obvious risk factor for AIDS), or smoking "free base" or "crack" cocaine. Each of these methods rapidly produces euphoria, a sense of power and clarity of thought, and increased physical vigor. The drug's effects last from minutes to an hour, depending on the dose and the route of administration into the body. After the initial high, users tend to experience a letdown ("crash") and an intense craving for more of the drug.

Cocaine increases heart rate and blood pressure. Continued use of the drug can result in appetite and weight loss, malnutrition, sleep disturbance, and altered thought and mood patterns. Frequent cocaine sniffing can inflame the nasal passages and cause permanent damage to the nasal septum. An overdose can cause seizures or death (see Chapter 14). Pregnant women who ingest cocaine risk giving birth to cocaine-addicted babies, who may be permanently disabled or even die in infancy.

Cocaine does produce tolerance, physical dependence, and withdrawal. The potential for psychological dependence is great, probably the greatest among all psychoactive drugs. Some people develop such a strong craving for the drug that their lives are consumed by their cocaine habit.

Amphetamines

Amphetamines are manufactured chemicals that stimulate the central nervous system. The most common amphetamine substances are dextroamphetamine, methamphetamine, dextromethamphetamine, and amphetamine itself. Amphetamines are usually taken orally but they can also be injected ("mainlined") and smoked. The effects of an oral dose usually last several hours. Slang terms for amphetamines include dexies, footballs, orange, bennies, peaches, meth, speed, and ice.

Although amphetamines may be used medically to treat narcolepsy and attention deficit hyperactivity disorder, they are principally used (illegally) to produce feelings of euphoria, increased energy, and greater self-confidence; an increased ability to concentrate; increased motor and speech activity; a perception of improved physical performance; and appetite suppression. Besides being used by those wishing to experience an amphetamine high, these drugs are frequently abused by people who fight sleep, such as students cramming for exams, entertainers, and truck drivers.

Excessive amphetamine use can cause headaches, irritability, dizziness, insomnia, panic, confusion, and delirium. The user often experiences a "crash," which occurs when the stimulants wear off, during which he or she usually is very depressed and tired and sleeps for long periods.

Prolonged use of amphetamines can lead to tolerance, especially for the euphoric effects and for appetite suppression. Amphetamines can cause mild physical dependence, and create a psychological dependence and a particular pattern of use called the "yo-yo," which is a cycle of amphetamine use for the stimulatory effect followed by use of a depressant to sleep, followed by more amphetamines the next day to get going. Chronic use can cause an amphetamine psychosis, consisting of auditory and visual hallucinations, delusions, and mood swings.

A particularly dangerous form of amphetamine is "ice"—a smoked form of pure methamphetamine hydrochloride. The inhaled drug reaches the brain almost immediately, producing a high that can last for several hours. Because the drug can be so easily inhaled, the potential for compulsive use, tolerance, and abuse is also very great. This amphetamine is manufactured at clandestine laboratories; the purity of the drug varies considerably from one laboratory to another, which adds to the risks of abusing it.

Amphetamines used illegally by some college students to promote alertness when studying, preparing assignments, or taking tests are the prescription medications Adderall and Ritalin. Adderall is a combination of amphetamine and dextroamphetamine; Ritalin is an amphetamine derivative, methylphenadate. These drugs are medically indicated for the treatment of attention deficit hyperactivity disorder (ADHD). Several million prescriptions for them are written for children and young adults diagnosed with ADHD, so these drugs are widely available. Patients or their siblings sell ADHD medicine to other students, who tend to use it periodically rather than chronically. That they are medicines may lead users to believe incorrectly that they are harmless. These drugs are potent stimulants with unpleasant side effects, and in high doses (such as when snorted), they can cause irregular heartbeat, stroke, and death.

Caffeine

Caffeine is a natural stimulant found in a variety of plants used in coffee, tea, chocolate, and soft drinks (**Table 16.5**). These beverages and foods are an integral part of American eating habits and may be enjoyed partly for their psychoactive properties.

The effects of caffeine are familiar to most people. They include decreased drowsiness and fatigue (especially when performing tedious or boring tasks), faster and clearer flow of thought, and increased capacity for sustained performance (for example, typists work faster with fewer errors). In higher doses, caffeine produces nervousness, restlessness, tremors, and insomnia and may have a negative effect on performance of complex tasks. In very high doses (10 grams, or about 100 cups of coffee), it can produce convulsions, which can be fatal.

In the past, caffeine was prescribed for a variety of complaints, but it is rarely used medically any more. However, it is still a key ingredient in more than a thousand over-the-counter drugs. For example, many "energizers" and "stay-awake" products are pure caffeine.

Table 16.5

Caffeine Content of Beverages and Chocolate

Item	Amount	Caffeine content (milligrams)
Coffee, generic brewed	8 oz	133 (range: 102–200)
Starbucks brewed coffee (grande)	16 oz	320
Starbucks vanilla latte (grande)	16 oz	150
Espresso, generic	1 oz	40 (range: 30–90)
Tea, brewed	8 oz	53 (range: 40–120)
Snapple fruit teas	16 oz	42
Arizona iced tea, green	16 oz	15
Vault	20 oz	118
Jolt Cola	12 oz	72
Diet Coke	12 oz	47
Dr. Pepper	12 oz	42
7-Up, regular or diet	12 oz	0
Fanta, all flavors	12 oz	0
Mug Root Beer, regular or diet	12 oz	0
Spike Shooter	8.4 oz	300
Rip It, all varieties	8 oz	100
SoBe No Fear	8 oz	83
Red Bull	8.3 oz	80
Häagen-Dazs coffee ice cream	8 fl. oz	58
Jolt caffeinated gum	1 stick	33
Hershey's chocolate bar	1.55 oz	9
Hot cocoa	8 oz	9 (range: 3–13)
NoDoz (maximum strength)	1 tablet	200
Vivarin	1 tablet	200
Excedrin (extra strength)	2 tablets	130
Anacin (maximum strength)	2 tablets	64

Source: Data from Center for Science in the Public Interest. Available: http://www.cspinet.org/new/cafchart.htm

---

Pain relievers, cough medicines, and cold remedies contain caffeine to counteract the drowsiness produced by other ingredients in these medications. Caffeine is also put into weight control and menstrual pain products because it increases urine output and water loss.

Psychological dependence may result from chronic use of caffeine, and tolerance to the stimulant effect

---

TERMS

amphetamines: synthetic drugs that stimulate the central nervous system and sometimes produce hallucinogenic states

caffeine: a natural stimulant found in a variety of plants; commonly found in tea, coffee, chocolate, and soft drinks

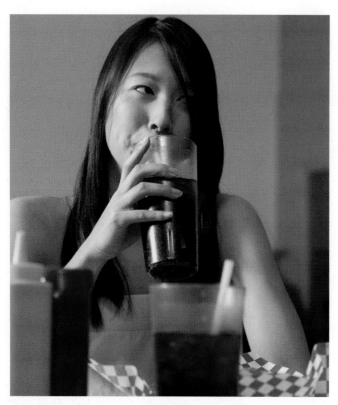

Most Americans consume more soft drinks than glasses of water. This can mean a significant daily intake of caffeine.

may gradually develop. Mild withdrawal symptoms, such as headache, irritability, restlessness, and lethargy, may occur when caffeine use is stopped.

Club Drugs

Club drugs consist of several psychoactive chemicals that are used at parties, dances, festivals, and raves to enhance social experiences and increase sensory stimulation. These include Ecstasy, GHB, ketamine, and Rohypnol. Compared to marijuana, amphetamines, hallucinogens, and opiates, club drugs are believed to give a sense of emotional closeness and euphoria (so-called entactogens), carry little or no risk for addiction, and, because they are ingested orally, no risk of contracting HIV/AIDS from injection. Despite these seeming benefits, club drugs can be dangerous, especially when taken together with alcohol or other drugs. Also, something sold as a club drug often is some other substance unknown—and possibly dangerous—to the user.

Ecstasy

Ecstasy is 3-4 methylenedioxymethamphetamine, or **MDMA**. Some of its common nicknames are "Adam," "XTC," "Clarity," and "Essence." Ecstasy is a synthetic chemical; that is, it does not occur naturally in plants. The substance has a chemical structure similar to the

stimulant methamphetamine and the hallucinogen mescaline, and it can produce both stimulant and psychedelic effects. Ecstasy is most often available in tablet form and is taken orally. It also is available as a powder; it is sometimes snorted and occasionally smoked, but rarely injected.

Ecstasy increases levels of the neurotransmitter serotonin in the brain, producing a high that lasts from several minutes to an hour. The drug's rewarding effects vary with the individual taking it and with the dose, purity, and the environment in which it is taken. Ecstasy can produce stimulant effects, such as an enhanced sense of pleasure and self-confidence and increased energy. Its psychedelic effects include feelings of peacefulness, acceptance, and empathy. Users claim they experience feelings of closeness with others.

The risks associated with using Ecstasy are similar to those found with the use of amphetamines and cocaine:

- Confusion, depression, sleep problems, drug craving, severe anxiety, and paranoia during and sometimes weeks after taking the drug
- Muscle tension, involuntary teeth clenching, nausea, blurred vision, rapid eye movement, faintness, and chills or sweating
- Increases in heart rate and blood pressure
- Long-term damage to serotonin-producing nerve cells in the brain
- Liver damage with long-term use

Ecstasy-related fatalities have been reported. The stimulant effects of the drug, which enable the user to dance for extended periods, combined with the hot, crowded conditions usually found at raves, or parties, can lead to dehydration, hyperthermia, and heart or kidney failure. Some researchers claim that Ecstasy can cause both short- and long-term damage to the dopamine (a neurotransmitter) system in the brain.

A content analysis of Ecstasy pills collected anonymously from people attending raves and other events in several American cities showed that 63% contained some Ecstasy or a close chemical relative; 21% contained the cough suppressant chemical dextromethorphan; 8% contained either caffeine, pseudoephedrine, ephedrine, or aspirin; and 9% contained no identifiable drug (Baggott et al., 2000). The amount of dextromethorphan in fake "Ecstasy" pills was two to four times the amount recommended for cough suppression, which could produce toxic symptoms, including lethargy, hyperexcitability, racing heart rate, dizziness and loss of balance, and PCP-like psychosis. MDMA and dextromethorphan block the drug-degrading system in the liver, which increases the risk of toxicity.

GHB

GHB is **gamma-hydroxybutyrate.** Its street names include "Georgia home boy," "liquid ecstasy," and "grievous bodily harm." GHB is ingested as a white powder or a clear, bitter-tasting liquid, which is often mixed with sweet alcoholic beverages to mask the bitter taste. This is often the way GBH is "slipped" into an unsuspecting person's drink. The drug's effects begin about 30 minutes after ingestion and can last several hours.

At low doses (~10 mg/kg body weight), GHB produces light sedation, increased sexual interest, relaxation, and short-term amnesia—the mental state sought in much of club drug use and that which increases the risk of sexual assault ("date rape"). At moderate doses (~20 mg/kg) users become lethargic. At large doses (~60 mg/kg), users can become comatose and stop breathing. More than half of the users of GHB at low doses experience unconsciousness, vomiting, and profuse sweating.

After more than 60 deaths were reported from GHB use, in 2000 the U.S. government classified the drug as a schedule I controlled substance. Even though distribution of GHB is illegal without a doctor's prescription, chemical precursors sold as dietary supplements (GBL, gamma-butyrolactone, and BD, 1-4-butane diol) are converted naturally to GHB in the body.

Ketamine

Ketamine is an anesthetic. Its street names include "K," "special K," "vitamin K," and "black hole." Mixing ketamine with MDMA (Ecstasy) is called "kitty flipping"; mixing it with MDMA and marijuana is called "EGK" (Ecstasy, ketamine, marijuana). "Trail mixes" are ketamine mixed with other drugs, such as methamphetamine, cocaine, Viagra, or heroin.

As a recreational drug, ketamine is generally ingested orally as a white powder or intranasally with an inhaler (called a "bumper"). It can also be administered by injection. After oral ingestion, drug effects occur after about 30 minutes and last up to three hours. At very low doses, ketamine can produce an out-of-body dissociative state and hallucinations (called "k-land"). At high doses, ketamine can produce muscular rigidity, bizarre behavior, psychosis, and social withdrawal (being in the "k-hole"). Overdose leads to vomiting (and possible fatal aspiration of vomitus) and respiratory depression.

Rohypnol

Rohypnol is a powerful tranquilizer. It reduces anxiety, inhibition, and muscular tension. At higher doses it can cause unconsciousness. Its effects are dangerously compounded when taken with alcohol or other sedating drugs. Chronic use can produce dependence and withdrawal symptoms.

Depressants

Depressants comprise a vast number of drugs whose common effects include a reduced level of arousal, motor activity, and awareness of the environment and increased drowsiness and sedation. The depressants include alcohol (see Chapter 18) and drugs that affect sleep: sedatives, hypnotics, and opiates. A number of other drugs, such as antihistamines and some medications used in the treatment of high blood pressure or heart disease, may also act as depressants. In low doses, depressants produce a mild state of euphoria, reduce inhibitions, or induce a feeling of relaxation. In high doses, they may impair mood, speech, and motor coordination.

Depressants are dangerous. All carry the potential for physical and psychological dependency, tolerance, unpleasant withdrawal symptoms, and toxicity from continual use or overuse. Acute overdoses may produce coma, respiratory or cardiovascular collapse, and even death. Aggravating the potential for lethal overdose are the synergistic actions of depressants. That is, when taken together, two or more different depressants can produce a much stronger effect than the sum of both drugs. The most common synergistic effect occurs when people drink alcohol while taking depressant medications such as barbiturates or tranquilizers.

Sedative and Hypnotic Drugs

A **sedative** is a drug that promotes mental calmness and reduces anxiety. A **hypnotic** is a drug that promotes sleep or drowsiness. Because of their potential for inducing dependence, almost all sedatives and hypnotics are highly regulated and are available only by prescription. Nevertheless, sedative-hypnotics are among the most widely used drugs in the United States.

The most common sedative-hypnotics are drugs called benzodiazepines, more popularly known as **tranquilizers.** Medically, these drugs are used to relieve anxiety, promote relaxation, induce sleep, alleviate muscle

---

TERMS

club drugs: psychoactive chemicals used at parties, dances, festivals, and raves to enhance social experiences and increase sensory stimulation

Ecstasy (MDMA): a club drug with both stimulant and pleasurable effects

gamma-hydroxybutyrate (GHB): a dangerous club drug with unpleasant side effects

hypnotics: central nervous system depressants used to induce drowsiness and encourage sleep

ketamine: an anesthetic used as a club drug

sedatives: central nervous system depressants used to relieve anxiety, fear, and apprehension

Rohypnol: a powerful tranquilizer used as a club drug

tranquilizers: central nervous system depressants that relax the body and calm anxiety

spasm and lower back pain, treat convulsive disorders, and lessen the discomfort of alcohol and opiate withdrawal. Benzodiazepines are most helpful when used on a short-term basis (a few weeks) as an adjunct to psychotherapy or medical therapy. Long-term use (more than four months) increases the risk of both dependence and of not confronting and overcoming issues and symptoms for which the benzodiazepines were originally prescribed.

Barbiturates are sedative-hypnotic drugs that include barbituric acid and its derivatives: amobarbital (Amytal), pentobarbital (Nembutal), phenobarbital (Luminal), secobarbital (Seconal), and Tuinal (50% amobarbital plus 50% secobarbital). Because they are less safe than benzodiazepines, barbiturates tend not to be prescribed for medical conditions that call for sedative-hypnotic drug therapy.

Opiates

The **opiates** are a group of chemically related drugs that depress the central nervous system. These substances (e.g., morphine, heroin, codeine, Demarol, Fentanyl, Oxycontin, Percodan, Vicodin) cause physical dependence, habituation, and tolerance and produce serious withdrawal symptoms. Opiates are derived from the opium poppy, *Papaver somniferum*, extracts of which have been used for thousands of years in a variety of cultures to produce euphoria, to relieve pain, and to treat various diseases.

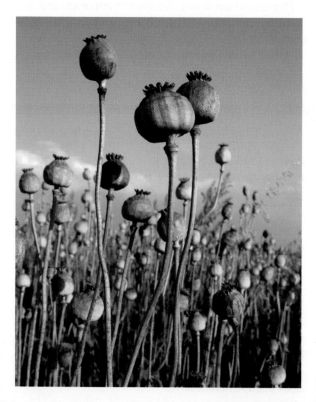

Opium poppies *(Papaver somniferum)*, from which morphine is obtained.

Medically, opiates are used for pain relief, cough suppression, and treatment of diarrhea. They can be taken by mouth, injection, snorting, and smoking. Heroin is converted to morphine in the body, and the morphine is eventually excreted in urine, saliva, sweat, and the breast milk of lactating women (which means that nursing infants can become addicted). Because morphine crosses the placenta, a developing fetus may become addicted even before birth and may experience withdrawal symptoms after it is born.

Opiates are commonly abused substances, taken for their pain-relieving and psychoactive effects. The psychological sensations produced by opiates include feelings of warmth and belonging, relaxation, and mellowness. Regular use of opiates can produce tolerance to the psychological effects, constipation, loss of appetite, depression, loss of interest in sex, constriction of the pupil of the eye, disruption of the menstrual cycle, and drowsiness. Very large doses or prolonged use can be fatal because of respiratory failure.

Marijuana

Marijuana is another name for the plant *Cannabis sativa*, which grows in temperate climates all over the world. Species of this plant have been cultivated for thousands of years as a source of hemp fiber used to make clothing and rope or for a substance that, when ingested, produces euphoria, a sense of relaxation, mood elevation, and altered perceptions of space and time, and heightened sensory awareness. Marijuana ingestion also produces increased hunger (the "munchies") and dry mouth.

The principal psychoactive ingredient in marijuana is a chemical called delta-9-tetrahydrocannabinol (THC). This substance is found in the plant's leaves, buds, seeds, and resins. THC can be ingested by smoking the dried and crushed flowers and leaves or by eating food that has been prepared with marijuana as an ingredient. THC is chemically similar to natural substances in the brain, called *endocannabinoids*, that modulate appetite, pain sensation, mood, memory, and other processes by binding to specific receptors in brain tissue. THC binds to the same cannabinoid receptors.

Hashish (a resin generally smoked in a special pipe) is a highly potent derivative of marijuana obtained from the sticky resin found on the flowers and leaves of marijuana plants. *Ganja,* another derivative of marijuana, consists of the dried tops of female plants. *Bhang* (called "ditch weed") is made from parts of the plant that contain lesser amounts of THC. *Sinsemilla* (from the Spanish word "without seeds") is a potent form of marijuana derived exclusively from female plants. All male plants are removed from the plot to prevent seed formation and to allow more of the female plant's energy to be directed into the growth and formation of psychoactive compounds.

Besides its intended psychoactive effects, marijuana ingestion may evoke confusion, anxiety, panic, hallucinations, and paranoia. Speech and short-term memory may be impaired, which may be interpreted as humorous changes in one's normal mental state. However, because perception, motor coordination, and reaction time are also impaired, driving a car or operating other machines while intoxicated with THC is unsafe (Bédard Dubois, & Weaver, 2007). Marijuana use may also aggravate an existing mental health problem, particularly schizophrenia (Kristensen & Cadenhead, 2007).

Some of the possible health dangers of long-term marijuana use include the risk of bronchitis caused by marijuana smoke, increased heart rate and blood pressure, and possibly a slight depression of immune system functions. Marijuana smoke, like tobacco smoke, contains carcinogens (see Chapter 13).

Regular use of marijuana can lead to marijuana abuse, defined as repeated instances of use under hazardous conditions (e.g., driving a car); repeated impairment of social, occupational, or educational functioning; or legal problems associated with marijuana use. Long-term regular use of marijuana can produce marijuana dependence in 7% to 10% of users (Kalant, 2004), characterized by increased tolerance to the drug, compulsive use, impaired control, and continued use despite physical and psychological problems caused or made worse by use.

Brain imaging studies support a body of psychological research showing an association between heavy marijuana use and impairment in short-term memory and attention, loss of internal control, and reduced learning while a person is intoxicated but not beyond the time of marijuana use (Lundqvist, 2005). Heavy, extended marijuana use is associated with lower performance in school and at work, lower educational attainment, and other illicit drug use (Ferguson & Boden, 2008).

Several states have legalized the use of marijuana for medical purposes, such as nausea caused by cancer chemotherapy; anorexia or wasting caused by cancer, AIDS, or other diseases; chronic pain; muscle spasms caused by multiple sclerosis or other neurologic disorders; and glaucoma. However, in 2005, the U.S. Supreme Court ruled that the federal government has the power to arrest and prosecute patients and their suppliers even if marijuana use is permitted under state law for medical conditions. Moving beyond the legal wrangling over medical marijuana, researchers are uncovering the neurobiological and neurochemical bases of marijuana's actions with the hope of developing new drugs that provide smokable marijuana's therapeutic effects without the potential for respiratory illness that results from smoking (Nicoll & Alger, 2004). Also, researchers are developing alternative marijuana delivery systems that do not involve smoking.

One of the major arguments for keeping marijuana illegal is that early use of marijuana leads to the use of other illegal drugs, the so-called gateway hypothesis. A number of scientific studies have addressed this question, but the results are conflicting and it still cannot be concluded that use of marijuana, especially by adolescents, inevitably leads to the use of other, more dangerous drugs (Maccoun, 2006).

> Insanity is doing the same thing over and over again and expecting a different outcome.
>
> *Albert Einstein*

Despite the confusions and caveats over the use of marijuana, as of 2008 12 states had legalized medical marijuana use: Alaska, California, Colorado, Hawaii, Maine, Montana, Nevada, New Mexico, Oregon, Rhode Island, Vermont, and Washington. Patients in these states with a variety of ailments and conditions can obtain a prescription from a physician authorizing them to use marijuana to alleviate their symptoms. Depending on the state, patients can grow a certain number of marijuana plants for personal use or can obtain ready-to-smoke marijuana from dispensaries. In California alone it is estimated that at least 200,000 people have physician-sanctioned prescriptions for medical marijuana use, and there are several hundred dispensaries scattered over the state (Samuels, 2008). A report based on U.S. government statistics estimates that, in 2006, the California marijuana crop was valued at about $14 billion, making the marijuana crop more valuable than the annual production of corn in the United States.

Hallucinogens

The **hallucinogens** comprise a variety of chemical substances derived from as many as 100 kinds of plants as well as by chemical synthesis in the laboratory (**Table 16.6**). Despite their chemical differences, hallucinogens share the ability to alter perception, thought, mood, sensation, and experience. The similarity of their effects to

TERMS

hallucinogens: psychoactive substances that alter sensory processing in the brain, producing visual or auditory sensations that are not real (i.e., that are hallucinatory)

hashish: the sticky resin of the *Cannabis* plant

marijuana: a psychoactive substance present in the dried leaves, stems, flowers, and seeds of plants of the genus *Cannabis*

opiates: central nervous system depressants derived from the opium poppy

Table 16.6

Substances Considered to Be Hallucinogenic or Psychedelic

Substance or active ingredient	Common name
D-Lysergic acid diethylamide	LSD
Trimethoxyphenylethylamine	Mescaline (peyote)
2,5-Dimethoxy-4-methylamphetamine	STP
Dimethyltryptamine	DMT
Diethyltryptamine	DET
Tetrahydrocannabinol	Marijuana (cannabis)
Phencyclidine	PCP
Psilocybin	Mushrooms

psychotic hallucinatory experience is one reason they are called hallucinogens, but in many respects the psychedelic drug experience is not the same as a psychotic hallucination. Psychotic hallucinations are generally auditory and frightening, and the hallucinator believes them to be real. Drug-induced hallucinations tend to be visual, usually are enjoyable, and the individual is aware that the experience is unusual and is not part of his or her normal state of consciousness.

Hallucinogens are most often ingested orally, either by eating the plant itself or by ingesting powder containing the active chemical. Normally, a hallucinogenic drug begins to take effect in 45 to 60 minutes. The first effects are physical: sweating, nausea, increased body temperature, and pupil dilation. These symptoms eventually subside, and the psychological effects become manifest within an hour or two of ingestion. Depending on the particular substance and the amount ingested, the "trip" lasts anywhere from 1 to 24 hours. Perhaps the most commonly used hallucinogen is **LSD** (D-Lysergic acid diethylamide), commonly called "acid."

A common feature of the hallucinogenic experience is the suspension of the normal psychic mechanisms that integrate the self with the environment. The distortion of self–environment interactions makes the user extremely open to conditions in the surroundings. For this reason, experience in any particular drug episode is highly influenced, for better or worse, by the environmental setting in which the trip takes place and by the "psychic set"—the expectations and attitudes—of the user.

Phencyclidine (PCP)

Phencyclidine, also known as **PCP,** angel dust, hog, crystal, and killer weed, was developed originally for medical use as an animal anesthetic. But because of the drug's many adverse effects, it was removed from legal sale and became an illegal recreational drug. In the 1960s, phencyclidine was called the PeaCePill—a serious misnomer in view of the drug's effects.

The effects of PCP are variable: Depending on the dose and the route of administration, it can be a stimulant, a depressant, or a hallucinogen. Some of the intended effects are heightened sensitivity to external stimuli, mood elevation, relaxation, and a sense of omnipotence. Some of the common unintended effects are paranoia, confusion, restlessness, disorientation, feelings of depersonalization, and violent or bizarre behavior. In high doses, the drug can cause coma, interruption of breathing, and psychosis.

Many admissions to psychiatric emergency rooms are for PCP intoxication. The drug impairs perception and muscular control, and users are prone to accidents such as falling from heights, drowning, walking in front of moving vehicles, and collisions while driving under the influence of the drug. PCP does not induce tolerance or physical dependence, but because it is eliminated slowly from the body, chronic users may experience the drug's effects for an extended period.

The effects of PCP are unpredictable and frequently unpleasant, if not terrifying and life-threatening. PCP produces more unwanted and dangerous symptoms of drug intoxication than any other psychoactive substance. Drug dealers often surreptitiously mix PCP with marijuana or cocaine or sell PCP while claiming it to be LSD, DMT, or some other drug. Because PCP is relatively easy to manufacture, it is one of the more readily available and dangerous of the illegal recreational drugs.

Inhalants

Inhalants are a wide variety of chemical substances that vaporize readily and when inhaled produce various kinds of depressant effects similar to those of alcohol. Like alcohol, inhalants are depressants of the central nervous system. Generally, their intended effect is loss of inhibition and a sense of euphoria and excitement. Unintended effects include dizziness, amnesia, inability to concentrate, confusion, impaired judgment, hallucinations, and acute psychosis.

Inhalants commonly used for recreational purposes include the following:

1. Commercial chemicals, such as model airplane glue, nail polish remover, shoe polish, paint thinner, and gasoline, and substances such as acetone, toluene, naphtha, hexane, and cyclohexane
2. Aerosols—found in aerosol spray products
3. Anesthetics, such as amyl nitrite, nitrous oxide ("laughing gas"), diethyl ether, and chloroform

Because they are vaporous, these substances enter the body rapidly. The fumes are usually inhaled from plastic bags. The intoxicant effects are often felt within minutes, and the high lasts less than an hour. Regular users tend to be preteens and others without the money to

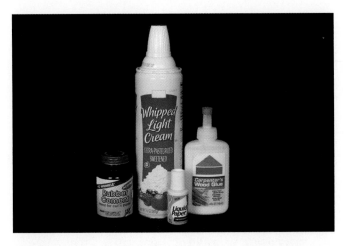

Inhalants are dangerous but unfortunately often readily available to kids looking for a "rush."

buy other drugs. Some adults use amyl nitrite ("poppers") during sexual relations, believing that the drug enhances the sexual experience. Some medical personnel are frequent users of nitrous oxide, or "laughing gas," because it is easily available.

The inhalant chemicals do not produce tolerance or withdrawal, nor do they induce physical dependence. However, they are dangerous. In addition to any harm resulting from uncontrolled behavior (such as driving while intoxicated), these chemicals damage the kidneys, liver, and lungs and can upset normal heartbeat.

About 2 million adolescents between the ages of 12 to 17 use inhalants, some beginning as young as age 7. Signs of inhalant use that adults can watch for include paint stains on clothing, red and runny eyes, chemical breath odor, sores around the mouth, and a drunken demeanor.

Anabolic Steroids

Anabolic steroids are synthetic derivatives of the male hormone testosterone. These derivatives of testosterone promote the growth of skeletal muscle and increase lean body mass (see Chapter 7). Anabolic steroids were first abused by elite athletes seeking to improve performance. Today, athletes and nonathletes use steroids to enhance performance and also to change physical appearance.

Anabolic steroids are taken orally or injected, typically in cycles of weeks or months rather than continuously. Users frequently combine several different types of steroids to maximize their effectiveness while minimizing negative side effects, a process known as stacking. Anabolic steroids produce increased lean muscle mass, strength, and ability to train longer and harder. Side effects of anabolic steroid use include liver tumors,

jaundice, fluid retention, high blood pressure, severe acne, and trembling. Shrinking of the testicles, reduced sperm count, infertility, baldness, and development of breasts have been observed in males. In females, growth of facial hair, changes or cessation of menstrual cycle, enlargement of the clitoris, and deepened voice are among the side effects.

Reducing Drug Use

Almost everyone takes drugs of one kind or another at one time or another. People take drugs to relieve headaches, heartburn, tension, cramps, fatigue, and anxiety. Drugs are used to get to sleep and to stay awake. They are used for body problems and emotional problems. When used appropriately, drugs can play a vital role in the treatment and prevention of disease.

However, as a society we are overmedicated and overly dependent on drugs. The healthiest approach is to be as free of drugs as possible. Wellness is not achieved by taking drugs. No drug should ever be taken casually, whether prescribed, over the counter, or offered in a social setting. Each person should learn when drugs are necessary to maintain or restore health and when the benefits of the drug outweigh the risks.

All drugs are dangerous, and illegal recreational drugs are especially so because you cannot be sure of either the quality or the strength. The use of most recreational drugs is illegal, and if caught, users and sellers are prosecuted as criminals. Still, many people in American society, especially young people, experiment with one or more illegal drugs. Experimenting with drugs is just that: You are taking a chance of getting caught, or getting high and causing an accident, or getting the wrong dose and dying.

> TERMS
>
> inhalants: vaporous substances that, when inhaled, produce alcohol-like intoxication
>
> LSD: a powerful hallucinogenic chemical; ingestion alters brain chemistry and produces a variety of hallucinogenic and behavioral effects
>
> phencyclidine (PCP): drug that, depending on the route of administration and dose, can be a stimulant, depressant, or hallucinogen; originally developed as an animal anesthetic

Critical Thinking About Health

1. The accompanying graph shows the results of a test of a new drug. Four groups of patients were involved. Group 1 received placebo; group 2, 20 mg of the drug; group 3, 40 mg; and group 4, 80 mg.

   a. Do the data support the hypothesis that the drug is effective? Why or why not?

   b. What percentage of people get well without the drug? What's a likely explanation?

   c. What's the maximum percentage of people that can be expected to get well from taking the drug?

   d. If 80 mg produces the desired effect in the largest number of people, why didn't the experimenters report the effects of 100 mg?

2. Bob Kozlo came home from work early one day. Upon hearing his dad's car pull up in the driveway, Jamie, Bob's 16-year-old son, quickly disposed of the joint he and his friend Max were sharing. Mr. Kozlo, who as a teenager also had experimented with marijuana, smelled the telltale odor and knew immediately what Jamie and Max had been up to.

   a. Should Mr. Kozlo ignore this situation or take some kind of action, and if so, what should he do?

   b. Should he tell Max's parents?

   c. What is your opinion of teenagers experimenting with marijuana or any other drugs, including alcohol and tobacco?

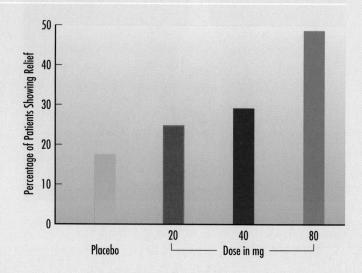

3. Why are some drugs illegal? What characteristics distinguish a legal drug from an illegal one? If you had unlimited power and resources, what would you do to solve the illegal drug problem in the United States?

4. In what ways has substance use and abuse touched your life?

Health in Review

- People have been ingesting drugs throughout recorded history for a variety of reasons, including curing illness and facilitating social interaction.

- A drug is a chemical substance capable of producing a change in physiology. Most drugs react by binding to receptor sites in or on cells, which alters biological activity.

- Legal or illegal, medical or nonmedical, drug use in the United States is widespread. Drug use is encouraged by extensive advertising by the pharmaceutical industry.

- The Food and Drug Administration requires the testing of new drugs for safety and efficacy before they are approved for sale.

- Drug abuse is the overuse of a drug, often to the point of loss of control. Many drugs of abuse are psychoactive, meaning that they alter thoughts, feelings, and perceptions. Many psychoactive drugs cause physical dependence; some cause psychological dependence.

- Tolerance is the adaptation of the body to repeated drug use so that ever-increasing doses of the drug are required to produce an effect.

- The most commonly used psychoactive drugs in the United States include stimulants (cocaine, amphetamine, caffeine), depressants (sedatives, tranquilizers, hypnotics), opiates, marijuana, hallucinogens, cocaine, and Ecstasy.

- The medical use of marijuana has been legalized in several states but is illegal by federal law.

Health and Wellness Online

The Web contains a wealth of information about health and wellness. By accessing the Internet using Web browser software, you can gain a new perspective on many topics presented in *Health and Wellness*, Tenth Edition. Access the Jones and Bartlett Publishers Web site at **health.jbpub.com/hwonline**.

References

Baggott, M., et al. (2000). Chemical analysis of Ecstasy pills. *Journal of the American Medical Association, 284,* 2190.

Bédard, M., Dubois, S., & Weaver, B. (2007) The impact of cannabis on driving. *Canadian Journal of Public Health, 98,* 6–11.

Boden, W. E., & Diamond, G. A. (2008). DTCA for PTCA— Crossing the line in consumer health education? *New England Journal of Medicine, 358,* 2197–2200.

Bohannon, J. (2007, April 6). Hard data on hard drugs, grabbed from the environment. *Science,* 42–44.

Classen, D. (2003). Medication safety. *Journal of the American Medical Association, 289,* 1154–1156.

Compton, W. M., et al. (2007). Prevalence, correlates, disability, and comorbidity of DSM-IV drug abuse and dependence in the United States. *Archives of General Psychiatry, 64,* 566–576.

Fergusson, D. M., & Boden, J. M. (2008). Cannabis use and later life outcomes. *Addiction, 103,* 969–976.

Hennessey, S., & Strom, B. L. (2007). PDDUFA reauthorization: Drug safety's golden moment of opportunity? *New England Journal of Medicine, 356,* 1703–1704.

Horvitz, A. V. (2009). Book review. *New England Journal of Medicine, 360,* 841–844.

Kalant, H. (2004). Adverse effects of cannabis on health: An update of the literature since 1996. *Progress in Neuropsychopharmacology and Biological Psychiatry, 5,* 849–863.

Kravitz, R. I., et al. (2005). Influence of patients' requests for direct-to-consumer advertised antidepressants. *Journal of the American Medical Association, 293,* 1995–2002.

Kristensen K., & Cadenhead, K. S. (2007). Cannabis abuse and risk for psychosis in a prodromal sample. *Psychiatry Research, 151,* 151–154.

Lasser, K. E., et al. (2002). Timing of new black box warnings and withdrawals for prescription medications. *Journal of the American Medical Association, 287,* 2215–2220.

Leibowitz, J. (2008). This pill not to be taken with competition: How collusion is keeping generic drugs off the shelves. Retrieved August 31, 2008, from http://www.ftc.gov/speeches/leibowitz/080225CephalonOpEd.pdf

Lundqvist, T. (2005). Cognitive consequences of cannabis use. *Pharmacology, Biochemistry, and Behavior, 81,* 319–330.

Maccoun, R. J. (2006). Competing accounts of the gateway effect: The field thins, but still no clear winner. *Addiction, 101,* 473–474.

Nakamura, Y. (2008). Pharmacogenetics and drug toxicity. *New England Journal of Medicine, 359,* 856–858.

Nicoll, R. A., & Alger, B. E. (2004, December). The brain's own marijuana. *Scientific American,* 68–75.

Samuels, D. (2008, July, 28). Dr. Kush. *The New Yorker,* 49–61.

Schweitzer, S. O. (2008). Trying times at the FDA. *New England Journal of Medicine, 358,* 1773–1777.

Shurin, S., & Nabel, E. G. (2008). Pharmacogenetics: Ready for prime time? *New England Journal of Medicine, 358,* 1061–1063.

Sprull, W. M., & Cunningham, M. L. (2005). Strategies for extending the life of patents. BiopharmInternational.com. Retrieved August 27, 2008, from http://biopharminternational.findpharma.com/biopharm/article/articleDetail.jsp?id=150834

Steinbrook, R. (2008). Disclosure of industry payments to physicians. *New England Journal of Medicine, 359,* 559-561.

Steinman, M. A., et al. (2007, April). Characteristics and impact of drug detailing for gabapentin. *PLoS Medicine, 4,* e134.

Suggested Readings

Alterm, J. (2001, February 12). The war on addiction. *Newsweek*, 35–54. A series of articles by *Newsweek* reporters on various aspects of the "war on drugs" in America.

Angell, M. (2005). *The truth about drug companies: How they deceive us and what to do about it.* New York: Random House. Discusses the effect of the current system of drug development and marketing on American society.

Avorn, J. (2005). *Powerful medicines: The benefits, risks, and costs of prescription drugs.* New York: Vintage. Suggests policy reforms to improve the current system of drug development.

Bass, A. (2008). *Side effects.* New York: Algonquin Books. A prosecutor, a whistleblower, and a best-selling antidepressant are on trial. An exposé of how regulatory agencies and drug companies both tried to cover up serious side effects of Prozac.

DeGrandpre, R. (2007). *The cult of pharmacology: How America became the world's most troubled drug culture.* Durham, NC: Duke University Press. A critical examination of the meaning that society places on drugs.

Erickson, C. K. (2007). *The science of addiction: From neurobiology to treatment.* New York: W.W. Norton. A noted professor of pharmcology, toxicology, and addiction science reviews the biology of addiction and its treatment.

Gray, M. (2000). *Drug crazy: How we got into this mess and how we can get out.* New York: Routledge. A scathing account of America's decades-long war on drugs, which has benefited only two groups of people: professional antidrug advocates and drug lords.

Hanson, G., Venturelli, P. J., & Fleckenstein, A. (2009). *Drugs and society* (10th ed.). Boston: Jones and Bartlett Publishers. A useful text.

Interlandi, J. (2008, March 3). What addicts need. *Newsweek*. Examines the interrelationships of biological, psychological, social, and spiritual aspects of addiction.

Iversen, L. L. (2007). *The science of marijuana.* New York: Oxford University Press. A well-known neuropharmacologist summarizes the historical and recent research on marijuana.

Kaiser Family Foundation (2007). Prescription drug trends. Available: http://www.kff.org/rxdrugs/3057.cfm. A summary of major trends in the use of prescription drugs, focusing primarily on cost trends.

Karch, S. B. (2006). *A brief history of cocaine: From Inca monarchs to Cali cartels—500 years of cocaine dealing.* Boca Raton, FL: CRC Press.

Klam, M. (2001, January 21). Experiencing Ecstasy. *New York Times Magazine*, 38–79. The author describes his experiences with Ecstasy and reasons for not using the drug in the first place.

Langreth, R. (2004, November 29). Just say no! *Forbes*, 102–112. Discusses the backlash building against the costs, risks, and benefits of prescription medications.

Nicoll, R. A., & Alger, B. E. (2004, December). The brain's own marijuana. *Scientific American*, 68–75. Explains the neurobiology of naturally occurring marijuana receptors and endogenous cannabinoids.

Recommended Web Sites

Please visit **health.jbpub.com/hwonline** for links to these Web sites.

Prevention Online (Prevline)

The Substance Abuse and Mental Health Service Administration's National Clearinghouse for Alcohol and Drug Information on preventing alcohol and drug abuse in families, schools, and the workplace.

Public Citizen Health Research Group

A nonprofit organization that publishes a monthly magazine, *Worst Pills—Best Pills*, that warns of dangerous prescription drugs. The organization also reports on FDA actions and the drug industry.

U.S. National Institute of Drug Abuse

A division of the National Institutes of Health dedicated to improving drug abuse and addiction prevention, treatment, and policy.

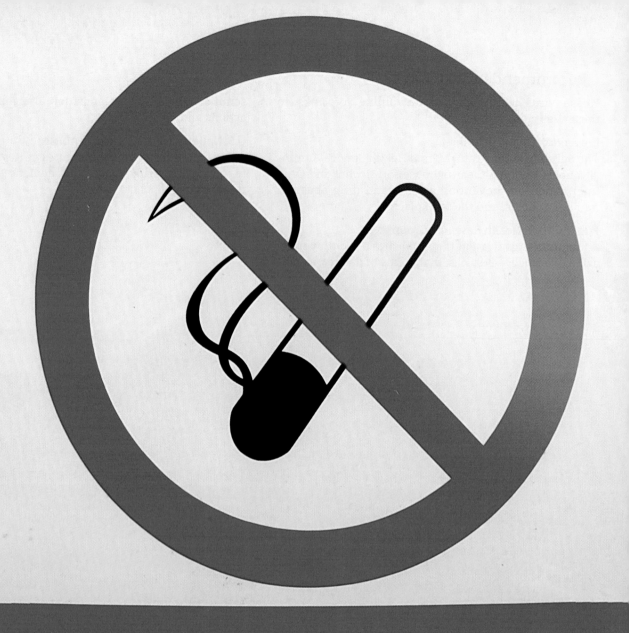

No smoking

Chapter Seventeen

Eliminating Tobacco Use

Learning Objectives

1. Describe the hazards of cigarette smoking.
2. Identify and explain the physiological effects of tobacco.
3. Describe the hazards of smokeless tobacco use.
4. Discuss the effects of smoke on nonsmokers, including children.
5. Explain why some people smoke.
6. Identify ways to quit smoking.
7. Describe the various ways to limit tobacco's damage to society.

"Warning: The Surgeon General Has Determined That Cigarette Smoking Is Dangerous to Your Health." By now, this message and other warnings about the dangers of smoking have reached just about everyone. Despite the warnings, however, about 45 million Americans aged 18 and older are cigarette smokers, making nicotine the most used addictive drug in the United States.

> Cigarettes are the only legal product that, when used as intended, cause death.
>
> *Louis W. Sullivan,* former secretary of Health and Human Services

The health costs of smoking are enormous. About 10 million people in the United States have diseases caused or made worse by smoking, including chronic obstructive lung disease, heart disease, stroke, type 2 diabetes, erection problems, high blood pressure, premature aging of the skin, baldness, and cancer of the lung, breast, esophagus, larynx, mouth, bladder, cervix, pancreas, and kidney. Each year about 443,000 Americans die as a result of smoking (**Figure 17.1**); this accounts for one in five deaths in the United States annually. Included in this total are approximately 1,300 children who die from in-home fires caused by cigarettes. Worldwide, about 5 million people die from smoking each year. On average, smokers die about 7 years earlier than nonsmokers. Tobacco use is the single most preventable cause of death in the United States.

The economic costs of smoking are staggering as well. Cigarette smoking costs the United States more than $200 billion in health care costs and lost productivity annually. About $35 billion of those costs are covered by smokers themselves in the form of cigarette taxes, direct costs, and health insurance. The remaining smoking-related costs are borne by nonsmokers. On average, each pack of cigarettes sold costs American society about four dollars in smoking-related health expenses.

Tobacco Use in the United States

About 25 million American men and 20 million American women smoke cigarettes. The prevalence of smoking among adult Americans has declined in recent years as the social views of cigarette smoking have become more and more negative (**Figure 17.2**). Unfortunately,

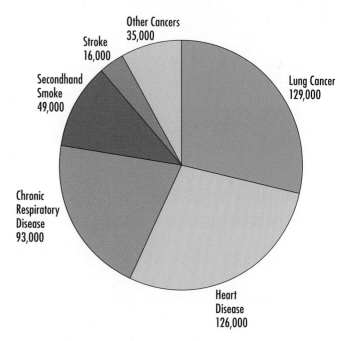

■ **Figure 17.1**

Annual Deaths Attributable to Cigarette Smoking in the United States

Source: Centers for Disease Control and Prevention.

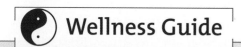

Wellness Guide

Smoking and Health: Not Only Lung Cancer

Here are a few lesser known facts about the health hazards of smoking:

Impotence: Studies of more than a thousand men showed that smoking was a significant contributor in erectile dysfunction or impotence. Men in their 40s who smoked were three times more likely to have difficulties in getting and maintaining an erection. The more they smoked, the more likely they were to be impotent.

Dental caries: Environmental tobacco smoke (passive smoke) increases the risk of cavities in young children as well as the risk of other diseases. Tooth decay is the most common chronic disease of childhood; health costs are estimated at $4.5 billion (Aligne et al., 2003).

Lung cancer risk: Filtered cigarettes claiming to contain medium tar, low tar, or very low tar, carry the same risks for lung cancer. Smokers who use unfiltered cigarettes have a higher risk for developing lung cancer (Harris et al., 2004).

Low test scores: Children exposed to environmental tobacco smoke (secondhand smoke) score lower on math, reading, and problem-solving tests. Kids exposed to little or no smoke scored about 7 points higher on standardized tests as compared with kids who were exposed to tobacco smoke. About 33 million children are at risk of lower scores because of exposure to secondhand smoke.

about 30% of the decline in cigarette smoking in the past decade has been offset by increased use of other tobacco products, such as moist snuff, waterpipes, and small cigars (Connolly & Alpert, 2008).

About 20% of American college students use tobacco at least occasionally (American College Health Association, 2008); about 8% of student smokers smoke daily. About 6% smoke cigars at least occasionally, and 3% use smokeless tobacco. Waterpipe smoking has become popular among college students in recent years, with prevalence estimates ranging from 20% to 40%. The popularity of waterpipe use is associated with the perception that the practice is safer and much more acceptable among one's peers than is smoking cigarettes. Although the health risks of waterpipe smoking have yet to be determined, the practice is known to deliver quantities of carbon monoxide and nicotine of the magnitude of cigarette smoking (El-Nachef & Hammond, 2008; Neergard et al., 2007). Smoking among Americans under age 18 increased during the 1990s but has declined since

then (**Figure 17.3**). Smoking among youth is particularly troublesome because adolescence is when regular use and dependence on tobacco begin. Among adults who smoke daily, three-fourths had done so by age 18.

What Is Tobacco?

Tobacco used for smoking, chewing, or snuff is the processed product of the leaves of the plant *Nicotiana tabacum*. This plant is indigenous to the western hemisphere, where it grows best in semitropical climates.

Tobacco was introduced to European societies in the sixteenth century by the Spanish returning from voyages to the Americas. The Spanish had learned about smoking from Native Americans, who used tobacco much as it is used today. In fact, the word "tobacco" is an Indian word referring to the pipe used to smoke the minced or rolled leaf of the tobacco plant.

The smoking habit spread quickly in Europe, fueled by tobacco imports from Spain's colonies. By the nineteenth century, changing social customs had caused tobacco smoking to be replaced largely by tobacco chewing; even more popular was the habit of sniffing tobacco in the form of snuff. Not until the 1880s, when the cigarette-making machine was invented in the United States, did cigarette smoking become the predominant form of tobacco use worldwide. Camel cigarettes, introduced in 1913, ushered in the modern era of smoking in the United States. By coincidence, the American Cancer Society was established in the same year.

Processing tobacco for consumption involves harvesting the tobacco leaves and curing them by any one of several drying methods. The cured tobacco leaves are shredded, and various types of leaves are blended into commercially desirable mixtures. Often flavorings and

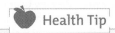

Health Tip

Smoking: Playing the Odds

If you like to gamble, here are the odds on dying from lung cancer for smokers as compared to nonsmokers.

	Increased risk	
Cigarettes per day	Men	Women
1 to 4	3-fold	5-fold
5 to 9	11-fold	12-fold
10 to 14	17-fold	18-fold
15 to 19	10-fold	20-fold

Overall, 90% of lung cancers are caused by cigarette smoking.

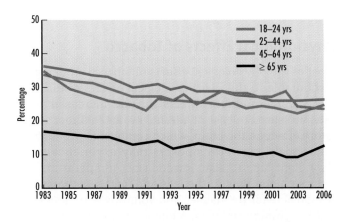

■ **Figure 17.2**

Percentage of Americans Who Smoke Cigarettes, by Age Group, 1983–2006

Source: National Health Interview Survey.

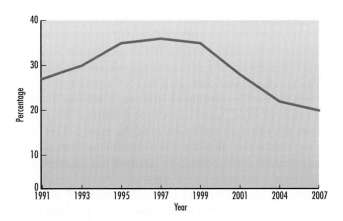

■ **Figure 17.3**

Prevalence of Smoking Among U.S. Youth
Smoking among U.S. teens peaked in the mid-1990s and has been declining since. The graph shows the percentage of high school students who admitted smoking in the last month.

Source: U.S. Centers for Disease Control and Prevention.

🌐 Global Wellness

The Global Burden from Cigarette Smoking

Nations around the world are working to come to grips with the catastrophic health consequences of cigarette smoking among their citizens. Experiencing a massive loss of customers in North America and Europe in the 1990s, American and European tobacco companies have now successfully shifted their attention to Asia, Africa, and Latin America to convert millions of poor, uneducated people into smokers. Eighty-four percent of smokers now live in emerging economies. Currently, nearly 6 million people worldwide die from tobacco smoking; over 1 million of those deaths occur in China, and about 1 million more occur in India. Without a massive antismoking intervention, the World Health Organization estimates that by 2020 over 10 million people will die each year of smoking-related causes; 70% of those deaths will be in developing countries.

In 2005, almost all of the countries of the world signed a treaty called the Framework Convention on Tobacco Control (FCTC) to combat this global health crisis (Indonesia, Russia, and the United States are exceptions). The treaty states, "Every person should be informed of the health consequences, addictive nature, and mortal threat posed by tobacco consumption and exposure." The treaty calls for all countries to take action to protect people from tobacco smoke and children and nonsmokers from exposure to secondhand smoke. Some actions taken by countries to rein in tobacco consumption include the following:

- *Controlling or banning cigarette advertising and promotion.* Cigarette companies rely heavily on advertising to recruit new smokers, especially among young people. Ads associate smoking with glamour, adventure, and (believe it or not) health. Cigarette ads are also associated with wealth, power, slimness, emancipation and sophistication for women, and independence and sexual attraction for teens. Cigarettes and logo-branded smoking paraphernalia are given away at sports and music events, and actors, celebrities, and film makers are paid to show particular brands of cigarettes. Some countries totally ban smoking advertising and promotion, especially to children. The United States opposes this position on the ground that it violates the constitutional right to free speech.
- *Health warnings and content disclosure.* Many countries require that one-third to one-half of a cigarette packet carry health warnings and images showing the consequences of smoking. They also ban the use of the works *light*, *low tar*, and *mild* in cigarette ads because these words deceive consumers into thinking that products labeled as such are not dangerous. Also, cigarette companies add a variety of chemicals to their products, some of which are toxic. These additives are required to be listed on the product label so consumers can know what they are being exposed to.

Besides controlling advertising and promotion and insisting on health warnings on packets, countries can reduce tobacco use by taxing tobacco products. A 10% price increase reduces consumption by about 4% in high-income countries and by 8% in low-income countries. Some countries also try to limit the importation of cigarettes. Despite these actions, cigarette companies are eager to supply those interested in smoking with tobacco products. But neither smokers nor tobacco companies want to take responsibility for the staggering economic and social costs resulting from cigarette smoking.

---

colorings are added, as well as chemicals that facilitate even burning. Finally, the mixture is used to manufacture cigarettes, pipe tobacco, and chewing tobacco, or is wrapped in specially cured tobacco leaves to make cigars.

The most familiar chemical constituent of tobacco is **nicotine,** but when tobacco is burned, approximately 4,000 other chemical substances are released and carried in the smoke. These chemicals include acetone, acrolein, carbon monoxide, methanol, ammonia, nitrous dioxide, hydrogen sulfide, traces of various mineral elements, traces of radioactive elements, acids, insecticides, and other substances. Besides these chemical compounds, tobacco smoke also contains countless microscopic particles that contribute to the yellowish brown residue of tobacco smoke known as **tar,** a documented cause of lung cancer. Forty-three of the chemicals in tobacco are known to cause cancer.

Bidis—hand-rolled cigarettes from India—are falsely believed to be less harmful than commercial American cigarettes. Whereas bidis contain about half the tobacco content of a standard cigarette, they contain 25% more nicotine per gram of tobacco. One bidi does deliver less tobacco smoke and nicotine than a standard American cigarette, but as with smokers of "light" cigarettes, bidi smokers are likely to make up the difference by smoking more cigarettes.

Physiological Effects of Tobacco

Most of the physiological effects of tobacco smoking are attributable to the pharmacological effects of nicotine. The most prominent effects include increased heart rate, increased release of adrenaline, and a direct stimulatory effect on the brain, which combine to produce the mild "rush" cigarette smokers may experience when they light up. It also lowers skin temperature and reduces blood flow in the legs and feet. Nicotine is also responsible for the nausea and vomiting experienced by most beginning smokers. Addiction to nicotine is largely responsible for perpetuating a smoker's habit.

Some harmful cardiovascular effects of cigarette smoking probably result from nicotine and carbon monoxide, which are believed to contribute to the development of heart and blood vessel disease. A host of other harmful chemicals contributes to the development of cancer and diseases of the respiratory tract. Among these chemicals are benzo-a-pyrene, aza-arenes, N-nitrosamines, and radioactive polonium. Polonium is a product of the breakdown of radioactive lead, a natural constituent of soil. Radioactive particles in the soil become deposited on sticky tobacco leaf hairs and eventually become part of tobacco smoke. Radon, a radioactive gas, is also present in tobacco smoke inhaled both by the smoker and nonsmoker via secondhand smoke. These radioactive substances can become trapped in tiny air sacs in the lungs, where they induce cancerous changes in lung tissue.

Smokeless Tobacco

Smokeless tobacco is available in two main forms: **chewing tobacco** and **snuff**. Chewing tobacco is processed into three different forms: loose leaf, firm/moist plug, and twist/rope chewing tobacco. A portion of chewing tobacco is either chewed or placed in the mouth and held in place between the lower lip and gum. Snuff is made from powdered or finely cut tobacco leaves and is available in two forms, dry and moist. In many European countries dry snuff is inhaled through the nose. However, in the United States a pinch of snuff is placed in the mouth and held in place between the cheek and gum, referred to as "snuff dipping." Dipping snuff is highly addictive and exposes the body to levels of nicotine equal to those of cigarettes. **Moist snuff** is made from air- and fire-cured tobacco leaves that are processed into fine particles, flavored, and packaged in moist form in round, flat containers. Moist snuff is considered the most hazardous form of smokeless tobacco because of the methods used in processing it.

Tobacco for chewing and sniffing has been used for many centuries. Smokeless tobacco use by both men and women flourished until the end of the nineteenth century. At this time, scientists discovered that bacteria and viruses could survive in saliva and be spread by air. Spitting into spittoons and onto barroom floors became unacceptable and even unlawful in many public places. Cigarettes replaced chew and snuff.

Chewing tobacco became fashionable again in the 1970s when the dangers of cigarette smoking became clear. Cigarettes were publicized as carcinogenic, and advertisers promoted smokeless tobacco as being a healthy alternative to cigarette smoking, which it is not. Smokeless tobacco creates dependence on nicotine just as cigarette smoking does. It leads to cancer of the mouth, lip, and gum.

It also causes other diseases of the mouth, such as hard white patches on the gums (leukoplakia) and inflammatory lesions of the gum (gingivitis). The majority of these lesions are benign, but about 2% to 6% of cases develop into cancer. Some users show a marked increase in blood pressure, which is a major factor in heart disease.

Smokeless tobacco has also been linked to other health problems. Taste-enhancing sugars and sweeteners found in loose chewing tobacco may lead to tooth decay. Abrasive ingredients found in tobacco cause receding gums in areas where the tobacco is held for long periods between the teeth and lower lip or the teeth and the cheek. Tobacco users often experience halitosis or a loss of taste and smell.

Social consequences of using smokeless tobacco include yellow and brown stains on the teeth, clothing, and automobile; the tobacco may cling to teeth, lips, tongue, and clothing. Spitting tobacco juice disgusts others.

The health risks of smokeless tobacco have become increasingly apparent, and various steps have been taken to alert the public to this problem. In 1986, the Comprehensive Smokeless Tobacco Health Education Act was passed. This bill banned all smokeless tobacco ads on television and radio, and mandated that health hazard warnings be placed on all tobacco packages. However, advertisements in print media and at car races and rodeos have increased the use of smokeless tobacco among young people. Male athletes are particularly at risk because of intensive marketing targeted to adolescent males, distribution of free smokeless tobacco to college players, promotions by professional athletes, and the convenience of using smokeless tobacco during games.

Cigars

Because cigar smokers generally do not inhale cigar smoke, it is often mistakenly assumed that cigar smoking is not harmful. However, compared with nonsmokers, cigar smokers who do not inhale have 3 times the risk of dying of lung cancer, and cigar smokers who inhale have

---

TERMS

chewing tobacco: a form of shredded smokeless tobacco; chewed or placed in the mouth between the lower lip and gum

moist snuff: a form of snuff made from air- and fire-cured tobacco leaves; most hazardous form of smokeless tobacco

nicotine: an addicting chemical in tobacco that produces rapid pulse, increased alertness, and a variety of other physiological effects

snuff: a form of smokeless tobacco; made from powdered or finely cut leaves

tar: the yellowish brown residue of tobacco smoke

11 times the risk of death from lung cancer. Cigar smokers, whether they inhale or not, have a greater risk of death from cancer of the lip, tongue, mouth, throat, esophagus, larynx, pancreas, and bladder. Because cigars have more tobacco than cigarettes, and because they often burn for much longer, they give off greater amounts of secondhand smoke. In general, secondhand smoke from cigars contains many of the same poisons (toxins) and cancer-causing agents (carcinogens) as cigarette smoke but in higher concentrations. It was not until the year 2000 that health warnings became required on cigar packages.

Smoking and Disease

Almost from the beginning of tobacco use in Europe and America, people have been concerned about the possible harmful effects of smoking (**Figure 17.4**). Several articles in the medical literature of the eighteenth and nineteenth centuries claimed tobacco smoking as a cause of cancer of the lip, tongue, and lung. Modern research on the health consequences of cigarette smoking has provided overwhelming evidence that among smokers as a group, the incidence of certain diseases is greater, sometimes much greater, than among nonsmokers. Smoking has been established as a factor in the development of coronary artery disease; lung cancer; bronchitis; emphysema; cancer of the larynx, lip, and oral cavity; cancer of the bladder and stomach; duodenal ulcer; and allergies.

Overwhelming data demonstrate that the death rate from cancer, heart disease, and respiratory diseases is higher among cigarette smokers than among nonsmokers. In fact, smoking decreases a person's life expectancy by an average of seven years. Smokers between the ages of 35 and 70 have death rates three times higher than those who have never smoked.

Effects of Parental Smoking on Children

Parental smoking harms children, beginning in pregnancy and continuing throughout a child's life. Smoking is a risk factor for spontaneous abortion, newborn death, and sudden infant death syndrome (SIDS). A pregnant woman exposed to environmental tobacco smoke (ETS) risks giving birth to a low-birth-weight infant. Compared to children raised in a nonsmoking environment, children exposed to ETS have a higher risk of bronchitis, pneumonia, and other respiratory tract infections. They also are at higher risk for asthma and ear infections.

Health Effects of Tobacco Use

Smoking kills more people than AIDS, poor diet and sedentary lifestyles, car accidents, alcohol, homicides, illegal drugs, suicides, and fires combined. It contributes substantially to deaths from cancer (especially cancers of the lung, esophagus, oral cavity, pancreas, kidney, and bladder), cardiovascular disease (i.e., coronary disease, stroke, and high

blood pressure), lung disease (i.e., chronic obstructive pulmonary disease and pneumonia), burns, and problems in infancy caused by low birth weight.

Lung Cancer

Lung cancer is responsible for more deaths among men and women than any other type of cancer. Each year approximately 197,000 persons receive a diagnosis of lung cancer and about 160,000 people die of this disease. Smoking is responsible for almost 90% of lung cancers among men and more than 70% among women. In

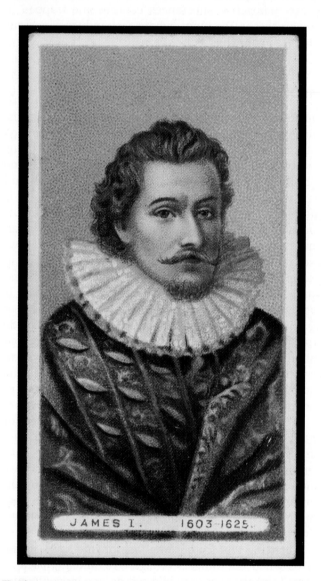

JAMES I.   1603-1625.

■ **Figure 17.4**

"A custom loathsome to the eye, hateful to the nose, harmful to the braine, dangerous to the lungs, and in the blacke, stinking fume thereof, nearest resembling the horrible Stigian smoke of the pit that is bottomlesse." So concluded James I of England in his *Counterblaste to Tobacco,* published in 1604. Sir Walter Raleigh had promoted and popularized the habit of smoking in the court of Queen Elizabeth of England in the late sixteenth century. But James I, who became king when Elizabeth died in 1603, was strongly opposed to the habit. He eventually had Raleigh beheaded for political reasons, but perhaps Raleigh also had smoked too much in the king's presence.

recent years, among American men, lung cancer incidence and death rates have declined, reflecting several decades of decline in active smoking and exposure to environmental tobacco smoke that together cause about 90% of lung cancer. In contrast, among American women, lung cancer incidence and death rates have increased, although the rate of increase has slowed in recent years. It is hoped that female lung cancer incidence and death rates will soon begin to decline as they have for men.

The increase in lung cancer deaths is the principal reason that the overall cancer death rate continues to rise. If lung cancer death rates are excluded from the statistics, the death rate from cancer has been falling steadily for many years, principally because of preventive efforts and improved diagnosis and treatment (see Chapter 13). This situation is ironic as well as tragic, for lung cancer is one of the most preventable of all diseases. People simply need to stop (or never start) smoking cigarettes.

A complete biological explanation of how smoking causes lung cancer (and contributes to cancer at other sites) is not yet available. There are 43 known **carcinogens** found in tobacco smoke that are thought to cause the cellular changes leading to cancer, probably by damaging genes in lung cells such that lung tissue function and/or cancer-protection systems are damaged.

Heart Disease

Smoking cigarettes increases the risk of heart disease (see Chapter 14). Smoking can increase tension in the heart muscle walls, speed up the rate of muscular contraction, and increase the heart rate. As the heart's workload increases, so does the need for oxygen and other nutrients. Smoking also reduces the amount of high-density lipoprotein (HDL) cholesterol (i.e., the "good" cholesterol), facilitating plaque formation and blood clotting.

Bronchitis and Emphysema

Bronchitis and **emphysema** are respiratory diseases sometimes classified with asthma as **chronic obstructive pulmonary diseases (COPD)**. Each of these diseases is associated with breathing difficulty caused by obstruction or destruction of some part of the respiratory system. Often persons suffer from more than one of these conditions at the same time.

Bronchitis is an inflammatory condition of the upper part of the respiratory tract, principally the **trachea,** the main airway. Bronchitis is characterized by excessive production of mucus by cells that line the airways, which causes the major symptoms of bronchitis, such as a continual cough (smoker's cough) and the production of large amounts of sputum. Some affected people also experience shortness of breath, particularly during exertion.

Apparently, excessive production of mucus by the glands of the bronchi is a reaction to irritation caused by cigarette smoke. Fortunately, the pathology that produces the symptoms of bronchitis can be almost completely reversed by quitting smoking, reducing exposure

to polluted air, or both. However, many people "live with" their persistent cough for many years and are not concerned with the message their body is giving them. If the disease is left to run its course, sufferers increase their vulnerability to other respiratory illnesses, and the airways may become irreversibly damaged.

Smoking is the primary cause of emphysema, which results from the destruction of the tiny air sacs deep in the lungs called **alveoli** (**Figure 17.5**). Each lung contains millions of alveoli; across their thin membranes the function of breathing is accomplished—the exchange of the respiratory gases, oxygen and carbon dioxide.

Emphysema is a disabling condition in which the walls of the air sacs in the lungs lose their elasticity and are gradually destroyed. The lungs' ability to obtain oxygen and remove carbon dioxide is impaired, requiring the heart to work harder, which results in the heart becoming enlarged. Emphysema involves a slow, irreversible process of alveolar destruction; as the disease progresses, affected people have greater and greater trouble breathing.

As with lung cancer, the exact mechanism by which tobacco smoking or air pollution contributes to emphysema is unknown. One hypothesis suggests that cells in the lung (macrophages and leukocytes produced by the immune system; see Chapter 12) normally engaged in the destruction of material foreign to the body release enzymes that inadvertently destroy lung tissue, thereby causing emphysema. Normally, a protein called *alpha-1-antitrypsin* (AAT) inhibits the activities of destructive enzymes in the lungs. The inhibitory protein blocks the action of the enzyme elastase, which, if not properly regulated, destroys alveoli and results in emphysema. Some people have low levels of the inhibitor because of a defective gene, and they are particularly at risk for emphysema.

TERMS

alveoli: tiny air sacs in the lungs that exchange oxygen and carbon dioxide

bronchitis: inflammation of the bronchi of the lungs as a result of irritation; often accompanied by a chronic cough

carcinogens: substances that can cause cancer in people and other animals

chronic obstructive pulmonary diseases (COPD): diseases that restrict the ability of the body to obtain oxygen through the respiratory structures (bronchi and lungs); includes asthma, bronchitis, and emphysema

emphysema: a progressive degeneration of the lung alveoli, causing breathing and oxygen assimilation to become more and more difficult

trachea: upper part of respiratory tract

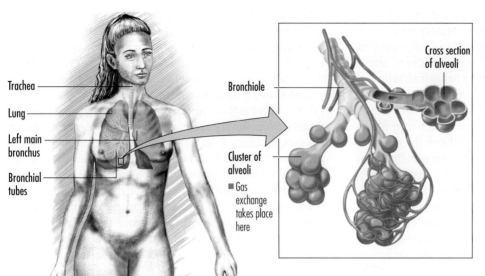

Trachea

Lung

Left main
bronchus

Bronchial
tubes

Bronchiole

Cross section
of alveoli

Cluster of
alveoli

■ Gas
exchange
takes place
here

■ **Figure 17.5**

Respiratory System
Provides oxygen and removes carbon
dioxide. Oxygen enters and carbon dioxide
leaves via tiny air sacs in the lungs called
alveoli. The rest of the respiratory system
facilitates gas exchange in the alveoli.

Tobacco Smoke's Effects on Nonsmokers

Nonsmokers who are exposed to tobacco smoke run a
significant health risk. People who work or live in environments heavily laden with tobacco smoke inhale the
same smokeborne substances as do smokers. In fact,
about two-thirds of the smoke from a burning cigarette
enters the environment.

Environmental tobacco smoke (ETS), also called secondhand smoke, contains the same 4,000 chemicals that
inhaled tobacco smoke does, but the concentration is
greater because ETS is unfiltered. Annually, about 3,000
nonsmoking American adults die of lung cancer and
about 50,000 die from heart disease as a result of exposure to ETS. Also, breathing ETS increases the severity of
asthma in nearly 1 million American children and is
responsible for several hundred thousand cases of bronchitis and pneumonia in children younger than 18
months.

A nonsmoker in a smoke-filled room can inhale in
one hour the equivalent of a cigarette's worth of nicotine, carbon monoxide, and carcinogenic substances.
Also, many people are allergic to tobacco smoke, which
can produce eye irritation, headache, cough, nasal congestion, and asthma. Nonsmokers forced to inhale
tobacco smoke for long periods, such as workers in
enclosed smoke-filled workplaces, can suffer impaired
lung function equivalent to that of smokers who inhale
while smoking 10 cigarettes a day. A study showed that
exposing healthy volunteers to secondhand smoke for
just 30 minutes compromised the lining of their coronary arteries to the same degree as habitual smokers
(Glantz & Parmley, 2001). Evidence for the damaging
effects of secondhand smoke on healthy nonsmokers
and children is overwhelming despite claims by tobacco
companies to the contrary. This is the reason that many
countries, states, and cities increasingly are banning
smoking in public places.

Health Tip

Smoking and Periodontal Disease

Periodontal disease (unhealthy gums and teeth) leads to
loosening of teeth; receding, swollen, or bleeding gums;
and eventually tooth loss. About 4% of the U.S. population
suffers from periodontal disease. Until recently, periodontal
disease was thought to be due to plaque buildup resulting
from poor dental hygiene and to inflammation of the gums
caused by bacteria (*gingivitis*). However, new studies
suggest that as much as 50% of periodontal disease may be
due to the effects of smoking tobacco or marijuana (Hujoel,
2008). Smoking cigarettes and marijuana reduces oxygen
supply to the gums, leading to inflammation and
destruction of gum tissue. If you have been looking for a
really good reason to stop smoking, the possibility of
destructive periodontal disease, loss of teeth, and
thousands of dollars in dental bills should do the trick.

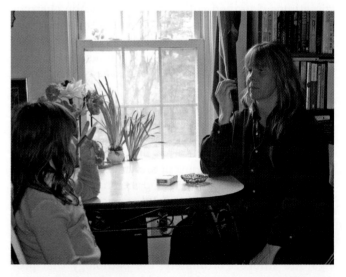

Children who live in homes where adults smoke have more respiratory
problems than children who are raised in smoke-free environments.

Why People Smoke

Most people begin to smoke in their teen years, emulating friends, parents, celebrities, film stars, or cigarette ad models. Teenagers also smoke to attain acceptance in their peer group. About half of those who experiment with smoking continue the habit into adulthood. Despite the unpleasant taste, the initial adverse physiological reactions to smoke and nicotine, and the knowledge that tobacco smoke causes cancer and other life-threatening diseases, some continue to smoke because of an unusually high susceptibility to nicotine addiction (DiFranza, 2008). Other factors that contribute to the development and maintenance of smoking include the following:

- *Stimulation.* Some people experience a psychological lift from smoking. They say that smoking helps them to wake up in the morning and organize their energies. They often report that smoking increases their intellectual capacities.
- *Handling.* Some people enjoy the mere handling of cigarettes and smoking paraphernalia, such as lighters.
- *Pleasurable relaxation.* Some smokers say they smoke simply because they like it. Smoking brings them true pleasure and relaxation and is often practiced to enhance other pleasurable sensations, such as the taste of food and alcoholic beverages. However, smoking actually dulls the taste buds.
- *Reducing negative feelings (crutch).* Approximately one-third of smokers say they smoke because it temporarily helps them deal with stress, anger, fear, anxiety, or pressure.
- *Craving.* Some people crave cigarettes and have no other explanation for their habit except that they have a frequent need to smoke, regardless of the tension-relieving effects that smoking might bring.

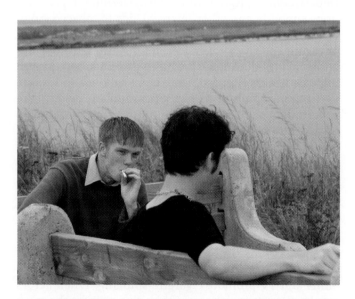

Smoking begins at an early age when peer acceptance is highly sought after.

- *Habit.* Some smokers light up only because of habit. They no longer receive much physical or psychological gratification from smoking; often they smoke without being aware of whether they really want the cigarette.

The question that still eludes a definitive answer is: What distinguishes people who smoke from those who do not? The list of suggested answers includes a biological susceptibility to dependence on nicotine; a variety of personal, sociological, and environmental traits; and a need to deal with stress. In the final analysis, however, smoking, like any other habitual, health-threatening behavior, is a matter of choice. In the case of smoking, the choice can ultimately be—and often is—fatal.

Quitting Smoking

Mark Twain once quipped, "Giving up smoking is easy. I've done it a hundred times."

Whereas that little joke is intended to show how difficult stopping smoking can be, it also confirms research that shows stopping smoking is a process, not an event. Often, people think about stopping for a period of time before they even consider trying, and sometimes people go through one or more cycles of stopping and starting up again before they quit permanently. These tries and retries are part of the stopping process.

The smoking habit is part biological (addiction to nicotine), part psychological (smoking alters mood and provides pleasure), and part social (smokers smoke with other smokers). Because smoking involves several parts of a smoker's life, quitting successfully generally requires examining how smoking is integrated into one's life,

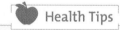
Health Tips

Benefits of Quitting Smoking

- 20 minutes after quitting: heart rate drops.
- 12 hours after quitting: carbon monoxide levels in blood drop to normal.
- 2 weeks to 3 months after quitting: lung function improves, risk of heart attack drops.
- 3 to 9 months after quitting: coughing and shortness of breath decrease.
- 1 year after quitting: risk of a heart attack is half that as compared to a smoker.
- 5 years after quitting: risk of a stroke is the same as for a nonsmoker.
- 10 years after quitting: risk of lung cancer is half that of a smoker's. Risk of other cancers also decreases.
- 15 years after quitting: risk of heart disease is the same as that of a nonsmoker.

Source: U.S. Centers for Disease Control and Prevention.

> A good plan executed right now is better than a perfect plan executed next week.
>
> *General George S. Patton*

then planning and adopting alternative experiences that meet the biological, psychological, and social needs that smoking satisfies.

Most smoking cessation plans center on a **quit date**—the day that the smoker stops smoking completely. Prior to the quit date, the smoker can prepare for stopping by

- Cutting back on the number of cigarettes smoked each day
- Identifying which cigarettes will be the hardest to give up (e.g., first of the day; after a meal) and planning alternative activities for after the quit date
- Identifying and preparing to do without the benefits of smoking and finding alternative activities to meet the needs that smoking provides (e.g., stress management)
- Asking friends and family to offer support while quitting
- Seeking professional smoking cessation counseling and support from smoking cessation groups. Nationwide telephone counseling is available at 1–800-QUIT NOW.
- Planning to stay away from smoking stimuli (e.g., not going to bars, not hanging out with friends who smoke, not smoking at breaks with coworkers, not smoking in the car)
- Investigating the possibility of using **nicotine replacement therapy** (nicotine patch, gum, or nasal spray) to lessen the effects of nicotine withdrawal, and prescription drugs such as buproprion and varenicline, that lessen the urge to smoke.

People stop smoking for a variety of reasons: to reduce the risk of early death from heart or lung disease; to enjoy, once again, the unpolluted taste of food; to please nonsmoking loved ones; to eliminate the ever-present ashes and smell of cigarette smoke from their homes and cars; and to fulfill a simple, yet important, commitment to be healthy. Frequently, a positive change in other aspects of life leads to cessation of smoking. For example, many people who take up meditation, t'ai chi ch'uan, jogging, or other physical activity lose the desire to smoke and stop smoking.

The War of Words

A long-standing war of words exists between public health professionals and the tobacco industry (tobacco growers and other businesses involved in the production and sale of smoking products). At stake is influencing the behavior of millions of smokers and prospective smokers, especially teens. The health groups try to persuade people not to smoke; the tobacco industry encourages them to smoke more and more.

The health war of words takes place in relative obscurity compared with tobacco advertising. Each year in the United States the tobacco industry spends billions of dollars to promote its products and to recruit new smokers. Perusal of many major magazines and newspapers reveals that cigarette advertising relies heavily on imagery portraying smoking as enjoyable and smokers as attractive, sexy, slim, and of high social status. Tobacco advertising in magazines for women and African Americans has increased in recent years, as has advertising of smokeless tobacco, with the erroneous implication that this form of tobacco consumption is safe. Besides print advertising, tobacco companies promote their products by sponsoring rock concerts, sporting events, and travel excursions. Some tobacco companies even support health research and smoking cessation programs, not only for the public relations benefits, but also to obtain scientific information that can appease regulators and consumers without harming sales.

> We must always follow somebody looking for the truth, and we must always run away from anyone who finds it.
>
> *Andre Gide*

Tobacco is the only legal consumer product that causes disability and death when used as intended. To replace the thousands of adult tobacco users who die each day, tobacco companies must recruit new users, generally from youth. Thus, a major tobacco company promotional tactic is offering price discounts to retailers, which reduces the price of tobacco products and thus makes them more available to youth. Another youth-recruiting tactic is the marketing of candy- and fruit-flavored cigarettes and smokeless tobacco.

The U.S. government plays a paradoxical role in the smoking war. It supports both sides. Through the Department of Agriculture, the government provides price supports and other financial aids to tobacco growers and the tobacco industry. Through the Department of Health and Human Services, the government supports antismoking educational programs and finances research into the health effects of smoking. Many health experts and others opposed to cigarette smoking believe the government should do more to combat the use of tobacco and confront the tobacco companies. An opponent of cigarette advertising points out that "Since billions of dollars are being spent to try to prevent terrorists from killing an unknown number of Americans, the nation ought to be able to at least match that amount to make significant reductions in the 440,000 deaths caused by tobacco every year" (Morrison, 2002).

Smoking in Films and on TV

Films and TV promote cigarette smoking. When actors smoke cigarettes on screen, they give viewers the message that smoking and smokers are cool. Nearly 80% of

Wellness Guide

Stages of the Quitting Process

Quitting smoking is a process involving five stages. The more one knows about the quitting process, the more likely one is to stop smoking and to have the confidence to remain tobacco free. The five stages of the quitting process are as follows.

Precontemplation Stage
Smokers in the precontemplation stage spend little time thinking about their smoking and may not see it as a problem. They see more negatives about quitting than positives, resulting in low motivation for stopping, even though they know that smoking carries serious health risks.

Contemplation Stage
Smokers in the contemplation stage are aware of the benefits of stopping and think about their smoking—and even about quitting—but they feel ambivalent about actually stopping. They may think about the negative aspects of smoking and the positive aspects associated with quitting, yet doubt that the long-term benefits associated with quitting will outweigh the short-term costs. Such ambivalence is a normal part of the quitting process and may last several months or even years.

Preparation
Smokers in the preparation stage have made the decision to quit and are taking steps to get ready to stop smoking. They

see the cons of smoking as outweighing the pros and say things like "I've got to do something about this—this is serious," or "Something has to change. What can I do?"

Action Stage
Smokers in the action stage are actively trying to stop smoking. They may try several different techniques, believe they have inner strength to quit, and tend to seek help and support. They develop plans to deal with both personal and external pressures that may lead to slips (i.e., smoking a cigarette), and they use short-term rewards to sustain their motivation.

Maintenance Stage
Smokers in the maintenance stage have learned to anticipate and handle temptations to smoke. They remain aware that what they are striving for is personally worthwhile and meaningful and are patient with themselves, recognizing that it often takes a while to let go of old behavior patterns and adopt new ones. They see "slipping" not as failure but as a learning experience and remind themselves of how much progress they have made.

American middle schoolers and nearly 90% of American high schoolers report seeing actors on TV and on film using tobacco (U.S. Centers for Disease Control and Prevention, 2005). Among American adolescents, the greater the exposure to smoking in films, the greater the risk for initiating smoking (Sargent et al., 2007). In 1998, the film industry instituted a self-imposed ban on accepting money from tobacco companies to have their products appear in films. This was after the disclosure that Sylvester Stallone had accepted $500,000 to smoke a particular brand of cigarettes in three of his movies. Tobacco companies even paid to have their brands of cigarettes placed in *Who Framed Roger Rabbit* and *The Muppet Movie*. Between 1999 and 2004, the overall percentage of films showing recognizable tobacco brands fell from 21% to 10%. However, during that same time period, the percentage of films rated PG-13 with recognizable tobacco brands remained at about 6% (Adachi-Mejia, 2005).

To determine the extent and type of tobacco use in movies, the American Lung Association asked more than 200 teenagers to review 50 top box office movies annually between 1991 and 1998. Teen reviewers found that many of the movies showed scenes in which tobacco use could be interpreted as sexy, exciting, powerful, sports-related, sophisticated, or celebratory; movies also included scenes in which tobacco use could be con-

sidered relaxing and in which tobacco use demonstrated independence or rebellion. A few movies included anti-tobacco messages, including no-smoking signs, comments by actors, and visual clues such as coughing or waving smoke away.

Reducing Tobacco's Damage to Society
In 1998, 46 states and seven large tobacco companies (Philip Morris Inc., R.J. Reynolds Tobacco Company, Brown and Williamson Tobacco Corporation, British American Tobacco Company, Lorillard Tobacco Company Inc., American Tobacco Company Inc., and the United States Tobacco Company) settled the states' lawsuits to recover their tobacco-related health care costs. The settlement, called the Master Settlement Agreement (MSA), totaled $206 billion, to be paid to the states over 25 years.

TERMS

nicotine replacement therapy: using nicotine-containing gum, skin patches, nasal sprays, or inhalers to temper the symptoms of nicotine withdrawal when quitting smoking

quit date: the day a smoker designates as the one on which she or he will stop smoking completely

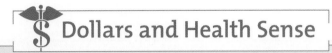

Dollars and Health Sense

Stop Your Financial Future from Going up in Smoke!

The smoking habit costs smokers a lot of money. A pack-a-day smoker spends about $1,750 a year just on cigarettes (estimated pack cost plus taxes = $5.00). If that money were invested at a 7.5% annual return, before taxes it would total:

- After 1 year . . . $1,750
- After 5 years . . . $10,164
- After 10 years . . . $28,757
- After 20 years . . . $75,783
- After 30 years . . . $180,948

Source: Hugh Chou. Stop smoking and save calculator. Available: http://www.hughchou.org/calc/smoking.cgi.

In addition to the MSA payments, the cigarette companies had to pay $5.15 billion over 12 years into a trust fund to compensate tobacco farmers and others for anticipated financial losses resulting from the implementation of the MSA. The states also signed a separate agreement with the leading smokeless tobacco company, United States Tobacco, that contains many of the same public health provisions as the MSA.

The MSA provides numerous restrictions and prohibitions on the tobacco industry, including bans on the following:

- The use of cartoons in tobacco advertisements
- The targeting of youth in advertising, promotions, or marketing, including free sampling
- The use of most outdoor advertisements, including billboards and signs and placards in arenas, stadiums, shopping malls, and video game arcades
- The distribution of apparel and merchandise with brand-name logos
- Payments to promote tobacco products in films, TV, and theater productions
- Distributing free samples of cigarettes any place where underage persons may be present
- Tobacco company lobbying against any proposed laws that limit youth access to tobacco
- Tobacco industry attempts to limit or suppress research on the health effects of smoking

It was hoped that the MSA money would help states devise antismoking programs and take other steps to reduce smoking. However, most states use most of their MSA money for general services and use only a small percentage on tobacco control.

Tobacco industry secret documents have revealed that for more than 40 years, tobacco companies misled and lied to the public about the harmful, addictive effects of tobacco. It is clear that they targeted and manipulated young people into starting smoking. And, despite the MSA, they continue to do so. In 2001, R.J. Reynolds was sued by the states of Arizona and California for mailing free cigarettes. The MSA prohibits tobacco companies from giving away free samples where children might gain access. In 1999, the United States Tobacco Company, the largest distributor of smokeless tobacco, was sued by the state of California for advertising with a discount coupon for one of its products in the San Diego State University student newspaper. Moreover, after the MSA, cigarette advertising increased in 19 magazines for which youth readers (between 12 and 17 years old) make up at least 15% of the readership (Massachusetts Department of Public Health, 2000). These magazines included *Sports Illustrated, TV Guide, Rolling Stone, Glamour,* and *Vogue.* Advertising for Marlboro, by far the most popular brand of cigarette among youth, increased by 25% in such magazines. In 1999, the advertising of tobacco products on billboards was banned, but tobacco companies simply moved their ads inside retail stores and increased giveaways of branded objects such as clocks and other items.

Because 90% of new smokers begin the habit before reaching age 18, the tobacco industry targets youth with its advertising and promotional messages. The tobacco industry knows that today's teenager is tomorrow's potential regular customer. As the Campaign for Tobacco-Free Kids points out, the tobacco industry is addicted to advertising to children.

In addition to the MSA, which was initiated and prosecuted by states, in 1999 the federal government sued the tobacco industry to recover Medicare funds used to treat tobacco-related illness, to establish smoking cessation treatment for smokers who want to quit, and to stop tobacco companies from denying that smoking kills and that nicotine is addictive, from manipulating the chemistry of tobacco to sustain addiction, from suppressing information on the ill effects of tobacco use, from marketing of "light" cigarettes, and from marketing to children and youth. The federal lawsuit (the largest civil litigation in U.S. history) went to trial in 2004, and during closing arguments in 2005, the U.S. Justice Department—over the objections of the lead staff attorneys prosecuting the case—unexpectedly reduced the amount of money requested as penalty for tobacco company wrongdoing from $130 billion to $10 billion. Many members of Congress and the public health community

Wellness Guide

Women and Cigarette Advertising

For over 80 years, advertising by American tobacco companies has enticed women to smoke by associating cigarettes with sexiness, slimness, elegance, fun, independence, social and economic success, and even health! Tobacco advertising targeting women began in the 1920s, with messages such as "reach for a Lucky instead of a sweet" to establish an association between smoking and slimness. In the first year of this ad campaign, sales of Lucky Strike cigarettes increased 300%, mirroring the general rise in smoking among American women. In 1923, women consumed 5% of all cigarettes sold. By 1929, the number had grown to 12%, and by 1933, it was 18%. Currently, about 20% of American women smoke.

Between 1965 and 1977, the percentage of women who smoked peaked at 34%, in no small part due to the advertising cunning of the Virginia Slims ad campaigns. Not only did the name of the product and the body shapes of the models promoting it associate smoking with slimness, but also the product's advertising slogan, "You've come a long way, Baby," co-opted women's desires for social and economic equality, emancipation from rigid gender role stereotyping, and empowerment. These same themes are common today. To counter women's concerns about the health risks of smoking, cigarette advertising uses images of models engaged in exercise or pictures of white-capped mountains against a background of clear blue skies.

Besides advertising, the tobacco industry has targeted women by offering the following:

- Cigarette brand clothing and other accessories
- A yearly engagement calendar and a catalog featuring clothing, jewelry, and accessories coordinated with the themes and colors of a product's print advertisement and product packaging
- Gifts, including mugs and caps, bearing a product's label in colors coordinated with the advertisement and packaging
- Discounts on turkeys, milk, soft drinks, and laundry detergent with the purchase of tobacco products
- Color-coordinated items in multiple-pack containers
- Free tickets to films and concerts

About 175,000 American women die from cigarette-caused diseases each year. Lung cancer has surpassed breast cancer as the leading cause of cancer deaths among women. And if that's not enough, the beauty editor of *Harper's* points out that "smokers' skin wrinkles up to 10 years sooner than that of nonsmokers."

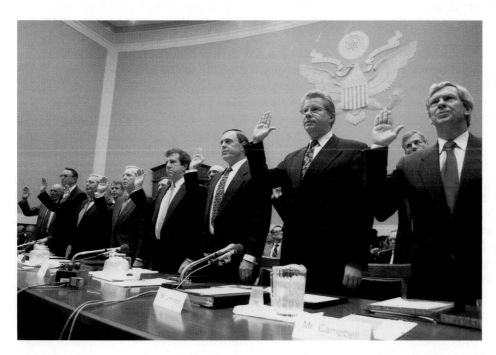

In the mid-1990s, the chief executives of the seven major U.S. tobacco companies were called before Congress to explain their business practices. Each of the executives testified under oath, "I do not believe smoking is addicting."

believe that the Justice Department's sudden decision to halt vigorous prosecution of the case represented political influences (tobacco companies are large campaign donors) and a lack of commitment to the public health (Fiore, Keller, & Baker, 2005).

There are other ways to reduce tobacco's damage to society in addition to litigation against tobacco companies to stop fraudulent and deceptive business practices and marketing tobacco products to youth. For example, every 10% increase in the price of cigarettes reduces consumption

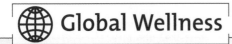

Global Wellness

Ireland Bans All Smoking in the Workplace

On March 29, 2004, Ireland became the first country in the world to ban any form of smoking in the workplace. This includes in restaurants, clubs, and pubs—anyplace that employs workers. The only place left for people who smoke is the privacy of their homes and the outdoors. And, in the freezing cold of an Irish winter, it is the hardy smoker indeed who wants to step outside to light up. After years of effort, the Irish government secured the support of all political parties, labor unions, and industry executives in banning all workplace smoking. Reports documenting the extreme hazards of secondhand smoke, especially to children, helped unite the country in banning smoking.

Of course, there were protests. Some bars held smoke-ins but won little support. Organized groups claimed that basic rights were being violated, that the tourist industry would collapse, that social life would erode, that the law was unenforceable. None of these arguments prevailed, however, and Ireland now enjoys a smoke-free workplace. Now that Ireland is committed to protecting citizens from the health hazards of tobacco, will other European countries have the courage to follow (McElvaney, 2004)? And what action will the United States take to protect its citizens from secondhand smoke?

by 4%. Thus, raising taxes on cigarettes and other tobacco products is a very effective way to reduce tobacco consumption, especially among youth.

Other ways to reduce tobacco's damage to society include the following:

- Create more smoke-free public places, including work sites, restaurants, and bars (see the Global Wellness feature "Ireland Bans All Smoking in the Workplace"). Five states and hundreds of local municipalities have banned smoking in essentially all public places.
- Provide comprehensive smoking cessation programs for all smokers who want to quit (about 70% of current smokers).
- Support strict advertising and marketing rules on tobacco products in accordance with the Framework Convention on Tobacco Control.

Tobacco use is the single most preventable cause of illness and death in the world. And yet, in the United States, the manufacture, marketing, and sale of tobacco products are virtually unregulated. Autos, airplanes, appliances, household products, all foods, and all drugs are regulated by the federal government to ensure public safety. Tobacco is not, despite the fact that smoking is responsible for over 440,000 deaths per year and nicotine in cigarettes is one of the most addictive substances.

Because nicotine is a legal drug, health professionals and some members of Congress want the tobacco industry to be regulated by the Food and Drug Administration (FDA). In 2009 the U.S. Congress passed the Family Smoking Prevention and Tobacco Control Act. The provisions of this new law are:

- Tobacco-product manufacturers must list the ingredients and additives they put into tobacco products so consumers could know what they are being exposed to. Any harmful chemicals and additives would themselves be liable to regulation.
- Cigarettes with fruit, spice, and other flavorings that appeal to youth would be banned. One exception is menthol, an ingredient in 25% of all cigarettes sold and 75% of all cigarettes sold to African Americans. Menthol could be banned if found to be harmful.
- The FDA would have the authority to regulate the use of words such as *light*, *mild*, and *low* in promotional materials and on packages, because they incorrectly imply that such products are less harmful than regular tobacco products.
- Warning labels about the dangers of tobacco would be larger and more prominently displayed on promotional materials and on packages.

Critical Thinking About Health

1. Smoking takes a toll on everyone—those who smoke and those who do not. Government officials estimate that cigarette smoking costs the nation about $100 billion a year in health care costs and lost productivity. These costs are borne equally by nonsmokers and smokers.
   a. Should nonsmokers pay for the health care expenses of people who smoke? Why or why not?
   b. Should cigarettes be taxed by the government to cover their full cost to society, which could lessen tobacco consumption, put tobacco growers out of business, and drastically reduce tobacco companies' profits?

2. Purchase a popular magazine and count the number of cigarette ads in that issue. Review each ad and respond to the following questions:
   a. Who is the ad targeting? (e.g., women, men, young, old)
   b. How is the ad appealing to its target audience? (e.g., sex, friends)
   c. Besides the warning label (which is required by law) does the ad mention any other negative effects of smoking?
   d. What does the ad imply will happen if you smoke that brand of cigarette?

3. Over the last three decades cigarettes have been shown to be hazardous to one's health. Smokeless tobacco was once thought to be a substitute for cigarette smoking, and its popularity increased during the 1970s and 1980s. You have been asked to return to your high school to discuss the negative consequences of tobacco.
   a. Identify two primary reasons for a young person not to begin using tobacco products.
   b. Respond to the following young athlete's question: "I don't smoke cigarettes because they are nasty. I use chew instead—my grandpa told me it wasn't bad. What can happen to me? I'm not inhaling tobacco."

4. Visit or call your local health department and ask them for a list of restaurants in your community that are smoke free.
   a. What percentage of your community's eating establishments are smoke free?
   b. What can you do to promote smoke-free eating establishments within your community?
   c. Should all public places—indoor and outdoor—be smoke free?

Health in Review

- No public health message is disseminated as widely as that on every package of cigarettes and in every cigarette advertisement: "Warning: The Surgeon General Has Determined That Cigarette Smoking Is Dangerous to Your Health."
- Despite the overwhelming evidence that cigarette smoking is associated with higher death rates from cancer, heart disease, and respiratory diseases, approximately 46 million American adults smoke. Smoking also is associated with a higher risk of emphysema and bronchitis.
- Cigarette smoking is responsible for 440,000 American deaths per year, far more than AIDS, auto accidents, and drug use combined. Smoking increases the risk for heart disease, lung cancer, respiratory diseases, and cancers of all kinds.
- Smoking tobacco comes from the processed leaves of *Nicotiana tabacum*. Tobacco smoke contains more than 4,000 chemicals, including nicotine—which is responsible for many of tobacco's drug effects, including physical dependence—and 43 others that are known to cause cancer.
- Smokeless tobacco is not a healthy alternative to smoking tobacco; it causes cancers of the lip and mouth. Cigar smoking also is harmful.

- Children are harmed by breathing parents' tobacco smoke. Pregnant women who smoke risk the health of their babies.
- Environmental tobacco smoke contains the same 4,000 chemicals and 43 carcinogens that inhaled tobacco smoke does, thus affecting the health of nonsmokers.
- People smoke cigarettes because of physical dependence on nicotine and a variety of psychological and social rewards that come from smoking.
- Smokers can stop smoking either on their own or with the help of a stop-smoking program.
- The advertising of cigarettes largely is aimed at young people and contributes to recruiting them to the smoking habit. In 1998, 46 states won a $206 billion settlement (Master Settlement Agreement) with the tobacco industry. This settlement is intended to help pay for smoking-related health costs and forbids tobacco companies from promoting tobacco products to youths under age 18.

Health and Wellness Online

The Web contains a wealth of information about health and wellness. By accessing the Internet using Web browser software, you can gain a new perspective on many topics presented in *Health and Wellness*, Tenth Edition. Access the Jones and Bartlett Publishers Web site at **health.jbpub.com/hwonline**.

References

Adachi-Mejia, A. M. (2005). Tobacco brand appearances in movies before and after the Master Settlement Agreement. *Journal of the American Medical Association, 293*, 2341–2342.

Aligne, C. A., et al. (2003). Association of pediatric dental caries with passive smoking. *Journal of the American Medical Association, 289*, 1258–1264.

American College Health Association. (2008). National college health assessment. Retrieved September 14, 2008, from http://www.acha-ncha.org/

Connolly, G. N., & Alpert, H. R. (2008). Trends in the use of cigarettes and other tobacco products, 2000–2007. *Journal of the American Medical Association, 299*, 2629–2630.

DiFranza, J. R. (2008, May). Hooked from the first cigarette. *Scientific American, 298*, 82–87.

El-Nachef, W. N., & Hammond, S. K. (2008). Exhaled carbon monoxide with waterpipe use in U.S. students. *Journal of the American Medical Association, 299*, 36–38.

Fiore, M. C., Keller, P. A., & Baker, T. B. (2005). The Justice Department's case against the tobacco companies. *New England Journal of Medicine, 353*, 972–975.

Glantz, S. A., & Parmley, W. W. (2001). Even a little secondhand smoke is dangerous. *Journal of the American Medical Association, 286*, 462–463.

Harris, J. E., et al. (2004). Cigarette yields in relation to mortality from lung cancer in the cancer prevention study II prospective cohort, 1982–8. *British Medical Journal, 328*, 72–76.

Hujoel, P. P. (2008). Destructive periodontal disease and tobacco and cannabis smoking. *Journal of the American Medical Association, 299*, 547–575.

Massachusetts Department of Public Health. (2000). Cigarette advertising expenditures before and after the Master Settlement Agreement.

McElvaney, N. G. (2004). Smoking ban—Made in Ireland, for home use and export. *New England Journal of Medicine, 350*, 2231–2232.

Morrison, A. B. (2002). Counteracting cigarette advertising. *Journal of the American Medical Association, 287*, 3001–3003.

Neergard, J. et al. (2007). Waterpipe smoking and nicotine exposure: A review of the current evidence. *Nicotine and Tobacco Research, 9*, 987–994.

Sargent, J. D., et al. (2007). Exposure to smoking depictions in movies: Its association with established adolescent smoking. *Archives of Pediatrics and Adolescent Medicine, 161*, 849–856.

U.S. Centers for Disease Control and Prevention. (2005). Tobacco use, access, and exposure to tobacco in media among middle and high school students—United States, 2004. *Morbidity and Mortality Weekly Report, 54*, 297–301.

Suggested Readings

Brandt, A. M. (2007). *The cigarette century.* New York: Basic Books. A thorough history of changing attitudes toward smoking in the United States and the scientific discoveries that exposed the dangers of smoking and the litigations against tobacco companies that followed.

Fiore, M. C., et al. (2004). Preventing three million premature deaths and helping five million smokers quit: A national action plan for tobacco cessation. *American Journal of Public Health, 94,* 205–210. In-depth discussion of programmatic strategies to help smokers quit.

Gostin, L. O. (2007). Global strategies for tobacco control. *Journal of the American Medical Association, 298,* 2057–2059. Presents a thorough analysis of various ways to control the international sale of tobacco products.

Kessler, D. (2001). *A question of intent: A great American battle with a deadly industry.* New York: Public Affairs. The former director of the FDA describes the agency's battle to regulate the tobacco industry and to document the deadly consequences of smoking.

U.S. Surgeon General. (2004). 2004 Surgeon General's report: The health consequences of smoking. Available: http://www.cdc.gov/tobacco/data_statistics/sgr/sgr_2004/index.htm

U.S. Surgeon General. (2006). The health consequences of involuntary exposure to tobacco smoke: A report of the Surgeon General. Available: http://www.surgeongeneral.gov/library/secondhandsmoke/

Recommended Web Sites

Please visit **health.jbpub.com/hwonline** for links to these Web sites.

Clearing the Air
Smoking cessation guide from the National Cancer Institute.

Quit Smoking Program
From the Canadian Lung Association.

The Quit Net
A quit-smoking Web site produced by the Boston University School of Public Health.

U.S. Centers for Disease Control Tobacco Information and Prevention Source (TIPS)
Everything you ever wanted to know about smoking and tobacco use.

You Can Quit Smoking
A guide from the U.S. National Institutes of Health.

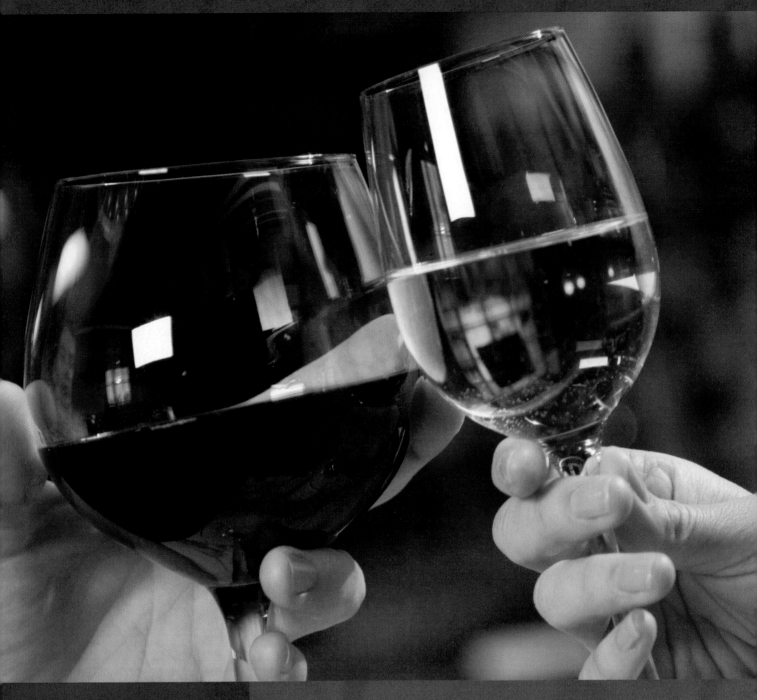

Chapter Eighteen

Using Alcohol Responsibly

Learning Objectives

1. Discuss the prevalence of drinking, types of drinking, reasons for drinking, and attitudes toward drinking among college students.

2. Explain the effects of alcohol on the body.

3. Describe how alcohol is absorbed into the body and how this absorption relates to blood alcohol concentration.

4. Discuss the effects of alcohol on behavior, including sexual behavior.

5. Describe the long-term effects of alcohol overconsumption.

6. Define *alcohol abuse*, *alcohol addiction*, and *alcoholism*.

7. Explain the phases of alcoholism.

8. Describe how alcohol affects one's significant others and the help that is available for both the family and the alcoholic.

Alcohol use and abuse are among the most significant health-related drug problems in the United States and in many other countries. Although cocaine and other illegal drugs receive much more attention from governments and the news media, these drugs affect far fewer people and cause far fewer health problems than alcohol. In the United States:

> See, the problem is that God gave man a brain and a penis, but only enough blood to run one at a time.
>
> *Robin Williams*

- About 50% of adults drink more than 12 drinks a year
- About 79,000 people die each year from alcohol-related diseases
- 25% of high school seniors have drunk five or more drinks at one time in the prior two weeks
- In any two-week span, 81% of college students drink some alcohol and 41% drink five or more drinks on an occasion
- 7% of persons age 12 and over drink five or more drinks per day five or more times a month
- About 14,000 Americans die each year from alcohol-related traffic collisions

- About 79,000 Americans are addicted to alcohol, including 1,300 children
- Approximately 1.4 million drivers are arrested for driving intoxicated
- It is estimated that alcohol abuse costs the U.S. economy $180 billion per year

Excessive alcohol use is also associated with thousands of divorces, as many as 80% of the incidents of family violence, 40% of crimes, and millions of hours of school and job absenteeism. In addition, alcohol abuse is linked to a long list of medical problems (**Figure 18.1**).

Alcohol use has long been a part of social events, such as parties, dinners, weddings, ball games, and picnics. The liquor industry encourages alcohol use by advertising in newspapers and magazines and on radio and television. No direct link between advertising alcoholic products and alcohol abuse has been established. However, public health authorities and organizations such as the American Medical Association are concerned that advertising that associates drinking with athletic prowess, material wealth, social prestige, and sex encourages irresponsible drinking behavior. Breweries and liquor distributors are especially active on college campuses, spending millions of dollars each year on advertising in campus newspapers and promoting their

■ **Figure 18.1**

Medical Problems Associated with Alcohol Abuse

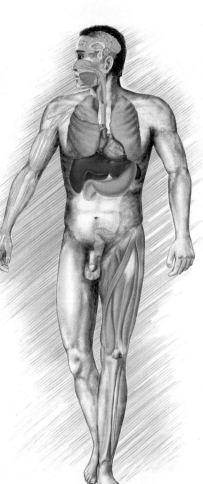

Brain Wernicke's syndrome, an acute condition characterized by ataxia, mental confusion, and ocular abnormalities; Korsakoff's syndrome, a psychotic condition characterized by impairment of memory and learning ability, apathy, and degeneration of the white brain matter

Esophagus Esophageal varices, an irreversible condition in which the person can die by drowning in his own blood when the varices open

Liver An acute enlargement of the liver, which is reversible, as well as irreversible cirrhosis of the liver

Muscles Alcoholic myopathy, a condition resulting in painful muscle contractions

Blood and bone marrow Coagulation defects and anemia

Eyes Tobacco-alcohol blindness; Wernicke's ophthalmoplegia, a reversible paralysis of the muscles of the eye

Pharynx Cancer of the pharynx is increased tenfold for drinkers who smoke

Heart Alcoholic cardiomyopathy, a heart condition

Lungs Lowered resistance is thought to lead to greater incidences of tuberculosis, pneumonia, and emphysema

Spleen Hypersplenism

Stomach Gastritis and ulcers

Pancreas Acute and chronic pancreatitis

Rectum Hemorrhoids

Testes Atrophy of the testes

Nerves Polyneuritis, a condition characterized by loss of sensation

products by sponsoring "pub nights," giving away items with product logos, and underwriting some of the costs of college athletic events.

Alcohol's positive public image makes many people doubt that they need to learn about alcohol use and abuse. Most people who drink believe that they can "hold their liquor" and that alcoholic beverages, especially beer, are no more harmful to health than soft drinks. As with so many other aspects of health, for most people responsible and moderate alcohol consumption is more desirable than overzealous adherence to a single course of action. Everyone can benefit from knowing more about the effects of alcohol.

History of Alcohol Use

It is likely that humans have been drinking alcohol since someone accidentally noticed the psychological effects of drinking fermented liquids. Archaeological evidence indicates that Stone Age people drank the fermented juice of berries. Perhaps this first fruit wine was produced when some berry juice was left too long in a covered earthen jar and yeasts began fermentation, converting the sugar in the juice to alcohol. The first

recorded use of alcohol dates from the Mesopotamian agrarian cultures of around 2000 B.C.

Through the ages, drinking fermented grains (beer); fermented berries, grapes, and fruits (wine); and the distilled products of natural fermentation ("hard" liquors) has been commonplace in many human societies. Alcohol is used in some religious ceremonies; is taken as medicine; is used to seal contracts, agreements, and treaties; and is offered to display hospitality. Alcohol consumption has been an integral part of American life since the landing of the *Mayflower* at Plymouth Rock. Yet over the years, many people have come to regard drinking as a social evil and drunkenness as a sin. The United States government tried to legislate alcohol use out of American lives in 1919 by the Volstead Act, a constitutional amendment that prohibited the sale and consumption of alcoholic beverages ("Prohibition"). This attempt to control alcohol consumption failed, however, and in 1933, Prohibition was repealed by another amendment to the Constitution.

Today, alcoholic beverages are available in many varieties. Not only are there the old standbys of beer, wine, and traditional hard liquors, but beverage manufacturers also market a variety of premixed cocktails, often sweetened with sugar and containing various flavors; wine coolers; and malt liquors.

Approximately 61% of U.S. adults have at least one drink per year, 14% are former drinkers, and 25% are lifetime abstainers. Most of those who consume alcohol engage in moderate drinking. Approximately 9% of the U.S. population's drinking behavior puts them at risk for alcohol-related health and social problems (**Table 18.1**).

Drinking on Campus

Each year several college students die from alcohol poisoning as a consequence of ingesting massive quantities of alcohol. In its coverage of these tragic occurrences, the national media remind Americans that drinking is as much a part of going to college as is going to class. Indeed, American college students spend more money on alcoholic beverages each year than they do on textbooks and soft drinks combined.

About 80% of American college students aged 18 to 29 years drink alcohol at least once in a while, which is about the same rate as their noncollege age peers (Dawson et al., 2004). Most of these students reserve their drinking for weekly "partying"—attending social events at which one is expected to "let loose," drink alcohol to excess

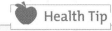

Health Tip

Signs of Alcohol Poisoning

No one expects to die from partying, but it can happen. Alcohol is a potent central nervous system depressant, and too much of it can inhibit the brain's respiratory center, leading to death or irreversible brain damage. Also, alcohol is toxic, so when too much has been consumed, the body vomits it out. However, alcohol can inhibit the gag reflex, so instead of going out of the body, vomit gets sucked into the lungs and causes death from asphyxiation. Even if someone has passed out from ingesting too much alcohol, alcohol in the intestines continues to be absorbed into the body, increasing the risk of death. Don't assume the person will be fine by sleeping it off. Know the signs of alcohol poisoning:

- Confusion, stupor, coma, or the person cannot be roused
- Vomiting
- Seizures
- Slow breathing (fewer than eight breaths per minute)
- Irregular breathing (10 seconds or more between breaths)
- Low body temperature, bluish skin color, paleness

If you suspect alcohol poisoning, don't try to sober the person up with black coffee, a cold bath or shower, or walking it off. Those methods don't work. Call 911 right away. You don't want to feel responsible for an alcohol-related tragedy. And don't worry that your friend may become angry or embarrassed afterward. Remember, you cared and did the right thing.

Source: College Drinking Prevention. Available: http://www .collegedrinkingprevention.gov/students/risky/alcoholpoisoning.aspx

> O God, that men should put an enemy into their mouths to steal away their brains!
> That we should with joy, pleasure, revel, and applause, transform ourselves into beasts.
>
> *Shakespeare,* Twelfth Night

Table 18.1

Criteria for Moderate and At-Risk Alcohol Use

Moderate drinking

Men: ≤ 2 drinks/day*

Women: ≤ 1 drink/day

Over 65 (men and women): ≤ 1 drink/day

At-risk drinking

Men: >14 drinks/week, or >4 drinks/occasion

Women: >7 drinks/week, or >3 drinks/occasion

Alcohol abuse

Significant impairment or distress in a 12-month period, including

- Failure to meet obligations at work, school, or home
- Recurrent use of alcohol in hazardous situations
- Legal problems related to alcohol
- Continued use despite alcohol-related social or interpersonal problems

Alcohol dependence

Significant impairment or distress in a 12-month period, including

- Tolerance to alcohol
- Withdrawal symptoms with abstinence from alcohol
- Use of larger amounts over a longer period than intended
- Persistent desire for alcohol (craving)
- Unsuccessful attempts to cut down or control use
- Important social, occupational, or recreational activities given up because of drinking
- Use despite knowledge of alcohol-related problems (denial)

*One drink = 12 g of alcohol, which is the equivalent of 150 ml (5 oz) of wine, 360 ml (12 oz) of beer, or 45 ml (1.5 oz) of 90-proof distilled spirits.

Source: U.S. National Institute on Alcohol Abuse and the American Psychiatric Association.

Table 18.2

Some Consequences of High-Risk College Drinking

1,700 deaths from alcohol-related unintentional injuries, including motor vehicle crashes

600,000 unintentional injuries

696,000 assaults by another student who has been drinking

97,000 victims of sexual assault or date rape

400,000 students have unprotected sex and more than 100,000 are too intoxicated to know if they consented to having sex

150,000 students develop an alcohol-related health problem

2,100,000 drove under the influence of alcohol

110,000 arrested for an alcohol-related violation such as public drunkenness or driving under the influence

Source: College drinking: A snapshot of annual high-risk college drinking consequences. Available: http://www.collegedrinkingprevention.gov/StatsSummaries/snapshot.aspx

(becoming "hammered" or "wasted"), and behave atypically (e.g., doing something "outrageous"; having sex with a stranger). More than 50% of students have at least three drinks when partying; 35% have five or more drinks (American College Health Association, 2008).

Participants view partying as a way to release the tensions of academic stress, meet new people, prove one's social competence, and simply have fun. However, nonparticipants view partying, especially the emphasis on excessive alcohol consumption, as foolishly dangerous (**Table 18.2**). They point out that excessive alcohol consumption—called **dangerous**, **high-risk**, or **binge drinking**—impairs one's judgment, thus increasing the risks for being involved in a motor vehicle crash, of an unintended pregnancy, acquiring a sexual infection, and being either a perpetrator or victim of sexual assault. As one researcher put it, "Alcohol is the AIDS virus of injury control [because it] lowers the defenses and immunity to injury" (Foege, 1987).

College students who drink to excess regularly are more likely

- To miss class
- To get behind in schoolwork
- To do something they regret
- Not to use protection when engaging in sex

- To engage in unplanned sexual activity
- To get into trouble with campus police
- To damage property
- To get injured
- To engage in dangerous driving behaviors
- To disturb, insult, quarrel with, or assault others
- To require care from others while being sick from drunkenness

Compared with nonathletes, college athletes are much more likely to engage in both heavy and binge drinking (Yusko et al., 2008). Because athletes are so visible on campus, their drinking behaviors contribute to the overall campus atmosphere regarding drinking and students' perceptions and expectations of campus norms regarding alcohol use.

The behaviors of excessive drinkers can affect non–binge drinkers and alcohol abstainers. So-called **secondhand binge effects** include the following:

- Being interrupted while studying
- Being awakened at night
- Having to take care of a drunken fellow student
- Being insulted or humiliated by a drunken student
- Being pushed, hit, or assaulted by a drunken student
- Being the victim of sexual assault

Although the majority of college students either do not drink or limit their drinking behavior to partying, about 7% abuse alcohol to a degree that it adversely affects their academic progress, personal relationships, and health. About 9% of college students meet criteria for alcohol dependence (Slutske, 2005).

In general, the cultural attitude of the campus regarding alcohol use has a tremendous influence on student drinking behavior. A campus culture that encourages legal and responsible alcohol use and discourages underage drinking, binge drinking, and alcohol-induced antisocial behavior promotes responsible behavior among the students (Wechsler & Nelson, 2008).

The opposite is true for a campus that has few or no student alcohol-use policies and at which students perceive that just about anything goes with regard to alcohol use. College students who drink heavily tend to view campus attitudes toward drinking as liberal. Students with the most enthusiastic attitudes toward drinking are typically the heaviest drinkers.

Given the extraordinary efforts of manufacturers of beer and other alcoholic beverages to market their products to college students, it's a wonder that so many college students drink responsibly. A typical campus newspaper usually contains advertisements for alcoholic beverages and bar events. Slogans such as "Think when you drink," "Know when to say when," and "Friends don't let friends drive drunk" only masquerade as responsible drinking messages. Their real message is to drink as much as you can and institute backup precautions for when you are drunk.

To reduce the degree of excessive drinking, college campuses are working to change the campus climate regarding alcohol use. Irresponsible drinking is not viewed as a rite of membership in campus organizations (e.g., clubs, athletic teams, fraternities, sororities), as an acceptable way to lessen social anxiety in party or other social situations, as the definition of partying, as an acceptable means to deal with academic stress, or as a rite of passage to adulthood and independence from parental control.

How Alcohol Affects the Body

Composition of Alcoholic Beverages

The alcohol in beverages is a chemical called **ethyl alcohol (ethanol)**. There are many other kinds of alcohol, such as **methyl alcohol** and **isopropyl alcohol**. Most alcohols are poisonous if ingested in small amounts. In large amounts, even ethanol is toxic, but the body has ways to detoxify and eliminate it, given enough time.

The amount of ethanol in a commercial alcoholic product usually is listed on the product label (beer is the exception). The amount of alcohol in beer and wine is usually given as the percentage of the total volume. Beer, for example, is generally about 4% alcohol, although some beers contain more or less (so-called light beers have nearly the same alcohol content as regular beers). Wine is about 12% alcohol. The amount of alcohol in distilled liquors (e.g., scotch, vodka, bourbon, tequila, rum) is given in terms of **proof,** a number that represents twice the percentage of alcohol in the product. Thus, an 80-proof whiskey is 40% alcohol; 100-proof vodka is 50% alcohol.

Most standard portions of alcoholic drinks contain about the same amount of alcohol (**Figure 18.2**). For example, a 12-ounce beer that is 5% alcohol contains 0.6 ounces of alcohol. The same amount of alcohol is in a 5-ounce glass of wine. The alcohol content of a mixed

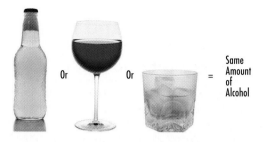

■ **Figure 18.2**

A bottle of beer, glass of wine, and a mixed drink have about the same amount of alcohol. So don't be fooled by the type of drink.

drink made of 1.5 ounces of 80-proof spirits (40% alcohol) contains 0.6 ounces of alcohol. So, a can of beer, a glass of wine, and a mixed drink contain approximately the same amount of alcohol. Thus, the perception that a beer is less alcoholic than a glass of wine or a mixed drink is wrong. Note that some malt liquors and ales are 6% to 8% alcohol; fortified wines, such as sherry and port, are 18% alcohol; and some distilled liquors are 100 proof (50% alcohol).

How Alcohol Is Absorbed, Excreted, and Metabolized

After alcohol is ingested, it is readily absorbed into the body through the gastrointestinal tract. About 20% of ingested alcohol is absorbed by the stomach and the rest by the small intestine. The alcohol is then carried through the bloodstream to all the body's tissues and organs. Although not strictly a food (it contains no protein, vitamins, or minerals), alcohol does contain calories—in fact, 7 calories per gram (almost twice as many calories per gram as sugar).

Several factors affect the rate at which alcohol is absorbed into the body tissues. For example, food in the stomach—especially fatty foods or proteins—slows the absorption of alcohol. Nonalcoholic substances in beer,

TERMS

dangerous (high-risk or binge) drinking: drinking behavior that results in unintended or undesirable harmful consequences for oneself and others

ethyl alcohol (ethanol): the consumable type of alcohol that is the psychoactive ingredient in alcoholic beverages; often called grain alcohol

isopropyl alcohol: rubbing alcohol, sometimes used as an anesthetic

methyl alcohol: wood alcohol or methanol

proof: a number assigned to an alcoholic product that is twice the percentage of alcohol in that product

secondhand binge effects: negative experiences caused by another's binge drinking

Dollars and Health Sense

Marketing Alcohol to Youth

Alcohol use is a major health issue among youth. Several thousand middle and high school students report getting drunk every day. Between 20% and 25% of high schoolers report consuming five drinks in a row during the prior two weeks. Alcohol use is responsible for over 5,000 deaths per year among persons younger than 21 years. Americans spend about $130 billion on alcohol each year; underage drinking accounts for about $23 billion of alcohol sales (Foster et al., 2003).

To help curtail alcohol use by youth, the Institute of Medicine, a division of the National Academy of Sciences, and Congress's Sober Truth on Preventing Underage Drinking Act (STOP ACT), want to reduce exposure of youth to alcoholic beverages and alcohol advertising and marketing directed at them. For example, in the mid 1990s, many large American and European alcohol companies created "alcopops," also called clear malts, flavored malt beverages, malternatives, or RTDs (as in "ready to drink"), that combine sweet flavors with the kick of malt liquor, vodka, or rum to create a taste that is less bitter than that of other alcoholic drinks.

The market for alcopops is supposed to be women between the ages of 21 (the legal age for alcohol consumption in the United States) and 30. However, it is evident that teen girls are also pursued as customers (American Medical Association, 2004). Teen girls report seeing or hearing more alcopops ads on TV, radio, billboards, the Internet, and in magazines than women 21 or older do. About one-third of teen girls have tried alcopops, preferring them to any other alcoholic beverage, whereas women over 21 prefer alcopops *least* among alcoholic beverages. These statistics support the argument that the alcohol industry is using alcopops as a gateway for teen women to the world of real alcohol consumption.

Youth (ages 12–20) are exposed to a large number of alcohol advertisements on TV, radio, and in magazines (Center for Alcohol Marketing and Youth, 2008). The average TV-watching 12- to 20-year old sees about 300 alcohol advertisements per year, principally on cable TV. About 40% of TV ads are placed on programs with a large youth audience. The U.S. Surgeon General and a variety of youth health advocates want alcohol companies not to advertise in programming in which youth represent more than 15% of the audience.

Beverage companies that claim they are not contributing to the underage drinking problem and helping to develop a new generation of alcoholics are doing just what the cigarette companies did for decades—deny everything as long as the product is legal and profitable.

wine, and cocktails can also slow absorption of alcohol. The presence of carbon dioxide in beverages, such as champagne, sparkling wines, beer, and carbonated mixed drinks, increases the rate of alcohol absorption. That is why people feel intoxicated more quickly when drinking champagne or beer, especially on an empty stomach. The higher the alcohol content in a drink, the faster it is absorbed.

The concentration of alcohol in the blood is called the **blood alcohol content (BAC),** which is measured in grams of alcohol per deciliter of blood. A simple way to estimate BAC is to assume that ingesting one standard drink per hour (one beer, one glass of wine, one mixed drink), which contains approximately one-half ounce of ethyl alcohol, produces a BAC of 0.02 in a 150-pound male. Thus, the BAC of an average-sized man who drinks five beers during the first hour at a party will be 0.10; this level of alcohol in the blood violates the drinking-and-driving laws of most states. This shorthand method of approximating BAC changes depending on a person's body size, body composition (e.g., muscle, fat), and sex. All other things being equal, after ingesting the same amount of alcohol, the BAC of a large person is less than that of a smaller person because the alcohol is diluted more in the large person's tissues. Women tend to have a higher BAC from the same number of drinks as men because they generally weigh less than men, have pro-portionately more body fat (which does not absorb alco-

hol as readily as muscle and other tissues), have sex hormones that tend to increase alcohol absorption and decrease its elimination, and tend to absorb more alcohol from the stomach.

Alcohol is eliminated from the body in two ways. About 10% is excreted unchanged through sweat, urine, or breath (hence the use of breath analyzers to test for drinking). The portion of alcohol that is not excreted (about 90%) is broken down primarily by the liver (metabolized), ultimately winding up as carbon dioxide and water. The liver detoxifies alcohol at a rate of about one-half ounce per hour; there is no way to speed up the process. Sobering-up remedies, such as drinking a lot of coffee, taking a cold shower, or engaging in vigorous exercise, do not accelerate the rate at which the liver removes alcohol from the body.

The Hangover

An occasional consequence of drinking alcohol is a **hangover,** which may involve stomach upset, headache, fatigue, weakness, shakiness, irritability, and sometimes vomiting after drinking too much. The frequency and severity of hangovers vary. The particular factors in alcohol that cause a hangover are unknown, but several causes have been suggested:

- When alcohol is present in the body, normal liver functions may slow to break down the alcohol. This slowdown may reduce the amount of sugar the

Table 18.3

Behavioral Effects of Alcohol in a 150-Pound Male

Number of drinks	Ounces of alcohol	BAC* (g/dl)	Approximate time for removal	Effects
1 beer, glass of wine, or mixed drink	1/2	0.02	1 hour	Feeling relaxed or "loosened up"
2½ beers, glasses of wine, or mixed drinks	1¼	0.05	2½ hours	Feeling "high"; decrease in inhibitions; increase in confidence; judgment impaired
5 beers, glasses of wine, or mixed drinks	2½	0.10	5 hours	Memory impaired; muscular coordination reduced; slurred speech; euphoric or sad feelings
10 beers, glasses of wine, or mixed drinks	5	0.20	10 hours	Slowed reflexes; erratic changes in feelings
15 beers, glasses of wine, or mixed drinks	7½	0.30	15–16 hours	Stuporous, complete loss of coordination; little sensation
20 beers, glasses of wine, or mixed drinks	10	0.40	20 hours	May become comatose; breathing may cease
25–30 beers, glasses of wine, or mixed drinks	15–20	0.50	26 hours	Fatal amount for most people

*BAC, blood alcohol content

liver releases into the blood, resulting in temporary hypoglycemia and its resultant fatigue, irritability, and headache.

- Alcohol may inhibit REM sleep, resulting in fatigue, irritability, and trouble concentrating.
- **Congeners,** which are chemical substances in an alcoholic beverage, or the breakdown products produced in the liver may cause a hangover.
- **Acetaldehyde,** a toxic substance produced when the liver breaks down alcohol, may be responsible for hangover symptoms.

The best way to deal with a hangover is to sleep, to drink juice to replace lost body fluid and blood sugar (alcohol increases urine output), and perhaps to take an analgesic for a headache. Ingesting more alcohol will only prolong the hangover symptoms.

The Effects of Alcohol on Behavior

Pharmacologically, alcohol acts as a central nervous system depressant, which means that it slows certain functions in some parts of the brain. In moderate amounts, alcohol may affect the parts of the brain that control judgment and inhibitions, which is why many people have a drink or two at a party to help "loosen up" or to become less shy and more able to interact freely with others. While some people may talk or laugh more than usual, others may become boisterous, argumentative, irritable, or depressed.

The behavioral effects of alcohol depend on the BAC (**Table 18.3**). At a BAC of 0.02, the "loosening-up" effects of alcohol become manifest. At a BAC of 0.10, the depressant effects of the drug become pronounced, the person may become sleepy, and motor coordination is affected. Speech may become slurred and postural instability may become noticeable.

Alcohol's effects on motor skills, judgment, and reaction times make driving after drinking extremely dangerous. Even after just one or two drinks, although an individual may not be legally drunk, reaction time, perception, and judgment are impaired. Approximately 40% of the nearly 40,000 highway fatalities each year involve people who are intoxicated. Highway accidents are among the 10 leading causes of death in the United States. The prevalence of driving after drinking is highest among full-time college students (34%), followed by part-time students (32%), and nonstudent young adults (28%) (Paschall, 2003).

Each year there are more than 120 million episodes of alcohol-impaired driving in the United States (Liu et al., 1997). Men in the 21 to 34 age group have the highest frequency of alcohol-impaired driving; men in the 18 to 20 age group have the second-highest frequency, despite the fact that all states prohibit drinking for persons under age 21. By contrast, the rate of alcohol-impaired driving among women in the same age groups is one-fourth that of their male peers. The frequency of alcohol-impaired driving declines as people become middle-aged.

TERMS

acetaldehyde: a toxic substance produced when the liver breaks alcohol down

blood alcohol content (BAC): the amount of alcohol in the blood

congeners: flavorings, colorings, and other chemicals present in alcoholic beverages

hangover: unpleasant physical sensations resulting from excessive alcohol consumption

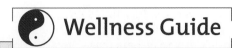

Wellness Guide

One Student's DUI Experience

Early in the morning last summer, I was arrested for driving under the influence of alcohol.

It's not easy to recall what actually happened—I see it through a fog, as if I was watching someone else.

The actual arrest is the blurriest. I was running for those few moments on pure adrenalin and fear. For awhile, I don't even think I was breathing.

It's hard to explain the exact emotions.

It's hard to explain what it feels like to want more than anything to be sober.

It's hard to explain losing complete control of your life for even a short time.

It is hard to explain the feeling of handcuffs.

It's hard to explain what it feels like to sit in a holding cell and bite your lip in the hope of not going to sleep.

One thing for sure is that when those flashing lights appeared in my rearview mirror, all the rationalizations that got me into that car vanished. "It's just around the corner," "I need

to get a friend home," or "No one is on the road at this hour"—none of them mean a thing—zero.

At the jail, it took what seemed like days to be fingerprinted and photographed and to fill out the required forms. Each step was just a little more humiliating than the last.

I am still overwhelmed at how a single, incredibly poor judgment could affect so many parts of my life.

The ramifications will be with me in various ways for the next 3 years—which is as far ahead as I have ever cared to plan.

These shock waves include probation for 3 years, an exorbitant increase in the cost of my car insurance, a restricted driver's license for 90 days (which was agreed upon in lieu of 2 days in jail), and a $600 fine, to name a few.

Many of the ramifications cannot be quantified. There was the call home, a couple of days of generally feeling lousy, and the unshakable sense that I had proven myself a fool.

Through all of it, however, I have some things to be thankful for.

On the top of that very short list is the fact that I didn't kill anyone.

Having struggled to come to terms with the arrest, it is impossible to imagine . . . for that there is no atonement.

Also on that list is the discovery of some very supportive people in my life, all of whom said not that what happened was okay, but that I was going to be okay. I turned to my parents and friends for help, and no one turned away—I am thankful.

Whether this column will keep anyone from driving drunk is doubtful. If I had read this column before my arrest, I would have thought of a hundred reasons why it would never have applied to me—but I would have been wrong.

Weight	Drinks (2-hour period) $1\frac{1}{2}$ oz. liquor or 12 oz. beer											
100	1	2	3	4	5	6	7	8	9	10	11	12
120	1	2	3	4	5	6	7	8	9	10	11	12
140	1	2	3	4	5	6	7	8	9	10	11	12
160	1	2	3	4	5	6	7	8	9	10	11	12
180	1	2	3	4	5	6	7	8	9	10	11	12
200	1	2	3	4	5	6	7	8	9	10	11	12
220	1	2	3	4	5	6	7	8	9	10	11	12
240	1	2	3	4	5	6	7	8	9	10	11	12

Be careful driving
BAC = up to 0.05%

Driving will be impaired
BAC = 0.05% – 0.08%

Do not drive
BAC = 0.08 – 0.10%

Effects of Drinking on Driving

Source: The Aggie (April 10, 1990). University of California, Davis. Reprinted with permission.

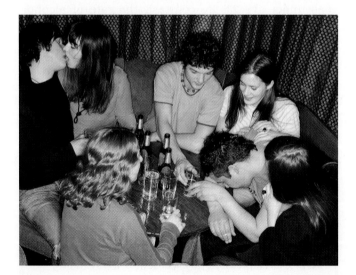

Drunkenness at parties can lead to actions and feelings that one regrets the next day—and sometimes for much longer.

Besides impaired driving, alcohol consumption contributes to arguments, fights, jeopardized relationships, employee absenteeism, school failure, and lost jobs. According to the National Institute on Drug Abuse, 30% of all drinkers aged 18 to 25 reported that they had become "aggressive" while drinking; 19% had been in "heated arguments"; and 11% had been absent from school or work as a result of drinking. Most homicides, assaults, robberies, sexual offenses, and incidents of domestic violence are alcohol-related (Brewer & Swahn, 2005).

Sexual Behavior

The effects of alcohol on sexual desire and performance vary from person to person, and depend on the BAC. In some individuals, small amounts of alcohol may dispel uncomfortable feelings about sex and may facilitate sexual arousal. Higher amounts of alcohol (a BAC of 0.10 or more) may cause problems for males, such as difficulty getting and maintaining an erection or ejaculating, and for females, such as inadequate vaginal lubrication and difficulty reaching orgasm. Even at moderate BACs, some individuals are too intoxicated to give and receive sexual pleasure effectively.

Alcohol consumption may contribute to a variety of undesired consequences of sexual behavior. While intoxicated, people can forget to use a birth control method or simply ignore the practice altogether and thus become unintentionally pregnant. Not using condoms or having sex with a stranger increases the risk of transmission of STDs and AIDS. Alcohol can blur one's judgment and can lead to unintended sexual experiences.

Acquaintance rape has been linked to alcohol consumption on college campuses (see Chapter 23). A sexual assault study revealed that 26% of men who acknowledged committing sexual assault on a date reported being intoxicated; 29% reported being slightly intoxicated. In this same study, 21% of the women who were victims of sexual aggression on a date reported being intoxicated; 32% were slightly intoxicated. A woman's alcohol consumption may prevent her from realizing that her friendly behavior is being perceived as seductive; men may be inclined to perceive friendly cues from a woman as a sign of sexual interest.

Other Effects of Alcohol

Alcohol can impair the functioning of body organs other than the brain. Alcohol can irritate the organs of the gastrointestinal (GI) tract—the esophagus, stomach, intestine, pancreas, and liver—causing upset or irritation, nausea, vomiting, or diarrhea. Alcohol can also dilate arteries and cause bloodshot eyes. Dilation of arteries in the arms, legs, and skin can cause a drop in blood pressure and decrease body heat, explaining why people occasionally feel flushed when they drink. Giving alcohol to people to "warm them up" actually produces the opposite physiological effect.

Alcohol should not be ingested simultaneously with other central nervous system depressants such as tranquilizers, sedatives, and antihistamines, which are found in cold medicines. In many instances, the depressant effects of alcohol and the other drug interact so that the combined effects of the two drugs is greater than the simple additive effects of either drug taken separately. Seemingly reasonable amounts of alcohol taken with another depressant drug can dangerously suppress brain function and respiration (**Table 18.4**).

Long-Term Effects

Long-term heavy drinking can affect immune, endocrine, and reproductive functions and can cause neurological problems, including dementia, blackouts, seizures, hallucinations, and peripheral neuropathy. Various cancers associated with heavy drinking include cancers of the lip, oral cavity, pharynx, larynx, esophagus, stomach, colon, rectum, tongue, lung, pancreas, and liver. Long-term heavy drinking can also increase the risk of chronic gastritis, hepatitis, hypertension, cirrhosis of the liver, and coronary heart disease.

Chronic alcoholic men may become "feminized," with breast enlargement and female body hair patterns. Chronic alcoholic women may experience menstrual disturbances, loss of secondary sex characteristics, and infertility. Women who drink heavily experience more gynecological problems and have surgery more often than women who do not.

Fetal Alcohol Syndrome

Alcohol can harm the health of anyone, man or woman, young or old. Even a fetus can be damaged by alcohol. Numerous kinds of birth defects and mental retardation may result from ingestion of alcohol by pregnant women—a condition known as **fetal alcohol syndrome** (see Chapter 15). Fetal alcohol syndrome is estimated to be the third leading cause of birth defects and mental retardation among newborns. Because the harmful effects on the fetus are believed to occur during the first few weeks of prenatal development, a time during which much of the nervous system is being formed, women should refrain from drinking if they are trying to become pregnant or if they suspect they are pregnant. Studies have also shown that the level of alcohol in the fetus's blood may be 10 times greater than the

Table 18.4

Alcohol and Drugs That Don't Mix

Alcohol should not be consumed when taking drugs such as these.

Drug	Dangerous interaction
Acetaminophen (Tylenol, Anacin-3)	Moderate use plus alcohol can cause liver damage.
Aspirin (Anacin, Excedrin)	Heavy use plus alcohol can cause bleeding of stomach wall and GI tract.
Antihistamines (Chlor-Trimeton, Benadryl)	Drowsiness and loss of coordination increased by alcohol.
Tranquilizers, sedatives (Valium, Dalmane, Miltown)	Alcohol increases their effects.
Painkillers (codeine, Percodan, morphine)	Alcohol increases sedation and reduces ability to concentrate.
Barbiturates (Amytal, Seconal, phenobarbital)	Potentially fatal. *Never* use with alcohol.

TERMS

fetal alcohol syndrome: birth defects and mental disabilities caused by ingestion of alcohol by the mother during pregnancy

BAC of the mother. This explains why even a couple of drinks early in pregnancy can endanger normal fetal development.

Health Benefits of Alcohol

A variety of studies have shown an association between consuming a small amount of alcohol (about a drink per day) and a lower risk of heart disease and stroke (Klatsky, 2008). The benefits of alcohol consumption were first reported among people in France, where it was noted that despite a diet high in fat, the rate of heart disease is low. This anomaly became known as the "French paradox." At first the French paradox was explained by the fact that red wine is widely consumed in France, and that substances in red wine, called flavonoids, were antioxidants that produced the heart-healthy effects. However, several studies have shown that the healthful effects of drinking are not specific to the type of drink, and hence it is concluded that such effects are caused by ethanol. The reasons for the protective effects of alcohol have not yet been elucidated. Alcohol consumption is related to increased blood levels of high-density lipoproteins (HDL, so called good cholesterol). Alcohol consumption also may reduce the risk of blood clots.

The enzyme responsible for detoxifying alcohol in the body is called *alcohol dehydrogenase*. It comes in three different forms, depending on a person's genetic makeup. The people who have the slow oxidizing form of the enzyme experience the benefits of moderate alcohol consumption in preventing heart attacks (Heidrich et al., 2007), so moderate drinking is not necessarily beneficial for everyone.

Alcohol Abuse and Alcoholism

Alcohol abuse and alcoholism are major drug problems in the United States. Approximately 61% of Americans of different ages, religions, races, educational backgrounds, and socioeconomic status have had problems with alcohol. More than 3 million American teenagers between ages 14 and 17 have a drinking problem. More than a third of all suicides involve alcohol. The American Psychiatric Association defines **alcohol abuse** as alcohol-related impairment or distress occurring within a 12-month period, characterized by one or more of the following:

> I don't even know what street Canada is on.
>
> *Al Capone*

- Failure to fulfill major obligations at work, school, or home
- Recurrent alcohol use in situations that are physically hazardous (e.g., driving an automobile or operating a machine)
- Recurrent alcohol-related legal problems (e.g., arrests for substance-related disorderly conduct)

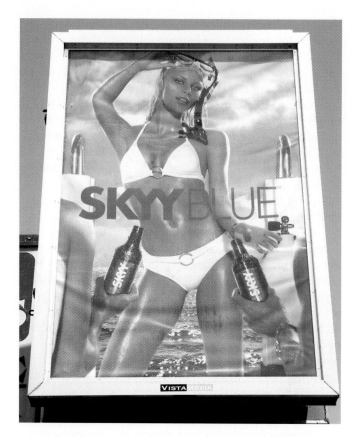

Alcohol advertisements, like cigarette ads, emphasize the connections among drinking, sex, and fun.

- Persistent or recurrent social or interpersonal problems caused or exacerbated by the effects of alcohol

Alcoholism is characterized by an intense craving for alcohol, an inability to control one's drinking, and physical dependence on alcohol. Withdrawal symptoms, including **delirium tremens (DTs),** characterized by hallucinations and uncontrollable shaking, may occur when a person affected by alcoholism is deprived of alcohol. About 61% of Americans have abused alcohol at some point in their lives; about 4.8% currently do so. Alcoholism has affected about 12.5% of Americans at some point in their lives—3.8% currently (Hasin et al., 2007).

Problem drinking can cause numerous negative consequences. Job and school performance can be impaired, family relationships and friendships can be destroyed, and drunk driving may cause financial problems, injuries, legal problems, and fatalities. Because alcohol supplies calories, alcoholics are rarely hungry. They may have vitamin deficiency syndromes, which result in mental confusion and loss of muscular coordination.

Researchers at the U.S. National Institute on Alcohol Abuse and Alcoholism (Moss, Chen, & Yi, 2007) have found that alcohol dependence displays three distinct patterns, as follows:

- Young adults, who rarely seek help for drinking problems, and who have moderately high levels of periodic heavy drinking, relatively low rates of

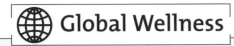

Global Wellness

Alcohol Abuse Is a Worldwide Problem

The World Health Organization (WHO) estimates that 2 billion people worldwide consume alcoholic beverages and that 76.3 million people have alcohol use disorders. The amount of alcohol consumed varies considerably around the world (Table 18.5).

Alcohol misuse is responsible for 1.8 million annual deaths worldwide (3.2% of total deaths), more than sanitation problems and high cholesterol (**Figure 18.3**). It is the leading risk factor for disease in low-mortality developing countries and the third largest risk factor in developed countries. Alcohol problems include intoxication (drunkenness), dependence, and causation of dozens of types of injuries and chronic diseases,

including esophageal cancer, liver cancer, cirrhosis of the liver, homicide, epileptic seizures, motor vehicle accidents, assault, domestic violence, homicide, and suicide.

Recognizing that alcohol-related problems are the result of a complex interplay between individual use of alcoholic beverages and cultural, economic, physical environment, political, and social forces, many countries are adopting measures to control supply and/or affect the demand for alcoholic beverages, attempting to alter hazardous drinking patterns, and implementing health services to treat problem drinkers. For example, countries can limit alcohol use by instituting high alcohol taxes, restricting alcohol advertising, and limiting availability by outright prohibition, rationing, and state monopolies; they can promote beverages with low or no alcohol content and regulate the density of outlets, hours, and days of sale, drinking locations, and minimum drinking age; they can institute health promotion campaigns and school-based education. Also, countries can set strict drinking-and-driving laws to reduce alcohol-related car crashes, injuries, and deaths. For example, in most European countries, the legal limit for alcohol in the blood (blood alcohol content, or BAC) is 0.05%; in some countries it is zero. (In the United States it is 0.08%.) In Germany, failing a breathalyzer test for blood alcohol content results in immediate suspension of one's driver's license. In Norway, two DUIs within a five-year span result in loss of one's driver's license for life. That's also the penalty for the first DUI in Russia.

Table 18.5

Adult Alcohol Consumption in Regions of the World

Region	Beverages mostly consumed	Total consumption (liters/yr)
Eastern Mediterranean (e.g., Afghanistan, Pakistan)	Spirits and beer	0.6
Eastern Mediterranean (e.g., Iran, Sudan)	Spirits and beer	1.3
Southeast Asia (e.g., India, Bangladesh)	Spirits	2.0
Southeast Asia (e.g., Indonesia, Thailand)	Spirits	3.1
Africa (e.g., Nigeria, Algeria)	Fermented beverages	4.9
Western Pacific (e.g., China, Philippines, Vietnam)	Spirits	5.0
Americas (e.g., Bolivia, Peru)	Spirits and beer	5.1
Africa (e.g., Ethiopia, South Africa)	Fermented beverages	7.1
Europe (e.g., Bulgaria, Poland, Turkey)	Spirits	8.3
Western Pacific (e.g., Australia, Japan)	Beer and spirits	8.5
Americas (e.g., Brazil, Mexico)	Beer and spirits	9.0
Americas (e.g., Canada, Cuba, U.S.A.)	Beer and spirits	9.3
Europe (e.g., Germany, France, U.K.)	Wine and beer	12.9
Europe (e.g., Russia, Ukraine)	Spirits	13.9

Source: Data from World Health Organization, Status Report on Alcohol, 2004.

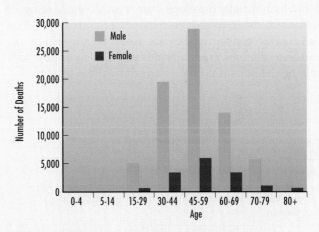

■ **Figure 18.3**

Global Deaths from Alcohol Use Disorders, 2001

Source: Data from World Health Organization, Global Status Report on Alcohol, 2004.

coexisting mental and physical illness, and a low rate of alcohol dependence in their families
- Adults with considerable alcohol dependence in their families, coexisting mental illness and other drug use disorders, low levels of psychosocial functioning, and high degrees of help-seeking
- Adults who develop alcohol dependence late in life and have low rates of periodic heavy drinking,

┃TERMS┃

alcohol abuse: frequent, continued use of alcohol; binge drinking

alcoholism: loss of control over drinking alcohol

delirium tremens (DTs): hallucinations and uncontrollable shaking sometimes caused by withdrawal of alcohol in alcohol-dependent individuals

medium/low levels of mental or physical illness, moderate levels of help-seeking, and high psycho-social functioning

It is hoped that delineation of these patterns will enhance understanding of the causes, best treatments, and prevention of alcohol dependency.

The cause or causes of problem drinking and alcoholism are unknown, although hypotheses abound. Before the advent of modern psychology and medicine, alcohol abuse was thought to be a manifestation of immorality and irreligiousness. Some people still hold that view, but many professionals (and problem drinkers) interpret alcohol abuse as a behavioral disorder or a medical disease. For example, some people may drink to feel better about themselves or to try to cope with life's adversities. Instead, they may add a drinking problem to their other problems.

Some evidence indicates that, at least for some people, alcoholism may have a biological basis, either because people metabolize alcohol differently or because their brains respond differently to alcohol. Some experts resist considering alcohol abuse a disease because doing so may remove the sense of personal and social responsibility for problem drinking. Others argue that calling alcohol abuse a "disease" fosters successful treatment because it removes the stigma, lessens guilt, and offers a supervised and presumably scientifically based plan for treatment.

The Phases of Alcoholism

Alcoholism usually develops from a prealcoholic stage of needing to drink to relieve tensions and anxieties. The prealcoholic phase may last for years, during which tolerance to alcohol gradually develops. Progression to a state of alcoholism is characterized by three phases:

- *The warning phase.* In this first stage of alcoholism, problem drinkers increase tolerance for alcohol and become more preoccupied with drinking. For example, when invited to a party they may ask what alcoholic beverages will be served rather than who is going to be there. In this stage problem drinkers may sneak drinks often and may deny that they are drinking too much. **Blackouts** may also occur. Blackouts are periods in which others observe the drinker as behaving normally or abnormally, but the drinker has no recall of events that happened while drinking.

- *The crucial phase.* This phase of alcoholism is characterized by loss of control over how much alcohol is consumed. The person may not drink every day, but cannot control the amount of alcohol consumed once drinking has begun. In this stage, the problem drinker may rationalize drinking behavior and actually believe that there are good reasons for heavy drinking. Alcoholics may still carry out responsibilities (e.g., housework, job, schoolwork) for some time, and they may employ a series of strategies to keep the family from rejecting them, including promises to stop drinking. Often alcoholics' extravagant measures to prove they do not have a drinking problem appear successful, but eventually they begin drinking heavily again. At this point the problem with alcohol is sometimes blamed on the kind of drinks preferred or on the usual place of drinking; as a result, problem drinkers may change to a different form of alcoholic beverage or to a different place in which to drink.

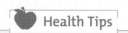 Health Tips

Are You a Problem Drinker?

The CAGE questionaire is a diagnostic tool for alcohol problems.

C = Concern by the person that there is a problem

A = Apparent to others that there is a problem

G = Grave consequences

E = Evidence of dependence or tolerance

Answer these questions:

1. Have you ever felt that you should **C**ut down on your drinking?
2. Have you ever become **A**nnoyed by criticism of your drinking?
3. Have you ever felt **G**uilty about your drinking?
4. Have you ever had a morning **E**ye opener to get rid of a hangover?

One "yes" response indicates possible alcohol abuse.

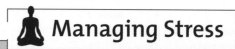 Managing Stress

Breaking Addictive Behaviors

It's a little known fact, but it was psychologist Carl Jung who inspired the Alcoholics Anonymous program. Frustrated with a client unable to change his alcoholism, Jung suggested that his only hope for recovery was to purposefully have a spiritual experience to rid himself of this addictive habit. So, Roland H. did just that. After conquering his addiction, he went on to share this experience with Edwin T., then Bill W., who then went on to co-found Alcoholics Anonymous.

In response to a letter from Bill W., Jung wrote, "His craving for alcohol was the equivalent, on a low level, of the spiritual thirst of our being for wholeness, expressed in medieval language: the union with God. You see alcohol in Latin is *spiritus,* and we use the same words for the highest religious experience as well as for the most depraving poison. The helpful formula therefore is: *Spiritus contra spiritum.*" (Spiritual crises require spiritual cures.)

- *The chronic phase.* In this phase, the alcoholic is dependent on the drug, and drinking behavior consumes all aspects of life. Friends and family have resigned themselves to the problem and may be angry or ignore the alcoholic. At this stage of alcoholism the person may miss work or school occasionally. The health consequences of alcohol abuse may intensify and the person may need medical attention and even hospitalization. When physical addiction to alcohol occurs, continual drinking is needed to prevent withdrawal symptoms. Drinking for days at a time (a **bender**) may take place. The great majority of alcoholics do not wind up on "skid row," but instead struggle with their problem within their families and communities.

The Effects of Alcoholism on the Family

Alcoholism can severely disrupt marital and family relationships. One family member's drinking problem can put stress on all the other members, causing them mental and emotional suffering and sometimes financial hardship. Alcoholism is costly to many people, not just the alcoholic. Seventy-six million Americans, about 43% of the population, have been exposed to alcoholism in the family.

Close relatives of a problem drinker can experience a variety of emotions, ranging from joy and relief when the problem drinker stops drinking for a time to feelings of failure and depression when the problem drinker begins drinking again. In between the highs and lows, family members can feel anger, shame, guilt, pity, and constant anxiety. They may try to cope with the situation in different ways. Some may try to assume responsibility for the problem; others may be designated as scapegoats and blamed for it, while some family members blame others (i.e., other family members, other people) for the drinker's problem. Some may withdraw in silence, whereas others try to maintain their sense of humor. These behaviors are all defenses against the family's psychological pain.

Like the problem drinker, family members may deny the problem, try to rationalize it, isolate themselves from friends and relatives, and, in some cases, actually feel responsible for the other's drinking problem. This **enabling,** or protection process, keeps the alcoholic from feeling responsible for his or her drinking—which is part of the paradox experienced by families of alcoholics. In their attempts to protect the alcoholic, family members may unwittingly contribute to the drinking problem; they may try to protect the alcoholic from serious social consequences of excessive drinking, for instance, making excuses for absenteeism from work or school.

Family members of alcoholics can attend Al-Anon, an organization that helps spouses, families, and friends of alcoholics. Alateen is a similar organization that helps children of alcoholics. Al-Anon and Alateen help family members understand how alcoholism has affected their lives and help them to explore the family relationships that contribute to the alcohol problem. Family therapy (with or without the problem drinker's participation) may help a family find ways to cope with the problem and regain harmony in their family life.

Children of Alcoholics

The National Clearinghouse for Drug and Alcohol Information estimates that there are 28 million children of alcoholics (COAs) in the United States, 11 million of whom are under the age of 18. Adult children of alcoholics (ACOAs) and COAs grew up in families in which one or both parents had a drinking problem. As children, many of these individuals experienced neglect, emotional deprivation, an unstable family environment, and sometimes violence and abuse. As a result, they may have developed ways of thinking and behaving that impair personal and relationship harmony in adulthood. Children of alcoholics are at a high risk of becoming alcoholics themselves.

To numb the emotional pain stemming from parental alcoholism, many COAs learn as children to block from their awareness the truth of their situation—both the fact of a parent's alcoholism and also the emotional pain resulting from it. This tendency is referred to as **denial.** The consequences of denial go beyond issues of parental alcoholism to become a generalized way of approaching life. As adults, many COAs are constricted in their capacities to see the world as it really is and also to experience emotional fulfillment.

Many COAs have a negative self-image and a tendency to be hypercritical of themselves. As children, they believe themselves to be the cause of their parents' erratic, violent behavior. Indeed, sometimes the troubled parents reinforced this assumption by blaming their children for their problems. The children not only come to believe themselves to be "bad," but also they tend to believe they are responsible for everyone else's emotions. Thus, they become so other-focused, that they have no lives of their own, a characteristic called **codependency.**

TERMS

bender: several days of binge drinking

blackout: failure to recall normal or abnormal behavior or events that occurred while drinking

codependency: a relationship pattern in which the nonaddicted family members identify with the alcoholic

denial: refusal to admit you (or someone else) have a drinking problem

enabling: denial of, or excuses for, the excessive drinking by an alcoholic to whom one is close

Another consequence of growing up in an alcoholic family is the tendency to try to control situations and other people. Because family life was unstable and painful, many ACOAs come to believe that their interpersonal environment is likely at any moment to become emotionally painful, violent, or disruptive. Thus, ACOAs tend to be constantly anxious and hypervigilant for signs of danger. To minimize the threat (experienced as criticism, abandonment, or abuse), ACOAs tend to be compliant and agreeable and actively try to please. Believing that others cannot be trusted and that the world must be made safe, ACOAs also try to be totally self-reliant and in control of their lives.

Denial, a negative self-image, the tendency to take responsibility for others, the need to control oneself and the environment, and other characteristics help a COA survive childhood in an alcoholic family. Unfortunately, in adulthood these same "survival" mechanisms limit the opportunity to grow and develop unique individual qualities and to experience healthy interpersonal relationships. Fortunately, these self-limiting beliefs and behaviors can be changed through counseling, 12-step programs such as Codependents Anonymous, and various spiritual practices.

Seeking Help: Treatment Options

The situation of problem drinkers and alcoholics is serious but not hopeless. Recovery is possible if the person is strongly motivated to stop drinking. Moreover, as in other aspects of health, "an ounce of prevention is worth a pound of cure."

Sometimes the motivation to stop drinking comes in the form of a threat—a drinking-related legal problem or illness, severe disruption of family life, the loss of a job. The motivation to stop drinking can also come from the person's own resolve to stop his or her self-destructive behavior and to stop feeling helpless, hopeless, and confused.

Alcoholics Anonymous (AA), the worldwide non-profit self-help organization, has assisted many people to get on the road back to wellness and enjoyment of life. AA bases its program on total sobriety, anonymity, and a step-by-step program of recovery. The environment at AA meetings is relaxing, caring, and open. Members share their experiences, strengths, and hopes with each other, with the goal of helping new and old members identify and learn more about their own problems with alcohol. Practical tips on how to remain sober are shared, and telephone numbers are exchanged so that a member can contact another member if stressful situations arise that previously led to drinking.

Alcoholics Anonymous emphasizes that sobriety is a state of mind, which means that recovering from a drinking problem involves changing values, attitudes, and lifestyles. The AA program helps problem drinkers honestly examine their feelings, recognize their limitations, and accept responsibility for past wrongs. For problem drinkers, remaining sober is an ongoing process, which involves finding new ways to satisfy emotional, spiritual, and social needs.

Besides AA, problem drinkers can receive help from individual and group psychotherapy. Many therapists are trained specifically to help problem drinkers and their families recover. Also, certain medicines may help. Disulfuram (Antabuse) causes uncomfortable physical and mental feelings when alcohol is ingested. Naltrexone can help reduce the craving for alcohol. Acamprosate reduces withdrawal symptoms. Several other drugs are being tested to help with alcohol addiction (Miller, 2008).

Responsible Drinking

Each person has the option of drinking or abstaining from alcohol. Each of you has the responsibility for determining the occasions for drinking and the amounts of alcohol that you consume. If you drink, here are some guidelines to remember:

- Make sure that alcohol use improves your social interactions and does not harm or destroy them.
- Drink slowly and avoid mixing alcohol with other drugs.
- Be sure that using alcohol enhances your general sense of well-being and does not make either you or other persons feel disgusted with your actions.
- If you plan to drink, decide beforehand that you will not drive and designate someone who will not drink to be the driver.

In addition to being responsible for your own drinking habits, you can also help others to drink responsibly. Respect the wishes of the person who chooses to abstain from drinking and don't push drinks on people at parties. If you are giving a party, be sure to provide alternatives to alcohol. You may also offer places to sleep for those who have been drinking and should not drive home. Remember to eat when you drink and to provide food at your parties.

There is no evidence to indicate that total abstinence from alcohol is necessary for health and wellness. On the other hand, there is a great deal of evidence showing that excessive alcohol use can destroy personal health and family relationships, can cause traffic deaths and suicides, and can produce birth defects in newborns. We believe that you can significantly improve your health and happiness by developing responsible drinking habits while you are young and maintaining moderate drinking habits throughout life.

Critical Thinking About Health

1. After about a month it was clear that inviting Chris to be their roommate had been a brilliant move. With a 3.9-plus GPA, Chris was a fountain of help with every subject from history to chemistry. Getting into law school was a foregone conclusion. The real question was how to get Chris on "Jeopardy!"

   When midterm exams rolled around, the roommates noticed that Chris was coming home every day with a 12-pack of beer—six cans would disappear before dinner and the rest disappeared as the night's studying progressed. Although Chris showed no signs of impairment from ingesting this quantity of alcohol, the roommates were concerned.
   a. What concerns might the roommates have? If you were Chris's roommate, would you be concerned?
   b. Given Chris's obvious success in school and the fact that Chris shows no outward sign of impairment, would you agree or disagree that Chris has a problem with alcohol?
   c. Do you think Chris's roommates should try to change Chris's drinking behavior, or is it none of their business?

2. "I don't like alcohol all that much. And it's never fun to wake up and find that you vomited all over yourself and don't remember doing it. There have been times I don't know how I got home, and I only hope that whoever drove the car wasn't as wasted as I was. Still, you need it. There's no better way to destress after a hard week of school. And you need to drink so you can be loose at a party. No one wants to dance with a loser, much less have sex with them."

   What's your opinion on this person's attitude? If you disagree with this student's philosophy, explain your reasons.

3. Every summer, State U. invites the parents of incoming students to "Parents' Day," a chance to visit the campus and talk to faculty, students, and administrators. Last summer, Dr. Meredith, one of the university's newest faculty members, gladly volunteered to give a "sample lecture" on paleontology to the parents and to chat with them at the luncheon in the Faculty Dining Room.

   A father of an incoming female student engaged Dr. Meredith in conversation about his daughter's likely experiences living in the college dormitory and swimming on the swim team.

   "My daughter's never been away from home before," said the father. "I want to be sure she'll be OK."

   Dr. Meredith silently gulped hard, for he knew that the dormitories had the reputation for massive illegal drinking during the first month or two of the school year, and that the swim coach would drink beer with the team members after swim meets.
   a. Does the father have anything to be concerned about?
   b. Should Dr. Meredith tell the father about alcohol use at the college?
   c. To avoid having to encounter another parent with similar concerns, Dr. Meredith vowed never again to help out at Parents' Day. What else could Dr. Meredith do to avoid such unpleasant experiences? Remember that Dr. Meredith is new at the university and without tenure.
   d. What is the campus climate toward tolerating alcohol use among students on your campus?

4. A college needs an electronic scoreboard for its football stadium, and a beer company is willing to buy it in exchange for exclusive advertising rights on the scoreboard and in the football game programs. The college president is against this deal, arguing that it promotes drinking on campus. However, the athletic director and the president of the alumni association favor it, arguing that it's vital to have the new scoreboard and besides, "beer and college always have gone together and always will, and there's nothing wrong with it."
   a. Do you favor or object to the scoreboard deal?
   b. Do you agree or disagree with the college president about the fact that advertising promotes drinking?
   c. Do you agree or disagree with the athletic director and alumni president that beer and college always have and always will go together?

Health in Review

- Alcohol abuse is a major drug problem in the United States. Consumption of alcohol is responsible for almost half of all highway fatalities and for numerous social, family, and health problems.
- Alcoholic beverages contain ethyl alcohol, which is produced by the action of yeast on sugar (fermentation) in grains and the juices of berries and fruits. Beer and wine are direct products of fermentation; "hard" liquor, such as whiskey, vodka, rum, and brandy, is made from distilled fermented liquids. Most standard portions of alcoholic beverages contain one-half ounce of ethyl alcohol.
- Social and normative influences on drinking behavior are evident in specific drinking patterns among college students. Drinking on campus increases the risk of violence, including sexual assault.
- Alcohol enters the bloodstream within minutes after ingestion. The physical and behavioral effects of alcohol depend on the blood alcohol content (BAC). A BAC of 0.02 produces a "loosening up"

effect. A BAC of 0.10 seriously impairs motor coordination and judgment; in most states it is illegal to drive with a BAC of 0.10.
- Frequent and constant use of alcohol can lead to physical dependence and tolerance for the drug (alcoholism). Alcoholism develops in stages, starting with the inability to control drinking and advancing to complete physical dependence.
- Alcoholics may encounter severe health problems, and their personal lives, family relationships, and friendships may be disrupted. Millions of children who grew up in families where one or both parents were alcoholics experience personal problems as adults that stem from their childhoods.
- Organizations such as Alcoholics Anonymous and individual or group psychotherapy can help people recover from problem drinking and alcoholism. Alcohol abuse can be prevented by taking responsibility for one's drinking behavior.

Health and Wellness Online

The Web contains a wealth of information about health and wellness. By accessing the Internet using Web browser software, you can gain a new perspective on many topics presented in *Health and Wellness*, Tenth Edition. Access the Jones and Bartlett Publishers Web site at **health.jbpub.com/hwonline**.

References

American College Health Association. (2008). National college health assessment. Retrieved September 18, 2008, from http://www.acha-ncha.org/

American Medical Association. (2004). Teenage girls targeted for sweet-flavored alcoholic beverages. Retrieved November 7, 2005, from http://www.alcoholpolicymd.com/press_room/Press_releases/girlie_drinks_release.htm

Brewer, R.D., & Swahn, M.H. (2005). Binge drinking and violence. *Journal of the American Medical Association, 294,* 616–618.

Center for Alcohol Marketing and Youth. (2008). Youth exposure to alcohol advertising on television, 2001 to 2007. Retrieved September 18, 2008, from http://camy.org/research/tv0608/

Dawson, D. A., et al. (2004). Another look at heavy episodic drinking and alcohol use disorders among college and noncollege youth. *Journal of Studies on Alcohol, 65,* 477–488.

Foege, W.H. (1987). Highway violence and public policy. *New England Journal of Medicine, 316,* 1407–1408.

Foster, S.E., et al. (2003). Adult consumption and expenditures for underage drinking and adult excessive drinking. *Journal of the American Medical Association, 289,* 989–995.

Hasin, D. S., et al. (2007). Prevalence, correlates, disability, and comorbidity of DSM-IV alcohol abuse and dependence in the United States. *Archives of General Psychiatry, 64,* 830–842.

Heidrich, J., et al. (2007). Alcohol consumption, alcohol dehydrogenase, and risk of coronary heart disease. *European Journal of Cardiovascular Prevention and Rehabilitation, 14,* 769–774.

Klatsky, A. (2008). Alcohol, wine, and vascular disease: An abundance of paradoxes. *American Journal of Physiology Heart and Circulatory Physiology, 294,* H582–H583.

Liu, S., et al. (1997). Prevalence of alcohol-impaired driving. *Journal of the American Medical Association, 277,* 122–125.

Miller, G. (2008). Tackling alcoholism with drugs. *Science, 320,* 168–170.

Moss, H. B., Chen, C. M., & Yi, H.Y. (2007). Subtypes of alcohol dependence in a nationally representative sample. *Drug and Alcohol Dependence, 91,* 149–158.

Paschall, M.J. (2003). College attendance and risk-related driving behavior in a national sample of young adults. *Journal of Studies on Alcohol, 64,* 43–49.

Slutske, W. S. (2005). Alcohol use disorders among U.S. college students and their non-college-attending peers. *Archives of General Psychiatry, 62,* 321–327.

Wechsler, H., & Nelson, T. F. (2008, July). What we have learned from the Harvard School of Public Health College Alcohol Study. *Journal of Studies on Alcohol and Drugs, 69,* 481–490.

Yusko, D. A., et al. (2008). Risk for excessive alcohol use and drinking-related problems in college student athletes. *Addictive Behaviors, 33,* 1546–1556.

Suggested Readings

Accoella, J. (2008, May 26). A few too many. *The New Yorker,* 32–37. An informative article about the effects of alcohol on the brain and body and why there is still no cure for the hangover.

Brown, S., & Lewis, V. (2002). *The alcoholic family in recovery: A developmental model.* New York: Guilford. Explains how families deal with abstinence and establish a more stable, yet flexible, family system.

Caetano, R., & Cunradi, C. (2002). Alcohol dependence: A public health perspective. *Addiction, 97,* 633–645. Examines epidemiological research on alcohol dependence and proposes a public health approach that emphasizes prevention and group-level interventions to lower the prevalence of alcohol abuse.

Cook, P. J. (2007). *Paying the tab: The costs and benefits of alcohol control.* Princeton, NJ: Princeton University Press. A comprehensive, in-depth analysis of two centuries of American alcohol-control policies, focusing on the role of taxation as an effective control measure.

Klatsky, A. (2003). Drink to your health. *Scientific American, 288,* 75–83.

Nurnberger, J. I., Jr., & Bierut, L. J. (2007, April). Alcoholism and our genes. *Scientific American,* 46–53. A discussion of the genetic–neurobiological correlates of alcohol dependence.

Sher, K.J., Grekin, E.R., & Williams, N.A. (2005). The development of alcohol use disorders. *Annual Review of Clinical Psychology, 1,* 493–523. Focuses on recent developments in the biological, psychological, and social etiology of alcohol use disorders.

Vallee, B.L. (1998, June). Alcohol in the Western world. *Scientific American,* 80–85. A distinguished scientist examines the history of the role of alcohol in Western civilization.

Wechsler, H., & Wuethrich, B. (2002). *Dying to drink.* New York: Rodale. A thorough discussion of drinking on college campuses.

Recommended Web Sites

Please visit **health.jbpub.com/hwonline** for links to these Web sites.

Alcohol Problems and Solutions
Information compiled by Professor David Hanson, SUNY Potsdam.

Alcohol and Public Health
The U.S. Centers for Disease Control and Prevention's online resource for information on alcohol use and abuse.

College Drinking: Changing the Culture
Research-based information on the nature and extent of dangerous drinking among students.

Getting Help
Links to Alcoholics Anonymous, Al-Anon, Alateen, and other alcohol-problem resources.

U.S. National Institute on Alcohol Abuse and Alcoholism
A reliable source of information on treatments for alcoholism and ongoing research on alcohol abuse.

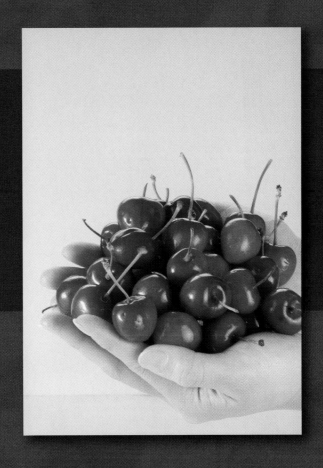

Making Healthy Choices

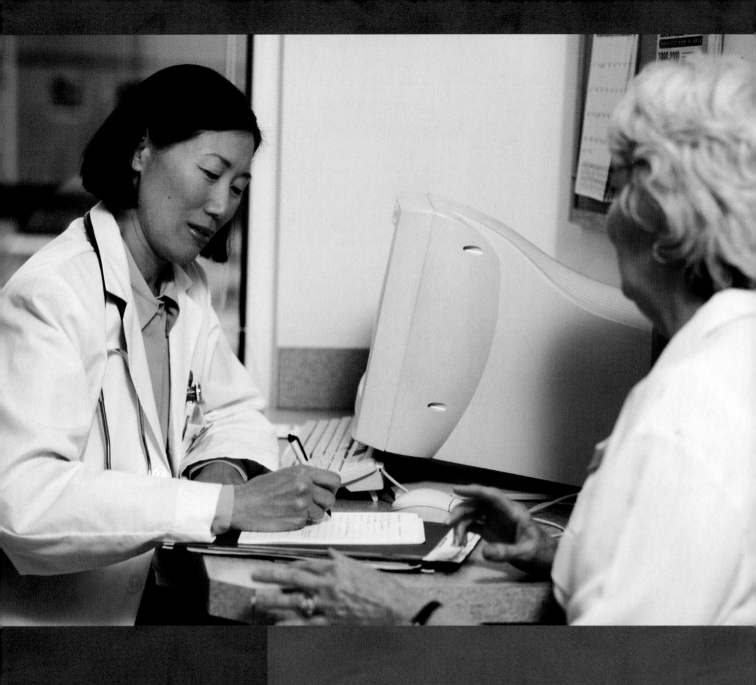

 Health and Wellness Online: **health.jbpub.com/hwonline**

Study Guide and Self-Assessment

Chapter Nineteen

Making Decisions About Health Care

Learning Objectives

1. Describe what you need to know to be an intelligent health care consumer.

2. Discuss the roles of several kinds of health care providers.

3. Compare the four main kinds of private health insurance available in the United States.

4. Discuss several reasons why health care costs have risen so dramatically in the United States in recent years.

5. Explain which populations are served by Medicare and Medicaid.

6. Compare health care and health insurance in Canada and the United States.

7. Discuss some of the problems with the quality of U.S. health care and frequency of medical errors.

8. Discuss the disparities of medical care based on patients' sex, race, and ethnicity.

9. Compare the pros and cons of organ transplants for donors and recipients.

10. List five kinds of cosmetic surgeries that are commonly performed.

Everyone will need health care at some time. People need to go to health care professionals for vaccinations, physical exams, and diagnostic tests and for treatment when sick. Occasionally people need to be hospitalized for serious illness, injury, or surgery. Quality health care and the cost of medical services are among people's most important concerns. Both state and federal governments have been trying to ensure that all citizens have some form of health insurance and can receive health care when needed, but about 46 million people in the United States still do not have health insurance.

> God heals and the doctor takes the fee.
> *Ben Franklin*

Modern medicine has become highly technical and expensive. The consumer of health care services must be able to evaluate the risks and benefits of diagnostic tests, treatments, recommended drugs, or surgery if he or she is to maintain control of decisions that affect health. Understanding your rights as a patient and knowing how to communicate your concerns and needs to health professionals will help you stay healthy and help in the healing process when you become sick.

Being a Wise Health Care Consumer

Making wise decisions about your health is part of self-care and self-responsibility. As health care consumers, we need to make important decisions about the health products we purchase, the health services we select, and the information we receive.

Behaviors that can help protect you from health fraud and unnecessary medical procedures include the following:

- Being well informed and knowing how to make healthy decisions
- Seeking reliable sources of information
- Being skeptical about health claims appearing in news media or advertising
- Avoiding unlicensed practitioners
- Selecting practitioners with great care and asking questions about fees, diagnoses, treatments, and alternative treatments
- Reporting health care fraud and wrongdoing to government regulating agencies

Being a wise health care consumer starts with three basic principles: (1) working in partnership with your health care provider, (2) sharing in health care decisions, and (3) becoming skilled at obtaining health care.

Communication is extremely important in a physician–patient relationship. It is the policy of the American Medical Association that "the patient has the right to receive information from physicians and to discuss the benefits, risks, and costs of appropriate treatment alternatives." Unfortunately, many physicians do not feel that they are obliged to fully inform patients of their options. A physician may feel that her or his religious beliefs or moral values justify not being fully open with patients regarding their options (Curlin et al., 2007). Alternatively, physicians also may recommend unnecessary tests and procedures to boost profits for themselves or their employers or to avoid being sued for medical malpractice. For all of these reasons, you should choose a health care provider in whom you have complete confidence and trust.

As a partner in your own health care, you are responsible for managing minor health problems. At the first sign of a serious health problem, you should observe and record symptoms to share with your health care provider, so that you and your health care provider can better manage problems. When visiting your health care provider, be prepared; you only have a limited time with him or her. Prepare a checklist of questions you want to ask, as well as a list of your symptoms. During your visit state your concerns, describe the symptoms, and ask questions regarding prescribed drugs, the diagnosis, and treatment recommendations. Be open and honest when asked about sexual activity, amount of smoking and drinking, use of prescription or illegal drugs, or other questions you might feel too embarrassed to answer. Being truthful with health care providers is essential if you want your health restored.

The second principle in being a wise health care consumer is shared decision making. In partnership with your health care provider, you should participate actively in every medical decision. You have this right except in the emergency room, where informed consent is not necessary. There are numerous ways to share in health care decisions: (1) Let your doctor know what you want, (2) do your own research, (3) ask why a test or treatment is recommended, (4) ask about alternatives, (5) consider watchful waiting, (6) state your health care preferences, and (7) accept responsibility.

Being skilled at obtaining health care is the third principle. By communicating and partnering with your health care provider, you can become skilled in purchasing health care services. There are many ways to cut the cost of health care without affecting the quality: (1) Exercise self-care and self-responsibility, (2) seek health care from a primary health care provider, (3) reduce unnecessary medical tests, (4) reduce drug use, (5) use specialists only when necessary, (6) use emergency services only for real emergencies, and (7) use hospitals only when recommended by a physician.

Choosing a Health Care Provider

Today's health care system is extraordinarily complex. For most people "going to the doctor" is the most obvious choice. But the doctor is one component of a medical system that includes nurses, physician assistants, physical therapists, paramedics, and a broad range of

Managing Stress

Health Care Professionalism Versus Religious Belief—Why You Need to Know Your Health Care Provider

A physician has a professional obligation to provide all patients nondiscriminatory access to medical services. A pharmacist has a professional obligation to fill all prescriptions for patients without discrimination. These tenets may seem obvious, but they are not practiced all of the time. Claiming violations of their "conscience," some physicians refuse to perform an abortion or refer a patient to another physician who will perform it. Some pharmacists refuse to fill a prescription for emergency contraception brought in by a rape victim and even refuse to return the prescription so that she can take it to another pharmacy (Charo, 2005).

At least 45 states now have "laws of conscience" that allow health care professionals to refuse any service that violates their conscience. Besides not performing an abortion, the list of health care services that could be denied includes:

- Refusing to counsel a patient about the availability of emergency contraceptive pills or even to write a prescription for such pills even for a rape victim
- Refusing to counsel infertile couples as to their options using new reproductive technologies (see Chapter 9)

- Refusing patients' requests that the use of painful or futile treatments be withheld or stopped
- Refusing to vaccinate a child for chicken pox (or even to tell parents about its availability) because the vaccine was developed with the use of tissue from aborted fetuses
- Refusal of a pharmacist to fill any prescription for birth control pills
- Refusal to counsel patients as to their end-of-life options or to follow their health directives

There was a time when health care professionalism meant doing the utmost in every situation to relieve suffering and to help others in distress. Are we entering a period when personal autonomy is more important than relieving suffering, and when "conscience" overrides professional ethics? The author C. S. Lewis wrote: "Of all tyrannies, a tyranny sincerely exercised for the good of its victims may be the most oppressive. It would be better to live under robber barons than under omnipotent moral busybodies. The robber baron's cruelty may sometimes sleep, his cupidity may at some point be satiated; but those who torment us for our own good will torment us without end for they do so with the approval of their own conscience" (Charo, 2005).

technical specialists—people who take blood and x-rays, perform invasive diagnostic tests, change dressings, make casts for broken bones, assist in rehabilitation, and many other functions. Besides doctors and other medical specialists, there are other health care providers that use alternative medicines, sometimes in conjunction with conventional, Western medicine. These include chiropractors, naturopaths, massage therapists, acupuncturists, herbalists, and many others (see Chapter 20). Deciding what kind of health care provider you need for your particular problem is the first step in being a wise health care consumer.

All physicians are trained in and practice modern (Western) medicine that is based on modern scientific principles, experimentation, and clinical trials that determine the efficacy of treatments or medicines. Traditional medicines (mostly Eastern) are based on thousands of years of observation and theories of the universe and of human biology that differ from modern science. Traditional medicine practiced in China, India, Tibet, and other Asian countries is based on herbal remedies and the balancing of human physiology with the elements of nature (see Chapter 20). Most Asian countries now use a mixture of Western and traditional medicines. In the United States, some physicians now incorporate elements of alternative medicines into their practices. People choose health care providers for many different reasons—past experience, knowledge, cultural preferences, affordability, and personal convictions.

Health Care Providers

The delivery of health care to the U.S. population is carried out by an enormous number of people trained in many different specialties (see **Table 19.1**). Physicians, of course, are the primary source of medical advice and care, but their tasks would be impossible to carry out without the help of others. A description of some important health care providers is presented here.

Physician Assistants

Physician assistants (PAs) are trained in many aspects of patient care. They work independently and with the supervision of a physician. PAs supervise other members of the physician's health team and perform complex diagnostic and therapeutic procedures. In busy offices, most patients spend more time interacting with the office PA than with the doctor. The PA can spend more time with the patient than the physician does and usually can answer most of the patient's questions regarding medications or operations.

Nurses

Registered nurses (RNs) are trained to promote health, advise patients on how to prevent disease, and assist in the care of patients. Hospital RNs are in frequent contact with sick patients and monitor their progress, administer medications, and record progress and problems. RNs assist physicians during treatments, surgeries,

Table 19.1

Selected Medical Specialties

After receiving their M.D. degree, physicians can specialize. This involves several additional years of training. Medical specialty boards certify physicians in a specialty by examination. Some medical specialties are described below.

Specialty	Specific focus
Allergy and immunology	Prevention, diagnosis, and treatment of allergic disease
Anesthesiology	Administration of drugs to prevent pain or to induce unconsciousness during surgical operations or diagnostic procedures
Cardiology	Diagnosis and treatment of diseases of the heart and blood vessels, including such problems as heart attacks, hypertension, and stroke
Dermatology	Diagnosis and treatment of skin diseases
Endocrinology	Deals with medical problems that result from abnormalities in the endocrine (hormone) system in the body
Family practice	General medical services for patients and their families
Geriatrics/gerontology	Concerned with problems of the elderly
Hospitalist	A physician who cares only for patients admitted to a hospital
Internal medicine	Diagnosis and nonsurgical treatment of internal organs of the body
Neurology	Diagnosis and nonsurgical treatment of diseases of the brain, spinal cord, and nerves
Obstetrics and gynecology	Care of pregnant women and treatment of disorders of the female reproductive system
Oncology	Diagnosis and treatment of all forms of cancer
Ophthalmology	Medical and surgical care of the eye, including prescription eyeglasses
Orthopedics	Diagnosis and treatment of abnormalities in bone and muscle, especially injuries resulting from sports activities
Pathology	Examination and diagnosis of organs, tissues, body fluids, and excrement
Pediatrics	Medical care of children, usually up to teenage years
Preventive medicine	Prevention of disease through immunization, good health care, and concern with environmental factors
Psychiatry	Treatment of mental and emotional problems
Public health	Subspecialty of preventive medicine that deals with promoting the general health of the community
Radiology	Use of radiation for the diagnosis and treatment of disease
Urology	Treatment of male reproductive system and urinary tract and treatment of female urinary tract

and examinations. Nurses may specialize in such areas as surgical, cancer, maternity, or emergency room care. Other areas of specialization include home health nurses, occupational health nurses, and public health nurses.

Nurse practitioners are RNs with additional training and skills that enable them to provide many primary care services. They take medical histories and perform physical exams. They also counsel patients and make preliminary diagnoses before referring patients to a physician.

Emergency Medical Technicians

Emergency medical care is delivered at home and accident sites by emergency medical technicians (EMTs) and paramedics. EMTs work in hospitals and with police and fire departments. Paramedics have more advanced training that enables them to perform a variety of emergency procedures for sick or injured people needing immediate attention. A trained paramedic will recognize a heart attack victim and begin cardiopulmonary resuscitation (CPR). EMTs and paramedics are trained in ways to safely move seriously injured people and can communicate with hospital physicians to determine the best course of emergency treatment.

Physical Therapists and Occupational Therapists

Physical therapists (PTs) are trained to restore function, improve mobility, and relieve pain of patients suffering from an injury or disease. They try to maintain, restore, and promote overall fitness. Physical therapists usually work in hospitals or medical clinics and work with patients who are referred by a physician for physical therapy. PTs help patients regain mobility and strength and train them in exercises that can further hasten their recovery.

Occupational therapists (OTs) help people in the workplace perform their daily tasks even if they have some disability or injury. They can help workers who spend long hours at a computer or checkout counter to avoid physical and mental stress and avoid a repetitive motion injury (see Chapter 21). They are trained counselors and often work with PTs to help workers recover from illness or injury.

Sports Medicine

Sports medicine involves the coordinated efforts of many different kinds of health care providers and specialists. Because sports or exercise injuries can derive from physiological, psychological, or environmental causes, a variety of specialists is needed for prevention, treatment, and rehabilitation of injuries sustained in physical activities. Surgeons, trainers, coaches, physical therapists, psychologists, and other health care providers are all involved.

Sports medicine originated in ancient Greece and Rome where athletic training and contests were a part of everyday life. Modern sports medicine dates from 1928

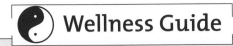

Wellness Guide

How to Have a Successful Interaction with Your Physician

- You should choose a physician you trust and in whose medical skills you have complete confidence. Take the time to find a primary care physician who can satisfy your medical needs. He or she should be someone to whom you can openly express your health concerns.

- Clear and open communication between you and your physician is essential. You should understand the nature of your medical problems and the reasons for any tests that are ordered. You should feel free to ask about different treatment options. You are entitled to all the information pertaining to your condition in language you can understand.

- You should feel confident enough to share with your physician any emotional problems you may have or any stress in your life. This information may be important in arriving at an accurate diagnosis and treatment recommendation. If you are upset in your interaction with a physician, the art of healing is not being practiced.

- Before going to a physician's office, try to relax your mind and body by practicing a meditation or image visualization exercise. This will help calm you when you are discussing your problems with the physician.

- Always remember how suggestible your mind is during a medical consultation. What the physician says about your condition can be as important in the healing process as the treatment. If the physician is positive and encouraging, the likelihood of a cure is increased.

- Although negative statements made by the physician cannot be ignored, try not to let your mind be unduly influenced by them. For example, statements regarding complications, adverse effects, chance of permanent disability, and probable duration of the sickness are general comments derived from statistical data collected from thousands of patients. You are not a statistic but an individual, and averages need not apply to you. Negative statements that are believed tend to produce negative effects on the body.

---

when an Olympic Committee organized the first congress of sports medicine. Today's specialties include cardiology, orthopedic surgery, biomechanics, and traumatology, as well as dietary, drug, and psychological counselors.

Most sports injuries such as abrasions, blisters, and localized tenderness usually are minor and heal without medical attention. However, if they do not heal or if you experience any of the following symptoms, you may need to consult a sports medicine specialist:

- *Comparative weakness:* When one side of the body feels weaker than the other does.
- *Muscle cramps:* A sudden, intense pain caused by a muscle locked in spasm.
- *Numbness:* Loss of sensation in some part of the body; may also be recognized by a tingling or prickling sensation.
- *Reduced range of motion:* Inability to move some part of your body through its normal range of motion.
- *Sprains:* These vary in severity but involve pain, swelling, and torn muscles or ligaments.

Seeing the Doctor

The majority of people who go to a doctor have minor complaints, have come for a routine follow-up of some chronic problem, or may simply need some kind of reassurance. In general, patients fall into three categories: (1) those who think they are sick and are, (2) those who think they are well but are actually sick, and (3) the "worried well" who come for reassurance that they are not sick. This last group may account for as many as half of all patients who are seen by family practice physicians.

Although some physicians encourage annual check-ups, most studies show that frequent medical exams for people who are basically healthy are unnecessary. How often you see a physician depends on your personal needs, but many people go to a physician for minor complaints and illnesses that usually do not require medical attention (**Table 19.2**). Often people are asking more from their doctors than just medicine.

Patient satisfaction with health care usually depends on what occurs in the physician's office. The quality of health care depends to a great degree on the interaction between the physician and the patient. Anxiety about what may be wrong, long waits to see the physician, and a seemingly endless number of tests can contribute to patients' stress. You can increase the chance of a successful encounter with your health care provider if you have a clear understanding of what you want to accomplish during your office visit.

Diagnosis is separate and distinct from treatment. In any illness, there are two important choices: first, admitting that you are sick and finding out what is wrong, which is the process of the **diagnosis**; and second,

TERMS

diagnosis: the cause of a disease or illness as determined by a physician

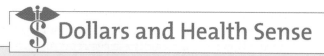

$ Dollars and Health Sense

No More Medicare Payments for Medical Mistakes

When a car mechanic botches an engine job or fails to install brakes properly, he or she doesn't get paid until the repair is completed to the customer's satisfaction. When a doctor makes a mistake, he or she not only gets paid for the original procedure but also gets paid for all procedures and care needed to rectify the original mistake. For example, if an artery becomes clogged again after insertion of a stent, the procedure must be repeated and paid for a second time. However, for some errors the practice is changing, at least for Medicare payments.

As of 2008, eight mistakes that commonly occur in hospitals are no longer reimbursed by Medicare:

- Object left in the body during surgery
- Air embolism
- Blood incompatibility during transfusion
- Catheter-associated urinary tract infection
- Pressure ulcers from lying in one position
- Vascular catheter-associated infection
- Infections at the surgical site after coronary artery bypass graft surgery
- Hospital-acquired injuries—fractures, dislocations, burns, and other injuries

Under previous payment rules, hospitals with poor performance records actually made more money from their mistakes than hospitals with high-performance records. For example, each year at least one million hospitalized patients acquire a urinary tract infection from having a catheter in place as part of their treatment. These hospital-acquired infections cost the health care system more than $400 million a year (Wald & Kramer, 2007).

Table 19.2

The 20 Most Common Reasons for Doctor Visits

One in eight persons goes to the doctor without any complaint or symptom.

Rank	Reason	Rank	Reason
1	Progress visits	11	Gynecological exam
2	Physical exam	12	Visit for medication
3	Pain, etc.—lower extremity	13	No medical reason
4	Pregnancy exam	14	Headache
5	Throat soreness	15	Fatigue
6	Pain, etc.—upper extremity	16	Pain in chest
7	Pain, etc.—back region	17	Well-baby exam
8	Cough	18	Fever
9	Abdominal pain	19	Allergic skin reaction
10	Cold	20	All other symptoms

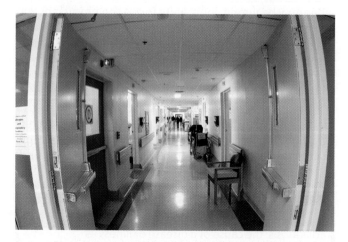

For many people, the hospital is an impersonal and confusing place. Developing good communication with health care providers and knowing your rights as a consumer can help combat those feelings.

deciding what is the best course of treatment, based on the diagnosis.

For example, suppose you have had a slight pain in your chest and the diagnostic tests indicate that you have partial blockage of a coronary artery. One physician might recommend dietary changes, exercises, and a drug to control the pain. Another physician might insist on immediate surgery to correct the condition. Only by obtaining as much information as possible can you make a decision that feels right to you.

Hospitals

At some time in your life you will need to use a health care facility, whether a hospital for planned surgery, an emergency room, or, as you, your parents, or friends become older, nursing home facilities. To make wise decisions concerning health care facilities, it is important to understand the types of facilities available and whether they meet your needs.

Most Americans will be admitted to a hospital at some time during their lives. For many people the hospital experience is confusing and frightening. To cope with this unpleasant reality, one should understand a hospital patient's rights.

On admission to a hospital, a patient is required to sign a consent form delegating all decisions regarding his or her care to the hospital and physicians. In most instances, physicians obtain informed consent for any invasive procedure, either diagnostic or therapeutic, before proceeding. But the amount of information that is given to the patient and how well a patient understands the proposed treatment usually depend on many factors that affect communication between the patient and the physician. The American Hospital Association publishes a Patient's Bill of Rights covering the situations and questions most often encountered by hospital patients. You are entitled to ask for a list of patients' rights in the hospital in which you are a patient.

The most frustrating and anxiety-producing situations for a patient are not understanding what is going to happen and, even worse, not knowing what is happening while being subjected to unfamiliar and uncomfortable procedures. Except in the case of a life-threatening emergency that demands immediate action, you have the right to be fully informed of all medical procedures and the reasons for them. As a patient, you have the responsibility for deciding what you want done. Once you have made that decision, you should understand how to cooperate fully to gain the most benefit.

Understanding Health Insurance

Many kinds of health insurance are available in the United States depending on a person's age, employment status, medical history, and financial resources. Large employers generally supply health insurance for their employees and dependents. The U.S. government provides health insurance for federal employees, members of the armed services, and veterans and their dependents. Federal, state, and local governments provide health insurance for the elderly and the disabled. However, the U.S. government does not provide universal health insurance for all citizens as is the case in all other industrialized nations. Approximately 46 million Americans have no health insurance of any kind.

Health insurance plans fall into two broad categories: (1) fee-for-service plans (also called indemnity plans), and (2) some form of **managed care** plan, which includes health maintenance organizations (HMOs), preferred provider organizations (PPOs), and point-of-service (POS) plans. More than half of all Americans who have health insurance are enrolled in some kind of managed care plan. One of the primary goals of all managed care plans is to control costs of health care. Important features of each health insurance plan are outlined in the following subsections.

Fee-for-Service Plans

Fee-for-service (indemnity) plans are the traditional health insurance plans. These plans allow a person complete freedom in choosing a physician or a hospital. For a fixed monthly fee, these plans will pay some fraction of the patient's medical costs, usually 80%.

Although this type of plan gives a person great flexibility in choosing health care providers, most plans restrict the kinds of services they will pay for. Most will not pay for routine physical exams, immunizations, drug abuse programs, and mental health services. You must understand what health care is covered and what is not and be sure it fits your needs. Also, paying 20% of the costs may be no hardship for minor health care needs. However, if a major illness requires surgery and hospitalization, costs can run into hundreds of thousands of dollars; 20% of such a large sum may be more than most people can afford.

Health Maintenance Organizations

Health maintenance organizations (HMOs) are prepaid health insurance plans that are an alternative to private insurance. The growth of HMOs has surged during the last two decades. HMOs are characterized by four principles defined by Congress in the Health Maintenance Organization Assistance Act of 1973: (1) an organized system of health care that accepts the responsibility to provide health care, (2) an agreed-upon set of comprehensive health maintenance and treatment services, (3) a voluntarily enrolled group of people in a specific geographic region, and (4) reimbursement through a prenegotiated and fixed payment schedule on behalf of the enrollee. An example of a large, successful HMO is the Kaiser-Permanente Medical Care Program, in which physicians emphasize early detection of illness and disease prevention.

Some HMOs have experienced criticism. In contracts between physicians and HMOs, physicians often are prohibited from recommending certain expensive procedures that are not covered by the HMO; they also may receive bonuses for not recommending referrals or for other services. Physicians also are prohibited from disclosing the conditions of their contracts; this so-called gag rule has been severely criticized and has generated a backlash against some HMOs. Although managed health care is well established, some health care analysts believe that eventually health care will have to evolve into some form of more equitable, universal coverage for all Americans.

Choosing the best HMO for your needs is difficult, especially if choices are limited by your place of employment or financial resources. However, some guidelines may help. Some independent organizations attempt to rate the quality of HMOs. Check carefully what each HMO offers, especially for emergency care or for chronic conditions. If you are enrolled in an HMO, find a physician that you trust and with whom you can communicate freely. If you are not satisfied with a diagnosis or treatment, consult another doctor or ask for a second opinion.

TERMS

health maintenance organization (HMO): an organization (either nonprofit or for-profit) of physicians, hospitals, and support staff that provides medical services to members

managed care: systems of health care in which the primary goal is to reduce costs

Preferred Provider Organizations

Preferred provider organizations (PPOs) are a combination of the traditional fee-for-service health care plan and an HMO. Employers or insurance companies negotiate low fee-for-service rates with selected hospitals and health care providers in a specific geographic region. Participants in PPOs must use one of the "preferred" providers if they want their medical bills paid. If a participant opts for care from a nonprovider, he or she will be charged a substantial fee. Group health insurance costs are reduced for both an HMO and PPO in exchange for a guaranteed pool of patients.

Point-of-Service Plans

This is a twist that some HMOs offer. Usually a primary care physician in an HMO is required to refer you to a specialist who is also a member of the same HMO. However, in a point-of-service (POS) plan, you can be referred to a physician who is not a member and still receive coverage. However, if you choose to go to an outside physician without a referral, then you will have to pay all or part of the costs.

Choosing a health insurance plan requires time and thought. Take into account your particular health needs. Don't be afraid to ask questions. Any plan that includes drug coverage will be considerably more expensive than one that does not include such coverage.

How the Federal Government Supports Health Care

It is only in the past 50 years that the U.S. government has become involved in supplying health care insurance to citizens other than veterans. In 1965, Congress enacted legislation creating Medicare, which provides health insurance for people over age 65, for people under age 65 who are disabled, and for persons with permanent kidney failure. Congress also established Medicaid, which provides health insurance for people who are economically disadvantaged and cannot pay for medical care. In 2009, spending on health care in the United States amounted to about $7,500 per person. This amount represents about 17% of the gross domestic product (GDP). By 2016, health care spending per person is projected to be almost $13,000, which will represent almost 20% of the GDP. Despite spending more on health than any other country in the world, 46 million Americans, including at least 10 million children, still have no health insurance. The Institute of Medicine estimates that about 18,000 Americans die each year because of lack of some kind of health insurance.

All eligible Medicare beneficiaries, on reaching age 65, automatically are enrolled in Medicare, Part A, which covers hospital costs, rehabilitation in a skilled nursing facility, and hospice care for the terminally ill. Enrollment in Medicare, Part B, is voluntary, but most beneficiaries choose to enroll. Part B pays for 80% (after a $100 deductible) of physicians' services, emergency room visits, laboratory fees, diagnostic tests, and other medical expenses.

In 1966, during its first year, Medicare had 19 million enrollees; by 2000 the number had increased to about 40 million and is expected to jump to 77 million by 2030 (Centers for Medicare and Medicaid Services, 2008). Medicare now insures one in every seven Americans; that ratio will increase to one in every five by 2030. In 2006, Medicare instituted Part D, a convoluted and expensive program for covering the costs of prescription drugs for persons on Medicare and Medicaid. It is estimated that Part D will cost between $750 billion and $1 trillion by 2015. Something must be done both to improve coverage and to lower costs of health care in the United States, but no solution is yet in sight.

Medicaid provides health insurance for certain poor people in the United States. To be eligible for Medicaid benefits, an individual must be on welfare, have dependent children, or receive supplementary security income for persons who are aged, blind, or disabled. In addition, Medicaid covers nursing home care for many elderly Americans.

Health Care Costs

Why Health Care Costs Continue to Rise

Anyone who has been to a physician, filled a prescription, paid a health insurance premium, or been admitted to a hospital realizes how expensive medical care has become. In 1994, the cost of medical care exceeded $1 trillion; that was the year former President Clinton tried and failed to pass comprehensive health care legislation that would have reformed the health care system, expanded Medicare and Medicaid coverage, and restrained cost increases. However, agreement could not be reached, and the legislation failed to pass in Congress.

Many factors contribute to the dramatic increases in the costs of health care in the United States: physician salaries and fees, cost of prescription drugs, malpractice insurance, cost of hospital rooms and emergency services, and cost of health insurance. Another significant factor is the aggressive marketing of medical technologies, new drugs, and tests to physicians and also directly to patients. The overzealous use of diagnostic technologies distinguishes U.S. medical care from that in other major industrialized countries. The United States leads the world in organ and bone marrow transplants, coronary artery bypass surgeries, and **magnetic resonance imaging (MRI)** use. Although MRI is an important diagnostic tool for many medical problems, ownership of an expensive MRI machine by a hospital demands frequent use to pay for it. Also, to stay competitive, almost every hospital must have one.

$ Dollars and Health Sense

Advertising Medical Devices and Procedures on TV

The U.S. Food and Drug Administration (FDA) has the authority to regulate the sale of prescription drugs and their advertisement in the media. This form of advertising is called direct-to-consumer advertising (DTCA). For years, TV viewers have been barraged with 30- and 60-second spots touting drugs for enlarged prostate, arthritis, depression, fibromyalagia, and, of course, erectile dysfunction (see Chapter 16). The effectiveness and profitability of DTCA is well documented; 10 of 12 drugs that used DTCA had sales in excess of $1 billion.

However, in 2007, a medical device and procedure were promoted to potential consumers in a TV advertisement for the first time. This ad is viewed as crossing the line in DTCA (Boden & Diamond, 2008). The ad was aimed at selling drug-eluting stents for clogged arteries, a subject the vast majority of viewers probably have never heard of or thought about. The surgical procedure used to insert the stents, percutaneous transluminal coronary angioplasty (PTCA), is hardly a household word among TV viewers. Nor could they be expected to know that drug-eluting stents are themselves controversial medical devices. Yet this ad ran during a Thanksgiving Day football game (New York Jets vs. Dallas Cowboys) watched by millions of people. How many people who watched this ad and who subsequently are diagnosed with a blocked artery are going to tell their surgeon they want the blocked-artery device they saw advertised on TV? The surgeon will then have to try to explain why a drug-eluting stent is not the proper device for their condition. Most physicians and surgeons do not appreciate having to counteract the misleading or controversial information their patients receive via DTCA, especially with regard to controversial medical devices.

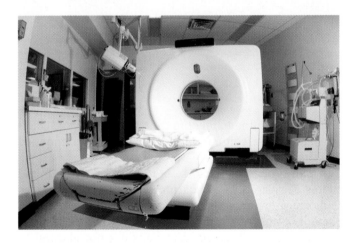

Computed tomographic (CT) scans and magnetic resonance imaging (MRI) help physicians make the correct diagnosis of an injury or disease.

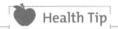

Health Tip

Whole-Body CT Scan—Unnecessary for Healthy People

Whole-body computed tomography (CT) scans have become a popular diagnostic tool for healthy Americans. They are a drain on soaring health care costs—and they may be dangerous. Such scans cost at least $1,000 and may be ordered by physicians even for mild complaints. Studies show that these scans may help in the diagnosis of disease in about 2% of male patients. But a whopping 90% of the men will have a false-positive result requiring further tests costing thousands of dollars more. In addition, multiple CT scans increase the risk of cancer as a result of exposure to ionizing radiation.

Other factors contributing to rising health care costs are unhealthy lifestyles and an aging population. The epidemic of obesity contributes to a bevy of chronic diseases, the most notable being type 2 diabetes. Diseases caused by smoking or alcohol are costly and preventable in principle. And, as the population ages, older Americans acquire chronic ailments that require more medical attention and costly drugs.

Medical Tourism

Because of the extraordinarily high cost of medical and dental procedures in the United States, thousands of patients now seek treatment in other countries, combining travel, vacation, and health care in one trip. Some estimates put the number of so-called *medical tourists* from the United States as high as 150,000. Thailand, India, Argentina, Costa Rica, and other countries now aggressively advertise for medical tourists. A comparison of prices for some common surgeries in the United States and in four other countries shows why medical tourism has become so popular (**Table 19.3**).

TERMS

magnetic resonance imaging (MRI): use of a strong magnetic field to produce images of internal parts of the body; especially useful for soft tissues

preferred provider organization (PPO): physicians who belong to the organization provide medical care at reduced costs that are negotiated by the organization

Table 19.3

Medical Tourism—Surgery Cost Estimates

Procedure	United States	India	Thailand	Singapore
Coronary bypass	$176,000	$10,000	$12,000	$20,000
Spinal fusion	90,000	5,500	7,000	9,000
Angioplasty	82,000	11,000	13,000	13,000
Knee replacement	58,000	8,500	11,000	13,000
Mastectomy	43,000	7,500	9,000	9,000

Source: Adapted from J. A. Unti. (2008). Medical tourism report to the American College of Surgeons Patient Safety and Quality Improvement Committee. Available: http://www.surgicalpatientsafety.facs.org/news/medicaltourism.html.

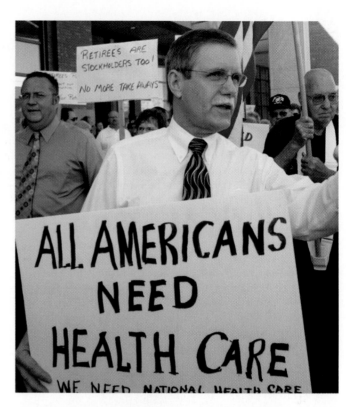

There are an estimated 46 million Americans without health insurance who gamble daily that they won't suffer a major illness or injury that could cost more than they could pay to treat.

Many hospitals overseas are accredited by a U.S. organization called the Joint Commission International (www.jointcommissioninternational.com). This non-profit agency checks hospitals every three years and uses the same standards used to accredit American hospitals. Also, many surgeons working overseas have been *board certified*, which means that their qualifications are the same as surgeons working in U.S. hospitals. The American Board of Medical Specialties (www.abms.org) lists thousands of surgeons working in other countries who are board certified.

All medical procedures entail risks, whether done in the United States or other countries. Patients should do as much research as possible by checking sites on the Internet and talking with patients who have undergone procedures overseas. It is important to ask questions about follow-up care. Communicate with the overseas surgeon if possible. Sometimes it is wise to work with an overseas travel company that can make all of the medical arrangements.

Health Care Costs in Other Countries

Other industrialized nations, such as Canada, Great Britain, France, Germany, and Japan, spend about half as much as the United States on health care costs and still manage to provide health insurance for all of their citizens (**Table 19.4**). Some claim that the United States has the best health care in the world, which justifies the high cost. This may be true if you are a kidney dialysis patient or need a heart transplant. But the United States also has a lower life expectancy and a higher infant mortality rate than Canada and many other industrialized countries do.

Some critics of U.S. health care advocate adopting Canada's model to provide universal health care for all citizens. There are arguments for and against this position. The most compelling reason is to provide everyone with basic health care. However, under the Canadian system, people must wait for some diagnostic tests and many kinds of elective surgery. People with conditions that are not immediately life threatening, such as colon cancer, usually wait a month or more for recommended treatment and surgery.

Many Canadian doctors opt to practice in the United States because they can earn more money; this creates a shortage of surgeons and other medical specialists in Canada. Also, Canada is experiencing a severe physician shortage partly because physicians are not allowed to have a private practice outside of the National Health Care system.

Canada saves considerable money because its health care administration costs are much less than administration costs in the United States (Woolhandler, Campbell, & Himmelstein, 2003). On average, the United States spends $752 more annually per citizen in administrative costs for health care than is spent in Canada. In 1999, approximately 27% of health care workers in the United States were involved in administration; in Canada, only 19% were involved in administration. The U.S. health care system is in need of a drastic overhaul, but there is no agreement among the various parties involved on what to do to make health care universally available and less expensive (Kutter, 2008).

Quality of Medical Care

Despite complaints about the cost of health care, the American health care system is often referred to as

Table 19.4

Comparison of Health Care Costs in Industrialized Countries

Country	Expenditure per capita, U.S. $ (2003)	Description
United States	5,711	Employers and private citizens purchase health insurance. State and federal governments provide health insurance for the elderly and the poor. About 45 million citizens have no health insurance.
United Kingdom	2,389	The National Health Service provides free health care for all citizens. People desiring medical care outside the system can purchase private insurance.
Japan	2,244	Workers get health insurance through their employers. All others are covered by a national health insurance plan.
Canada	2,989	Universal health coverage. Physicians are not allowed to have private practices or accept money outside the system.
Germany	3,001	Everyone is enrolled in government-approved health plans financed by employee and employer contributions. Wealthy people can buy private insurance.
France	2,902	Universal health care funded through Social Security. Private insurance also available.

Source: Adapted from Kelley, E. (2007). Health, spending, and the effort to improve quality in OECD countries. *Journal of the Royal Society for the Promotion of Health, 127,* 64–71.

Table 19.5

Health Status Rank of the United States Among 29 Other OECD Countries

Health status measure	U.S.	U.S. rank in OECD
Infant mortality (all races)	6.8 deaths/1,000 live births	25
Maternal mortality during birth (all races)	9.9 deaths/100,000 live births	22
Life expectancy from birth		
All women	80.1 years	23
All men	74.8 years	22
Life expectancy from age 65		
All women	19.8 years	10
All men	16.8 years	9

The OECD is the Organization for Economic Cooperation and Development. The following countries are in the OECD: Australia, Austria, Belgium, Canada, Czech Republic, Denmark, Finland, France, Germany, Greece, Hungary, Iceland, Ireland, Italy, Japan, Korea, Luxembourg, Mexico, the Netherlands, New Zealand, Norway, Poland, Portugal, Slovak Republic, Spain, Sweden, Switzerland, Turkey, United Kingdom, and United States.

Source: Data from OECD. (2007). *Health at a glance: OECD indicators.* Paris, France: OECD Publishing.

being the best in the world. But is it? Thirty developed countries, including the United States, make up the Organization for Economic Cooperation and Development (OECD). On the standard measures of health status of citizens in these countries, the United States ranks near the bottom in almost all categories (**Table 19.5**). Among 192 nations, the United States ranks 46th in average life expectancy from birth and 42nd in infant mortality (Schroeder, 2007). The United States also ranks near the bottom for low-birth-weight babies and neonatal deaths and for years of potential life lost (excluding accidents and other external causes). The United States does not meet many basic health needs as well as other countries that spend far less on health care.

In 1999, the Institute of Medicine (IOM) published a report titled "To Err Is Human: Building a Safe Health System." This report concluded that medical errors were directly responsible for between 44,000 and 98,000 deaths each year in the United States. Medical errors rank as the eighth leading cause of death—ahead of AIDS, breast cancer, and motor vehicle accidents (Altman, Clancy, & Blendon, 2004). The study found that Americans died from various kinds of medical errors, including unnecessary surgery, errors in medications given in hospitals, other hospital errors in patient care, hospital-acquired (nosocomial) infections, and adverse effects of prescribed medications.

The IOM report created an outcry for change in the public and among government officials. On December 7, 1999, President Clinton signed an executive order giving federal agencies 90 days to develop plans and changes that would ensure patient safety. Private sector physicians, hospitals, and insurers also implemented strategies to improve patient safety. To improve patient safety, the U.S. Congress enacted legislation in 2005 that set up a national network for reporting, analyzing, and correcting medical errors. It was hoped that this legislation would not only increase patient safety but also reduce medical costs by preventing frivolous medical malpractice suits. However, in its latest report, the Institute of Medicine estimated that the average hospital patient is subjected to at least one medical error per day. It also estimated that each year more than 1.5 million patients experience injuries resulting from preventable adverse drug effects (Burke, 2007).

Almost everyone agrees that the quality of U.S. health care needs to be improved. It makes no sense that receiving health care carries the same risk of death that bungee jumping and mountain climbing do (about 100 deaths per 100,000 encounters). The U.S. Department of Health and Human Services provides information on how well hospitals care for patients with certain medical conditions or surgical procedures as well as results from a survey of patients about the quality of care they received during recent hospital stays. Information on the quality of care hospitals provide is available at http://www.hospitalcompare.hhs.gov.

Inequities in Health Care

Socioeconomic status and race play crucial roles in health and health care. Level of education, amount of income, and type of job all contribute to a person's health (Jemal et al., 2008). People earning less than $9,000 a year die at a rate three to seven times greater than those earning more than $25,000 a year. African Americans and Hispanic Americans generally have lower incomes than white Americans, experience more health problems, and are less likely to receive medical care. Poor people smoke more cigarettes, drink more alcohol, use more illegal drugs, and are exposed to violence more than people with high incomes.

Lack of health insurance and access to medical care takes its toll not only on health but also on length of life. Compared to adult African-American men in urban areas, adult white men living in the rural plain states live an average 11 years longer (77 years vs. 66 years). The gap in life expectancy between urban African Americans and urban and suburban whites in the entire country is approximately 7 years (Murray et al., 2006). Urban African Americans have life expectancies that are similar to some low-income developing countries. That is why many people around the world are beginning to realize that the right to health is just as basic as other human rights.

> At one time I had ambitions, but I had them removed by a doctor in Buffalo.
>
> *Tom Waits*

Many studies have shown that African Americans are less likely to receive a wide range of medical services as compared with white Americans with the same conditions and problems, including ones requiring surgery (Egede & Bosworth, 2008). The federal government has set the goal of eliminating racial and ethnic differences in medical care in six major areas, including treatment of cardiovascular disease. However, surveys show that de facto segregation still is widely prevalent in U.S. hospitals and physicians' offices (Blustein, 2008).

Even among people enrolled in Medicare, significant disparities in health care exist. Surgical treatment for osteoarthritis of the knee was found to vary dramatically according to sex, race, ethnicity, and geographic section of the country (Gornick, 2008).

Organ Transplants

The medical technology for transplantation of organs from one person to another has made great advances in the past decade. Most major human organs now can be transplanted, including kidney, liver, heart, lung, and pancreas, as well as eye and skin tissues. Organs can be transplanted from cadavers (people who have died suddenly, usually in accidents) and from living donors as well. The number of U.S. transplant operations set a new record in 2006: almost 29,000 patients received organs, according to government figures. But the supply of organs is still far below demand; about 62,000 patients in the United States are currently waiting for a kidney transplant, but only about a quarter of them will live long enough to receive one (Steinbrook, 2005).

More than 71,000 people in the United States have donated an organ to another person, often a family member. Kidney donations are the most frequent because everyone has two kidneys, and one kidney can be donated without serious effect—providing the remaining kidney continues to function normally. So, there is always an unknown element of risk. If the kidney donor is a young person, in his or her 20s or 30s, for example, the donor may lose the remaining kidney to infection or injury later in life and have to go on a waiting list for a kidney transplant. Because of this possibility, some hospital transplant centers prefer to transplant organs from older persons, but this also means the donor is at additional risk from the transplantation procedure, especially if she or he is not in the best of health.

No federal guidelines or state laws regulate who can donate and who can receive an organ. Each hospital or organ transplant center makes its own rules. Critics of live organ transplants argue that, because of the lack of official guidelines or standards, a person really cannot give informed consent. For example, no data are kept on the subsequent health or medical problems of living donors. Some hospital records indicate that from 15% to 67% of live liver donors experience infections or other complications following the transplantation. But there are no laws requiring that records be kept on the fate of live donors. Some live donors feel that they were inadequately informed before the donation and received insufficient medical care afterward.

Because there are not nearly enough cadaver donors available to meet the burgeoning demand from people with failing organs, live donors will continue to play an important role. A parent at age 70 may be quite comfortable donating a kidney to save a child. But a young person considering donating an organ to save a much older person should carefully contemplate the risks and benefits to both parties. Each potential live donor presents a unique situation that can be resolved only by discussions among everyone involved, including doctors, spouses, family members, and others who may be affected by the decision.

Medicalization of Human Behaviors and Traits

Medicalization refers to medical consideration of conditions, behaviors, or traits that generally were not regarded as illnesses or medical problems. Once medicalized, these conditions are deemed to require treatment of some kind, such as psychotherapy, medication, or surgery. Once a condition has been medicalized, payment to doctors by health insurers is permissible.

The first significant human behavior to the medicalized was homosexuality (Conrad, 2007). For years homosexuality was stigmatized in the United States and other countries as a "disease" that required treatment with drugs, psychotherapy, and other methods. Homosexuality was officially demedicalized in the United States in the 1970s and is now viewed as a normal variation in a human trait, just as variation exists in intelligence and athletic ability. But medicalization of other human behaviors, conditions, and traits has increased markedly in recent years.

For centuries, people considered personal choice to be the reason for smoking tobacco and drinking alcohol, even to the point of undesirable health and personal consequences. Although many still hold this view, in recent decades both smoking and the overuse of alcohol have been medicalized; smokers and heavy drinkers now are encouraged to seek treatments for these unhealthy behaviors.

Drug companies have been quick to see the potential profit in medicalizing human conditions and traits. For years human growth hormone (hGH) was in short supply, but now it is available in unlimited amounts thanks to modern biotechnology. Children who are at the low end of the average distribution in height are now diagnosed with "idiopathic short stature" and are eligible to be treated with injections of hGH for years, provided that their parents can afford the expense of such injections. Children who are completely normal thus become stigmatized by the medicalization of their shortness. The psychological harm that is done to these children may far outweigh the maximum of 2 inches in height that they may gain from the treatments.

Drug companies have made enormous profits from the medicalization of "male aging problems" such as sexual impotence and baldness. These conditions and their drug solutions are presented daily to TV viewers as permitted by direct-to-consumer advertising (see Chapter 16). The advertising of prescription drugs directly to consumers is banned in all countries except for the United States.

Hyperactive children in classrooms are diagnosed with attention deficit hyperactivity disorder (ADHD) and are treated with stimulant drugs that help many of them quiet down for reasons that are not understood scientifically. In any case, parents and teachers benefit from the calmer classroom and home environments. The diagnosis of ADHD has been extended to older populations who are said to suffer from "adult ADHD," which expands the potential for drug therapy enormously.

Obesity is a serious health problem for a large segment of the American population. Most often, obesity results from overeating and a lack of physical activity. The causes of obesity are rooted in individual lifestyle choices, social forces that promote sedentary living, and the mega-industrialization of the food supply that provides products for consumption that increase the risk of overweight and obesity. Because changing lifestyle, social, and economic forces is difficult, obesity has been medicalized. Pharmaceutical researchers are competing to find drugs that can stop weight gain or promote weight loss. Increasingly, the recommended medical treatment for obesity is bariatric surgery, which removes a portion of the stomach to prevent a person from overeating.

Individuals are still free to take responsibility for their health. They do not have to accept being medicalized for some behavior or condition that requires them to be treated. We urge all of our readers to accept responsibility for their health and to adopt behaviors and attitudes that foster health and well-being.

Cosmetic Surgery

For people who can afford it, **cosmetic surgery** is used to improve appearance, enhance beauty, or correct the visible effects of aging. Cosmetic surgery is a growth industry in the United States. In 2007, about 11.7 million cosmetic surgical and nonsurgical procedures were performed in the United States (Table 19.6). In addition to cosmetic surgeries, about 5.2 million reconstructive plastic surgical procedures were performed. Women received 91% of all cosmetic surgeries, and men the remainder. Botox injections to remove wrinkles and age lines on the face are the most popular nonsurgical procedures among both men and women.

Large HMOs such as Kaiser and other health insurance organizations are now offering cosmetic surgery to their members for a fee, usually discounted from fees charged by private physicians. Cosmetic surgery is seen as a way to make money that can finance other medical

---

TERMS

cosmetic surgery: surgery performed not for any medical condition but solely to enhance appearance or correct visible effects of aging

medicalization: medical treatment of conditions, behaviors, or traits that generally were not regarded as illnesses or medicals problems

Table 19.6

Surgical and Nonsurgical Cosmetic Surgeries for Men and Women in 2007

Surgical		Nonsurgical	
Women	**Men**	**Women**	**Men**
Breast augmentation	Liposuction injection	Botox injection	Botox injection
Lipoplasty	Eyelid surgery	Hyaluronic acid	Laser hair removal
Eyelid surgery	Rhinoplasty	Laser hair removal	Microdermabrasion
Abdominoplasty	Breast reduction	Microdermabrasion	Hyaluronic acid
Breast reduction	Hair transplant	IPL laser treatment	IPL laser treatment

Procedures are listed in the table according to frequency. IPL, intense pulsed light.

services. Dermatologists and plastic surgeons perform the majority of the cosmetic surgeries, but many physicians now offer botox and collagen injections to their patients. As the population continues to age, it is anticipated that the boom in cosmetic surgeries will also grow.

Most cosmetic surgeries are safe, especially if performed by a board-certified physician. However, complications such as infections, scarring, and undesirable outcomes also occur. Liposuction is one of the more popular procedures; nearly 400,000 were performed on women and about 58,000 were performed on men in 2007. Liposuction is used to remove subcutaneous fat from various parts of the body to sculpt it into a more attractive shape. A variety of complications can result from liposuction, some of which can be serious or fatal, so it is not a procedure to undergo lightly and without considerable investigation of possible undesirable outcomes.

Critical Thinking About Health

1. Congressman John Sockittoim from Arkansas has been working on a bill to solve the Medicare financial crisis. In trying to generate more funds for Medicare and Medicaid, he has proposed a 10% tax on all cosmetic surgeries that are not done out of medical necessity (such as breast reconstruction after mastectomy) but solely for enhancing physical appearance. He argues that people who can afford cosmetic surgery can also afford to support the basic medical needs of people less fortunate. Decide whether you approve or disapprove of this tax and discuss your reasons.

2. Have you ever been hospitalized for an illness or injury? Describe the condition that caused you to be hospitalized, and discuss the care and tests that you experienced in the hospital. What things were the most positive and healing in the hospital? What things were the most distressing and unhealthy about your hospital experience? Suggest ways (based on your experience) that hospitals might improve the care they provide to patients.

3. The Medicare program, like the Social Security program, will face a fiscal crisis in the near future. The money that is collected by these two federal programs will not cover their costs unless they are restructured. Congress has proposed a new Medicare system for retired persons in which each worker would be required to put away a percentage of earnings during working years to pay for medical needs after retirement. This means that workers would now have to contribute additional money for future health care. Discuss whether you think this is the proper solution to solve Medicare's financial problems. Can you propose any other alternatives to provide the Medicare program with the money that is needed and that you think would be fair? Or do you think the federal government should not be involved in providing health care for retired persons at all?

4. Joe Windam is in the hospital with liver failure. Joe is only 32 years old but has been a heavy drinker most of his life, just like his father. He also contracted a hepatitis C infection several years ago that has contributed to his liver disease. Joe has been out of work for over a year and does not have any health insurance. The only hope that Joe has is a liver transplant; without a new liver, Joe will probably die in a few months. Do you think Joe should be given a high priority for a liver transplant because of his young age? Who should pay the several hundred thousand dollars in hospital and doctor bills? How should the priority for liver transplants be assigned, since there are not enough livers available for all the patients who need them?

Health in Review

- Everyone needs medical care at some time in his or her life. Knowing what to ask and what to expect from your physician is essential.
- The physician's responsibility is to find the cause of illness. The patient's responsibility is working in partnership with the health care provider, sharing in health care decision making, and becoming skilled at obtaining health care.
- Admission to a hospital is often an unsettling experience. Patients should be aware of their rights and ask questions that will ease their concerns and reduce errors.
- Health care is increasingly provided by large organizations of physicians and hospitals, called preferred provider organizations or health maintenance organizations.
- The costs of medical care in the United States have grown so rapidly that some form of health care reform is needed. Forty-five million Americans lack health insurance and access to health care.
- Drug, hospital, and medical errors account for thousands of deaths in the United States each year. Medical errors are the eighth leading cause of death.
- Health care providers include physicians, nurses, physical therapists, occupational therapists, physician assistants, and specialists in sports-related injuries.
- Disparities in health care exist depending on a patient's sex, race, ethnic origin, or geographical location in the country.
- Organ transplants from live donors are becoming more frequent and pose problems for donors and recipients.
- Medicalization of human behaviors such as smoking, drinking, and overeating has transferred responsibility for the resulting health problems from individuals to physicians. The normal human trait of short stature also has been medicalized.
- Millions of Americans spend billions of dollars each year on various kinds of surgical and nonsurgical cosmetic procedures to improve appearance.

Health and Wellness Online

The Web contains a wealth of information about health and wellness. By accessing the Internet using Web browser software, you can gain a new perspective on many topics presented in *Health and Wellness,* Tenth Edition. Access the Jones and Bartlett Publishers Web site at **health.jbpub.com/hwonline.**

References

Altman, D.E., Clancy, C., & Blendon, R.J. (2004). Improving patient safety—five years after the IOM report. *New England Journal of Medicine, 351,* 2041–2043.

Blustein, J. (2008). Who is accountable for racial equity in health care? *Journal of the American Medical Association, 299,* 814–816.

Boden, W. E., & Diamond, G. A. (2008). DTCA for PTCA—Crossing the line in consumer health education? *New England Journal of Medicine, 358,* 2197–2200.

Burke, J. B. (2007). Preventing medication errors. *New England Journal of Medicine, 357,* 624–625.

Centers for Medicare and Medicaid Services. (2008). 2008 Medicare trustees report. Retrieved October 24, 2008, from http://www.cms.hhs.gov/ReportsTrustFunds/

Charo, R. A. (2005). The celestial fire of conscience—Refusing to deliver medical care. *New England Journal of Medicine, 352,* 2471–2472.

Conrad, P. (2007). *The medicalization of society: On the transformation of human conditions into treatable disorders.* Baltimore: Johns Hopkins University Press.

Curlin, F. A., et al. (2007). Religion, conscience, and controversial clinical practices. *New England Journal of Medicine, 356,* 593–600.

Egede, L. E., & Bosworth, H. (2008). The future of health disparities research: 2008 and beyond. *Journal of General Internal Medicine, 23,* 706–708.

Gornick, M. E. (2008). A decade of research on disparities in Medicare utilization: Lessons for the health and health care of vulnerable men. *American Journal of Public Health, 98,* S162–168.

Jemal, A. (2008). Mortality from leading causes by education and race in the United States, 2001. *American Journal of Preventive Medicine, 34,* 1–8.

Kutter, R. (2008). Market-based failure—A second opinion on U.S. healthcare costs. *New England Journal of Medicine, 358,* 549–551.

Murray, C. J. L., et al. (2006). Eight Americas: Investigating mortality disparities across races, counties, and race-counties in the United States. *PLoS Medicine, 3,* e260. DOI: 10.1371/journal.pmed.0030260

Schroeder, S. A. (2007). We can do better—Improving the health of the American people. *New England Journal of Medicine, 357,* 1221–1228.

Steinbrook, R. (2005). Public solicitation of organ donors. *New England Journal of Medicine, 353,* 441–449.

Tremain, K. (2007, January/February). Beyond the silver bullet. *California Magazine,* 39–42.

Wald, H. L., & Kramer, A. M. (2007). Nonpayment for harms resulting from medical care. *Journal of the American Medical Association, 298,* 2782–2784.

Woolhandler, S., Campbell, T., & Himmelstein, D.U. (2003). Costs of health care administration in the United States and Canada. *New England Journal of Medicine, 349,* 768–774.

Suggested Readings

Annas, G. J. (2004). *The rights of patients: The authoritative ACLU guide to the rights of patients.* Carbondale: Southern Illinois University Press. The country's foremost expert on medical ethics describes tragic cases and the need for patients to exercise their rights as patients.

Farmer, P. (2003). *Pathologies of power: Health, human rights, and the new war on the poor.* Berkeley: University of California Press. A powerful critique of how globalization, financial institutions, and despotic leaders result in poor health for the poor of the world.

Gawande, A. (2007, December 10). The checklist. *The New Yorker,* 86–95. Describes how enforcing hand washing and hygiene in intensive care units (ICUs) could dramatically reduce infections and save lives.

Groopman, J. (2003, August 11). Sick with worry. *The New Yorker,* 28–34. An article that describes the large number of patients who have nothing wrong but who demand treatment.

Groopman, J. (2007, January 29). What's the trouble? *The New Yorker,* 36–41. An article describing how difficult it is sometimes for a doctor to arrive at the correct medical diagnosis.

Merck manual of medical information—Home edition. (2005). New York: Merck Publishing Group. A very helpful guide to understanding diseases and drugs. This book is based on the book doctors use when they leave the examining room to figure out what is going on.

Relman, A. S. (2007). *A second opinion: Rescuing America's health care.* New York: Public Affairs. Essential reading for persons interested in the problems of health care in America. Relman's basic premise is that the U.S. health care system puts profits over patients and that health care should be nonprofit.

Sapolsky, R. (2005, December). Sick of poverty. *Scientific American,* 93–99. An article showing that poverty affects not only quality of life but length of life also.

Steinbrook, R. (2005). Public solicitation of organ donors. *New England Journal of Medicine, 353,* 441–449. An important article to read for anyone thinking about becoming a living organ donor.

Recommended Web Sites

Please visit **health.jbpub.com/hwonline** for links to these Web sites.

A Consumer Guide for Getting and Keeping Health Insurance
Guidelines for all states and the District of Columbia, from the Georgetown University Health Policy Institute.

Guide to Health Insurance
Discusses the basic forms of health coverage and includes a checklist to help compare plans.

Kaiser Family Foundation
Provides facts, analysis, and explanation on health policy issues to policymakers, the media, and the public.

Medicare
The U.S. government's health insurance program for seniors and persons with disabilities.

Organ Donors
Living Donors Online provides information for prospective organ donors.

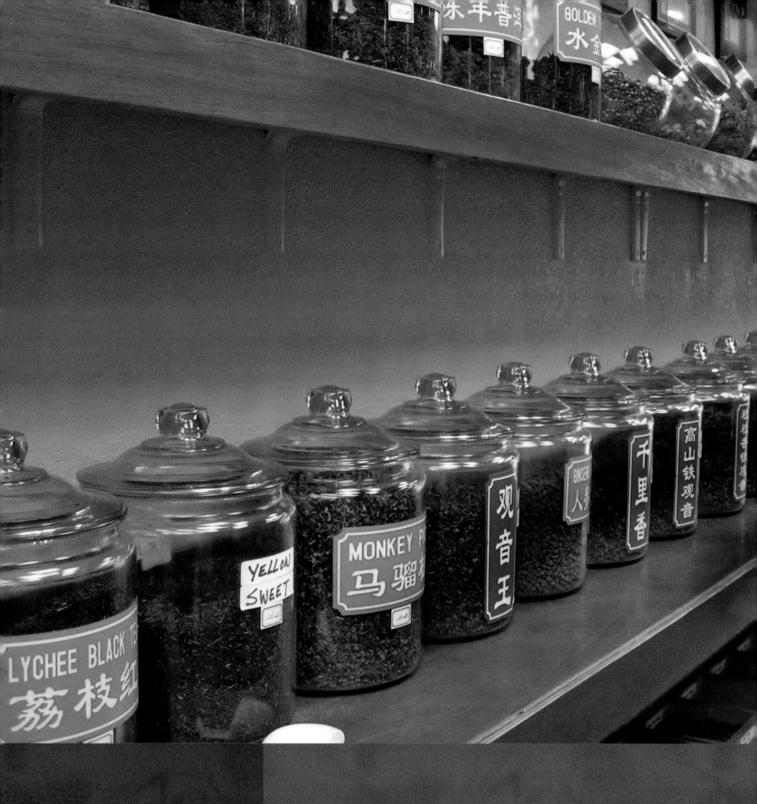

Chapter Twenty

Exploring Alternative Medicines

Learning Objectives

1. Describe the main differences between modern medical care and alternative medicines.

2. Define the four categories of alternative medicines.

3. Discuss the philosophy and method of treatment in acupuncture, chiropractic, herbal medicine, and homeopathy.

4. Discuss the reasons why some people choose an alternative medicine in addition to, or instead of, modern medicine.

5. List reasons why herbal remedies may be dangerous.

6. Explain how biomagnetic therapy might help certain health problems.

7. Explain how you can protect yourself from being victimized by health fraud.

Although most people in the United States elect to visit a physician when they are sick, many seek alternatives to modern medicine for a variety of reasons. One important reason is cultural; persons raised in cultures that rely on herbal remedies and tribal healers to treat sickness often continue to use their own remedies even if they move to another country.

Some people who use **alternative medicine** do so because Western, scientific medicine has failed to relieve their suffering or cannot cure their disease. For example, people with terminal cancer for which no further treatments are available will often turn to some alternative medicine that offers hope, however faint, for prolonging life. People with chronic diseases such as arthritis, chronic fatigue syndrome, depression, or persistent allergies who do not respond satisfactorily to medical treatments often turn to alternative medicines for relief.

> You cannot teach a person anything. You can only help him to find it for himself.
>
> *Galileo*

Some surveys indicate that one-third to one-half of patients with serious medical problems use some form of alternative medicine in addition to conventional treatment. The alternative medicines that people use most frequently are herbal remedies, massage, megavitamin therapy, energy healing, and homeopathy. Some physicians in the United States have begun to address their patients' needs and preferences for alternative medicines. If an alternative medicine is used in conjunction with a conventional treatment, it is referred to as **complementary medicine** to indicate that both treatments complement one another. For example, a person with lower back pain might receive medications for pain and muscle relaxation as well as being referred to a chiropractor or a massage therapist. A few doctors prescribe homeopathic remedies as well as prescription drugs for a variety of symptoms.

Sometimes the terms *complementary medicine* and *alternative medicine* are used interchangeably. Because many newly certified physicians incorporate some alternative medicines in their practices, these physicians are said to practice **integrative medicine**. Physicians practicing integrative medicine can offer patients advice on herbs, vitamins, homeopathic remedies, and many other alternative medicines. Today, many of the most prestigious medical schools in the United States have departments of integrative medicine that offer courses in complementary and alternative medicines.

Patients should always discuss with their physicians any alternative medicine that they are using because some herbs or treatments may interfere with any conventional therapy or prescribed drug that the patient is using. For example, some herbs are dangerous because they contain toxic substances; others interfere with the actions of prescribed drugs, thereby reducing the medicine's effectiveness. Also, many alternative medicines have not been scientifically tested in clinical trials or proven to be safe and effective. Finally, some practitioners of alternative medicines are not well trained and many practitioners are unlicensed. Anyone contemplating using an alternative medicine for a serious medical problem should obtain as much information as possible and discuss the problem with a qualified health practitioner.

In recognition of the growing use of alternative medicine, Congress established the Office of Alternative Medicine (OAM) in 1992. The task of OAM was to fund research that would test the validity and effectiveness of many alternative medicines, such as acupuncture, massage, hypnosis, biofeedback, yoga, macrobiotic diets, and others. In 1998, the National Institutes of Health turned the small OAM into a full-fledged research agency called the National Center for Complementary and Alternative Medicine (NCCAM). The annual budget jumped from about $2 million to more than $100 million. Medical schools quickly established departments of complementary and alternative medicine (CAM), and more than two-thirds of American medical schools began to offer CAM courses.

The goal of NCCAM is to test alternative therapies that have a plausible scientific basis and that can help patients' unmet needs. To this end, NCCAM has funded large clinical trials of chondroitin sulfate and glucosamine in treatment of osteoarthritis, vitamin E and selenium in the prevention of prostate cancer, and the effect of *Ginkgo biloba* on slowing dementia and memory loss.

Even if scientific studies "prove" certain alternative therapies to be of no value, it is not certain that the public will heed the results. For example, the very principles of homeopathy (discussed later) preclude its being tested scientifically, and most of its medicines contain no active ingredients. Yet homeopathy is being used more and more around the world, and millions of people attest to its therapeutic value in treating many diseases.

Defining Alternative Medicine

Alternative medicine can be divided into four broad categories based on the method of healing or intervention: (1) spiritual, psychic, or mental approaches, including prayer, meditation, hypnotherapy, and faith healing; (2) nutritional therapies, including change in diet, fasting, and the use of supplements; (3) therapies using herbs or other substances derived from natural sources, such as homeopathy, herbal medicine, or immune system boosters; and (4) physical therapies, such as chiropractic, acupuncture, massage, and yoga. **Table 20.1** presents a partial list of the hundreds of different alternative medicines.

Table 20.1

Partial List of Alternative Medicines and Healing Methods

Physical and nutritional	Mental and spiritual
Acupuncture	Ayurveda
Alexander technique	Biofeedback
Ayurveda	Christian Science
Feldenkrais technique	Co-counseling
Herbal medicine	Guided imagery
Kinesiology (touch for health)	Hypnosis
Macrobiotics	Meditation
Massage	Past lives therapy
No nightshade diet	Primal scream therapy
Qigong	Progressive relaxation
Reflexology	Psychic healing
Shiatsu	Magnetic therapy
T'ai chi ch'uan	Psychodrama
Yoga	Rebirthing

Some alternative medicines, such as acupuncture and herbal remedies, have been used for thousands of years and would not have survived if people had not benefited. Other alternative medicines, such as homeopathy and chiropractic, are of recent origin and emerged partly as a response to the extraordinarily harsh practices of conventional medicine in the eighteenth and nineteenth centuries.

Before this century, irritants of all kinds were used to purge the body of unknown causes of illness. Bleedings, cuppings, leechings, enemas, and emetics (vomiting inducers) were all commonly used by doctors to treat diseases of which they had no real understanding. These treatments generally weakened the patient and often interfered with the natural processes of healing.

Today, patients with chronic diseases and pain still seek treatments that offer the promise of relief and which do little harm. The problem for the health consumer is knowing which alternative medicines might be of help and which ones are safe. To help you understand how to choose, some of the more widely used alternative medicines are described here.

Alternative Medicines

Ayurveda

Ayurveda refers to one of the world's oldest medical systems, which has been practiced in India for more than 4,000 years. Like other Asian medical practices, **Ayurvedic medicine** embodies a holistic approach to health; it teaches that health results from a balance of mind, body, and spirit, as well as a balance between people and the environment and their relationship to the cosmos. The word *Ayurveda* is from the Sanskrit and is a combination of two words: *ayur,* which means "life," and

veda, which means "knowledge." Thus, health is knowledge of life. Ayurveda has been primarily practiced in the past by Buddhists or Hindus, but it is becoming increasingly popular in Western countries.

Ayurveda sees nature and people as being made of five elements or properties—earth, water, fire, air, and space; each element consists of both matter and energy. It is the interaction of these basic elements that gives rise to the universe and to human beings, who are viewed as being a microcosm or reflection of the macrocosm. Each element is associated with specific properties. For example, the earth element is dense and hard. Solid structures in the body, such as the skeleton, are derived from the earth element. The air element is cold and mobile. In the body, this element governs breathing and movement in the digestive tract. Thought, desire, and the will to do things also are under the control of the air element. The water element is fluid and soft and regulates the blood, secretions, and cerebrospinal fluid. The fire element is hot and light and regulates body temperature and all aspects of digestion. Space plays a unique role in Ayurveda because it permits us to perceive sound and also regulates vibrations that affect the body. Harmony among these five elements in each individual (and in the world) produces health; disharmony in any of the elements produces disease.

The interaction of the body with the environment is further defined by the *doshas,* which mediate the functions of the body tissues and waste products. When the doshas are in balance, people experience health on all levels—physical, emotional, and spiritual. In holistic terms, these individuals are not just free of disease but experience optimal health. They have an abundance of energy and are intelligent and competent in all that they do. They enjoy good relations with other people and

TERMS

alternative medicine: a therapy or healing procedure that is used *instead of* Western, scientific medical treatments

Ayurvedic medicine: a traditional form of preventive medicine and healing, involving mind, body, and spirit, practiced in India for thousands of years. Ayurveda is spreading to Western countries.

complementary medicine: an alternative therapy that is used *along with* conventional medicine. Usually there is some scientific evidence for the effectiveness and safety of the complementary medicine

integrative medicine: physicians who combine the practice of scientific, Western medicine with alternative medicines that they feel are safe and effective for their patients

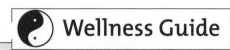

Wellness Guide

Sources for Information on Alternative Medicines

Alternative Medicines
The NCCAM Web site (http://nccam.nih.gov/) is a reliable source of information on all forms of alternative medicines. This site provides up-to-date information on recent research and news.

Chiropractic
Treatment usually involves direct spinal manipulation. Chiropractors contend that the spine is literally the backbone of health, and misalignment sabotages it. Practitioners diagnose with palpation and x-rays.
Information: Foundation for Chiropractic Education and Research, 380 Wright Road, Norwalk, IA 50211; 515-981-9888. http://www.fcer.org/

Homeopathy
Treatments aim to stimulate the body's defenses with tiny doses of substances that, in larger amounts, would cause the disease's symptoms.
Information: National Center for Homeopathy, 801 North Fairfax Street, Suite 306, Alexandria, VA 22314; 703-548-7790. http://www.homeopathic.org/

Aromatherapy
"Essential oils" distilled from plants and herbs are massaged into the skin, inhaled, or placed in baths in an attempt to treat stress, anxiety, and other conditions.
Information: National Association for Holistic Aromatherapy, 3327 W. Indian Trail Road PMB 144, Spokane, WA 99208; 509-325-3419. http://www.naha.org/

Ayurveda
Disease, says this ancient practice from India, is caused by an imbalance of movement, structure, and metabolism. Herbs, diet, meditation, and yoga are treatments.
Information: National Institute of Ayurvedic Medicine, 584 Milltown Road, Brewster, NY 10509; 845-278-8700. http://niam.com/corp-web/index.htm

Herbal Medicine
Plants or plant-based substances are used to treat a wide range of illnesses and enhance physical functions.
Information: American Botanical Council, P.O. Box 144345, Austin, TX 78714-4345; 800-373-7105. http://www.herbalgram.org/

Mind–Body Connection
Negative effects of stress are treated with exercise, meditation, and concentration.
Information: Center for Mind-Body Medicine, 5225 Connecticut Avenue, N.W., Suite 414, Washington, DC 20015; 202-966-7338. http://www.cmbm.org/

Chinese Medicine
Ancient healing says an imbalance of vital force, *chi,* causes disease. Diet, herbs, and acupuncture are preventive treatments.
Information: Alternative Medicine Foundation. http://www.amfoundation.org/tcm.htm

---

with the environment, and they are emotionally stable and happy. Spiritually, they are attuned with the cosmos. Imbalance in any of the doshas can produce mental, emotional, or physical illness. The goal of Ayurvedic medicine is to restore the balance of the doshas that is correct for each person.

An Ayurvedic physician diagnoses the patient's disease by a technique called pulse diagnosis, which is a highly developed skill in taking a pulse. Also, signs of illness are found by examination of the tongue, urine, and aspects of the body such as the condition of the nails, skin, and lips. Once the nature of the imbalance is determined, the physician provides various remedies. As with modern medicine, nutrition and exercise are among the primary recommendations. Ayurvedic medicine, however, does not define nutrition in terms of fats, proteins, vitamins, minerals, or food groups. Ayurveda recognizes six "tastes": salty, sweet, sour, pungent, bitter, and astringent. These tastes not only are sensations on the tongue but also effects on the body. Each taste is associated with a physiological function, such as elimination,

condition of mucous membranes, amount of stress, and so on. The diet is adjusted to restore a balance of the tastes. Exercises such as yoga and t'ai chi are recommended; today, jogging may be included. Other techniques employed by Ayurvedic practitioners include massage, meditation, and herbal remedies. The success of Ayurvedic medicine is attested to by its long history and the increasing number of people who embrace its principles.

People who use Ayurvedic medicines need to use caution in making purchases. Most Ayurvedic medicines are made in Southeast Asia without regulation and sold in Asian grocery stores in the United States. About one in five products purchased in the Boston area were found to contain potentially harmful levels of heavy metals such as lead, mercury, and/or arsenic (Saper et al., 2008). At present, consumers have no way of knowing which products are safe and which ones contain heavy metals.

> Words are the most potent drug that mankind uses.
> *Rudyard Kipling*

Homeopathy

Of all the alternative medicines, **homeopathy** is the most widely used in America and around the world. Many physicians in the United States use some form of homeopathy in their practice of medicine. Homeopathy also is used by nurse practitioners, dentists, naturopathic doctors, chiropractors, acupuncturists, and veterinarians. Between 2 and 3 million Americans take homeopathic remedies each year and spend upward of $200 million on homeopathic preparations. In European countries, homeopathy is widely used by physicians, and in India, there are more than 100,000 homeopathic practitioners.

Homeopathy is only about 200 years old and was founded by Samuel Hahnemann, a German pharmacologist and physician. The word *homeopathy* derives from two Greek words: *omoios,* meaning "similar," and *pathos,* meaning "feeling." Homeopathy is primarily a self-healing system that is assisted by very small doses of medicines or remedies. Hahnemann believed that tiny doses of a substance (a medicine) that evoked symptoms *similar* to the disease symptoms could, in some way, stimulate the body's natural defenses and promote healing. According to Hahnemann, homeopathy is based on four principles:

1. Substances that produce the same symptoms as the disease in an individual as the disease will cure that individual (Law of Similars).
2. Substances are tested by giving them to healthy subjects and observing symptoms (Law of Proving).
3. Smaller doses are more potent than undiluted solutions (Law of Potentiation or Law of Infinitesimals).
4. Vital forces must be released in the treated individual, which will result in reestablishing harmony (homeostasis) in the body.

For example, the substance *belladonna,* which is extracted from a poisonous plant, causes flushing and flulike symptoms when ingested by a healthy person. Thus, a homeopathic practitioner might use diluted doses of belladonna to treat the flu or high fever. The recommended dose of belladonna might be listed as 30×; this refers to the number of times that the original extract has been diluted. Practically, this means that one drop of the original extract is added to nine drops of water; then one drop of this solution is added to nine drops of water (or alcohol) and so on until 30 tenfold dilutions are reached. Statistically, the final solution is unlikely to have any molecules of belladonna in it. This is the primary reason that homeopathy is dismissed today as bogus by conventional medicine and Western science. Nonetheless, 200 years of experience and observation by patients and physicians show that it does help many patients suffering from many kinds of diseases.

Homeopathy began to be practiced extensively around 1830, a time when conventional medicine was particularly ineffective in treating epidemics of infectious diseases such as cholera, typhus, and scarlet fever. During this period, homeopathic doctors were significantly more successful in treating people than conventional doctors because the remedies worked, because people believed that they worked, or a combination of both. By 1890, at least 15% of conventional physicians used homeopathy and there were 22 homeopathic medical schools and more than 100 homeopathic hospitals operating in the United States.

In the 1800s, the American Medical Association (AMA) offered to include homeopaths in its organization. However, homeopaths chose to remain outside mainstream medicine, and the AMA began to harass and threaten physicians who practiced any form of homeopathy. In 1914, the AMA became the exclusive organization for licensing physicians to practice medicine; as a result, homeopathic medicine disappeared from the American scene for more than 50 years. In the 1970s, along with a general resurgence in alternative medicine, homeopathy again emerged as the choice of many sick people, either as a sole therapy or as an adjunct to conventional medical care.

Homeopathic practitioners use their remedies to evoke symptoms so that the body can recognize them and initiate a healing process from within. Homeopathy is used to treat both acute (infections, injuries) and chronic (arthritis, allergies, high blood pressure) conditions. It does not generally treat structural diseases or those stemming from long-term organic damage, such as cirrhosis, diabetes, chronic obstructive lung diseases, inherited diseases, neurological diseases, or cancer.

Homeopathic remedies are derived from plant, animal, microbial, and mineral sources. Examples of plant remedies include herbs, spices, foods, fragrances, and extracts from mushrooms and lichens. Mineral remedies include solutions of metals (copper, gold, tin, zinc), dilute solutions of acids, and substances derived from ores and rocks. Remedies derived from animal substances include venom from insects, spiders, and crustaceans, hormone extracts, and material taken from diseased tissues.

Chiropractic

Chiropractic was founded in the United States around 1900 by Daniel David Palmer, who had no scientific or medical training, but who believed throughout his life

---

TERMS

chiropractic: an alternative medicine that uses manipulation of the spine and joints for healing

homeopathy: an alternative medicine that administers very dilute solutions of substances that mimic the patient's symptoms

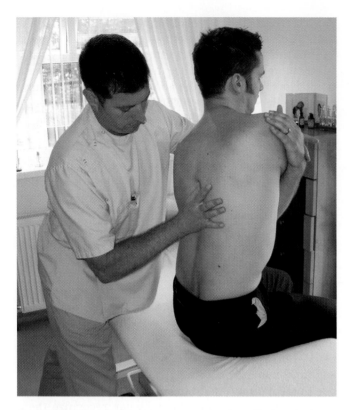

Chiropractic manipulations help many people who suffer from back pain and other musculoskeletal disorders.

that he had a "calling" to heal people. At age 50, Palmer cured Harvey Lillard of deafness by manipulating his spine. Lillard had been deaf for 17 years after working stooped over in a mine. Palmer found a misaligned vertebra, which he manipulated; this allowed Harvey to straighten up for the first time in years and simultaneously restored his hearing. After several other cures by spinal manipulation, Palmer concluded that virtually all diseases are caused by *subluxed* (misaligned) vertebrae.

Palmer coined the name "chiropractic" (from the Greek *cheir,* meaning "hand," and *praktikos,* meaning "practical"; the two words are usually interpreted to mean "done by hand"). Two years later he opened the Palmer School for Chiropractic in Davenport, Iowa. In 1906, Palmer and his son, Bartlett Joshua (or B.J. Palmer), were arrested for practicing medicine without a license. Palmer was tried, convicted, and jailed. His son's case never came to trial.

B.J. Palmer took over the chiropractic practice and turned it into a multimillion-dollar business. B.J. was a genius at commercializing chiropractic, and he was the first to come up with the idea of mail-order diplomas. B.J.'s philosophy of chiropractic was summed up in his description of the spine: "The principal functions of the spine are to support the head, to support the ribs, and to support the chiropractor." Shortly after B.J. took over, chiropractic split into two distinct schools, which still exist today. One group, "the straights," adheres to the original idea that almost all diseases are caused by subluxion of the vertebrae. The other group was founded by John Howard, who believed that other factors also are involved in disease processes. This group became known as the "mixers," and practitioners of this philosophy include nutrition, relaxation, exercise, and other techniques, along with spinal manipulation, in their chiropractic practices.

Although chiropractors treat a wide range of diseases, 90% of patients seeking chiropractic help do so because of back pain, neck pain, or headaches. When the spine is in complete alignment, energy flows freely to all tissues and organs in the body and is the basis for health. **Subluxation** of vertebrae is the principal cause of disease according to chiropractic theory; subluxation can be caused by genetic disorders, falls, injuries, improper sleeping habits, poor posture, obesity, stress, or occupational hazards.

A number of research studies have demonstrated both short-term and long-term benefits of chiropractic for chronic, disabling lower back pain. Other studies have concluded that chiropractic is cheaper and more effective in treatment of back pain and musculoskeletal disorders than conventional medicine. However, claims that chiropractic is effective in reducing blood pressure or relieving allergies or ulcers have not been substantiated by research.

Osteopathy

Osteopathy, like chiropractic, is basically treatment by manipulation of the spine and other structural parts of the body. Osteopathic physicians, called doctors of osteopathy (D.O.), undergo training that is as rigorous as the education of physicians, and generally osteopaths have the same medical privileges of prescribing drugs and performing surgery as do physicians. However, most practitioners of osteopathy rely primarily on physical manipulation and exercises for their patients' conditions.

Osteopathic medicine was founded in the United States by Andrew Taylor Still, who was born in Virginia in 1828. His father was a preacher–physician, and Andrew grew up observing his father treat patients. He eventually developed his own methods of healing, which depended heavily on manipulation. Today, there are hundreds of osteopathic hospitals in the United States and thousands of doctors of osteopathy.

Acupuncture

Acupuncture is an integral part of traditional Chinese medicine, and the use of acupuncture goes back at least 5,000 years. The accumulated knowledge of acupuncture was passed down over the centuries and recorded in a text called *The Yellow Emperor's Classic of Internal Medicine* written in the second or third century B.C. Although acupuncture has been used in China and other Asian countries for centuries, it became popular in the West

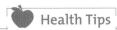

Health Tips

Treating a Headache with Acupressure

Many people experience headaches caused by tension in the muscles of the neck and head. Often the tension alters blood supply to the brain, which causes a headache. Pressing acupressure points at two different locations may relieve the headache pain. The points are located just below the base of the skull, at the back of the head, just to the right and left of center.

Cup the back of your head with your fingers and use your two thumbs to press quite firmly just under the skull on either side of center. The thumbs should be an inch or so apart and away from the centerline of the skull. Press hard for up to a minute or until your thumbs become tired. Repeat the pressure two or three times. Breathe deeply while pressing. Notice if the pain has lessened or disappeared.

Two other acupressure points for headache relief are located on the back of each hand in the soft part between thumb and index finger. Using the thumb and index finger (or middle finger) of the opposite hand, press firmly on the acupressure point. This point may be sensitive, so press only as hard as is comfortable. Repeat on the opposite hand. Press these points for up to a minute and repeat several times. Notice if the headache pain has subsided.

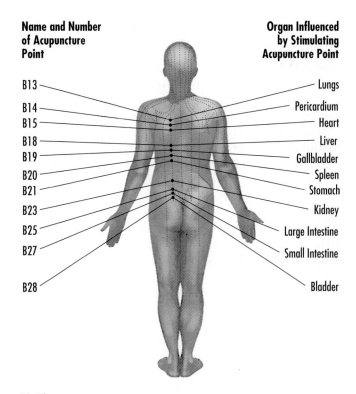

Name and Number of Acupuncture Point

Organ Influenced by Stimulating Acupuncture Point

B13 — Lungs
B14 — Pericardium
B15 — Heart
B18 — Liver
B19 — Gallbladder
B20 — Spleen
B21 — Stomach
B23 — Kidney
B25 — Large Intestine
B27 — Small Intestine
B28 — Bladder

■ **Figure 20.1**

Acupuncture points supposedly influence the functions of internal organs.

only after President Nixon's visit to China in the 1970s. A *New York Times* reporter, James Reston, who was covering Nixon's trip, became ill and underwent an emergency appendectomy. He later wrote an article describing his acupuncture anesthesia, and American physicians began traveling to China to learn more about acupuncture. Today, acupuncture is the most widely used and thoroughly researched alternative medicine.

The underlying principle of acupuncture is the existence of *qi* (pronounced *chi*)—the vital life force that circulates throughout the body and is carried by channels called **meridians.** There are 12 major meridians that connect all of the major organs, as well as a network of minor meridians. The meridians intersect with the surface of the body at many positions; these are the acupuncture points that are "needled" to restore balance to the qi to cure illness or relieve pain. According to Chinese medicine, an organ that is diseased or not functioning properly will manifest symptoms or signs on a corresponding meridian. These may include pain or ache, a change in temperature, sensitivity to touch, or a change in skin texture or color along the affected meridian. Thus, the acupuncturist must first diagnose the cause of the illness by locating the affected meridians; then the correct acupuncture points can be treated.

In acupuncture treatment, very thin metal needles are inserted just under the skin at specific acupuncture points (**Figure 20.1**). Traditional Chinese medicine describes about 365 acupuncture points located along 14 meridians in the body. Usually no more than a dozen or so needles are used. These remain in place for about a half hour, during which they may be twirled or connected to low-voltage generators to increase effectiveness in balancing qi. Sometimes heat is applied to the acupoint in a process called moxibustion. A small piece of an herb, *Artemisia vulgaris* (commonly known as mugwort), is either burned on the tip of the needle or placed on the acupoint.

In 1997, a scientific panel at the National Institutes of Health concluded that traditional acupuncture is

TERMS

acupuncture: an ancient Chinese alternative medicine that uses thin needles inserted into specific points on the body to produce healing energy

meridians: the channels along the body where energy flows and where acupuncture points are located

osteopathy: an alternative medicine that uses manipulation and medicines for healing; osteopaths receive training comparable to that of physicians and can prescribe drugs

subluxation: misalignment of a vertebra from its correct position

effective in relieving postoperative dental pain and in controlling nausea caused by surgery, chemotherapy, or pregnancy. Other conditions listed for which acupuncture may be effective include drug and smoking addiction, lower back pain, stroke rehabilitation, menstrual cramps, tennis elbow, headache, and carpal tunnel syndrome. Although there is no research to substantiate claims of effectiveness, acupuncture also is used to treat neurological disorders (Ménière's disease, trigeminal neuralgia), gastrointestinal disorders (ulcers, colitis, diarrhea), and respiratory disorders (asthma, rhinitis, sinusitis, bronchitis), as well as arthritic conditions.

Acupuncture is effective in reducing the pain of osteoarthritis of the knee (Selfe & Taylor, 2008). More than 20 million Americans suffer from this condition, which is caused by degenerating cartilage. The director of NCCAM, Dr. Stephen Straus, recommended that physicians seriously consider treating knee osteoarthritis with acupuncture to reduce pain and increase mobility.

Acupuncture is also widely used to treat migraine and chronic tension headaches. However, a study showed that real acupuncture was no better than sham acupuncture in reducing the frequency of migraine headaches (Alecrim-Andrade et al., 2008). About 50% of the migraine patients in both the treated and untreated group showed significant reduction of migraine attacks, suggesting that acupuncture also exerts a powerful placebo effect. In both the acupuncture treated group and the control group, about 50% of patients had fewer headaches. Most double-blind placebo-controlled clinical trials show that 40% to 50% of all patients in the placebo group experience as much relief as patients in the treated group (see Chapter 2).

Lest one think that the research cited previously resolves the issue, another study came to the opposite conclusion (Davis et al., 2008). In this large study, patients with chronic headaches, many of whom suffered from migraines, were given either acupuncture treatments or standard medications. The group treated with acupuncture experienced fewer headaches over a 12-month period than patients treated with conventional medicines did.

These two studies highlight the problem of sorting out the scientific research on alternative medicines. Experimental designs are usually different, and conditions of the experiment vary from one research setting to another. Thus, the patient seeking relief for a condition usually acts on the recommendation of another person or on his or her own convictions about the effectiveness of an alternative medicine.

Herbal Medicine

Herbs have been used as medicines for centuries to treat every conceivable form of ailment. Ancient Chinese, Greek, and Roman societies compiled extensive *Pharmacopoeia* describing the uses and preparation of herbal remedies. One herbal compilation published by Nicholas Culpepper in the seventeenth century has gone through countless printings and lists more than 3,000 herbal remedies.

Herbal medicines consist of materials derived from plants and can be prepared as pills, teas, extracts, tinctures, salves, and other forms. In the 1780s, an English physician noted that one of his patients was cured of dropsy by drinking tea made from dried, powdered foxglove leaves. The physician, William Withering, made the connection between dropsy and heart disease. Subsequently, the chemical digitoxin in foxglove leaves was identified as the ingredient that helps heart functions.

Herbs and other plants have been the source for extracting and purifying modern drugs such as ephedrine, digitalis, atropine, reserpine, quinine, and most recently tamoxifen, used to treat breast cancer, and artemisinin, to treat malaria. Herbal medicines often contain a mixture of herbs, so it is difficult to know what component is involved in alleviating symptoms or in healing. Only with the advent of modern chemistry could plant materials be broken down into individual chemical components that can be tested for medicinal properties. Many herbal remedies are used for a variety of ailments and conditions (**Table 20.2**).

Herbal remedies can have the same potential for side effects and harm as prescription drugs. Some plants

Table 20.2

Herbs Used for Common Ailments

Herb	Use
Aloe	Burns, skin irritations
Black cohosh	Menstrual cramps, PMS, menopause
Chamomile	Digestion
Echinacea	Immune system stimulant
Feverfew	Reduces fever, helps migraine
Foxglove	Controls heart rhythm, angina
Garlic	Digestion, protects against high blood pressure
Ginger root	Motion sickness, cough
Ginkgo biloba	Dilates blood vessels, dementia
Ginseng	Reduces stress
Hawthorn	Lowers blood pressure, dilates blood vessels
Milk thistle	Protects damaged liver, prevents toxins from entering liver
Peppermint	Indigestion
St. Johns' wort	Depression
Saw palmetto	Enlarged prostate, improves urinary flow, anti-inflammatory agent
Senna	Strong laxative
Tea-tree oil	Skin and vaginal infections, acne
Valerian root	Mild sedative
Willow bark	Headache

contain toxic chemicals along with the beneficial ones; the concentrations of both kinds of chemicals will vary from plant to plant and from one season to the next. Thus, one batch of herbs may be safe and effective whereas another batch may be toxic, ineffective, or both. Without rigorous testing (which is required for prescription drugs), the safety and efficacy of herbal remedies cannot be assured. Problems, side effects, and risks associated with some commonly used herbs are listed in **Table 20.3**.

An herb that helps reduce depression is *St. John's wort*. Clinical studies indicate that extracts of *St. John's wort* are as effective in treating moderate to severe depression as the prescription antidepressant drug *paroxetine* (Szegedi et al., 2005). However, a major problem with this herb is that it reduces the effectiveness of birth control drugs, so that unanticipated pregnancies have occurred among depressed women taking St. John's wort. The herb also reduces the effectiveness of other prescription antidepressants, AIDS drugs, and anticoagulants. In fact, research shows that the herb can reduce the effectiveness of as many as 50% of all prescription drugs (Markowitz et al., 2003). Using this herb carries sufficient risk that it should be used only on the advice of a physician who is familiar with its many effects.

Kava kava (or simply kava or awa) is an herbal drink used for thousands of years by people indigenous to islands of the Pacific such as Micronesia, Fiji, and Hawaii. Among these peoples, kava is imbibed mostly on ceremonial occasions, but kava beverages are also widely drunk in social settings as a relaxant and for stress reduction. In recent years, the use of kava in Europe, Canada, and the United States has blossomed into a major industry. Kava is sold as a drink, a tea, and as a powdered supplement in pill form. In 2002, a number of kava users, primarily in Europe, suffered severe liver damage and some died. Shortly thereafter, kava was banned in most European countries and Canada. It is still legal to sell and use kava in the United States, but the Food and Drug Administration advises against its use. It is likely that the traditional preparation and use of kava, which is made by squeezing liquid from the bark on roots of the kava bush, is safe. However, in the West, extracts and pills are made from the bark as well as the roots of the plant. It appears that the bark contains toxic chemicals that are not present in the roots. In any event, drinking kava or taking kava supplements involves health risk and should be avoided.

Ephedra is a potent drug present in a Chinese herb called *ma huang*. It is widely added to dietary supplements as a stimulant to help people lose weight and is used by athletes to enhance performance (Shekelle et al., 2003). Ephedra raises blood pressure and heart rate and causes psychiatric symptoms and gastrointestinal problems. As a consequence of its effect on the heart, it

---

Table 20.3

Risks and Side Effects Associated with Some Herbs

Echinacea
Allergic reactions, including rashes, increased asthma, and anaphylaxis (a life-threatening allergic reaction), especially if already allergic to related plants in the daisy family (ragweed, chrysanthemums, marigolds, and daisies)

Ephedra
Stroke, heart attack, and sudden death; worsening of cardiovascular disease, kidney disease, sleep disorders, and diabetes; nausea, anxiety, headache, psychosis, kidney stones, tremors, dry mouth, irregular heart rhythms, heart damage, high blood pressure, restlessness, sleep problems, irritation of the stomach, and increased urination

Garlic
Breath and body odor, heartburn, upset stomach, and allergic reactions; reduced ability of blood to clot (may be a problem during or after surgery and dental work)

Ginkgo biloba
Headache, nausea, gastrointestinal upset, diarrhea, dizziness, or allergic reactions; reduced ability of blood to clot (may be a problem during or after surgery and dental work)

Ginseng
Headaches, sleep, gastrointestinal problems, allergic reactions, lower levels of blood sugar (more likely to occur in people with diabetes)

Green tea
Contains caffeine, which can cause insomnia, anxiety, irritability, upset stomach, nausea, diarrhea, or frequent urination; contains small amounts of vitamin K, which can make anticoagulant drugs, such as warfarin, less effective

Kava
Drowsiness (avoid driving and operating heavy machinery), liver damage and (sometimes fatal) liver failure, abnormal muscle spasms or involuntary muscle movements; may interact with several drugs, including drugs used for Parkinson's disease

St. John's wort
Increased sensitivity to sunlight; anxiety, dry mouth, dizziness, gastrointestinal symptoms, fatigue, headache, and sexual problems; may increase or decrease the effects of other drugs, such as antidepressants, hormonal contraceptives, digoxin, warfarin, indinavir, and drugs used in organ transplantation

Valerian
Headaches, dizziness, upset stomach, and tiredness the morning after its use

Source: National Center for Alternative and Complementary Medicine. Available: http://nccam.nih.gov/health/herbsataglance.htm.

---

can cause palpitations that may result in heart attacks and stroke in susceptible persons. Between 1997 and 2001, the U.S. armed forces documented 30 deaths among service personnel using ephedra products. In

TERMS

herbal medicines: materials derived from plants and other organisms that are made into teas, powders, and salves to treat diseases and injuries

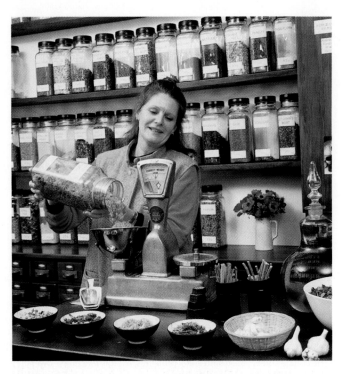

Herbal remedies are continuing to increase in popularity among Americans with a variety of ailments.

recent years, the deaths of several high-profile professional athletes were linked to ephedra supplements. In addition to deaths, thousands of people using ephedra products have reported adverse effects.

In April 2004, the Food and Drug Administration (FDA) issued a rule that banned the sale of herbal and dietary supplements containing ephedra (Rados, 2004). This was the first time that the FDA banned a supplement under the procedures provided in the Dietary Supplement Health and Education Act (DSHEA) passed by Congress in 1994. This act gives the FDA the power to ban a supplement when there is compelling evidence of its potential health dangers.

The scientists at the FDA felt that they had a strong case; however, in April 2005, a federal court judge overturned the ephedra ban. In the ruling, the judge said that the evidence presented by the FDA on the dangers of ephedra at low doses (10 mg per daily dose) was not convincing, and ordered that the ban on ephedra sales be lifted. The FDA appealed that ruling. In the meantime, ephedra supplements still can be purchased in stores and over the Internet. Congress is considering a new dietary supplement law that would give the FDA more power to regulate the manufacture and sales of herbal and dietary supplements.

Manufacturers are also marketing ephedra-free weight-loss supplements in anticipation of an ephedra ban. The new supplements contain *synephrine* (also called bitter orange). This compound also affects heart rate and

blood pressure, and products containing it may be just as dangerous as ones with ephedra. At least one case of stroke has already been reported from use of synephrine. Supplements containing ephedra or synephrine are dangerous and should not be used by anyone concerned about his or her health.

Vitamin and herbal supplements are a multibillion-dollar industry in the United States, and suppliers of these products are opposed to any legislation that would dampen sales. For example, *ginkgo biloba* is one of the best-selling herbs; it is used as a memory booster and to help ward off senility in the elderly. In 2002, *ginkgo biloba* sales exceeded $175 million. However, taking *ginkgo biloba* can be quite dangerous if you are also taking a blood thinner medication for heart disease.

Scientific studies defining the risks and benefits of dietary and herbal supplements are not available for most supplements that people take. Manufacturers are not required to carry out tests that establish the safety and efficacy of a product before they sell it. Most vitamin and mineral supplements are safe if taken in reasonable amounts, and many Americans take them to supplement a diet that may be deficient in essential nutrients for one reason or another. However, herbal medicines pose a significant risk. Herbs contain chemicals that act as drugs, but the actual amounts of the active chemicals in most herbal medicines are often not known or may be misrepresented or underrepresented on the label. Anyone planning on using an herbal medicine should consult a knowledgeable health care provider about its risks and benefits. Any adverse reactions to an herbal medicine should be reported to health authorities.

Many herbs are now being added to foods to increase marketability and sales. Herbs are added to sodas, fruit drinks, cereals, and many other kinds of foods. Remember that food is for eating enjoyment and maintaining health. Herbs are for treating ailments or diseases. Do not confuse the functions of food and herbs, and do not consume any herb in food "just because it might help me feel better."

Naturopathy

Naturopathy is a uniquely American approach to health that arose in the late nineteenth century. The term was introduced by Dr. John Sheel in 1895; the principles of naturopathy as a system of healing and way of living were formulated by Benedict Lust in 1902. In the early 1900s, more than 20 naturopathic schools of medicine trained naturopathic doctors (N.D.). But with the rise of conventional medicine, naturopathy all but disappeared from the American health scene. However, it experienced a revival in the 1970s, along with other alternative medicines.

Naturopathy's approach to health emphasizes the prevention of disease and the individual's responsibility for a healthy lifestyle. Naturopathy draws on all available alternative medicines, as well as aspects of conventional medicine. However, it does reject the use of surgery and drugs. If there is a single unifying concept to naturopathy, it is that the body possesses the "energy" or "intelligence" to heal itself. In that sense it is similar in philosophy to Ayurvedic and Chinese medicine.

The eight basic principles of naturopathy are as follows:

- The human body possesses an innate ability to heal itself.
- It is the duty of the naturopathic practitioner to find and treat the underlying cause of illness, not simply the symptoms.
- The naturopathic practitioner is first and foremost a teacher who must educate the patient on how to prevent illness and restore health.
- The naturopathic practitioner must employ therapies that "do no harm." Surgery and drugs are not recommended.
- The focus is mainly on prevention of illness. The patient's lifestyle is examined in detail, and recommendations are made to reduce health risks and to foster health.
- Good nutrition is an essential goal of naturopathy. Without a healthy diet, the body invites illness.
- The treatment must involve the whole person, not just an organ or part of the body. A person's physical, mental, emotional, and spiritual states must be evaluated and altered as necessary to promote health.
- The ultimate goal of naturopathy is optimal health, not just the absence of disease.

These principles of naturopathy are essentially those of modern holistic medicine. The emphasis of the medicine of the future should be to prevent disease by educating patients in the health benefits of good nutrition and in helping them reduce destructive health behaviors such as smoking, drinking, or using recreational drugs. Also, people must find ways to reduce stress, anxiety, and emotional turmoil if they are to enjoy optimal health. In the modern world, these are difficult tasks even for a motivated individual.

Naturopathic doctors receive training that is as complete as a medical school that awards the M.D. degree. A naturopathic doctor who has graduated from one of the half dozen schools offering degrees in naturopathy is well equipped to diagnose and treat a wide range of diseases. It is the approach to healing that distinguishes the N.D. from the M.D., although many physicians with an M.D. practice naturopathic medicine even though they also can prescribe drugs and recommend surgery. Because naturopathy eschews the use of surgery and drugs, naturopathic doctors do not treat acute illness or conditions that require emergency care. People usually consult a naturopathic doctor to construct a lifestyle that will prevent illness and promote overall optimal health.

Therapeutic Massage

Therapeutic massage is a hands-on therapy in which touch is used to heal. Cave paintings dating back approximately 15,000 years depict injured people being treated with what looks like massage. The use of massage to heal is described in ancient Chinese, Greek, and Roman texts. Seemingly miraculous cures have been reported over the centuries by the "laying on of hands" by people believed to have divine powers, such as priests, shamans, and holy persons. Despite its effectiveness as an alternative medicine, some people still regard massage as a guise for sexual stimulation. However, therapeutic massage administered by a trained and licensed professional is a highly effective form of therapy for many conditions.

Human touch is essential to normal development of infants and children and to health in general. Americans tend to touch one another much less than people in other cultures. Psychologists who observe the number of times people touch one another in cafes or other public places report that, on average, Americans touch one another less frequently than almost any other culture in the world. In similar situations, Parisians touch one another more than 100 times per hour and Puerto Ricans almost 200 times per hour! Cultural anthropologists report that cultures that are more physically affectionate toward infants and children have lower rates of adult violence such as domestic and sexual abuse.

The most immediate effect of therapeutic massage is improved blood circulation. As the skin is stretched and the muscles are kneaded, the amount of blood returning to the heart is increased, and toxins released into the blood can be excreted more readily. Enhanced circulation also supplies more oxygen to tissues and to the brain. Massage benefits digestion and elimination, and it hastens wound healing. Massage also eases muscle pain caused by strain or injury; it may stimulate the release of endorphins and enkephalins, pain-relieving chemicals synthesized in the body.

There are certain conditions and diseases in which therapeutic massage should *not* be used because of the

---

TERMS

naturopathy: an alternative medicine that uses nutrition, herbs, massage, and other techniques to promote healing

therapeutic massage: promotes relaxation and healing by massage of the skin and muscles

possibility of causing further damage to tissues or organs. These are as follows:

- Recent bone fractures or severe sprains
- Herniated disk in the spine
- Excessive blood pressure
- Areas of the body in which hemorrhage has occurred
- Any acute inflammation of the skin or joints
- Blood conditions such as phlebitis and thrombosis
- Severe varicose veins
- Certain kinds of cancer

Therapeutic massage involves five basic kinds of manipulation of a person's skin and muscles. The first is an extended gliding stroke with the whole hand or thumb. This warms the skin and relaxes muscle tension. The next is a kneading motion in which muscles are grabbed and lifted. This relieves soreness and improves circulation. Friction manipulation is used around joints and thick muscles. Repeated circular movement of the hands can help break up adhesions. The hands also can be used in a chopping or tapping motion to stimulate the skin and muscles; this chopping is used when muscles are spastic or cramped. Finally, the fingers or flattened hands are pressed into muscles and "vibrated" for a few seconds. This vibration stimulates nerves and circulation in the area.

Massage therapists are required to pass a licensing exam in most states. Many people claim to be massage therapists who are not licensed or who have limited training. Making sure a therapist is licensed and talking to people who have benefited from that therapist are good ways to ensure that your experience will be helpful. Even if you do not have a specific medical condition that needs massage therapy, getting a massage is relaxing and refreshing.

Some specific forms of massage are these:

Swedish massage: uses long strokes, kneading of muscles, and friction techniques on the outer layers of the body. Also uses active and passive movement of joints.

Shiatsu and acupressure massage: both techniques use pressure on specific points of the body to treat pain and improve body functions. In Shiatsu, pressure may be applied with fingers, elbows, or feet. In acupressure, fingers are used.

Lomi lomi massage: an ancient Hawaiian healing art that is a form of spiritual massage used to restore mind–body harmony.

Rolfing: developed by Ida Rolf to realign the body by deep (and often painful) massage of underlying myofascial tissues. Rolfing is also called structural integration.

Rosen massage: uses gentle touch and verbal communication to relieve suppressed emotions locked into musculature from past traumatic incidents.

Trigger point massage: uses finger pressure on "trigger points" in painful or inflamed areas of muscle to break the cycles of spasm and pain.

Aromatherapy

Aromatherapy is a centuries-old alternative medicine in which the essential oils of plants (many of which are fragrant) are administered so that chemicals contained in the oils are absorbed into the body and act as drugs. In that sense, aromatherapy is similar to herbal medicine or to conventional drug therapy. Since the 1980s, aromatherapy has increased in popularity among Americans seeking alternative medicines, and now is a more than $300 million annual business.

Priests and healers in the ancient world used oils and perfumes to treat illnesses and as a prevention against disease. In the Egyptian Ebers Papyrus, which dates to about 1500 B.C., there are descriptions of more than 800 plant and herbal remedies, many of which are fragrant oil extracts. The modern medicinal use of plant oils and fragrances, as well as the term *aromatherapy*, derives from a French chemist who began to study the healing power of plant oils in the 1930s. He became interested after burning his hand in his family's perfume factory. He plunged his burned hand into a vat of lavender oil for relief and discovered that the burn healed rapidly and without scarring.

Some of the most popular aromatherapy oil extracts are derived from the following:

- The leaves of eucalyptus and peppermint
- The fruits and blossoms of oranges and lemons
- The flowers of lavender and roses
- Woods such as camphor and sandalwood
- Cinnamon bark, lemongrass, fennel, and rosemary
- Dried spices such as clove and fresh garlic bulbs

Essential oils made from plant extracts are very concentrated and contain hundreds of chemicals that can act as drugs. Thus, only minute amounts of oils are used, and a person practicing aromatherapy needs to be knowledgeable about the kinds of chemicals present in different extracts and their effects on the body. Aromatherapists treat people by prescribing oils that can be inhaled directly, applied to the skin as part of a massage, or added to a hot bath, in which case the oils are both absorbed and inhaled. Aromatherapy is used to treat infections, pain, arthritis, skin disorders, headaches, digestive disorders, and other conditions.

Although aromatherapy has been used for thousands of years, there is no scientific evidence that it cures any disease. It is critical that patients using aromatherapy (or other alternative medicine) inform their physicians as to what oils, herbs, or supplements they are using to avoid serious complications from drug–drug or drug–herb interactions.

Biomagnetic Therapy

Biomagnetic therapy (also called magnetic therapy) involves the use of static magnetic fields or pulsed magnetic fields created by electrical currents to treat a wide variety of ailments, especially pain. Biomagnetic therapies have been used for thousands of years, primarily in

$ Dollars and Health Sense

Marketing "Miracle" Health Juices

In recent years a multibillion-dollar business has developed—primarily on the Internet—in marketing exotic juices that proponents claim can cure almost any disease as well as boost longevity and energy. The juices are primarily derived from such fruits as pomegranate, mangosteen, goji, and noni. Pomegranates are probably familiar to most people, but the other plants are of Asian origin and rarely seen in U.S. markets. The fruits of these plants contain antioxidants (as do many fruits and vegetables), which are advertised as cures for cancer, diabetes, heart disease, macular degeneration, Alzheimer's, and other serious diseases.

The current health fad in exotic fruit juices began in 2003 with the mass marketing of POM, a mixture of pomegranate and grape juice that sold for $5 for a 16-ounce bottle. Pomegranates contain phytochemicals that act as antioxidants; cranberries, blueberries, and strawberries also contain significant amounts of phytochemicals. Marketers recommended that people drink at least 8 ounces of pomegranate juice a day, which would mean spending $75 a month or more for this juice.

For centuries, people in Asia have been using the fruit and bark of the *mangosteen* to treat stomach and skin problems. In the United States, shrewd marketers set up a pyramid scheme of salespersons and multiple Web sites to hype the benefits of mangosteen juice. (It is usually mixed with nine other juices.) The brain behind the sales of mangosteen products is a company called XanGo; in 2005 its sales topped $200 million. Health claims for mangosteen juice include boosting the immune system, enhancing physical performance, improving the respiratory system, and supporting the health of bone and cartilage. (Such claims do not violate any laws because they do not refer to specific diseases.)

Another popular tropical fruit product is *noni*, which grows in the wild on most Pacific islands, including Hawaii. When ripe, noni fruits soften rapidly and exude a foul-smelling and equally foul-tasting liquid. Proponents of noni claim that it will cure almost anything. Tahitian Noni, the largest of the noni marketers, claims to have sold over $2 billion worth of noni juice between 1996, when it was introduced, and 2006. A 32-ounce bottle costs between $40 and $50, and it is recommended that people drink 1 to 3 ounces a day for whatever ails them. Scientific studies to date do not support any of the health claims posted on noni Web sites.

The most recent addition to the booming business in functional health juices is *goji* juice, which is derived from small berries that grow in mountainous regions of China and Tibet. For centuries extracts of goji berries have been used in Chinese herbal remedies for a variety of conditions, including poor vision and cough. In contrast to noni's unpleasant taste and smell, goji juice is delicious, with a delightful blend of sweet and sour flavors. It is as easy to drink as a glass of lemonade. But at $40 to $50 a bottle for wild-berry juice, it's a rich person's drink. And, with the current craze for goji juice, the Himalayan plants are rapidly becoming extinct. The best thing that can be said for all these "antioxidant" juices is that they probably do no harm to health. These fruit juices do not cure cancers or extend life, as many of their proponents claim, but they are making some companies and salespeople very rich.

---

non-Western countries, to treat pain, inflammation, stress, fractures, and other health problems. The ancient Greeks discovered lodestone, a naturally magnetized substance, and thought that it had healing properties.

The earth has a magnetic field, and because all life developed in the earth's magnetic field, it is argued that the functions of damaged cells can be improved with biomagnetic therapies. Most of the evidence for the effectiveness of biomagnetic therapies comes from testimonials, which do not constitute scientific proof. In general, it is difficult to design randomized, placebo-controlled studies using magnets to treat specific conditions. However, a few positive studies have been carried out. The use of high-energy, pulsed magnetic fields to treat severe depression has met with some success. Also bone healing has been accelerated with the use of electrical currents and magnetic fields, and some people claim to have experienced pain relief using small electrical generators.

However, despite numerous claims, use of static field magnets to treat a wide variety of health concerns has not been substantiated by scientific studies. Mag-nets are put under beds to reduce pain and stress or to cure other conditions. Magnets placed in shoes are used to treat pain. Magnetic bracelets are worn for many health reasons. And magnetized water is a booming business. Americans spend more than $300 million each year on various forms of biomagnetic therapies. Yet scientific studies showing that biomagnetic therapies are effective are rare and usually negative. Treatment of plantar heel pain by inserting magnets into shoes gave no evidence of benefit (Winemiller, 2003). Also, no benefit was found in the use of magnets to reduce muscle strain or pain after exercise.

TERMS

aromatherapy: use of fragrant extracts of plants to promote healing

biomagnetic therapy: use of magnetic fields to treat pain, ailments, and diseases

The use of magnets may produce benefits by virtue of the placebo effect (see Chapter 2). Anything that a person believes in strongly can produce a healing effect through the mind's capacity to alter chemistry and physiology in distant parts of the body. Biomagnetic therapies, especially ones using static magnetic fields, do no harm. People spend money on many kinds of health aids to find relief from pain and other problems. Whether money spent on biomagnetic therapies is well spent is a matter of personal choice.

Medical Quackery

Quackery is a term that refers to the sale of useless potions, devices, or other substances that promise to heal or cure the buyer of whatever ails him or her. People (quacks) who sell bogus medical products may actually believe in the products' worth and, consequently, are not committing fraud, which involves knowledge of the worthlessness of the products. Legally, it is difficult to separate quackery and fraud.

Quackery has a long history, and during the eighteenth and nineteenth centuries, traveling entertainers sold all sorts of nostrums and potions in towns all over America. Some of these potions actually contained "feel good" substances such as opium or cocaine. Quackery in the United States was dealt a serious blow with the passage of the Pure Food and Drug Act in 1906, which made the sale of worthless medicines illegal. But over the years, sales of useless health products have grown continuously. Ten years ago, the FDA estimated that 38 million Americans purchased a fraudulent health product in the previous year. The most prevalent fraudulent products listed by the FDA are the following:

- Fraudulent arthritis products
- Fake cancer clinics
- Bogus AIDS cures
- Instant weight-loss schemes
- Fraudulent sexual aids
- Useless baldness remedies
- False nutritional schemes
- Useless muscle stimulators
- Candidiasis hypersensitivity cures

Why do people buy useless and/or dangerous health products? Why are people easily fooled by quackery? There is no easy answer to these questions. If you want to safeguard your health and your pocketbook, you should check on any product or treatment that is not provided by a licensed health care provider. A reliable source of information about fraudulent products can be found at www.quackwatch.com.

Choosing an Alternative Medicine

Many people are satisfied with the care they receive from modern medicine and the physicians who treat them. However, many Americans also seek alternative medicines to complement conventional treatments. And some persons choose to rely on alternative medicines exclusively. For many kinds of chronic sickness, alternative medicines may provide relief and healing.

> There is no medicine that cures stupidity.
> *Japanese proverb*

It often is wise to begin with the least invasive form of treatment before undergoing surgery or taking drugs that can also do harm. Our society is gradually coming to the view that healing can be accomplished by both conventional and alternative medicine. And, as we have pointed out repeatedly, the belief of the patient in a particular treatment, physician, acupuncturist, or chiropractor may be what heals.

TERMS

quackery: promotion and sale of unapproved and worthless products, especially for medical problems and health enhancement

Critical Thinking About Health

1. Suppose that you have been in an auto accident and have a whiplash injury to your neck. It is some months since the accident and your doctor says that your neck has healed and that she cannot find anything wrong. However, you still have pain and difficulty moving your head. What alternative medicines would you now consider to relieve your symptoms? Discuss the rationale behind your choice of alternative medicine(s). If you have actually experienced such an accident, describe the healing process that you went through.

2. Describe any herbal remedy that you are now taking and the condition for which it is being used. Answer each of the following questions and discuss your reasons for taking this remedy and how you think it has helped you (if it has).
   a. Have you investigated whether this herbal remedy has been studied in clinical trials and found to be effective?
   b. Have you investigated whether there are any dangers associated with taking this herb?
   c. Have you discussed taking this herbal remedy with a physician?

3. Therapeutic touch (TT) is a technique widely used by nurses to alleviate suffering and promote healing in patients with a wide variety of ailments, including cancer. TT claims that nurses achieve healing and relief by sensing and manipulating a "human energy field" that is felt above the patient's body. A recent scientific study of TT found that, under controlled laboratory conditions in which nurses had to sense the presence of the experimenter's hand over one of their own without being able to see the person on the other side of a screen, nurses were unable to score significantly above chance (i.e., they had a 50% chance of being correct). The scientists concluded that nurses who practice TT are unable to detect a human energy field, that TT is bogus, and that further professional use of TT is unjustified.
   a. Do you agree with the scientists' conclusions?
   b. Think of reasons why the experiment might not be a valid test of TT and explain your criticisms in detail.
   c. Can you devise an experiment that you think would be better in proving or disproving that TT had beneficial effects on patients?

4. Studies of acupuncture have consistently shown that it is more effective when used on Chinese patients in China than when it is used on patients in the United States. In addition to being more effective on individual patients, more diseases respond to acupuncture treatments in China than when the same diseases are treated with acupuncture in the United States.
   a. Make a list of as many reasons that you can think of that would explain these observations (e.g., American acupuncturists are not as proficient as Chinese acupuncturists).
   b. Discuss each of the items on your list and describe how it would explain the observed difference.
   c. Pick one of the items that you have identified and design a scientific experiment that would prove whether your hypothesis is true or not.

Health in Review

- Alternative medicine consists of hundreds of methods for dealing with sickness and disease in ways that are different from modern medical care performed by physicians.
- The broad categories of alternative medicine include spiritual and mental therapies, nutritional therapies, herbal remedies, and physical therapies.
- Homeopathy administers very dilute solutions of substances that are supposed to mimic the symptoms of sick persons and help the body cure itself of the disease.
- Chiropractic and osteopathy use manipulation of the spine and joints to treat musculoskeletal disorders and other diseases.
- Ayurveda and aromatherapy are ancient healing techniques.
- Acupuncture involves inserting very thin needles into specific points on the body to restore harmony to the functioning of tissues and organs.
- Herbal medicine uses mixtures of herbs in the form of pills, powders, teas, and tinctures to help the healing process. Some widely used herbs are ineffective.
- Some herbal remedies contain toxic chemicals, and some interact with prescription drugs to make them either more or less effective.
- There is little scientific evidence for the effectiveness of biomagnetic therapy in the treatment of disease, but many people use it for pain relief and for other health problems.
- Americans spend hundreds of millions of dollars each year on fraudulent health products and treatments; many are victims of quackery.
- Consumers of alternative medicine need to guard against fraudulent claims and unscrupulous persons who advertise therapies of unproved safety and of dubious value.

Health and Wellness Online

The Web contains a wealth of information about health and wellness. By accessing the Internet using Web browser software, you can gain a new perspective on many topics presented in *Health and Wellness*, Tenth Edition. Access the Jones and Bartlett Publishers Web site at **health.jbpub.com/hwonline**.

References

Alecrim-Andrade, J., et al. (2008). Acupuncture in migraine prevention: A randomized sham controlled study with 6-months posttreatment follow-up. *Clinical Journal of Pain, 24,* 98–105.

Davis, M. A., et al. (2008). Acupuncture for tension-type headache: A meta-analysis of randomized, controlled trials. *Journal of Pain, 9,* 667–677.

Markowitz, J. S., et al. (2003). Effect of St. John's wort on drug metabolism by induction of cytochrome P450 3A4 enzyme. *Journal of the American Medical Association, 290,* 1500–1504.

Rados, C. (2004, March/April). Ephedra ban: No shortage of reasons. *FDA Consumer,* 6–7.

Saper, R. B., et al. (2008). Lead, mercury, and arsenic in US- and Indian-manufactured Ayurvedic medicines sold via the Internet. *Journal of the American Medical Association, 300,* 915–923.

Selfe, T. K., & Taylor, A. G. (2008). Acupuncture and osteoarthritis of the knee: A review of randomized, controlled trials. *Family and Community Health, 31,* 247–254.

Shekelle, P. G., et al. (2003). Efficacy and safety of ephedra and ephedrine for weight loss and athletic performance. *Journal of the American Medical Association, 289,* 1537–1545.

Szegedi, A., et al. (2005). Acute treatment of moderate to severe depression with hypericum extract WS5570 (St. John's wort): Randomized controlled double blind non-inferiority trial versus paroxetine. *British Medical Journal, 330,* 567–571.

Winemiller, M. H. (2003). Effect of magnetic vs sham-magnetic insoles on plantar heel pain. *Journal of the American Medical Association, 290,* 1474–1478.

Suggested Readings

Bausell, R. B. (2007). *Snake oil science: The truth about complementary and alternative medicine.* New York: Oxford University Press. The author gently debunks most alternative medicines but also believes that most of them *do* work because of the placebo effect.

Ernst, E., Pittler, M. H., Stevinson, C., & White, A. (Eds.). (2001). *The desktop guide to complementary and alternative medicine: An experience-based approach.* St. Louis: Mosby. Primarily for physicians, this medical text provides the evidence for using some alternative medicines.

Gold, P. E., Cahill, L., & Wenk, G. L. (2003, April). The lowdown on ginkgo biloba. *Scientific American,* 86–91. Discusses the evidence that this herb and other substances may be of help in improving memory and slowing the effects of dementia.

Rados, C. (2004, March/April). Science meets beauty: Using medicine to improve appearances. *FDA Consumer,* 30–35. Discusses various cosmetic procedures and possible dangers.

Raloff, J. (2003, June 7). Herbal lottery. *Science News,* 359–361. The article explains that most herbal remedies do not contain what the labels say.

Ruggie, M. (2004). *Marginal to mainstream: Alternative medicine in America.* New York: Cambridge University Press. A good overview of the pros and cons of alternative medicines.

Recommended Web Sites

Please visit **health.jbpub.com/hwonline** for links to these Web sites.

Alternative Medicine Home Page
Resources and links maintained by the University of Pittsburgh Medical Library.

MedlinePlus on Alternative Medicine
This site is useful for checking on the validity or dangers of alternative medicines or therapies.

National Center for Complementary and Alternative Medicine
Education and resources from the U.S. National Institutes of Health.

Quackwatch.com
Good place to check for fraudulent products and treatments.

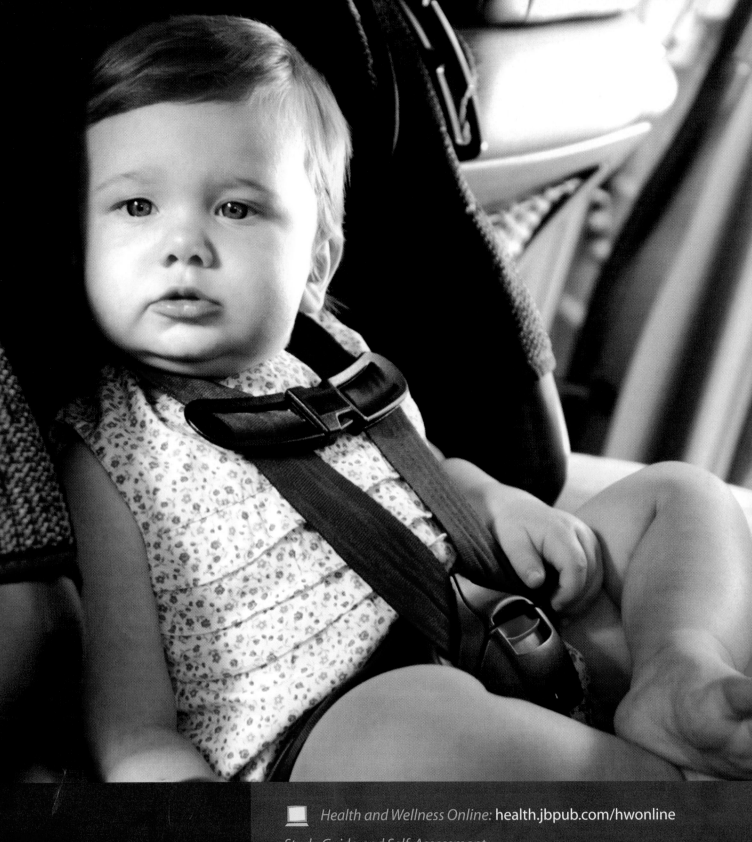

Chapter Twenty-One

Accidents and Injuries

Learning Objectives

1. Define *safety*, *accidents*, and *unintentional injuries*.

2. Describe various strategies to prevent unintentional injuries.

3. Use the epidemiological triad to identify unintentional injury risk factors.

4. Describe the Haddon matrix and explain why it was developed.

5. Discuss various ways to prevent motor vehicle crashes, motorcycle accidents, bicycle accidents, and pedestrian accidents.

6. Describe various strategies to improve home and work safety.

7. Describe ways to prevent firearm injuries.

8. List the major sports with the highest risk of injury for boys and girls.

Injuries affect the health and well-being of millions of Americans every year. Unintentional injuries and accidents of various kinds are a far greater source of ill health and death than most people realize. Safety warnings and increased public awareness measures have reduced the number of unintentional injury deaths significantly since 1900 (**Figure 21.1**). In 2006, the number of unintentional injury deaths from all causes in the United States was estimated at 120,000. Over the past 50 years, deaths from unintentional injuries in the United States have ranged from a high of 120,000 in 2006 to a low of 86,777 in 1992. However, because the U.S. population has been increasing steadily, the overall rate of deaths from unintentional injuries has been declining, except for a period in the 1960s and early 1970s. The increased death rate in this period prompted Congress to pass legislation designed to improve safety equipment for automobiles and mandate the use of seat belts.

> The best way to avoid something is to cause that which is to be avoided, to avoid you of its own accord.
>
> *Sufi proverb*

Despite the encouraging reduction in unintentional injury deaths, the adverse health consequences of unintentional injuries are still too high and should be reduced further. In the United States, unintentional injuries are the leading cause of death among all persons aged 1 to 34 and the fifth leading cause of death among people of all ages.

Many people believe accidents are chance occurrences over which people have no control. Whereas it is true that some accidents are the result of bad luck, a vast number of accidents and the injuries resulting from them are caused by social and economic conditions—unsafe roads and automobiles, unsafe homes and work sites—and personal factors—poor judgment, lapses in attention, recklessness, loss of emotional control, and mental states that are imbalanced by alcohol and drugs. Insofar as the environment can be made safer and individuals become more cautious, the number of unintentional injuries from accidents can be reduced.

Unintentional Injuries and Accidents

What is **safety?** The word *safety* is used in a wide context with various meanings to different individuals. Few experts or safety agencies can agree on a universal definition. "Is this a safe part of town to be in late at night?" "He is not a very safe motorcycle driver." "My daughter's safety has been a concern of mine since she obtained her driver's license." "Is that old ladder safe to use?" As you can see, the word *safe* or *safety* may be used in a variety of situations.

One way to tie all these different scenarios together is the word **accident.** As defined by the National Safety Council, an accident "is that occurrence in a sequence of events which produces unintended injury, death, or property damage. Accident refers to the event, not the result of the event."

Each year one in four individuals will sustain some type of serious injury that requires medical attention and that is a result of an accident. Injuries are a serious problem, but many individuals lack the necessary knowledge and skills to help themselves if a serious accident does occur. Injuries are the leading cause of disability in young people and cause more deaths in children than all the infectious diseases combined.

Unintentional injury refers to the *result* of an accident and its health consequences. Deaths from unintentional injuries result from motor vehicle accidents, home accidents (falls, fires, poisonings), workplace accidents, firearm accidents, and other causes (**Table 21.1**). The greatest number of deaths occur as a result of motor vehicle crashes, falls, and poisonings. However, the age groups that are most likely to die in these kinds of accidents differ significantly. Teenagers and young adults are most likely to die in motor vehicle crashes, middle-aged persons by poisoning, and the elderly by falls (**Figure 21.2**).

Unintentional injuries are the fifth leading cause of death overall, exceeded only by heart disease, cancer, stroke, and chronic obstructive pulmonary disease. The five leading causes of death from unintentional injury are motor vehicle accidents, falls, poisoning by solids and liquids, fires and burns, and drowning: These have

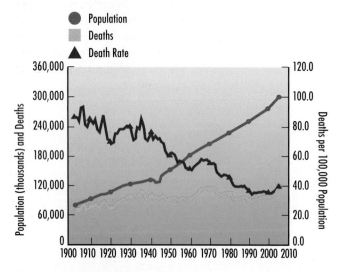

■ **Figure 21.1**

Unintentional Injury Deaths , Population Increase, and Death Rates in the United States, 1903–2006

The total number of deaths from unintentional injuries has remained relatively constant over the past century. However, because the population has increased dramatically, the death rate has declined significantly.

Source: National Safety Council, *Injury facts,* 2008. Reprinted with permission.

been the same since 1970. For most of the twentieth century, the rate of death from accidents steadily dropped because of increased safety and health efforts. However, in the last few years, there has been an increase in total deaths from unintentional injury, which should be a warning that greater attention to increased safety efforts is needed to reverse this trend.

The causes of death from unintentional injury change with age. Poor diet, sedentary lifestyle, arthritis, decreased mobility, poverty, chronic diseases, or lack of access to primary medical care may contribute to injuries and accidental death as people get older. Persons over age 75 are at highest risk of death compared to

younger age groups from virtually all kinds of accidents—pedestrian and motor vehicle accidents, falls, choking, fires, and exposure to unusual natural heat or cold.

Reducing Your Risk of Accidents

When considering accidents, their prevention, and their consequences, public health professionals focus on **accident mitigation**—methods to reduce damage caused by unplanned events—and **accident prevention**—ways to eliminate the occurrence of unintended injuries. Accident mitigation and prevention can be viewed in two contexts: (1) individual or personal and (2) environmental or community.

Many factors are involved in unintentional injury: knowledge, attitudes, beliefs, and behaviors; economic and social conditions; ability level of the performer of tasks; conditions of the environment; and alcohol and other drug use. Positive changes in these factors will reduce injuries, but more attention should be directed to prevention strategies. Even though unintentional injuries have decreased by more than half over the past century, the cost is still staggering (**Figure 21.3**).

Attitudes and beliefs may be the most significant factor involved in unintentional injuries. Your individual attitude toward safety precautions greatly influences the likelihood of an injury. You may believe that safety precautions are a waste of time because you have no control over the situation (what will happen, will happen), or you may have a reckless attitude (you like to take risks).

Lack of knowledge and skills also plays a role in unintentional injury. In special circumstances, especially when performing a new procedure or task, lacking the proper knowledge or skills could result in unintentional injury (e.g., operating a new power tool before reading the instructions, operating a motorcycle the first time, or using a new kitchen appliance).

Table 21.1

Leading Causes of Unintentional Injury Deaths in the United States in 2006

Cause of death is ascribed to a single category even though many factors contribute to an accident.

Cause of death	Number of deaths
Motor vehicle crashes	44,700
Poisoning by solids and liquids	25,300
Falls	21,200
Choking	4,100
Drowning	3,800
Fires, flames, and smoke	2,800
Mechanical suffocation	1,100
Natural heat or cold	800
All others (includes firearms, lightning, railroads, machinery)	16,200
Total unintentional injuries	**120,000**

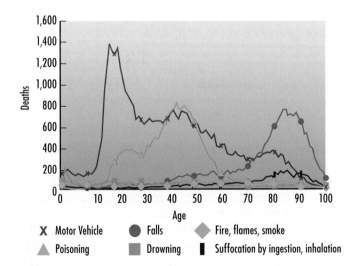

Legend:
X Motor Vehicle   ● Falls   ◆ Fire, flames, smoke
▲ Poisoning   ■ Drowning   ▮ Suffocation by ingestion, inhalation

■ **Figure 21.2**

Leading Causes of Death by Unintentional Injury According to Age in the United States, 2004

People of different ages have very different risks of accidental death from different causes.

Source: National Safety Council, *Injury facts,* 2008. Reprinted with permission.

TERMS

accident: sequence of events that produces unintended injury, death, or property damage; refers to the event, *not* the result of the event

accident mitigation: methods to reduce damage caused by unplanned events

accident prevention: ways to eliminate the occurrence of unintended injuries

safety: an ever-changing condition in which one attempts to minimize the risk of injury, illness, or property damage from the hazards to which one may be exposed

unintentional injury: preferred term for accidental injury; result of an accident

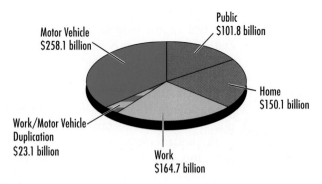

■ Figure 21.3

Costs of Unintentional Injuries by Classification, 2006

Total cost of unintentional injuries was more than $607.7 billion; the greatest cost is from motor vehicle injuries and property damage.

Source: National Safety Council, *Injury facts,* 2008. Reprinted with permission.

Socioeconomic factors also play a role in unintentional injury. Some individuals may lack the necessary funds to replace unsafe or old equipment. Some may even lack the necessary funds to obtain proper training in safety-related matters. Safety training can be received through a local National Safety Council office on such topics as proper storage of household cleaning items, tool safety, and safety tips for the babysitter. Local health departments may also provide educational workshops on safety issues.

Some social settings may lend themselves to accidents. Attitudes and beliefs as well as the social setting can raise or lower the probability of an unintentional injury. For example, alcohol and drug use definitely affect the frequency of unintentional injuries. Prescribed medications, especially ones with a sedative effect, can increase the likelihood of an accident while operating a motor vehicle, motorcycle, or power tool.

The ability of the individual performing a task or activity may affect the probability of an unintentional injury. The person may be a child who is too young to perform a task competently. At the other end of the spectrum, an elderly individual may not be strong enough or steady enough to perform a simple task like sawing a piece of wood.

The environment can be the most unpredictable risk factor in unintentional injuries. Environmental risks include appropriate maintenance of streets, safe power transmission and sewage treatment, and laws that regulate the hazards of appliances and tools. Natural disasters such as floods, hurricanes, earthquakes, or tornadoes are also environmental risks. The devastation caused by natural disasters may affect us at some point in our lifetime. In 2004, hundreds of thousands of people died in Indonesia from a tsunami that followed an earthquake. In 2005, the Gulf Coast of the United States was devastated by Hurricane Katrina, and the city of New Orleans was flooded. In 2008, a cyclone in Burma killed more than 10,000 people and an earth-

quake in China killed approximately 70,000 people, many of them children. Natural disasters can strike anyone and anywhere.

Stress and fatigue contribute greatly to higher rates of unintentional injuries. Stress may interfere with your concentration when performing even a simple task or may distract you while you are engaged in an activity. Fatigue causes you to be less alert or have slower reaction times; fatigue affects your coordination, and, at worst, can cause you to fall asleep. It is not wise to attempt difficult tasks while you are fatigued or under stress.

> He who feels punctured must have been a bubble.
> He who feels unarmed must have carried arms.
> He who feels belittled must have been consequential.
> He who feels deprived must have had privilege.
> *Lao Tzu,* The Way of Life

Analysis of Unintentional Injury

Scientific studies of unintentional injury try to uncover why injuries occur, what factors play a role, and who or what age group is most at risk. Analysis of unintentional injury provides us with data that are necessary before effective educational, preventive, or enforcement strategies can be implemented.

Injury epidemiology, used to investigate risk factors that cause unintentional injuries, is analogous to the epidemiological model for disease. For injuries to result, three factors are involved: (1) the agent or source of energy exchange (i.e., mechanical, chemical, electrical, or thermal), (2) the vehicle for the transmission of mechanical energy (i.e., a car, truck, motorcycle, powerline, or poison), and (3) a host or object (i.e., a person, school building, or house) (**Figure 21.4**).

Most unintentional injuries involve many factors; interactions among risk factors affect the likelihood of an accident. For example, cutting trees with a chain saw on a windy or rainy day may increase the risk of accident, whereas choosing a dry, calm day might reduce the chance of an accident.

The Haddon matrix is one of the scientific models used in unintentional injury analysis. Developed by William Haddon Jr. in the 1960s, this model was used originally to investigate motor vehicle risk factors and to develop and implement programs to prevent or reduce the occurrence of car accidents.

According to some estimates, "every two miles, the average driver makes 400 observations, 40 decisions, and one mistake. Once in every 500 miles, one of these mistakes leads to a near collision, and once in every 61,000 miles, one of these mistakes leads to a car crash" (Gladwell, 2001). The Haddon matrix analyzes accidents in three phases:

- *Phase 1: Pre-event phase.* Includes factors that may determine whether an accident will happen; lack of

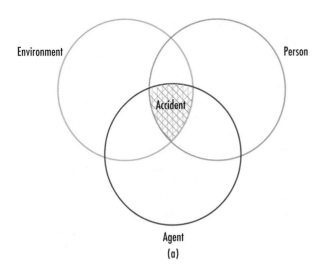

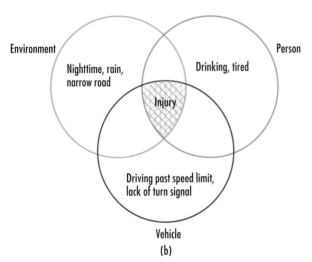

■ Figure 21.4

Epidemiological Model for Unintentional Injuries
The model shows that (a) the environment, a person, and an agent (car)
interact to create conditions for an accident. Part (b) shows the
environmental factors that increase the likelihood of an injury.

knowledge or skills and alcohol use are the most
significant factors.

- *Phase 2: Event phase.* Occurs when the host comes
  into contact with forces of energy. Many preventive
  measures, such as the use of helmets, seat belts, or
  protective goggles, are associated with this phase.

- *Phase 3: Postevent phase.* Includes emergency
  procedures provided after the injury has occurred.
  Preventive signaling devices, smoke and carbon
  monoxide detectors, or fire alarms will increase the
  speed with which help reaches an injured person.
  Emergency transportation and care of an injured or
  sick person occurs in this phase.

All approaches to unintentional injury reduction
include (1) educational and prevention strategies, (2)
stricter laws and regulations (e.g., mandates to enforce
seat belt and helmet compliance), and (3) better product

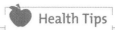

Health Tips

Ways to Avoid Having a Motor Vehicle Accident

Resolve to do the following each time you drive:
- Wear the seat belt.
- Don't drink and drive.
- Don't use a cell phone while driving.
- Don't speed or drive aggressively.

Remember: A motor vehicle accident injury occurs once
every 13 seconds; a death occurs once every 12 minutes.

design and automatic protection devices (e.g., air bags,
child-proof car door locks, child-proof safety caps on
medicines).

Motor Vehicle Safety

Even though motor vehicle death rates have been
declining, the number of deaths is still very high. Motor
vehicle travel is the primary means of transportation in
the United States, and it provides an unprecedented
degree of mobility. Yet, for all its advantages, injuries
resulting from motor vehicle crashes are the leading
cause of death. Each year, approximately 41,000 Americans are killed in motor vehicle crashes, and about 2.5
million suffer disabling injuries.

The National Highway Traffic Safety Administration
(NHTSA) estimates that alcohol was involved in 41% of
fatal crashes and 7% of all traffic accidents, fatal and
nonfatal. Approximately 3 in every 10 Americans will be
involved in an alcohol-related traffic accident some time
in their lives. Alcohol involvement in fatal crashes during the day is 18% but rises to 61% at night. More than
one million drivers are arrested for driving under the
influence of alcohol or other drugs every year. Another
important statistic to be aware of is that in almost half
of pedestrian fatalities in which someone was hit by a
car, either the driver, the pedestrian, or both were intoxicated. Heed the warning: *Do Not Drink and Drive.* Do not
ride with any driver who has been drinking. And do not
go walking on busy roads if you have been drinking.

Many accidents involving young persons occur after
dark, after parties, and after drinking. Alcohol in the
blood and brain impairs a driver's judgment, coordination, and reaction time. The effects of alcohol vary considerably from one person to another, so even small

TERMS

injury epidemiology: the study of the occurrence,
causes, and prevention of injury

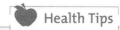

Driving Defensively

Driving defensively means not only taking responsibility for yourself and your actions but also keeping an eye on "the other guy." The National Safety Council offers the following guidelines to help reduce your risks on the road:

- Don't leave the driveway without securing each passenger in the car, including children and pets. Seat belts save thousands of lives each year!
- Remember that driving too fast or too slow can increase the likelihood of collisions.
- Don't kid yourself. If you plan to drink, designate a driver who won't drink. Alcohol is a factor in almost half of all fatal motor vehicle accidents.
- Be alert! If you notice that a car is straddling the center line, weaving, making wide turns, stopping abruptly, or responding slowly to traffic signals, the driver may be impaired.
- Avoid an impaired driver by slowing down, letting the driver pass, pulling onto the shoulder, or turning right at the nearest corner. If it appears that an oncoming car is crossing into your lane, pull over to the roadside, sound the horn, and flash your lights.
- Notify the police immediately after seeing a motorist who is driving suspiciously.
- Follow the rules of the road. Don't contest the "right of way" or try to race another car during a merge. Be respectful of other motorists.
- While driving, be cautious, aware, and responsible.

amounts of alcohol may impair driving skills and cause an accident. New laws have been proposed that set a zero tolerance for blood alcohol for persons under age 21.

Teenagers between the ages of 16 and 17 have more car accidents than any other group, whether based on age or miles driven. For this reason, a majority of states have instituted a graduated driver licensing system (GDL) in an attempt to reduce the number of accidents among the youngest drivers. At least 43 states employ a three-stage GDL system for licensing teenage drivers. The system involves driver education classes, supervised driving lessons, restricted night driving, and prohibition on carrying teenage passengers. The results of GDL systems vary from state to state, and safety experts are still studying which aspects of the system are most effective in reducing accident risks among first-time drivers.

Many factors other than alcohol use contribute to motor vehicle fatalities and injuries, such as road conditions and speeding. The interaction between these two factors is particularly risky. In all severe accidents, rural and urban, exceeding the posted speed limit was the most common factor. Defects in a vehicle, such as faulty tires, brakes, headlights, or steering system, also contribute to the risk of motor vehicle accidents.

Driving can be difficult even when you are concentrating on the road and your surroundings. But driving while you dial or talk on a cellular phone can be distracting and potentially dangerous. Cell phones may be convenient, but if not used properly, they are a danger to the user and everyone on the road. At 55 miles per hour, a vehicle travels the length of a football field in 3.7 seconds, less time than it takes to dial a phone number.

Anything that takes a driver's concentration off the road increases the possibility of an accident. America's growing enchantment with cellular phones in automobiles brings with it the need for renewed emphasis on safe driving practices. Studies show that carrying on a conversation over a cell phone is much more distracting than having a conversation with someone in the car or listening to the radio. Doing business or having an argument with someone in a cell phone conversation increases the risk of an accident. Inattention to the task of driving is a contributing factor in about 80% of all motor vehicle accidents. The National Safety Council has recommended that "the best practice is to not use electronic devices, including cell phones, while driving. When on the road, drivers shall concentrate on safe and defensive driving and not on making or receiving phone calls, delivery of faxes, using computers, navigation systems, or other distracting influences."

Seat Belts

Lap/shoulder seat belts are the best protection against fatal injury in a crash. Seat belts are estimated to reduce the risk of fatal injury to front seat occupants by 45%; between 1975 and 2005, it is estimated that 211,128 lives were saved by the use of seat belts.

Seat belt use is at a record high. The national average for seat belt use in 2007 was 82%. Twelve states averaged over 90%, the highest being Hawaii, with 97% of drivers using seat belts. Only three states were below 70%: Arkansas, Massachusetts, and New Hampshire. Despite the increased use of seat belts, more than two-thirds of teenagers who died in crashes that occurred at night were not using seat belts. A national program called *Click It or Ticket* implemented in recent years has helped boost the use of seat belts across the nation. The value of consistent seat belt use by both drivers and passengers is incontrovertible; everyone should buckle up whenever riding in a car or truck.

Air bags provide additional protection, but are not very effective by themselves except in a head-on collision; they should always be used in conjunction with a lap/shoulder seat belt.

Government regulations, use of lap/shoulder seat belts and child safety seats, and installation of air bags have helped reduce the number of motor vehicle fatalities and injuries.

Americans are addicted to speed. Studies show that more and more Americans are driving faster than ever.

Wellness Guide

Protect Your Kids in the Car

The type of child safety seat to buy and how you position it depend on the child's age, weight, and size. Every state and the District of Columbia have child protection laws. The safest place for any child aged 12 and younger is in the back seat. Every child should be buckled into a child safety seat or a booster seat or a lap shoulder belt, if it fits. A few pointers:

Riding with Babies

- Infants up to about 20 pounds and up to age 1 should ride in a rear-facing child seat. The child seat must be in the back seat and face the rear of the car, van, or truck.
- Babies riding in a car must never face front. In a crash or sudden stop, the baby's neck can be hurt badly.
- Infants in car seats must never ride in the front seat of a car with air bags. In a crash, the air bag can hit the car seat and hurt or kill the baby.
- Never hold your baby in your lap when you are riding in the car. In a crash or sudden stop, your child can be hurt badly or killed.

Riding with Young Kids

- Kids over 20 pounds and older than 1 year should ride in a car seat that faces the front of the car, van, or truck.
- It is best to keep kids in the forward-facing car seat for as long as they fit comfortably in it.
- Older kids over 40 pounds should ride in a booster seat until the car's lap and shoulder belts fit them correctly. The lap belt must fit low and snug on their hips. The shoulder belt must not cross their face or neck.
- Never put a shoulder belt behind a child's back or under a child's arm.

Remember . . .

- All kids are safest in the back seat, in a safety seat or seat belt.
- Always read the child seat instructions and the car owner's manual. Test the child seat to ensure a snug fit by pulling the base to either side or toward the front of the car.

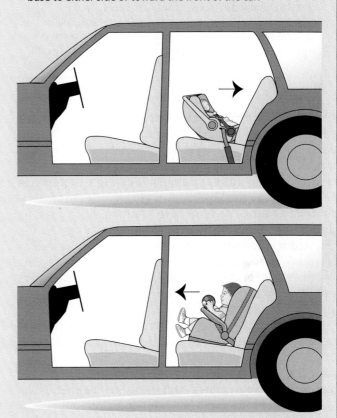

Source: National Highway Traffic Safety Administration, U.S. Department of Transportation, *Protect your kids in the car,* August 1997.

Many Americans believe that speeding is a basic right, regardless of the posted speed limit. Automobile manufacturers build big, fast, heavy cars that can easily go over 100 mph, and many drivers get "high" by driving fast. Race car drivers are heroes to many Americans, and millions of Americans engage in the "sport" of racing modified cars on highways and freeways. Speeding takes the lives of many young drivers as well as the lives of innocent passengers and drivers of other cars.

Motorcycle Safety

Motorcycles appeal to many individuals for various reasons: low cost to purchase, repair, and operate; the exciting feeling of open-air riding; and association with fellow motorcycle riders. However, higher risks include less crash protection than an automobile, and less

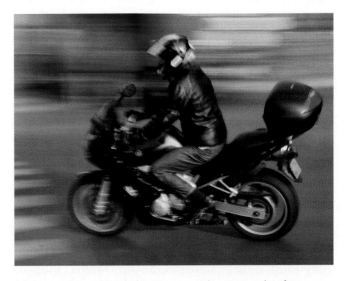

A helmet and protective clothing are essential to motorcycle safety.

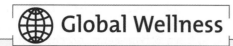

Global Wellness

Driving: The Rising Cost Worldwide

One of the leading (and often overlooked) causes of death and injuries worldwide is motor vehicle accidents. Each year about 1.2 million people are killed and another 10 million seriously injured or disabled in motor vehicle accidents.

In developing countries such as China and India, millions of people are acquiring their first automobile. They want to drive somewhere, anywhere in their new car. Roads are poor, traffic lights and rules are often ignored, people are in a hurry, and the frequency of accidents is exceptionally high.

It is paradoxical that we blithely accept the fact of millions of motor vehicle deaths and injuries but will devote enormous resources to curing diseases that cause many fewer deaths each year.

---

visibility by other drivers. Motorcycle operators can ensure a safer ride by securing proper training in operational procedures and by using a helmet and proper protective clothing. Less than 10% of all motorcycle operators receive any formal training. Wearing a motorcycle helmet reduces the likelihood of fatal injuries in an accident by about 37%. Protective clothing, such as long sleeves and pants, jackets, and boots, may lessen the chance for abrasions should an accident occur as well as protect from bad weather.

In 1966, Congress mandated that motorcycle riders and passengers use helmets in all states. If states did not enforce this mandate, they would lose federal highway funds. Only three states at first adopted helmet laws. However, by 1975, 47 states had helmet laws in force. During this 10-year period (1966–1975), fatal motorcycle accidents declined from 12.8 to 6.5 deaths per 100,000 riders. Only four states still have no helmet laws: Colorado, Iowa, Illinois, and New Hampshire. All motorcycle helmets sold in the United States are required to meet federal guidelines, which establish the minimum level of protection helmets must afford each user.

Riding a motorcycle is significantly more dangerous than riding in a passenger vehicle. Although motorcycles represent only 3% of registered motor vehicles, motorcycles are involved in 11% of fatal accidents. Motorcycles are fun but, even with training, helmets, and protective clothing, are still a very risky activity.

All-Terrain Vehicles

Another popular vehicle, especially among the 16 and under age group, is the all-terrain vehicle (ATV). These can be driven by anyone off road and almost anywhere they can be made to go. In addition to causing significant environmental damage to park lands, beaches, hiking trails, and pristine areas normally accessible only on foot, they also are responsible for many deaths and injuries. In 2005, 136,000 accidents were reported; approximately one-third of them occurred to persons younger than age 16 (Scelfo, 2007). Despite the growing number of serious accidents among youths, sales of ATVs continue to increase each year.

Some states have tried to legislate the use of ATVs but with little success. Kids can take their parent's vehicles without permission and can ride on public lands where roads are not policed.

Powered Scooters

Almost every kid wants to be on something that goes fast. If they cannot talk their parents into an ATV, then maybe they will settle for a powered scooter. Those kids you see whizzing through shopping malls and zipping by pedestrians on sidewalks are riding gasoline- or electric-powered scooters. Most powered scooters are made to go no faster than 20 mph; however, with modifications they can be made to go as fast as 50 mph.

Between 2002 and 2006, about 16,000 youngsters who were riding a power scooter and had an accident wound up in an emergency room (Griffin, 2008). Many scooter accidents are caused by faulty machines—loose handlebars, wobbly wheels, and brake failures. The companies that make scooters have recalled hundreds of thousands because of dangerous defects.

Some communities have banned the use of power scooters on city streets, but most cities and towns do not regulate the use of power scooters. In any case, laws governing the use of power scooters are difficult, if not impossible, to enforce. Parents who are concerned about their child's safety should encourage other physical activities that are healthier and less risky than power scooter riding. If a child is using a power scooter, the same protective gear that is recommended for skateboards should be used.

Pedestrian Safety

In 2006 in the United States, about 70,000 pedestrians were injured in motor vehicle accidents and about 6,000 were killed. About 80% of all pedestrian deaths and injuries involve children aged 5 to 9 who are either crossing or entering a street. Among young children, implementation of preventive strategies and educational efforts addressing safety procedures in traffic areas may reduce accidents. Many young children don't know what traffic signals or signs mean. Young children are also unable to judge the distance and speed of vehicles, which puts them in danger when trying to cross a busy intersection. Close supervision by adults helps prevent accidents; education of child-care workers is another preventive strategy.

The elderly are especially at risk for pedestrian injuries, as a result of failing eyesight, hearing, and mobility problems. Some pedestrian injuries occur when individuals dart into a busy street or are unable to see oncoming traffic because their view is blocked by a parked vehicle. Many pedestrian injuries involve joggers, runners, and walkers. Bright-colored clothes, especially reflective clothes, offer protection for pedestrians during both day and night. Also, just as alcohol impairs the judgment of motor vehicle operators, it impairs the judgment of pedestrians.

Whether an intersection is marked with a crosswalk does not seem to make a difference in pedestrian deaths among persons aged 65 and older. The important factor seems to be whether the intersection has a stop sign or signal. Pedestrians should always walk to a corner that has a stop sign or signal light; crossing in the middle of a block is dangerous even if there is a marked crosswalk.

Other preventive strategies can also help reduce the number of pedestrian injuries and deaths. Underpasses and overpasses in high-traffic areas, well-marked crosswalks, and pedestrian guardrails all offer protection for the pedestrian. Limiting traffic during peak hours of pedestrian traffic—for instance, before and after school or church—is also beneficial.

Bicycle Safety

Bicycle safety concerns have been increasing as more bicycles are used for exercise, recreation, and commuting to school or work. Few bicyclists wear a protective helmet every time they ride their bike, yet the single most important factor in reducing bicycle deaths is the use of protective helmets. The use of a helmet can reduce the chance of head and brain injuries by more than 80% should an accident occur. Only 21 states currently require the use of bicycle helmets by all riders. A total of 55,000 bicyclists were injured and 1,100 were killed in collisions with motor vehicles in 2006.

Bicycle riders are required to follow the same rules of the road as automobile operators. But many bicycle riders lack knowledge of these rules, do not use proper hand signals, or ride on the wrong side of the street, contributing to bicycle injuries and fatalities. Also, lack of skill in handling a bicycle increases the risk of an accident. Individuals who purchase a new bicycle should be familiar with all its devices before riding it. Many young bicycle riders are unaware of the rules of the road or are too small to see over motor vehicles.

Bicycle riders need to wear bright, reflective clothing, and the bicycle itself should be properly equipped with reflectors and lights. A recent and dangerous phenomenon is wearing headphones while riding. Inability to hear the sounds of traffic, the honk of a horn, or a shout of warning may contribute to an accident. Construction of more bicycle paths, underpasses, overpasses, and guardrails along with defensive riding skills can reduce bicycle injuries and deaths.

Home and Community Safety

Accidental deaths in the home are gradually declining but are still a major source of injury and death. Accidents in the home take a special toll on both young and elderly persons. As the elderly population continues to grow, accidents in the home and community will increase. The main categories of home accidents include falls, poisonings, fires, suffocation, and drowning (**Figure 21.5**).

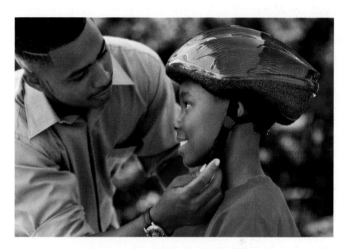

Appropriate helmet and reflector use is crucial to bicycle safety.

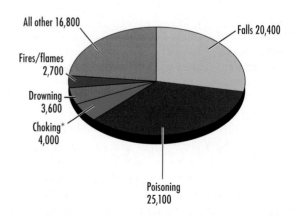

■ **Figure 21.5**

Unintentional Injury Deaths at Home and in the Community, United States, 2006

*Inhalation and ingestion of food or other objects that obstructs breathing.
Source: National Safety Council, *Injury facts,* 2008. Reprinted with permission.

Between 1912 and 2001, deaths caused by unintentional home and community injuries were reduced by 57%. Disabling injuries are more frequent in the home than in the workplace and in motor vehicle accidents combined. In 2006, disabling injuries of various kinds in the home numbered about 28 million and had an estimated cost of $252 billion. Clearly, taking steps to reduce accidents at home and in the community should be an important priority, especially if young or elderly people are involved.

Falls

People of all ages fall, but most fatal injuries occur among elderly persons. Falls are the leading cause of deaths from unintentional injuries in the home and community. Children often fall because of their strenuous activities, but usually the injuries are minor and heal rapidly. However, children also fall down stairs, out of trees, from open windows, and from the backs of trucks. They fall while climbing, jumping, or running. People responsible for watching children at play must be alert to the danger of a fall.

Falls are an especially serious problem for the elderly. Each year, one in three Americans over age 65 and one in two over age 75 fall and suffer an injury. Two-thirds of those who fall will suffer another fall within six months of the first fall. About 40% of all nursing home admissions result from injuries suffered in falls. It is no wonder that many older people have a fear of falling. When an elderly person falls, it can result in hospitalization and permanent loss of independent living.

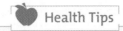

Health Tips

Don't Fall at Christmas

Every year several thousand Americans suffer injuries from falls while decorating a Christmas tree. Be extra cautious during the holiday season and remember these tips when decorating a tree:
- Make sure any ladder you use is stable. If leaned against a wall, observe the 4 to 1 rule: if you climb 4 feet the base of the ladder should be 1 foot from the wall; for 8 feet the base should be 2 feet from the wall.
- Do not lean backward or sideways from the ladder. Keep feet in the center of each step.
- Do not overload the top of the tree with ornaments or lights.
- Do not place candles on or near the tree. A Christmas tree is a match waiting to be lit.
- Make sure Christmas tree lights are in good condition and will not spark or cause a wire to become hot. Test before stringing lights on trees.

Enjoy the holiday season and avoid accidents.

The elderly need to take specific actions to avoid falls. Being physically active is important. Performing daily strength and flexibility exercises is helpful. Paying attention to balance and using canes or other walking aids may help avert a fall. Move slowly and carefully around the house and in the community. If an area is unfamiliar, an older person who is unsteady should ask someone to hold his or her arm for extra support.

Certain areas in the home are hazardous for falls. The kitchen, bathroom, and laundry room are dangerous because they often have wet floors. Stairs are also hazardous; a person may stumble while walking up or down, particularly if he or she is distracted or if the stairs are not well lit. Bumping into furniture or tripping over the legs of tables, chairs, or loose rugs are also common causes of falls. Climbing ladders may be an invitation for a fall if a person is careless or the ladder is weak or unstable. When performing any activity in which a fall is possible, take extra safety measures, such as having someone hold the ladder that you are climbing. After motor vehicle accidents, falls cause the greatest number of unintentional injury deaths.

Poisonings

A **poison** is any chemical substance that causes illness, injury, or death. Poisons enter the body by being ingested (medicines, drugs, mushrooms, shellfish, chemicals), inhaled (carbon monoxide, hydrogen sulfide), injected (bee sting, snake bite), or by contact with the skin (poison ivy, solutions that burn). Toxins arising from bacteria-contaminated foods are not considered poisons medically; illness and death resulting from them are considered diseases. Chemical poisons such as pesticides disturb essential biological reactions in the body and cause a variety of symptoms, even death. Some poisons cause only transitory symptoms; the body returns to normal once the poison is eliminated. However, some poisons cause permanent and irreversible damage.

Many cultivated and wild plants, trees, and bushes contain poisonous compounds. Eating the berries, seeds, roots, or leaves of unfamiliar plants can produce mild or severe symptoms of poisoning. Many common household plants are also poisonous, even the Christmas poinsettia. Collecting and eating wild mushrooms can be dangerous unless you are knowledgeable about what species are edible.

Young children, especially once they have learned to crawl or walk, are particularly susceptible to poisoning accidents. Children are curious, active, and adventurous, and it is natural for young children to put things in their mouths, including nonfood items such as paint chips, dirt, marbles—almost any small object. When children are hungry, thirsty, or just curious, they are likely to ingest whatever is closest to hand—medicines, pills, household products, pesticides. Children between ages one and five suffer the greatest number of accidental poisonings.

Precautions by manufacturers of drugs, solvents, paints, and other products have markedly reduced the number of accidental childhood poisonings. Child-resistant lids, tamper-proof caps, and internal seals help to prevent children from ingesting harmful substances. Precautions by parents and other child caregivers are essential to reduce the risk further. All household products and medicines should be kept out of reach of small children. Dangerous substances should be kept in locked cabinets. Small children should not be left unsupervised in areas like bathrooms, kitchens, and garages, where dangerous household products are stored.

There are several hundred poison control centers across the country. Should a poisoning accident occur, someone at a poison control center can give you immediate expert advice. Keep the number of a poison control center near the phone in case of emergency.

Acetaminophen (known as Tylenol in the United States and paracetamol in other countries) is one of the most widely used drugs for pain, headache, colds, and other symptoms. It also is the most common cause of poisoning worldwide. Acetaminophen poisoning is estimated to have caused about 300 deaths and 70,000 hospital admissions in the United States in 2005 (Heard, 2008). Acetaminophen poisoning can occur from either excessive doses or too frequent doses of the drug. It also is used in some attempted suicides.

Poisoning by gases and vapors is mainly caused by carbon monoxide. Carbon monoxide results from incomplete combustion in cooking stoves, heating equipment, and standing running motor vehicles. Most deaths are the result of suicide, but many are accidental. The largest number of carbon monoxide fatalities occurred in the group aged 15 to 24; males commit suicide with carbon monoxide three times as often as females. Most carbon monoxide deaths occurred in stationary motor vehicles, although fireplaces, stoves, and appliances using natural or liquid propane gas were responsible for 10% of all unintentional carbon monoxide fatalities. Regulations that have lowered carbon monoxide emissions have contributed significantly to reducing the rates of unintentional carbon monoxide fatalities.

Drowning

Drowning accounts for many unintentional injuries and fatalities in the home; young children are especially vulnerable. Young children can drown in five-gallon buckets or in toilet bowls. About half of all drownings occur during June, July, and August, when many people are engaged in summer water activities. Recreation in large bodies of water, rivers, and streams provides the opportunities for accidental drowning.

When a person is under water and inhales water instead of air, an automatic muscular contraction of the

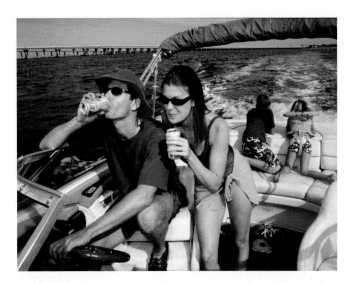

Many boating accidents are associated with drinking alcohol while having fun on the water.

larynx occurs that is called **laryngospasm.** This muscular reflex closes the body's main airway in an attempt to keep water from entering the lungs. The spasm continues as long as the person is under water and within a few minutes can lead to death by suffocation. Once the laryngospasm relaxes, water enters the lungs. Only about 10% of people survive not breathing under water for as long as 6 minutes, and these victims will survive only if artificial respiration is applied immediately. Few people recover if breathing has stopped for as long as 10 minutes.

Scientific evidence does not support the widely held belief that swimming shortly after eating induces stomach cramps, thereby increasing the risk of drowning. However, it is true that after eating, blood is diverted to the stomach to assist digestion and consequently less oxygen may be available for muscles, which can lead to muscle spasms. This sequence poses no problem for a healthy person, but if a person is in poor health, is overweight, or has existing heart disease, the risk of drowning may be increased.

Knowing your swimming ability and avoiding swimming in dangerous waters are ways to reduce the risk of accidental drowning. Using a personal flotation device (commonly called a life jacket) while you engage in water sports can also reduce the risk of drowning.

TERMS

laryngospasm: spasm of the larynx caused by inhaling water

poison: any chemical substance that causes illness, injury, or death

Alcohol and other drugs may be the biggest predisposing factor in drowning for individuals aged 15 and older. Impairment of the individual's judgment may lead to the death of others as well, for example, operating a boat with passengers while intoxicated or supervising children who are in or near the water while drinking.

Choking and Suffocation

Choking to death as a result of an object lodged in the airway passage occurs more often than one might expect. Each year in the United States more than a thousand people die because a piece of food or a foreign object became stuck in their throats and caused them to stop breathing. Food that is swallowed without being chewed sufficiently is a common cause of choking and blockage of the air passage. Small bones from fish or chicken also can be swallowed inadvertently and become stuck in the airway. Sometimes dentures, fillings, or crowns become loose, are accidentally swallowed, and may cause the person to choke. Being intoxicated also increases the risk of swallowing improperly.

When the airway is completely blocked, a choking victim is unable to speak, breathe, or cough. A choking person often clutches his or her throat. If the object is not removed quickly, the victim may become unconscious and death may follow rapidly from lack of oxygen.

Mechanical suffocation is another type of unintentional injury, occurring most frequently in young children up to four years old. A small child can get into tight spaces and become trapped or wedged, resulting in suffocation. As infants become more mobile and inquisitive, the risk of entrapment and suffocation increases. Long cords dangling from appliances, draperies, or blinds should be placed well out of the way of a curious infant or toddler. Bulky bedding materials have been responsible for the suffocation of young children, especially fluffy comforters or infant bean bag cushions, and some household items, such as the bean bag cushion, have been recalled because of suffocation risks.

Anything stuck in the throat blocking the air passage can stop breathing and cause unconsciousness and death within minutes. Do not interfere with a choking person who can speak, cough, or breathe, but if a conscious person cannot speak, cough, or breathe, perform the following procedure immediately:

- Stand behind the person and wrap your arms around his or her middle just above the navel. Clasp your hands together in a double fist. Press in and up in vigorous thrusts. Repeat several times. This is called the *Heimlich maneuver*.

If the object is dislodged, take the person to a hospital immediately even if he or she seems all right. This is especially important if the swallowed object is a chicken or fish bone that may not have been completely dislodged. Also, if a bone has been swallowed, it can cause serious damage as it passes through the digestive system.

Fires

Two catastrophic fires in nightclubs in Chicago and Rhode Island in 2002 and 2003 focused the nation's attention on the deaths and injuries that can occur from fires. The fires in these two clubs spread rapidly, and exits were either locked or blocked. Hundreds of people were trapped in the buildings and died from burns or suffocation; hundreds more were seriously burned or injured.

House fires caused about 2,500 deaths in 2006 in the United States. Those at highest risk include the elderly, minority, and low-income populations (Shai, 2006). Fires in the home may be attributed to many factors: fireplaces, wood stoves, kerosene or space heaters, improper placement of appliances, faulty wiring of the house or

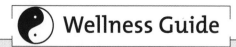

Wellness Guide

Smoke Detectors Guard You from Fires

Most deaths and injuries in fires result from inhalation of smoke and toxic gases that reach victims before the flames do. Survival depends on an early warning system that gives you time to vacate the premises at once. The best warning system available is a smoke detector that cuts your risk of dying in a fire in half. The U.S. Consumer Product Safety Commission offers these suggestions about smoke detectors:

- Many localities require that you have a smoke detector in your home, so buy one—at least one. They're inexpensive and are available at most hardware stores and supermarkets. Check your local codes and regulations; they may require you to purchase a specific kind.
- Read the instructions that come with the detector for advice on where to install it. You should purchase at least one for every floor in your house. Preferably you should place one outside every bedroom.
- Manufacturers know what is best for their products and tell you how to care for them. Follow their instructions. Detectors can save lives, but only if you install and maintain them properly.
- Never disconnect a fire detector. If it goes off at wrong times because of heat from a stove or steam from a bathroom, move it to another location.
- Replace the battery annually (January 1 is an easy day to remember) or when you hear a "chirping" sound. And press the test button regularly to be sure the batteries work.
- Keep your detector clean. Dust, grease, or other materials can interfere with efficient operation. You may want to vacuum the grill work on the detector.

appliances, grease fires in the kitchen (loose sleeves dangling over open flames), improper storage of combustible materials, or a careless smoker in the house.

Death rates from fires or burns have markedly decreased since the 1950s. Smoke detectors, portable ladders, and fire extinguishers have helped reduce fatalities. Also, many elementary school students are receiving annual training from local fire departments concerning fire safety. Prevention and education are, once again, the best strategies to eliminate unintentional injuries from fires and burns. Each household should have a planned escape route, smoke detectors placed at key locations throughout the home, and posted emergency phone numbers. Everyone should know how to operate a fire extinguisher and know exactly where it is kept, and in two-story houses, a portable ladder should be readily accessible.

Fire Retardants   Fire retardants are chemicals added to clothing, drapes, furniture, bedding, and other fabrics to help prevent the spread of a fire should one start. Most fire retardant chemicals are toxic—they usually are carcinogenic when tested on laboratory animals, and they can pollute land and water and harm the environment. The amount of fire retardant chemicals added to fabrics and furniture is considerable—up to 5% of the fabric's weight. In the 1970s, two fire retardants (called *brominated tris* and *chlorinated tris*) that had been added to children's sleepwear for years were finally banned. These chemicals are carcinogenic and are absorbed into the body from pajamas and other bedding containing fire retardant chemicals. These substances are still added to the foam and fabrics used in furniture. The risk to health and to the environment far outweighs the risk of a fire in a home spreading from furniture. This is especially true now that most homes have smoke detectors. Also, 22 states require that all cigarettes be fire-safe (Blum, 2007).

Firearms

Many Americans view ownership of guns as a constitutional right; others believe that it is a privilege and that ownership should be restricted and regulated. One aspect of firearms is incontrovertible—they cause thousands of deaths and injuries each year.

Firearm-related deaths fall into three categories: unintentional, intentional, and undetermined. Studies show that having access to a firearm increases the risk of a firearm-related injury or death. If you keep one or more firearms in your home, you should be trained in their use and take all possible safeguards to prevent against intentional or unintentional injury or death. All firearms should be locked away. Guns should never be stored loaded. Ammunition should be kept locked in a separate location.

Nonpowder guns such as pellet rifles (BB guns) and paintball guns are thought to be harmless by most Americans. These guns, powered by compressed air, are often given to children as gifts and are regarded as "toys." However, they are far from harmless. Each year, about 20,000 Americans are treated in hospital emergency rooms for nonpowder gun injuries; most of those injured were children between the ages of 5 and 14 years. The power of many of these guns can equal that of a 22-caliber rifle; when they are shot at someone at close range, they can kill, and several such deaths occur each year. Parents are advised not to let their children possess or use nonpowder rifles or pistols.

> The hour of departure has arrived and we go our separate ways—I to die and you to live. Which is better, God only knows.
>
> *Socrates*

Work Safety

During the past century, unintentional injury deaths in the workplace were reduced by 90%. For 2006, the U.S. Occupational Health and Safety Administration reported that there were 3.2 million disabling workplace injuries and 4,988 deaths. Occupational injuries occur most often in manufacturing industries. Agriculture has the highest incidence of skin diseases and disorders, which may be attributed to agricultural workers' close contact with hazardous chemicals. Common occupational illnesses include skin disorders, respiratory conditions caused by inhalation of toxic substances, disorders associated with repeated trauma, poisonings, and dust-related diseases of the lungs. The incidence is suspected to be higher than reported because many workers do not seek medical attention for their illnesses or injuries.

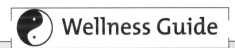

Wellness Guide

Prevent Computer-Related Injuries

Anyone who spends 30 to 40 hours a week in front of a computer screen risks some form of repetitive motion injury. Most injuries occur in the neck and shoulders; the elbow and wrist are the second most vulnerable areas. These injuries are due to the repetitive motions used to watch the screen and operate the keyboard.

People who spend many hours at a computer day after day should take precautions to reduce the risk of injury. Using an ergonomic chair and having the monitor and keyboard at comfortable positions and heights are important. Taking frequent breaks is also helpful. A recent study showed that forearm support boards can significantly reduce injuries to the neck and shoulders. Computer users should take all available measures to reduce the risk of musculoskeletal disorders.

Carpal tunnel syndrome is one of a group of injuries known as **repetitive motion disorders** (also called repeated trauma), caused by stress of a body part, resulting from repetitive motion for long periods (**Table 21.2**). Symptoms of carpal tunnel syndrome are burning, numbness, tingling, and stiffness of the hand, fingers, or wrist. Dentists, dental hygienists, supermarket cashiers, seamstresses, musicians, factory workers, computer keyboard operators, and surgeons are at risk for carpal tunnel syndrome. Better product design, correct positioning of the operator and the tool, and limiting time spent at the same task are being investigated as possible solutions to the rising incidence of cumulative trauma disorders.

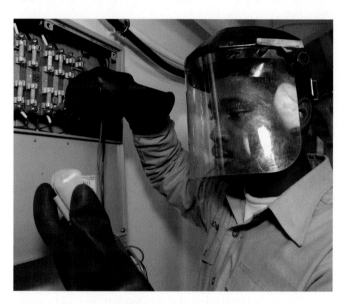

Workers should always wear the appropriate safety equipment while on the job.

Table 21.2

Repetitive Motion Disorders

These injuries affect muscles, tendons, and nerves.

Cervical radiculopathy:

People who look up to a computer screen or who balance a phone on their shoulder are at risk.

Pronator syndrome:

Mechanics, baseball pitchers, and barbers are at risk.

Carpal tunnel syndrome:

Typists, computer programmers, and potters are at risk.

Thoracic outlet syndrome:

Violinists and other musicians are at risk.

Cubital tunnel syndrome:

Truck drivers or other persons who keep their arms in fixed, flexed positions are at risk.

Distal ulnar neuropathy:

Meat packers, assembly line workers, and machine operators are at risk.

Sick building syndrome consists of a variety of symptoms reported by workers in modern office buildings. Recent investigations have found a correlation between pollutants in or near the building or a poor ventilation system and sick building syndrome. Much of the evidence of these symptoms is self-reported by the workers or documented by physicians. Symptoms include asthma, lung infections, dizziness, nausea, throat and eye irritations, fatigue, cough, and shortness of breath. Based on limited research to date on sick building syndrome, ventilation alone was not a significant factor. Possibly the combination of the ventilation system and volatile organic substances used in many new building products may be the determinants.

Sports and Recreational Injuries

Millions of American youths engage in some kind of sport or physical activity, either with a school team, with organized leagues, in pick-up games, or just for fun. Playing sports is both fun and healthy. However, each year close to 4 million children, teenagers, and young adults wind up in hospital emergency rooms as a result of a sport or recreational injury. Approximately one-fourth of all emergency room admissions of persons aged 5 to 24 are due to a sport or recreational injury.

The most common sports injuries among boys result from playing basketball, football, or cycling. Among girls, basketball, soccer, and cycling cause the most injuries. The numbers do not indicate which sport is the most dangerous, because the number of people engaging in each sport is not known. Children between the ages of 5 and 14 are the most susceptible to injury; as children become older, the chance for injury declines. Boys are twice as likely as girls to visit an emergency room with a sport injury, but as more and more girls engage in sports, their number of visits is increasing. Coaches and parents have the obligation to see that protective gear is worn at all times and that recklessness is not a part of any game. It is useless (although all parents do it) to tell kids to be careful when they are playing sports or just having fun, but reasonable precautions should be taken by coaches and volunteers to prevent injuries, especially with young children.

In the past few years, activities called "extreme" sports have become very popular. Extreme sports include inline skating, snowboarding, mountain bicycling, rock climbing, kickboxing, skateboarding, and ultra-endurance racing. All of these activities, however fun and enjoyable, carry increased risk for injury. Everyone engaging in an extreme sport needs to weigh the risks against the enjoyment of engaging in extreme sports.

Concussion

A **concussion** results from a head injury involving a temporary loss of consciousness and a period of amnesia upon awakening. Blows to the head that cause a person to "see stars" or feel dazed momentarily are regarded as milder forms of a concussion. A grade 1 concussion involves feeling dazed or confused for less than 15 minutes. If mental confusion persists for more than 15 minutes, the concussion is classified as grade 2. Any blow to the head involving loss of consciousness is a grade 3 concussion.

Concussions are among the most common kinds of injuries people experience, especially while engaging in strenuous physical activities. Sports and bicycle accidents account for the greatest number of concussions among children aged 5 to 14 years. About 150,000 grade 3 concussions are diagnosed each year in the United States (Ropper & Gorson, 2007).

Concussions involving loss of consciousness produce two kinds of amnesia upon regaining consciousness. *Retrograde amnesia* involves loss of memory of events just prior to the blow to the head, although sometimes the retrograde amnesia may extend hours or even days into the past. The extent of memory loss correlates roughly with the length of unconsciousness. *Anterograde amnesia* refers to the inability to retain new information for some time after awakening from a concussion. A brief, grade 3 concussion may be accompanied by a convulsion, but this is not a true "seizure" or epileptic fit and does not require medical treatment. A serious consequence of concussions is cranial bleeding, which can be detected by x-ray images of the brain (CT scan). Fortunately, only about 10% of people who suffer a concussion have cranial bleeding. The harder the blow to the head is, the more likely is the risk of cranial bleeding and formation of a clot in the brain.

A concussion involves movement of the brain within the skull. All concussions represent potentially serious threats to health, and repeated concussions may have more serious consequences (**Table 21.3**). Proper

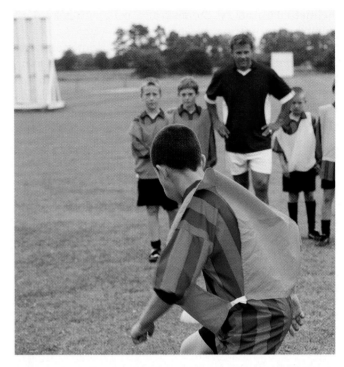

Soccer is a very popular children's sport. Teaching children proper techniques can prevent injuries.

TERMS

concussion: a blow to the head that causes injury, temporary loss of consciousness, and possibly a period of amnesia upon awakening

repetitive motion disorders: disorders caused by repeated stress to a body part; carpal tunnel syndrome is a repetitive motion disorder

sick building syndrome: collection of symptoms reported by workers in some modern buildings

Table 21.3

Managing Sports-Related Concussions

Symptoms	First concussion	Second concussion
Grade 1: no loss of consciousness; transient symptoms and mental confusion lasting less than 15 minutes	Remove from play Examine at 5-minute intervals May return to play after 15 minutes if all symptoms have resolved	May not play for 1 week May return after 1 week if symptom free at rest and with exertion
Grade 2: same as grade 1 but with symptoms on exertion	Remove from play for rest of day Examine for signs of cranial lesion May return after 1 week if medical tests are normal	May return after 2 weeks if no symptoms at rest or lasting more than 15 minutes May not play for rest of season if medical tests show any abnormality
Grade 3: any loss of consciousness	Requires neurological exam (and imagery if needed) May not play for 1 week if unconsciousness lasts seconds; for 2 weeks if minutes; may only play if all medical tests and symptoms are normal	May not play until 1 month after all symptoms have resolved and with medical clearance

helmets can reduce the risk of a serious head injury when biking, skating, or playing sports.

Traumatic brain injury (TBI) results from more serious blows to the head. These usually occur following physical assault, falls from a height, and from motor vehicle crashes. An estimated 5.3 million Americans have serious disabilities resulting from a TBI. Each year, approximately 50,000 Americans die from a TBI and another 80,000 are disabled for life (Morrison, 2007). In TBI, the brain is mechanically deformed, which results in immediate destruction of some brain cells and prolonged damage to others. At present there is no way to limit or treat the progressive brain damage that occurs. It is the latent brain damage from a TBI that makes these injuries so serious and tragic.

A football helmet is now available that is equipped with sensors that measure the magnitude, location, and direction of each blow to a player's head. The data are wirelessly transmitted to a computer on the sidelines that analyzes them and evaluates the likelihood that the player may have suffered a concussion. The helmet is not cheap (about $1,000), but a number of NCAA colleges have ordered them for their players.

First Aid and Emergencies

First aid and medical emergencies can be handled appropriately if you take a deep breath and tell yourself you can handle the situation until a qualified medical professional arrives to take over. First aid is defined as the immediate care given to an injured or ill person. First aid is temporary assistance given until a person has recovered or until a qualified medical person can provide assistance.

Knowledge about first aid and medical emergencies can literally mean the difference between life and death and can help prevent disability or permanent injury. Knowledge of first aid skills will increase your confidence in dealing with both minor and major emergencies and will be reassuring to an injured person.

Taking Risks and Preventing Accidents

Risks cannot be avoided in life; accidents and unintentional injuries are a consequence of the risks we take. As soon as a child learns to crawl, he or she begins to take risks to explore and understand the environment. At each stage of life we take risks to learn and to expand our capabilities and experiences. We take a risk when we cross the street in traffic, run to catch a bus, or swing from the branch of a tree. When we go hiking or climbing or engage in sports, we are taking risks.

The important question YOU need to ask is: "What risks are necessary and acceptable for me to live the way I want to?" The answer will also, to some extent, determine your risk of unintentional injury. People differ enormously in their need for risk-taking behaviors. Some people thrive on high-risk endeavors, such as mountain climbing, racing cars, or skydiving. However, even people who live more sedate lives may be at risk for unintentional injuries because of destructive behaviors or unhealthy mental attitudes.

Whatever your personal beliefs, a commitment to safe living can be made at any time. Why not make the commitment now? Eliminating or reducing the use of alcohol can reduce the risk of many kinds of injuries, especially motor vehicle accidents. Lowering your stress level will also contribute significantly to reducing unintentional injuries. Not keeping a loaded firearm in the house can eliminate the risk of an unintentional firearm injury. Reading and following the manufacturer's instructions and warnings before operating a new product will also help to reduce the risk of unintentional injury. Before undertaking any sport activity, climbing a ladder, or riding a bike, take a moment to consider essential safety measures. Observe posted safety rules and warning signs. Keep in good physical condition and have a positive mental attitude when undertaking a potentially dangerous activity.

Although unintentional injuries are usually not a laughing matter, one accident statistic does sound a humorous note. Saturday and Sunday are the two most dangerous days of the week for fatal accidents. Going out on the weekends just to have fun increases the risks of serious injuries. Maybe studying or reading on weekends is a good idea after all.

Critical Thinking About Health

1. Briefly explain a recent injury that happened to you, a friend, or family member using the epidemiologic triad presented in Figure 21.4.
   a. What were the human factors involved in the injury?
   b. What were the environmental factors (physical as well as social) involved in the injury?
   c. What were the vehicle (or agent) factors involved in the injury?
   Which factor(s) could have been modified in such a way that may have prevented the injury from occurring?
2. Alcohol is a contributing factor in about half of motor vehicle fatalities. What are your campus and community doing to help prevent people, both young and old, from driving while intoxicated? Some questions to consider:
   a. Are there educational programs? If so, what are they and who do they target?
   b. How would you design an educational program to keep your peers from drinking and driving?
   c. Are there seasonal programs that increase awareness about the dangers of drinking and driving (e.g., high school prom, Fourth of July)?
   d. What is the role of local law enforcement, both on and off campus, with regard to decreasing drinking and driving accidents and fatalities?
3. Federal, state, and local governments have written and passed laws and regulations that enforce certain safety behaviors that have an impact on the individual and/or community. Such laws regulate using a seat belt, restraining your child in a car seat, and wearing a helmet while riding a motorcycle or bicycle. Some people believe that the government (at any level) should not mandate laws regarding individual safety and injury prevention. Others believe that the government has a right to demand certain safe behaviors among its citizens for the public good. What's your opinion? Should the government be allowed to regulate individual safety behaviors? Explain why or why not.

Health in Review

- Unintentional injuries and deaths cost Americans billions of dollars in medical costs as well as costs as a result of loss of work each year. Unintentional injuries and deaths are preventable!
- Many factors contribute to unintentional injuries: knowledge, attitudes, beliefs, and behaviors; economic and social factors; competence; environmental conditions; and use of alcohol and other drugs.
- The Haddon matrix was developed to assess motor vehicle risk factors and is used to develop prevention programs.
- A multidimensional approach to injury prevention includes education, prevention strategies, stricter laws and regulations, and better product design.
- One motor vehicle death occurs every 12 minutes.
- Alcohol is involved in more than half of all motor vehicle accidents.
- Motorcycle, all-terrain vehicles, and bicycle safety rules and equipment are keys to preventing accidents. Wear reflective clothing and obey safety rules.
- Safety in the home includes preventing falls, poisonings, drownings, choking, and fires.
- Work-related injuries have decreased steadily; however, they still cost employers and employees large amounts of time and money. Injuries to the back are most frequent, followed by legs, arms, and trunk. Proper work safety procedures can prevent the majority of work-related injuries.
- Millions of young people go to emergency rooms each year with a sport- or recreation-related injury. The highest percentage of injuries occur in basketball, cycling, football, and soccer.
- Concussions are serious injuries to the head that cause loss of consciousness. Protective head gear should be worn in all sports with a high risk of head injury.
- Accidents and injuries are a consequence of the many risks we take. Although most of what we do has some degree of risk, we can decrease that risk by increasing safety knowledge and taking safety precautions for physical activities we engage in.

Health and Wellness Online

The Web contains a wealth of information about health and wellness. By accessing the Internet using Web browser software, you can gain a new perspective on many topics presented in *Health and Wellness,* Tenth Edition. Access the Jones and Bartlett Publishers Web site at **health.jbpub.com/hwonline.**

References

Blum, A. (2007). The fire retardant dilemma. *Science, 318,* 194.

Gladwell, M. (2001, June 11). Wrong turn. *The New Yorker,* 50–61.

Griffin, R., et al. (2008). Comparison of severe injuries between powered and nonpowered scooters among children aged 2 to 12 in the United States. *Ambulatory Pediatrics, 8,* 379–382.

Heard, K. J. (2008). Acetylcysteine for acetaminophen poisoning. *New England Journal of Medicine, 359,* 285–292.

Istre, G. R., et al. (2001). Deaths and injuries from house fires. *New England Journal of Medicine, 344,* 1911–1916.

McCartt, A. T. (2001). Graduated driver licensing systems: Reducing crashes among teenage drivers. *Journal of the American Medical Association, 386,* 1631–1632.

Morrison, B. (2007, January/February). The brain injury epidemic. *Technology Review,* 24–25.

National Safety Council. (2008). *Injury facts.* Itasca, IL: Author.

Ropper, A. G., & Gorson, K. C. (2007). Concussion. *New England Journal of Medicine, 356,* 166–172.

Scelfo, J. (2007, May 14). Accidents will happen. *Newsweek,* 59.

Shai, D. (2006). Income, housing, and fire injuries: A census tract analysis. *Public Health Reports, 121,* 149–154.

U.S. Occupational Health and Safety Administration. (2004). Workplace injury, illness and fatality statistics. Retrieved May 11, 2006, from http://www.osha.gov/oshstats/work.html

Suggested Readings

Ashley, S. (2001, October). Driving the info highway. *Scientific American,* 50–68. A discussion of all the electronic gadgets being used in automobiles and how they might affect safety.

Barss, P., Smith, G., Baker, S., & Mohan, D. (1998). *Injury prevention: An international perspective.* Cary, NC: Oxford University Press. Injuries are rapidly assuming epidemic proportions throughout the world. This book provides a worldwide overview of injury problems, including the epidemiology of injury, surveillance, and policy.

Gladwell, M. (2001, June 11). Wrong turn. *The New Yorker,* 50–61. An interesting look at why automobile safety measures may not be working as originally expected.

Recommended Web Sites

Please visit **health.jbpub.com/hwonline** for links to these Web sites.

MedlinePlus on Accidents
Information on household, motor vehicle, childhood, and other safety issues.

U.S. National Center for Injury Prevention and Control
Statistics, fact sheets, and other information to help reduce morbidity, disability, mortality, and costs associated with injuries.

U.S. National Highway Traffic Safety Administration
Information about motor vehicle safety.

U.S. National Institute of Occupational Safety and Health
Dedicated to workplace safety and health.

Part Seven

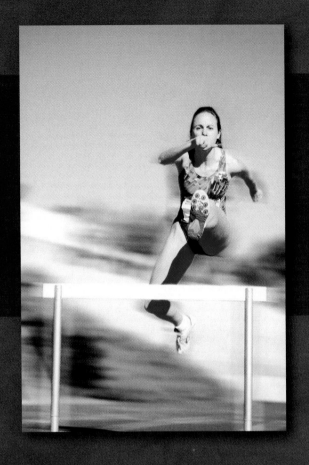

Overcoming Obstacles

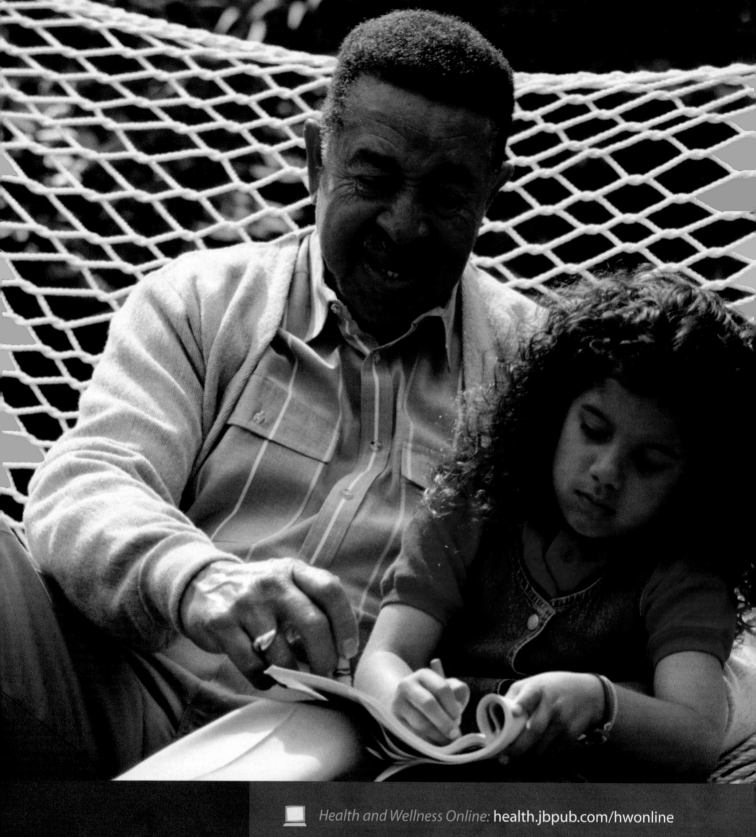

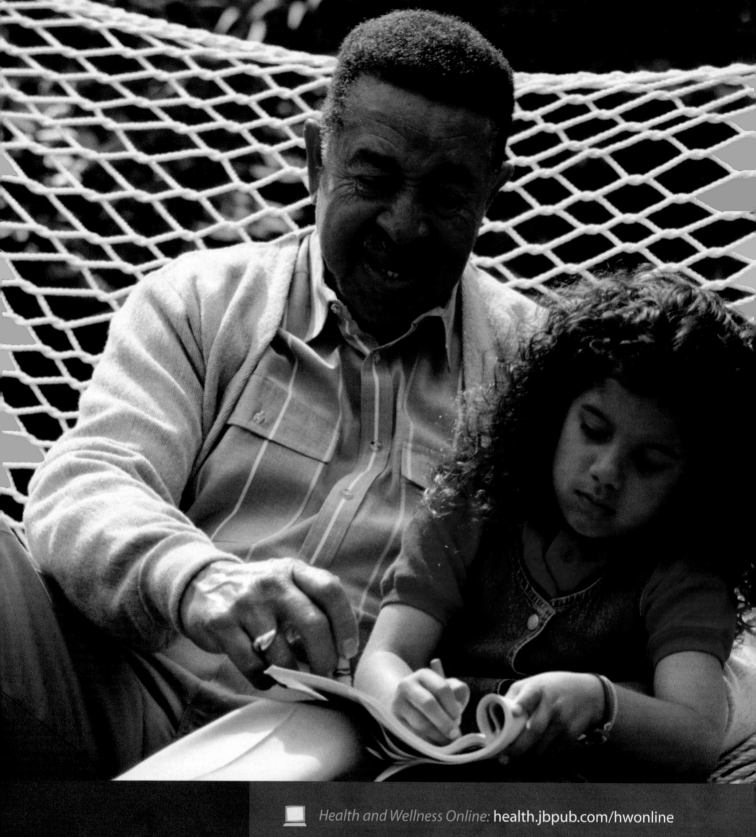
Health and Wellness Online: **health.jbpub.com/hwonline**

Study Guide and Self-Assessment

22.1   Healthy Aging

Chapter Twenty-Two

Understanding Aging and Dying

Learning Objectives

1. Describe some of the biological changes that occur with aging.

2. Define *aging*, *maximum life span*, *average life span*, *life expectancy*, *ageism*, and *gerontology*.

3. Discuss some of the health and social issues that stem from the "graying" of the American population.

4. Briefly explain two major theories of aging processes.

5. Explain how undernutrition affects the aging process.

6. Describe some of the symptoms of Alzheimer's disease and Parkinson's disease.

7. Describe measures you can take while young to reduce the risk of dementia later in life.

8. Describe some of the causes of vision and hearing loss.

9. Describe several ways to reduce the risk of osteoporosis.

10. Discuss the stages of dying as explained by Kübler-Ross.

11. Explain the role of the two documents that constitute advance directives.

12. Briefly define the terms *physician-assisted suicide*, *hospice*, and *palliative care*.

13. Indicate steps you can take while young to help ensure a healthy old age.

Everything in the universe—plants, animals, mountains, planets, and stars—changes over time and eventually dies (plants and animals) or disintegrates and disappears (planets and stars). Our planet is aging in the sense that its resources are being used up and the environment is changing. The nuclear reactions that fuel the sun will eventually slow down, and the sun is expected to explode about 5 billion years from now.

Many people associate aging with sickness, disability, loneliness, and increased inactivity. However, such negative views of aging are exaggerated; many older persons today are sexually and physically active and continue to work well into their 80s or even 90s. George Burns, comedian and movie star, performed on stage and in movies until he was nearly 100 years old.

> I don't want to achieve immortality through my work. I want to achieve immortality by not dying.
>
> *Woody Allen*

In America, negative views about aging are still prominent in movies, television, and, especially, advertising. The ideal American is portrayed as eternally young, active, attractive, and wrinkle-free. Advertisements exhort people to retard the noticeable signs of aging by using face and body creams, dyes for graying hair, and special herbs or vitamins, or by resorting to Botox injections or various kinds of cosmetic surgery.

The normal processes of aging are not caused by disease, so aging cannot be cured. The noticeable effects of aging result from wear and tear on organs, bones, and tissues in the body that change and become less efficient over the years—muscles weaken, immune system functions decrease, and sex drive is reduced. Even the healthiest body wears out slowly. However, by developing healthy habits while young and by understanding aging processes, most people can remain vigorous and healthy until the very end of life.

Life expectancy in the United States is at an all-time high. In 2005, the average life expectancy for Caucasian men was 75.7, and for Caucasian women it was 80.8 years (life expectancy for African Americans is 69.5 years for men and 76.6 years for women). Between 1950 and 2001, the average life expectancy for Americans increased by about 9 years. However, to attain the average or better-than-average life expectancy, it is vital to adopt healthy behaviors and lifestyles while young.

America's Aging Population

Aging refers to the normal changes in body functions that occur after sexual maturity and continue until death. In an idealized situation, everyone would survive close to the **maximum life span** for the species; for human beings, maximum life span is about 120 years

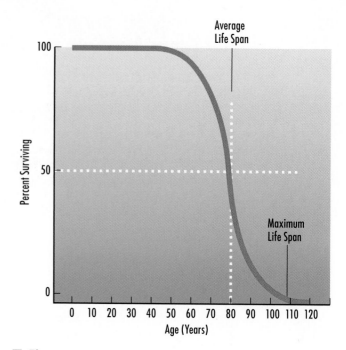

■ **Figure 22.1**

Survival as a Function of Years in an Idealized Aging Human Population

(**Figure 22.1**). The oldest person whose age has been reliably documented is Jeanne Calment, who died in Arles, France, on August 4, 1997. At the time of her death she was 122 years and 164 days old. She also had a brother who lived to 97 and other long-lived relatives, which suggests that her genetic makeup played a role in her longevity. The **average life span** is defined as the age at which half of the members of a population have died. Insurance companies use data based on actual populations to determine what insurance premiums are necessary to pay survivor benefits. **Life expectancy** is the average length of time that members of a population can expect to live. The average life expectancy at birth in the United States has increased by almost 30 years since 1900.

Genes are not the primary cause of aging. Although genes play a significant role in aging processes, studies show that the genes one inherits account for much less than half of the differences in life span among individuals. Evidence supporting this comes from the observation that identical twins who share identical genes often die at quite different ages.

It seems counterintuitive but average life expectancy cannot be increased significantly by curing the major causes of death such as heart disease and cancer. Complete elimination of one or even both of these diseases would add only a few years to the average life expectancy after age 50 (**Figure 22.2**). Although curing major diseases is of inestimable benefit to those who die prematurely from them, their elimination has only a small effect on the average life expectancy of the entire U.S. population. However, slowing the aging processes

Global Wellness

Japan's Aging Society

The proportion of children in Japan's population has been declining for more than 30 years and reached an all-time low of 13.5% in 2008. By comparison, in the United States, the proportion of children in the total population is about 20%. Among 31 major industrialized nations, Japan has the fewest number of children under 14 years and the highest proportion of elderly. Currently about 22% of Japan's population is 65 or older; by 2040, the number of elderly persons is expected to outnumber children by 4 to 1.

Today Japan is one of the world's largest economies, but by 2050, the country is expected to lose 70% of its workforce. A government report projects that Japan's population, now about 127 million, will shrink by one-third within 50 years and by two-thirds within a century. With a rapidly aging and shrinking population, Japan faces daunting economic and social problems in the coming years. To care for its elderly, the government is subsidizing the development of robotic caregivers.

Although Japan is at the forefront of countries with aging and shrinking populations, other major industrialized countries are expected to have similar problems to varying degrees. One solution is to increase immigration of young workers from underdeveloped countries, but this creates other social and economic problems.

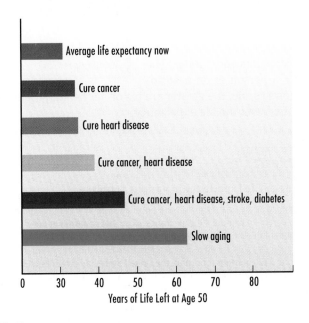

■ Figure 22.2

Increase in Average Life Expectancy After Age 50 Resulting from Curing Major Diseases or from Slowing Aging Processes
Eliminating cancer or heart disease as causes of death adds only a few years to the average life expectancy of the U.S. population. However, if ways could be found to slow aging processes, as much as 60 years could be added to the average life expectancy after age 50.

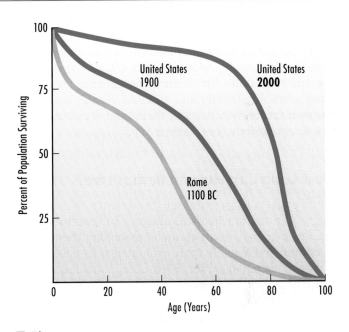

■ Figure 22.3

Approximate Survival Curves for Various Populations
The U.S. population is beginning to approximate the idealized curve.

can have a dramatic effect, allowing most people to live almost 60 years beyond age 50. That is why scientists are studying the mechanisms of aging in the hope of finding ways to slow aging processes.

Because of disease, accidents, and other factors, populations in the real world do not survive according to the idealized situation but have followed various paths throughout history (**Figure 22.3**). The average U.S. life span has increased dramatically in the last century. Because of this, the average age of the U.S. population is rapidly increasing.

TERMS

aging: normal changes in body functions that begin after sexual maturity and continue until death

average life span: the age at which half the members of a population have died

life expectancy: average number of years a person can expect to live

maximum life span: the theoretical maximum number of years that individuals of a species can live

In 2000, the U.S. population was 282 million; in 2050, it is expected to increase to 420 million. The last of the baby boomers will turn 65 in 2011. By 2030, one out of every five Americans will be 65 years or older. This major demographic shift in population is expected to strain all areas of society—health care, Social Security, education, elder care, and voting patterns to name just a few.

The "graying" of America has caused social, medical, and economic problems. First and most important is the ability of the federal government to sustain Social Security payments in the future. At the present rate, the government has estimated that the Social Security system will run out of money within 30 to 40 years. To avoid this, Congress has begun to discuss ways to reform Social Security so that future retirees still will receive benefits. Although many older people are vigorous and healthy, a large number of people over age 65 have chronic illnesses and disabilities that require ongoing medical care, and some need expensive, long-term care. About 80% of older Americans have at least one serious chronic medical condition; about 20% have five or more chronic conditions. The costs of health care for the elderly are rising rapidly and will be a greater burden in the near future, which is why there is an urgent need for health care reform (see Chapter 19).

How Long Can Human Beings Live?

Some experts in **gerontology** (the science that studies the causes and mechanisms of aging) believe that populations in many countries are approaching the current maximum average life span, estimated at 85 to 90 years, although, as noted earlier, a few exceptional individuals live longer. One bit of evidence for a maximum average life span of 85 to 90 years comes from government estimates that show differences in the life expectancies of people in various countries (**Table 22.1**). Andorra, Hong Kong, and Japan top the list. At the bottom of the list are

countries in Africa, where life expectancy is less than 40 years. The rapid decline in life expectancy in some African countries is primarily a result of the spread of HIV infections and deaths from AIDS (see Chapter 12).

The average life expectancy at birth for male and female Americans combined is about 77 years, but there are significant differences between the sexes and races that result from socioeconomic factors, education, and access to health care. For example, Caucasian women outlive Caucasian men by 5.1 years (Caucasian male life expectancy is 75.7 years; Caucasian female life expectancy is 80.8 years). The difference in life expectancy between African Americans and Caucasian Americans is 5.6 years (average life expectancy for African American men and women combined is 73.2 years; for Caucasian men and women combined it is 77.8 years). Although many factors have been invoked to explain differences in life expectancies, studies suggest that socioeconomic factors are the strongest predictor (Marmot, 2004). The lower a person is on a socioeconomic scale, the greater are his or her health problems and the lower the life expectancy.

> The older we get, the fewer things seem worth waiting in line for.
>
> *Will Rogers*

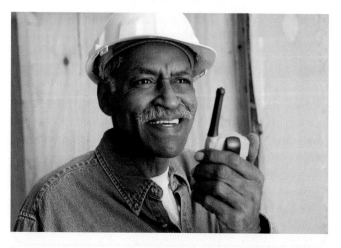

Many people continue to enjoy work long after the "normal" retirement age.

Table 22.1

Average Life Expectancy in Various Countries

Countries at the top of the list have populations that are approaching the average maximum life expectancy. Note that countries at the bottom of the list, primarily in Africa, have populations with life expectancies that are 40 to 50 years less than countries at the top. Among 212 countries reporting, the United States ranks number 43 in life expectancy at birth.

Country	Life expectancy at birth
Andorra	83.51
Hong Kong	81.59
Japan	81.25
Switzerland	80.51
Canada	80.22
Italy	79.81
France	79.73
Israel	79.46
Germany	78.80
United Kingdom	78.54
United States	77.85
Mexico	75.41
China	72.58
Russia	67.08
India	64.71
Haiti	53.23
Kenya	48.93
South Africa	42.73
Zimbabwe	39.29
Botswana	33.74

Source: CIA World Factbook, 2007.

A slightly different picture of aging emerges from studies of people between the ages of 85 and 100—a group known as the "oldest old." Statistical studies of oldest old Scandinavians suggest that in the absence of disease, senescent death (death from old age) could occur as late as 110 years. However, whether the maximum life expectancy for most people in the absence of disease is 85, 100, or 110 years, no human being is going to live to be as old as Methuselah, the biblical patriarch who is said to have lived for 967 years.

Theories of Aging

Biological Clocks Regulate Aging

Theories of aging fall into two broad categories. One ascribes aging to biological and genetic mechanisms that are specific for each species of animal and determine its maximum life span and rate of aging. The other theories focus on environmental factors that affect aging, such as nutrition, susceptibility to diseases, and exercise. Evidence for a "biological clock" that determines the maximum life span comes from measuring the amount of energy per gram of body weight consumed per day by mammals of different species. This energy consumption per day, called the **specific metabolic rate,** shows a striking correlation with the maximum life span of different species (**Figure 22.4**). Mammals that have the highest specific metabolic rate have the shortest life span; human beings have the slowest metabolic rate and the longest life span.

Longevity also has been associated with the number of heartbeats in individuals of different species. It is esti-mated that the total number of heartbeats for any mammal of any species is limited to about 1.5 billion beats before the heart wears out. In this model, longevity is determined by the rate of heartbeats. For example, shrews live only a few years and have hearts that beat thousands of times a minute. At the other extreme are elephants, whose hearts beat about once every three seconds and who live for more than a hundred years. It is not clear whether a person's resting heart rate is a predictor of longevity, because many other environmental and lifestyle factors also must be taken into account.

Further evidence for a biological clock that governs aging comes from studying the growth of cells in the laboratory. Conditions have been established in which cells from various tissues of different animals can be grown under fixed laboratory conditions. The surprising result of these experiments is that cells grow and divide in a laboratory medium for a fixed number of generations and then die. The number of generations of growth

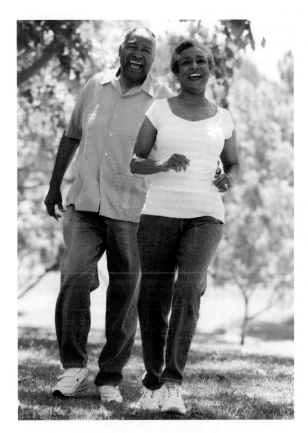

Shared activities are healthful at any age.

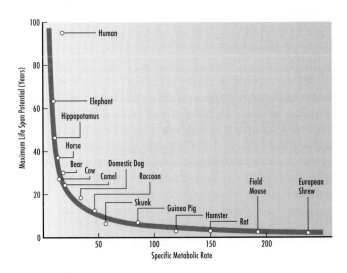

■ **Figure 22.4**

Correlation Between the Rate of Energy Consumed and Maximum Life Span Potential

Rate of energy consumption is calculated as energy per gram of body weight per day. Life span of various mammalian species is shown. The correlation suggests that the maximum human life span is a function of human biology and ultimately of human genes.

TERMS

gerontology: science that studies the causes and mechanisms of aging

specific metabolic rate: the amount of energy per gram of body weight consumed per day

🧘 Managing Stress

Giving Up Driving Is a Hard Decision

One of the hardest choices older people have to make is deciding when to give up driving. Driving a car is a sign of independence; being able to come and go as one pleases often depends on driving. Having to stop driving means becoming more dependent on other people.

Even if a person is basically healthy, driving skills decline as we get older. The American Association of Retired Persons (AARP) lists these signs that it may be time to stop driving:

- Do I get nervous at intersections or when making left turns?
- Do I have trouble scanning far down the road to anticipate problems?

- Do I fail to notice red lights or traffic signs?
- Do cars suddenly seem to come out of nowhere?
- Do I generally feel nervous while driving?
- Do I have trouble looking over my shoulder when changing lanes?
- Do I have trouble seeing the sides of the road when looking straight ahead?
- Have I had a "close call" while driving in the past six months?

is related to the maximum life span of the animal from which the cells were taken. Mouse cells only divide a few times, but human cells divide many times before dying. The inescapable conclusion from these experiments is that built into the cells of every animal is a genetically controlled clock that determines how many times cells can grow and divide before a signal tells them to stop (Hayflick, 1997).

A distinguishing feature of cancer cells is that they are immortal when grown under the same laboratory conditions used for growing normal cells. Cancer cells grow and divide indefinitely as long as fresh nutrients are provided; cells taken from human tumors more than 50 years ago are still kept growing in the laboratory. Thus, cancer cells have lost the ability to regulate normal growth and aging both in people and in the laboratory (see Chapter 13).

Mutations discovered in specific genes in research animals such as worms and flies have produced individuals that live about twice as long as usual. More important, such long-lived worms and flies are healthy and active even as they pass the age at which the control population dies. Thus, it seems possible that when more is understood about how genes affect aging, people also may live longer, healthier, and more active lives.

Environmental Factors Affect Aging

Although genetic factors contribute to aging, environmental factors play an even greater role. The longer we live, the more we are exposed to radiation and chemicals that can damage DNA in cells and, over time, may cause the death of essential cells in the body. For example, most cells possess enzymes that repair damage to their DNA; loss of these cellular repair enzymes with age could lead to widespread cell death. This has been called the "error

> I don't believe in aging. I believe in forever altering one's aspect to the sun.
>
> *Virginia Woolf*

catastrophe" theory of aging. Accumulated damage to the chromosomes in cells may be responsible for development of cancer and also for aging.

Another effect of exposure to radiation and chemicals is the production of very reactive molecules in cells, called free radicals (see Chapter 14). These substances are normally inactivated in cells, but as we age, our cells may be less able to cope with the damaging effects of free radicals. Free radicals also increase the damage to mitochondria, the complex structures in all cells that provide the energy for cellular growth and function. Without enough energy, cells become weak and possibly die; if too many cells die, organs function less efficiently and the person ages more rapidly. The mitochondrial error theory of aging is supported by animal studies. Mice have been genetically engineered so that the mitochondria in their cells accumulate mutations at a rapid rate. These mutations adversely affect essential mitochondrial functions. These mice age prematurely and die young (Krishnan et al., 2007).

Other scientists have found in laboratory experiments that the normal decline in the functions of mitochondria in cells can be reversed or slowed. Adding two naturally occurring compounds, acetyl L-carnitine and alpha lipoic acid, to mitochondria improves their capacity to manufacture the chemical energy required by cells. Both of these substances are synthesized in the body, but the amount declines with age.

In other studies, rats were fed the two compounds and, according to the researchers, the older rats were much more energetic than comparable rats that were not fed the supplements. Clinical trials in people have not been carried out, so any anti-aging benefits from these nutritional supplements are still speculative.

Immune system function also becomes less efficient with age, so that we become more susceptible to infections and autoimmune diseases. Overall, aging is a complicated process brought on by a combination of genetic and environmental factors.

Calorie (Energy) Restriction Slows Aging

A large body of evidence shows that **caloric restriction** allows laboratory animals to live longer. For example, a laboratory rat usually has a maximum life span of about 40 months; rats whose caloric intake is restricted have a maximum life span of about 57 months. Moreover, the older rats in the calorie-restricted group are healthier and act younger than old rats in the control group who have been well fed. The laboratory animals that live longer are not starved or deprived of any essential nutrients. Only the total amount of food that they are allowed to eat each day is restricted. Calorie-restriction studies similar to those performed with rats also extend life in other animal species.

One problem with caloric restriction is knowing when to begin restricting the amount of food. Young animals (including young children) require abundant nutrition for physical growth and for brain development. In the rat studies, it was shown that caloric restriction is of no value in prolonging life if it is begun too late in the animal's life.

A detailed evaluation of the effects of caloric restriction on people concluded that the risks outweigh the possible benefits (Fontana & Klein, 2007). Although some people might benefit from caloric restriction accompanied by adequate nutrient intake, lean people might be harmed by caloric restriction.

At present not enough is known about calorie restriction and life span to make any recommendations to people, except that everyone should consume a varied and healthy diet and not become overweight.

Alzheimer's Disease and Senile Dementia

In the absence of disease, normal mental functions can be maintained to age 100 or longer. However, many of the elderly have some loss of normal cognitive functions. The medical term for impairment or loss of cognitive functions in elderly persons is **senile dementia.**

The symptoms of senile dementia include the following:

- Loss of memory that increases over time
- Feeling confused
- Loss of problem-solving skills
- Suffering from delusions and agitated behavior
- Becoming lost in familiar settings
- Loss of interest in daily activities

Many conditions can cause dementia. A common cause is small strokes that gradually destroy cognitive functions in the brain. Neurodegenerative diseases such as Parkinson's disease, Huntington's disease, and Alzheimer's disease also cause dementia. In addition, viral and bacterial infections that cause HIV/AIDS, syphilis, tuberculosis, and meningitis also can give rise to symptoms of dementia.

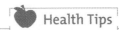 Health Tips

Steps You Can Take to Reduce the Risk of Dementia

Generally speaking, actions that promote good health also reduce the risk of Alzheimer's disease and other forms of dementia later in life. Some research supports the following risk-reduction strategies:

Physical exercise: Moderate exercise such as walking several times a week.

Omega-3 fatty acids: Consuming more of these fatty acids that are found in fish.

Mental activity: Staying mentally active, even doing crossword puzzles or playing challenging games such as chess.

Healthy diet: Eating healthfully; maintaining normal weight.

B vitamins: Supplementing B vitamins, especially folic acid.

The most common cause of dementia in the elderly is **Alzheimer's disease** (AD), which accounts for more than half of all cases of dementia. AD is caused by damage to neurons in the brain, resulting in loss of cognitive functions, memory, mobility, and eventually death. Currently, about 5.2 million Americans suffer from AD. Approximately 12% of Americans over age 65 have been diagnosed with AD. The percentage increases with age, and more women than men suffer from AD. The current cost of medical and nursing home care for AD patients is estimated at $148 billion and is expected to rise as the overall population continues to age. There is no cure for AD, nor is the cause known. However, anything that can delay the onset or slow the progression of AD can generate significant benefits for patients and society (**Figure 22.5**).

The disease is named for Alois Alzheimer, a German physician who, in 1907, described the abnormal brain structures he observed under the microscope in tissues obtained from patients who died from senile dementia. Alzheimer's findings at autopsy revealed what are still

TERMS

Alzheimer's disease: a common cause of senile dementia and other symptoms, eventually leading to death

caloric restriction: restricting the daily caloric intake of an animal or person while maintaining adequate nutrient intake

senile dementia: loss of cognitive functions in elderly people

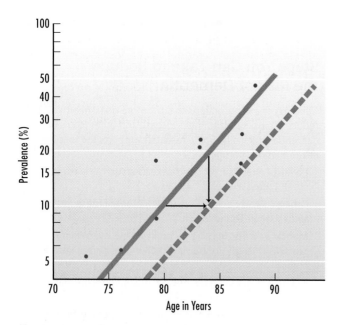

■ **Figure 22.5**

Benefits of Slowing Onset of Alzheimer's Disease (AD)
Approximately 10% of the U.S. population over age 65 and at least 20% by age 85 will have Alzheimer's disease. AD shows a linear increase with increasing age. If the onset of symptoms could be delayed by only five years, the prevalence of the disease would be only half as great. This marked reduction in the number of persons with symptoms of dementia would be of enormous benefit to society and save a substantial amount of health dollars.

Source: Courtesy Robert Katzman, University of California, San Diego.

the diagnostic criteria for the disease: (1) the presence of bundles of tangled nerve fibrils in certain areas of the brain; and (2) the presence of a specific protein called **amyloid protein,** which is localized in certain areas and blood vessels of the brain. How these changes affect the brain to produce loss of cognitive functions is still not understood.

Two forms of Alzheimer's disease are recognized, familial AD and sporadic AD. Familial AD, also known as early onset AD, is a rare form of the disease and usually develops in susceptible individuals who are less than 60 years old. This form probably has a strong genetic basis and often occurs in families in which many members suffer from AD at an early age. The sporadic form of AD probably is caused largely by environmental factors, which are undetermined as yet. The primary risk for sporadic AD is age. After diagnosis, AD can progress rapidly or slowly; the average time until death after diagnosis is 8 to 10 years.

Several drugs have been approved for treating the memory and cognitive losses that accompany Alzheimer's disease. Three of the drugs are known as cholinesterase inhibitors; these are the drugs donepezil, rivastigmine, and galantamine. The other approved drug, memantine, blocks the attachment of a specific neurotransmitter to cells. Clinical trials showed a very modest effect on symptoms of patients with moderate dementia, and only a minority of patients benefited at all. As one physician observed, "You can name 11 fruits in a minute instead of 10. Is that worth 120 bucks a month?" Still, many family members, caregivers, and physicians who are desperate to do something to slow the ravages of Alzheimer's disease are willing to pay the price. As AD progresses and behaviors become more agitated, antipsychotic drugs also are prescribed.

Despite the current research emphasis on finding defective genes linked to Alzheimer's disease risk, environmental factors appear to be very important. Epidemiological studies show that people with more education (college graduates) are much less likely to develop Alzheimer's disease than are people with little or no education. A study of Catholic nuns who died between ages 76 and 100 has confirmed the importance of education.

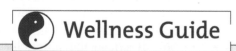

Wellness Guide

Spice Up Your Mind

Curry is a staple component of food in India and other Asian and Middle Eastern countries. The spice that gives curry its aroma, flavor, and color is turmeric. Recently, scientists have discovered that a particular chemical in turmeric called *curcumin* may be effective in preventing and treating Alzheimer's disease. An estimated 24 million people worldwide have Alzheimer's disease, and the number is increasing as the world's population ages. Several drugs are available for treating Alzheimer's disease, but they only mitigate cognitive problems; they do not slow progression of the disease.

In Pennsylvania, the prevalence of Alzheimer's disease among persons aged 65 and older is 17.5 per 1,000 individuals; in southern India where curry dishes are eaten daily, the prevalence is 4.7 per 1,000 individuals (Barry, 2007). In the

laboratory, adding curcumin to cells that contain amyloid protein plaques (found in the brains of Alzheimer's patients after death) rids the cells of the harmful protein. The evidence is thus building that curcumin really does have therapeutic potential for treating Alzheimer's disease. Although years of research lie ahead before curcumin or some derivative can be approved as an effective drug for Alzheimer's disease, its potential seems strong.

Taking curcumin as a supplement is not advised because dietary supplements are not regulated or tested for purity. Eating more curry dishes may be a good idea, however. Stick with yellow curry powder, which contains more turmeric than red curry powder does.

All of these Catholic nuns were college-educated and had a much lower prevalence of Alzheimer's disease than the general population. And among the few who did develop the disease, it could be shown by studying their brains after death that stroke was a primary trigger of the clinical symptoms of Alzheimer's disease.

It is not simply the level of education that helps to prevent the development of Alzheimer's disease. The key is to use the brain throughout life. Keep learning new things, explore new ventures—even doing crossword puzzles may help. It is now clear that brain cells continue to grow and establish new connections throughout life and that brain growth and health are dependent on mental stimulation. Just as exercise is necessary to maintain the body's fitness at all ages, exercising the brain is necessary to maintain mental functions (Marx, 2005).

Parkinson's Disease

Parkinson's disease (PD) is the second most common cause of neurodegenerative disease (after Alzheimer's disease) among older persons. About 1 million Americans suffer from PD, and about 50,000 new cases are diagnosed every year. Like other major neurological diseases such as Alzheimer's or Lou Gehrig's disease (ALS), Parkinson's disease is chronic and progressively worsens despite treatments that alleviate symptoms. PD was first described in 1817 by an English physician, James Parkinson, who described the symptoms as "the shaking palsy."

The four defining symptoms of PD are:

- *Tremor:* The tremor of a person suffering from PD involves a rhythmic back-and-forth motion of the thumb and forefinger that appears as if the patient is rolling a pill between the fingers. Although the tremor usually is observed in a hand, it can also arise in a foot or in the jaw.
- *Rigidity:* A basic principle of all movements of the body is that all muscles have opposing muscles. Movement occurs when one set of muscles contracts and the opposite set relaxes. The signals that tighten or relax muscles originate in the brain and are transmitted automatically to the muscles so that we make the movement that we desire. In PD patients, the signals from the brain are not coordinated, and the delicate balance between muscle tension and muscle relaxation is lost. In PD, the muscles stay constantly tensed and contracted, and the patient feels stiff and achy.
- *Bradykinesia:* This is probably the most distressing symptom of PD. Bradykinesia refers to the slowing down and loss of spontaneous movement. One moment, a person with PD is moving normally—crossing a street, for example—the next moment, the patient is frozen and cannot move, possibly in the middle of the crosswalk. Daily activities such as washing or putting on clothes may take hours because routine movements cannot be performed rapidly or continuously.
- *Postural instability:* Because PD patients have impaired balance and coordination of movements, they develop a tendency to lean forward or backward and to fall easily. As the disease progresses, walking becomes increasingly difficult; a patient may freeze in midstep and topple over if someone is not there for support.

The most effective drug used to treat PD is L-dopa (L-3,4-dihydroxyphenylalanine). Discovered in the 1960s, L-dopa delays the onset of the symptoms described and gives patients a period of time during which they can function more or less normally. Not all patients with PD are helped to the same degree by L-dopa, and not all symptoms of PD improve to the same degree. Today, L-dopa usually is taken with another drug, carbidopa; this reduces the dose of L-dopa needed and increases its effectiveness. Although L-dopa therapy, in combination with other drugs, is effective for some time, eventually the drugs' effectiveness diminishes as the disease progresses. The hope for PD patients lies in new drugs that may be able to halt the loss of dopamine neurons in the brain or in direct replacement of neurons by transplantation of healthy tissues.

As with other neurodegenerative diseases, the causes of PD are both genetic and environmental. Several genes are linked to rare forms of PD, and studies using laboratory animals have implicated abnormalities in mitochondrial function, damage from free radicals, and the accumulation of abnormal proteins as biological causes of neuronal dysfunction and survival in PD (Thomas & Beal, 2007).

However, environmental factors such as exposure to pesticides and other chemicals that affect the functions of mitochondria, the energy-generating organelles in cells, also can result in PD. Studies with mice have shown that blocking mitochondrial functions with a specific chemical can cause the mice to develop symptoms that mimic those of PD. These preliminary results should further alert people to the potential serious, long-term dangers of pesticide exposure (see Chapter 24).

Parkinson's disease, Alzheimer's disease, and other forms of dementias affect millions of elderly people. These neurodegenerative diseases erode the quality of

---

TERMS

amyloid protein: an abnormal protein in the brain of patients with Alzheimer's disease

Parkinson's disease: a neurodegenerative disease in which brain functions that control movements of the body are gradually lost

life for millions of elderly people, create enormous medical bills for families, and strain the resources and lives of caregivers. Medicines can provide some relief and perhaps slow the progression of the disease, but, ultimately, all neurodegenerative diseases are fatal. Recently, a group of related genes called *sirtuins* has been shown to play crucial roles in the development of age-related neurodegenerative diseases (Dillin & Kelly, 2007). Both activation and inhibition of these genes have been shown to affect the accumulation of toxic proteins that are associated with the development of neurodegenerative diseases. With the discovery of genes and proteins that may be causally related to development of these diseases comes the possibility of developing drugs that counteract the effects of these genes. On several fronts, progress is being made in both understanding how to increase longevity and how to eliminate the age-related diseases that make becoming old so depressing for many people.

Osteoporosis

The skeleton provides a means of locomotion, protection of vital organs, and a readily available store of calcium and phosphorus. Only recently has it been recognized that the skeleton is a delicately balanced regenerating tissue, regulated as precisely as the destruction and synthesis of blood cells. The most common metabolic bone disease is **osteoporosis,** which results from many environmental factors such as poor diet, smoking, corticosteroid use, excess alcohol consumption, and lack of exercise. Genetic variation among individuals also may be an important factor in the development of osteoporosis in some individuals but not others.

Osteoporosis occurs because the rate of bone breakdown exceeds the rate of bone renewal; many factors contribute to this. In older women, estrogen loss following menopause contributes to loss of bone material. In both older men and women, aging results in bone loss and increases the risk of fracture, depending on how much bone mass is reduced (**Figure 22.6**). Generally, the bone loss in women caused by low estrogen levels is significantly greater than the bone loss caused by normal aging processes.

The risk of osteoporosis in older women can be lessened by replacing the lost estrogen with **hormone replacement therapy (HRT).** For many women HRT has been beneficial because it reduces the risk of osteoporosis later in life. However, some studies showing that HRT increases slightly the risks of heart attack, stroke, and breast cancer have persuaded many postmenopausal women to forgo HRT therapy. On the other hand, other studies show that very low doses of estrogen may help prevent osteoporosis while avoiding the risks of standard HRT therapy. Estrogen supplementation in postmenopausal women also reduces the risk of Alzheimer's disease by about half. Thus, the use of HRT or low-dose estrogen may benefit some postmenopausal women. Making an informed decision is difficult, but discussing all options with one's health provider is important.

The best way to avoid osteoporosis is to build up as much bone mass as possible while young through a healthy diet with sufficient calcium, vitamin D, and exercise. Only 10% of American children get enough calcium or vitamin D or exercise enough to prevent osteoporosis later in life. Even children can be diagnosed with low bone mass that will only worsen as time goes on. After maturity, calcium and vitamin D still are needed to maintain bone mass. Consuming at least a gram of calcium daily is recommended, but nutritional surveys indicate that half of all Americans do not consume that amount. Vitamin D is essential because it assists in the absorption of calcium and in bone formation. Milk is advocated as the best bone-building food. It contains

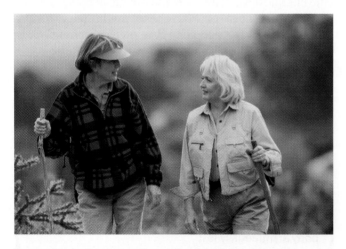

Regular exercise is important for reducing the risk of osteoporosis.

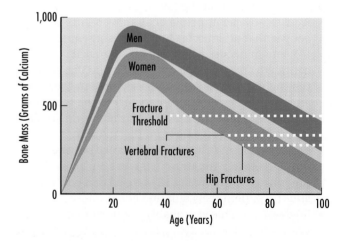

■ **Figure 22.6**

Changes in Bone Mass in Aging Men and Women
The risk of bone fracture from osteoporosis occurs when bone mass falls below a theoretical threshold and even a slight strain can cause a fracture.

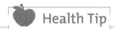
Health Tip

The Surgeon General's Recommendations for Preventing Osteoporosis

- Be sure you are getting the recommended daily amounts of calcium and vitamin D. High levels of calcium are found in milk, leafy green vegetables, soybean products, and cheese. Vitamin D is synthesized in the skin by sunlight exposure. People getting insufficient amounts of these substances should take supplements.
- The average adult younger than age 50 needs about 1 gram of calcium per day and 200 International Units (IU) of vitamin D. One cup of fortified milk provides 302 mg of calcium and 50 IU of vitamin D.
- Adults should maintain a healthy weight and exercise at least 30 minutes daily. Weight-bearing and balance exercises also are recommended.
- Take steps to reduce the risk of falls at home, at play, and at work.

  A copy of the Surgeon General's report on bone health and osteoporosis can be obtained by calling toll-free 1-866-718-BONE or on the Web at www.surgeongeneral.gov.

large amounts of calcium and is fortified with vitamin D to facilitate calcium absorption.

Osteoporosis can be treated in two different ways. Either the breakdown of bone can be slowed or the synthesis of new bone can be accelerated. In principle, both of these mechanisms can be treated with drugs, but in practice only one or the other is effective, not both. The class of drugs that reduces bone breakdown (also called remodeling or bone resorption) is bisphosphonates. These drugs have proved effective and result in an increase in bone mass in postmenopausal women by about 1% per year (Heaney & Recker, 2005). The drug that stimulates new bone formation is a fragment of the parathyroid hormone. This drug can increase bone mass by as much as 10% in a year, but it has some drawbacks. It must be taken daily, there are risks of side effects, and the regained bone mass is lost when the therapy is stopped. Clinical trials in which both drugs were used turned out to be less effective than using the parathyroid fragment alone.

In 2004, the U.S. Surgeon General issued a report documenting the impending public health crisis of osteoporosis. Currently, 10 million Americans over age 50 are suffering from osteoporosis and millions more are at risk. The report estimates that by the year 2020, just a few years from now, *half* of all Americans over age 50 will be at risk of life-threatening fractures caused by osteoporosis. At present, osteoporosis is the cause of more than 1 million fractures every year in people over age 50. The most frequent kinds of fractures are these:

- Hip fractures—300,000
- Vertebrae fractures—250,000
- Wrist fractures—250,000
- Other bone fractures—300,000

About 20% of senior citizens who have a hip fracture die from complications of the fracture; another 20% wind up in a nursing home. The direct costs of fractures in the elderly are estimated at $18 billion a year and are expected to rise sharply in the coming years.

It is difficult for young, active people to think about building up their bone mass while young. However, a healthy diet consisting of green leafy vegetables and milk (not soda) and lots of exercise will go a long way toward keeping your body strong and active later in life. The Surgeon General issued this report to alert the nation to adjust their lifestyles in ways that will ensure adequate bone mass throughout life.

Age-Related Vision Loss

Another major health problem for the elderly is loss of vision as a result of **age-related macular degeneration (AMD)**. The central portion of the retina consists of a structure called the macula, which contains specialized cells that give the eye the capacity to see fine detail. For reasons that are still undefined, these cells begin to die in some people as they age. AMD progresses slowly over years and eventually means that people can no longer drive, read normal print, watch television, recognize faces at a distance, or perform tasks involving small objects. Macular degeneration does not affect peripheral vision, so complete blindness does not occur and affected individuals can still be active in many ways.

About 8 million Americans over age 50 have vision loss caused by AMD (Jager, Mieler, & Miller, 2008). About 20% of people between the ages of 65 and 74 and about 40% of people over age 75 are affected. Because the U.S. population is expected to age rapidly in coming years, the number of older people with macular degeneration is expected to increase to 50% by the year 2020.

TERMS

age-related macular degeneration (AMD): loss of vision as a result of death of cells in a region of the eye called the macula; loss of vision progresses slowly over several years

hormone replacement therapy (HRT): administration of estrogen to menopausal and postmenopausal women to help prevent symptoms of menopause, osteoporosis, and heart disease

osteoporosis: a condition in older people, particularly women, in which bones lose density and become porous and brittle

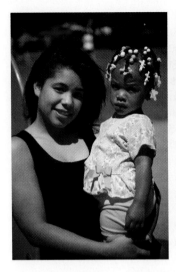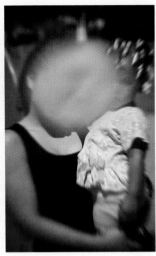

Macular degeneration.

Macular degeneration occurs in two forms: age-related dry macular degeneration is the most common, occurring in about 90% of patients. The other form is caused by proliferation of blood vessels in the macula; this form is called age-related wet macular degeneration. This is the most serious form because loss of vision progresses rapidly; occasionally the dry form may convert to the wet form. The wet form can be treated with laser surgery, which may be able to slow the progression of the damage. A drug, *ranibizumab*, also has been approved for treating the wet form of macular degeneration. However, the drug must be injected monthly, and each dose costs about $2,000. The injections must be continued indefinitely.

There are no approved treatments for the dry form of macular degeneration. However, in many people the loss of vision proceeds rather slowly so that many years pass after the initial diagnosis before legal blindness occurs. The progression of the dry form of macular degeneration can be significantly slowed by daily antioxidant supplements consisting of vitamin C, vitamin E, beta-carotene, zinc oxide, and copper oxide (van Leeuwen et al., 2005). Taking these antioxidants when damage to the macula is minimal substantially slowed the progression of the disease and preserved functional vision for a longer period of time than in a control group of patients who did not take daily antioxidants.

Other substances that may slow the progression of macular degeneration are lutein (a plant-derived antioxidant), zeaxanthin (a pigment in the macula), and bilberry extracts. Also, trace minerals such as zinc, selenium, and chromium may help. Some people are at higher risk for AMD because of inherited genes, some of which have been identified. Still, environmental factors such as smoking, exposure to UV radiation in sunlight, and high lipid levels in blood, as well as age and caucasian ancestry are the major causes of macular degeneration.

Age-Related Hearing Loss

Age-related hearing loss refers to hearing loss experienced by people as they get older and which interferes with understanding normal conversation. Hearing loss is the third most common chronic health condition among older Americans after high blood pressure and arthritis. About 4 million Americans over age 65 have hearing loss and difficulty hearing and understanding normal conversations. Some age-related hearing loss is inevitable as sensitive cells of the inner ear die or become less functional. However, much hearing loss is caused by exposure to noise and is referred to as noise-induced hearing loss (see Chapter 24). Even a single exposure to an extremely loud noise such as an explosion or a blast of sound from a loudspeaker can produce some permanent hearing loss. Lifetime exposure to loud noises such as driving in urban traffic, using power tools, listening to loud music, and working in noisy factories may also result in a gradual but permanent hearing loss.

Protecting your hearing while young is essential to preserving as much hearing as possible when you become old. Avoid explosions from firecrackers and guns or take precautions to protect your hearing. Always wear ear plugs or ear muffs designed to reduce environmental noise when operating any kind of noisy equipment. Even vacuum cleaners and hair dryers may exceed safe noise levels. Your hearing is precious; protect it at all times.

Physical Exercise May Slow Aging

Physical exercise has long been recommended for older people to help them remain physically fit and to prevent weight gain. In addition to maintaining physical vigor, exercise may actually have a beneficial effect on the structural integrity of chromosomes. Structures at the ends of chromosomes (called *telomeres*) are responsible for maintaining the integrity of each chromosome and prevent the loss of genes near the ends each time the chromosomes duplicate. Telomeres are like the leader on film, which protects the loss of scenes from the beginning of a film due to wear and tear each time the film is threaded through the machine.

Telomeres wear away little by little as we age; if telomeres become too short, cells die. If too many cells die, organs fail and we may die. Scientists have examined the length of telomeres in cells taken from older people who exercised and from people who were sedentary. The most active people had telomeres that were considerably longer than ones from people who did not exercise at all (Cherkas et al., 2008). The conclusion of the study was that exercise may slow aging by preventing chromosome destruction and consequent death of cells in the body.

Thinking About Aging

When you are young, thinking about aging usually is the last thing on your mind. You look at your parents and grandparents and cannot really imagine what it feels like to be 60 or 80 years old. Aging is something that happens to everyone irrespective of how successful they have been in living a "healthy" life. Of course, efforts that are implemented while you are young to care for your physical, emotional, mental, and spiritual health will help to maintain well-being when you are old. But there is no guarantee. Things happen. Life is a journey. Nothing in life is predictable. The main thing is to have the resiliency, understanding, and spiritual strength to cope with changes.

Acceptance of change is crucial to "successful" aging. When you get older, physical strength may diminish, but hopefully you no longer need to lift heavy objects. You walk more instead of being "on the run." Having time to

cook at home and being able to enjoy fresh foods are daily pleasures. You have time to read, think, and meditate. You have more time for art, gardening, reading, exercise, and socializing. Small things like watching a full moon rise from the ocean are special events. You are more aware of the spiritual side of nature and people.

Health and aging are lifelong processes, not goals that can be set and achieved with concentrated effort. Certainly, you can take steps that will improve your health now and later in life:

Physical health

- Enjoy a balanced, nutritious diet and maintain a healthy weight.
- Exercise; walk, run, jump, play; watch less TV.
- Do not take unnecessary risks such as diving into a shallow pond.
- Do not smoke or use tobacco.
- Use alcohol wisely; getting drunk is always dangerous. Drinking and driving can be lethal.

Mental, emotional, and spiritual health

- Take pleasure in healthy relationships with family and friends.
- Find time to cultivate a quiet mind. Practice meditation, yoga, or t'ai chi ch'uan.
- Engage in activities that bring pleasure and make you feel good.
- Stay positive and relate in positive, supportive ways with others.
- Manage your finances so that money worries do not create stress and worry. Renounce excess "consumerism."
- See adversity as a challenge and opportunity for changing some aspect of your life.
- Maintain awareness of your spirituality.

End-of-Life Decisions

With few exceptions, the media portray aging as a time of life beset with sickness, inactivity, and deterioration of physical, sexual, and mental functions. These negative views of aging are used to sell products and do not truthfully portray the experiences of most older Americans.

Of all human fears none is greater than the fear of death. When we are young, thoughts of death and dying are rare. Instead we are occupied with living, learning, and daily activities. We can't imagine that someday we will die. As we grow older and see parents, relatives, and

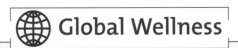

Global Wellness

Can Beliefs Influence Life Span?

Just how powerful are thoughts and feelings in influencing health? Can beliefs affect the duration of a person's life? A survey of the causes and ages of death among Chinese Americans shows that strongly held beliefs can affect the cause of death and how long a person lives (Phillips, Ruth, & Wagner, 1993).

In Chinese astrology, a particular phase—metal, water, wood, fire, or earth—is associated with the year of a person's birth. Also associated with each phase is susceptibility to particular diseases (see table). According to Chinese astrology and medicine, being born in a particular year makes a person more likely than usual to succumb to diseases associated with the phase of their birth year. An analysis of almost 30,000 death certificates of Chinese Americans showed that people with the predicted combination of birth year and disease susceptibility died two to five years before white Americans with the same diseases and phases.

The more traditional the Chinese lifestyle of the person, the shorter their life was once they contracted the disease associated with their birth year. The most plausible explanation of the findings is that Chinese Americans who believe in the predictions of Chinese astrology are the most likely to succumb to the disease that they expect will kill them. It appears that beliefs not only affect health through the onset of disease but also affect life span.

Birth year ends in	Phase	Susceptibility to
0 or 1	Metal	Pulmonary diseases
2 or 3	Water	Kidney disease
4 or 5	Wood	Cirrhosis of liver
6 or 7	Fire	Heart attack
8 or 9	Earth	Cancer, diabetes, ulcers

TERMS

age-related hearing loss: loss of hearing with advancing age; some loss of hearing may be caused by exposure to loud noise earlier in life

friends die, we become more aware of our own mortality. We may begin to ponder our own eventual death.

Fear of aging and death may lead to anxiety and stress that may hasten aging processes. A few of the many fears that people associate with aging are illness, poverty, being attacked or victimized, falling and being injured while alone, loss of responsibility for one's life, memory loss, and sexual inadequacy. Most of these fears are unfounded, but they diminish quality of life. Chronological age often does not correlate with biological age. Some people feel and act young even if old.

Steve Jobs, CEO of Apple Computer and Pixar Animation Studios, was incorrectly diagnosed with terminal pancreatic cancer in 2004. It turned out to be a very rare form of pancreatic cancer that was treatable. In an eloquent address to the Stanford University graduation class, Jobs described what this experience did for him.

> Remembering that I'll be dead soon is the most important tool I've ever encountered to help me make the big choices in life. Because almost everything—all external expectations, all pride, all fear of embarrassment or failure—these things just fall away in the face of death, leaving only what is truly important. Remembering that you are going to die is the best way I know to avoid the trap of thinking you have something to lose. (Jobs, 2005)

Death can strike without warning in the form of an accident or an unexpected heart attack. However, for most people, thoughts of death do not occupy their daily lives until old age. People in their 20s are too busy living to think about dying. But people in their 70s and 80s realize the inevitability of death and may modify their lives and affairs accordingly. Younger people who acquire a life-threatening disease such as cancer also are forced to face the reality of death.

Most people would prefer to die peacefully in their sleep after living a full, satisfying life. Some may be fortunate to die like this, but others may have to endure considerable pain and suffering for years. In addition to wondering how they are going to die, people usually wonder what will happen to them after death. Christianity provides a heaven where one's "soul" can exist in the grace of God for all eternity. Buddhism embraces a belief in reincarnation; after a series of deaths and rebirths a person can attain "Buddhahood," a perpetual state of enlightenment.

In our society, death is not discussed openly, although this is beginning to change. Dying people are often isolated in hospitals and their care is left to physicians who may perform unwanted or unnecessary treatments. Sterile, impersonal death in a hospital or nursing home has increased many people's fears of death and the process of dying.

Stages of Dying

People have different attitudes toward death and dying. In conversations with many persons who were facing death, Elisabeth Kübler-Ross (1975) identified five distinct stages in the process of dying. Not all persons experienced all stages, but most experienced some of them. These stages of dying are (1) denial and isolation, (2) anger, (3) bargaining, (4) depression, and (5) acceptance.

The work of Kübler-Ross has found widespread acceptance, especially among counselors and those who help dying patients, but it has also received criticism. The main objection is that the studies were not conducted scientifically but were based on personal observation and interpretation. Another criticism is that because the stages of dying that Kübler-Ross proposed have been widely accepted and publicized, some dying patients may feel obliged to follow the stages she described.

More and more it is recognized that dying, like living, is an individual, personal matter. People can do as poet Dylan Thomas recommended and "Rage, rage against the dying of the light." Or they can embrace the idea that "with a better understanding of aging, it will become easier to accept the fact that life ends" (Campion, 1998).

Advance Directives

In 2005, the widely publicized case of Terri Schiavo created a national controversy. On February 25, 1990, Terri Schiavo suffered a heart attack that was triggered by complications of an eating disorder. The heart attack interrupted the flow of blood to her brain. Although she was kept alive, she suffered extensive, permanent brain damage and survived in what is medically described as a "persistent vegetative state," a condition in which no detectable cognitive brain function remains.

Terri Schiavo was kept alive for 15 years by means of a feeding tube that supplied nutrition and water. Her husband, Michael Schiavo, insisted that his wife would not have wanted to be kept alive in this way and wanted the feeding tube removed. Terri Schiavo's parents were adamantly opposed to this action and insisted that their daughter be kept alive by all means. The battle over Terri Schiavo ultimately involved the governor and legislature of the state of Florida, the U.S. Congress, the Supreme Court, and President George W. Bush (Bloche, 2005). In the end, the courts allowed the feeding tube to be removed and Terri Schiavo died on March 31, 2005 (Annas, 2005).

The Terri Schiavo case made millions of Americans realize the importance of executing **advance directives** so that family and health providers know exactly what your wishes are regarding medical care should you become unable to function on your own behalf. Advance directives are particularly important for the elderly but should be executed by young people as well. Terri Schiavo was only 26 when she suffered her heart attack.

Advance directives typically consist of two distinct documents. A **living will** explicitly states your desires for or rejection of specific treatments should you become unable to communicate. A living will should indicate your wishes with respect to artificial ventilation, CPR (cardiopulmonary resuscitation), tube feeding, and do-not-resuscitate (DNR) orders as well as other treatments. A living will is signed and witnessed, and copies are given to your personal physician as well as to family members and others that you trust.

A living will should be as detailed as possible but may not cover all circumstances in a medical emergency. If you suffer a heart attack and someone calls 911, paramedics are required by law to administer CPR irrespective of what is stated in a living will. Only after you reach a hospital can the provisions in a living will be respected by physicians and hospital staff.

Another important document is a **health care power of attorney** in which you designate a spouse, family member, or close friend as the person responsible for health decisions in the event you are unable to make such decisions. The person you designate must be 18 years or older and cannot be one of your health care providers. Together, a living will and health care power of attorney make up your advance directive.

States differ considerably in the forms and terminology of advance directives. Help in understanding and completing advance directive forms can be obtained at a number of Web sites. Forms and instructions for each state can be obtained at www.compassionandchoices.org.

Everyone should execute advance directives to avoid the tragedy of Terri Schiavo. Filing advance directives with your physician and family does not mean that you give up the right to make your own health decisions. Advance directives are used only if you become incapacitated and are unable to communicate.

Physician-Assisted Suicide

In 1997, Oregon passed the Death with Dignity Act, which legalized **physician-assisted suicide** in that state. In the first year after the bill passed, 23 persons received prescriptions for lethal medications, and 15 actually took the medicine and died. In 1999, physicians prescribed lethal medications to another 33 patients, but some died before they could take the drugs. In the years from 1998 to 2007, 341 terminally ill patients in Oregon died from physician-prescribed drugs. It is clear from these numbers that, so far, there has not been a rush among terminally ill patients in Oregon to end their lives.

In 2001, U.S. Attorney General John Ashcroft ruled that the Oregon law regarding physician-assisted suicide violated the federal Controlled Substances Act (CSA). In January 2006, the U.S. Supreme Court upheld the Oregon Death with Dignity Act. Specifically, the U.S. Supreme Court held that "the CSA does not allow the Attorney General to prohibit doctors from prescribing regulated drugs for use in physician-assisted suicide under state law permitting this procedure."

In physician-assisted suicide, a terminally ill patient who is mentally competent must express a desire to die on a number of occasions. Then a second physician would be consulted. Finally, if both physicians agree that the patient is mentally competent (not clinically depressed) and has an incurable, painful disease, one physician would supply the patient with the drugs needed to commit suicide or otherwise help the patient end his or her life.

Physician-assisted suicide also has been practiced in the Netherlands for a number of years, even though it is officially illegal. In the Netherlands, several thousand seriously ill patients die each year with the help of their physicians; the criteria for physician-assisted suicide in that country include the following:

- The patient must repeatedly and explicitly request the desire to die.
- The patient's decision must be well informed and free.
- The patient must be suffering from severe physical or mental pain with no prospect of relief.
- All other options for therapy must have been exhausted.
- The physician must consult at least one other physician.

Despite growing public support for physician-assisted suicide in the United States, there is still great resistance to its use among physicians, clergy, and members of right-to-life activist movements. In 2008, voters in Washington state approved a physician-assisted suicide law similar to the one enacted in Oregon. As of 2009, Oregon and Washington are the only two states that permit physician-assisted suicide for terminally ill patients. Thirty-four other states still have laws that explicitly criminalize any form of assisted suicide; Washington previously was in this group.

There is general agreement that end-of-life care needs to be improved substantially. Studies show that of the more than 2 million people that die each year in the United States, almost half of hospitalized patients suffer serious pain in the days preceding death. And only about one-third of patients in nursing homes receive adequate pain relief. Two national health care organizations have proposed that

---

TERMS

advance directive: legal documents that express your desires regarding treatments should you be unable to communicate. A living will and health care power of attorney constitute an advance directive

health care power of attorney: designates someone to make health care decisions for you if you are unable to communicate

living will: a legal document that expresses your wishes regarding treatment if you become unable to make your own medical decisions

physician-assisted suicide: a form of active euthanasia in which a physician helps a patient who no longer desires to live because of pain or an incurable illness to commit suicide

every physician attending to a dying patient should make the following six promises:

- You will have the best of medical treatment, aiming to prevent exacerbation, improve function and survival, and ensure comfort.
- Your care will be continuous, comprehensive, and coordinated.
- You and your family will be prepared for everything that is likely to happen in the course of your illness.
- Your wishes will be sought and respected, and they will be followed whenever possible.
- We will help you consider your personal and financial resources and we will respect your choices about their use.
- We will do all we can to see that you and your family will have the opportunity to make the best of every day.

The public discussion over end-of-life treatments and legal options and problems has been active in the United States for more than a quarter of a century and is still far from being resolved. In 1990, the U.S. Supreme Court did rule that withholding or withdrawal of life support to dying patients who can no longer be helped medically is legal.

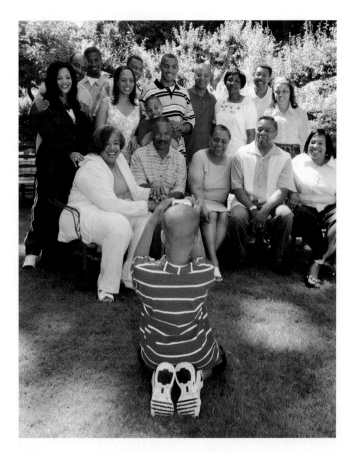

Strong family ties are healthy for young and old alike.

Palliative Care

Palliative care is a newly recognized branch of medicine that focuses on noncurative treatments for the dying. The World Health Organization (WHO) defines palliative care as follows:

- Affirms life and regards dying as a normal process
- Neither hastens nor postpones death
- Provides relief from pain and other distressing symptoms
- Integrates the psychological and spiritual aspects of patient care
- Offers a support system to help patients live as actively as possible until death
- Offers a support system to help families cope with the patient's illness and death

When a person elects palliative care, the emphasis of treatment shifts from prolonging life to enhancing the quality of life that remains, preserving a person's dignity, and relieving suffering. Usually, a team of health professionals, in consultation with the patient and family, will decide if palliative care is appropriate.

Many opponents of physician-assisted suicide embrace the concept of palliative care and believe that it is more in accord with the ethics of medical practice. Now that palliative care is seen as a reimbursable form of therapy by many health insurance programs, eventually all terminally ill patients may have access to such care and no longer have to fear prolonged pain and suffering.

The Hospice

The term **hospice** originally applied to medieval Christian hospitals caring for the poor, the aged, and the sick. Hospices also provided refuge for people on religious pilgrimages. Providing physical necessities, medical care, and spiritual comfort was the primary purpose of the early religious hospices. In the United States today there are more than 2,000 hospices offering comprehensive care for terminally ill patients. The goal of a hospice is to meet the total health needs—physical, psychological, and spiritual—of patients who have weeks or months to live. Medications are given to ease pain, but heroic treatments are not attempted. Family and friends are free to visit with the patient in a comfortable setting, whether it is in a patient's home or a hospital with a hospice attached.

The hospice philosophy is that dying is part of living and should not be resisted with every weapon in the modern medical arsenal. Hospice care is designed to control pain and make patients comfortable, but staff also are trained to discuss emotional and spiritual issues relevant to death. Counseling and social services are available in hospices, and close family members are encouraged to participate in daily activities.

In 1982, Congress passed the Medicare Hospice Benefit Act. This law ensures that Medicare will pay hospice costs for any terminally ill patient whose projected life expectancy is six months or less. In 2008, more than 3,000 hospices were enrolled in the Medicare plan. Overall, about one in three Americans now dies under hospice care either at home or in a hospice facility.

Healthy Aging Depends on a Healthy Lifestyle

With the dramatic upward shift in average life expectancy in the United States and other countries, finding ways to improve health in elderly people has become a major challenge. Generally, increasing age is associated with increasing disability and functional impairments, such as loss of mobility, sight, or hearing. One goal of gerontology is to find ways to minimize or postpone the disabilities that accompany aging so that quality of life extends to, or close to, the end of life.

The scientific evidence is now quite overwhelming that most of the disability and long-term medical care in elderly persons results from major chronic diseases that were already present in midlife. The most significant predictors of a healthy old age are low blood pressure and low serum glucose levels, not being obese, and not smoking cigarettes while young. These factors are also important in predicting such diseases as cardiovascular

disease, cancer, and diabetes. Thus, the evidence points to the importance of developing healthy habits while young if the "golden years" are going to be enjoyed with one's physical and mental abilities intact.

Persons surviving to age 55 today can expect to live, on average, another 25 years; those surviving to age 75 can expect to live another 10 to 12 years. Many of these older people are relatively healthy and the length of time that they will be disabled before death is short. In general, people who live to the oldest ages without disabilities are those who have practiced good nutrition, were physically and mentally active, and did not use tobacco or drink alcohol excessively.

More and more attention is being paid to the role of nutrition in healthy aging. Increased consumption of fresh fruits and vegetables is thought to slow the aging

---

TERMS

hospice: a place for terminally ill patients to spend the time before death in an environment that attends to their physical, emotional, and spiritual needs but does not administer any further treaments; hospice care also can be given in a patient's home

---

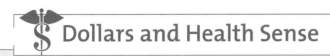

$ Dollars and Health Sense

Anti-Aging Hormones

In recent years, the search for the "fountain of youth" has focused on hormones that might halt or reverse the aging processes. Human growth hormone (hGH), which is responsible for the growth spurt during adolescence, declines about 12% per decade after middle age in both men and women (Stewart, 2006). Estrogen production declines abruptly in postmenopausal women, and testosterone levels fall, although more slowly, as men age. The adrenal gland produces a sex hormone, *dehydroepiandrosterone* (DHEA), that progressively declines after age 30; at age 60 the level of DHEA is about half of what it was during youth. Some studies have hinted at an association between the declining levels of these hormones and age-related changes such as loss of bone density and fractures, cognitive impairment, increased fat deposition, and increased risk of cardiovascular disease. However, no scientific studies have established a causal link between any hormone decline and aging disabilities. Despite the lack of evidence of benefit, companies are aggressively marketing these hormones as solutions to aging problems as well as to athletes for performance enhancement.

The use of hGH is approved only for short-stature problems in children and for certain indications in adults. Studies have shown that it does not spur growth of muscles in healthy individuals, nor does it alter any of the changes that occur

during aging in the elderly. Despite this evidence, an enormous illicit industry engages in marketing hGH for unapproved purposes. In January 2007, the Food and Drug Administration (FDA) published an alert emphasizing that use of hGH for anti-aging, bodybuilding, or sport performance enhancement is dangerous (Olshansky & Perls, 2008). But the FDA has little enforcement power. A driving force for the illegal market is the enormous amounts of money that can be made. An investigation in New York revealed that a pharmacy in that state would purchase 25 grams of hGH overseas for $75,000. It would repackage it in small doses and sell it for more than $1 million. The documented adverse effects of using hGH are edema (swelling), carpal tunnel–like symptoms, gynecomastia (male breast enlargement), and increased risk of developing diabetes.

The effects of administering the adrenal hormone DHEA have been studied in both elderly men and women. No beneficial effects were observed in body composition, physical strength, or utilization of insulin. In younger, healthy women, administration of DHEA does increase libido slightly, but there were no physical benefits. Also, no benefits were observed when testosterone was given to elderly men or women (Nair et al., 2006).

processes; those containing antioxidant chemicals are regarded as particularly potent anti-aging foods. These include avocado, berries, broccoli, cabbage, carrots, citrus, grapes, onions, tomatoes, and spinach. Coffee and tea also contain significant amounts of antioxidants. But according to believers in the antioxidant theory of aging, supplements still are needed to ensure that you are getting sufficient amounts of antioxidant vitamins and minerals.

Every age of life provides opportunities for growth and satisfaction. Even though we have no way of knowing when serious illness or death will confront us, we do have control of how we live each day and the satisfactions we find in life. The way we choose to live when we are young will greatly affect our health later. For example, smoking while young increases the likelihood of developing cancer and heart disease later. Drinking alcohol to excess and taking unnecessary chances invite accidents that can cause death or permanent disability. Although each person's life span is partly determined by genes, environmental factors, such as nutrition, exercise, and lifestyle, are also important not only in determining how long we live, but how well we live.

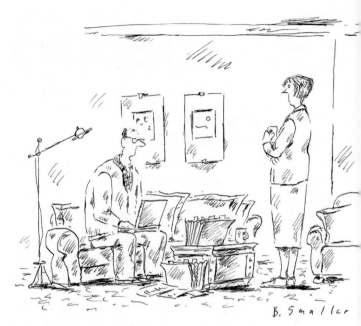

"If we take a late retirement and an early death, we'll just squeak by."

© The New Yorker Collection 2003 Barbara Smaller from cartoonbank.com. All rights reserved.

Critical Thinking About Health

1. Since the breakup of the former Soviet Union, the life expectancy of people in Russia has been declining dramatically. Make a list of all the factors you can think of that would contribute to a shorter life expectancy in Russia now compared with previously. Discuss each factor and how important you think it is in contributing to the decline. Also indicate whether any of the factors you have discussed for the decline of life expectancy in Russia are important in explaining the difference in life expectancy between Caucasian and African Americans discussed in this chapter.

2. Imagine that you have just learned that your mother is suffering from terminal cancer that cannot be treated. The physician estimates that death can occur at any time within a few months and that your mother's pain will be considerable. Although drugs can alleviate some of the pain, the doctor honestly does not know how effective the pain relief will be. Your mother is 75 years old and is aware of her condition. When you and she discuss her condition, she expresses a strong desire not to suffer to survive a few weeks or months. She asks you to help her obtain drugs that she can use to end her life peacefully whenever she chooses.

   Describe how you would feel in such a situation and what actions you would take. Would you discuss the problem with her physician, with a religious counselor, or with someone else? Would you be concerned about legal problems if you did obtain the lethal drugs and give them to your mother? Would you tell your mother that you want to keep her alive at all costs and you will do all that you can to reduce her suffering? Make a list of all the steps you would take in this situation, and explain your reasons for each action.

3. Make a list of all the health-related factors in your life that you think might play a role in how healthy you will be at age 70 (e.g., you smoke cigarettes, you are significantly overweight). After thinking about the list you have made, ask yourself if some behaviors or lifestyle factors are worth changing to help ensure that you will enjoy a healthy old age. Or perhaps you feel that it is not worth worrying about old age now and that the important thing is how to enjoy life at the present time. Discuss these different views and try to develop a personal philosophy of aging that is right for you.

4. Because both of your grandmothers have Alzheimer's disease, the other members of your family are very concerned over their own future mental health, even though both of your parents are only in their 50s. Having read that a particular gene contributes to the risk of Alzheimer's disease and that doctors can test for the presence of this gene, your mother and father have been discussing the advisability of getting the test. They also have asked if you would like to be tested for the Alzheimer's gene. What advice would you give them? Would you want to be tested for the Alzheimer's susceptibility gene? Discuss in detail the reasons for your advice to them and the decision you would make for yourself.

Health in Review

- Aging and dying are natural stages of life. People should strive to remain physically, emotionally, mentally, and spiritually active at all stages of life regardless of chronological age.
- The maximum human life span is approximately 115 years; the average life span in many countries is 80+ years, which means that half of the people in those countries will live to be 80 years of age or older.
- The average age of the population in the United States is rising rapidly, increasing health care costs and causing problems for the Social Security system.
- Aging is partly determined by genes and partly by environmental factors that cause cellular damage. Caloric restriction slows aging in laboratory animals but is impractical in people.
- Loss of cognitive abilities in the elderly is called senile dementia; the major cause of mental deterioration is Alzheimer's disease.

- Parkinson's disease is a neurodegenerative disease that affects movement.
- Bone loss in the elderly causes osteoporosis.
- The major cause of vision loss in the elderly is macular degeneration.
- Advance directives consist of executing a living will and a health care power of attorney.
- Palliative care is treatment that does not cure but relieves pain and suffering of dying patients and deals with the distress of family members.
- Hospice care provides terminally ill patients with medical, emotional, and spiritual support during the final weeks or months of their lives.
- Successful aging depends on maintaining a healthy weight; eating a nutritious, balanced diet; getting lots of exercise; and keeping mentally active.

Health and Wellness Online

The Web contains a wealth of information about health and wellness. By accessing the Internet using Web browser software, you can gain a new perspective on many topics presented in *Health and Wellness,* Tenth Edition. Access the Jones and Bartlett Publishers Web site at **health.jbpub.com/hwonline.**

References

Annas, G. J. (2005). "Culture of life" politics at the bedside—The case of Terri Schiavo. *New England Journal of Medicine, 352,* 1710–1715.

Barry, P. (2007, September 15). Curry powder. *Science News,* 167–168.

Bloche, M. G. (2005). Managing conflict at the end of life. *New England Journal of Medicine, 352,* 2371–2373.

Campion, E. W. (1998). Aging better. *New England Journal of Medicine, 338,* 1064–1066.

Cherkas, L. F., et al. (2008). The association between physical activity in leisure time and leukocyte telomere length. *Archives of Internal Medicine, 168,* 154–158.

Dillin, A., & Kelly, J. W. (2007). The yin-yang of sirtuins. *Science, 317,* 461–462.

Fontana, L., & Klein, S. (2007). Aging, adiposity, and caloric restriction. *Journal of the American Medical Association, 297,* 986–994.

Hayflick, L. (1997, January). Myths of aging. *Scientific American,* 110–113.

Heaney, R. P., & Recker, R. R. (2005). Combination and sequential therapy for osteoporosis. *New England Journal of Medicine, 353,* 624–625.

Jager, R. D., Mieler, W. F., & Miller, J. W. (2008). Age-related macular degeneration. *New England Journal of Medicine, 358,* 2606–2616.

Jobs, S. (2005). Graduation address at Stanford University, June 12, 2005.

Krishnan K. J., et al. (2007). Mitochondrial DNA mutations and aging. *Annals of the New York Academy of Science, 1100,* 227–240.

Kübler-Ross, E. (1975). *Death: The final stage of growth.* Englewood Cliffs, NJ: Prentice Hall.

Marmot, M. (2004). *The status syndrome: How social standing affects our health and longevity.* New York: New York Times Books.

Marx, J. (2005). Preventing Alzheimer's: A lifelong commitment? *Science, 309,* 864–867.

Nair, K. S., et al. (2006). DHEA in elderly women and DHEA or testosterone in elderly men. *New England Journal of Medicine, 355,* 1647–1653.

Olshansky, S. J., & Perls, T. T. (2008). New developments in the illegal provision of growth hormone for "anti-aging" and bodybuilding. *Journal of the American Medical Association, 299,* 2792–2794.

Phillips, D. P., Ruth, T. E., & Wagner, L. M. (1993, November 6). Psychology and survival. *Lancet, 342,* 142–145.

Rosen, C. J. (2003, March). Restoring aging bones. *Scientific American,* 71–77.

Stewart, P. M. (2006). Aging and fountain-of-youth hormones. *New England Journal of Medicine, 355,* 1724–1726.

Thomas, B., & Beal, M. F. (2007). Parkinson's disease. *Human Molecular Genetics, 16,* R183–R194.

van Leeuwen, R., et al. (2005). Dietary intake of antioxidants and risk of age-related macular degeneration. *Journal of the American Medical Association, 294,* 3101–3107.

Suggested Readings

Casses, C. K. (2002). Use it or lose it: Activity may be the best treatment for aging. *Journal of the American Medical Association, 288*, 2333–2335. Discusses the latest research on slowing the effects of aging. Exercise comes out on top.

Fins, J. J. (2006). *A palliative ethic of care: Clinical wisdom at life's end*. Sudbury, MA: Jones and Bartlett. An excellent discussion of palliative care and end-of-life decisions.

Gawande, A. (2007, April 30). *The way we age now. The New Yorker*, 48–57. An intimate portrait of how one elderly person copes with aging.

Goodwin, J. S. (1999). Geriatrics and the limits of modern medicine. *New England Journal of Medicine, 340*, 1283–1285. A thoughtful article about how we have "medicalized" many of the problems of old age and should be less aggressive in treating people in their 80s and 90s.

Holliday, R. (2007). *Aging: The paradox of life*. Dordrechtt, The Netherlands: Springer. A renowned expert on aging presents a slew of fascinating facts about why we age and possible interventions to prolong life.

Nuland, S. B. (2007). *The art of aging: A doctor's prescription for well-being*. New York: Random House Publishing. A famous physician, now in his 70s, offers advice on how to age successfully.

Rados, C. (2005, May/June). Sound advice. *FDA Consumer*, 20–27. An excellent article about the causes of hearing loss and what can be done to protect hearing and restore it.

Sinclair, D. A., & Guarente, L. (2006, March). Unlocking the secrets of longevity genes. *Scientific American*, 48–57. An interesting article that describes the genes that have been discovered so far that increase the normal life span in animals.

Travis, J. (2004, July 10). Dying before their time. *Science News*, 26–28. This article explains why aging is now thought to result from damage to mitochondria in cells. Also describes chemicals that might slow the processes of aging.

Recommended Web Sites

Please visit **health.jbpub.com/hwonline** for links to these Web sites.

Compassion and Choices
Offers help and advice on end-of-life decisions. Provides advance directives tool kit. Helped to design Oregon's Death with Dignity Act.

HospiceNet
Information and education about hospice and other death and dying issues, including bereavement and end-of-life caretaking.

My Health Directive.com
This site also provides information and help with advance directives.

National Right to Life
The National Right to Life Committee supplies living wills that instruct physicians to use all techniques available to preserve life.

NIH Senior Health
Health information for older Americans from the U.S. National Library of Medicine.

U.S. Administration on Aging
General information on aging.

U.S. National Institute on Aging
Information on research on aging problems.

POLICE LINE — DO NOT CROSS

Health and Wellness Online: health.jbpub.com/hwonline

Study Guide and Self-Assessment

23.1 Do I Protect Myself from Crime?

Chapter Twenty-Three

Violence in Our Society

Learning Objectives

1. Describe the different kinds of interpersonal violence.

2. Explain ways that violence affects health.

3. List the kinds of violence and abuse that can lead to posttraumatic stress disorder.

4. Describe the different forms of child abuse.

5. Define *sexual assault*, *forcible rape*, and *acquaintance rape*.

6. Discuss the reasons that underlie forcible rape and acquaintance rape.

7. Define *elder abuse* and the factors that contribute to it.

8. List and describe the different kinds of hate crimes.

9. Discuss some of the ways that firearms increase the risk of homicide and suicide among young people.

10. Discuss how media violence contributes to aggression and violence among children.

11. Discuss some of the effects terrorism has had on people's lives and on American society.

Anger, aggression, hostility, and violence are inherent to all animals, including humans. Their major biological roles are to aid in the acquisition of food, mates, territory, and other resources, and to ward off danger to self and offspring and, in some species, family and community as well. As intelligent as humans are, they seem unable to control biologically rooted rage and violent behavior. Compared to other animals, modern humans have sophisticated weapons and ways to assault, vanquish, and kill, sometimes out of need, but most often out of greed. In addition, we kill others and ourselves, not for self-defense or the acquisition of material wealth, but because of ideas, beliefs, prejudices, insults, and a host of hurts that are conjured up in our minds. The goal of modern societies—as yet unrealized—is to develop ways to prevent and control human aggression and violence.

> In war, truth is the first casualty.
> *Aeschylus (525–456 B.C.)*

Violence is a physical or verbal behavior in which the intent is to harm, injure, or destroy someone or something. Human beings are unique in understanding the future possibility of injury and death and so will fight for many reasons, including being threatened by loss of personal freedom. People also have many intangible things to fear—fear of being hungry, fear of being poor, fear of being attacked, and fear of being unwanted or unloved are examples. All of these fears can provoke violent behavior.

Some people use violence as a means of gaining power over others. In its simplest form, power is the ability to satisfy one's needs. Power and its accompanying violence manifest in society in a variety of ways—as rape, domestic violence, child abuse, elder abuse, homicide, suicide, terrorist attacks, gang fights, and wars between nations.

More than 20,000 persons die in the United States every year from homicide, and more than 2 million persons are injured in violent attacks. Homicide is the second leading cause of death among persons aged 15 to 24, and suicide is the third in the same age group. The consequences of violence in society are broken families, battered women, abused children, and countless unnecessary injuries and deaths.

To treat the effects of violence on the minds and bodies of people is expensive, difficult, and often unsuccessful. The only solution to violent human behavior, as with other serious diseases, is prevention. Although some people believe that violence in human societies is inevitable, many others do not and choose to live nonviolent lives and work to end violent behaviors.

Intimate Partner Violence

Intimate partner violence (IPV) refers to physical, sexual, or psychological harm by a current or former intimate partner or spouse. Women are the most likely victims of IPV, but both heterosexual and homosexual men also are affected. Until recently, the public generally viewed intimate partner violence as rare. However, IPV and other forms of domestic violence are now recognized as major public health problems. IPV is regarded as one of the most serious, preventable public health problems, affecting a total of more than 32 million Americans at one time or another in their lives.

Several categories of IPV are recognized by health experts:

Physical violence: the intentional use of physical force on another person that has the potential for causing injury, disability, or death. Physical violence may include scratching, pushing, kicking, punching, grabbing, biting, choking, and use of weapons.

Sexual violence: (1) use of physical force to compel another person to engage in a sexual act against his or her will; (2) any sexual act against a person who is unable to understand the act or to indicate unwillingness to engage in a sexual act, for example, a person might be too drunk or intimidated to prevent the act; and (3) abusive sexual contact.

Threats of physical or sexual violence: use of words, gestures, or weapons to communicate the intent to cause physical injury or death.

Psychological or emotional violence: use of acts, threats of acts, or coercive measures that cause the victim to feel humiliated, embarrassed, diminished, or frightened; denying a victim access to friends, money, or food.

Stalking: behavior that causes victims to feel a high level of fear of physical or sexual violence.

Studying IPV is difficult because it often is not discussed openly by family members or even by abused individuals. It is estimated that fewer than half of all cases of family violence are reported to authorities, but the extent of physical and sexual attacks on women in the United States is alarming (**Table 23.1**). More women are treated in hospital emergency rooms for IPV injuries each year than for muggings, rape, and traffic accidents combined. And battering during pregnancy is the leading cause of birth defects and infant mortality.

In trying to reduce the epidemic of intimate partner violence, the federal government has declared each October as National Domestic Violence month. Extra efforts are made during this period to increase public awareness of domestic violence and to educate people on how to prevent it.

Women who experience battering or rape by a partner or acquaintance not only have medical problems but also may suffer from anxiety, depression, chronic pelvic pain, gastrointestinal upset, substance abuse, obesity, or headaches. Assaulted women may also develop symp-

Table 23.1

Violence Against Women

Number	Violent acts
5.3 million	Number of times American women are stalked or abused by an intimate partner each year.
555,000	Number of American women who suffer serious injuries from domestic abuse each year; 73% of all domestic abuse goes unreported.
145,000	Number of American women who are hospitalized each year from domestic abuse.
1,200	Number of women killed each year; 31% of all female homicides in the United States are committed by husbands or boyfriends.

Source: U.S. Department of Justice.

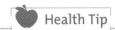
Health Tip

Hotline for Domestic Violence Help

If you or someone you know is subject to domestic or interpersonal violence of any kind, professional help should be obtained as quickly as possible. Advice and assistance can be obtained by calling the following hotline:

U.S. Government's National Domestic Violence Hotline: 800-799-SAFE (7233)

---

toms of *posttraumatic stress disorder (PTSD)* (see Chapter 3) and its variants, battered women's syndrome or rape trauma syndrome. Many long-term health consequences associated with battering, rape, and sexual abuse are associated with PTSD. For example, traumatized individuals tend to be more susceptible to arousal by stimuli that makes it difficult for them to differentiate normal aches, pains, and sensations from signals of disease, leading to increased incidence of seeking help from health professionals. Also, emotional upset and guardedness can produce painful muscle tension and skeletal misalignment. Chronic anxiety can lead to gastrointestinal upsets. Alcohol, nicotine, and other drugs may be used to block out memories of abuse and to alleviate uncomfortable emotions and physical sensations that accompany memories of the assault or abuse.

Recovering from the trauma of relationship violence requires patience and support. Victims are encouraged to seek psychological counseling from professionals who specialize in helping victims of relationship violence and to join support groups of other assaulted individuals. Support can hasten healing and recovery and help restore the trust that is shattered by assault. Support groups can also provide a place to stay if the victim needs to escape the abuser, or the group can offer companionship if the victim is afraid to be alone.

Symptoms of PTSD include the following:

- Reexperiencing the traumatic event(s) through recurrent intrusive images, thoughts, dreams of the trauma, and "flashbacks"—having a sense of reliving the trauma, including reexperiencing the disturbing emotions.
- Intense reactions to things that symbolize the traumatic experience. For example, in recovering from a rape, victims may intensely fear being in locales that resemble the scene of the assault.
- Some women may experience nausea when thinking of the rape, and some may have difficulties with sexual relations.

- Being unable to recall the trauma (denial), or being able to "make the mind go somewhere else" to avoid the pain associated with the memory of the trauma (dissociation). Victims may feel detached or estranged.
- Manipulation of others and the environment as a way to keep things calm and under control. Victims may become compliant as a way to avoid real or imagined abuse.
- Persistent arousal symptoms, such as difficulty falling or staying asleep, being edgy, jumpy, irritable, and sometimes irrationally angry. Victims may have difficulty concentrating, be hypervigilant to their surroundings, and have an exaggerated startle response.

Causes of Domestic Violence

There is no single cause of domestic violence, but contributing factors include the following:

- A high level of conflict and stress in the family
- Male dominance and the view that women and children are men's property
- Cultural norms that permit family violence
- Displays of violence on TV and in other media
- Being raised in a violent family
- Alcohol and drug abuse
- Victim-blaming ("people get what they deserve")
- Denying the existence of physical violence or sexual abuse

TERMS

intimate partner violence (IPV): physical, sexual, or psychological harm by a current or former intimate partner or spouse

stalking: behavior that causes victims to feel a high level of fear of physical or sexual violence

violence: a physical or verbal behavior in which the intent is to harm, injure, or destroy someone or something

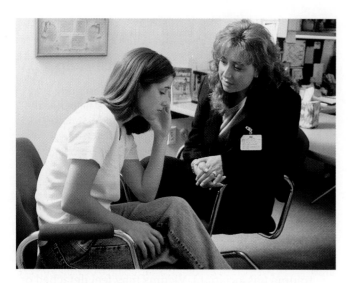

Being able to tell an understanding person what happened helps.

Table 23.2

Symptoms of Parental Violence in Children

Children who are exposed to parental violence are subject to a variety of symptoms.

Behavioral symptoms

Aggression	Tantrums	Immaturity	Delinquency

Emotional symptoms

Anxiety and depression	Low self-esteem	Anger	Withdrawal

Cognitive symptoms

Poor performance in school	Poor language skills		

Physical symptoms

Eating disorders	Poor motor skills	Sleep problems	Retarded growth
Psychosomatic disorders			

Women who are at the greatest risk for serious injury from domestic violence include those with male partners who abuse alcohol or drugs, are unemployed or intermittently employed, have less than a high school education, and are former husbands or boyfriends of the women.

Ways to prevent domestic violence include providing shelters, safe houses, and other protective environments for abused women; reducing contributing social and economic factors (unemployment, poverty, and racism); holding the abusers accountable for their actions; training law enforcement and health care professionals to recognize and intervene in cases of domestic violence; training everyone in nonviolent conflict resolution; and reducing the amount of violent imagery on TV, in films, and in popular music. Physicians also are receiving more training in recognizing, treating, and helping victims of domestic violence, most of whom are women, find shelter and support.

Domestic violence does not only affect adults who are in an abusive relationship; children who share the abusive environment also suffer (**Table 23.2**). Resolution of conflicts between parents or partners is essential to the long-term health of children. And children who grow up in physically or sexually abusive environments are much more likely to find themselves in abusive relationships as adults.

The Brain Controls Violent Behavior

Although personal experiences, social environment, and cultural norms all contribute to the expression of violent behavior, it is also a fact that there are specific areas of the brain that govern violent, antisocial behaviors. Neurological and biological factors, as well as environmental influences, contribute to the development of what is regarded as acceptable personality and behavioral traits. The brain's intimate control of behavior was demon-strated by a bizarre accident that occurred more than 150 years ago.

On September 13, 1848, a 25-year-old railroad construction foreman named Phineas P. Gage was setting blasting charges in rock to level terrain for the laying of railroad ties. Holes were drilled in the rocks, and a powder charge was inserted and tamped down with an iron rod. On this day, Gage was tamping down a charge when it went off prematurely. The steel tamping rod, one inch thick and a yard long, shot through his face, through his brain, and emerged from his skull and landed yards away. Remarkably, within moments after the accident, Gage regained consciousness, was able to talk, and able to walk away with the help of his men (Damasio et al., 1994).

Gage survived the catastrophic injury with all his intelligence and physical abilities intact. His speech was unaffected. His memory was complete and accurate. However, Gage was a different man. Before the injury he had been responsible, socially well adjusted, and popular with his peers and bosses. After the accident he became profane, argumentative, and irreverent. He lost all respect for social conventions. He could not be trusted or relied on in any assignment. His employers, who had called him "the most efficient and capable" man in their employ, had to dismiss him. Gage spent the remaining 15 years of his life wandering around, largely unemployed, and unaccepted in any company. His family wound up caring for him until his death.

Twenty years after the accident, a scientist named John Harlow postulated that the behavioral and personality changes observed in Gage after the accident resulted from damage to a particular area of the brain. This was the first scientific insight that acceptable personal and social behavior, what we commonly refer to as rationality, is controlled by the brain. In effect, there is a neural basis not only for intelligence, but for ethical, moral, and social behaviors as well.

Modern neurological experiments have confirmed Harlow's insight. Other patients have also been identified who have suffered damage to their frontal lobes and who exhibit deficits in rational behaviors and in the processing of emotions. Future research may elucidate how neurons in the frontal lobe function to generate socially acceptable behaviors—or their opposite.

Maltreatment of Children

In the 1990s, **child abuse,** physical, mental, or sexual maltreatment or neglect of a child, gained widespread public attention when numerous clergy were prosecuted for sexual abuse and molestation of youths in their care and who were involved in church activities. Hundreds of sexually abused victims broke years of silence to describe how they were sexually maltreated by clergy when they were young. Many described how seriously their lives had been damaged by their traumatic childhood experiences. In addition, some day care operators were also charged with child abuse, but, in some cases, the charges turned out to be unfounded. Young children have vivid imaginations and can easily be led by an investigator into agreeing with things that the investigator describes. However, confirmed cases of child abuse indicate that the problem of maltreatment of children is as serious a problem as intimate partner violence.

Each year in the United States, almost 1 million documented cases of child abuse occur. (Many more cases occur but are not reported). Among these cases, about 20% are physical abuse, 10% are sexual abuse, 5% are mental abuse, and 61% are harmed by neglect. More than 1,000 American children die each year from neglect and physical abuse. In 2008, a report from the Centers for Disease Control and Prevention (CDC) concluded that about 2% of infants in the United States under the age of 1 suffer from neglect or abuse, often in the first few weeks of life. A large number of these cases is related to drug abuse by the mother.

A particularly disturbing form of child abuse is **shaken-baby syndrome (SBS)** in which infants are violently shaken by adults either to punish them or to stop them from crying. SBS affects as many as 1,400 infants each year. Shaken infants can be identified by physicians and trained personnel by a collection of symptoms that result from the violent shaking. Any kind of violent shaking of an infant is a crime.

Child abuse involves several forms of maltreatment, all of which invariably lead to serious harm.

Physical Abuse When intentional force of any kind that results in injury is used on a child, the child has suffered physical abuse. Injuries can also result from accidents, which are not the result of physical abuse. For example, a child may fall and be bruised while running during play. This is understood by the child to be an accident and may lead to more careful behavior. It may also be something the child is proud of and can be "brave" about.

However, physical force that is used to discipline or control a child or adolescent can cause serious physical and psychological injury. Often a parent is venting anger over some other issue that is irrelevant to the child's behavior; the child is the unwitting victim of the anger and knows that the punishment is unjust. The younger the child, the more likely a serious injury will result from the use of physical force. Shaking a baby repeatedly to get it to stop crying, or for any other reason, can cause death.

Emotional Abuse Psychological abuse can cause severe emotional distress and can produce illness and violent behavior that may lead to suicide or homicide. Being screamed at repeatedly and told that one is worthless, stupid, or defective can permanently damage psychological and social development.

Sexual Abuse This is another form of maltreatment of children. Sexual contact between adults and children is forbidden by both cultural taboos and by criminal law. Although it is difficult to determine with accuracy the prevalence of child sexual abuse in this country, some surveys find that as many as 15% of women and 6% of men have experienced sexual abuse as children. Because this subject is not one that most people are willing to discuss, the prevalence of child sexual abuse may be higher than reported. Sexual abuse of children may result in depression, anxiety, and general dysfunction later in their lives.

Neglect This is probably the most common form of maltreatment of children. Neglect includes failure to provide a child with adequate nourishment, proper clothing, and prescribed medications or to oversee a child's hygiene. Neglected children are left to their own devices for long periods without adult supervision, and many neglected children engage in self-destructive behaviors.

Although it is true that males are the usual perpetrators of violence on children, especially female children, mothers also abuse their children both physically and sexually. Women who inflict serious injury on their

> T E R M S
>
> child abuse: physical or mental injury, sexual abuse or exploitation, maltreatment, or neglect of a child by a person who is responsible for the child's welfare
>
> shaken-baby syndrome (SBS): a form of child abuse in which an infant is violently shaken by an adult

children are often mentally ill and may suffer from *dissociative identity disorder,* formerly known as multiple personality disorder.

Child abuse affects children not only physically (e.g., broken bones, burns, or even death) but emotionally as well (e.g., they may become abusive themselves, suicidal, or withdrawn). Effects are both short- and long-term and invariably devastating to all victims. As the abused child reaches age 10 and older and becomes more independent, he or she may feel in a hopeless situation and may run away from home. The consequences for many runaways are dismal: teenage prostitution, illicit drug and alcohol use, higher rates of juvenile crimes, and higher school dropout rates. Child abuse is costly to society and directly or indirectly affects everyone.

Social Aspects of Child Maltreatment

Because many cases of child abuse go unreported, reliable data are difficult to obtain; also, abusers and the abused usually do not offer information freely. As a result, much information on child abuse has been incorrect or misleading.

For whatever reasons, males tend to abuse their children at a higher rate than females. However, no unique factors have been found that distinguish male abusers of children from female abusers. Male children are abused more frequently and seen by parents as more deserving of harsh treatment than female children. Male children even blame themselves more than female children do for their own maltreatment.

Two-thirds of all abused children are between the ages of 5 and 17. Younger children are abused more frequently because they lack both physical strength to resist child abuse and knowledge about what is normal and abnormal behavior. Infants are attacked less frequently than older children by abusive parents, but are at greater risk of death than older children, especially when shaken. As children pass the age of 15, they are more likely to be abused by peers than by family members.

Children with physical or mental disabilities such as blindness, deafness, mental retardation, or cerebral palsy are at a greater risk for child abuse than others. It is unclear if the physical disability itself provokes the abuse or if stress created by caring for such a child is the underlying cause of the abuse. Children who are temperamental, impulsive, aggressive, depressed, or hyperactive are also at a higher risk for being abused. These behaviors create parental stress that may contribute to child abuse.

Cultural Aspects of Child Maltreatment

Lack of knowledge and skills about child care may predispose parents to child maltreatment, possibly because of frustration and stress created by the needs of a child and its apparent lack of cooperation. Males who are primary caregivers usually have received little or no training regarding child care.

The same holds true for adolescent mothers and mothers with low levels of education, for example, high school dropouts. They, too, lack the knowledge and skills necessary for adequate child care. This lack places them in a stressful situation in which abuse is more likely to occur. These mothers feel they have no one to turn to for help, and they may not even know where to obtain help. In frustration, they abuse their children.

If the family lives in an unsafe neighborhood, family members may feel afraid to venture out to seek help for their problems. This fear results in even more isolation and may exacerbate family conflicts and abuse. Other reasons for child abuse are social isolation, lack of friends, dangerous neighborhoods, or lack of access to transportation.

Child Maltreatment Prevention

There are child abuse prevention programs that can help parents reduce the stress that is a risk factor in child abuse. These programs emphasize educating parents on how to care for their children and how to avoid abuse.

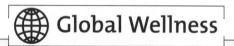

Global Wellness

Forced Labor Around the World

The United Nations estimates that, worldwide, at least 12.3 million people are subjected to forced labor in violation of human rights (Doyle, 2006). Forced labor is broken down into three categories: economic, state imposed, and sexual. The regions of the world most involved in forced labor are Asia, the Pacific Islands, Latin America, and Africa. Profits from the use of forced labor were estimated to be $44 billion in 2005.

Companies in the United States are also guilty of human rights abuses from the use of forced labor, particularly in agribusiness. Research studies estimate that, at any given time,

the United States has about 10,000 workers who are forced to endure primitive and unhealthy working and living conditions and are given almost no pay. The forced labor populations come mostly from Mexico and China; the states most likely to have forced labor camps are California, Florida, Texas, and New York.

Sexual exploitation of young girls in poor countries accounts for almost half of all forced labor. Many young girls are recruited by being promised good jobs or marriages; they are then transported and sold. In most countries, laws prohibiting forced labor are usually too weak or too vague to be enforced.

Different stress reduction programs have been developed for adolescent mothers, young parents, fathers who have never been in charge of child care before, working mothers, single parents, step parents, and siblings who are in charge of child care. Stress management programs are particularly important in communities where unemployment rates are high.

Conflict resolution programs can also help prevent child abuse. If people are able to manage conflict without using physical force, the risk of child abuse is lower. Both anger mediation programs and conflict resolution programs have been shown to help lower rates of child abuse. Training in life and social skills for all individuals involved with child abuse is recommended. Training in parenting skills for both males and females of all ages is also strongly suggested. This training also educates them about resources for assistance.

Coping with Anger

Anger. The word itself brings to mind images of pounding fists, yelling, and violent behavior. But anger is as natural a human emotion as love. Anger is a survival emotion; it's the fight component of the fight-or-flight response. We use anger to communicate our feelings, from impatience to rage. We employ anger to communicate boundaries and defend values. Although feeling angry is within the normal limits of human emotions, anger is often mismanaged and misdirected. Unfortunately, we have been socialized to suppress our feelings of anger. As a result, it either tears us apart from the inside or promotes intermittent eruptions of verbal or physical violence, which can be seen played out in local and national headlines. In most cases, we do not deal with our anger wisely.

Research reveals four very distinct ways in which people mismanage their anger.

1. **Somatizers:** People who never show any signs of anger and internalize their feelings until eventually there is major bodily damage (i.e., temporomandibular joint syndrome, colitis, migraine headaches).
2. **Exploders:** Individuals who erupt like a volcano and spread their temper like hot lava, destroying anyone and anything in their path with either verbal or physical abuse. This type of mismanaged anger style is what makes the news headlines.
3. **Self-Punishers:** People who neither repress their anger nor explode, but rather deny themselves a proper outlet of anger because of feelings of guilt. Examples of their behavior include excessive sleeping, eating, and shopping.
4. **Underhanders:** Individuals who sabotage or seek revenge against someone through barely socially acceptable behavior (e.g., sarcasm, tardiness, not returning phone calls).

When anger is mismanaged and left unresolved it becomes a control issue, if not a control drama.

Here are some ways to deal with anger sensibly or creatively:

1. Take a "time-out" from the situation, followed by a "time-in" to resolve the issue.
2. Communicate your feelings diplomatically.
3. Think of the consequences of your anger.
4. Plan several options to a situation.
5. Lower personal expectations.
6. Most important, learn to forgive—"make past anger pass."

Although anger is an emotion we all experience and should recognize when it arises, it is crucial to manage anger. Sometimes just writing down what frustrates you can be the beginning of the resolution process. Above all, make a habit of resolving your angry feelings once they arise. Learn to let go of your feelings of anger before they become toxic to your mind, body, and spirit.

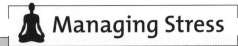 Managing Stress

Check Your Anger Level

Answer the questions below using the following scale:

Almost never	1 point
Sometimes	2 points
Often	3 points
Almost always	4 points

1. I am quick tempered. _____
2. I would say that I have a fiery temper. _____
3. I am a hotheaded person. _____
4. I get angry at others' mistakes. _____
5. I feel annoyed when my work is not recognized. _____
6. I fly off the handle easily. _____
7. When I get angry, I say nasty things and swear. _____
8. It makes me furious when I am criticized in front of others. _____
9. When I am frustrated, I feel like hitting someone. _____
10. I get angry when I do a good job and get a poor evaluation. _____

A score of 22 points or more indicates a high anger level. To double-check your score, ask one or more friends to take the same test and mark the answers as if they were you. If your anger score remains high, you may want to consider anger counseling. Anger often leads to violence against another person.

Sexual Violence

Every two to three minutes in the United States a woman is sexually assaulted. In a national survey, 28% of college women reported that they had suffered from rape or attempted rape since the age of 14. Women who are sexually assaulted suffer from a variety of symptoms, often for a long time after the assault. Symptoms include headache, fatigue, sleep disturbances, recurrent nausea, eating disorders, menstrual pain, sexual dysfunction, and suicide. Coping with the anguish of the sexual assault also often leads to substance abuse.

Rape, incest, attempted rape, and unwanted sexual touching are called **sexual violence.** There has been a significant increase in public recognition of sexual crimes against women, including intense media scrutiny of rape issues in high-profile rape trials such as the one involving basketball star Kobe Bryant. The legal definition of **forcible rape** varies from state to state. However, rape is generally viewed as penetration by force or threat of force of a body orifice, including the mouth, rectum, or vagina. Penetration includes the use of objects or other body parts, such as fingers. Forced sexual activity can occur between men and women, men and men, women and women, and married and unmarried people. Regardless of the identity of the victims and perpetrators, sexual assault is a criminal activity; it is not sex and has nothing to do with sex. Sexual assault is an act of violence, an attempt to humiliate a victim. Whether the term is *sexual assault* or *forcible rape,* the end result is physical and psychological violence to the victim.

Some men try to deny the fact of sexual assault with statements such as "women enjoy being raped," "she asked for it," and "I didn't think she meant no." These kinds of statements are heard repeatedly; however, the facts of sexual assault are plain:

- Sexual assault is an act of power and control—*not* an act of sex or passion.
- Most sexual assaults go unreported.
- Most sexual assaults do not occur on impulse or in remote areas.
- In 80% of all sexual assaults, according to some estimates, the assailant was a casual acquaintance, friend, or relative of the victim.
- Sexual assailants come from *all* socioeconomic and ethnic backgrounds.
- Rapists are not sexually deprived people.
- Women do not secretly want to be raped.
- Forced sexual contact in a dating situation also is sexual assault.

Acquaintance Rape

Acquaintance rape, or date rape, occurs when a person known to the victim uses verbal or physical force to coerce the victim into having sex. About half of all cases of sexual violence against women are committed by a friend or acquaintance; about one-quarter are committed by an intimate partner. Acquaintance rape carries

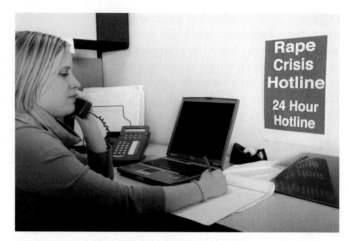

Many communities have crisis centers for rape victims.

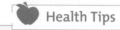 Health Tips

How to Prevent Date Rape

Be wary of a relationship that is operating along classic stereotypes of dominant male and submissive, passive female. The dominance in ordinary activities may extend to the sexual arena.

Be wary when a date tries to control behavior or pressure you in any way.

Be explicit with communication. Don't say "no" in a way that could be interpreted in any way as a "maybe" or "yes."

Avoid ambiguous messages with both verbal and nonverbal behavior. Saying "no" and permitting heavy petting creates confusion or ambiguity.

First dates with an unknown companion may be safer in a group.

Avoid remote or isolated places where help is not available.

Avoid becoming intoxicated while on a date.

the same legal penalties as sexual assault committed by a stranger.

Women of high school and college age are the most vulnerable to acquaintance rape. Every year, more than 100,000 forcible rapes are reported in the United States. This number is probably low because many rapes are not reported by the victim.

Cultural views on sexual relationships between men and women play a significant role in acquaintance rape. Many young women who are victims of attacks that meet the legal definition of rape do not know that what happened to them was sexual assault. Victims may believe that a sexual assault can be committed only by a stranger or they may blame themselves for the act. A rapist may not realize that the victim's refusal really means NO. Aggressive males mistakenly believe that when women say no, men should insist. In a survey conducted by *MS.* magazine, 84% of men whose actions came under the legal definition of sexual assault believed they had not committed sexual assault.

Table 23.3

Reactions and Feelings of Significant Others of Sexual Assault Victims

Anger	Concern	Guilt	Embarrassment	Vulnerability
• At assailant for committing crime • At system for letting "those kinds of people" run the streets • At victim for engaging in "risky behavior"	• For the victim's well-being and safety • About how the relationship between victim and significant other will change • For the victim's rights	• For not having prevented assault ("I should have been with her" OR "I should have given her a ride home") • For not having been there to protect victim	• Worry about gossip (myth and stigma hold strong effect) • Embarrassed for victim	• Realization that it can happen to me as well • Intensely heightened awareness of environment

Table 23.4

Feelings Reported by Sexual Assault Victims

Fear	Embarrassment	Shame	Guilt	Anxiety
• Fear of death • Fear of rapist	• Embarrassed to discuss details • Embarrassed about their bodies	• Destruction of self-esteem, self-worth, self-respect • Ashamed at having the medical exam • Ashamed at having to perform a sexual act to stay alive	• Feelings of shame and of having provoked the rape • Feeling of blame for the assault	• Shaking • Nightmares • Difficulty sleeping or sleeping all the time • Constantly reminds self what "should or shouldn't have" been done
Stupidity	**Vulnerability**	**Concern**	**Anger**	**Loss of control**
• Feels stupid for engaging in risk-taking behavior(s) • Feels stupid for being too trusting	• General fear of people • Paranoid feelings • Intensely heightened awareness of environment	• Will the rapist get psychiatric help? • What will happen to offender if rape is reported?	• Toward assailant • Toward self • Toward men and women in general, especially if they resemble assailant	• Small decisions seem monumental • Unsure about self or actions

Consequences of Acquaintance Rape

Victims of acquaintance rape often suffer serious, long-term psychological effects. Compared with victims of stranger rapes, acquaintance rape victims tend to blame themselves for what happened. They often have difficulty trusting people in later relationships. It may take acquaintance rape victims longer to recover, particularly if the rape involved physical violence. Acquaintance rape victims are less likely than other rape victims to seek crisis services, tell someone, report the incident to the police, or seek counseling. Family and friends may not provide the same support for acquaintance rape victims as they might offer victims of stranger rape. If victims tell friends or family, the severity of the attack may be minimized or the victim may be blamed for the sexual assault (Table 23.3).

If a woman has had too much to drink or has been drugged and is unconscious, she cannot consent to any sexual act. Having sex with a woman who is unconscious or semiconscious is defined as an act of rape. Certain substances are known as "date rape drugs." Rohypnol (also called "Roofies," "rope," "activesex") is an odorless, tasteless compound that can be added to a person's drink that will render the person unconscious. People who commit rape on drugged victims are sentenced to long terms in prison if convicted.

Rape victims usually have two types of behavioral reactions: expressed or controlled. Those who express their feelings usually manifest fear, anger, and anxiety. They may display these emotions through crying, tension, nervousness, restlessness, and hysteria. Those who control their feelings may appear calm or quiet, but either reaction indicates that the victim is in a state of shock (Table 23.4). Expressed or controlled feelings may occur at any time and often come and go more than once after the incident. Acknowledging or recognizing these feelings is a normal part of the healing process.

TERMS

acquaintance rape: (also known as "date rape") sexual assault occurring when the victim and the rapist are known to each other and may have previously interacted in some socially appropriate manner

forcible rape: sexual assault using force or threat of force and involving sexual penetration of the victim's vagina, mouth, or rectum

sexual violence: violent actions that include rape, incest, attempted rape, and unwanted sexual touching

What to Do After a Sexual Assault

A person who has been sexually assaulted is advised to do the following:

- Contact a rape-crisis hotline.
- DO NOT shower, bathe, douche, change or destroy clothing, or straighten up the area where the sexual assault occurred (if indoors) because these actions would destroy important evidence.
- Go to the nearest hospital emergency room.
- Notify the police.
- Seek professional counseling.

Each person's reaction to being sexually assaulted is different, and it is natural that each victim's pain and needs are unique. All victims of sexual assault should seek counseling from someone they trust.

Elder Abuse

We are an aging society, and with increasing frequency adult children are required to care for disabled or demented elderly parents and grandparents. It is only within the last generation that the problem of elder abuse has been recognized and documented. Studies now indicate that more than 1 million elderly persons are victims of abuse each year in the United States. In addition to abuse by their adult children, elderly persons also are abused frequently by their spouses or care-givers. The magnitude of elder abuse in the United States is now only slightly less than that of child abuse.

Elder abuse is defined as the physical, sexual, or emotional maltreatment or financial exploitation of an adult aged 60 or older. The abuse or neglect may be by any caregiver—spouse, child, relative, or friend—and occurs in a domestic setting. Self-neglect is also included in the definition because almost half of the cases of elder abuse involve self-neglect.

Self-neglect may result from physical or mental disability of the elder person. He or she may not be able to obtain essential food, clothing, shelter, or medical care. Quite often the financial affairs of a neglected elder person are in disarray. Despite increased public attention to the problems of elder abuse, much maltreatment of elders still remains hidden to a large extent.

A variety of abusive methods are used by caregivers in the domestic setting to control the elder persons under their care. These include screaming and yelling (the most frequent form of abuse), physical restraint, forced feeding or medicating, blows and slaps, and threats to send the person to a nursing home.

However, the abuse is not all one way. Elder persons who are disabled or immobilized also use abusive methods to control their caregivers. Elder persons scream and yell, pout and withdraw, refuse food and medication, cry or become emotional, throw objects, and threaten to call the police. As with other forms of abuse, the reasons for the abusive behaviors by both persons in the relation-ship are many. Alcohol plays a role in many situations, and emotional illness contributes, as does mental impairment on the part of one or both parties.

The reason why much elder abuse remains hidden or undocumented is that many elderly people are concerned about the family's privacy and fear public exposure and embarrassment. The victim also may feel shame at having raised the child who has now become abusive. If the child is stealing money, the elderly parent may fear that the child will be sent to jail if the abuse is reported. And, despite the abusive treatment, the elder person may feel that the situation is preferable to being sent to a nursing home. Elder abuse is likely to become an even greater problem in the future, as more and more people live to be age 80 or older and as the number of people with dementia increases (see Chapter 22).

Firearm Violence

Year after year in the United States, firearms kill and injure thousands of people both by design and by accident (see Chapter 21). In 2005, more than 30,000 Americans died from gunshot wounds; more than half of these deaths were suicides. In addition, another 70,000 people received treatment for gunshot wounds in hospital emergency rooms. Gun violence in the United States costs about $2 billion in medical costs and an estimated $100 billion in other intangible costs. Living in a house where there are guns increases the risk of homicide by as much as 170% and the risk of suicide by as much as 460% (Wintemute, 2008). States with the most liberal gun ownership laws also have the highest rates of firearm-related deaths; states with stringent gun control laws have the lowest rates of firearm-related deaths.

> Every gun that is made, every warship launched, every rocket fired signifies, in the final sense, a theft from those who hunger and are not fed, those who are cold and are not clothed.
>
> *President Dwight D. Eisenhower (1953)*

Firearms are the second leading cause of death among young people between the ages of 10 and 24. A national survey found that 1 student in 12 admitted to carrying a firearm within the past month, either for defense or for fighting. People living in homes in which guns are kept have a risk of suicide that is five times greater than for people living in homes without guns. Surveys also show that the vast majority of teenage suicides are accomplished with guns.

Americans have a long-standing love–hate relationship with firearms, and many people believe strongly in the constitutionally guaranteed right to carry and use firearms. Their views are defended with money and lobbying by the National Rifle Association (NRA), which works to prevent passage of laws limiting or regulating the purchase and use of guns by civilians. The NRA is opposed by physicians, health organizations, and law enforcement agencies, including the Federal Bureau of Investigation (FBI), which supports stricter gun control laws.

In 1993, in response to the escalating number of homicides, suicides, and assaults, 11 states, including New York, New Jersey, and California, passed gun control laws. In addition, the U.S. Congress passed a gun control law known as the Brady Bill. (Jim Brady was permanently disabled in the assassination attempt on President Ronald Reagan in 1981.) The Brady Bill imposes a five-day waiting period for the purchase of handguns and requires local police agencies to determine whether the prospective buyer has a criminal record. However, years later the U.S. Supreme Court invalidated the background check of prospective gun buyers required by the original Brady Bill.

Violence and the use of firearms in the United States have become some of society's most pressing concerns. Juveniles under 21 years now account for about one-quarter of all arrests for the possession or use of a gun. African American youths are three times more likely to be arrested for a gun violation than are white American youths, and about half of all homicide victims are African Americans. Most homicides are not racially motivated, however, because 94% of victims are killed by members of their own race, and 83% of white American murder victims are killed by other whites.

No one knows what causes a person to commit suicide (see Chapter 4), but the ready availability of guns is a factor: About 60% of suicides are accomplished with a gun. Although the reasons and causes behind a suicide are complex, genetics plays a significant role. The child of a parent who has attempted suicide is six times more likely to attempt suicide than is a child whose parents have never attempted suicide. Also, 13% of identical twins of a parent who died by suicide eventually took their own lives, as compared with 0.7% of nonidentical twins with the same background. One day researchers hope to be able to genetically identify persons who are at high risk for suicide and develop prevention strategies for those at risk.

Youth Gangs

Youth gangs exist in nearly every major city in the United States. Surveys indicate that more than 200,000 adolescents and young adults are members of almost 4,000 gangs. Previously, gangs were primarily focused in major cities, such as Los Angeles, Chicago, and New York, but they have since spread to most large cities in the Midwest, Northwest, South, and Southwest. The sale of drugs

> War is but a spectacular expression of our daily conduct.
>
> *Krishnamurti*

has been a key factor in the movement of gangs to more and more cities. In most cities with gangs, it is not only poor areas that are affected; gang activities have also spread to suburbs and to schools.

A number of factors contribute to a teenager or young adult deciding to join a gang: poverty, failure at school, substance abuse, dysfunctional family life, and family violence. Easy access to illegal drugs and the lure of financial rewards from drug dealing are both powerful attractants for a young person with no money, no education, no job, and no future. For them, gang life is exciting and rewarding.

Gang recruits often have a poor self-image, low self-esteem, and no adult to provide counseling and support. Some gang members are the children of gang members and are following in their parents' footsteps. Gang members often gain recognition from other gang members and from a society that fears them—in this way they gain attention and respect.

Drugs and guns are an integral part of gang acceptance. Often a recruit is not deemed fit until he or she has obtained a gun—and used it, either on a rival gang member or in committing a crime. About half of the juvenile inmates of prisons report that their gang regularly bought and sold guns and that gun theft was an important gang activity. Thus, the ready accessibility of guns in America directly contributes to gang activities and the destruction of the lives of thousands of young people.

Hate Crimes

Hate crimes are a special category of crime; a **hate crime** is an unlawful act committed against a person, group, or place that is motivated by hate or bias. Bombing a church, synagogue, or mosque because it represents places of worship of particular faiths is a hate crime. Attacking a gay person because of his or her sexual orientation is a hate crime. Attacking a person because of his or her gender or nationality is a hate crime. In general, any act of violence that is committed in whole or in part by a person's race, religion, ethnicity, gender, sexual orientation, disability, or age is a hate crime.

In 1990, the U.S. Congress recognized the increasing frequency and seriousness of such crimes and required the FBI to keep statistics on the number and kinds of hate crimes in the country. Hate crimes are prosecuted first as a particular crime and, in addition, as a hate crime. Additional penalties are added if the person is

> **TERMS**
>
> **elder abuse:** physical, sexual, or emotional maltreatment or financial exploitation of an adult aged 60 or older
>
> **hate crime:** any unlawful act committed against a person, group, or place that is motivated by hate or bias

convicted of a hate crime. Shooting someone is homicide; shooting the person because he or she is African American or Jewish or Latino is both a homicide and a hate crime.

Sometimes there is a thin line between freedom of speech and a hate crime. Freedom of speech, no matter how offensive, is protected under the U.S. Constitution. Biased views and verbal attacks cannot be prosecuted as hate crimes, but sometimes the line between the two is not obvious to everyone. In 2005, former Secretary of Education William Bennett stated on his talk show in response to a caller, "If you wanted to reduce crime, if that were your sole purpose, you could abort every black baby in this country, and your crime rate would go down. That would be an impossible, ridiculous, morally reprehensible thing to do, but your crime rate would go down." Millions of Americans were offended by Bennett's comment, but such views are protected as freedom of speech.

However, if the speech advocates the committing of a crime, such as incitement to riot, to destroy property, or actually to hurt someone, then the person has committed a crime. Hate crimes, unfortunately, are a worldwide phenomenon. Nazi war crimes were hate crimes. Genocide in Rwanda was a hate crime. Killing of Muslims of one sect by Muslims of another sect is a hate crime. Hate in any guise is destructive both to the people who are hated as well as to those who hate.

School Violence

In the past two decades, an epidemic of shootings by teenage boys in schools across the United States has brought tragedy and horror into the affected families and communities. The worst shooting on record and the most publicized occurred on April 20, 1999, at Columbine High School in Littleton, Colorado. Two teenage boys at the school shot and killed 12 fellow students and a teacher and wounded 24 other students. When their shooting rampage ended, they shot and killed themselves.

In 2005, a 16-year-old teenager stole his grandfather's gun and killed his grandfather and his companion. He then went to his high school on an Indian reservation in Minnesota. He shot and killed an unarmed security guard, a teacher, five students, and then himself.

School killings focus on the controversy over the right of citizens to own firearms in this country, a right that many argue is guaranteed by the U.S. Constitution. The National Rifle Association persistently argues that ownership of guns has nothing to do with violence and killings. After the killings in Springfield, Oregon, in 1998, a spokesman for the NRA stated, "Lawful arms ownership has nothing to do with this tragedy." In refuting this, a prominent physician pointed out that:

> Children and adolescents are by definition immature and may lack judgment. Life's embarrassments, rejections, and torments may send them into fits of

> temper, even rage, and may prompt a desire for revenge. Impulsively, some children lash out at others and at themselves. Nonetheless, they are only murderous when they have the means, and a loaded gun is the "perfect" tool. (Kassirer, 1998)

One out of every three U.S. households contains one or more guns (Cole & Johnson, 2005). Storing guns so that children and adolescents cannot get to them or use them can prevent many homicides, suicides, and school shootings.

Despite years of research and studies by educators, counselors, psychologists, and other health experts, no one can really say what the underlying factors are that cause teenage boys to go on shooting rampages. However, three facts are common to almost all school shootings over the past 20 years:

- The gunman was 16 years of age or younger.
- The boy had easy access to a firearm at home.
- The boy had experienced long-term harassment and marginalization by fellow students before he snapped.

Recognizing that harassment and bullying of particular students play an important role in inciting violence, many school districts have instituted "no bullying" policies. The rules encourage students to report instances of bullying or any form of verbal or physical abuse. However, most bullying and teasing goes on outside the classroom; this is where the aggression must be stopped.

Every day 24 million children are bused to and from school (Harrison, 2005). The children are unsupervised and often engage in verbal and physical violence against any student who is "different" or unpopular for any reason or who is regarded as an easy target for abuse. The bus driver has to concentrate on driving even if he or she observes fights and violence among the students. Some school districts have begun to place adult monitors on buses, but this is an added expense that most schools cannot afford. Discussing and teaching tolerance in classrooms can provide a powerful antidote to the poisons of intolerance and violence expressed by children and adolescents.

Violence in the Media

A major contributor to violent and aggressive behaviors by children and adolescents is exposure to violence on TV and in the movies. Use of firearms to threaten and kill is rampant on both TV shows and in movies. In 2005, the Surgeon General issued a detailed report on youth violence in America that concluded: "A diverse body of research provides strong evidence that exposure to violence in the media can increase children's aggressiveness in the short term. Some studies suggest that long-term effects exist, and there are strong theoretical reasons why this is the case."

Efforts to reduce media violence have been largely unsuccessful. As with newspapers, violence sells TV shows and movies. Parents are urged to control what their children see, but in this electronic world of video games, computers, TV, movies, and DVDs, it is virtually an impossible task.

Media violence also causes a confusion of values in children and acceptance of aggressive behavior as a way of dealing with problems. TV advertising also encourages children to demand material objects, and many children become angry and aggressive when their demands are not met.

Terrorism and Violence

The nature of violence in the United States (and the world) changed forever on September 11, 2001. On that day, four commercial airplanes were hijacked and crashed into the World Trade Center in New York, the Pentagon in Washington, DC, and a field in Pennsylvania by suicidal terrorists. More than 3,000 people in the planes and on the ground were killed. The World Trade Center towers in New York collapsed, leaving a smoldering ruin in lower Manhattan.

In addition to the people killed in the terrorist attacks, tens of thousands of people fled in panic and fear from the sites of the attacks. Millions around the country watched in horror as the events unfolded. The horror of that day and of subsequent events affected the mental health and well-being of countless persons at the scene and at home who witnessed the events. It is estimated that as many as 35% of persons directly exposed to the events of September 11 will eventually suffer from posttraumatic stress syndrome (see Chapter 3) that will require treatment and counseling (Yehuda, 2002).

The violence that has been unleashed in the world has heightened people's stress and fears. Agencies of the government at the federal and local levels are struggling to cope with the new threats to public health and safety. Security at airports and public events has been increased enormously. In efforts to stop world terrorism, wars have been fought in Afghanistan and Iraq.

In this time of violence, each individual must continue to strive to reduce the level of anger and stress in his or her personal life and in the world at large. Understanding, compassion, and patience are what we must strive for to reduce violence in these troubled times of uncertainty and heightened security.

The Threat of Bioterrorism

Shortly after the September 11 airplane hijackings, lethal anthrax spores were sent in letters to offices in Florida, New York, and Washington, DC. Several people died from inhalation of the deadly spores, many others became ill, and thousands had to take antibiotics as a precaution against possible infection. Buildings had to be closed and decontaminated. The postal system was forced to revise the way mail was processed, delivered, and opened. Bioterrorism with anthrax was used to

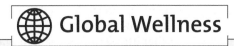

Global Wellness

Homicide in Countries Around the World

The ultimate measure of human violence is homicide, the killing of another person. In this regard countries vary enormously in the rate of homicide (see accompanying table). The two most violent countries in the world are Swaziland in Africa and Colombia in South America. Relative to these and some other countries, the rate of homicide in the United States seems low, but it still is higher than in any other industrialized nation. The rate of homicide in the United States is about three times greater than in Canada and about six times greater than in Japan.

Compared with other industrialized nations, the United States also leads in all forms of interpersonal violence, such as domestic violence, child abuse, and rape. The United States also imprisons a higher percentage of its population than any other industrialized nation. Many scholars have searched for the reasons for the high levels of violence in the United States, but no clear answers have emerged.

Homicide Rates by Country, 2006	
Country	Homicide rate (per 100,000 population)
El Salvador	58.07
Ecuador	18.07
Paraguay	12.33
Mexico	10.97
Lithuania	8.13
Thailand	7.92
Kenya	5.72
United States	5.62
Argentina	5.24
Philippines	3.82
India	2.82
Canada	1.86
Jordan	1.75
England and Wales	1.41
Italy	1.06
Greece	0.98
Holland	0.97
Germany	0.88
Norway	0.71
Spain	0.77
Lebanon	0.57
Singapore	0.39

Source: Data from *Tenth United Nations Survey of Crime Trends and Operations of Criminal Justice Systems.* Vienna, Austria: UN Office on Drugs and Crime.

attack politicians and media personnel and to disrupt basic American services and business operations. In 2008, the scientist thought to have prepared and sent the anthrax spores was finally identified but committed suicide before he could be arrested and tried. Fortunately, no further acts of bioterrorism have been reported, but fear of other attacks remains high and the federal government has taken steps to prepare for possible attacks using biological material.

In addition to anthrax, deadly biological agents include smallpox and, to a lesser degree, other bacterial and viral agents. Because smallpox was eliminated from the world in 1997, people are no longer vaccinated for it and are unprotected (Brennan & Henderson, 2002). It is believed that some governments retained laboratory stocks of smallpox and that such material could fall into the hands of terrorists. The U.S. government has developed new supplies of the smallpox vaccine and has begun protecting military and medical personnel by vaccination. However, widespread vaccination of the U.S. population against a hypothetical smallpox attack is highly controversial. If widespread vaccination for smallpox were instituted, a small number of persons would sicken and some would die. Furthermore, experience gained from the eradication of smallpox in the 1970s suggests that any outbreak could be quickly contained. Still, that would be of little comfort to those who might contract the deadly disease.

Violence Is Not Inevitable

Many people believe that violence among people and in societies is inevitable; that is, violence is biologically determined and cannot be changed. At best, society can try to limit the amount of violence and punish offenders. This belief is not substantiated by cultural studies of societies around the world that have little or no violence as long as their traditional lifestyle is not disrupted. Examples of nonviolent societies include the Semai Senoi people of Malaysia, Mabuti pygmies of Zaire, the Inuit of Canada, the Zuni Pueblo Indians of New Mexico, and the Ladakh people of northwestern India. The Ladakh, in particular, is a Buddhist culture whose doctrines identify greed, hate, aggression, lust, envy, jealousy, and pride as the ultimate sources of human unhappiness.

We believe that the point to remember about violence is that it is a personal decision to be violent or not, just as it is a personal decision to exercise or not. The fact that nonviolent societies do exist and that people may choose to live nonviolent lives should encourage everyone who abhors violence to reduce the level of violence in their lives. In so doing, the violence in society is reduced.

Critical Thinking About Health

1. Imagine that you are in a debate in school over this question: "Should all Americans over 21 years of age be allowed to own (a) a handgun, (b) a rifle, (c) a semi-automatic weapon, or (d) an automatic weapon?"

   Take a position on this issue with respect to owning or not owning guns in general. If you favor the ownership of guns, give your reasons for owning or not owning each of the four categories of guns. If you do not favor the ownership of guns, explain your reasons. Whatever side of the issue you are on, discuss whether you believe that ownership and availability of guns contribute to violence and crime in America.

2. You and Jennifer have been close friends for more than 15 years (since you both were in high school). Jennifer has recently divorced and has a 5-year-old son, Timmy, who is a "handful" in your view. You and Jennifer have shared many thoughts and feelings over the years. One day after work you stop by to see how Jennifer is doing. You notice that Timmy is limping and has several bruises on his legs. When you comment on Timmy's limp, Jennifer looks at the boy sharply and says, "You fell out of a tree. Isn't that right, Timmy?" The boy mumbles, "Yes" and limps from the room. Jennifer seems tense and doesn't want to talk. You soon leave but not before you smell alcohol on her breath.

   Do you think that this might be a case of child abuse? If so, what do you think your actions should be? In your discussion, indicate whether you are a male or female. Do you think a male or female friend of Jennifer's would act differently in this situation?

3. Volunteer to help at a retirement or nursing home in your community. Ask the older persons what they enjoy and dislike most about being elderly. Observe how many of the persons living there are mentally incompetent in your judgment and to what degree. Make a report of your findings and observations. Describe how your views of the elderly have changed as the result of your volunteer work.

4. By all statistical measures, the United States is the most violent society among all industrialized countries in the world by a large margin. The United States has more forcible rapes, more battered women, more homicides, and more suicides than any other industrialized nation on a per capita basis. Discuss why you think our society is so violent and what could be done to change its violent nature.

Health in Review

- Domestic violence includes relationship abuse and child abuse. Violence refers to use of force and power.
- Child maltreatment encompasses physical abuse, emotional abuse, sexual abuse, and neglect.
- Women who have been assaulted may experience anxiety, depression, substance abuse, headaches, and other medical problems. These are symptoms of posttraumatic stress disorder (PTSD). Many long-term consequences of sexual abuse are associated with PTSD.
- Acquaintance rape, or date rape, occurs when a person known to the victim uses force or power to coerce the victim into having sex. Women of high school and college age are most vulnerable to acquaintance rape.
- Child maltreatment is a form of domestic violence that reaches across all social, economic, racial, ethnic, geographic, and educational barriers.
- Education is the key to all forms of violence prevention, including firearm violence, relationship abuse, acquaintance rape, and child abuse.
- The United States exceeds all other developed nations in the per capita rate of rapes, homicides, and suicides and in the percentage of its population in prisons.
- Violence and the presence of handguns in schools mirror our communities and generate fear.
- Since September 11, 2001, the United States and other countries have become engaged in a war against terrorism around the world.
- Violence is not an essential part of human behavior, and many societies in the world are nonviolent.

Health and Wellness Online

The Web contains a wealth of information about health and wellness. By accessing the Internet using Web browser software, you can gain a new perspective on many topics presented in *Health and Wellness*, Tenth Edition. Access the Jones and Bartlett Publishers Web site at **health.jbpub.com/hwonline**.

References

Brennan, J. G., & Henderson, D. A. (2002). Diagnosis and management of smallpox. *New England Journal of Medicine, 346*, 1300–1308.

Cole, T. B., & Johnson, R. M. (2005). Storing guns safely in homes with children and adolescents. *Journal of the American Medical Association, 293*, 740–741.

Damasio, H., et al. (1994). The return of Phineas Gage: Clues about the brain from the skull of a famous patient. *Science, 264*, 1102–1105.

Doyle, R. (2006, January). Modern slavery. *Scientific American, 30*.

Harrison, M. M. (2005, Fall). Bully on the bus. *Teaching Tolerance Magazine*, Southern Poverty Law Center.

Kassirer, J. P. (1998). Private arsenals and public peril. *New England Journal of Medicine, 338*, 1375–1376.

Wintemute, G. J. (2008). Guns, fear, the Constitution, and public health. *New England Journal of Medicine, 358*, 1421–1424.

Yehuda, R. (2002). Post-traumatic stress disorder. *New England Journal of Medicine, 346*, 108–114.

Suggested Readings

Baumeister, R. F. (2001, April). Violent pride. *Scientific American*, 98–101. A psychologist explains why he believes that violent behaviors stem not from low self-esteem but from egotism, pride, and inflated self-esteem.

Gellert, G. A. (1997). *Confronting violence: Answers to questions about the epidemic destroying America's homes and communities*. Boulder, CO: Westview Press. A thoughtful and comprehensive discussion of all aspects of violence in America. The best source for persons who want to know more about specific kinds of violence and what to do about them. The author was working two miles from the blast that killed 169 people in Oklahoma City on April 19, 1995.

Guilleman, J. (2005). *Biological weapons: From the invention of state-sponsored programs to contemporary bioterror-ism*. New York: Columbia University Press. Carefully discusses the history of bioterrorism attacks in Russia and China and the current race to develop biological weapons and deterrents to their use.

Miller, G. (2008). The roots of morality. *Science, 320*, 734–737. Scientists are studying the biological bases of human morality by seeking answers in genes and in brain structures. Such understanding may help reduce violence.

Muscari, M. (2002). *Not my kid: 21 steps to raising a nonviolent child*. Scranton, PA: Ridge Row Press/University of Scranton. Discusses how media violence influences children and how parents can reduce their children's exposure to violent media.

Recommended Web Sites

Please visit **health.jbpub.com/hwonline** for links to these Web sites.

Center for the Prevention of Hate Violence
Provides a training program that teaches ways to reduce hate and hate crimes.

Centers for Disease Control and Prevention
Resources on violence facts and prevention.

Initiatives Related to Domestic Violence
Legal and educational references for families, justice professionals, and mental health and social service professionals.

Minnesota Center Against Violence and Abuse
Research, education, and access to violence-related resources, from the University of Minnesota.

National Domestic Violence Hotline
Information and resources available from the telephone hotline (800-799-7233).

Tolerance.org
Provides information and advice on how to reduce hate crimes, school violence, and other violence problems in society.

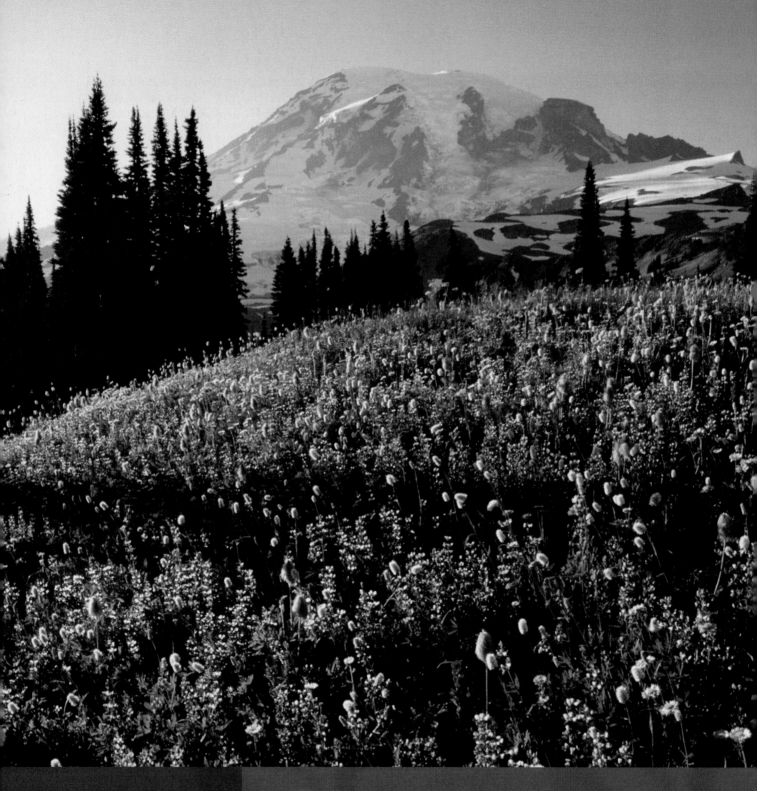

Health and Wellness Online: **health.jbpub.com/hwonline**

Study Guide and Self-Assessment

24.1   Environmental Awareness Questionnaire
24.2   How Environmentally Friendly Is My Car?
24.3   How Healthy Is My Drinking Water?

Chapter Twenty-Four

Working Toward a Healthy Environment

Learning Objectives

1. Discuss the relationship between environment and health.

2. Describe the health effects of air pollution, including smog and the hole in the ozone layer.

3. Explain the greenhouse effect and the predicted consequences of global warming.

4. Describe the effects of lead on children's health and intelligence.

5. Describe substances that pollute water in the United States.

6. Discuss the impact of land pollution on food production and health.

7. Describe sources of pesticide contamination and their effects on health.

8. Explain the effects of endocrine disruptors.

9. Identify the potential health problems associated with noise pollution and EMFs.

10. Discuss how human population growth will affect global health and environmental issues.

The term **environment** refers to all external physical factors that affect us. To survive, all animals, including human beings, require a certain amount of high-quality air, water, food, and shelter. If people are deprived of any essential environmental factors, or if the environment is polluted with toxic substances, health is adversely affected. Anyone who has experienced difficulty breathing smoggy, dusty, or smoke-filled air realizes the unhealthy effects of polluted air. Anyone who has become sick from consuming contaminated food or water knows the importance of sanitation and uncontaminated food in maintaining health.

> More than any other time in history mankind faces a crossroads. One path leads to despair and utter hopelessness; the other to total extinction. Let us pray we have the wisdom to choose correctly.
>
> *Woody Allen*

To achieve optimal health, we must live in a high-quality environment. Unfortunately, the quality of many aspects of the environment is deteriorating from pollution, degradation, depletion of natural resources, and extinction of species. The effects of environmental pollution are long lasting and often irreversible. People and nations are beginning to appreciate the serious consequences of ongoing air, water, and land pollution that adversely affect health. Dramatic changes in personal lifestyles and industrial technology are likely to be required to reduce existing pollution and prevent future destruction of the environment.

Environmental problems are not restricted to the United States or even to industrialized countries; environmental problems are global. Worldwide problems include:

- Global warming from increased amounts of carbon dioxide and other pollutants in the atmosphere. Global warming could alter climate patterns, raise the sea level and flood coastlines, imperil the world's food supply, increase the frequency and distribution of infectious diseases, and create extremes in the weather.
- Land degradation caused by deforestation, desertification, and soil erosion. Land degradation undermines the ability of populations to grow food and protect fresh water supplies.
- Fresh water shortages caused by overpopulation, lack of modern sanitation in parts of the world, and outmoded irrigation practices.
- Air pollution from the burning of fossil fuels by industry and cars and trucks. Pollutants foul the air and cause respiratory disease, destruction of forests and lakes by acid rain, and destruction of atmospheric ozone, which increases the risk of cancer and other biological damage.
- Exposure to toxic industrial and agricultural chemicals, which can cause cancer and disrupt normal biological functions in humans, animals, microorganisms, and plants.
- Extinction of species from global warming, destruction of tropical rain forests, overhunting and overfishing, habitat destruction from human activity, and the introduction of nonnative species into new environments.
- Nuclear, chemical, and biological terrorism and warfare.

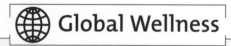

Global Wellness

Gaia: Is the Earth Alive?

Life on Earth depends on a very precise range of climatic and chemical conditions. On a global scale, the temperature and the chemical composition of air, land, and water, as well as other natural processes we take for granted, must be relatively constant for life to survive. Since the dawn of the Industrial Revolution over 200 years ago, human activity has been altering the chemical balance of the earth, and it remains to be seen if Earth can tolerate these alterations.

In 1979, James E. Lovelock, an English chemist and engineer, published a book called *Gaia: A New Look at Life on Earth*, which proposed that a special, interdependent relationship exists between life (particularly human beings) and all the physical and chemical processes of the planet required to sustain biological life. Lovelock suggested that, in a sense, Earth was "alive" and chose the name of the Greek goddess of earth, *Gaia*, to express the idea of a living planet. Lovelock described Gaia "as a complex entity involving the earth's biosphere, atmosphere, oceans, and soil; the totality constituting a feedback or cybernetic system which seeks an optimal physical and chemical environment for life on this planet" (Lovelock, 1979).

The idea that Earth is a self-regulating system may be correct; however, there is little indication that people will alter their mistreatment of the earth any time soon. So, in a way, the Gaia hypothesis will be tested and all the world will see the results. Either Earth can adapt to the effects of human activity, or it cannot. And if it cannot, it is not unreasonable to predict that humans will become extinct. Extinction has been the fate of virtually all the species that ever existed on Earth; even the dinosaurs, who survived for about 150 million years, eventually became extinct.

The dilemma for people today is whether they want to test the limits of Earth's adaptive capacities or learn to live in harmony with her.

Environmental health hazards stem from many different causes. Through the enactment and enforcement of environmental laws and regulations, the United States made progress in reducing environmental pollution and its negative health consequences. The United Nations and the World Health Organization carry out research and sponsor programs to stop environmental degradation and its health consequences. However, governments and other organizations alone cannot solve environmental problems. Each individual must strive to reduce or eliminate air, water, and land pollution and to take steps to create a healthy environment. People's activities are at the root of almost *all* environmental pollution and consequent health problems.

Outdoor Air Pollution

Pure air is a requirement for life. Each of us breathes about 35 pounds of air per day—more than 6 tons over the course of a year. Fresh, clean air consists of about 21% oxygen, 78% nitrogen, and trace amounts of seven other gases. It is the oxygen in air that is essential for human life. If the oxygen content of the air drops below 16%, body and brain functions are impaired. If breathing stops for even a few minutes, a person becomes unconscious and will die unless breathing is quickly restored.

Since the beginning of the Industrial Revolution in the nineteenth century, the burning of fossil fuels (coal, oil, and natural gas) to power transportation and industry has progressively polluted the air with carbon dioxide, oxides of nitrogen and sulfur, soot, and small particles, some of which cause health problems. A variety of chemical substances used in modern societies pollute the air as well (e.g., chlorofluorocarbons, dioxin). Thus, technological advances over the past 200 years have created, as a by-product, pollution of the air we breathe and of Earth's atmosphere.

Smog

Everybody has heard of **smog,** a term first used in England to describe a hazardous combination of sulfurous chemicals emitted into the air from the burning of coal and water vapor in fog. Smog causes breathing problems, coughs, bronchitis, and asthma, and can even result in death among people with lung diseases. In most U.S. cities, smog is not associated with fog but results from the action of sunlight on various chemicals and particles in the air that come from automobiles, oil refineries, electricity generating plants, and other industrial sources. This is why it is called **photochemical smog.** Photochemical smog consists of ground-level ozone, carbon monoxide, sulfur dioxide, nitrogen oxides, particulates, and volatile organic compounds (**Table 24.1**).

Ground-Level Ozone   Ozone (O_3) consists of three atoms of oxygen, as compared with the oxygen we breathe, which consists of two atoms of oxygen (O_2). Whereas ozone in the upper atmosphere benefits life on Earth by shielding it from harmful ultraviolet radiation from the sun, high amounts of ozone at ground level are a major health hazard. Ground-level ozone is not emitted

TERMS

environment: all external physical factors that affect us

photochemical smog: air pollution from the action of sunlight on emissions from motor vehicles and industrial sources

smog: air polluted by chemicals, smoke, particles, and dust

Table 24.1

Major Air Pollutants and Their Health Effects

These pollutants affect breathing, damage lungs, and cause a wide range of health problems. The primary sources of these air pollutants are industrial emissions, automobiles and trucks, and coal and oil burning in industry and homes.

Pollutant	Health effects and symptoms
Carbon monoxide gas	Low levels cause dizziness, headache, and fatigue. High levels lead to coma and death. Especially dangerous for persons with asthma and heart disease.
Nitrogen oxide gas	Causes a smelly brown haze that irritates the eyes, nose, and lungs.
Sulfur dioxide gas	Sulfur dioxide gas is poisonous and irritates the eyes, nose, throat, and lungs. It kills plants and rusts metals.
Particulate matter (particles from dust and smoke that are less than 10 microns in diameter)	Causes throat irritation and permanent lung damage. Some industrial soot particulates may cause cancer.
Ozone (O_3)	In the stratosphere ozone protects us from UV light. Can be formed at ground level from nitrous oxides and organic compounds. Causes eye irritation, cough, and breathlessness.
Volatile organic compounds	Smog-forming chemicals, such as benzene, toluene, methylene chloride, and methyl chloroform. All VOCs can cause serious health problems.

directly into the air from polluting vehicles or industries. Instead, it is formed when sunlight acts on two other pollutants, volatile organic compounds (VOCs) and oxides of nitrogen (nitrogen oxide and nitrogen dioxide).

Ozone can damage lung tissue, reduce lung function, and sensitize the lungs to other irritants. Exposure to even relatively low amounts of ozone for several hours can induce respiratory inflammation in healthy people during exercise. This decrease in lung function generally is accompanied by chest pain, coughing, sneezing, and pulmonary congestion. Ozone's effects on people with impaired respiratory systems, such as asthmatics, is usually more severe.

Carbon Monoxide Carbon monoxide (CO) is a colorless, odorless, poisonous gas produced by incomplete burning of carbon-containing fuels. Three-fourths of CO emissions in the United States are from transportation sources, mostly motor vehicle exhaust. Other major CO

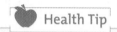

Health Tip

The Next Time You Buy a Car, Go Hybrid

When you buy a fuel-efficient, low-emissions vehicle, you enhance your health (and the health of your children and their children) and help the environment by making the air cleaner and reducing the amount of climate-warming carbon dioxide in the atmosphere. A 5 miles-per-gallon improvement in fuel efficiency reduces the annual amount of carbon dioxide a car produces by about 2,800 pounds.

Before you buy, use the EPA's Web site to assess and compare cars and trucks for gas mileage, greenhouse gas emissions, annual fuel costs, air pollution ratings, and safety information (http://www.fueleconomy.gov).

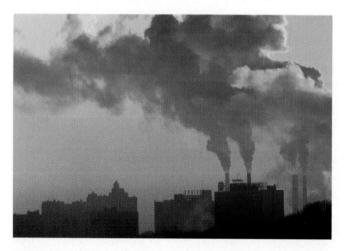

Polluted, "smoggy" air over many large cities contributes to respiratory problems and other diseases.

sources are wood-burning stoves, incinerators, and industries.

When CO enters the bloodstream, it reduces the amount of oxygen that can be delivered to the body's organs and tissues. Exposure to high levels of CO can cause impairment of visual perception, manual dexterity, learning ability, and performance of complex tasks. If the air contains 80 parts per million (ppm) of CO, the oxygen supplied to the body is reduced by 15%. In heavy freeway traffic, the levels of carbon monoxide may reach 400 ppm. It is no surprise that many commuters in large cities who get stuck in traffic jams arrive home with headaches. Car mechanics and parking garage attendants, who are exposed to high levels of carbon monoxide for long periods, may develop health problems. Health threats from CO are most serious for those with heart disease.

Sulfur Dioxide Sulfur dioxide (SO_2) is produced when gasoline, diesel fuel, and coal or oil, all of which contain sulfur, are burned in cars, trucks, power plants, and industrial and home heating systems. Sulfur dioxide also is produced by active volcanoes. Sulfur dioxide can mix with water vapor to form sulfuric acid, a highly corrosive substance that can erode stone, pit metal, and damage living tissue. Exposure to SO_2 makes breathing difficult and aggravates existing respiratory and cardiovascular diseases. Sulfur dioxide in the air can combine with water to form acid rain (discussed later in this chapter), which damages aquatic ecosystems and forests in many parts of the world.

Nitrogen Oxides The major sources of nitrogen oxides are from transportation, electric power plants, and industrial boilers. Nitrogen oxides consist principally of nitrogen oxide (NO) and nitrogen dioxide (NO_2). In photochemical smog, nitrogen oxide is converted to NO_2, which is a brownish, highly reactive gas that can irritate the lungs, opening the way for bronchitis, pneumonia, and other respiratory infections. Nitrogen oxides also contribute to ground-level ozone and acid rain, and they may alter both terrestrial and aquatic ecosystems.

Particulate Matter Particulate matter (PM) is microscopic particles that arise principally from the burning of diesel fuel and coal. These particles are released into the air, causing the haze associated with photochemical smog and damaging soil and structures in the process. When inhaled, particulate matter damages the respiratory system and impairs breathing; the particles also aggravate existing respiratory and cardiovascular diseases.

The ports of Los Angeles and Long Beach in California handle 40% of all the goods shipped into the United States. Diesel engines power the ships, trucks, and trains that move these goods. Southern Californians breathe air that contains more than half of all the diesel particulate matter emitted in the United States each year. It is estimated that about 2,400 lives are shortened each year from breathing particulate-polluted air.

The evidence that particulate matter is a serious threat to health is now quite compelling. The Environmental Protection Agency (EPA) estimates that thousands of elderly Americans with heart and respiratory problems die each year as a result of breathing dusty air—air that meets EPA standards for particulate matter. The EPA monitors PM10 particles (particles in the size range of 10 microns) and PM 2.5 particles (particles in the size range of 2.5 microns). However, ultrafine particles smaller than 0.1 microns are present in polluted air and are more dangerous to health; they also are a major source of air pollution in urban areas. It is estimated that worldwide, more than 500,000 people die each year from breathing particulate matter in polluted air (Eftim, 2008).

In the aftermath of the World Trade Center tragedy on September 11, 2001, thousands of rescue workers and people living in the area developed "World Trade Center cough." The dust cloud created by the collapse of the buildings and the ensuing cleanup contained millions of tons of dust and particulate matter. Breathing the polluted air caused some firefighters to become permanently disabled from lung damage and left thousands of others with a persistent cough (Chen & Thurston, 2002). The pulverized concrete from the collapse of the buildings also generated tons of alkaline dust, which damages the esophagus. Many workers exposed to this corrosive alkaline dust developed gastrointestinal reflux disease (GERD), otherwise known as severe heartburn, due to acid in the stomach being regurgitated into the esophagus. Even short-term exposure to particulate matter in air increases hospital admissions for cardiovascular and respiratory diseases (Bell et al., 2008).

In considering healthy lifestyle changes, we usually think about giving up smoking and alcohol, or improving our diet and losing weight. But we rarely think about the quality of the air we breathe. When you think of moving away to go to school or to take a job, check into the quality of air in the area in which you choose to live. Although healthy young people can breathe polluted air for years without noticeable effects, eventually they may develop asthma, diminished lung capacity, heart disease, and other health problems.

Volatile Organic Compounds   Volatile organic compounds (VOCs) are chemical substances that exist in the air as gases. About 50% of VOCs come from industrial and commercial processes such as oil refining, printing, painting, and dry cleaning. Another 40% of VOCs come from motor vehicle exhaust. Five percent come from power generation, and the rest from miscellaneous sources. In the presence of sunlight, some VOCs (called "ozone precursors") easily combine with other air pollutants to form ground-level ozone. Besides contributing to photochemical smog, some VOCs are harmful to

human health and are known as hazardous air pollutants or air toxics.

Children and Air Pollution   Children who live in smoggy cities such as Los Angeles and Mexico City suffer a 10% to 15% decrease in lung function as compared with children who grow up where the air is less polluted. Early exposure to polluted air can damage the respiratory tract and can increase the risk of respiratory disease in adult life. Children are much more likely than adults to develop smog-related lung damage because they inhale several times more air than adults, and they breathe faster, particularly during strenuous physical activity. In addition, they spend more time outdoors than any other segment of the population. The lungs in children and adolescents undergo steady development, with peak lung capacity reached between the ages of 20 and 25. Lung capacity remains stable for another 10 years and then gradually declines with age. Breathing polluted air while the lungs are still developing can decrease lung function later in life and contribute to the development of asthma, chronic obstructive lung disease, and cardiovascular disease.

Prior to the 2008 summer Olympics in Beijing, the Chinese government took unprecedented steps to reduce the severe air pollution that covers the city almost constantly. In the years prior to the Olympics, the government planted millions of trees in and around the city. In the months leading up to the Olympics, the government ordered the shutdown of air-polluting industries for hundreds of miles around the city. Construction in Beijing was halted and traffic was sharply curtailed. Although not producing crystal clear air, these efforts did significantly improve air quality during the 2008 Olympics.

The world's automobile "population" is exploding along with its human population. In 1950, there were about 50 million cars worldwide; by 1990, the number had increased to 400 million. As nations such as India and China, which together constitute 38% of the world's population, continue to progress economically, the car population in these and other less-developed countries also will increase. Car manufacturers will rejoice, but the effects on air and land pollution will be devastating.

A modern U.S. car with a catalytic converter to reduce emissions still produces about 20 pounds of carbon dioxide for every gallon of gas that is burned; this is a significant factor in global warming. Over an average 10-year life, each American car spews 50 tons of carbon dioxide into the atmosphere. If mileage standards were increased and cars were made more fuel efficient, CO_2 emissions could be reduced significantly.

One major victory in the battle against air pollution was the elimination of lead in gasoline in the United States. The phaseout of leaded gasoline, which began in 1984, has markedly reduced the blood levels of lead in the U.S. population. The battle to eliminate lead in gasoline took more than 10 years to accomplish, which shows the amount of time and effort that goes into changing just one factor in air pollution. Efforts are ongoing to develop less-polluting fuels and vehicles.

When it passed the Clean Air Act and Clean Water Act in the 1970s, the U.S. Congress established the Environmental Protection Agency (EPA) to carry out the mandates of those and other environmental laws. When Congress and the presidential administration are pro-environment, the EPA tends to lock horns with industry, which resists changes in the design and manufacture of products intended to provide a clean environment on the ground that the costs of doing so will weaken the U.S. economy. Often, industry tries to bolster its resistance by attempting to find flaws in scientific research.

The evidence that particulate matter in air is a health hazard is overwhelming, but industries argue that other air pollutants underlie the health problems and that particulates are not responsible. It required more than 10 years of heated debate and legal wrangling to prove that lead from gasoline was damaging the brains of young children. Many years of effort and research were devoted to showing that chlorofluorocarbons (CFCs) were destroying the ozone layer that protects the earth's surface from harmful UV irradiation. Eventually, both lead in gasoline and CFCs were banned. These two examples show that improving air quality can be accomplished with long-term effort.

A dramatic example of the air pollution caused by electricity-generating plants was provided by the August 2003 blackout that affected much of the Midwest and northeastern United States. Air samples collected over Pennsylvania a day after the shutdown of all plants in the region showed a 90% reduction in sulfur dioxide and a 50% reduction in ozone. Visibility increased by 25 miles. Suddenly, the air was no longer hazy. Finding cleaner ways to generate electricity is another urgent problem that needs to be solved.

Acid Rain

Acid rain is rainwater containing large amounts of sulfur dioxide and nitrogen oxides that have been released into the atmosphere. When these gases combine with water, they produce sulfuric acid and nitric acid, which are dispersed in the rain. Acid rain harms forests, and raises the acidity of lakes and rivers to levels that kill fish and vegetation. Acid rain is a global problem.

Canada and the United States began to monitor the extent of acid rain damage to lakes and streams in the 1970s, and both countries have since reduced their emissions of sulfur dioxide gas significantly. A revised Clean Air Act was passed by Congress in 1990. As a result of the air standards mandated by this act of Congress, many of the lakes in the northeastern United States have been returned to a state in which fish and vegetation can again thrive.

Solutions to the acid rain problem involve difficult economic and political decisions. Acid rain can fall hundreds of miles from the source of the sulfur dioxide emission, making it difficult to determine the exact source and responsibility. Acid rain does not observe national boundaries, so countries must cooperate if the problem is to be solved. Like other atmospheric pollution problems, acid rain is likely to continue far into the future.

Carbon Dioxide and Global Warming

Along with the gases oxygen (O_2) and nitrogen (N_2), carbon dioxide (CO_2) is a natural component of Earth's atmosphere. Plants use carbon dioxide to manufacture more plant material, and in the process, they give off oxygen that animals breathe. Carbon dioxide in air also is absorbed into oceans, where it forms carbonate-containing rocks.

Before humans began burning coal, oil, and natural gas in vast quantities to fuel the Industrial Revolution, the level of carbon dioxide in the atmosphere was fairly constant at about 290 parts per million (ppm) (**Figure 24.1**). By 1920, the level of atmospheric CO_2 rose to about 300 ppm, and by 1950 it rose further to about 315 ppm. In 2007, atmospheric CO_2 levels reached an all-time high of about 390 ppm. The rate of increase in CO_2 levels during 2007 was the highest ever recorded, which increased fears of catastrophic climate change in the future. Also, for the first time in a decade, the amount of methane gas in the atmosphere increased. Methane is about 25 times more potent than CO_2 in causing global warming. However, because there is much less of it in the atmosphere as compared with CO_2, its contribution to global warming is still minimal. As the levels of these two gases in Earth's atmosphere continue to increase, so too will global warming.

In 1861, an English scientist pointed out that carbon dioxide is a good absorber of infrared radiation. When sunlight lands on the earth's surface, some of the energy in the light is radiated back toward space as infrared radiation or heat. Carbon dioxide absorbs the infrared radiation and thereby traps heat in the atmosphere. Because this process is analogous to how a garden greenhouse works, this phenomenon is called the **greenhouse effect (Figure 24.2)**.

TERMS

acid rain: rain, snow, fog, mist, and the like, with a pH lower than 5.6

greenhouse effect: the ability of atmospheric carbon dioxide to reflect heat radiated from the earth back to the earth and to thereby raise the earth's temperature globally

Over the past 20 years it has become clear that the increase of atmospheric CO_2 (and other "greenhouse gases" such as methane, nitrogen oxides, etc.) would, in fact, heat up the atmosphere like the inside of a greenhouse and lead to global warming. It became apparent in the 1990s that the earth's temperature is increasing (**Fig-** **ure 24.3**) and that it is *not* due to natural fluctuations in the global climate; nearly all climate scientists now believe that the rise in global temperature is caused by human activity (Collins et al., 2007). If humans continue to pump greenhouse gases into the atmosphere even at reduced rates, it is predicted that sometime in this

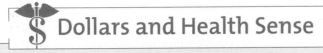

■ **Figure 24.1**

Carbon Dioxide (CO₂) Levels in the Atmosphere
Data prior to 1953 are from CO_2 measured in ice cores. Data after 1953 are direct measurements in the atmosphere.

Source: National Oceanic and Atmospheric Administration.

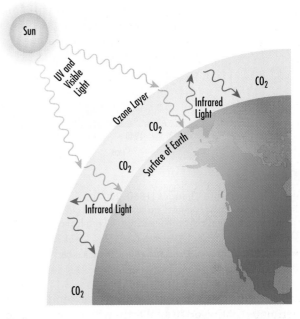

■ **Figure 24.2**

Greenhouse Effect
Carbon dioxide (CO_2) in the earth's atmosphere acts like the glass roof in a greenhouse. Carbon dioxide is transparent to the radiation from the sun and lets it pass to the ground, which warms up.

$ Dollars and Health Sense

The United States Is the World's Biggest Energy User

The United States is the third most populous country in the world after China and India, but still contains less than 5% of the world's population. However, Americans consume about 21% of the world's energy, largely in the form of gasoline. (China is the world's second-largest energy user, at 16%; Russia is third, at 6.2%.) There are about 600 million cars in the world; about one-fourth of that number is registered in the United States.

In 2005, the EPA reported virtually no change in the average fuel economy of the U.S. car/light truck fleet for the past 20 years. Cars average about 24.5 miles per gallon (mpg) and light trucks average about 17.8 mpg. Sport utility vehicles (SUVs) are the main reason for this situation because they make up about 30% of the American automobile fleet.

If cars got better mileage, there would be less air pollution, less lung disease, and a reduced threat from global warming. In 1976, the U.S. Congress tried to deal with the problem of excessive energy use by automobiles when it passed the Energy Policy and Conservation Act, a law that requires car and truck manufacturers to meet certain standards for fuel efficiency. These standards, called *corporate average fuel economy* (CAFE), apply to a manufacturer's entire fleet of vehicles. When first issued, CAFE standards were 27.5 mpg for cars and 20.5 mpg for trucks.

In 2005, the CAFE standards for the nation's fleet of SUVs, minivans, and light trucks were raised to 22 mpg. Because they are built on a truck chassis, small trucks, minivans, and SUVs are classified as trucks and thereby qualify for the lower mileage standard. Of course, everyone knows that these vehicles are purchased almost exclusively for use as passenger vehicles and rarely are they used as working trucks.

In 2007, Congress mandated a new fleet standard 35 mpg, to be achieved by 2020. In 2009, the EPA increased fuel economy standards to 35.5 mpg, to be achieved by 2016. New passenger cars would be required to get 39 mpg, and light trucks would be required to get 30 mpg. The new standards are projected to save 1.8 billion barrels of oil over the life of the program as well as to reduce greenhouse gas emissions by approximately 900 million metric tons.

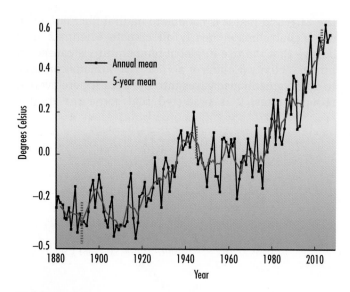

Figure 24.3

Global Temperature Changes (1880–2007)
Almost all atmospheric scientists are convinced that global warming is real
and that temperatures will continue to rise as a result of current and future
CO_2 emissions.

Source: U.S. National Aeronautics and Space Administration, 2008.

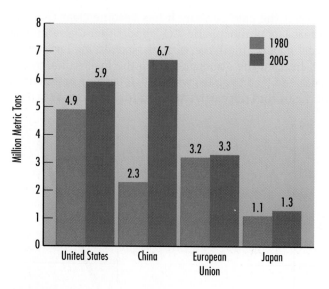

Figure 24.4

**Comparison of Carbon Emissions into the Atmosphere
by Various Countries in 1980 and 2005.**

Source: Netherlands Environmental Assessment Agency, 2008.

> It ain't what we don't
> know that gives us
> trouble, it's what we
> know that ain't so
> that gives us trouble.
> *Will Rogers*

century the temperature of Earth will increase 5 to 10 degrees Fahrenheit. Five to 10 degrees may not seem like much, but in climatic terms it is a tremendous change (Haines & Patz, 2004). Some of the predicted effects of such global warming include:

- A rise in sea level from the melting of ice masses in the Arctic, Antarctic, and on mountaintops sufficient to flood coastal and low-lying regions all over the world. A 3-degree increase in global temperature will raise sea level 1 to 3 feet. People would be forced to relocate, possibly resulting in massive refugee problems. During the past century, sea level rose 4 to 10 inches. The Arctic Ocean and tundra no longer are completely covered with ice during winter. Chunks of ice as large as Delaware have broken off the Antarctic ice shelf and melted in the southern oceans.

- A massive change in the earth's climate. Some tropical regions will become deserts while some temperate regions will become more tropical. In some parts of the world rainfall will increase, whereas in others it will decrease. Winters may become a bit more temperate with less snow, and summers may be hotter and more humid. Global climate change certainly will affect food production throughout the world in a variety of ways. Already, the natural habitats of many land- and water-living plants and animals have changed.

- Many diseases, particularly insectborne diseases, will spread to new regions. Dengue fever, previously unknown in South America, is now prevalent and has spread as far north as Texas. Malaria will spread widely to warmer areas, particularly those subject to large annual increases in rainfall from tropical storms, cyclones, and hurricanes. Increased weather variability has already contributed to the emergence of both hantavirus pulmonary syndrome and West Nile virus infections. Increased summer temperatures and humidity will threaten people who cannot take refuge in air-conditioned buildings.

- The number and intensity of violent storms—hurricanes, cyclones, drought, blizzards, and wildfires—will increase globally. Since 1992, record-setting storms have struck countries around the world and produced weather changes, including record rainfall, drought, hurricanes, and tornados in regions of the United States.

At an international conference on global warming in Kyoto, Japan, in December 1997, a historic treaty was proposed to dramatically reduce the global emissions of CO_2 by all of the industrialized nations. The United States, which produces about 25% of the world's CO_2 emissions, agreed to reduce levels to 7% below the 1990 levels by the year 2012. However, in early 2001, President Bush repudiated the Kyoto agreement, arguing that the commitment to curtail CO_2 emissions will harm the coal, petroleum, automotive, electricity-generating, and other major industries in the United States and thus harm the country's economy.

Global Wellness

Wind-Based Electrical Power

The answer, my friend, is blowin' in the wind.

—*Bob Dylan*

The world uses more and more electrical energy every year. The bulk of this energy is supplied by coal- and oil-fired generating plants that emit enormous amounts of pollutants into the atmosphere. These plants also are a major contributor to global warming and create health problems for people breathing polluted air.

Researchers at Stanford University studied sustained wind speeds at 8,000 locations around the world. They concluded from their study that wind-based power generation is sufficient to meet the *entire* global demand for electrical power. It was estimated that the United States alone could use wind turbines to produce 14% of the world's total output of electrical energy.

Spain is currently the world leader in promoting and producing electrical energy with wind turbines. In 2007, Spain generated about 10% of its total electrical energy with wind. On a gusty day in March, 2008, Spain produced 28% of its electrical energy with wind turbines.

Using wind to generate a large percentage of electrical energy appears to be feasible with existing technologies.

For decades, the United States was the world's largest emitter of carbon dioxide (**Figure 24.4**). However, in 2007, China's total carbon dioxide emissions surpassed those of the United States. As the economies of China, India, Mexico, and Russia grow, global warming and climate change are expected to continue to increase for the foreseeable future.

Reducing Your Carbon Footprint

Anxiety over global warming and its consequences for human health has prompted people to search for ways to reduce their individual contributions to CO_2 emissions. Your "carbon footprint" is a measure of how your lifestyle adds to CO_2 emissions and global warming. Some lifestyle changes that help curb further increases in global warming are obvious: Drive less and walk or ride a bicycle whenever possible. If you buy a new car, buy one with high fuel efficiency. Replace incandescent light bulbs with compact fluorescent light bulbs, and reduce electrical power use wherever possible.

Other lifestyle changes are not as obvious. Changing your diet and where you buy food can lessen your carbon footprint. For example, about 15% of all CO_2 emissions due to human activities come from the transport of goods. Thus, the global economy is a major contributor to global warming. Buying goods, especially food, that are manufactured near where you live can reduce your carbon footprint. Changes in diet also have an impact. The food and agriculture industries account for about one-third of greenhouse gases. Eating meat and dairy products contributes considerably to global warming. The digestive systems of cattle emit tons of methane gas into the atmosphere, and methane is many times more potent than CO_2 in causing global warming. (Are you ready to eat fewer or no cheeseburgers to reduce your carbon footprint?) Reducing your carbon footprint may help in a small way to solve the problem of global warming. At the very least, reducing your carbon footprint may help you make dietary and lifestyle changes that make you healthier.

The Ozone Layer

The **ozone layer** consists of ozone molecules (i.e., three atoms of oxygen bonded together: O_3) that form a layer in the outermost region of the earth's atmosphere. The ozone layer absorbs much of the dangerous ultraviolet (UV) light that is radiated from the sun and protects us from excessive exposure to UV radiation that can increase the risk of skin cancer and cataracts in the lens of the eye. The ozone in the ozone layer is the same chemical produced in photochemical smog. However, in the upper reaches of the atmosphere ozone protects life, whereas at ground level it is a toxic irritant.

A class of chemicals called **chlorofluorocarbons (CFCs)** has been widely used as refrigerant and propellant gases in cans during the 20th century. These CFCs escape into the atmosphere and rise to the ozone layer, where they destroy ozone molecules. In the 1970s it was discovered that the ozone layer was thinning over the Antarctic and that an **ozone hole** appears during the Antarctic spring (September to October). Ozone disappears completely in that region at that time. The ozone hole reached its largest size in 2000—about three times the size of the United States. In 2008, the ozone hole over the Antarctic was observed to be larger in size as

TERMS

chlorofluorocarbons (CFCs): chemicals formerly used as coolants that are released into the atmosphere and are responsible for destroying stratospheric ozone

ozone hole: an ozone-deficient portion of the atmosphere above Antarctica that has been steadily growing since the problem was first reported in 1985

ozone layer: a layer of ozone molecules located in the stratosphere in a diffuse band extending from 10 to 30 miles above the earth's surface

compared to 2007 and earlier years. The hole also contained less ozone than in previous years. The decrease in ozone raises the intensity of UV radiation reaching Earth and increases the risk of skin cancer. The ozone hole has now spread over populated areas of Asia and northern Europe. The intensity of UV radiation in these areas is increasing, exposing people to a higher risk of skin cancer and cataracts.

When the seriousness of the thinning of the ozone layer was realized, 31 industrialized countries agreed in 1987 to phase out the use of CFCs. Even though CFC use has now dropped significantly, the large amounts of these chemicals already in the atmosphere will persist for many decades.

Evaluating the Risks of Air Pollution

In evaluating the health hazards of toxic air pollutants, two important factors must be evaluated separately. **Emission** refers to the amount of a substance that is released into the atmosphere from an automobile or other source of air pollution. **Exposure** refers to the amount of the substance to which people are exposed. Frequently, emission can be high, while exposure is low. Alternatively, emission can be low, while exposure is high.

For many air pollutants, such as carbon monoxide, benzene, and chloroform, the major sources of emissions are automobiles, industry, and sewage treatment plants, respectively. However, the major health risks from these substances are *not* from the sources of highest emission, but from gas stoves, cigarettes, and chloroform in shower water, respectively (**Table 24.2**).

To regulate all of the possible pollutants of the air is impossible, so it is important to identify both the sources of greatest emission and the sources of greatest exposure. For example, benzene is an important chemical used in many industrial processes; it also can cause leukemia in people who are exposed to it. Of all the ben-

zene released into the air, 50% comes from automobiles. However, although cigarettes emit only a tiny amount of benzene compared with automobiles, at least half of the total population's exposure to benzene comes from smoking cigarettes (**Figure 24.5**). Even nonsmokers get most of their exposure to benzene from secondhand cigarette smoke as opposed to benzene from automobile exhausts. The most serious indoor air pollutant is cigarette smoke.

Indoor Air Pollution

Cigarette smoke is not only harmful to the person who smokes, but the secondhand smoke that is produced is harmful to others who breathe it (see Chapter 17). The carbon monoxide levels in smoke-filled rooms can rise to hazardous levels. For example, in bars and conference rooms where many people are smoking, the air may contain levels of carbon monoxide as high as 50 ppm. This level is sufficient to produce headache, nausea, impaired judgment, and other symptoms (**Table 24.3**). Cigarette smoking has been banned in public buildings and most workplaces for many years. Most major cities such as San Francisco and New York have also banned smoking in restaurants and bars. No smoking is allowed in flight by any airline in the world. These represent significant improvements in air quality and health for millions of people.

Table 24.2

Major Sources of Emission of a Pollutant Versus Major Sources of Exposure to It

Pollutant	Major emission sources*	Major exposure sources
Benzene	Industry; automobiles	Smoking
Tetrachloroethylene	Dry-cleaning shops	Dry-cleaned clothes
Chloroform	Sewage treatment plants	Showers
p-Dichlorobenzene	Chemical manufacturing	Air deodorizers
Particulates	Industry; automobiles; home heating	Smoker at home
Carbon monoxide	Automobiles	Driving; gas stoves
Nitrogen dioxide	Industry; automobiles	Gas stoves

*For many hazardous airborne pollutants, the health risk is not related significantly to the major source of emission (as shown in Figure 24.5).

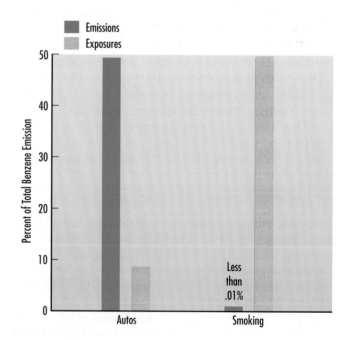

■ **Figure 24.5**

Benzene Emissions
Automobiles emit the greatest amount of benzene into the air—about 50% of the total. However, in terms of the amount of benzene that people inhale, most exposure comes from cigarette smoking.

Table 24.3

Symptoms of Carbon Monoxide (CO) Poisoning

CO blood level (%)	Symptoms
0–2	No symptoms.
2–5	No symptoms in most people, but sensitive tests reveal slight impairment of arithmetic and other cognitive abilities. Levels of 2–5% are found in light or moderate smokers.
5–10	Slight breathlessness on severe exertion. Levels of 5–10% are found in smokers who inhale one or more packs of cigarettes per day.
10–20	Mild headache, breathlessness on moderate exertion. These levels are sometimes seen in smokers who are exposed to additional CO from other sources.
20–30	Throbbing headache, irritability, impaired judgment, defective memory, rapid fatigue.
30–40	Severe headache, weakness, nausea, dimness of vision, confusion.
40–50	Confusion, hallucinations, ataxia, hyperventilation, and collapse.
50–60	Deep coma with possible convulsions.
Above 60	Usually results in death.

Radon

Another form of indoor air pollution is **radon,** a radioactive gas that is invisible and odorless. Radon is naturally produced in the ground in areas that contain uranium ore. In New Jersey, for example, some homes built on top of rocks that contain uranium ore have over 100 times the safe level of radon in air inside the house. Homes also may be constructed from bricks or building materials that contain radioactive minerals, one of the decay products of which is radon gas. The radon is slowly released into the house over many years.

Long-term exposure to radon increases the risk of lung cancer. Uranium miners exposed to radon for years have a much higher risk of lung cancer than average. Cigarette smoking seems to act synergistically with radon; smokers who also are exposed to radon get lung cancer at rates much higher than individuals whose exposure is limited solely to cigarette smoke or solely to radon. The EPA estimates that radon exposure in homes is responsible for as many as 30,000 deaths from lung cancer a year. It is possible to test one's home for the presence of radon and to reduce the amount of radon if it is found.

Heavy Metal Pollution

Lead Lead is a heavy metal that is a serious threat to the health of millions of Americans, especially children. Lead contaminates air, land, water, and houses that still contain lead-based paints. Early symptoms of **plumbism** (lead poisoning) are loss of appetite, weakness, and anemia (**Table 24.4**). Lead poisoning also causes brain damage and is responsible for an enormous number of learning problems among children.

Recent research suggests that high lead levels in children not only cause learning and behavior problems but are also associated with criminal activity and arrest later in life (Wright et al., 2008). Studies involving children who had blood lead levels ranging from 4 to 37 micrograms per deciliter (µg/dl) showed that arrests and the violence of the crimes increased in proportion to the

Table 24.4

Effects of Lead in People

Lead blood level (µg/dl)	Observable effects
10	Enzyme inhibition, learning disabilities
15–40	Red blood cells affected
40–50	Anemia, infertility (men)
50–60	Central nervous system effects, cognitive disabilities
60–100	Permanent brain damage, death

childhood blood lead level. The crimes were committed when the subjects were aged 19 to 24 years. Any parent whose child is diagnosed with learning, behavior, or cognitive disabilities should have the lead level in the child's blood measured.

Over the past 50 years, the U.S. Centers for Disease Control and Prevention (CDC) has repeatedly lowered the figure given as an acceptable level of lead in people's blood. In 1960, the acceptable level was 60 µg/dl; in 1970, the level was lowered to 40, then to 20, and now the acceptable level is 10 µg/dl of blood. Is that level safe? No. Studies show that children's performance on IQ tests is inversely related to the levels of lead in their blood and that any level of lead is likely to have some

TERMS

emission: amount of substance that is released into the atmosphere

exposure: actual amount of the substance people are exposed to

plumbism: disease caused by lead poisoning

radon: a radioactive gas found in some homes that can increase the risk of cancer

adverse effect (Lanphear et al., 2005). These studies indicate that the brains of many more young children are affected by environmental lead than previously thought.

The good news is that blood levels of lead continue to drop; the most recent report shows that only 1.6% of American children under the age of 5 years have blood lead levels that exceed the current acceptable limit of 10 micrograms per deciliter (**Figure 24.6**). This dramatic decline in children's blood lead levels over the past 25 years is almost entirely the result of the elimination of leaded gasoline.

Poor children are at highest risk for having elevated blood lead levels because they live in old buildings that still contain lead-based paints. The paint flakes off walls and the lead becomes a component in house dust. Also, very young children like to eat paint flakes, which further elevates their blood lead levels.

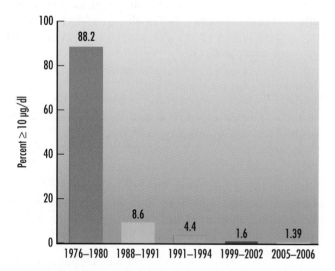

■ **Figure 24.6**

Percentage of U.S. Children Ages 1–5 with Blood Lead Levels Equal to or Greater Than 10 Micrograms per Deciliter

Source: Environmental Protection Agency (EPA).

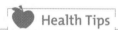

Dispose All Mercury Thermometers Safely

Many medicine cabinets in American homes still contain mercury thermometers. If one of these thermometers breaks and the mercury spills, dangerous levels of mercury may be inhaled as the mercury vaporizes, and the contaminated spot will release mercury for months or years.

If you have mercury thermometers, they must be disposed of at a hazardous waste site. Call local government officials to find out how to dispose of hazardous waste in your area. If mercury has spilled in your home, you should contact a hazardous waste expert to arrange a cleanup.

Unfortunately, neurological damage from lead poisoning cannot be reversed by detoxification. The best way to prevent learning disabilities in children caused by lead pollution is to clean up the environment.

Lead is important to many industries, particularly the battery industry, so it is still an uphill battle to further reduce the amount of lead released into the environment and to clean up all sources of lead contamination. Despite the progress society has made in reducing lead contamination of the environment, the neurological development of millions of children is still at risk from lead toxicity.

Mercury In 1953, an epidemic of methylmercury poisoning occurred in several villages around Minamata Bay in Japan. Since that epidemic, mercury poisoning has become known as "Minamata disease." High levels of mercury in any form, but especially methylmercury, cause a variety of severe neurological symptoms, including blindness, deafness, coma, and death. Symptoms of low levels of mercury poisoning include hair loss and chronic fatigue. In 1970, high levels of methylmercury were found in Lake St. Clair in Canada, where a chemical plant had been discharging wastes. As a result, the U.S. Food and Drug Administration began testing lakes and rivers for mercury contamination. Based on these findings, sport fishing restrictions were implemented by many states because of high levels of methylmercury

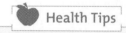

Compact Fluorescent Light Bulbs Contain Mercury

Compact fluorescent light bulbs (CFLs) use about one-fourth the amount of electricity as standard incandescent light bulbs and last 10 times longer. Some countries already have laws requiring that all standard light bulbs be replaced by CFLs by 2010 or shortly thereafter. The United States is expected to also ban standard light bulbs soon. In 2007, two billion CFLs were sold in the United States.

The downside of CFLs is that they contain mercury, a dangerous neurotoxin. Two billion CFLs contain 10 metric tons of mercury (Appell, 2007). If all the bulbs sold in the United States were CFLs, the mercury content would be 200 metric tons. Obviously, CFLs must not be disposed in the usual ways if a pollution disaster is to be avoided. Never throw a CFL into the trash! Some companies and stores already have recycling programs. Many states are expected to pass laws mandating recycling as standard bulbs are phased out.

If you break a CFL, open windows to help dissipate the mercury vapor. Use gloves and sticky tape to pick up glass fragments and powdery residue. Vacuum the area. Double-bag all the contents and dispose in a hazardous waste pickup if possible. For information on recycling CFLs, go to http://www.energystar.gov/index.cfm?c=cfls.pr_cfls.

found in fish taken from contaminated streams and lakes.

Methylmercury is a worldwide environmental pollutant found in fresh water, land, and oceans Methylmercury contamination of fish in both fresh water and oceans is now common (Balshaw et al., 2007). Because fetal development is especially sensitive to damage by mercury compounds, the EPA and FDA jointly issued the following consumer advisory to limit fish consumption by pregnant women, women who plan to become pregnant, and nursing mothers:

- Do not eat shark, swordfish, king mackerel, or tilefish.
- Limit consumption of commercial fish to 12 ounces per week (about 2 meals).
- Fish with the lowest levels of mercury include shrimp, canned light tuna, salmon (wild), pollock, and catfish. (Albacore tuna has higher levels of mercury than light tuna.)

In the United States, coal-fired power plants are responsible for 40% of all mercury pollution. Mercury and other heavy metals are released into the air by the plant's smokestack and are carried around the world by air currents. Rain washes mercury from the air into lakes, rivers, and oceans, where it is transformed by bacteria into hazardous methylmercury. In 2005, the EPA ruled that, as a group, the nation's coal-fired power plants must reduce their combined amount of mercury pollution by 30% by 2010 and 70% by 2018. Rather than requiring all coal-fired power plants to conform to the reduction targets, the EPA allows the worst polluters not to reduce mercury pollution if cleaner coal-fired power plants offset the mercury the worst plants would produce. This system reduces the overall level of mercury emissions, but it creates "hot spots" of mercury pollution near the worst coal-fired power plants. People living near these "dirty" plants (especially children) are at risk for neurological damage.

Water Pollution

After air, water is the body's most essential requirement. We can survive without air for only a few minutes and without water perhaps for several days. The human body is composed of about 60% water, which is essential to every function carried out by organs in the body.

Agriculture, cities, and industry in this country are enormous consumers of water. For example, producing a gallon of gasoline requires five gallons of water; brewing a barrel of beer consumes a thousand gallons; a ton of newspaper takes about 50,000 gallons; a ton of steel requires 25,000 gallons; and irrigating an acre of orange trees requires almost a million gallons of water a year. A family of four uses about 600 gallons of water daily.

Water is continuously recycled in the environment by evaporation and rain. However, as more and more water becomes polluted from pesticides, chemicals, oil spills, and sewage, less and less water is suitable for human consumption and agricultural use. Of special concern is the chemical contamination of rivers, lakes, and underground water supplies, which provide most of our water needs. Around the world, safe, sufficient water supplies are stretched to the limit (Perkins, 2002). Worldwide, it is estimated that about 1.2 billion people lack safe, unpolluted drinking water.

Waterborne diseases, such as cholera, typhoid fever, and dysentery, have been virtually eliminated in North America through sanitation and water treatment methods. In many communities, the water supplied to homes is purified by sedimentation, filtration, or chlorination. The addition of chlorine to water kills dangerous bacteria; however, it may create other health hazards. Interaction of chlorine with other chemicals in the water produces toxic substances, such as chloroform and chloramines, which are cancer-causing agents. The widespread use of detergents, herbicides, pesticides, fertilizers, and other chemicals also has contributed to increased water pollution.

Drinking Water

In the early 1970s, the Environmental Protection Agency found that the water supplies of many towns and cities were dangerously contaminated with pathogenic organisms and toxic chemicals. As a result of these findings, Congress passed the Safe Drinking Water Act of 1974, which covers 58,000 community water supply systems and another 160,000 private systems. The act requires that these systems meet federal drinking water safety standards; but it is one thing to pass such a law and another thing to enforce it.

In 1996, Congress renewed the Safe Drinking Water Act of 1974. Under the new act, consumers must be notified whenever contaminants are found in drinking water and not merely when the water does not meet federal standards for contamination and safety. Community water systems in the United States must be tested for 80 contaminants. Each year, about 7% of community water systems report exceeding federal safety levels for at least one contaminant, which may be why so many people are buying and drinking bottled water.

The most dangerous and ubiquitous chemical found in drinking water is arsenic. This chemical, which occurs naturally in soils and water supplies around the world, is a well-known poison. In low doses, arsenic increases the risk of cancer; at higher doses that may occur in well water, arsenic causes skin eruptions, vomiting, diarrhea, pain, and death. Globally, at least 50 million people are at risk of arsenic poisoning from drinking arsenic-contaminated water.

Americans generally take for granted their (seemingly) endless supply of safe, clean water for daily needs (Table 24.5). Most of the people in the world, particularly in developing countries, are not so fortunate. More than

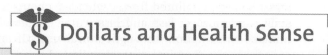

$ Dollars and Health Sense

Bottled Water Battles

In 2007, U.S. consumers bought more than 8 billion gallons of bottled water. Bottled water is the fastest-growing area of the vast soda industry. The water bottled by the two largest distributors (Aquafina by Pepsi and Dasani by Coke) is actually reprocessed tap water. But tap water in the United States is the safest and purest in the world. Still, millions of Americans needlessly spend billions of dollars a year on bottled water.

There are many problems with bottled water. First, the bottled water may not be as pure or safe as people think. Some companies actually bottle tap water without any purification. The plastic bottles may leach cancer-causing and reproduction-harming chemicals such as phthlates and bisphenol-A. About 50 billion plastic water bottles are used each year, and only about 10% get recycled; the rest clutter streets and lots, pollute the oceans and waterways, or wind up in landfills. It takes an estimated 1.5 million barrels of oil to manufacture the plastic water bottles used each year, and then there is the energy used to transport the bottles to markets around the country.

Maybe it's time to stop the bottled water craze. Buy a reusable bottle, fill it with tap water, and carry it with you. Enjoy.

Table 24.5

Water Use

Average water use per person in the United States

Toilet	19 gallons/day
Shower	12 gallons/day
Bath	70 gallons/day
Faucets	11 gallons/day
Leaks	10 gallons/day
Garbage disposal	5 gallons/day
Washing machine	50 gallons/load
Dishwasher	10 gallons per load

Ways to conserve water

Check and fix leaks in faucets and toilets.

Install low-flush (1.6 gallon) toilets.

Install low-flow shower heads (2.5 gallons/minute).

Do not overwater lawn and gardens.

Do not leave hose running when washing car.

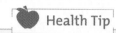 Health Tip

Good Riddance to the Plastic Bag

In March, 2007, San Francisco passed a law banning the use of plastic grocery bags. But the United States is just catching up to the rest of the world; Ireland, Australia, Uganda, Kenya, and Taiwan have already banned their use.

More than a trillion plastic bags are used and discarded every year worldwide. The plastic bag is arguably the most environmentally destructive item ever invented. Plastic bags clog sewers and kill fish and seabirds of all kinds (seabirds pick up bits of plastic on the ocean surface to feed to chicks; when the chicks' stomachs are full of plastic, they die). Plastic bags and other debris destroy coral reefs. Discarded plastic bags collect water and provide a breeding ground for mosquitoes and diseases. In China, plastic bags are called "white pollution." Civilized societies may finally have had it with plastic bags as more cities and nations move to ban them. Beat the crowd. Carry reusable cotton, hemp, or sisal bags with you every time you shop.

a billion people in the world do not have access to safe, clean water. Those who do often must carry it in buckets from sources a long way from where they live. If rivers or wells run dry, they will die within days if they cannot find water.

Worldwide, including in the United States, water is becoming increasingly scarce. Vast underground water aquifers in the American West and South are being depleted. At least 36 states anticipate water shortages by 2013. The water table under Beijing, China, has sunk more than 200 feet in just the last 20 years (Specter, 2006).

The average American uses 100 or more gallons of water a day, more than people anywhere else in the world. It is estimated that, just to survive, a person needs about 10 to 15 gallons a day for drinking, cooking, and washing. In large cities such as New Delhi, India, about one-third of all the water is lost before it reaches consumers due to leaky, broken underground pipes. Many cities in the American West lose a comparable amount of water due to aging water pipes that leak. Water for drinking, agriculture, manufacturing, and other needs is going to become more difficult to obtain in the years ahead.

Land Pollution

Until relatively recently, little attention was paid to the disposal of garbage and solid wastes in landfills around the country. Now, however, we are beginning to run out of space to dump the stuff we want to get rid of. Each year in the United States, we junk about 8 million cars and trucks; 100 billion cans, bottles, and jars; and more than 200 million tons of garbage. The average American

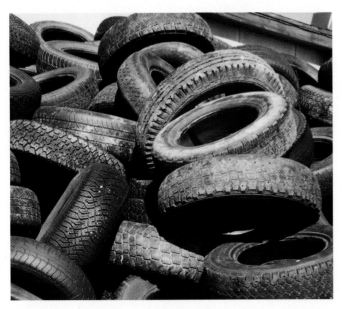

Do you ever think about what happens to your old tires? It's not a pretty picture, but it's a problem we have to solve.

generates more than twice as much garbage as citizens of other industrialized countries.

Many old, abandoned solid waste disposal sites are dangerous to health because they contain hazardous materials that may be corrosive, flammable, or contain toxic chemicals (Table 24.6). In 1980, Congress passed the Superfund Act, which provides for the cleanup of the most dangerous waste sites. By 2008, only 317 Superfund sites had been cleaned up. Over 1,200 toxic waste sites await attention. It is estimated that 11 million Americans live within a mile of one of these Superfund sites, and their health is at some risk from exposure to toxic substances. You can find out where Superfund sites are located and whether you live near one of the listed sites. Go to http://www.epa.gov/superfund/sites/npl/npl.htm. Enter your zip code to find out if you are living close to a Superfund site that is on the priority list for cleanup.

Americans are big consumers and big discarders. Every year millions of cars, tires, appliances, computers, TVs, paints and solvents, construction materials, and other objects, large and small, wind up in landfills or toxic waste disposal sites. To the extent that we continue to pollute the land we live on, the environment and our health will be adversely affected. Many items can be recycled with a little effort. Many communities have recycle programs for bottles, cans, plastic, and paper. Many organizations have recycle programs for old computers, cell phones, batteries, solvents used in printers, and other machines that contain toxic substances. Think of the environment when you consume and when you discard.

Pesticides

Soil, water, foods, and people have become increasingly contaminated with chemicals used to control weeds, insects, and plant diseases in the environment. Any chemical capable of killing a plant or animal is called a **pesticide**. Specific kinds of chemicals that destroy specific organisms are **insecticides** (to kill insects), **fungicides** (to kill molds and fungi), **herbicides** (to kill weeds), and **rodenticides** (to kill rats and mice). Pesticides are important to the agriculture industry, which has claimed over the years that the abundance and quality of food grown in the United States depend on the use of chemicals to destroy crop pests. Although pesticides may contribute to agricultural productivity (this is contested by people who practice organic farming), widespread

TERMS

fungicide: a chemical that kills fungi and molds
herbicide: a chemical that kills weeds
insecticide: a chemical that kills insects
pesticide: a chemical that kills unwanted plants and animals
rodenticide: a chemical that kills mice and rats

Table 24.6

Hazardous Wastes That Escape into the Environment Cause Many Health Problems

Millions of tons of these substances are discarded every year in the United States.

Substance	Source	Health effects
Mercury	Sludge from chloralkali plants; electrical equipment, fluorescent lights	Tremors, mental retardation, loss of teeth, kidney damage, neurological damage
Arsenic	Arsenic trioxide from coal combustion and from metal smelters	Diarrhea, vomiting, paralysis, skin cancers
Cadmium	Waste from electroplating industry; paint containers, nickel-cadmium batteries	Lung diseases
Cyanide	Electroplating industry waste	Poisoning, interferes with cellular energy metabolism
Pesticides	Solid wastes and wastes in solutions	Multiple effects including rashes, respiratory and gastrointestinal symptoms, neurological disorders, hemorrhages

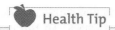

Health Tip

Precautions for Pesticide Use

- Before you buy a pesticide product, read the instructions for use and any health and safety warnings. When mixing, do not increase the concentration of the pesticide above the label-recommended amount. Do not purchase the product if you can't use the pesticide properly (you may not have the right equipment). If you don't understand or feel completely comfortable with the health and safety information provided, get more information before you buy the product. Also, consider whether you have adequate storage space for the pesticide. A bigger bottle may be cheaper, but can you store it safely?
- Use the least toxic pesticide available for your pest control problem. Try to strike a balance between effective pest control and the safety of people, pets, and other nontarget organisms. Minimize skin and respiratory contact with pesticides. Wear rubber gloves. When you select gloves, consider both the solvent used in the pesticide formulation and the possibility that the pesticide itself can penetrate skin. You may want to use a respirator to guard against inhaling pesticide spray or dust.
- Use pesticides only for the uses for which they are intended. For instance, some wood preservatives are meant for outside use only, so don't use them inside the house!
- Don't leave seemingly empty pesticide containers where children can get them. Children have been poisoned by drinking from "empty" containers that actually contained leftover pesticide.
- Never smoke, eat, or drink while using pesticides.

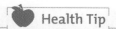

Health Tip

Avoid Pesticide-Contaminated Fruits and Vegetables

Listed below are fruits and vegetables that are most highly contaminated with pesticide residues and ones that are relatively free of pesticides.

Most contaminated	Least contaminated
Peaches	Onions
Apples	Avocados
Bell peppers	Sweet corn
Celery	Pineapples
Nectarines	Mangos
Strawberries	Asparagus
Cherries	Sweet peas
Pears	Kiwifruit
Imported grapes	Bananas
Spinach	Cabbage
Lettuce	Broccoli
Potatoes	Papaya

dissemination of pesticides in the environment has created health problems for people and animals.

Many pesticides have been found to be so dangerous that their use has been banned by the EPA, the federal agency that regulates pesticide use. One of the most widely used pesticides, DDT, was found to be carcinogenic and was banned by the EPA only after vast amounts had been released into the environment.

Pesticides such as heptachlor, kepone, dieldrin, mirex, and toxophene also have been banned, and these chemicals have been off the market in the United States for a number of years. The quandary faced by the EPA is balancing the legitimate use of chemicals by agriculture and other industries while safeguarding public and environmental health. Many of the banned pesticides are still in use in other countries around the world.

Most of the pesticides that accumulate in the bodies of young children come from the food that they eat. The good news is that switching the children's diet to organic foods lowers the concentration of agricultural pesticides in their bodies within a few days. Researchers measured the levels of various commonly used agricultural pesticides in children's urine samples. Within a few days of switching to organic fruits, vegetables, and grains, no pesticides could be detected in urine samples. Switching to foods grown without pesticides can substantially reduce the amount of potentially harmful chemicals absorbed into the body.

Generally, the health effects of pesticides on people and other animals are subtle. For the most part, pesticides do not cause sudden, severe sickness or death unless the amount of exposure is extremely high. The amount of pesticide capable of causing death varies widely depending on the specific chemical, as well as on individual susceptibility.

As a society, we are not ready to abandon the use of pesticides. However, as individuals we should restrict our use of pesticides as much as possible to protect ourselves and the environment. To achieve this goal, many people now grow their own vegetables without the use of pesticides. Others shop at stores that sell organic fruits and vegetables grown without the use of pesticides and herbicides.

Endocrine Disruptors

Endocrine disruptors are chemical substances, usually pesticides, in the environment that enter the body and interfere with the action of one or more hormones. Some endocrine disruptors mimic the effects of a hormone, causing overstimulation of a normally regulated biological process. Other endocrine disruptors block the actions of normal hormones, thereby lessening or completely inhibiting a biological process. Because hormones are present in the body in very small amounts,

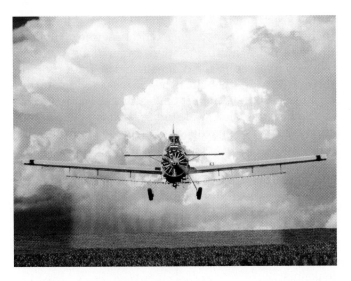

Large amounts of pesticides are routinely sprayed on major food crops.

only a small amount of an endocrine disruptor can affect hormone signaling.

Many large animals, birds, and fish now have high levels of endocrine-disrupting pesticides in their tissues. For example, in a lake in Florida, 80% to 95% of alligator eggs have failed to hatch in recent years, a mortality rate 10 times normal. The alligator eggs contain abnormal levels of estrogen and testosterone, which are essential reproductive hormones in all animals. The few male and female alligators that do survive are reproductively abnormal, and males have abnormally small penises. A pesticide called dicofol, similar to DDT in structure, is present in the lake as a result of dumping by a chemical company that used to operate on its shore. Dicofol mimics the action of estrogen and causes abnormalities in reproduction and in sexual development.

The evidence for negative health effects of pesticide endocrine disruptors continues to grow. A study in India showed that chronic exposure to the pesticide *endosulfan* delays the onset of puberty in adolescent boys. This pesticide is widely used on squash, melons, strawberries, and other crops around the world. In the United States, more than a million pounds of endosulfan is used every year. In 2009, the Environmental Protection Agency ordered pesticide manufacturers to test chemicals in their pesticides to determine if they adversely affect the endocrine systems of laboratory animals. Testing will focus on whether the pesticides mimic or interfere with the actions of estrogen, androgen, and thyroid hormones.

Toxic Plastics

Plastic products are essential to virtually every aspect of modern-day life. Think of an object, and it is probably made of some type of plastic: eating utensils, tools, packaging, toys, bottles, shelving, pipes, and so on. In recent years, two chemicals used in the manufacture of

plastics have been implicated in a number of developmental defects in animals and humans and in a variety of health problems.

Phthalates are used in the manufacture of plastic flooring, medical devices, cosmetics, and coatings on drugs. Phthalates are everywhere in the environment, and about 75% of human urine samples show significant levels of phthalate metabolites. Some male infants who were prenatally exposed to phthalates show genital abnormalities (Trubo, 2005). In a survey of girls with premature breast development, about 76% of those affected had high levels of phthalates in their blood (Colon et al., 2000). In older men, high phthalate levels in the blood have been associated with low sperm counts and low testosterone levels. There is also speculation that phthalates in people may be contributing to the dramatic rise in obesity and diabetes.

Bisphenol-A (BPA) is a chemical used in the manufacture of polycarbonate plastic, a clear, hard plastic identified by the number 7 imprinted somewhere on the product. BPA has been linked to miscarriages, birth defects, and abnormal brain development in fetuses.

BPA was first synthesized in the 1930s in an effort to develop a synthetic estrogen but was abandoned in favor of diethylstilbestrol (DES), which proved to be a more effective estrogen. Subsequently, chemists discovered that BPA could be used to make polycarbonate plastic. Today, polycarbonate plastics are used in canned goods, water bottles, baby bottles, microwave cookware, and many other products. As polycarbonate plastics age or when they are heated or exposed to strong detergents, BPA leaches out. Surveys show that 92% of Americans have significant amounts of BPA in their bodies.

Pregnant women and nursing mothers should avoid products made of polycarbonate plastic as much as possible. Do not use polycarbonate plastic water bottles or, if you do, do not wash them in hot water with detergent. Do not use baby bottles or baby gadgets that are made of polycarbonate plastic. Do not heat food in polycarbonate plastic containers. In general, try to avoid any food or beverage that is packaged in polycarbonate plastic.

> TERMS
>
> endocrine disruptors: chemical substances in the environment that interfere with the actions of one or more of the body's hormones
>
> phthalates: chemicals used in the manufacture of various plastics; may cause abnormal genital development in males and premature breast development in girls
>
> bisphenol-A (BPA): chemical used to manufacture polycarbonate plastics; may cause abnormal brain development in fetuses and birth defects

The U.S. Food and Drug Administration has been reluctant to ban the use of polycarbonate plastics for food and beverage containers despite the mounting scientific evidence of the health hazards of BPA. Pressure from manufacturers and political concern about economic impacts have, so far, outweighed health concerns regarding BPA (Schardt, 2008).

To monitor the effects of environmental chemical pollution on human health, the Centers for Disease Control and Prevention (CDC) has been measuring the chemical load in a cross section of Americans every two years since the late 1990s. In its third National Report on Human Exposure to Environmental Chemicals, the CDC measured the levels of 148 chemicals in blood and urine samples taken from people of all ages (U.S. Centers for Disease Control and Prevention, 2005). The CDC publishes updates to the third National Report on its Web site (www.cdc.gov/exposurereport).

The measurement of environmental chemicals that are detectable in the body is called **biomonitoring**. Chemicals enter the body from air, water, food, dust, soil, or consumer products. Although the sensitivity of chemical tests has improved in recent years, the health effects of many environmental chemicals that accumulate in the body are unknown; more research must be done. The most recent report shows that levels of lead and *cotinine* (a chemical that measures exposure to secondhand cigarette smoke) have declined significantly, especially among children. However, the levels of organophosphate pesticides, phthalates, and other compounds known to cause health problems are increasing.

Electromagnetic and Microwave Radiation

Electric power lines, appliances, motors, TV sets, microwave ovens, and power tools all emit very low-frequency **electromagnetic fields (EMFs)**. Except for the earth's electromagnetic field, all EMFs come from electricity that is generated by electrical devices of all kinds (**Table 24.7**). Only in the past few generations have people been exposed to the magnetic fields. Until recently, these EMFs were thought to be too weak to affect living organisms, so their impact on health was ignored.

Some epidemiological studies have found an association between the incidence of childhood leukemia and brain tumors and exposure to EMFs. Families that live close to high-voltage power lines or electrical distribution boxes tend to experience more sickness and more cancers. However, a very careful study of the risks of childhood leukemia and exposure to EMFs showed that the risk of cancer was not increased. On the other hand, studies suggest that exposure to EMFs among adult railway workers is associated with a higher risk for leukemia.

All of us are exposed to EMFs every day. An electric shaver or hair dryer puts out a strong EMF, although users are exposed for only a few minutes a day (**Figure 24.7**). If a person lives near a high-voltage transmission line, exposure to EMFs may be considerable depending on the distance between the house and the wires. And the exposure goes on day and night. Calculating EMF exposure, at best, yields crude approximations, one reason why the evidence regarding EMFs and harmful health effects is conflicting.

Cellular Phones

Digital cellular phones emit pulses of microwave radiation. About 200 million Americans use cell phones, often for several hours a day. Any possible health consequences from long-term cell phone use by hundreds of millions of people around the world are as yet uncertain. Another uncertainty is the health consequences of working in modern offices that are filled with microwave radiation from a variety of electronic devices. People who use cell phones extensively should use a headset to keep the phone away from the head.

Table 24.7

Strength of Electromagnetic Fields from Household Sources

Many electrical appliances, especially ones with motors, produce very strong magnetic fields, but the strength of the field falls rapidly with increasing distance from the appliance.

Source	Intensity (milligauss) at distance from source	
	At 4 cm	At 20 cm
100-watt bulb	2.5	—
Refrigerator (back)	11	5
200-watt stereo	27	5
80-watt fluorescent bulb	34	18
Coffeemaker	90	7
Electric drill	600	6
Hair dryer	1,000	0.1

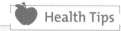 Health Tips

Ways to Reduce Your Exposure to EMFs

- Don't use an electric blanket or water bed heater unless it is a newer model with reduced EMFs.
- Use battery-operated shavers and hair dryers. Battery-operated appliances and toys do not put out EMFs.
- Don't sit too close to computers, TVs, fans, or light fixtures.
- If your work requires long exposure to EMFs, look for ways to reduce it. Do not sit too close to computer screens for long periods.
- If you rent or buy a house, choose one that is not near a high-voltage line or distribution transformer.

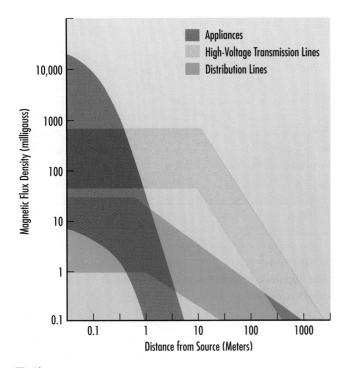

Figure 24.7

Strength of Magnetic Fields from Sources of Electromagnetic Fields (EMFs)

Small appliances produce strong fields, but the strength disappears within a few feet. High-voltage lines produce less dense magnetic fields, but they cover a large area.

Source: Adapted from H. K. Florig. (2001). Alternative goals and policy mechanisms for radiation protection. *Health Physics, 80,* 397–400.

Some cancer researchers believe that long-term use of a cell phone might increase the risk of getting a brain tumor. Other scientists believe that the ubiquitous microwave towers scattered throughout the landscape may also be a health hazard.

Based on current research, the risk to health from exposure to EMFs and cell phone radiation must be regarded as small compared with the risks of chemical pollutants in air, soil, water, and food. Moreover, our lives are so dependent on electricity and the gadgets that make life more comfortable that major changes in electrical use are not anticipated.

Noise Pollution

Have you ever been kept awake at night by a dripping faucet or a neighbor's party? Does the sound of sirens and horns put you on edge? Have you ever found yourself thinking, "If that noise doesn't stop, I'm going to scream"? Everyone is sensitive to noise, and excessive noise produces stress and can cause health problems. Noise interferes with sleep and over periods of time can cause fatigue, irritability, tension, and anxiety.

Sound activates the nervous system, thereby affecting functions of the endocrine, cardiovascular, and

Table 24.8

Noise Levels Produced by Daily Activities and Machines

A noise level above 85 dB can damage hearing and cause hearing loss over time.

Source of noise	Sound level (dB)
Firearms	140 to 170
Jet engines	140
Rock concerts	90 to 130
Amplified car stereos	140 (at full volume)
Portable stereos (e.g., iPods)	115 (at full volume)
Power mowers	105
Jackhammers	100
Subway trains	100
Video arcades	100
Freeway driving in a convertible	95
Power saws	95
Electric razors	85
Crowded school buses	85
School recesses or assemblies	85
Hair dryer	60 to 90
Normal conversation	40
Quiet room	10

reproductive systems. Noise is a "stressor" and can increase blood pressure, alter hormone levels, constrict blood vessels, and cause intense pain at high levels.

Sound levels are measured in **decibels** (dB). The danger zone for hearing loss begins at about 85 dB, a level present on school buses crowded with kids or driving in freeway traffic with the window open (**Table 24.8**). Many daily activities expose us to sound levels that can permanently damage hearing. Millions of people in the United States are exposed to dangerous levels of sound every day that can cause hearing loss.

Rock musicians and people who listen to loud rock music are particularly at risk for hearing loss. Members of many famous rock bands suffer from **tinnitus,** a persistent ringing in the ears, or have lost a significant amount of their hearing. Children are especially prone to turning up the volume and to listening to music with

TERMS

biomonitoring: measurement of environmental chemicals present in the body that may harm health

decibel: a measure of noise level

electromagnetic fields (EMFs): a form of radiation produced by electrical power lines and appliances that may increase the risk of cancer

tinnitus: persistent ringing in the ears, often caused by repeated or sudden exposure to loud noises

> We have met the enemy and he is us.
>
> *Walt Kelly,*
>
> Pogo

earphones at dangerously high sound levels. In 1999, the World Health Organization (WHO) reported that worldwide, noise-induced hearing impairment is the most prevalent irreversible occupational hazard. WHO estimated that 120 million people worldwide have disabling hearing loss (Babisch, 2005).

Many people live and work amid the din of urban life and have forgotten the rest and peacefulness that come with silence. If you have the good fortune to spend time at isolated spots in remote woods or mountains, you become aware of the beneficial effects of quiet. The human need for stillness was expressed eloquently in 1854 by Chief Seattle, after whom the modern city in Washington is named:

> There is no quiet place in the white man's cities. No place to hear the unfurling of leaves in spring or the rustle of insects' wings. But perhaps it is because I am a savage and do not understand. The clatter only seems to insult the ears. And what is there to life if a man cannot hear the lonely cry of the whippoorwill or the arguments of the frogs around a pond at night?

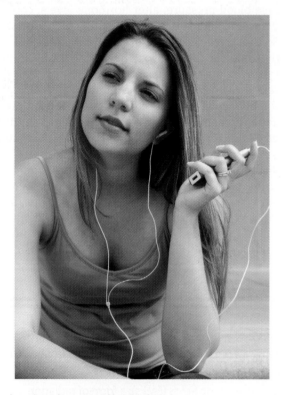

Keep the volume low to avoid hearing loss.

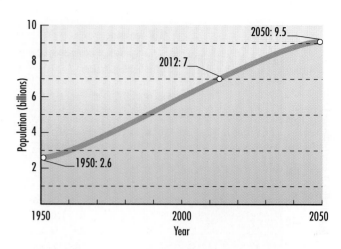

■ **Figure 24.8**

World Population from 1950 to 2050 (estimate)

Source: U.S. Bureau of the Census.

How Human Population Growth Affects Us

In 1960, the world's population was about 3 billion people. By 1999, in just 40 years, the population had doubled to about 6 billion people. By 2050, the world's population is expected to reach 9 or 10 billion people (**Figure 24.8**). Young people aged 10 to 19 currently make up the largest age group in the world, accounting for about 20% of the world's total population. Virtually all of the population increase in the next 40 years is expected to take place in underdeveloped nations, especially in the world's poorest countries (**Table 24.9**). In contrast, the developed, industrialized nations are expected to be near zero population growth, except for the United States.

Of the more than 6 billion people living today, it is estimated that 1 billion have no access to clean water, 2 billion have inadequate sanitation, and 1.5 billion breathe polluted, unhealthy air. Human activities are resulting in the extinction of almost 10,000 plants and animals a year. A few hundred years ago, the rate of extinction was about 10 species per year.

Deforestation; loss of native species of plants and animals; depletion of natural resources; and air, water, and land pollution are all related to too many people needing too many scarce resources. The demand for modern lifestyles and products adds to the destruction and pollution of the environment. Indeed, as one close observer of nature has observed, "Our world is a spectacularly beautiful, interesting, and diverse place. Only by attending to its problems will it remain so" (Pimm, 2003).

The actions, needs, and goals of people are at the root of all environmental problems and the ongoing

Table 24.9

Countries Projected to Have the Largest Populations in 2050

By 2050, the world's population is predicted to increase to 9 or 10 billion people. Most of the population increase will occur in the poorest and least developed countries in Africa and Southeast Asia. The population of the United States is expected to increase by about 50%, while the populations of most European countries will decline.

Country	Population 2000	2050
India	1.0 billion	1.6 billion
China	1.3 billion	1.5 billion
United States	275.5 million	403.9 million
Indonesia	224.7 million	337.8 million
Nigeria	123.3 million	303.5 million
Pakistan	141.5 million	267.8 million
Brazil	172.8 million	206.7 million
Bangladesh	129.1 million	205.0 million
Ethiopia	64.1 million	187.9 million
Republic of Congo	52.0 million	181.9 million

Source: United Nations, 2007.

destruction of nature. As the economies of nations become stronger and the aspirations of people around the globe increase, so does the rate of environmental destruction. Political and economic solutions to the population problem are discussed, but many nations are unable or unwilling to undertake the measures that might curb population growth. Some countries have family planning programs, but the success of these pro-grams depends on educating people and in raising their standard of living so that they understand that large families are not in their best interest. Most of the world's population is opposed to any form of birth control, so the world's population is expected to continue to increase for at least the next 50 years.

The United States has made progress in slowing damage to the environment. Thanks to legislation, environmental lawsuits, and improved technology, air quality has improved, many waterways are cleaner than they were 20 years ago, and disposal of hazardous wastes into the environment has declined dramatically. While all this is good news, we have a long way to go in solving environmental and population problems. Most observers of the world's population growth are not optimistic about the future well-being of human beings and other wildlife on the planet (Cohen, 2005). More than 99% of all plant and animal species that ever lived on Earth have become extinct.

The dinosaurs survived for about 150 million years and disappeared about 65 million years ago, presumably as a result of the earth being hit by a giant meteor that changed the climate drastically. According to anthropologists, the modern human species has been around for only about 3.5 million years. At the rate we are destroying habitat, using up Earth's resources, and polluting the environment, we may be hastening our own disappearance.

> What we call the beginning is often the end
> And to make an end is to make a beginning.
> The end is where we start from.
>
> —*T. S. Eliot*
> Four Quartets

Critical Thinking About Health

1. Check around your house or apartment, and make a list of all pesticides or herbicides that are stored anywhere. Decide which ones you really need to keep and which ones can be discarded. (Check with your local waste management authorities for proper disposal of pesticides and herbicides.) Make a list of how and when you use pesticides and what precautions you take when you use them. After doing this, write a report on how you can reduce your use and exposure to pesticides and herbicides.

2. The United States has made a commitment to lower carbon dioxide (CO_2) emissions dramatically in the next few years. To accomplish this, society must make major readjustments in the use of energy and transportation and in industrial output. Everyone will have to contribute to this effort. Begin by making a list of how you can:

   a. Reduce your electricity use by 30%. What appliances use the most electrical energy and what changes can you make to reduce their use?

   b. Reduce the use of your automobile by 30% or more. What changes in your lifestyle can you make that will reduce your dependence on car transportation?

   c. Find out what industries release the most CO_2 in manufacturing their products. Are these products essential to your life, or would you be able to live without some of them?

3. The major global threats to the environment are (a) nuclear, chemical, and biological warfare; (b) depletion of the ozone layer; (c) global warming; (d) land and ocean degradation; and (e) extinction of species of plants and animals. Indicate which of these global environmental problems is of the most concern to you personally. What can you personally do about the problem? What do you think governments should do about the problem? Discuss any effects that you think this problem will have on your life now and in the future.

4. If you had the option of living anywhere in the world, where would you choose to live? Is your choice largely determined by job opportunities, environmental concerns, access to a favorite sport (e.g., surfing), or by some other variable? Discuss your choice in detail, and explain the things that are most important to you in making your selection. Do you think your choice will be the same 10 years from now? Why might it change?

Health in Review

- To maintain good health, people require adequate unpolluted air, water, food, and shelter.
- The air we breathe is often polluted with ozone, carbon monoxide, hydrocarbons, nitrogen and sulfur oxides, lead, cigarette smoke, and other contaminants.
- Global warming is expected to cause serious environmental disruptions in this century.
- The greenhouse effect and the ozone hole are examples of global environmental problems caused by human activities.
- Pollution of air, land, and water from heavy metals, such as lead, is particularly hazardous to health. Children with even small amounts of lead or mercury in their bodies may suffer from learning deficits and growth retardation.
- Drinking water may be contaminated with chemicals or microorganisms that can cause disease.
- Pesticides, some of which are endocrine disruptors, can harm health, especially reproduction.
- Noise pollution can cause a wide range of health problems, including stress, tinnitus, and hearing loss.
- World population is expected to increase by 3 billion people in the next 50 years, severely taxing an already depleted environment and creating more health and environmental problems.

Health and Wellness Online

The Web contains a wealth of information about health and wellness. By accessing the Internet using Web browser software, you can gain a new perspective on many topics presented in *Health and Wellness*, Tenth Edition. Access the Jones and Bartlett Publishers Web site at **health.jbpub.com/hwonline**.

References

Appell, D. (2007, October). Toxic bulbs. *Scientific American,* 30–31.

Babisch, W. (2005). Noise and health. *Environmental Health Perspectives, 113,* A14–A15.

Balshaw, S., et al. (2007). Mercury in seafood: Mechanisms of accumulation and consequences for consumer health. *Reviews in Environmental Health, 22,* 91–113.

Bell, M. L., et al. (2008). Seasonal and regional short-term effects of fine particles on hospital admissions in 202 U.S. counties, 1999–2005. *American Journal of Epidemiology, 168,* 1301–1310.

Chen, L.C., & Thurston, G. (2002). World Trade Center cough. *The Lancet, 360,* s37–s38.

Cohen, J.E. (2005, September). Human population grows up. *Scientific American,* 48–55.

Collins, W., et al. (2007, August). The physical science behind climate change. *Scientific American,* 64–71.

Colon, I., et al. (2000). Identification of phthalate esters in the serum of young Puerto Rican girls with premature breast development. *Environmental Health Perspectives, 108,* 895–900.

Eftim, S. E., et al. (2008). Fine particulate matter and mortality: A comparison of the six cities and American Cancer Society cohorts with a Medicare cohort. *Epidemiology, 19,* 209–216.

Haines, A., & Patz, A. J. (2004). Health effects of climate change. *Journal of the American Medical Association, 291,* 99–103

Lanphear, B. P., et al. (2005). Low-level environmental lead exposure and children's intellectual function: An international pooled analysis. *Environmental Health Perspectives, 113,* 894–899.

Lovelock, J. E. (1979). *Gaia: A new look at life on Earth.* New York: Oxford University Press.

Muscat, J. E., et al. (2000). Handheld cellular telephone use and risk of brain cancer. *Journal of the American Medical Association, 284,* 3001–3007.

Perkins, S. (2002). Crisis on tap? *Science News, 162,* 42–43.

Pimm, S. L. (2003). *The world according to Pimm: A scientist audits the earth.* New York: McGraw-Hill.

Schardt, D. (2008, April). Hard questions about hard plastics. *Nutrition Action Health Letter,* 8–11.

Specter, M. (2006, October 23). The last drop. *The New Yorker,* 60–71.

Trubo, R. (2005). Endocrine-disrupting chemicals probed as potential pathways to illness. *Journal of the American Medical Association, 294,* 291–293.

U.S. Centers for Disease Control and Prevention. (2005). National report on human exposure to environmental chemicals. Retrieved April 5, 2006, from http://www.cdc.gov/exposurereport

Wright, J. P., et al. (2008). Association of prenatal and childhood blood lead concentrations with criminal arrests in early adulthood. *PLoS Medicine, 5,* e101.

Suggested Readings

Cohen, J.E. (2005, September). Human population grows up. *Scientific American,* 48–55. A comprehensive discussion of the problems associated with continued human population growth.

Duncan, D. E. (2006, October). The pollution within. *National Geographic,* 118–149. Hundreds of toxic chemicals in our bodies can now be measured. How bad are they for our health?

Gore, A. (2006). *An inconvenient truth: The planetary emergency of global warming and what we can do about it.* New York: Rodale Press. Former Vice-President Gore's views about global warming were also made into a documentary. Gore shared the 2008 Nobel Prize with the United Nations for increasing public awareness of the potential catastrophic consequences of global warming.

Johns, C. (Ed.). (2004, September). Global warming [Special issue]. *National Geographic,* 2–75. An entire issue of the magazine devoted to the problems of global warming and climate change.

Kolbert, E. (2007, January 22). Mr. Green. *The New Yorker,* 34–39. An interesting article about Amory Lovins, who probably knows more about saving energy than anyone.

Pearce, F. (2006). *When the rivers run dry: Water—the defining crisis of the twenty-first century.* Boston: Beacon Press. The author believes the battle for water in the coming years will cause conflicts and create a global crisis.

Specter, M. (2008, February 25). Big foot. *The New Yorker,* 44–53. Discusses the science and morality of leaving a carbon footprint.

Recommended Web Sites

Please visit health.jbpub.com/hwonline for links to these Web sites.

Environmental Defense
Information and education about, and advocacy for, a clean environment.

History of Lead Industry Advertising
The Cincinnati Children's Hospital depicts the lead industry's advertising campaign to counter the evidence implicating lead paint in children's deaths.

Intergovernment Panel on Climate Change
Expert analysis from the World Meterological Organization (WMO) and the United Nations Environment Programme (UNEP) on the scientific, technical, and socioeconomic information relevant for the understanding of the risk of human-induced climate change.

National Report on Human Exposure to Environmental Chemicals
Presents the findings of the CDC's third report on the level of 148 potentially harmful chemicals that were measured in people's blood and urine.

National Safety Council
Fact sheets on the health effects of more than 80 toxic chemicals.

Rocky Mountain Institute
The Rocky Mountain Institute provides independent analyses of energy policies.

U.S. Center for Environmental Health
Information from the Centers for Disease Control and Prevention about environmental health topics.

U.S. Department of Energy Efficiency and Renewable Energy
The official site of the U.S. Department of Energy Efficiency and Renewable Energy.

U.S. Environmental Protection Agency
Information about air, water, land, and other types of pollution.

APPENDIX

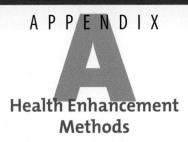

Health Enhancement Methods

This appendix contains several methods for enhancing health and well-being. The techniques include mental imagery (Experiencing the Peacefulness of a Mountain Lake and Open Heart and Compassion Meditation), muscular stress reduction (Progressive Muscular Relaxation), and mind–body harmony exercises (Hatha Yoga Postures and T'ai Chi Movements). You may want to record the instructions on an audiotape so that you can listen to the instructions while focusing on the exercise. A selection of relaxation exercises in mp3 format are available from Jones and Bartlett Publishers at http://health.jbpub.com/hwonline/10e.

Exercise 1
Experiencing the Peacefulness of a Mountain Lake

Imagine yourself walking alone in the early morning along a path leading to some nearby mountains. All around you are trees rustling in the breeze; the path is covered with soft leaves and pine needles. The air is cool but not cold; your body feels relaxed as you walk slowly through the woods. You become aware of the quietness of the surroundings, how different from the constant noise of city life. As you stroll along you hear the calls of different songbirds. You breathe in the cool air tinged with the fragrance of pine and eucalyptus. You walk through patches of sunlight and see the mountain peaks in the distance.

As you gradually walk higher, you notice the subtle sound of water cascading over rocks, and the sound mixes with the wind moving through the branches of the tall trees. Up ahead, a chipmunk is perched on an old stump of a tree, frozen in the moment as it decides which way to jump. Suddenly it is gone and you notice yellow, brown, and orange insects buzzing around the flowers on the bushes. The path begins to level off and the air turns slightly cooler. Now the path is more rocky, and as you come around a bend, a deep blue mountain lake comes into view. You climb onto a boulder weathered smooth by water, wind, and time. You sit down on the boulder to see the entire lake.

Near the shore of the lake are tall green grasses, and spreading back from the shore are clusters of spruce, pine, aspen, and birch. You see a large bird perched on top of one tree in the distance. As you watch, the bird spreads its wings and swoops down over the lake, soars up again, and is gone. The peaks of the mountains surrounding the lake are mixtures of gray and white snow. As your eyes move from the lake to the peaks and back to the lake again, you become aware of the harmony of nature, how each part seems to be in balance with the other parts of the scene.

The sky is dotted with small puffs of white clouds that circle the peaks. The rock you are sitting on radiates the sun's warmth, and you feel your body relaxing, melting into the comfortable saddle of the rock. Your eyes return to the surface of the lake and now you notice the evenly spaced ripples moving across its surface.

As you become more aware of the wind-induced ripples on the otherwise still surface of the lake, you imagine that the ripples on the lake are the tensions in your body. You want your body to become as quiet and relaxed as the stillest part of the lake. As the cessation of the breeze causes the ripples to cease, so the cessation of thoughts in your mind causes the tension to disappear. As you watch the surface of the lake, all of your attention is focused on the ripples as they form, move toward the shore, and disappear.

Breathe slowly and deeply from your diaphragm and continue to focus on the stillness of the beautiful, clear mountain lake that you have created in your mind. Notice that you can make the surface of the lake as smooth as a mirror; as you do this, all of your tensions, thoughts, and worries also disappear, and your mind and body become fully relaxed. Hold onto this feeling of calm and relaxation for as long as you desire. Remind yourself that this is a place you can come back to in your mind time and time again whenever you feel tense, stressed, or angry. It's your personal safe haven that will always induce a feeling of calmness and relaxation.

Note: You can record this image-visualization exercise yourself or have a friend read it into a voice recorder so that you can simply listen to the instructions whenever you feel the need for some mental and physical relaxation. Also, the details of the image can be changed to suit your own experiences or imagination.

Exercise 2
Open Heart and Compassion Meditation

The heart is vital to life, and heart disease is still the number one cause of death in most industrialized countries. The heart is a pump; it circulates blood through the body. But symbolically, we think of the heart as the center of feeling; love flows from the heart. However, we also think of a *hardened heart,* one that may express mean, hateful, destructive, indifferent, and inconsiderate sentiments. What we feel in our heart symbolically can be manifested as stress and in physiological changes that may eventually produce illness. Fear, anger, or hate may contribute to heart disease as well as other ailments. A healthy goal is to rid the heart of acrimonious, destructive feelings and to develop feelings of love and compassion for others, even those who hurt us either deliberately or unwittingly. The following suggestions are designed to help you open your heart to feeling love and compassion for others.

- Sit quietly for a few minutes in a comfortable position on a chair or on the floor, and pay attention to your breathing. Feel the air come in through your nose and flow down into your lungs as the lungs expand and your diaphragm moves outward. Breathe in slowly and exhale slowly to a count of ten. Repeat this a number of times while noticing your body becoming more relaxed with each breath. It may help to repeat silently in your mind, "My body is calm and relaxed."
- After your breathing has become slow and even, focus your attention on the left side of your chest where your heart is located. Picture there a symbol you associate with love, such as a flower or some other object. If you visualize a flower, imagine it starting out as a bud and opening up into a full blossom.
- As you breathe in and out, see the flower or other object symbolic of your heart radiating love outward through your chest.
- Imagine some person to whom you want to send your love or deep feeling of compassion. Use your imagination to surround that person with the rays of your love and caring.
- Make the feeling of love or compassion as profound as you can. Feel the warmth of it in your chest.
- Realize that this love can be sent both to people whom you truly love as well as to people with whom you feel angry or frustrated. Use your imagination to beam your love and caring feelings to the person whose image you have in your mind. You may want to visualize the person at work or at home and see how the person responds to the feelings you are sending.
- Feeling and sharing love and compassion with others help to keep you emotionally and spiritually well.

Exercise 3
Progressive Muscular Relaxation

The following is a slight variation of a stress reduction technique developed by a physician, Edmund Jacobson, in 1929 in Chicago. Our technique involves deliberately tensing various muscles in the body to varying degrees. For each area of the body listed in this exercise, tense the muscles for about 5 seconds (1) as hard as you can, (2) about half as hard as the first time, and (3) just the slightest tension. In so doing, you train your mind to recognize varying degrees of tension in different parts of the body and, more important, how to relax the tension. After performing these exercises for a while, your mind automatically recognizes tension building up in different parts of your body, and that awareness leads to relaxation of the tension.

In this exercise we describe how to tense and relax various parts of the body that most commonly accumulate tension. After you have practiced progressive muscle relaxation exercises for a while, you can apply the same principles to any area of your body that needs to learn how to relax.

Jaws

Take a moment to feel the muscles of your jaws. Notice any tension, even the slightest amount. The jaw muscles can harbor a lot of undetected muscle tension. Now consciously tense the muscles of your jaws really tight, as tight as you can and hold it, even tighter, hold it. Now relax these muscles, exhale, and sense the tension disappear completely. You may even feel your mouth begin to open a little. Feel the difference between how these muscles feel now, compared with what you just experienced at 100% contraction. Feel the absence of tension. Now, contract these same muscles, but at half the full intensity, a 50% contraction. Hold the tension, keep holding, and now relax again. Feel how relaxed these muscles are. Compare this feeling of relaxation with what you felt before. By comparing the difference in tension levels, a greater sense of relaxation will surface. Once again, contract these same muscles, but with only a 5% contraction. A 5% contraction is a very slight twinge, with no motion whatsoever, just the acknowledgment that these muscles can contract. Now hold it, keep holding, and relax. Release any remaining tension so that these muscles are completely loose and relaxed. And sense just how relaxed these muscles are. To enhance this feeling of relaxation, take a comfortably slow, deep breath and sense how relaxed your jaw muscles have become.

Shoulders

Concentrate on the muscles of your shoulders and isolate these from the surrounding neck and upper arm muscles. Take a moment to sense these muscles. The shoulder muscles can hold a lot of undetected muscle tension resulting in stiffness. Symbolically, your shoulders carry the weight of all your thoughts, the weight of your worries and concerns. Now, consciously tense the muscles of your shoulder really tight, as tight as you can and hold it, even tighter, hold it. Now relax these muscles and sense the tension disappear completely. Sense the difference between how these muscles feel now compared with what you just experienced at 100% contraction. Once again, contract these same muscles, but this time only half as tight, a 50% contraction. Hold the tension, keep holding, and now completely relax these muscles. Sense how relaxed your shoulder muscles are. Compare this feeling of relaxation with what you felt before. By comparing the difference in tension levels, a greater sense of relaxation will surface. Finally, contract these same muscles at only 5%. A 5% contraction is a very slight twinge, with no motion whatsoever— just the acknowledgment that these muscles can contract, just a sense of the clothing touching the shoulder muscles. Now hold it, keep holding, and relax. Release any remaining tension so that these muscles are completely loose and relaxed. To enhance this feeling of relaxation, take a slow, deep breath and sense how relaxed your shoulder muscles have become.

Hands and Forearms

Concentrate on the muscles of your hands and forearms. Take a moment to feel these muscles, including your fingers, palms, wrists, and forearms. Notice the slightest bit of tension. Now consciously tense the muscles of each hand and forearm really tight by making a fist as tight as you can and hold it, as if you're going to punch something. Now release the fist and relax these muscles. Sense the tension disappear completely. Open the palm of each hand slowly, extend your fingers, and let them recoil just a bit. Sense the difference between how relaxed these muscles feel now compared with what you just experienced at 100% contraction. They should feel very relaxed. Now contract these same muscles at half the intensity, a 50% contraction. Hold the tension, keep holding, and now relax again. Sense how relaxed these muscles are. Compare this feeling of relaxation with

what you felt before. By comparing the difference between tension and relaxation, a more profound sense of relaxation will surface. Now, barely contract these same muscles. A slight contraction is like holding an empty, delicate eggshell in the palm of your hand. Try to imagine that. Now hold it, keep holding, and relax. Release any remaining tension so that hand and arm muscles are completely relaxed. To enhance this feeling of relaxation, take a slow, deep breath and sense how relaxed your forearm and hand muscles have become.

Abdominals

Really focus your attention on your abdominal muscles. Take a moment to sense any residual tension in either the muscles or organs of the abdomen. Now consciously tense your abdominal muscles really tight as if someone is about to punch you in the stomach and you want to block that punch. Contract as tight as you can and hold it, even tighter, hold it. Now relax these muscles and sense the tension disappear completely. Feel the complete absence of tension. Compare the difference between how these muscles feel now with what you just experienced at 100% contraction. Once again contract these same muscles, this time at half the full intensity. A 50% contraction is like preparing for a false stomach punch. You know they won't make contact, but just in case you want to be ready. Hold the tension, keep holding, and now relax again. Feel how relaxed these muscles are. Compare this feeling of relaxation with what you felt before. When you compare the difference between tension levels and this current state of relaxation, a greater sense of relaxation will follow. Finally, contract these same muscles so slightly you barely feel the clothing over your stomach area. Now hold it, keep holding, and relax. Release any remaining tension so that these muscles are completely relaxed. Sense just how relaxed these muscles have become. To enhance this feeling of relaxation, take a slow, deep breath and feel how relaxed your abdominal region has become.

Feet

Focus your attention on the muscles of your feet. Typically the muscles of the feet are not tense, but standing can produce a lot of tension. In addition, in the confinement of shoes, feet muscles become tense. Now consciously contract the muscles of your feet by scrunching your toes really tight, as tight as you can. Hold it, even tighter, hold it. Now relax these muscles and sense the tension disappear completely. You may even feel your feet become warm as they relax. Feel the difference between how these muscles feel now as compared with when they were tense. Once again contract these same muscles at half the tension. Hold the tension, keep holding, and now relax again. Compare this feeling of relaxation with the tension you felt at full tension. By comparing the difference in tension levels, a greater sense of relaxation will surface. Now, contract these same muscles only slightly. Now hold it, keep holding, and relax. Release any remaining tension so that these muscles are completely relaxed. Sense just how completely relaxed these muscles are. To enhance this feeling of relaxation, take a slow, deep breath and feel how relaxed your feet and whole body are now. Your whole body feels completely relaxed and calm.

Now lie still, and enjoy the complete feeling of relaxation.

Exercise 4
Hatha Yoga Postures *(Asanas)*

Yoga has been used for centuries as a way to relax the mind and body and to promote health and spiritual well-being. The following hatha yoga postures (or

asanas) were chosen and arranged to reflect a typical yoga class. Each position should be done slowly and without pain. Go only as far into the posture as you can while maintaining full complete breaths. It is very important to breathe through each posture. Hold each posture for at least 30 seconds. If you feel any pain (especially in your knees or lower back) ease out of the pose until the pain subsides. Do not judge yourself. Yoga is not about reaching an ideal or being competitive; it is about moving your body, listening to your body, and increasing your flexibility over time.

If you find these postures enjoyable and helpful in reducing tension, you may want to enroll in a yoga class, because it is very helpful to have an instructor. Also, DVDs are available that allow you to follow a course of instruction in your own home at your own convenience.

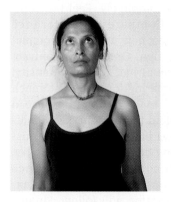
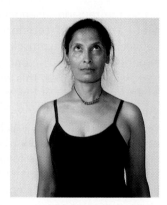
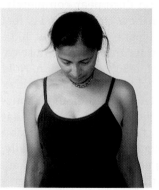
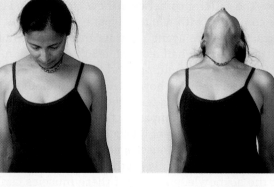
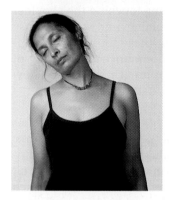
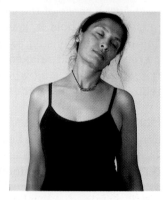

Eye Exercises Sitting comfortably on a chair or on the floor, lengthen the spine and relax the facial muscles. Be sure to breathe normally throughout the exercises. Without moving the head, move the eyes slowly and smoothly: (1) look up and keep looking up without blinking for a couple breaths and then look down and hold for a couple breaths; return to a neutral gaze; (2) look to the right and hold, and then to the left and hold; return to a neutral gaze; (3) slowly circle the eyes clockwise and then counterclockwise. Finish by rubbing the palms together quickly and vigorously to create heat and lightly cup the palms over closed eyes to soothe and relax them.

Neck Exercises (1) Keeping the torso upright, gently and slowly move the head forward, easing the back neck muscles long. Use the weight of the head to lengthen the muscles as you breathe easily in and out. Roll the head back up and tilt it on the top of the spine (which is at the level of the ears) as you gently ease the chin up toward the ceiling, allowing the head to tilt back only as far as is comfortable. Be careful not to crunch the neck; keep those muscles long. Roll back up and repeat forward and backward several times. (2) Tilt the head to the right, easing the right ear toward the right shoulder. Keep the shoulders level while you breathe through the stretch. Repeat to the left side.

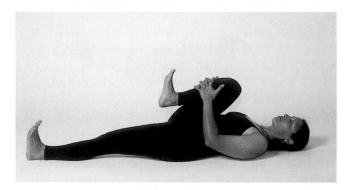

Wind Relieving Pose *(Pavanmuktasana)* Lie on your back, spreading your back along the floor. Bring the right knee toward the head and the right thigh toward the chest. Grasp the knee or behind the knee to pull the leg in closer, as you lengthen the left leg along the floor. Breathe easily in and out while you stay in this position. Bring the left knee up and in as you lengthen the right leg along the floor. Breathe easily in and out while you stay in this position.

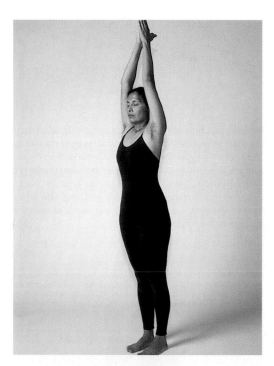

Mountain *(Tadasana)* Stand comfortably with your feet hip-width apart as you lengthen your head up off the top of the spine. Feel the weight of your arms dropping down and out to the sides of your body. Allow the arms to lengthen out wide to the sides as you float them up overhead, palms facing each other. (Be sure not to arch your back. If your back is arched, bring your hands out in front of you. Also, don't lock your knees.) Take a few easy sufficient breaths and gradually release the arms out and down to the sides.

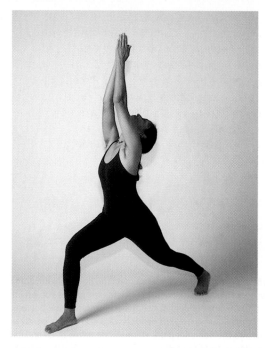

Warrior *(Virabhadrasana)* Come into Mountain pose and inhale an easy breath. Exhale on a "ha" sound as you step forward with your right leg into a lunge position. Check that your right knee is directly over your right foot (front to back and side to side). Straighten your left leg behind you as you ease the left heel toward the ground. Breathe easily a few times. If you feel comfortable, you can bring a slight arch in your back and look up at the ceiling. Lean forward over your right leg with your arms and trunk as you step your left foot forward to join your right and return to Mountain pose. Notice the sensations in your body as you allow the arms to float back down to your sides. Repeat with the left leg forward and the right leg behind.

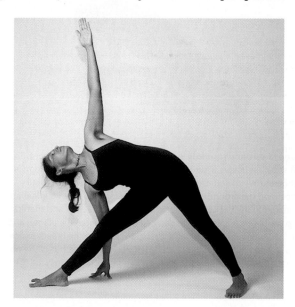

Triangle *(Trikonasana)* Come into Mountain pose. Step lightly to the right so your feet are about three feet apart and bring your arms out to the side at shoulder height, palms facing down. Rotate the right leg out from the hip joint to turn the knee and foot to the right. Inhale, and as you exhale, ease your hips to the left as you reach out with your right fingertips as far as you can. Find ease as you inhale. Exhale as you rotate the arms, the left up toward the ceiling and the right down toward your leg, palms facing forward. Turn the head to look up at your left hand. Continue to breathe. If you cannot breathe easily, bring your torso up a little. Return slowly to the upright position and repeat on the left side.

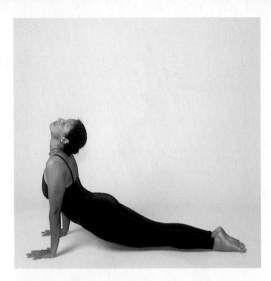

Cobra *(Bhujangasana)* Lie comfortably on the floor on your stomach, with your legs together. Soften your body into the ground as you breathe. Bring the palms to the floor under your shoulders, keeping wide between the shoulder blades. Lengthen your head forward and roll up, gently pressing the palms into the floor. Keep the elbows close to the body and ease the shoulders down, away from the ears. (Don't crunch the lower back. If you have any pain, be sure to come back down.) Breathe in and out a few times and ease down keeping the spine long.

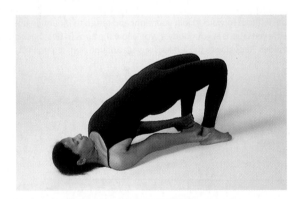

Bridge *(Setu bandhasana)* Lie on your back with your knees bent. Spread your shoulder blades wide and ease your lower back onto the floor. Slide your heels toward your buttocks, hip-width apart. Begin to lift your buttocks off the ground, sending your knees forward over your feet and gradually roll the back up off the ground toward the neck and shoulders. Clasp the hands underneath as you begin to straighten the elbows and ease the shoulder blades together behind you. Allow the breath to flow in and out with ease as you maintain this position. To come out of the pose, separate the hands, widen the shoulders and back, and slowly roll the back down onto the ground.

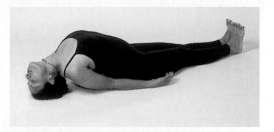

Fish *(Matsyasana)* Lie on your wide, long back with your legs together in front of you. Place your hands close together under your buttocks, palms down, arms straight, and elbows as close together as possible. Allowing the head to roll back, press your elbows into the ground as you expand your chest and torso forward and up, gently resting the crown of the head on the ground, and lengthening the front of your neck. Keep lengthening and expanding the torso as you breathe. Ease the heels of the feet forward and when you are ready, tuck the chin forward and slowly ease your back onto the ground. Release the arms out to the sides and rest, making note of the movement of your breath.

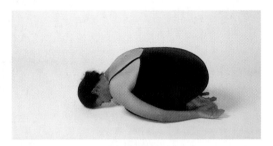

Child *(Gharbasana)* Come onto your knees and gently sit on your heels as you lengthen the spine. Lean forward as you allow your chest to come toward your knees. Rest your forehead on the ground or on a pillow. Allow your arms to lengthen in front of you, then let them rest on the ground. Soften the facial muscles, feel the massage of your organs against your thighs as you breathe. Spread your back wide and long. Stay for a couple of minutes, and when you are ready, gently and slowly support the torso with your hands as you return to kneeling.

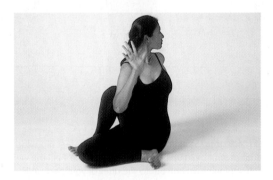

Spinal Twist *(Matsyendrasana)* Before you begin, sit with legs extended straight out in front of you. (If you can't sit comfortably, with your back straight, you may want to sit on the edge of a cushion or rolled up towel or blanket.) Then bend the left leg and put it to the right of your right knee. Bring the left knee as close to you as you can while keeping the foot on the floor. Grab the left knee in the crook of your right arm and pull on the arm to help bring your torso forward and up. Keep the right leg extended in front of you, opening the knee toward the floor, with the foot flexed. Inhale and bring the left arm out to the side at shoulder height and with palm down. As you exhale, take your arm, eyes, and head to the left, rotating slowly through the entire spine. Place the left arm down on the floor, close to your body, and support yourself into a more upright position. Follow the movement of your body as you breathe. Ease back out by unwinding the spinal rotation. Repeat on the other side, left leg down, right knee up, and twisting to the right.

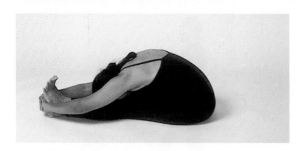

Stretch of the West *(Paschimottanasana)* Find comfort in sitting, with legs together and extended straight out in front of you. (If you can't sit comfortably, with your back straight, you may want to sit on the edge of a cushion or rolled up towel or blanket.) Put your fists on the floor next to your hips and press them into the ground as you lengthen your torso up. Keep the spine long and, without curving the back, ease your way forward by bending in your hip joints. Go only as far as you can with a straight back and be careful not to roll the shoulders forward. Open the backs of the knees into the floor, bring the toes toward you, and find ease in the body as you breathe. Notice where you feel sensation and slowly float the head and torso back up.

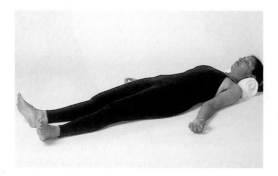

Corpse *(Savasana)* Slowly lower yourself onto your back. Resting on the floor, lengthen the neck muscles as you ease the head away from your feet. Wrap your arms around yourself and grasp your shoulder blades, easing them out to the sides. Lower the arms to the floor about 30 degrees out from the sides of the body, palms facing up. Gently press the lower back into the floor, then release it, allowing the natural curve of the spine to return. Lengthen the heels away from your torso, and let the heels roll out from the hips, feet opening out. Scan the body to find any areas of tension and let it go: in the face muscles, neck, shoulders, arms, torso, buttocks, abdomen and pelvis, legs, and feet. Rest here for at least 10 minutes as you follow the flow of your breath.

Exercise 5
T'ai Chi Movements

T'ai chi forms are sets of movements varying in length from five minutes to nearly one hour. The example illustrated here is an excerpt from a Yang style form. The orientation of the body is described in terms of north, south, east, and west directions. When starting, you should be facing north. Keep in mind that although the exercise is described as a series of steps, the movement is continuous.

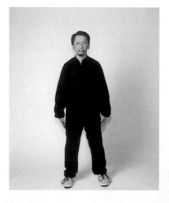

Starting Position Stand erect with feet shoulder-width apart, arms by your side, palms in toward the legs, chin up, and eyes looking directly ahead.

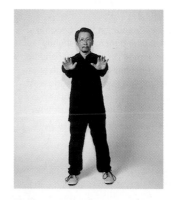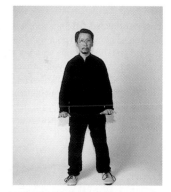

Beginning Position Leading with the wrists, raise your arms directly in front of the body to about shoulder level. Elbows should be slightly bent and shoulders relaxed. Leading with the elbows, slowly allow your arms and hands to return to starting position below waist level.

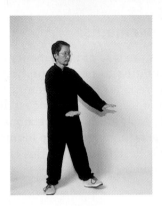
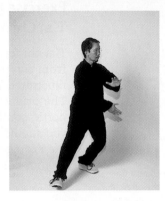
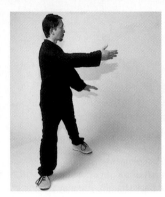

Right Hand Ward-Off With your weight on your right foot pivot your body left about 90 degrees. Keep your arms in front of you, palms down and at waist level. Once you've rotated your body, shift your weight to your left foot, bending at the knee. Bring your left hand up to mid-chest level, keeping the palm turned down. Keep your right hand at waist level but turn your palm up, keeping space between your hands. Step north with the right foot. Shifting your weight back to the right leg, extend your right arm and raise your right hand to shoulder level. Lower your left hand to waist level, keeping your palm down and your arm extended.

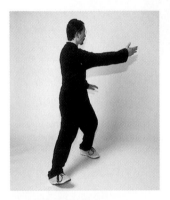
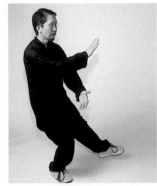
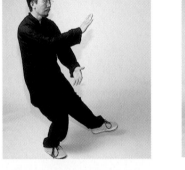

Left Hand Ward-Off Shift your weight back to your left foot, bending at the knee. Pivoting on your right heel, bring your right foot in slightly toward your body. Move your right arm, bringing your arm and hand up to chin level and keeping your arm outstretched. Shift your weight to your right leg, bending at the knee. Set the left foot on its heel, pointing west. Turn the palm of your right hand outward and start pulling your arm in toward your chest, bending at the elbow. Pull your left arm across your body so that it is underneath your right arm, and turn the palm inward.

Grasp the Bird's Tail Shift your weight forward to your left foot. While doing this movement, bring your left arm, still curved, across your body with the palm facing inward at chin level. Keep your right hand in front of you, palm facing outward. Turn the left hand out to face forward while pushing outward with both arms.

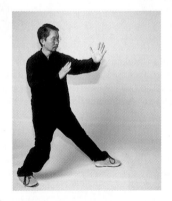
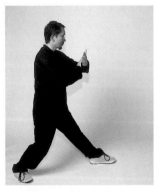
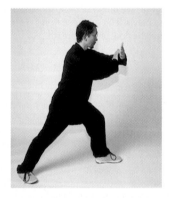

Rollback and Press Shift your weight backward onto your right leg, bending at the knee, and rotate your body to the right. Pull your right arm back toward your chest, bending at the elbow and keeping your palm facing the same direction as your body and at shoulder height. Rotate your body to the left, keeping your right arm close to your chest. Pull your left arm across your body and bring your palm toward your right hand as if the two were touching. As you shift your weight forward onto your left leg, push through the movement by pushing both arms forward in front of your body as if the right arm were pushing the left arm out at the wrist.

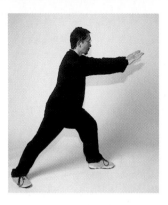 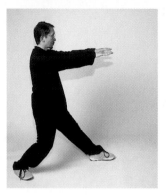 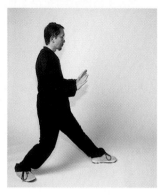 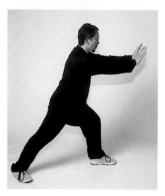

Push Continue to lean forward and extend your arms, turning both palms down with fingers pointing slightly upward. Release the wrists so the palms face down and pull back, shifting your weight to your right leg. Leading with your elbows, pull both arms down and toward your stomach. With your elbows bent, your forearms should be parallel to the floor with your palms facing forward. Shift your weight forward onto your left leg and extend your arms outward in front of you with palms continuing to face outward, as if you were pushing against a wall.

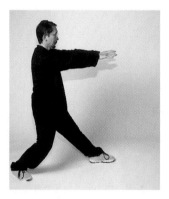 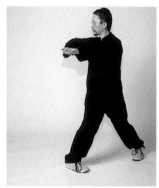

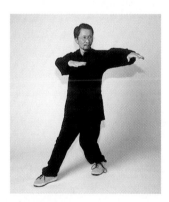 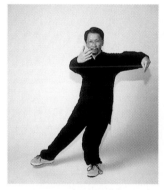 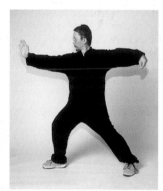

Holding a Single Whip With your arms still outstretched, release your wrists so your palms face the floor. Shift your weight back onto your right leg, bending at the knee. Keeping the right leg bent, pivot on your left heel, turning the foot in 90 degrees. Bend your right arm at the elbow and bring your right hand toward your chest, your palm continuing to face down. Keep your left arm extended out. Shift your weight to your left foot, bending at the knee, and pick up the right foot and step 45 degrees to the right. Keep your arms in the same position and rotate them around with your body. Your left hand points down toward the floor as you continue to shift your weight to your left foot, bringing the right foot off the floor and turning the leg outward (right foot points east). Turn the palm of your right hand to face toward you at chin level. Let the left wrist bend and the four fingers of the hand gather around the thumb to form a beak-hand. Shift your weight to the right onto your right leg and swing your right arm open so the palm faces outward. (The body and palm should now be facing east.) Keep your left arm out behind you.

APPENDIX B

Calendar of Events and Health Organizations

January

National Volunteer Blood Donor Month
American Association of Blood Banks
8101 Glenbrook Road
Bethesda, MD 20814
301-907-6977
www.aabb.org
Contact: Public Relations

February

American Heart Month
American Heart Association
7272 Greenville Avenue
Dallas, TX 75231
800-AHA-USA1
www.americanheart.org
Contact: Local chapters

National Children's Dental Health Month
American Dental Association
211 E. Chicago Avenue
Chicago, IL 60611
312-440-2593
www.ada.org
Contact: Public Information

National Child Passenger Safety Awareness Week
U.S. Department of Transportation
National Highway Traffic Safety Administration
400 Seventh Street, SW
Washington, DC 20590
202-366-0123
www.nhtsa.dot.gov

March

Hemophilia Month
National Hemophilia Foundation
116 West 32nd Street
11th Floor
New York, NY 10001
800-42-HANDI
www.hemophilia.org

National Kidney Month
National Kidney Foundation
30 E. 33rd Street, Suite 1100
New York, NY 10016
800-622-9010
www.kidney.org
Contact: Local chapters

National Chronic Fatigue Syndrome Awareness Month
National Chronic Fatigue Syndrome Association
3521 Broadway
Suite 222
Kansas City, MO 64111
816-931-4777

National Nutrition Month
American Dietetic Association
120 South Riverside Plaza
Suite 2000
Chicago, IL 60606-6995
800-877-1600
www.eatright.org

Red Cross Month
American Red Cross
National Headquarters
431 18th Street, NW
Washington, DC 20006
www.redcross.org
Contact: Public Inquiries

National Poison Prevention Week
Poison Prevention Week Council
4330 East West Highway
Bethesda, MD 20814
301-504-0580 x1184
Third full week in March

April

National Alcohol Awareness Month
National Council on Alcoholism and Drug Dependence
20 Exchange Place, Suite 2902
New York, NY 10005
212-269-7797
www.ncadd.org

Cancer Control Month
American Cancer Society
1599 Clifton Road, NE
Atlanta, GA 30329-4251
800-ACS-2345
www.cancer.org
Contact: Local chapters

National Child Abuse Prevention Month
National Committee to Prevent Child Abuse
2950 Tennyson Street
Denver, CO 80212
303-433-2541
www.childabuse.org

Alcohol-Free Weekend
Rhode Island Council on Alcoholism and Drug Dependence
500 Prospect Street
Pawtucket, RI 02860
800-622-7422

World Health Day
American Association for World Health
1825 K Street, NW
Suite 1208
Washington, DC 20006
202-466-5883
www.thebody.com/aawh/aawhpage.html

National Minority Cancer Awareness Week
National Cancer Institute
NCI Public Inquiries Office
Suite 3036A
6116 Executive Boulevard, MSC8322
Bethesda, MD 20892-8322
800-4-CANCER (Cancer Information Service)
http://nci.nih.gov

May

Clean Air Month
American Lung Association
61 Broadway, 6th Floor
New York, NY 10006
212-315-8700
www.lungusa.org

Mental Health Month
National Mental Health Association
2001 N. Beauregard Street, 12th Floor
Alexandria, VA 22311
703-684-7722
www.nmha.org

National High Blood Pressure Month
National Heart, Lung, and Blood Institute
P.O. Box 30105
Bethesda, MD 20824-0105
301-592-8573
www.nhlbi.nih.gov

National Physical Fitness and Sport Month
President's Council on Physical Fitness and Sports
200 Independence Avenue, SW
Humphrey Building, Room 738H
Washington, DC 20201
202-690-9000

Older Americans Month
Administration on Aging
One Massachusetts Avenue
Suites 4100 & 5100
Washington, DC 20201
202-619-0724
www.aoa.dhhs.gov

National Employee Health and Fitness Day
National Association for Health and Fitness
401 West Michigan Street
Suite 560
Indianapolis, IN 46202-3233
317-955-0957
www.physicalfitness.org
Third Wednesday in May

World No Tobacco Day
Coalition for World No Tobacco Day
P.O. Box 3543
New York, NY 10163
212-601-8245
www.wntd.com

June

Dairy Month
American Dairy Association
O'Hare International Center
10255 W. Higgins
Suite 900
Rosemont, IL 60018-5616
800-853-2479
www.dairyinfo.com

National Safety Week
American Society of Safety Engineers
1800 E. Oakton Street
Des Plaines, IL 60018-2187
847-699-2929
www.asse.org

July

National Therapeutic Recreation Week
National Therapeutic Recreation Society
22377 Belmont Ridge Road
Ashburn, VA 20148
703-858-0784
www.nrpa.org/index.cfm?publicationID=21

August

National Water Quality Month
Culligan International
One Culligan Parkway
Northbrook, IL 60062
847-205-6000
www.culligan.com

September

National Cholesterol Education Month
National Cholesterol Education Program
Program Information Center
P.O. Box 30105
Bethesda, MD 20824-0105
301-592-8573
www.nhlbi.nih.gov/cholmonth
Contact: Information Center

National Sickle Cell Month
Sickle Cell Disease Association of America
200 Corporate Pointe
Suite 495
Culver City, CA 90230-8727
800-421-8453

Treatment Works Month
**National Clearinghouse for Alcoholism and
   Drug Information**
P.O. Box 2345
Rockville, MD 20852
800-729-6686
www.health.org

October

Domestic Violence Awareness Month
National Coalition Against Domestic Violence
1120 Lincoln Street
Denver, CO 80203
www.ncadv.org

Family Health Month
American Academy of Family Physicians
11400 Tomahawk Creek Parkway
Leawood, KS 66211-2672
800-274-2237
www.aafp.org

National Breast Cancer Awareness Month
Susan G. Komen Breast Cancer Foundation
5005 LBJ Freeway
Suite 250
Dallas, TX 75244
972-855-1600
www.komen.org

National Collegiate Alcohol Awareness Week
**Interassociation Task Force on Campus Alcohol
   and Other Substance Abuse Issues**
P.O. Box 100430
Denver, CO 80250
Starts the third Sunday in October

World Food Day
National Committee for World Food Day
2175 K Street, NW
Washington, DC 20437
202-653-2404

American Heart Association's HeartFest
American Heart Association
7272 Greenville Avenue
Dallas, TX 75231
800-AHA-USA1
www.americanheart.org
Contact: Local chapters

National Adult Immunization Awareness Week
**National Coalition for Adult Immunization
   and National Foundation for Infectious Diseases**
4733 Bethesda Avenue
Suite 750
Bethesda, MD 20814-5278
301-656-0003
www.nfid.org/ncai
Last full week in October

November

National Alzheimer's Awareness Month

Alzheimer's Association
225 N. Michigan Avenue
Suite 1700
Chicago, IL 60601-7633
800-272-3900
www.alz.org

Great American Smokeout

American Cancer Society
1599 Clifton Road, NE
Atlanta, GA 30329-4251
800-ACS-2345
www.cancer.org
Contact: Local chapters

December

National Drunk and Drugged Driving Prevention Month

National Coalition Against Drunk Driving
8403 Colesville Road, Suite 370
Silver Spring, MD 20910
240-247-6004
www.ncadd.com

World AIDS Day

American Association for World Health
1825 K Street, NW
Suite 1208
Washington, DC 20006
202-466-5883
www.thebody.com/aawh/aawhpage.html

GLOSSARY

A

abortion: the expulsion or extraction of the products of conception from the uterus before the embryo or fetus is capable of independent life; abortions may be spontaneous or induced

accident: sequence of events that produces unintended injury, death, or property damage; refers to the event, not the result of the event

accident mitigation: methods to reduce damage caused by unplanned events

accident prevention: ways to eliminate the occurrence of unintended injuries

acetaldehyde: a toxic substance produced when the liver breaks alcohol down

acid rain: rain, snow, fog, mist, and the like with a pH lower than 5.6

acquaintance rape: (also known as "date rape") sexual assault occurring when the victim and the rapist are known to each other and may have previously interacted in some socially appropriate manner

acupuncture: an ancient Chinese medicine that uses thin needles inserted into specific points on the body to produce healing energy

addiction: physical and psychological dependence on a drug, substance, or behavior

adult attention deficit hyperactivity disorder (ADHD): difficulty focusing on activities, organizing and finishing tasks, managing one's time, following instructions, and/or being overly restless, "on the go," and perceived as not thinking before acting or speaking

advance directive: legal documents that express your desires regarding treatments should you be unable to communicate. A living will and a health care power of attorney constitute an advance directive

aerobic: biological energy production using oxygen

aerobic training: exercise that increases the body's capacity to use oxygen

afterbirth: placenta and fetal membranes

age-related hearing loss: loss of hearing with advancing age; some loss of hearing may be caused by exposure to loud noise earlier in life

age-related macular degeneration: loss of vision as a result of death of cells in a region of the eye called the macula; loss of vision progresses slowly over several years

agency: the belief that one can influence the nature and quality of one's life, rather than believing that one's fate is determined by reacting to circumstances not in one's control

aging: normal changes in body functions that begin after sexual maturity and continue until death

AIDS (acquired immune deficiency syndrome): a syndrome of more than two dozen diseases caused by HIV

AIDS antibody test: detects antibodies in blood that are produced in response to infection by HIV

alcohol abuse: frequent, continued use of alcohol; binge drinking

alcoholism: loss of control over drinking alcohol

allergens: foreign substances that trigger an allergic response by the immune system

alternative medicine: a therapy or healing procedure that is used instead of Western, scientific medical treatments

alveoli: tiny air sacs in the lungs that exchange oxygen and carbon dioxide

Alzheimer's disease: a common cause of senile dementia and other symptoms, eventually leading to death

amenorrhea: cessation of menstruation

amino acids: compounds containing nitrogen that are the building blocks of protein

amniocentesis: a procedure that involves aspiration of amniotic fluid from the uterus to detect certain abnormalities in the fetus

amnion: the inner membrane that forms a fluid-filled sac surrounding and protecting the embryo and fetus

amniotic fluid: fluid in the amniotic sac

amphetamines: synthetic drugs that stimulate the central nervous system and sometimes produce hallucinogenic states

amyloid protein: an abnormal protein in the brain of patients with Alzheimer's disease

anaerobic: biological energy production without using oxygen

anaphylactic shock: a severe allergic reaction involving the whole body that can cause death

androgenic anabolic steroids: synthetic male hormones used to increase muscle size and strength

anemia: a deficiency of red blood cells; often caused by insufficient iron

aneurysm: a ballooning out of a vein or artery

angina pectoris: medical term for chest pain caused by coronary heart disease; a condition in which the heart muscle doesn't receive enough blood, resulting in chest pain

anogenital warts: hard growths caused by an infection with human papillomavirus (HPV) that appear on the skin of the genitals or anus

anorexia nervosa: disorder occurring most commonly in adolescent females, characterized by abnormal body image, fear of obesity, and prolonged refusal to eat, sometimes resulting in death

antibodies: proteins that recognize and inactivate viruses, bacteria, and other organisms and toxic substances that enter the body

antigens: foreign proteins on infectious organisms that stimulate an antibody response

antioxidants: substances that in small amounts inhibit the oxidation of other compounds

anxiety: the fear of an imaginary threat

aorta: the large artery that transports blood from the heart to the body

aromatherapy: use of fragrant extracts of plants to promote healing

arteries: any one of a series of blood vessels that carry blood from the heart to all parts of the body

arteriosclerosis: hardening of the arteries

arthritis: a variety of chronic diseases involving inflammation, stiffness, and pain in joints of the body

artificial fats: chemicals added to packaged foods to provide the taste and texture of fat but few or no calories

artificial insemination: introduction of semen into the uterus or oviduct by other than natural means

asthma: a chronic disease involving inflammation and narrowing of the airways that makes it difficult to breathe

atherosclerosis: a disease process in which fatty deposits (plaques) build up in the arteries and block the flow of blood

atrial fibrillation: rapid, erratic contraction of the upper chambers of the heart

autogenic training: the use of autosuggestion to establish a balance between the mind and body through changes in the autonomic nervous system

autoimmune diseases: mistakes in the functioning of the immune system that cause it to attack tissues in the body

autonomic nervous system: the special group of nerves that control some of the body's organs and their functions

average life span: the age at which half the members of a population have died

Ayurvedic medicine: a traditional form of preventive medicine and healing, involving mind, body, and spirit, practiced in India for thousands of years. Ayurveda is spreading to Western countries

B

B-cells: cells of the immune system that produce antibodies

bacterial vaginosis (BV): vaginal infection from overgrowth of some kinds of vaginal bacteria

basal body temperature (BBT) method: uses daily body temperature readings taken immediately after waking to identify the time of ovulation; approximately 24 hours after ovulation, the BBT increases

basal cell carcinoma: a form of skin cancer that usually can be removed surgically

basal metabolic rate (BMR): the amount of energy needed per day to keep the body functioning while at rest

basal metabolism: the minimum amount of energy needed to keep the body alive

bender: several days of binge drinking

benign tumor: a tumor whose cells do not spread to other parts of the body

binge eating disorder: an uncontrolled consumption of large quantities of food in a short period of time, even if the person does not feel hungry

biofeedback: using an electronic device to "feed back" information about the body to alter a particular physiological function

biomagnetic therapy: use of magnetic fields to treat pain, ailments, and diseases

biomonitoring: measurement of environmental chemicals present in the body that may harm health

biopsy: removal of cells from a tumor for examination under a microscope

bipolar disorder: episodes of depression followed by episodes of mania

bisphenol-A (BPA): chemical used to manufacture polycarbonate plastics; may cause abnormal brain development in fetuses and birth defects

blackout: failure to recall normal or abnormal behavior or events that occurred while drinking

blood alcohol content (BAC): the amount of alcohol in the blood

body composition: the relative amounts of the body's major components

body dysmorphic disorder: a preoccupation with an imagined defect in one or more of one's body parts

body image: a person's mental image of his or her body

body mass index: a measure of body fatness, calculated by dividing body weight (in kilograms) by the square of height (in meters)

Braxton-Hicks contractions: normal uterine contractions that occur periodically throughout pregnancy

breasts: a network of milk glands and ducts in fatty tissue

bronchitis: inflammation of the bronchi of the lungs as a result of irritation; often accompanied by a chronic cough

bulimia: serious disorder, especially common in adolescents and young women, marked by excessive eating, often followed by self-induced vomiting, purging, or fasting

C

C-reactive protein (CRP): a protein in blood that is a measure of chronic inflammation and risk of a heart attack

caffeine: a natural stimulant found in a variety of plants; commonly found in tea, coffee, chocolate, and soft drinks

calendar rhythm: estimation of fertile, or unsafe, days to have intercourse

caloric restriction: restricting the daily caloric intake of an animal or person while maintaining adequate nutrient intake

calorie: the amount of energy required to raise 1 g of water from 14.5°C to 15.5°C

cancer: unregulated multiplication of cells in the body

cancer susceptibility gene: gene responsible for familial breast cancer and genes that cause susceptibility to colon cancer; increases the risk of a person developing cancer in his or her lifetime

capillaries: extremely small blood vessels that carry oxygenated blood to tissues

carbohydrates: the main source of biological energy; biological molecules consisting of one or more sugar molecules

carcinogens: substances that can cause cancer in people and other animals

cardiac catheterization: visualization of blocked coronary arteries using a catheter and monitoring blood flow in coronary arteries; a dye is injected through the catheter

cardiologist: a physician who specializes in diseases of the heart

cardiopulmonary resuscitation (CPR): an emergency lifesaving procedure used to revive someone who has stopped breathing or suffered cardiac arrest

cardiorespiratory fitness: the degree to which the body can supply sufficient fuel and oxygen to produce sustained, effortful physical activity

cardiovascular disease: any disease that causes damage to the heart or to major arteries leading from the heart

carotid endarterectomy: removal of fatty deposits in arteries in the neck to prevent a stroke

celibacy: sexual abstinence

cell-mediated immunity: the response of T-cells to infections

cellulose: a carbohydrate forming the skeleton of most plant structures and plant cells; the most abundant polysaccharide in nature and the source of dietary fiber

cervical cap: small latex cap that covers the cervix, used with spermicidal jelly or cream inside the cap

cervix: the lower, narrow end of the uterus

cesarean section (C-section): delivery of the fetus through a surgical opening in the abdomen and uterus

challenge situations: positive events that may involve major life transitions and may cause stress

chancre: the primary lesion of syphilis, which appears as a hard, painless sore or ulcer, often on the penis or vaginal tissue

chemical carcinogen: a chemical that damages cells and causes cancer

chemotherapy: use of toxic chemicals to kill cancer cells and treat some forms of cancer

chewing tobacco: a form of shredded smokeless tobacco; chewed or placed in the mouth between the lower lip and gum

chi: a Chinese term referring to the balance of energy in the body

child abuse: physical or mental injury, sexual abuse or exploitation, maltreatment, or neglect of a child by a person who is responsible for the child's welfare

chiropractic: an alternative medicine that uses manipulation of the spine and joints for healing

chlamydia: a sexually transmitted disease caused by the bacterium *Chlamydia trachomatis*

chlorofluorocarbons (CFCs): chemicals formerly used as coolants that are released into the atmosphere and are responsible for destroying stratospheric ozone

cholesterol: a fatlike compound occurring in bile, blood, brain, nerve tissue, liver, and other parts of the body

chorionic villus sampling (CVS): a method to detect biochemical disorders and chromosomal abnormalities in the fetus

chromosomes: threadlike structures in the nuclei of cells that carry an individual's genetic information

chronic disease: a disease that persists for years or even a lifetime

chronic obstructive pulmonary diseases (COPD): diseases that restrict the ability of the body to obtain oxygen through the respiratory structures (bronchi and lungs); includes asthma, bronchitis, and emphysema

cilia: microscopic hairs in the lining of the bronchial tubes

circumcision: a surgical procedure to remove the foreskin from the penis

clitoris: erotically sensitive structure located above the vaginal opening

cloning: the process of making genetically identical plants or animals

club drugs: psychoactive chemicals used at parties, dances, festivals, and raves to enhance social experiences and increase sensory stimulation

cocaine: a stimulant drug, obtained from the leaves of the coca shrub, that causes feelings of exhilaration, euphoria, and physical vigor

codependency: a relationship pattern in which the non-addicted family members identify with the alcoholic

cognition: the act or process of knowing

colostrum: yellowish liquid secreted from the breasts; contains antibodies and protein

combination hormonal contraceptives: pills, a skin patch, a vaginal insert, and injections that contain two kinds of synthetic hormones that are chemically similar to a woman's natural ovarian hormones, estrogen and progesterone

communicable disease: an infectious disease that is usually transmitted from person to person

complementary medicine: an alternative medicine that is used along with conventional medicine. Usually there is some scientific evidence for the effectiveness and safety of the alternative medicine

complex carbohydrates: a class of carbohydrates called polysaccharides; foods composed of starch and cellulose

concussion: a blow to the head that causes injury, temporary loss of consciousness, and possibly a period of amnesia upon awakening

condom: a latex or polyurethane sheath worn over the penis (male condom) or inside the vagina (female condom); can be both a barrier method of contraception and act as a prophylactic against sexually transmitted diseases

congeners: flavorings, colorings, and other chemicals present in alcoholic beverages

congenital (birth) defect: any abnormality observed in a newborn that occurred during development

conscious: being aware of one's thoughts, beliefs, and emotions

contact dermatitis: an allergic reaction of the skin to something that is touched

contraceptive sponge: a dome-shaped device coated with spermicide

contraindication: any medical reason for not taking a particular drug

coping: efforts to manage a stressful situation regardless of whether those efforts are successful

coping strategies: ways people devise to prevent, avoid, or control the emotional distress of unfulfilled needs

coronary arteries: two arteries arising from the aorta that supply blood to the heart muscle

coronary artery bypass surgery: surgery to improve blood supply to the heart muscle by replacing the damaged portion of the artery with a graft

cosmetic surgery: surgery performed not for any medical condition but solely to enhance appearance or correct visible effects of aging

Cowper's glands: small glands secreting drops of alkalinizing fluid into the urethra

creatine: a natural substance in skeletal muscle tissue required for muscle contraction, which can also be purchased as a dietary supplement

cross-training: incorporating more than one activity into a regular activity plan

cystitis: inflammation of the bladder

cytokines: small molecules that coordinate the activities of B-cells and T-cells

D

dangerous (high-risk or binge) drinking: drinking behavior that results in unintended or undesirable harmful consequences for oneself and others

decibel: a measure of noise level

defense mechanisms: mental strategies for avoiding unpleasant thoughts and emotions

defibrillator: an electrical device that can restart a heart that has stopped beating by delivering electrical shocks to it

delirium tremens (DTs): hallucinations and uncontrollable shaking sometimes caused by withdrawal of alcohol in alcohol-dependent individuals

denial: refusal to admit you (or someone else) have a drinking problem

deoxyribonucleic acid (DNA): a nucleic acid of complex molecular structure occurring in cell nuclei; carrier of the genes; present in all body cells of every species

depression: a mental state characterized by feelings of helplessness, hopelessness, and self-recrimination

diagnosis: the cause of a disease or illness as determined by a physician

diaphragm: a soft, rubber, dome-shaped contraceptive device worn over the cervix and used with spermicidal jelly or cream

diastole: the pressure in the arteries when the heart relaxes (the lower number)

dietary supplements: products that provide one or more of the 40 essential nutrients or nonessential vitamins, minerals, enzymes, amino acids, herbs, hormones, and nucleic acids

direct-to-consumer advertising (DTCA): the marketing of prescription drugs to consumers to stimulate demand for a drug

distress: stress resulting from unpleasant stressors

DNA (deoxyribonucleic acid): the chemical substance that carries all of a person's genetic information in chromosomes in cells

dose: amount of drug that is administered

double-blind: when neither the person receiving the drug nor the person administering the drug knows whether it is a placebo or the real drug

douching: rinsing the vaginal canal with a liquid; not an effective means of birth control or STD prevention

drug: a single chemical substance in a medicine that alters one or more of the body's biological functions

drug abuse: persistent or excessive use of a drug without medical or health reasons

drug hypersensitivity: an allergic reaction to a drug

dysmenorrhea: abdominal pain during menstruation ("menstrual cramps")

dysthymia: a long-lasting, mild form of depression

E

Ecstasy (MDMA): a club drug with both stimulant and pleasurable effects

ectopic pregnancy: a pregnancy occurring outside the uterus, usually in a fallopian tube

elder abuse: physical, sexual, or emotional maltreatment or financial exploitation of an adult aged 60 or older

electromagnetic fields (EMFs): a form of radiation produced by electrical power lines and appliances that may increase the risk of cancer

embryo: the developing infant during the first two months of conception

embryonic stem cells: cells derived from human fertilized eggs and grown in laboratory dishes; stem cells have the capacity to differentiate into many different tissues and organs

emission: amount of substance that is released into the atmosphere

emotion-focused coping: appraising and accepting a stressful situation as not immediately changeable and adopting an attitude that lessens anxiety and brings comfort

emotional wellness: understanding emotions and knowing how to cope with problems that arise in everyday life, and how to endure stress

emphysema: a progressive degeneration of the lung alveoli, causing breathing and oxygen assimilation to become more and more difficult

enabling: denial of, or excuses for, the excessive drinking by an alcoholic to whom one is close

endocrine disruptors: chemical substances in the environment that interfere with the action of one or more of the body's hormones

endometrium: the inner lining of the uterus

endurance: the ability to move an object without becoming quickly fatigued

energy balance: when energy consumed as food equals the energy expended in living

environment: all external physical factors that affect us

environmental model: modern analyses of ecosystems and environmental risks to health, such as socioeconomic status, education, and various environmental factors that affect health

ephedra: an herb that is a stimulant

epidemiology: a branch of science that studies the causes and frequencies of diseases in human populations

epididymitis: inflammation of the epididymis, a structure that connects the vas deferens and the testes

episiotomy: an incision in the perineum to facilitate passage of the baby's head during childbirth, while minimizing injury to the woman

ergogenic aids: substances used to increase strength and endurance

erythropoetin: a hormone that increases the number of red blood cells, thus increasing the body's ability to carry oxygen to tissues

essential amino acids: amino acids that cannot be synthesized by the body and must be provided by food

essential fat: necessary body fat required for normal physiological functioning

essential (primary) hypertension: high blood pressure that is not caused by any observable disease

essential nutrients: chemical substances obtained from food and needed by the body for growth, maintenance, or repair of tissues; not made by the body; must be obtained from food

ethyl alcohol (ethanol): the consumable type of alcohol that is the psychoactive ingredient in alcoholic beverages; often called grain alcohol

etiology: specific cause of disease

eustress: stress resulting from pleasant stressors

exposure: actual amount of the substance people are exposed to

F

failure rate: likelihood of becoming pregnant if using a birth control method for one year

fallopian tubes: the usual site of fertilization; a pair of tubelike structures that transport ova from the ovaries to the uterus

familial hyperlipidemia (FH): an inherited disease causing extremely high levels of cholesterol in the blood

fat-soluble vitamins: soluble in fat; there are four fat-soluble vitamins

fatty acids: naturally occurring in fats, either saturated or unsaturated (monounsaturated or polyunsaturated)

feedback: response of the receiver of a message to let the sender know the message was received

female athlete triad: combination of disordered eating, cessation of menstruation (amenorrhea), and weakened bones (osteoporosis)

fertility awareness methods: methods of birth control in which a couple charts the cyclic signs of the woman's fertility and ovulation, and/or uses basal body temperature, mucus changes, and other signs to determine fertile periods

fertility cycle: the near-monthly production of fertilizable eggs

fertilization: the fusion of a sperm cell and an ovum

fetal alcohol syndrome: birth defects and mental disabilities caused by ingestion of alcohol by the mother during pregnancy

fiber: a group of compounds that make up the framework of plants; fiber cannot be digested

fight-or-flight response: a defensive reaction that prepares the organism for conflict or escape by triggering hormonal, cardiovascular, metabolic, and other changes

first-stage labor: the beginning of labor during which there are regular contractions of the uterus

follicle-stimulating hormone: stimulates ovaries to develop mature follicles (with eggs); the follicle produces estrogen

food allergies: allergic responses to something that is eaten

Food Guide Pyramid: guidelines for a healthful diet based on grains, fruits, and vegetables

forcible rape: sexual assault using force or threat of force and involving sexual penetration of the victim's vagina, mouth, or rectum

foreskin: a fold of skin over the end of the penis

free radicals: oxidizing substances in the body that can damage blood vessels and tissues

fructose: a simple sugar found in fruits and honey

functional food: a food to which additional vitamins, minerals, herbs, or other substances are added to allow the manufacturer to make health claims

fungicide: a chemical that kills fungi and molds

G

galactose: a monosaccharide derived from lactose

gamma-hydroxybutyrate (GHB): a dangerous club drug with unpleasant side effects

gamma irradiation: nonchemical method of food preservation

gene therapy: a technique for replacing defective genes with normal ones in certain tissues of a person affected with a hereditary disease

general adaptation syndrome (GAS): a three-phase biological response to stress

generalized anxiety disorder: persistent and often nonspecific worry and anxiety

genetic counseling: information to help prospective parents evaluate the risks of having or delivering a genetically handicapped child

gerontology: science that studies the causes and mechanisms of aging

glucose: the principal source of energy in all cells; also called dextrose

glycogen: the form in which carbohydrate is stored in humans and animals

goiter: an enlargement of the thyroid gland resulting from lack of iodine, causing a swelling in the front part of the neck

gonorrhea: sexually transmitted disease caused by gonococcal bacteria (*Neisseria gonorrhoeae*)

greenhouse effect: the ability of atmospheric carbon dioxide to reflect heat radiated from the earth back to the earth and to thereby raise the earth's temperature globally

growth needs: human needs that include social belonging, self-esteem, and spiritual growth

H

habituation: psychological dependence arising from repeated use of a drug

hallucinogens: psychoactive substances that alter sensory processing in the brain, producing visual or auditory sensations that are not real (i.e., that are hallucinatory)

hangover: unpleasant physical sensations resulting from excessive alcohol consumption

harm-and-loss situations: stressful events that include death, loss of property, injury, and illness

hashish: the sticky resin of the *Cannabis* plant

hate crime: an unlawful act committed against a person, group, or place that is motivated by hate or bias

health: state of sound physical, mental, and social well-being

health care power of attorney: designates someone to make health care decisions for you if you are unable to communicate

health maintenance organization (HMO): an organization (either nonprofit or for-profit) of physicians, hospitals, and support staff that provides medical services to members

heart attack: death of, or damage to, part of the heart muscle caused by an insufficient blood supply

hemicellulose: substances found in plant cell walls that are composed of various sugars chemically linked together

hemophilia: a hereditary disease (primarily in men) caused by lack of an essential blood clotting factor; results in excessive bleeding in response to any scratch or injury

hepatitis: serious disease of the liver caused by hepatitis viruses B, C, or D; also caused by chemicals and alcohol

herbal medicines: materials derived from plants and other organisms that are made into teas, powders, and salves to treat diseases and injuries

herbicide: a chemical that kills weeds

hereditary (genetic) disease: any disease resulting from the inheritance of defective genes or chromosomes from one or both parents

herpes: sexually transmitted disease caused by herpes simplex virus, HSV

hierarchy of needs: a progression of human requirements, including physiological needs, safety, love, self-esteem, and self-actualization

high-density lipoprotein (HDL): the carrier of cholesterol from tissues to the liver for removal from the circulation; carrier of "good" cholesterol

histamine: a chemical released by cells in an allergic response; causes inflammation

histocompatibility: the degree to which the antigens on cells of different persons are similar

HIV (human immunodeficiency virus): the virus defined as the cause of AIDS

HLA (human leukocyte antigens): antigens that are measured to determine the suitability of an organ for transplantation from donor to recipient

holistic model: encompasses the physiological, mental, emotional, social, spiritual, and environmental aspects of health

homeopathy: an alternative medicine that administers very dilute solutions of substances that mimic the patient's symptoms

homeostasis: the tendency for body systems to interact in ways that maintain a constant physiological state

homocysteine: a substance derived from the amino acid methionine; high blood levels increase the risk of heart disease; blood levels are reduced with adequate intake of folic acid

hormone replacement therapy (HRT): administration of estrogen to menopausal and postmenopausal women to help prevent symptoms of menopause, osteoporosis, and heart disease

hormones: chemicals produced in the body that regulate body functions

hospice: a place for terminally ill patients to spend the time before death in an environment that attends to their physical, emotional, and spiritual needs but no further treatments are administered; hospice care also can be given in a patient's home

hostility: a personal trait characterized by an ongoing mistrust of others, cynicism, a personal emotional style of anger mixed with disgust and contempt, and a tendency to act out those feelings with overt aggression, snide comments, or criticism

human chorionic gonadotropin (HCG): a hormone produced during the first stages of pregnancy; it is used as a basis for pregnancy tests

human growth hormone: a naturally occurring pituitary hormone

human immunodeficiency virus (HIV): the virus that causes AIDS; it causes a defect in the body's immune system by invading and then multiplying within certain white blood cells

human papillomavirus (HPV): a genus of viruses including those causing papillomas (small nipple-like protrusions of the skin or mucous membrane) and warts

humoral immunity: the response of B-cells to infections

hypertension: high blood pressure

hypnotherapy: the use of hypnosis to treat sickness

hypnotics: central nervous system depressants used to induce drowsiness and encourage sleep

hypothalamo-pituitary-adrenal (HPA) axis: a coordinated physiological response to stress involving the hypothalamus of the brain and the pituitary and adrenal glands

hysterectomy: surgical removal of the uterus

I

I-statements: statements beginning with "I"; positive communication skill

image visualization: use of mental images to promote healing and change behaviors

immune system: an interacting system of organs and cells that protect the body from infectious organisms and harmful substances

immunizations: vaccinations to prevent a variety of serious diseases caused by both bacteria and viruses

immunosuppressive drugs: drugs to suppress the functions of the immune system (e.g., after organ transplants)

in vitro fertilization (IVF): a procedure in which an egg is removed from a ripe follicle and fertilized by a sperm cell outside the human body; the fertilized egg is allowed to divide in a protected environment for about two days and then is inserted into the uterus

incidence: the number of new cases of a particular disease

infarction: death of heart cells resulting from a blocked blood supply

infertile: unable to become pregnant or to impregnate

ingredients label: label on a manufactured food that lists the ingredients in descending order by weight

inhalants: vaporous substances that, when inhaled, produce alcohol-like intoxication

injury epidemiology: the study of the occurrence, causes, and prevention of injury

insecticide: a chemical that kills insects

insoluble fiber: cannot be dissolved in water

insomnia: prolonged inability to obtain adequate sleep

integrative medicine: physicians who combine the practice of scientific, Western medicine with alternative medicines that they feel are safe and effective for their patients

intellectual wellness: having a mind open to new ideas and concepts

intimate partner violence (IPV): physical, sexual, or psychological harm by a current or former intimate partner or spouse

intrauterine device (IUD): a flexible, usually plastic, device inserted into the uterus to prevent pregnancy

ionizing radiation: radiation, such as x-rays, that can damage cells and cause cancer; also used to treat cancer

ischemia: an insufficient supply of blood to the heart

isometric training: a type of strength training

isopropyl alcohol: rubbing alcohol, sometimes used as an anesthetic

K

karyotype: visual display of all of a person's chromosomes that can detect chromosomal abnormalities characteristic of inherited diseases

ketamine: an anesthetic used as a club drug

kilocalorie: unit of energy; the amount of heat needed to raise 1 kilogram of water 1°C, equivalent to 1,000 calories

L

labia majora: a pair of fleshy folds that cover the labia minora

labia minora: a pair of fleshy folds that cover the vagina

labor: the process of childbirth

lactase: enzyme secreted by glands in the small intestine that converts lactose (milk sugar) into simple sugars

lacto-ovo-vegetarian: one who excludes meats, poultry, and fish, but includes eggs and dairy products

lacto-vegetarian: one who excludes meat, poultry, fish, and eggs, but includes dairy products

lactose: a molecule of glucose and galactose chemically bonded together; found primarily in milk

laryngospasm: spasm of the larynx caused by inhaling water

Leading Health Indicators: ten categories of health goals that represent the major public health concerns in the United States

lecithin: an essential component of cell membranes

leukocytes: white blood cells that fight infections

life expectancy: average number of years a person can expect to live

lifestyle drugs: drugs prescribed for conditions that arise from certain living habits or from the natural process of aging

lightening: the positioning of the fetus for birth by descent in the uterus

linoleic acid: an essential fat that must be obtained from food

lipids: fats such as cholesterol and triglycerides

liposuction: surgery used to remove fat under the skin to reshape parts of the body

literal message: a message that is conveyed by symbols

living will: a legal document that expresses your wishes regarding treatment if you become unable to make your own medical decisions

low-density lipoprotein (LDL): the carrier of "bad" cholesterol in blood

lowest observed failure rate: likelihood of becoming pregnant if using a birth control method consistently and as intended

LSD: a powerful hallucinogenic chemical; ingestion alters brain chemistry and produces a variety of hallucinogenic and behavioral effects

lupus erythematosus: an autoimmune disease that mostly affects women

luteinizing hormone: anterior pituitary hormone that causes a follicle to release a ripened ovum and become a corpus luteum; in the male, it stimulates testosterone production and the production of sperm cells

Lyme disease: a serious, difficult-to-diagnose infectious disease caused by bacteria deposited by ticks when they bite

lymph nodes: nodules spaced along the lymphatic vessels that trap infectious organisms or foreign particles

lymphatic system: a system of vessels in the body that trap foreign organisms and particles; the immune system is part of the lymphatic system

M

macrophages: specialized cells that destroy and eliminate foreign particles and microorganisms from the body

magnetic resonance imaging (MRI): use of a strong magnetic field to produce images of internal parts of the body; especially useful for soft tissues

maintenance needs: human needs that include physical safety and survival requirements, such as food and water

major depression: a mental state characterized by feelings of hopelessness, helplessness, and self-recrimination

malaria: a disease of red blood cells that produces fever, anemia, and death

malignant tumor: a tumor whose cells spread throughout the body

mammogram: x-ray picture used to detect tumors in the breast

managed care: systems of health care in which the primary goal is to reduce costs

mandala: an artistic, religious design used as an object of meditation

mantra: a sound or phrase that is repeated in the mind to help produce a meditative state

manual vacuum aspiration: the most common abortion method, in which the uterus is emptied with the gentle suction of a manual syringe

marijuana: a psychoactive substance present in the dried leaves, stems, flowers, and seeds of plants of the genus *Cannabis*

masturbation: self-induced sexual stimulation

maximum life span: the theoretical maximum number of years that individuals of a species can live

medical abortion: nonsurgical abortion using medications to stop pregnancy

medical model: interprets health in terms of the absence of disease and disability

medicalization: medical treatment of conditions, behaviors, or traits that generally were not regarded as illnesses or medical problems

medicine: drugs used to prevent, treat, or cure illness; aid healing; or suppress symptoms

melanoma: a particularly dangerous form of skin cancer

menarche: the beginning of menstruation

menopause: the cessation of menstruation in midlife

menstrual cycle: the period of time from one menstruation to another

menstruation: the regular sloughing of the uterine lining via the vagina

mental health: a sense of optimism, vitality, and well-being, and intentional behaviors that lead to productive activities, fulfilling relationships with others, and the ability to adapt to change and cope with adversity

mental illness: alterations in thinking, emotions, and/or intentional behaviors that produce psychological distress and/or impaired functioning

meridians: the channels along the body where energy flows and where acupuncture points are located

mesothelioma: a form of lung cancer caused by asbestos

metabolic equivalents (METs): per-minute multiples of the amount of energy used while sitting or lying still

metabolic syndrome: a model embracing five risk factors that puts people who have at least three risk factors at risk for cardiovascular disease, diabetes, and premature death

metabolism: the process of obtaining energy and matter from the chemical breakdown of molecules obtained from food or from the body

metamessage: how the message is interpreted between sender and receiver

metastasis: the process by which cancer cells spread throughout the body

methyl alcohol: wood alcohol or methanol

minerals: inorganic elements found in the body both in combination with organic compounds and alone

mini-pill: a progestin-only contraceptive pill

moist snuff: a form of snuff made from air- and fire-cured tobacco leaves; most hazardous form of smokeless tobacco

mononucleosis: an infectious disease caused by the Epstein-Barr virus, common among college-age adults

monounsaturated fatty acid: carries one less than all the hydrogen atoms it possibly could

morbidity: the number of persons in a population who are ill

mortality: death rate: number of deaths per unit of population (e.g., per 100, 10,000, or 1,000,000) in a specific region, age range, or other group

multiple sclerosis (MS): an autoimmune disease that affects the central nervous system

mutations: permanent changes in the genetic information in a cell; only mutations in sperm and eggs are inherited

myelin: a substance that sheaths and insulates nerve fibers in the brain and spinal cord

myocardium: muscular wall of the heart that contracts and relaxes

myotonia: muscle tension

MyPyramid: an educational tool based on the principles of the 2005 Dietary Guidelines for Americans and other nutritional standards to help consumers make healthier food and activity choices

N

narcolepsy: extreme tendency to fall asleep during the day

naturopathy: an alternative medicine that uses nutrition, herbs, massage, and other techniques to promote healing

nicotine: an addicting chemical in tobacco that produces rapid pulse, increased alertness, and a variety of other physiological effects

nicotine replacement therapy: using nicotine-containing gum, skin patches, nasal sprays, or inhalers to temper the symptoms of nicotine withdrawal when quitting smoking

nitrates: preservatives containing any salt or ester of nitric acid. Some individuals are sensitive to nitrates and may suffer from headache, diarrhea, or urticaria after ingesting them

nitrites: preservatives containing any salt or ester of nitrous acid

nonessential amino acids: eleven amino acids required for protein synthesis that are synthesized by humans and are not specifically required in the diet

nutraceutical: a dietary supplement intended to prevent or treat an illness or disease

nutrition facts label: label on a manufactured food that lists the quantity of certain nutrients in the food and the percent daily value for those nutrients

nutritional calorie: unit of energy; often used interchangeably with the term *kilocalorie*

O

obesity: storage fat exceeding 30% of body weight

obsessive-compulsive disorder: persistent, unwelcome thoughts or images and the urgent need to engage in certain rituals

occupational wellness: enjoyment of what you are doing to earn a living and contribute to society

open-heart surgery: surgery performed on the opened heart while the blood supply is diverted through a heart–lung machine

opiates: central nervous system depressants derived from the opium poppy

opportunistic infection: any infectious disease in a patient with a weakened immune system; often occurs in AIDS patients

optimism: the thought process of imagining a high probability of attaining a goal

orgasm: the climax of sexual responses and the release of physiological and sexual tensions

osteopathy: an alternative medicine that uses manipulation and medicines for healing; osteopaths receive training comparable to that of physicians and can prescribe drugs

osteoporosis: a condition in older people, particularly women, in which bones lose density and become porous and brittle

ova: female eggs (singular, *ovum*)

ovaries: a pair of almond-shaped organs in the female abdomen that produce egg cells (ova) and female sex hormones

overload: the feeling that there are too many demands on one's time and energy from being confronted with too many challenges

over-the-counter (OTC) drugs: drugs that do not require a prescription

overuse injuries: injuries to muscles, tendons, ligaments, and joints resulting from too much exercise

ovulation: release of an egg (ovum) from the ovary

oxidation: the chemical term for the process of oxygen-present energy production

oxytocin: hormone that promotes release of milk; also can cause muscles in the uterine wall to contract

ozone hole: an ozone-deficient portion of the atmosphere above Antarctica that has been steadily growing since the problem was first reported in 1985

ozone layer: a layer of ozone molecules located in the stratosphere in a diffuse band extending from 10 to 30 miles above the earth's surface

P

pacemaker: an electrical device implanted in the chest to control irregular heartbeats

panic disorder: severe anxiety accompanied by physical symptoms

parasomnias: activities that interrupt restful sleep

Parkinson's disease: a neurodegenerative disease in which brain functions that control movements of the body gradually are lost

pathogen: a disease-causing organism

pathologist: a physician who specializes in the causes of diseases

pedometer: a step-counter

penicillin: an antibiotic produced by mold and capable of curing many bacterial infections

penis: the male's organ of copulation and urination

perceived social support: believing that support from one's social network is available if needed

percent daily value: percentage of the recommended daily amount of a particular nutrient found in a food

percutaneous transluminal coronary angioplasty (PTCA): a procedure to open blocked arteries

pessimism: the thought process of imagining a low probability of attaining a goal

pesticide: a chemical that kills unwanted plants and animals

pharmacogenetics: tailoring drugs to a particular individual to match his or her biology

phencyclidine (PCP): drug that, depending on the route of administration and dose, can be a stimulant, depressant, or hallucinogen; originally developed as an animal anesthetic

phobia: a powerful and irrational fear of something

photochemical smog: air pollution from the action of sunlight on emissions from motor vehicles and industrial sources

phthalates: chemicals used in the manufacture of various plastics; may cause abnormal genital development in males and premature breast development in girls

physical activity level (PAL): a measure of the amount of energy expended per day over and above that used for basal metabolism

physical dependence: a physiological state that depends on the continuous presence of a drug; absence of the drug may cause discomfort, nervousness, headaches, and sweating (withdrawal symptoms) and sometimes death

physical wellness: maintenance of your body in good condition by eating right, exercising regularly, avoiding harmful habits, and making informed responsible decisions about your health

physician-assisted suicide: a form of active euthanasia in which a physician helps a patient who no longer desires to live because of pain or an incurable illness to commit suicide

phytochemicals: chemicals produced by plants

Pilates: a system of stretching and strengthening exercises

placebo effect: healing that results from a person's belief in a treatment that has no medicinal value

placenta: the flat circular vascular structure within the pregnant uterus that provides nourishment to and eliminates wastes from the developing embryo and fetus and is passed as afterbirth after the baby is born

plaque: deposit of fatty substances in the inner lining of arteries

plumbism: disease caused by lead poisoning

poison: any chemical substance that causes illness, injury, or death

polyunsaturated fatty acid: carries at least two fewer hydrogen atoms than it would if saturated

posttraumatic stress disorder (PTSD): physical and mental illnesses resulting from severe trauma

preferred provider organization (PPO): physicians who belong to the organization provide medical care at reduced costs that are negotiated by the organization

premenstrual dysphoric disorder (PMDD): premenstrual symptoms severe enough to impair personal functioning

prevalence: the number of people within a population with a particular disease

probiotic therapy: ingesting beneficial bacteria to help treat digestive disorders or other problems

problem-focused coping: appraising a stressful situation as changeable and making and attempting a plan for changing something to improve things

progestin-only contraceptives: work by inhibiting ovulation and thickening of the cervical mucus; completely reversible

progestin-only implantation methods: inserting a 1.5-inch hormone-containing plastic rod under the skin, where it remains for three years

progestin-only injectable methods: injection of a 12-week supply of hormone, which is released at a steady rate

prolactin: a hormone produced by the anterior lobe of the pituitary gland that stimulates milk production

proof: a number assigned to an alcoholic product that is twice the percentage of alcohol in that product

prostate gland: gland at the base of the bladder providing seminal fluid

prostate-specific antigen (PAS) test: a blood test that detects a protein associated with abnormal growth of the prostate gland

protein: the foundation of every body cell; biological molecules composed of chains of amino acids

psychoactive: any substance that primarily alters mood, perception, and other brain functions

psychological dependence: dependence that results because a drug produces pleasant mental effects

psychosomatic illnesses: physical illnesses brought on by negative mental states such as stress or emotional upset

pubic lice: small insects that live primarily in hair in the genital and rectal regions

puerperium: the six weeks after childbirth, also called postpartum period

Q

quackery: promotion and sale of unapproved and worthless products, especially for medical problems and health enhancement

quit date: the day a smoker designates as the one on which he or she will stop smoking completely

R

radiation therapy: use of high-energy radiation, such as x-rays, to kill cancer cells and treat some forms of cancer

radon: a radioactive gas found in some homes that can increase the risk of cancer

range of motion: the amount of rotating, bending, or twisting allowed by the anatomy of a joint

rapid eye movement (REM) sleep: stage of sleep in which dreams occur

reactive hypoglycemia: occurring after the ingestion of carbohydrates, with consequent release of insulin

receptor: protein on the surface or inside of a cell to which a drug or natural substance can bind and thereby affect cell function

recommended [daily] dietary allowances (RDA): levels of nutrients recommended by the Food and Nutrition Board of the National Academy of Sciences for daily consumption by healthy individuals, scaled according to gender and age

relative perceived exertion: awareness of one's relative response to exercise

relaxation response: the physiological changes in the body that result from mental relaxation techniques

repetitive motion disorders: disorders caused by repeated stress to a body part; carpal tunnel syndrome is considered a repetitive motion disorder

RICE: an acronym for rest, ice, compression, elevation; the first aid measures for sports injuries

rodenticide: a chemical that kills mice and rats

Rohypnol: a powerful tranquilizer used as a club drug

S

safety: an ever-changing condition in which one attempts to minimize the risk of injury, illness, or property damage from the hazards to which one may be exposed

saturated fat: generally solid at room temperature; comes from animal sources

scabies: infestation of the skin by microscopic mites (insects)

schizophrenia: a mental disorder that involves a disturbance in thinking, in perceiving reality, and in functioning

scrotum: the sac of skin that contains the testes

seasonal affective disorder: depressive symptoms that appear in autumn or winter and remit spontaneously in spring

second-stage labor: the stage during which the baby moves out through the vagina and is delivered

secondary hypertension: high blood pressure caused by a recognizable disease

secondary sex characteristics: anatomical features appearing at puberty that distinguish males from females

secondhand binge effects: negative experiences caused by another's binge drinking

sedatives: central nervous system depressants used to relieve anxiety, fear, and apprehension

sedentary lifestyle: a pattern of living that lacks physical activity sufficient for good health

self-actualization: a state in which a person has achieved the highest level of growth in Maslow's hierarchy of needs

self-disclosure: sharing personal experiences and feelings with someone

self-efficacy: the belief that one can carry out the actions required to accomplish a goal

self-esteem: the judgment one places on one's self-worth

semen: a whitish, creamy fluid containing sperm

seminal vesicles: glands that secrete a fluid that is a component of semen

seminiferous tubules: convoluted tubules in the testicles that produce sperm

senile dementia: loss of cognitive functions in elderly people

sexual orientation: the propensity to be sexually and romantically attracted to a particular sex

sexual response cycle: the four-phase physiological response to sexual arousal in both men and women

sexual violence: violent actions that include rape, incest, attempted rape, and unwanted sexual touching

sexually transmitted diseases (STDs): infections passed from person to person by sexual contact

shaken-baby syndrome (SBS): a form of child abuse in which an infant is violently shaken by an adult

sick building syndrome: collection of symptoms reported by workers in some modern buildings

side effects: unintended and often harmful actions of a drug

simple sugars: a class of carbohydrates called monosaccharides; all carbohydrates must be reduced to simple sugars to be digested

sinoatrial node: the region of the heart that produces an electrical signal that causes the heart to contract

smegma: a white, cheesy substance that accumulates under the foreskin of the penis

smog: air polluted by chemicals, smoke, particles, and dust

snuff: a form of smokeless tobacco; made from powdered or finely cut leaves

social anxiety disorder: fear of being observed and evaluated by others in social situations

social support: resources that one receives from others, particularly people in one's immediate social network with whom one has emotional bonds and/or social ties

social wellness: ability to perform social roles effectively, comfortably, and without harming others

socialization: the process by which social groups confer attitudes and expectations upon individuals

soluble fiber: can be dissolved in water

somatization: occurrence of physical symptoms without any bodily disease or injury being present

specific metabolic rate: the amount of energy per gram of body weight consumed per day

spectatoring: observing one's own sexual experience rather than fully taking part in it

spermicide: a chemical that kills sperm; particularly foams, creams, gels, and suppositories used for contraception

spiritual wellness: state of balance and harmony with yourself and others

squamous cell carcinoma: cancer of the top layer of skin; most are curable if removed early

stalking: behavior that causes victims to feel a high level of fear of physical or sexual violence

starch: complex chain of glucose molecules

statins: a class of drugs that block synthesis of cholesterol in the liver and reduce the amount of cholesterol in the blood

sterility: the state of permanent infertility

stimulants: substances that increase the activity of the central nervous system

storage fat: also called depot fat; energy stored as fat in various parts of the body

strength training: the use of resistance to increase one's ability to exert or resist force for the purpose of improving performance

stress: the sum of physical and emotional reactions to any stimulus that disturbs the harmony of body and mind

stressor: any physical or psychological situation that produces stress

stroke: an insufficient supply of blood to the brain, resulting in loss of muscle function, loss of speech, or other symptoms

subluxation: partial displacement of a vertebra from its correct position

sucrose: common refined table sugar; a molecule of glucose and a molecule of fructose chemically bonded together

sulfites: used as preservatives for salad, fresh fruits and vegetables, wine, beer, and dried fruit; in susceptible individuals, especially those with asthma, they can cause a severe reaction

sympto-thermal method: using both the basal body temperature and the mucus methods at the same time

syphilis: a sexually transmitted disease caused by spirochete bacteria (*Treponema pallidum*)

systole: the pressure in the arteries when the heart contracts (the higher number)

T

T-cells: cells of the immune system that attack foreign organisms that infect the body

t'ai chi ch'uan: a Chinese martial arts system of movements that enhances freedom of movement and focus of mind

tar: the yellowish brown residue of tobacco smoke

target heart rate: the heart rate during strenuous exercise associated with inducing the training effect

teratogen: any environmental agent that causes abnormal development of a fetus

testes: a pair of male reproductive organs that produce sperm cells and male sex hormones

therapeutic massage: promotes relaxation and healing by massage of the skin and muscles

third-stage labor: the stage during which the afterbirth is expelled

threat situations: events that cause stress because of a perception that harm or loss may occur

tinnitus: persistent ringing in the ears, often caused by repeated or sudden exposure to loud noises

tolerance: a condition in which increased amounts of a drug or increased exposure to an addictive behavior are required to produce desired effects

trachea: upper part of respiratory tract

training effect: beneficial physiological changes as a result of exercise

tranquilizers: central nervous system depressants that relax the body and calm anxiety

trans-fatty acid: also trans fat, an artificial fat manufactured by chemically modifying monounsaturated and polyunsaturated fatty acids

triglyceride: a storage form of fat

tubal ligation: a surgical procedure in women in which the fallopian tubes are cut, tied, or cauterized to prevent pregnancy; a form of sterilization

tumor: a mass of abnormal cells

tumor viruses: viruses that infect cells, change their growth properties, and cause cancer

type A behavior: behaviors characterized by traits, such as time urgency or hostility, that contribute to the risk of heart disease

typical failure rate: likelihood of becoming pregnant considering all the potential problems associated with a birth control method

U

ulcers: open sores that occur in the stomach or small intestine from infection by the bacterium *H. pylori*

ultrasound scanning: use of sound waves to visualize the fetus in the womb

unconscious: mental activities outside of conscious awareness

unintentional injury: preferred term for accidental injury; result of an accident

universal donors: people whose blood is accepted by everyone during transfusion

universal recipients: people whose blood type is compatible with anyone else's blood

urethra: a tube that carries urine from the bladder to the outside

urethritis: an irritation or infection of the urethra caused by bacteria

urinary tract infection (UTI): inflammation and/or infection of the urethra and/or bladder, usually by bacteria

uterus: the female organ in which a fetus develops

V

vaccines: inactivated bacteria or viruses that are injected or taken orally; the body responds by producing antibodies and cells that provide lasting immunity

vagina: a woman's organ of copulation and the exit pathway for the fetus at birth

varicose veins: swelling of veins (usually in the legs) resulting from defective valves

vasectomy: a surgical procedure in men in which segments of the vas deferens are removed and the ends tied to prevent the passage of sperm

vasocongestion: the engorgement of blood in particular body regions in response to sexual arousal

vector: the carrier of infectious organisms from animals to people or from person to person

vegan: one who excludes all animal products from the diet, including milk, cheese, eggs, and other dairy products

vegetarian: one who consumes no meat, poultry, or fish

veins: blood vessels that return blood from tissues to the heart

violence: a physical or verbal behavior, in which the aim is to harm, injure, or destroy someone or something

virtual reality therapy: use of computers to create virtual worlds to engage the mind in overcoming pain and fear and to treat symptoms of posttraumatic stress disorder

vital statistics: numerical data relating to birth, death, disease, marriage, and health

vitamins: essential organic substances needed daily in small amounts to perform specific functions in the body

vulva: the female external genital structures

vulvovaginitis: inflammation of the vaginal region

W

water-soluble vitamins: soluble in water; there are nine water-soluble vitamins

wean: to discontinue breastfeeding, using other means to provide nutrients

Western blot: a test to determine the presence of specific HIV proteins; very accurate

withdrawal method: removing the penis from the vagina just prior to ejaculation; also called coitus interruptus or pulling out

withdrawal symptoms: uncomfortable and sometimes dangerous reactions that occur after a person stops taking a physically addicting drug

X

xenoestrogens: environmental chemicals that mimic the effects of natural estrogen; may cause cancer

Y

yoga: a system of exercises formulated in India thousands of years ago to unite one's mind and body

you-statements: statements beginning with "you"; negative communication skill

Z

zygote: the first cell of a new person, formed at fertilization

CHAPTER
1

1.1 My Definition of Health

Whatever you can do or dream you can do, begin it. Boldness has genius, power, and magic in it.
—Goethe

Directions

Write a one-paragraph response to these questions:

- What is your personal definition of health?

_____

_____

_____

_____

_____

_____

_____

_____

- How does your definition compare to the World Health Organization's definition of health (Chapter 1)?

_____

_____

_____

_____

_____

_____

_____

1.2 Health Issues Affecting My Academic Performance

You're good at what you practice.
—Sensei Mel Weitsman,
Berkeley Zen Center

Directions

1. Use the chart below to indicate how much each health issue affects you.

2. For any frequent health issue, describe how it affects your academic performance and offer strategies for lessening the frequency with which the issue occurs.

Health Issue	Affects My Academic Performance		
	Rarely/not at all	Sometimes	Frequently
Stress	_____	_____	_____
Cold/flu/sore throat	_____	_____	_____
Sleep difficulties	_____	_____	_____
Concern about family/friend	_____	_____	_____
Relationship difficulties	_____	_____	_____
Depression/anxiety	_____	_____	_____
Internet use/games	_____	_____	_____
Sinus infection	_____	_____	_____
Death of friend/family	_____	_____	_____
Alcohol use	_____	_____	_____

Study Guide and Self-Assessment

1.3 My Campus Health Environment

Even if you're on the right track, you'll get run over if you just sit there.
—Will Rogers

Directions

The following chart lists health goals for American colleges and universities for year 2010 and baseline data from year 2000. Rate *your perception* of your school's efforts toward achieving each of the listed 2010 health goals. Mark "thumbs up" if you perceive your school as working toward the 2010 health goal. Mark "thumbs down" if you perceive that it is not working toward the 2010 health goal.

Health Goal	Year 2000 Data	Year 2010 Goal	👍	👎
Increase the proportion of college students with health insurance.	83.3%	100%		
Increase the proportion of college students receiving information from their institution on each of 11 priority health-risk behavior areas.*	3.1%	17.4		
Increase the proportion of females who use contraception.	95.1%	100%		
Reduce unintentional pregnancies among college women.	25.3%	17.5%		
Increase the proportion of sexually active women/men who used condoms at last intercourse.	40/46.8%	60/60%		
Increase use of safety belts.	69.5%	94%		
Decrease the proportion of college students who have been in an emotionally abusive relationship (per 1,000).	124	93.9		
Reduce the annual rate of rape or attempted rape (per 1,000).	34.6	23.3		
Reduce sexual assault/unwanted sexual touching other than rape (per 1,000).	96	56.4		
Reduce physical assaults (per 1,000).	37	21.3		
Reduce the proportion of college students who report that they drove after drinking any alcohol at all during the previous 30 days.	30.9%	15.3%		
Reduce the proportion of college students engaging in high-risk (binge) drinking of alcoholic beverages during the past two weeks.	39%	20%		
Reduce tobacco use by college students.	25.1%	10.5%		
Reduce the rate of suicide attempts by adolescents and college students (12-month average rate).	1.5%	0.53%		
Increase the proportion of adults and college students who are at a healthy weight. Healthy weight is defined as a body mass index (BMI) equal to or greater than 18.5 and less than 25.	66.8%	75%		
Increase the proportion of college students who consume at least five daily servings of fruit and vegetables.	7.4%	25.5%		
Increase the proportion of adults and college students who use the oral health care system each year.	77%	92%		

*11 priority health-risk behaviors: tobacco use, alcohol use, sexual assault/relationship violence, violence prevention, injury prevention and safety, suicide prevention, pregnancy prevention, HIV/AIDS prevention, STD prevention, dietary behaviors and nutrition, physical activity and fitness

Source: American College Health Association - National College Health Assessment, 2003.

Study Guide and Self-Assessment

1.4 My Health and Wellness Assessment

We need a path, not to go from here to there, but to go from here to here.
—Jashuko Kwong

Directions

1. Complete the Health and Wellness Assessment on the following pages.

2. For each question, write the number (1 to 5) that corresponds to your response to each question in the Health and Wellness Assessment.

3. Calculate your scores for the six wellness categories (e.g., Emotional Health, Fitness and Body Care, etc.).

4. List two aspects of your personal health that you are the most pleased with and explain your reasoning.

   _____
   _____
   _____

5. List two aspects of your personal health that you are the least pleased with and explain your reasoning.

   _____
   _____
   _____

6. List three questions in the Health and Wellness Assessment that interested you and explain your reasons.

   _____
   _____
   _____

7. Indicate one or more aspects of your personal health that you would like to change and explain your reasons. Consider doing a Health Behavior Change project as a way to make a positive health change in your life.

   _____
   _____
   _____
   _____
   _____

8. Identify factors that prevent you from accomplishing your health goals.

   _____
   _____
   _____
   _____
   _____

Study Guide and Self-Assessment

Health and Wellness Assessment

Complete the following health and wellness inventory to gauge your present degree of wellness. For each of the questions, circle a number:

5 if the statement is ALWAYS true
4 if the statement is FREQUENTLY true
3 if the statement is OCCASIONALLY true
2 if the statement is SELDOM true
1 if the statement is NEVER true

1. I am able to identify the situations and factors that overstress me. 　5 4 3 2 1

2. I eat only when I am hungry. 　5 4 3 2 1

3. I don't take tranquilizers or other drugs to relax. 　5 4 3 2 1

4. I support efforts in my community to reduce environmental pollution. 　5 4 3 2 1

5. I avoid buying foods with trans-fats. 　5 4 3 2 1

6. I rarely have problems concentrating on what I'm doing because of worrying about other things. 　5 4 3 2 1

7. My employer (school) takes measures to ensure that my work (study) place is safe. 　5 4 3 2 1

8. I try not to use medications when I feel unwell. 　5 4 3 2 1

9. I am able to identify certain bodily responses and illnesses as my reactions to stress. 　5 4 3 2 1

10. I consider the necessity of diagnostic x-rays. 　5 4 3 2 1

11. I try to change personal habits that are risk factors for heart disease, cancer, and other lifestyle diseases. 　5 4 3 2 1

12. I avoid taking sleeping pills to help me sleep. 　5 4 3 2 1

13. I try not to eat foods with refined sugar or corn sugar as ingredients. 　5 4 3 2 1

14. I accomplish goals I set for myself. 　5 4 3 2 1

15. I stretch or bend for several minutes each day to keep my body flexible. 　5 4 3 2 1

16. I support immunization of all children for common childhood diseases. 　5 4 3 2 1

17. I try to prevent friends from driving after they drink alcohol. 　5 4 3 2 1

18. I minimize my salt intake. 　5 4 3 2 1

19. I don't mind when other people and situations make me wait or lose time. 　5 4 3 2 1

20. I climb four or fewer flights of stairs rather than take the elevator. 　5 4 3 2 1

21. I eat fresh fruits and vegetables several times a week (or daily). 　5 4 3 2 1

22. I use dental floss at least once a day. 　5 4 3 2 1

23. I read product labels on foods to determine if the ingredients are safe and not harmful to health. 　5 4 3 2 1

24. I try to maintain a normal body weight. 　5 4 3 2 1

25. I record my feelings and thoughts in a journal or diary. 　5 4 3 2 1

26. I have no difficulty falling asleep. 　5 4 3 2 1

27. I engage in some form of vigorous physical activity at least three times a week. 　5 4 3 2 1

28. I take time each day to quiet my mind and relax. 　5 4 3 2 1

29. I want to make and sustain close friendships and intimate relationships. 　5 4 3 2 1

30. I obtain an adequate daily supply of vitamins from my food or vitamin supplements. 　5 4 3 2 1

31. I rarely have tension or migraine headaches or pain in the neck or shoulders. 　5 4 3 2 1

32. I wear a safety belt when driving or when I am a passenger in the front seat. 　5 4 3 2 1

33. I am aware of the emotional and situational factors that lead me to overeat. 　5 4 3 2 1

34. I avoid driving my car after drinking any alcohol. 　5 4 3 2 1

35. I am aware of the side effects of the medicines I take. 　5 4 3 2 1

36. I am able to accept feelings of sadness, depression, and anxiety, realizing that they are almost always transient. 　5 4 3 2 1

37. I would seek several additional professional opinions if my doctor recommended surgery for me. 　5 4 3 2 1

38. I agree that nonsmokers should not have to breathe the smoke from cigarettes in public places. 　5 4 3 2 1

39. I think that pregnant women who smoke should stop in order to prevent harm to the developing fetus. 　5 4 3 2 1

40. I feel I get enough sleep. 　5 4 3 2 1

41. I ask my doctor why a certain medication is being prescribed and inquire about alternatives. 　5 4 3 2 1

42. I am aware of the calories expended in my exercise activities. 　5 4 3 2 1

43. I am willing to give priority to my own needs for time and psychological space by saying "no" to others' requests of me. 　5 4 3 2 1

44. I walk instead of drive whenever feasible. 　5 4 3 2 1

45. I eat a breakfast that contains about one-third of my daily need for calories, proteins, and vitamins. 　5 4 3 2 1

46. I prohibit smoking in my home. 　5 4 3 2 1

47. I remember and think about my dreams.   5 4 3 2 1

48. I seek medical attention only when I have symptoms
    or feel that some (potential) condition needs checking,
    rather than have routine yearly checkups.   5 4 3 2 1

49. I endeavor to make my home accident-free.   5 4 3 2 1

50. I ask my doctor to explain the diagnosis of my problem
    until I understand all that I care to.   5 4 3 2 1

51. I try to include fiber or roughage (whole grains, fresh
    fruits, vegetables, or bran) in my daily diet.   5 4 3 2 1

52. I can deal with my emotional problems without
    alcohol or other mood-altering drugs.   5 4 3 2 1

53. I check the calorie content of the packaged foods
    that I eat.   5 4 3 2 1

54. I require children riding in my car to be in infant
    seats or in shoulder harnesses.   5 4 3 2 1

55. I try to associate with people who have a positive
    attitude about life.   5 4 3 2 1

56. I try not to eat snacks of candy, pastries, and
    other "junk" foods.   5 4 3 2 1

57. I avoid people who are "down" all the time and
    who bring down those around them.   5 4 3 2 1

58. I am aware of the calorie content of the foods I eat.   5 4 3 2 1

59. I brush my teeth after meals.   5 4 3 2 1

60. (*for women only*) I regularly examine my breasts
    for any signs of cancer.   5 4 3 2 1

    (*for men only*) I am aware of the signs of
    testicular cancer.   5 4 3 2 1

How to Score

Enter the numbers you've circled next to the question number in the columns below and total your score for each category. Then use the wellness status key to determine your degree of wellness for each category.

Emotional Health	Fitness and Body Care	Environmental Health	Stress	Nutrition	Medical Self-Responsibility
6 _____	15 _____	4 _____	1 _____	2 _____	8 _____
12 _____	20 _____	7 _____	3 _____	5 _____	10 _____
25 _____	22 _____	17 _____	9 _____	13 _____	11 _____
26 _____	24 _____	32 _____	14 _____	18 _____	16 _____
36 _____	27 _____	34 _____	19 _____	21 _____	35 _____
40 _____	33 _____	38 _____	28 _____	23 _____	37 _____
47 _____	42 _____	39 _____	29 _____	30 _____	41 _____
52 _____	44 _____	46 _____	31 _____	45 _____	48 _____
55 _____	58 _____	49 _____	43 _____	51 _____	50 _____
57 _____	59 _____	54 _____	53 _____	56 _____	60 _____
Total _____	Total _____	Total _____	Total _____	Total _____	Total _____

My Wellness Status

To access your status in each of the six categories, compare your total score in each column to the following key: **0–34,** need improvement; **35–44,** good; **45–50,** excellent.

1.5 My Health Behaviors

He has half the deed done who has made a beginning.
—Horace

Health is a precious gift that you give yourself by living meaningfully and in harmony with your inner self and all that surrounds you. Researchers have found that the personal behaviors listed in the table below contribute to health.

Directions

1. List the behaviors in the table that are regular aspects of your life.

   _____

   _____

   _____

   _____

2. Identify one behavior that you would like to be part of your life right now and explain your reasoning. Consider doing a Health Behavior Change project (see workbook Exercise 1.7) to integrate one of these health behaviors into your life.

   _____

   _____

   _____

The Breslow Study	The Ornish Study
No smoking	No smoking
7–8 hours of sleep per night	No more than 10% of daily calories from fat
Body weight not less than 10% and not more than 30% of recommended for height and body frame	Daily meditation
Regular exercise	Daily exercise
Eating breakfast regularly	Vegetarian diet
Little between-meal snacking	Daily yoga
Little or no alcohol consumption (1–2 drinks per day)	Support group meetings twice a week

Note: The data in column 1 are from L. Breslow and J. E. Enstrom, 1980, "Persistence of health habits and their relationship to mortality," *Preventive Medicine, 9,* 469–483; T. C. Camacho and J. A. Wiley, 1983, Health practices, social networks, and change in physical health. In L. Berkman and L. Breslow, eds., *Health and Ways of Living: The Alameda County Study.* New York: Oxford University Press. Data in column 2 are from D. Ornish et al., 1998, "Intensive lifestyle changes for reversal of coronary heart disease," *Journal of the American Medical Association, 280,* 2001–2007.

Study Guide and Self-Assessment

1.6 My Personal Vital Statistics

Your health is bound to be affected if day after day you say the opposite of what you feel.
—Boris Pasternak, *Doctor Zhivago*

Enter the appropriate data about yourself. Date it and keep it for your personal records.

Height in inches (without shoes):_____

Weight in pounds (with clothes):_____

Highest adult weight:_____ pounds. At what age?_____

Lowest adult weight:_____ pounds. At what age? _____

Recommended weight for height (see text, Chapter 5):_____

Body Mass Index (see text, Chapter 5):_____

Resting heart rate (pulse): _____beats per minute (see Exercise 7.1)

Blood pressure: Systolic (top number): _____ Diastolic (bottom number): _____

Blood type: | A | B | O | AB | Rh− | Rh+ |

Total blood cholesterol:_____ LDL cholesterol: _____ HDL cholesterol: _____

1.7 Health Behavior Change Project

Everyone has the power for greatness, not fame, but greatness. Because greatness is determined by service.

—Martin Luther King, Jr.

Design, carry out, and evaluate a project for changing a personal health behavior (e.g.: stop smoking, learn a relaxation method, alter diet, begin an exercise plan).

The Health Behavior Change project has five steps:

Step 1.   Project Declaration: You state what you want to do. Address the following:

1. The reasons for your choice

2. What you hope to learn or achieve and why

3. Any prior experiences that are similar

4. Your start and stop dates

5. The ways you will determine progress

Step 2.   Research: You find four resources that provide information about your proposed Health Behavior Change project. Consult books, magazines, the Internet, or personal advisors to determine a way(s) to accomplish your goal(s). Because research in the health field is extensive, find resources that are no older than five years. For each of the four resources report the following:

- The title

- The author or writer

- The source: name of magazine, producer of video, affiliation of professional expert, Internet address

- Date of publication and pages on which the information appears

Step 3.   Project Plan: You develop and describe a plan for carrying out your Health Behavior Change project. Describe what you plan to do for your Health Behavior Change project and the ways you will determine progress.

Step 4.   Project Activity: You carry out your project for three weeks. Choose a start date. Keep a diary/journal of your activity. Note obstacles that get in the way of progress. At the end of each week, write a progress report that summarizes that week's experience, including obstacles you encounter.

Step 5.   Assessment: You write an evaluation of your experience by:

- Summarizing your project plan and the health principles it represented

- Describing the experience of trying to accomplish your goal(s)

- Listing at least two things about your topic that you learned

- Describing what doing the project helped you learn about yourself

- Describing what you learned about how to change a health behavior

- Stating whether the project was worthwhile and why

Study Guide and Self-Assessment

2.1 The Relaxation Response

Everything starts with clear intention.
—Yvonne Rand,
Buddhist priest and teacher

Many students live fast-paced, hectic lives that are full of time pressures and stress. Trying to accommodate to all of life's demands produces near continuous physiologic arousal, resulting in sleep disturbances, muscle tension, gastrointestinal symptoms, and an increased risk for cardiovascular disease. The Relaxation Response is an automatic physiological pattern opposing nervous system arousal. Do it for 10 to 20 minutes each day to keep yourself centered and calm.

Directions

1. Place yourself in an environment in which you are comfortable and can relax. Turn off cell phones, pagers, computers, and music. Lock the door.

2. Sit or lie comfortably. Breathe comfortably.

3. Silently repeat the word *one*. If your mind wanders, as soon as you notice, refocus your attention on silently repeating the word *one*. Do not become angry or frustrated because you "aren't doing it right."

4. Do the exercise for as long as you are able. Try to work up to 20 minutes per day.

2.2 Autogenic Training

An ounce of example is worth a pound of advice.
—Evan Esar

Autogenic training uses autosuggestion to balance and harmonize the mind and body. Autogenic training involves concentrating on one of six basic autogenic phrases for a few minutes each day for a week or more. After weeks or months of practice, you are able to attain a deep sense of relaxation, often within seconds. The six basic autosuggestions are as follows:

- My arms and legs are heavy.

- My arms and legs are warm.

- My heartbeat is calm and regular.

- My lungs breathe me.

- My abdomen is warm.

- My forehead is cool.

Directions

1. Place yourself in an environment in which you are comfortable and can relax. Turn off cell phones, pagers, computers, and music. Lock the door.

2. Sit or lie comfortably. Breathe comfortably.

3. Choose one of the autogenic phrases from the preceding list and silently (or aloud) repeat it seven times.

4. Open your eyes, stretch, and mentally note or "observe" the sensations in your body.

5. Repeat steps 3 and 4 five times, for a total of about 10 minutes.

6. After one week, carry out the exercise using a different autogenic phrase.

Note: The exact phrasing of any autogenic suggestion is not critical to its effectiveness. The words carry no particular power. Any suggestion can be rephrased so that it becomes comfortable, believable, and acceptable to you.

Study Guide and Self-Assessment

2.3 Anchoring

Ordinary men hate solitude, but the master makes use of it, embracing his aloneness, realizing he is one with the whole universe.

—Lao Tzu

Follow the directions below to learn how to Anchor. Then, on each of six consecutive days, practice Anchoring for 20 minutes. At the end of the six days, describe your experience. You can also check out the Chapter 2 Web exercises at http://health.jbpub.com/hwonline for an online anchoring tutorial.

Directions

Become comfortable: Sit straight, uncross your legs, place your feet flat on the floor. Place your hands in your lap and take two easy, deep breaths. Then breathe easily and naturally. Bring your shoulders down from your ears.

Step 1. Anchoring on the feet: Close your eyes for a few seconds and focus your awareness on the sensation of the bottoms of your feet touching the insoles of your shoes. After you open your eyes, note what your mind was doing while your eyes were closed.

Step 2. Anchoring on the back: Close your eyes for a few seconds and focus your awareness on the sensation of your back touching the chair. After a couple of seconds with your eyes closed, open your eyes, take an easy breath, and note what your mind was doing while your eyes were closed.

Step 3. Anchoring on the breath: Close your eyes for a few seconds and notice your breathing. Don't change your breathing rhythm or pattern, just notice the breath going in and out of your body.

Now you know three basic Anchoring postures: feet on the floor, back against the chair, and focusing on the breath. With a bit of practice, you will discover the Anchoring posture that is best for you.

Step 4. Anchoring for 30 seconds, and then 90 seconds: Become comfortable (see above). Choose one of the three Anchoring postures as your Anchor place. Close your eyes, and focus your awareness on your Anchor place for 30 seconds. While you're Anchoring, if you notice your mind wandering, refocus your awareness on your Anchor place. When you think the 30 seconds has elapsed, open your eyes and take a breath.

What did you notice while you were Anchoring? Did you hear sounds? Did your mind wander? Did you think about your to-do list? Did you tell yourself this was silly? Did you feel sleepy? Did you relax? All of these reactions are common. Whenever you Anchor, you can expect your mind to wander and to think. When you notice that it does, just notice, and refocus your awareness on your Anchor place. When you are ready, try Anchoring for 90 seconds.

Study Guide and Self-Assessment

2.4 Image Visualization

A wise man changes his mind. A fool, never.
—Spanish proverb

Your mind has the power to promote your personal wellness and to help healing. By dwelling on negative thoughts and images, such as "I feel lousy," you increase the chance that you will feel that way. On the other hand, thinking positive thoughts, such as "I feel great" or "Today is a good day," you can create positive feelings and positive behavioral outcomes. You can put healing suggestions into your mind, too. For example, you can suggest to yourself that a headache will go away in an hour or a cold will be mild.

Directions

Find a quiet, pleasant place where you can sit or lie down comfortably. Remove any uncomfortable clothing, eyeglasses, or contact lenses. Turn off the phone, TV, and computer. Give yourself permission to relax and decide what you are going to visualize. It's probably best to begin with something specific. You can visualize yourself being slimmer, giving up cigarettes, being successful in an upcoming job interview, or taking an exam while feeling confident and sure of the answers. You can visualize yourself becoming physically stronger or an area of your body becoming well.

Allow your eyes to close, and relax the muscles in the eyelids all the way—to the point where they are so relaxed and comfortable that you feel you are unable to pull your eyelids open. Then let your mind transfer that same comfortable, relaxed feeling to all the other parts of the body, one by one, from top to bottom—head, chest, arms, hands, back, stomach, legs, feet.

Imagine that you are floating on a white cloud bathed in warm sunlight. Everything is quiet and peaceful. You are warm and comfortable and serene. Allow your mind to visualize whatever scene or image it chooses

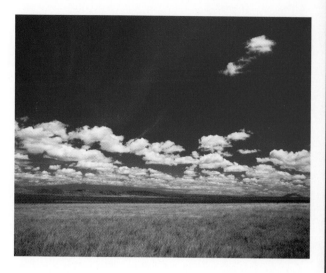

that is related to what you want to improve or heal. Accept your mind's images. They are helping you to change, to feel better. Allow yourself to remain in this relaxed state while your mind continues to create pleasant, positive, beneficial images. Begin to notice how relaxed your body is and how good it feels.

Whenever your mind decides it wants to return to a fully awake state, you will automatically open your eyes and be fully aware of your surroundings. Notice how refreshed and relaxed you feel!

Study Guide and Self-Assessment

2.5 Progressive Muscle Relaxation

Meditation is the action of silence.
—Krishnamurti

Developed by American physician Edmund Jacobson in 1938, Progressive Muscle Relaxation (PMR) involves tightening individual muscles or muscle groups for five seconds and slowly releasing to create a reflex relaxation.

Directions

On each of two consecutive days, practice PMR, following the directions below. You can start at your feet and progress toward your head or vice versa, whichever is most comfortable for you. Try voice-recording the directions so you don't have to refer to the printed page. *Note:* Some people experience muscle cramps while doing this exercise, especially in their feet. If a muscle cramps, either (1) straighten out the muscle, or (2) "breathe through" the muscle: close your eyes and imagine that air is entering your body through the tight muscle instead of your lungs. If cramping or any other aspect of this exercise is uncomfortable, you may stop.

PMR Exercise (15–20 minutes)
Phase 1: Sinking into the floor
> Put yourself in quiet, comfortable surroundings.
> Shoes off, clothes loosened.
> Lie on your back on a soft or padded surface.
> Set feet slightly apart with palms facing upward.
> Close eyes; breathe naturally.
> Observe thoughts without focusing on them.
> As if it were a sponge, imagine the surface on which you are lying drawing tension from your body. As tension leaves your body, notice that it feels as though you are sinking into the floor.
> Breathe naturally.
> Lie quietly for at least two minutes.

Phase 2: Lower-body PMR
> Focus your awareness on your feet. Breathe normally.
> Keeping your heel on the floor, point the toes on your left foot away from you as far as you can. Hold five seconds and slowly release.
> Repeat for right foot.
> Rest, breathe naturally, and observe the sensation that follows.
> Keeping your heel on the floor, point the toes on your left foot toward you as far as you can. Hold five seconds and slowly release.

> Repeat for right foot.
> Rest, breathe naturally, and observe the sensation that follows.
> With leg outstretched, tighten the thigh muscles of your left leg. Hold five seconds and slowly release.
> Repeat for right leg.
> Rest, breathe naturally, and observe the sensation that follows.
> Tense pelvic (butt) muscles. Hold five seconds and slowly release.
> Rest, breathe naturally, and observe the sensation that follows.

Phase 3: Upper-body PMR
> Tense stomach muscles. Hold five seconds and slowly release.
> Rest, breathe naturally, and observe the sensation that follows.
> With palms turned down and keeping your forearm on the floor, bend your left hand at the wrist and point the fingers back as far as they will go. Hold five seconds and slowly release.
> Repeat for right hand.
> Rest, breathe naturally, and observe the sensation that follows.
> With palms turned up and keeping your forearm on the floor, bend your left hand at the wrist and point the fingers toward your face as far as they will go. Hold five seconds and slowly release.
> Repeat for right hand.
> Rest, breathe naturally, and observe the sensation that follows.
> Tense muscles of the left upper arm. Hold five seconds and slowly release.
> Repeat for right arm.
> Rest, breathe naturally, and observe the sensation that follows.
> Tense the muscles in your back. Hold five seconds and slowly release.
> Rest, breathe naturally, and observe the sensation that follows.
> Tense the muscles in your shoulders.
> Hold five seconds and slowly release.
> Rest, breathe naturally, and observe the sensation that follows.

Phase 4: Head and neck PMR
> Tense the muscles in your neck. Hold five seconds and slowly release.
> Rest, breathe naturally, and observe the sensation that follows.
> Tense the muscles in your face. Hold five seconds and slowly release.
> Rest, breathe naturally, and observe the sensation that follows.
> Close your eyes and squeeze the lids tightly shut. Hold five seconds and slowly release.
> Rest, breathe naturally, and observe the sensation that follows.

Study Guide and Self-Assessment

2.6 Quiet Time Exploration

Men have become the tools of their tools.
—Henry David Thoreau

For three weeks, experiment with different methods of relaxation to find one(s) that suits you and that you can practice indefinitely to enhance your health and well-being.

During Week 1
Experiment with three of the following relaxation techniques (or others of your choosing).

- Mantra meditation

- Breathing meditation

- Walking

- T'ai chi ch'uan

- Image visualization

- Progressive muscle relaxation

- Hatha yoga

During Week 2
Choose one technique and practice it for at least 3 days for 10 minutes each time.

During Week 3
Practice your chosen technique for at least 6 days for 20 minutes each day. For each day record the following information:

- The name the relaxation activity you're doing

- The time you spent each day doing the activity

- What you experienced doing the activity

- Any obstacles that prevented you from carrying out a day's activity

- Strategies for overcoming any obstacles

2.7 The Power Write

Do not say a little in many words, but a great deal in a few.
—Pythagoras

You've probably heard of a power nap. How about a power write, a 5-minute exercise designed to focus your attention on something other than dealing with the stresses and hustle-and-bustle of daily life? When you realize that you're caught up in a whir of mental and physical activity that seems to separate you from yourself, power-write about any of the following:

- A message from your body to you. What's going on right now?

- A conversation with someone you admire.

- What is stressing you today.

- What you find meaningful in life.

- Some place you'd rather be right now and the reasons why.

2.8 Massage

I am not who I think I am.
I am not who you think I am.
I am who I think you think I am.
              —Anonymous

Everyone experiences tense muscles and soreness in parts of the body occasionally. Some parts of the body, such as the neck, shoulders, and back, are prime locations for accumulated tension. Mental and emotional distress can cause muscle tension and physical discomfort.

Massage is an excellent way to reduce physical tension and relax body muscles. In turn, a relaxed body facilitates a relaxed state of mind. All human beings need physical contact with other people. Babies and children are constantly seeking ways to be held, touched, and massaged by their caregivers. Mothers instinctively stroke and rub their infants. Unfortunately, as we grow older we tend to give and receive less physical contact.

Giving a Back Massage

Anyone can give a massage to another person. All that's required is the desire to make another person feel more comfortable and a willingness to be sensitive to another person's stiff muscles.

Learn by exchanging massages with friends and persons you are comfortable with and trust. The person being massaged can be sitting up or lying down. The area to be massaged should be free of clothing. Begin with the neck, using your thumbs to press the muscles on either side of the spine. Press firmly and smoothly away from the spine. Work down the back, always pressing down and away from the spine. Be sensitive to sore places or knots of tense muscles. Apply steady gentle pressure to these areas until you feel the person relax or the muscles soften. As you become more experienced, you can use the heels of your hands or your knuckles to knead tense muscles. Always be sensitive to what the other person is feeling.

It helps to use a small amount of massage oil on your hands to reduce friction. You may want to play soft music or encourage the person to relax while you are massaging him or her.

Giving a Foot Massage

A foot massage is a relaxing, pleasant experience. The foot is a sensitive part of the body and often has places that are stiff or sore. Most people feel greatly relaxed after receiving a foot massage.

Begin by washing the person's feet with warm water. Rub the whole foot and ankle with a small amount of massage oil. Massage each toe and between each toe. Gently pull each toe to stretch the muscles and joints. You may hear the joint make a small cracking sound; this is normal. Massage the foot with your thumbs, fingers, or knuckles from top to bottom. Do one foot and then the other. It's easier if you cradle the foot in your lap. Be sensitive and gentle. Ask the person to tell you if any part hurts. Spend more time in places that are sore by gently pressing, rubbing, and massaging the area.

Always give a massage with your whole being—not just your hands. Be gentle, caring, and sensitive to what the other person is experiencing. A massage is an ideal way for two persons to become more in touch with their bodies and to release physical tension.

2.9 Leaving It at the River

My religion is kindness.
—Dalai Lama

Directions

1. Read the story of "Two Monks and the River."

Two Monks and the River
   Two monks set out on their last day's journey to their monastery. At mid-morning they came upon a shallow river, and on the bank there stood a beautiful young maiden.
   "May I help you cross?" asked the first monk.
   "Why, yes, that would be most kind of you," replied the maiden.
   So the first monk hoisted the maiden on his back and carried her across the river. They bowed and went their separate ways.
   After an hour or two of walking, the second monk said to the first monk, "I can't believe you did that! I just can't believe it! We take vows of chastity, and you touched a woman. You even asked her! What are we going to tell the abbot when we get home? He's going to ask how our journey was, and we can't lie. What are we going to say?"
   Another couple of hours passed and the second monk erupted again. "How could you do that? She didn't even ask. You offered! The abbot's going to be incredibly angry."
   By late afternoon the two were nearing their home, and the second monk, now filled with anxiety, said, "I can't believe you did that! You touched a woman. You even carried her on your back. What are we going to tell the abbot?"
   The first monk stopped, looked at the second monk, and said, "Listen, it's true that I carried that maiden across the river. But I left her at the river bank hours ago. You've been carrying her all day."

2. Which monk was the most stressed and why?

   _____

   _____

   _____

3. Write a brief essay describing your interpretation of the story.

   _____

   _____

   _____

   _____

   _____

   _____

   _____

   _____

   _____

   _____

   _____

   _____

4. When you are stressed or upset, what can you do to "leave it at the river"?

   _____

   _____

   _____

   _____

   _____

   _____

   _____

   _____

Study Guide and Self-Assessment

3

3.1 My Stressors

Never look down on somebody else unless you're helping them up.
—Jesse Jackson

Directions

1. Use the chart below to indicate the degree to which each item affects you.

2. For any frequent stressor, describe how it affects your life and offer strategies for lessening the frequency with which it occurs.

	Affects My Life		
Stressor	Rarely/not at all	Sometimes	Frequently
Academic			
Competition	_____	_____	_____
Schoolwork (difficult, low motivation)	_____	_____	_____
Exams and grades	_____	_____	_____
Poor resources (library, computers)	_____	_____	_____
Oral presentations/public speaking	_____	_____	_____
Professors/coaches (unfair, demanding, unavailable)	_____	_____	_____
Choosing and registering for classes	_____	_____	_____
Choosing a major/career	_____	_____	_____
Time			
Deadlines	_____	_____	_____
Procrastination	_____	_____	_____
Waiting for appointments and in lines	_____	_____	_____
No time to exercise	_____	_____	_____
Late for appointments or class	_____	_____	_____
Environment			
Others' behavior (rude, inconsiderate, sexist/racist)	_____	_____	_____
Injustice: seeing examples or being a victim of	_____	_____	_____
Crowds/large social groups	_____	_____	_____
Fears of violence/terrorism	_____	_____	_____
Weather (snow, heat/humidity, storms)	_____	_____	_____
Noise	_____	_____	_____
Lack of privacy	_____	_____	_____
Social			
Obligations, annoyances (family/friends/girl-/boyfriend)	_____	_____	_____
Not dating	_____	_____	_____
Roommate(s)/housemate(s) problems	_____	_____	_____
Concerns about STDs	_____	_____	_____

Stressor	Affects My Life		
	Rarely/not at all	Sometimes	Frequently
Self			
Behavior (habits, temper)	_____	_____	_____
Appearance (unattractive features, grooming)	_____	_____	_____
Ill health/physical symptoms	_____	_____	_____
Forgetting, misplacing, or losing things	_____	_____	_____
Weight/dietary management	_____	_____	_____
Self-confidence/self-esteem	_____	_____	_____
Boredom	_____	_____	_____
Money			
Not enough	_____	_____	_____
Bills/overspending	_____	_____	_____
Job: searching for or interviews	_____	_____	_____
Job/work issues (demanding; annoying)	_____	_____	_____
Tasks of Daily Living			
Tedious chores (shopping, cleaning)	_____	_____	_____
Traffic and parking problems	_____	_____	_____
Car problems (breakdowns, repairs)	_____	_____	_____
Housing (finding/getting or moving)	_____	_____	_____
Food (unappealing or unhealthful meals)	_____	_____	_____

3.2 My Stress Reactions

We know what we are, but know not what we may be.
—Shakespeare, *Hamlet*

Many people experience particular physical reactions to excessive stress. Here's a list of some common stress reactions. Which ones do you frequently experience? Can you add some reactions that are not on the list?

Reaction	Once a day	Once every 2–3 days	Once a week	Once a month	Not in the last 2 months
Headaches	_____	_____	_____	_____	_____
Nervous tics and twitches	_____	_____	_____	_____	_____
Blurred vision	_____	_____	_____	_____	_____
Dizziness	_____	_____	_____	_____	_____
Fatigue	_____	_____	_____	_____	_____
Coughing	_____	_____	_____	_____	_____
Wheezing	_____	_____	_____	_____	_____
Backache	_____	_____	_____	_____	_____
Muscle spasms	_____	_____	_____	_____	_____
Itching	_____	_____	_____	_____	_____
Excessive sweating	_____	_____	_____	_____	_____
Palpitations	_____	_____	_____	_____	_____
Constipation	_____	_____	_____	_____	_____
Jaw tightening	_____	_____	_____	_____	_____
Rapid heart rate	_____	_____	_____	_____	_____
Impotence	_____	_____	_____	_____	_____
Pelvic pain	_____	_____	_____	_____	_____
Stomachache	_____	_____	_____	_____	_____
Diarrhea	_____	_____	_____	_____	_____
Frequent urination	_____	_____	_____	_____	_____
Dermatitis (rash)	_____	_____	_____	_____	_____
Hyperventilation	_____	_____	_____	_____	_____
Irregular heart rhythm	_____	_____	_____	_____	_____
High blood pressure	_____	_____	_____	_____	_____
Delayed menstruation	_____	_____	_____	_____	_____
Vaginal discharge	_____	_____	_____	_____	_____
Nail biting	_____	_____	_____	_____	_____
Heartburn	_____	_____	_____	_____	_____

Study Guide and Self-Assessment

3.3 How Susceptible Am I to Stress?

Forget injuries, never forget kindnesses.
—Confucius

Some persons are more susceptible to the harmful effects of stress than others. The following inventory can give you an indication of your susceptibility. Score each item from 1 (almost always) to 5 (never) as it applies to you. A total score lower than 50 indicates you are not particularly vulnerable to stress. A score of 50 to 80 indicates moderate vulnerability, and a score of more than 80, high vulnerability—time to make some changes.

_____ 1. I eat at least one hot, nutritious meal a day.
_____ 2. I get 7 to 8 hours of sleep at least four nights a week.
_____ 3. I am affectionate with others regularly.
_____ 4. I have at least one relative within 50 miles on whom I can rely.
_____ 5. I exercise to the point of sweating at least twice a week.
_____ 6. I smoke fewer than 10 cigarettes a day.
_____ 7. I drink fewer than five alcoholic drinks a week.
_____ 8. I am about the proper weight for my height and age.
_____ 9. I have enough money to meet basic expenses and needs.
_____ 10. I feel strengthened by my religious beliefs.
_____ 11. I attend club or social activities on a regular basis.
_____ 12. I have several close friends and acquaintances.
_____ 13. I have one or more friends to confide in about personal matters.
_____ 14. I am basically in good health.
_____ 15. I am able to speak openly about my feelings when angry or worried.
_____ 16. I discuss problems about chores, money, and daily living issues with the people I live with.
_____ 17. I do something just for fun at least once a week.
_____ 18. I am able to organize my time and do not feel pressured.
_____ 19. I drink fewer than three cups of coffee (or tea or cola drinks) a day.
_____ 20. I allow myself quiet time at least once during each day.

TOTAL
SCORE _____

Source: Adapted from a test developed by L. H. Miller, and A. D. Smith.

Study Guide and Self-Assessment

3.4 Warning Signs of Stress

Knock hard. Life is deaf.
—Mimi Parent

Do you have any of these warning signs of stress?

	No	Yes
Trouble falling asleep	_____	_____
Difficulty staying asleep	_____	_____
Waking up tired and not well rested	_____	_____
Fatigue	_____	_____
Changes in eating patterns	_____	_____
Craving sweet/fatty/salty foods ("comfort foods")	_____	_____
More headaches than usual	_____	_____
Short temper/irritable	_____	_____
Recurring colds and minor illness	_____	_____
Muscle ache or tightness	_____	_____
Trouble concentrating, remembering, or staying organized	_____	_____
Depression	_____	_____

3.5 My Life Changes and Stress

No bird flies too high if he flies with his own wings.
—William Blake

Directions

1. Mark any item in the Recent Life Changes Questionnaire (below) that has occurred in your life in the past one month.

2. Total the number of Life Change Units (LCUs) you have accumulated.

3. Refer to Chapter 3 of the text to determine if you are at risk for a health change.

Recent Life Changes Questionnaire

Life Event	Life Change Units		Life Event	Life Change Units	
	Women	Men		Women	Men
Death of son or daughter	135	103	Moderate illness	47	39
Death of spouse	122	113	Loss or damage of personal property	47	35
Death of brother or sister	111	87	Sexual difficulties	44	44
Death of parent	105	90	Getting demoted at work	44	39
Divorce	102	85	Major change in living conditions	44	37
Death of family member	96	78	Increase in income	43	30
Fired from work	85	69	Relationship problems	42	34
Separation from spouse due to marital problems	79	70	Trouble with in-laws	41	33
Major injury or illness	79	64	Beginning or ending school or college	40	35
Being held in jail	78	71	Making a major purchase	40	33
Pregnancy	74	55	New, close personal relationship	39	34
Miscarriage or abortion	74	51	Outstanding personal achievement	38	33
Death of a close friend	73	64	Troubles with coworkers at work	37	32
Laid off from work	73	59	Change in school or college	37	31
Birth of a child	71	56	Change in your work hours or conditions	36	32
Adopting a child	71	54	Troubles with workers whom you supervise	35	34
Major business adjustment	67	47	Getting a transfer at work	33	31
Decrease in income	66	49	Getting a promotion at work	33	29
Parents' divorce	63	52	Change in religious beliefs	31	27
A relative moving in with you	62	53	Christmas	30	25
Foreclosure on a mortgage or a loan	62	51	Having more responsibilities at work	29	29
Investment and/or credit difficulties	62	46	Troubles with your boss at work	29	29
Marital reconciliation	61	48	Major change in usual type or amount of recreation	29	28
Major change in health or behavior of family member	58	50	General work troubles	29	27
Change in arguments with spouse	55	41	Change in social activities	29	24
Retirement	54	48	Major change in eating habits	29	23
Major decision regarding your immediate future	54	46	Major change in sleeping habits	28	23
Separation from spouse due to work	53	54	Change in family get-togethers	28	20
An accident	53	38	Change in personal habits	27	24
Parental remarriage	52	45	Major dental work	27	23
Change residence to a different town, city, or state	52	39	Change of residence in same town or city	27	21
Change to a new type of work	51	50	Change in political beliefs	26	21
"Falling out" of a close personal relationship	50	41	Vacation	26	20
Marriage	50	50	Having fewer responsibilities at work	22	21
Spouse changes work	50	38	Making a moderate purchase	22	18
Child leaving home	48	38	Change in church activities	21	20
Birth of grandchild	48	34	Minor violation of the law	20	19
Engagement to marry	47	42	Correspondence course to help you in your work	19	16

Source: Adapted from Miller, M. A. and Rahe, R. H. (1997). Life changes scaling for the 1990s. *Journal of Psychosomatic Research, 43,* 279–292, with permission from Elsevier Science.

Study Guide and Self-Assessment

3.6 Prioritizing Tasks: First Things First

You must look into people as well as at them.
—Lord Chesterfield

Directions

1. Refer to your to-do list for today or create one for this exercise.

2. Sit or lie quietly for a few minutes to become mentally and physically relaxed (see note below).

3. Using a four-box chart, place each item on your to-do list in the appropriate box according to its *urgency* and *importance* (see example).

4. Carry out your tasks in this order: (1) urgent and important; (2) not urgent but important; (3) urgent but not important; and (4) not urgent and not important.

Note: Quieting yourself helps you distinguish the urgent/important tasks from the urgent/not important ones because urgency is a state of mind that makes tasks seem important even if they are not.

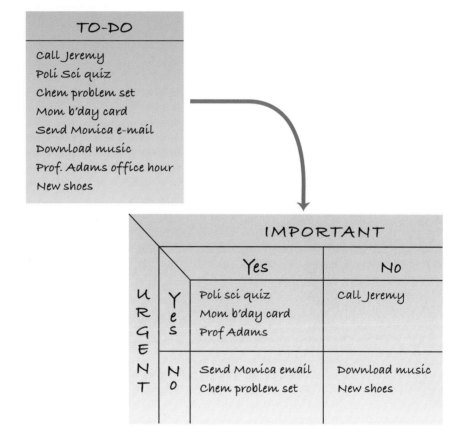

TO-DO

Call Jeremy
Poli Sci quiz
Chem problem set
Mom b'day card
Send Monica e-mail
Download music
Prof. Adams office hour
New shoes

		IMPORTANT	
		Yes	No
URGENT	Yes	Poli sci quiz Mom b'day card Prof Adams	Call Jeremy
	No	Send Monica email Chem problem set	Download music New shoes

3.6 Prioritizing Tasks: First Things First

3.7 Time Audit for Time Management

Half our life is spent trying to find something to do with the time we have rushed through life trying to save.

—Will Rogers

Directions

1. For three representative days in your life, keep a Time Diary (example below) in which you record your activities for every hour of the day. Make entries in your Time Diary two to three times a day. For example, at noon, record your activities since awakening; at 5:00 P.M. or so, record your activities since noon; at bedtime, record your activities since 5:00 P.M.

Time	Activity
6:00 A.M.	wake up
6:15 A.M.	shower/dress/eat
7:00 A.M.	go to school
8:00 A.M.	Chem lecture
9:30 A.M.	hang out in library/snack
10:30 A.M.	Psych lecture
12:00 noon	job
5:00 P.M.	go home

2. Calculate the average daily hours and percentage of a day's time spent in the following activities:

Time awake	_____ hrs.	_____ %
Time asleep	_____ hrs.	_____ %
Time traveling to and from work/school/activities	_____ hrs.	_____ %
Time spent at school	_____ hrs.	_____ %
Time spent studying/with schoolwork	_____ hrs.	_____ %
Time spent at job	_____ hrs.	_____ %
Time spent with family	_____ hrs.	_____ %
Time spent with friends	_____ hrs.	_____ %
Time spent with self	_____ hrs.	_____ %

3. Are you getting the recommended 7 to 8 hours of sleep per night? If not, what could you change to get more sleep?

_____

_____

_____

_____

4. Can you identify windows of time that you can devote to priority activities that now go neglected?

_____

_____

_____

_____

5. What did you learn from the Time Audit?

_____

_____

_____

_____

Study Guide and Self-Assessment

3.8 Are You a Procrastinator?

The journey of a thousand miles begins with the first step.
—Chinese proverb

Do you label yourself a procrastinator? Are you haunted by undone tasks? People who label themselves as procrastinators make the mistake of focusing on the end result of their activities (the end of the "journey of a thousand miles") instead of steps required to get to the end. Doing this can make getting to the end so difficult that they become stymied and put off moving toward their goal. And the more they put it off, the more formidable it seems because time is closing in. The way out of this is to focus on the first step instead of the end result.

Directions

1. Identify ONE task or goal that you cannot seem to do or move toward. Write it down here: _____.

2. Ask yourself, "What simple thing can I do today to move me toward my goal?" For example, if you are procrastinating about doing an assignment, take your textbook or lecture notes out of your backpack and make them visible. Write down here what step you could take: _____.

3. Do the step you wrote down in step 2.

4. When you are ready, ask yourself, "What step can I take now to move me toward my goal?" For example, you may decide to open your textbook or flip through your notes. Write it down here: _____

5. Do the step you wrote down in step 4.

6. Repeat steps 4 and 5 as many times as necessary to accomplish your goal. If all you can do is two steps, that's fine. At least you got started.

Note: Be alert for a voice in your head that tells you how lame you are for only doing a few steps or how lame this exercise is. This voice is trying to protect you from some harm it associates with accomplishing the goal. Sit quietly and "converse" with this voice (perhaps write out a dialogue) to lessen its effect on your behavior.

Study Guide and Self-Assessment

3.9 Minimizing In-class Listening Errors

*Besides the noble art of getting things done, there is a nobler art of leaving
things undone. The wisdom of life consists in the elimination of
nonessentials.*

—Lin Yutang

Ineffective learning skills are major contributors to academic stress. One
group of ineffective learning skills consists of in-class listening errors, which
are listed below. For each error on the list, indicate how likely you are to engage in that behavior using this scale:

1= never, 2 = infrequently, 3 = sometimes, 4 = often, 5 = frequently

For behaviors marked with a 4 or 5, think of ways to limit their frequency.

In-class Listening Errors

_____   1. Calling the subject or speaker uninteresting or boring. Doing
this allows you to "distance" yourself from the listening
experience—to lose focus—and to daydream, chat, or sleep.
 The Efficient Listener says, "As long as I'm here, I'll focus
on what's going on to gain as much as I can."

_____   2. Criticizing the speaker's delivery. This allows you to distract
yourself from the content of the message by focusing on the
presentation.
 The Efficient Listener, while possibly noting that the
speaker's delivery is sub par, nevertheless pays attention to
the content and reserves judgment until the talk is over.

_____   3. Getting worked-up with disagreements with the speaker's
message. If you allow yourself to get caught up in challenging
or contradicting the speaker (even silently in your mind), you
are talking to yourself and no longer listening.
 The Efficient Listener pays attention to gather all the
information before thinking about challenging what is said.

_____   4. Listening only for facts. This risks focusing on getting one fact
and losing getting others.
 The Efficient Listener listens for main ideas and themes
and notes facts that illustrate and support the main ideas. By
having a structure, more facts are remembered.

_____   5. Trying to outline the talk. This will work if the speaker's
remarks are themselves organized. If not, the main ideas and
themes can be lost while trying to find a pattern.
 The Efficient Listener notes main themes and ideas and
organizes them later.

_____   6. Faking attention. This is being present in body and not in
mind.
 The Effective Listener accepts that attention will
wander and learns to become aware of when attention is lost
and to refocus the mind.

_____   7. Tolerating or creating distractions. If someone is creating a
distraction, tell the person that the behavior is distracting. If
you cannot tell the person, raise your hand and ask the
speaker to ask for order. If you lose your focus and create
distractions, either take a deep breath to center yourself or
excuse yourself from the talk so as not to distract others.

_____   8. Evading or avoiding difficult material. This is a form of giving
up. If you do not understand the material, rather than tune
out, use your curiosity to try to learn something.

_____   9. Letting emotion-laden words throw you off focus. Responding
in your mind or verbally to emotionally charged ideas can
distract you from the content. If you have a reaction to what is
said, note it in your mind or jot down a word or two about it
and then refocus your attention.

_____ 10. Letting your mind wander. People process what they hear in
less time than it takes a speaker to talk. Don't let your mind
wander in that brief period of time.
 The Effective Listener learns to "be still" by quieting the
mind to keep focused during interims.

Source: The authors gratefully acknowledge Karen Halliday for this list.

Study Guide and Self-Assessment

3.10 Image Visualization for Exam Anxiety

It ain't what we know that gives us trouble. It's what we know that ain't so that gives us trouble.

—Will Rogers

Because of school pressures and exam anxiety, students' health often suffers. Students suffer from tension and migraine headaches, stomach upsets, frequent infections, and a host of other mental and physical symptoms that are brought on or made worse by stress. Exam anxiety is learned behavior and it probably began quite early in your school life. (You may be able to recall the first time you experienced exam anxiety in school.) Like any learned behavior, exam anxiety can be unlearned or the response to it can be changed. There is absolutely nothing frightening or dangerous in exams themselves. Rather, the anxiety you experience is directly related to the importance you attach to your success on the exam. Obviously, if you feel that your whole life and future hinge on how well you score on an exam, you are constructing a situation that can cause severe anxiety and such physical symptoms as headaches and diarrhea.

Image visualization can be a powerful technique for reducing the panic and physical symptoms of exam anxiety. By using image visualization prior to an exam, you can teach your mind and body how to relax.

Directions

Step 1. Find a comfortable place in your house or apartment and a time when it is quiet. Pick an environment in which you feel secure and where there are no disturbing distractions. Sit in a comfortable chair or lie down on a couch, bed, or floor. The main thing is to get physically comfortable. If music helps you relax, you can play some of your favorite instrumental music, but it should not be so loud that it becomes intrusive.

Step 2. Close your eyes and ask your mind to recall a place where you felt content and happy. Let it be a place where you had the kind of positive feeling that you wish you had all the time. Use your imagination to reconstruct the scene or place where you felt comfortable and happy. It might be a vacation spot or a time when you were lying on a beach or hiking in the mountains. The main thing is to let your mind freely choose a place or memory that feels the most comfortable and to let yourself become totally involved in that scene. It's like having a daydream except that you are constructing your own dream. While your mind is engaged in this pleasurable memory, your body automatically relaxes.

Step 3. After your mind and body have become comfortable and relaxed, you can refocus your attention on an upcoming exam. You can visualize in your mind taking the exam while remaining relaxed and confident. Because your mind and body have already been relaxed and because you are secure and comfortable in your own environment, your mind will associate these positive feelings with the inner visualization of the exam. Use your imagination to project your mind into the future when you are taking the exam, being calm and confident as you write down the answers to the questions or write your essay.

Let your imagination construct all of the details of the exam situation. Visualize the exam room and where you are sitting; notice that you can read and understand the questions without any effort. Pay attention to how you feel as you take the exam and note the absence of anxiety and the absence of uncomfortable physical symptoms. Continue with the visualization until you feel comfortable with the experience and with the exam. Repeat this exercise for several days prior to the actual exam. When you take the exam you will be surprised at the absence of nervousness or anxiety; you will be even more surprised and pleased at the improvement in your grades.

Study Guide and Self-Assessment

CHAPTER 4

4.1 Saying No

*Anyone can become angry. That is easy. But to be angry with the right person, to the right degree,
at the right time, and for the right purpose—this is not easy.*

—Aristotle

Many people have a hard time saying *no* to the requests and demands made by others and an equally hard time saying *yes* to themselves for something they want. To be generous with time and energy is thought to be a virtue; to accommodate your own wishes, selfish. There are times, however, when saying *no* to others and *yes* to yourself is highly appropriate. Your emotions tell you those times. The time to say *no* is when saying *yes* makes you feel angry, stressed, resentful, or unwell. The time to say *yes* to yourself is when it increases physical, emotional, and spiritual well-being.

Think about some recent times when you said *yes* to others when you really wanted to say *no*. Write them down like this: I would have liked to have said *no* when _____ asked me to _____.

Prepare yourself to say *no* to the same or other requests the next time they occur. Imagine yourself saying *no* to another and firmly and politely dealing with the other person's response.

Learning to say *no* may take practice, so don't get discouraged if at first you find it difficult.

4.2 My Definition of Mental Health

Success is getting up just one more time than you fall down.
—Barbara Milo Orbach

Directions

List and describe five characteristics of a mentally healthy person.

1. _____
   _____

2. _____
   _____

3. _____
   _____

4. _____
   _____

5. _____
   _____

If you were (are) a parent, how would you ensure that your child(ren) manifests the five characteristics on your list?

_____
_____
_____
_____
_____
_____
_____
_____
_____
_____
_____

4.3 Keeping a Journal

As long as you derive inner help and comfort from anything, keep it.
—Mahatma Gandhi

Our emotions tell us how well we are fulfilling our life needs and how well we are achieving our life goals, but sometimes it is difficult to understand why we feel a certain way at a certain time. One way to clarify thoughts and feelings is to record them in a journal or notebook, which is something like a diary except that thoughts and feelings are recorded instead of specific events. Practice keeping a journal of your thoughts and feelings for a two-week period. Set aside a particular time each day, perhaps just before you go to sleep, to check in with your feelings by writing how you feel at that moment or how you felt that day and explaining why those feelings may have occurred.

- Use a special notebook for your journal.

- Write in a quiet place.

- Keep your journal private so you can be honest with yourself.

- Write continuously. Don't worry about grammar or spelling.

- Be expressive. Don't worry about making sense.

4.4 My Fears and Phobias

Those who flow as life flows know they need no other force. They feel no wear, they feel no tear; they need no mending, no repair.

—Lao Tzu

Many health behaviors are reflections of beliefs and attitudes that operate beneath the level of conscious awareness. Because these beliefs and attitudes in the mind are similar to programs in a computer, they *can* be changed. Your mind can create new, health-promoting programs to replace old, health-destroying ones.

Health problems often arise from destructive mental programs that have their origins in frightening life experiences, especially ones encountered early in life. If you can become aware of how such frightening experiences have programmed your mind and have thereby influenced your subsequent behavior, you can take steps to reprogram your mind and eliminate both the fear and the unwanted behavior.

Directions

Step 1. Identify your fears and phobias using the chart below.

Step 2. Sit or lie down in a quiet, comfortable place and allow your mind to recall experiences that may have caused one of your present fears—perhaps the one that bothers you the most. Allow yourself to relax your mind and body as much as possible, then let the images just freely enter your mind. When you encounter a frightening situation, *imagine* it taking place in a manner that is *not* frightening—in your mind, any scene can be changed so that you feel safe and comfortable. Let the situation resolve itself in a positive way. Remember, because everything is going on in your mind, you have complete control of all actions and events in your imagined scene.

Step 3. Practice this positive imagery until you feel that your fear is less intense.

Frightening Situations or objects	No fear	Mild fear	Strong fear
Airplanes	_____	_____	_____
Birds	_____	_____	_____
Bats	_____	_____	_____
Blood	_____	_____	_____
Cemeteries	_____	_____	_____
Dead animals	_____	_____	_____
Insects	_____	_____	_____
Crowds of people	_____	_____	_____
Dark places	_____	_____	_____
Dentists or doctors	_____	_____	_____
Hospitals	_____	_____	_____
Dirt or germs	_____	_____	_____
Lakes or oceans	_____	_____	_____
Dogs or cats	_____	_____	_____
Other animals	_____	_____	_____
Guns	_____	_____	_____
Closets or elevators	_____	_____	_____
Heights	_____	_____	_____
Public presentations	_____	_____	_____
Loud noises	_____	_____	_____
Driving in a car	_____	_____	_____
Being shouted at	_____	_____	_____
Being rejected	_____	_____	_____
Walking alone at night	_____	_____	_____
Other fears	_____	_____	_____

Study Guide and Self-Assessment

4.5 My Sleep and Dream Record

Life is what happens when you're making other plans.
—Tom Smothers

Each morning for one week, assess your sleep behavior with the aid of a chart like the one below. Also record the details of your dreams in a journal or notebook. Hints for dream recording:

1. Keep a pen or a pencil and a pad of paper near your bed.

2. Remind yourself before going to sleep that you want to remember your dreams.

3. Write down your dreams immediately upon awakening.

	Sun	Mon	Tues	Wed	Thurs	Fri	Sat
Time to bed							
Time fell asleep (estimate on waking)							
Feelings before falling asleep							
Trouble falling asleep? (yes or no)							
Take sleeping aid? (e.g., milk or pills)							
Number of times awake in the night							
Time woke up							
Time got out of bed							
Feelings on awakening							
Dreams? (yes or no)							
Total sleep time							

4.6 How Can I Sleep Better?

What lies behind us and what lies before us are tiny matters compared to what lies within us.

—Oliver Wendell Holmes

College students are notoriously poor sleepers. Which of the healthy sleep habits listed below could you incorporate into your life? Explain your reasoning.

- *Establish a regular sleep time.* Give your own natural sleep cycle a chance to be in synchrony with the day–night cycle by going to bed at the same time each night (within an hour more or less) and arising *without being awakened by an alarm clock.* This will mean going to bed early enough to give yourself enough time to sleep. Try to maintain your regular sleep times on the weekend. Getting up early during the week and sleeping late on weekends may upset the rhythm of your sleep cycle.

- *Create a proper (for you) sleep environment.* Sleep occurs best when the sleeping environment is dark, quiet, free of distractions, and not too warm. If you use radio or TV to help you fall asleep, use an autotimer to shut off the noise after falling asleep.

- *Wind down before going to bed.* About 20 to 30 minutes before bedtime, stop any activities that cause mental or physical arousal, such as work or exercise, and take up a "quiet" activity that can create a transition to sleep. Transitional activities could include reading, watching "mindless" TV, taking a warm bath or shower, meditation, or making love.

- *Make the bedroom for sleeping only.* Make the bedroom your place for getting a good night's sleep. Try not to use it for work or for discussing problems with your partner.

- *Don't worry while in bed.* If you are unable to sleep after about 30 minutes in bed because of worry about the next day's activities, get up and do some limited activity such as reading a magazine article, doing the dishes, or meditating. Go back to bed when you feel drowsy. If you cannot sleep because of thinking about all that you have to do, write down what's on your mind and let the paper hold onto the thoughts while you sleep. You can retrieve them in the morning.

- *Avoid alcohol and caffeine.* Some people have a glass of beer or wine before bed to relax. Large amounts of alcohol, although sedating, block normal sleep and dreaming patterns. Because caffeine remains in the body for several hours, people sensitive to caffeine should not ingest any after noon.

- *Exercise regularly.* Exercising 20 to 30 minutes three or four times a week enhances the ability to sleep. You should not exercise vigorously within three hours of bedtime, however, because of the possibility of becoming too aroused to sleep.

Study Guide and Self-Assessment

4.7 How Do I Affect Others?

My granary has burned down—now I can see the sun.
—Japanese proverb

You can influence how others feel simply by your words and actions. When you sincerely say to someone, "You look terrific," you make that person feel good, thereby initiating a series of psychophysiological processes that begin in the mind and affect hormonal and nervous regulation of the body in such a way that his or her wellness is enhanced. On the other hand, when you say to someone, "You look terrible," you can initiate physiological responses that are correspondingly negative.

Directions

Step 1. For one week keep a record of the remarks you make to others that may affect their health and well-being, either positively or negatively. For example:

To John: "I liked the way you handled your anger in that situation. How'd you do it?"
To Sue (who is overweight): "You sure do pack away the food. I don't see where you put it all."

Step 2. For one week try to avoid remarks that can hurt a person's feelings or make a person feel bad. Say positive things to the people you interact with. Tell others how well they look and how well they are doing things. Show them that you care how they feel. As people around you feel better, so will you.

4.8 Disarming Your Internal Critic

I don't know the key to success, but the key to failure is trying to please everybody.
—Bill Cosby

The Internal Critic is mental self-criticism. The Internal Critic says things like, "You can't do that!" or "Don't do it that way, you'll embarrass yourself." The Internal Critic can stop us from doing things for fear of shame and embarrassment, and it can make us feel generally incompetent and bad about ourselves.

You can learn to identify and disarm your Internal Critic by being alert for it. When the Internal Critic is activated, someone facing a challenge might say, "I can't" or "I'm confused." Sometimes a student verbalizes the Internal Critic's message, as in, "I'm too stupid to understand this."

Disarming the Internal Critic

1. *Name and Voice It.* Write or say what the Internal Critic says. Be sure to add the Internal Critic's emotional tone.

2. *Defend Yourself.* Say to the Internal Critic, "Don't talk to me like that!"

3. *Talk Back to It.* Write or say, "I hear you, but I'm going ahead anyway."

4. *Ignore It.* Acknowledge that the Internal Critic has been activated and say to yourself, "There's that Internal Critic again," and shift your mental focus to the task at hand.

5. *Try to Understand It.* Sometimes the Internal Critic is trying to protect you from an imagined hurt. Write an imaginary conversation with your Internal Critic in which you discuss its motive(s).

Study Guide and Self-Assessment

4.9 Constructing Your Personal House

The unexamined life is not worth living.
—Socrates

Let the drawing of this house represent your personal life. Write a one paragraph description for each of these parts of your house:

Foundation: Your life governing principles
Walls: Your means of physical and emotional support
Roof: Ways you protect yourself physically and psychologically
Chimney: Ways you relieve stress
Attic: Your fears
Chest: Highly personal things you are willing to share with another
Window: Things you are proud of
Door: Physical and psychological things you have borrowed from others
Mirror: How you see yourself (self-image, self-esteem, strengths, weaknesses)
Trash can: Things you want to get rid of

The authors wish to acknowledge John Porter for this exercise.

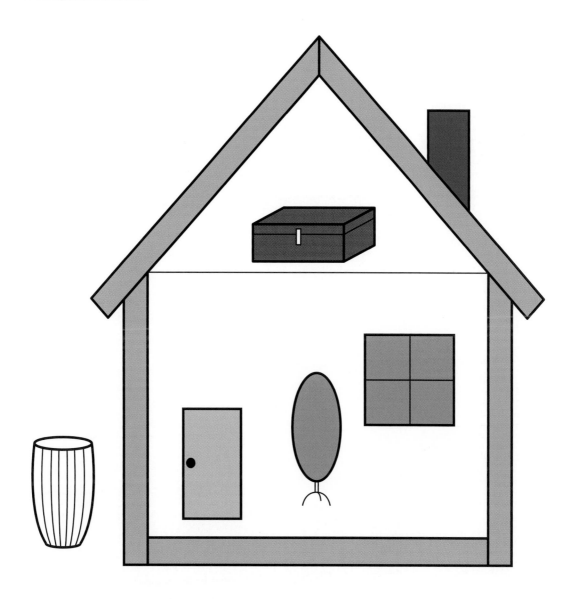

5.1 My Estimated Daily Calorie Requirement

There are two ways of being disappointed in life; one is not to get what you want and the other is to get it.

—George Bernard Shaw

Estimate your daily calorie requirement using steps 1–4 below.

Step 1. I am _____ feet _____ inches tall.

Step 2. Calculate your total body mass units:

- Women: Allow 100 body mass units for the first 5 feet of height + 5 body mass units for each additional inch.

- Men: Allow 106 body mass units for the first 5 feet of height + 6 body mass units for each additional inch.

My total body mass units = _____.

Step 3. My activity factor is:

Sedentary = 13
Active = 15
Very active = 17

Step 4. Calculate your estimated daily calories by multiplying your body mass units by your activity factor:

(Body mass units) × (Activity factor) = _____ (my estimated calories)

5.2 My Food Diary

If your stomach disputes you, lay down and pacify it with cool thoughts.
—Leroy "Satchel" Paige

Directions

For two days that are representative of your usual food consumption patterns, keep a list of *everything* you eat (see illustration below). Record:

- the name of each food item

- the quantity of each food item consumed

- the time of day each item was consumed

- whether consumption was part of a meal or as a snack

- whether you ate because of hunger or for other reasons

- your feelings at the time you ate

- the social circumstances surrounding eating (alone, with friends, with family, etc.)

Food	Quantity	Time of day	Meal or snack	Hungry? Other?	Feelings?	Social?
cereal	bowlful	6:30 AM	meal	hungry	sleepy	alone
banana	one					
milk, skim	cup					

Data Analysis

1. How close are you to the recommended Five-A-Day servings of fruits and vegetables?

   _____

   _____

   _____

   _____

2. Describe your snacking patterns.

   _____

   _____

   _____

   _____

3. Describe ways your feelings affect your food consumption.

   _____

4. Log on to the U.S. Department of Agriculture's nutritional analysis Web site (http://www.mypyramid.gov).

   - Click the My Pyramid Plan link and enter the appropriate data for your age, sex, and level of physical activity to determine your nutritional recommendations. Print the response.

   - On the Web page with your recommendations, click the Meal Tracking Worksheet link and analyze your diet by filling in the spreadsheet.

Study Guide and Self-Assessment

5.3 My Dietary Analysis

People are satisfied, not by the presence of food, but by the absence of greed.
—Gurdjieff

Refer to your Food Diary and consult the U.S. Department of Agriculture's MyPyramid Web site (http://www.mypyramid.gov) to analyze the nutrient content of your diet and to obtain recommendations for improving the nutrient quality of your diet.

Directions

1. Log on to MyPyramid.gov

2. Click the My Pyramid Plan link and enter the appropriate data for your age, sex, and level of physical activity to determine your nutritional recommendations. Print the response.

3. On the Web page with your recommendations, click the MyPyramid Tracker link and enter the foods from your Food Diary for a day that is typical of your dietary pattern.

4. Click the Analyze Your Food Intake tab and obtain an analysis of your diet and recommendations for a healthy diet by clicking (and printing out):

   • Meeting 2005 Dietary Guidelines

   • Nutrient Intakes

   • MyPyramid Recommendations

5. On a typical day, I consume:

   _____ grams of fiber

   _____ grams of total fat

   _____ grams of saturated fat

   _____ grams of cholesterol

   _____ milligrams of calcium

   _____ milligrams of iron

   _____ grams of sodium

6. How does your diet compare to the MyPyramid recommendations?

   _____

   _____

   _____

   _____

   _____

   _____

   _____

   _____

   _____

   _____

Study Guide and Self-Assessment

5.4 Fast-Food Restaurant Research

After dinner sit awhile. After supper walk a mile.
—English proverb

Each day approximately 20% of the U.S. population eats at a fast-food restaurant. The reasons for patronizing such establishments are convenience (they are everywhere), perceived lack of time to shop and prepare meals at home, fast food's taste and texture, the need to mollify nagging children, and cost. Since fast food is so popular and prevalent, it is healthful to know the nutrient content of the fast food you consume. So . . .

Directions

1. Go to your favorite fast-food restaurant and ask the serviceperson for a copy of the brochure listing the nutritional content of that establishment's foods. (If you do not patronize such establishments, do the assignment for someone you know who does and share the information with her or him.)

2. Choose a fast-food meal that is typical for you. Refer to the restaurant's brochure, and for each of the meal's components list the following information:

   - Total calories
   - Grams of protein
   - Total grams of fat
   - Total grams of saturated fat
   - mg of cholesterol
   - mg of salt
   - Grams of fiber

3. Calculate the dollar cost of the energy content of the meal (divide total calories by the total cost). This tells you how much bang (energy) you are getting for your buck.

4. What percentage of your estimated daily calories is contributed by this meal?

   _____

   _____

5. Describe your experience obtaining the company's brochure at the restaurant.

   _____

   _____

6. List the reasons you patronize this establishment.

   _____

   _____

7. How frequently do you patronize fast-food restaurants?

   _____

   _____

8. What did you learn from this assignment?

   _____

   _____

Note: Fast Food Facts (http://www.foodfacts.info) lists the nutrient composition of fast foods. Most fast-food corporations list nutrient composition of their products on the company Web site. Whereas it is possible to analyze the data for this assignment with that Web tool, it is more interesting and makes you a better health consumer if you go personally to the restaurant and ask for the data.

Study Guide and Self-Assessment

5.5 Can I Read a Food Label?

If A is success in life, then A equals x plus y plus z. Work is x, y is play, and z is keeping your mouth shut.

—Albert Einstein

Directions

1. Look at the Nutrition Facts Label on any commercial food product. The Percent Daily Values says that a person with a 2,000 calories per day energy requirement should not ingest more than how many grams of fat per day?

   _____

   _____

2. How many milligrams of cholesterol per day are recommended for someone with a daily calorie requirement of 2,000 calories? 2,500 calories?

   _____

   _____

3. Take the Food Label Quiz at the U.S. Food and Drug Administration's Center for Food Safety and Applied Nutrition Web site: http://www.cfsan.fda.gov/~dms/flquiz1.html. Find out the following information:

- Which muffins maximize fiber intake?

  _____

  _____

  _____

- Are these pretzels low in sodium?

  _____

  _____

- Which has less calories, the low-fat blueberry yogurt or the low-fat cherry yogurt?

  _____

  _____

- Which is the best source of calcium?

  _____

  _____

- Which packaged food has the least saturated fat?

  _____

  _____

Study Guide and Self-Assessment

5.6 Five-A-Day

If more of us valued food and cheer and song above hoarded gold, it would be a merrier world.
—J. R. R. Tolkien

Use your Food Diary (see Exercise 5.2) to determine the number of servings of fruits and vegetables you consume each day. For three weeks, try to increase by one (at most two) the number of servings a day of fruits and vegetables that you consume.

1. Keep a daily record of the number of servings of fruits and vegetables you consume.

2. Make a graph in which you record the number of servings of fruits and vegetables you consume each day over the three-week activity period.

3. Identify any obstacles that prevented you from carrying out a day's activity.

4. Develop strategies for overcoming any obstacles that keep you from increasing the number of servings you consume.

5.7 My Fiber Consumption

Failures are finger posts on the road to achievement.
—C. S. Lewis

1. Use your Food Diary (see Exercise 5.2) to determine the number of grams of fiber you typically consume per day.

2. Make a list of foods that you will consume to bring your total number of grams of fiber consumed to 20–30 per day.

3. For three weeks, try to consume 20–30 grams of fiber per day. Keep a diary in which you
   - Record the number of grams of fiber you consume and their sources
   - Identify obstacles that prevented you from achieving your goal
   - Identify and implement strategies for overcoming obstacles

4. Record on a graph the number of grams of fiber you consume daily over the three-week activity period.

5.8 Dietary Fat Consumption

Never go to excess, but let moderation be your guide.
—Cicero

Reduce fat consumption to 30% (or less) of daily calories.

1. Use your Food Diary and the U.S. Department of Agriculture's Nutrient Data Laboratory Web site (http://www.ars.usda.gov/ba/bhnrc/ndl) to determine the percentage of total calories from fat you typically consume each day.

2. Make a list of food exchanges that you will employ to lower your fat intake (e.g., piece of fruit for a candy bar, pasta for a hamburger, etc.).

3. For three weeks, alter your diet to lower your fat intake.

4. Keep a dairy in which you record the following information:
   - The amount of fat grams and fat calories you consume each day
   - Any obstacles that prevented you from carrying out a day's activity
   - Strategies for overcoming any obstacles

5. Make a graph in which you record the percentage of total daily calories derived from fat during the three-week action period.

5.9 My Soda Consumption

Respect yourself and others will respect you.
—Confucius

Soda is nutritionally inferior. Sodas with sugar contribute to weight gain. Try to limit or eliminate soda consumption using the following steps:

- For one week, keep a diary of your soda consumption; count how many sodas you consume each day.

- For the next 2–3 weeks, reduce soda consumption gradually by choosing alternative beverages, such as water, tea, or 100% juice (no sugary "juice drinks" or "energy drinks"). *Note:* Going "cold turkey" on sodas may produce caffeine withdrawal headaches for a couple of days. Cut back gradually.

- Continue to keep your soda consumption diary to record decreasing consumption. Record obstacles that get in the way of reducing soda consumption.

6.1 My Body Weight

People through finding something beautiful, think something else unbeautiful. Through finding one man fit, judge another unfit.

—Lao Tzu

My height in feet and inches (without shoes):_____

My weight in pounds now (with clothes):_____

My highest weight as an adult = _____ pounds, which I weighed when I was _____ years old

My lowest weight as an adult = _____ pounds, which I weighed when I was _____ years old

The recommended weight for my height and body frame is (see text Chapter 6):_____

My body mass index* is _____.
(See the chart on text page 139 or the online calculator at (http://nhlbisupport.com/bmi/.)

The circumference of my body at my waist† is _____.
The circumference of my body at my hips is _____.
The ratio‡ of my waist/hip circumferences is _____.

---

*The Body Mass Index (BMI) is the most common way doctors assess the relationship of body size and health. It is calculated by dividing a person's weight in kilograms by her or his height in meters squared: BMI = wgt/(hgt)(hgt). A BMI between 18 and 24.9 is not associated with an increased risk of weight-related illness. (*Note:* The health risks for a BMI over 25 are less reliable for people who are muscular or of a large body frame.)

†A waist circumference of more than 40 inches in men and 35 inches in women indicates overweight.

‡A waist-to-hip ratio of 0.95 in men and 0.80 in women indicates overweight.

6.2 Managing My Weight

Be true to yoru work, your word, and your friend.
—Henry David Thoreau

Develop a plan for weight loss/weight management.

1. Determine your healthy weight range by consulting the weight-for-height tables and BMI table in Chapter 6 of the text.

    My healthful body weight range is _____.

    My Body Mass Index is _____.

2. If you wish to lose weight, make a plan that combines increased exercise and moderate calorie reduction to produce the loss of not more than one pound a week until body weight is reduced by 10%. List the types and duration of exercise you will do, foods that you will limit, and the length of time you will devote to a weight loss regime.

    Exercise I will increase:

    _____

    _____

    _____

    Foods I will limit:

    _____

    _____

    _____

Time allotted to lose 10% of current body weight:

_____

_____

_____

3. Increase exercise and limit certain foods (e.g., junk and fast foods, sodas).

4. Keep a daily record of exercise and dietary changes. For each day record the following information:

    • The exercise changes you're doing

    • The food changes you make

    • What you experience

    • Any obstacles that prevented you from carrying out a day's plan

    • Strategies for overcoming any obstacles

5. Make a graph in which you record each day the number of minutes of exercise you do and the number of calories you don't consume.

Study Guide and Self-Assessment

6.3 My Body Image

Hope for the best, plan for the worst.
—Chinese proverb

Body image (more accurately, *body esteem*) is a self-appraisal of your body's size and shape.

Directions:

1. Do the Body Image questionnaire below.
    How do you feel about the appearances of these regions of your body?

    _____

    _____

	Quite satisfied	Somewhat satisfied	Somewhat dissatisfied	Very dissatisfied
Hair	❏	❏	❏	❏
Arms	❏	❏	❏	❏
Hands	❏	❏	❏	❏
Feet	❏	❏	❏	❏
Waist	❏	❏	❏	❏
Buttocks	❏	❏	❏	❏
Hips	❏	❏	❏	❏
Legs and ankles	❏	❏	❏	❏
Thighs	❏	❏	❏	❏
Chest or breasts	❏	❏	❏	❏
Posture	❏	❏	❏	❏
General attractiveness	❏	❏	❏	❏

2. Write an essay in which you respond to these questions:

    *   Which of your regular thoughts and actions are likely to enhance your body image?

        _____

        _____

    *   Which of your regular thoughts and actions are likely to be detrimental to your body image?

        _____

        _____

    *   How do social expectations of body size and shape affect your body image?

        _____

        _____

    *   How susceptible are you to media images of "ideal" body proportions for members of your sex?

        _____

        _____

    *   How could you become more satisfied with your body image?

        _____

        _____

        _____

Study Guide and Self-Assessment

7.1 Putting Exercise Into My Life

Give what you have. To someone, it may be better than you dare to think.
—Henry Wadsworth Longfellow

1. Use your Time Audit (see Exercise 3.7) to identify four "windows" of time during the week to exercise.

2. Choose an activity that interests you and schedule it for your four "exercise windows".

3. Keep a diary of your exercise sessions. For each day record the following information:

   - The activity

   - The time you spent doing the activity

   - What you experienced while doing the activity

   - Any obstacles that prevented you from carrying out a day's activity

   - Strategies for overcoming any obstacles

4. Make a graph in which you record the number of sessions of exercise and their length each week.

7.2 Walking for Health

Walking is man's best medicine.
—Hippocrates

Everyone knows that physical activity is good for health. Those who are not active frequently say that they don't have time to go to the gym and/or that they hate to sweat. Aerobic activity (the kind in which you breathe hard and sweat) and strength training, while good for health if done in moderation so as to avoid injury, are not the only ways to be active. The easiest and cheapest form of physical activity is to walk.

The current minimum recommendation is to walk for a total of 150 minutes a week, which is about 20 minutes a day (1 mile). Forty minutes to an hour a day is best (3 miles). And you don't have to do the whole 20–60 minutes at once. You can break it up into segments.

If you like to count or like to challenge yourself, you can get a pedometer, a device that counts your steps. Try to walk 10,000 steps a day in any way you can. Keep a "walking log" in which you record the number of steps you take each day.

7.3 My Target Heart Rate Zone

You should ask yourself every day why you are doing what you're doing.
—Robert Arneson

Your target heart rate zone is the level of activity that leads to maximum conditioning. Activity below the target heart rate zone conditions little; activity above the target heart rate zone may be dangerous for some people.

The pattern of the preferred exercise session is shown in the following figure:

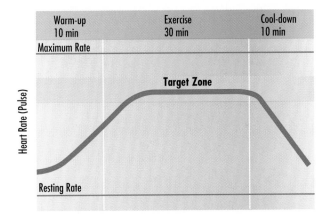

To compute your target heart rate zone:

1. Subtract your age from 220 (Example: For a 20-year-old person with resting heart rate of 80 beats/min: 220 − 20 = 200).

2. Subtract resting heart rate from number obtained in step 1 (200 − 80 = 120).

3. Multiply the result once by 0.65 and once again by 0.75 (120 × .65 = 78; 120 × .75 = 90).

4. Add resting heart rate to the results obtained in step 3 to give lower and upper heart rates of target zone (Lower limit: 78 + 80 = 158; upper limit: 90 + 80 = 170).

After your warm-up period and 10 minutes of activity, take your pulse and compare it to the heart rate for your target zone level of activity. If you are below your target zone heart rate, increase your activity. If above, slow down.

Measuring Heart Rate

Your heart rate, or pulse, is the number of times your heart beats per minute. When your heart beats, it pushes about a cup of blood into your circulatory system. At certain sites in the circulatory system you can feel when the blood from the most recent heartbeat arrives. These sites are where you measure your heart rate. The most commonly used are in the neck (carotid artery), the wrist below the thumb (radial artery), or the inner thigh (femoral artery). To measure your heart rate:

- Get a clock/watch that measures seconds.

- Place your first two fingers, not your thumb (it has a pulse and can confuse things), on one of the common measuring sites (neck, wrist, or inner thigh).

- Press a tiny bit to make solid contact with the tissue under the skin (including the artery).

- Move your fingers around until the sensation of the pulse is strongest.

- Look at your timing device and count the number of beats/pulsations in 15 seconds.

- Multiply the number of beats/pulsations in 15 seconds by 4 to get beats per minute.

Study Guide and Self-Assessment

7.4 My Fitness Index

*People measure their esteem of each other by what each has and not by
what each is. . . .   Nothing can bring you peace but yourself.*
—Ralph Waldo Emerson

The Harvard Step Test is a standardized measure of cardiorespiratory fitness.
To carry out the Harvard Step Test, you need to be comfortably dressed (athletic clothes are best); you need a chair, stool, or bench 12–18 inches high, a
stopwatch or clock with a second hand, a pencil and paper, and a metronome
or some other method to produce a rhythmic 100–120 beats per minute,
such as a recording of a march or some disco music. Once all this is assembled, you can begin.

1. Make a 15-second recording of your resting pulse and multiply by 4 to
   obtain your rate per minute.

2. Start the metronome or music; 120 beats per minute.

3. Step completely up on the bench with the left leg first, followed by
   your right leg, then step back down with the left leg first, followed by
   the right. The stepping should be done on a four-count: up-up-down-down; up-up-down-down. . . .

4. Continue the exercise for 3 minutes unless you are more than 30 years
   old and have been rather inactive for more than six months. In that
   case, do the test for only a minute or two, whichever you think you
   can do. If you are sure you cannot do the test for even a few seconds,
   don't.

5. When the 3 minutes of exercise are through, immediately take your
   pulse. Record the number of heartbeats between 15 and 30 seconds
   after exercising. Make another heart rate measurement between 60
   and 75 seconds; another between 120 and 135 seconds; another
   between 180 and 195 seconds; another between 240 and 255
   seconds; and a final measurement between 300 and 315 seconds.

6. Multiply each of the 15-second heart rates by 4 to give the beats per
   minute. Record your data on the graph provided.

7. Compute your Fitness Index: Add the per-minute heart rates for the
   first 3 minutes after exercise. Then divide that number into 30,000.

Fitness index	Rating
above 90	Excellent
80–89	Good
65–79	Average
55–64	Low Average
below 55	Poor

Harvard Step Test Data Record		
Time	Heartbeats per 15 Seconds	Heartbeats per Minute
At rest	_____ × 4 =	_____
15–30 sec.	_____ × 4 =	_____
60–75 sec.	_____ × 4 =	_____
120–135 sec.	_____ × 4 =	_____
180–195 sec.	_____ × 4 =	_____
240–255 sec.	_____ × 4 =	_____
300–315 sec.	_____ × 4 =	_____

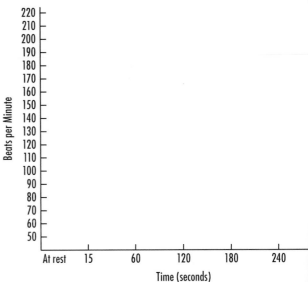

7.5 Increasing My Physical Fitness

I finally realized that being grateful to my body was key to giving more love to myself.

—Oprah Winfrey

1. Measure your level of fitness using the Harvard Step Test (see Exercise 7.4).

2. Measure your resting heart rate.

3. Determine your Target Zone heart rate (see Exercise 7.3).

4. Refer to your Time Audit to find at least four times per week when you can exercise for 30–60 minutes (see Exercise 3.7).

   My Fitness Index is _____.

   My resting heart rate is _____ beats per minute.

   My Target Zone heart rate is between _____ and _____ beats per minute.

5. Choose an aerobic activity that interests you and exercise at least four times a week for three weeks. Determine your heart rate at the end of each exercise session to see if you are exercising within your target zone.

6. Keep a diary of your activity. For each day record the following information:
   - The activity
   - The time you spent doing the activity
   - What you experienced doing the activity
   - Any obstacles that prevented you from carrying out a day's activity
   - Strategies for overcoming any obstacles

7. For each week record your resting heart rate and your Fitness Index.

8. Make a graph in which you record for the three-week period:
   - The number of sessions of exercise and their length
   - Your resting heart rate at the start and end of the project
   - Your Fitness Index at the start and end of the project

Study Guide and Self-Assessment

7.6 My Flexibility Index

You don't have to learn the lotus position or climb to the top of a mountain in Tibet to be able to sit down and relax your mind.
—College health student

Body flexibility is a fundamental aspect of feeling good and keeping your body healthy. Use this simple YMCA test to determine your degree of body flexibility, and continue to use it to determine your progress in becoming more limber.

1. Warm up with some stretching before the test.

2. Sit on the floor with your legs extended and feet a few inches apart.

3. With a piece of adhesive tape, mark the place where your heels touch the floor. Your heels should touch the near edge of the tape.

4. Place a yardstick on the floor between your legs and parallel to them. The beginning of the yardstick should be closest to you and the 15-inch mark should align with the near edge of the tape.

5. Slowly reach with both hands as far forward as possible. Touch your fingers to the yardstick to determine the distance reached. Do not jerk to increase your distance—this may cause damage to your leg muscles.

6. Repeat the exercise two or three times and record your best score.

	Inches reached		Rating
Men	Women		
22–23	24–27		Excellent
20–21	21–23		Good
14–19	16–20		Average
12–13	13–16		Fair
0–11	0–12		Poor

7.7 Increasing My Flexibility

So you see, imagination needs noodling—long, inefficient, happy idling,
dawdling and puttering.

—Brenda Ueland

Increase your flexibility by undertaking a regular regime of stretching or yoga.

1. Measure your flexibility by using the flexibility test (see Exercise 7.6).

2. Refer to your Time Audit (see Exercise 3.7) to find at least four occasions per week when you can stretch for 10–20 minutes each time.

3. Choose a stretching regime (see text Chapter 7) that interests you and carry it out at least four times a week.

4. Keep a diary of your activity:

   - Record the number of stretching sessions you do each week.

   - Record the time spent in each session.

   - Record your physical and psychological experiences before and after each session.

   - Identify any obstacles that prevented you from carrying out a day's activity.

   - Develop strategies for overcoming any obstacles.

5. Make a graph in which you record the number of sessions of stretching each week. Determine your flexibility index (inches reached) at the end of each week.

7.8 The Sun Salute

The best way to avoid something is to cause that which is to be avoided to avoid you of its own accord.
—Sufi saying

The sun salute, a Hatha yoga exercise, is a series of 12 postures, or asanas, intended to be done in one flowing routine. Each of the 12 postures is held for 3 seconds. The entire routine should be done at least twice in succession, alternating the legs. The Sun Salute is an excellent way to stretch the body every morning or any time you may need to relax tense muscles and restore deep, regular breathing. Try it.

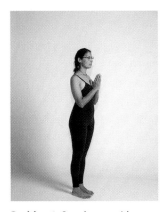

Position 1 Stand erect with your feet hip-width apart and palms together in front of your chest. Inhale and exhale slowly and calmly.

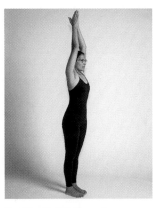

Position 2 Inhaling, raise your arms above your head, palms facing in. Lengthen through the spine, but do not arch your back.

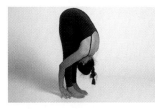

Position 3 Exhaling, bend forward from the hips, keeping your arms extended and your head hanging loosely between them. Keep your legs slightly bent and relax your neck and shoulders.

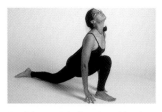

Position 4 Inhaling, bend both knees and place your palms flat an the floor by the outsides of your feet. Extend your left leg back. Stretch your chin toward the ceiling.

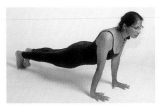

Position 5 Continue while holding the breath if you can—don't strain. Reach your forward leg back next to the other leg. Hold your body straight, supported by your hands and toes, with ankles, hips, and shoulders in a straight plane.

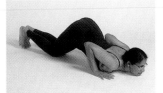

Position 6 Exhaling, lower your knees, chest, and chin or forehead to the floor, keeping your hips up and toes curled under.

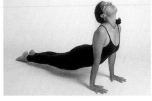

Position 7 Inhaling, bring the tops of your feet to the floor, straighten your legs, and come up to straight arms, opening the chest and stretching your chin toward the ceiling. Be careful not to overarch your lower back.

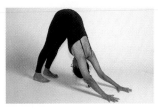

Position 8 Exhaling, curl your toes under and raise your hips into an inverted "V." Push back with your hands and lengthen your spine by reaching your hips upward. Keep your head hanging loosely.

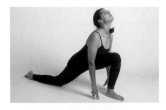

Position 9 Inhaling, lift your head and bring your left leg between your hands, keeping the right leg back. Raise your chin toward the ceiling.

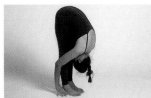

Position 10 Exhaling, bring your left foot forward so your feet are together. Bend forward from the hips, keeping your legs slightly bent and your upper body relaxed. If you can, touch your head to your knees and place your palms beside your feet.

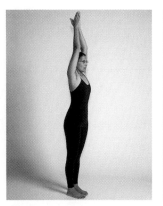

Position 11 Inhaling, slowly straighten up with your arms extended above your head. If you have any lower back pain, be sure to bend your knees.

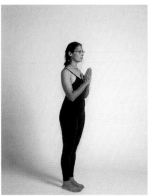

Position 12 Exhaling, bring your hands together in front of you. Close your eyes for a moment and feel the sensations in your body.

CHAPTER 8

8.1 Sexual Anatomy

You cannot live a perfect day without doing something for someone who will never be able to repay you.
—Coach John Wooden

Directions

On the following pages are silhouettes of the male and female pelvic regions and a page of drawings of the sexual/reproductive organs. Cut out the organs and attach them to the proper positions on the silhouettes found on pages 691–699, and label the female front view on page 700.

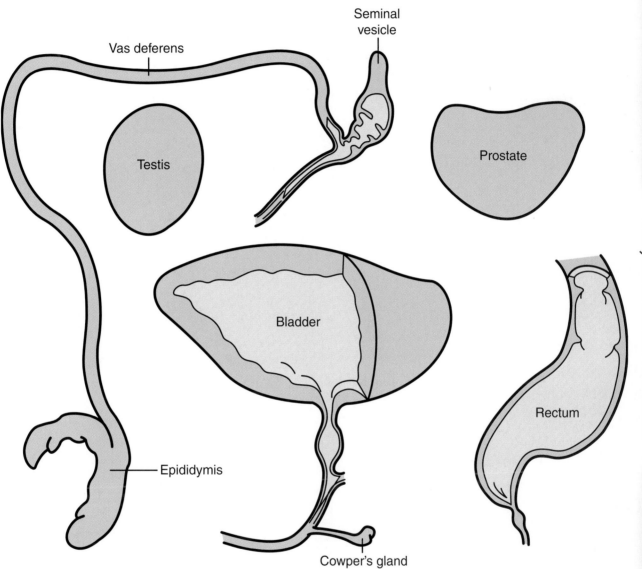

Male side

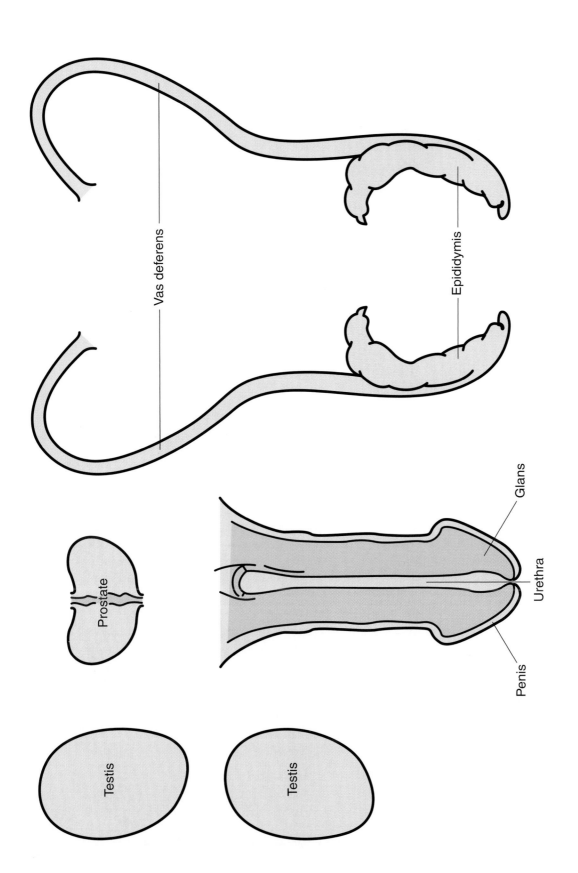

Vas deferens

Epididymis

Prostate

Glans

Urethra

Penis

Testis

Testis

Male front

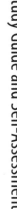

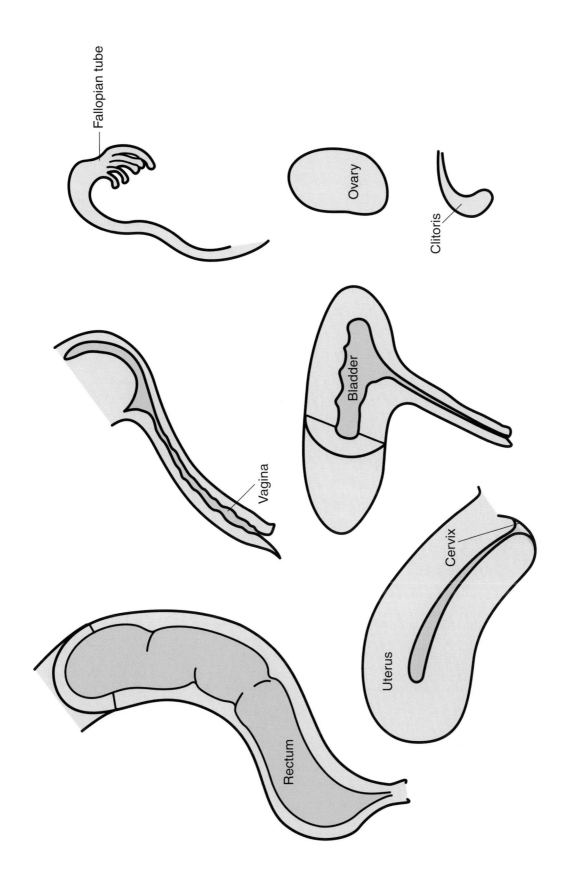

Female side

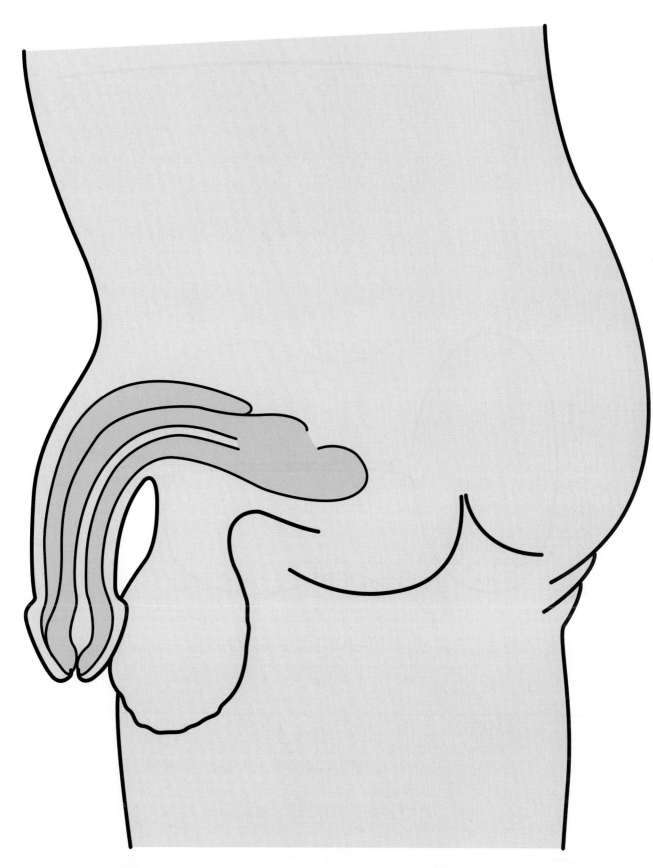

Male side

Study Guide and Self-Assessment

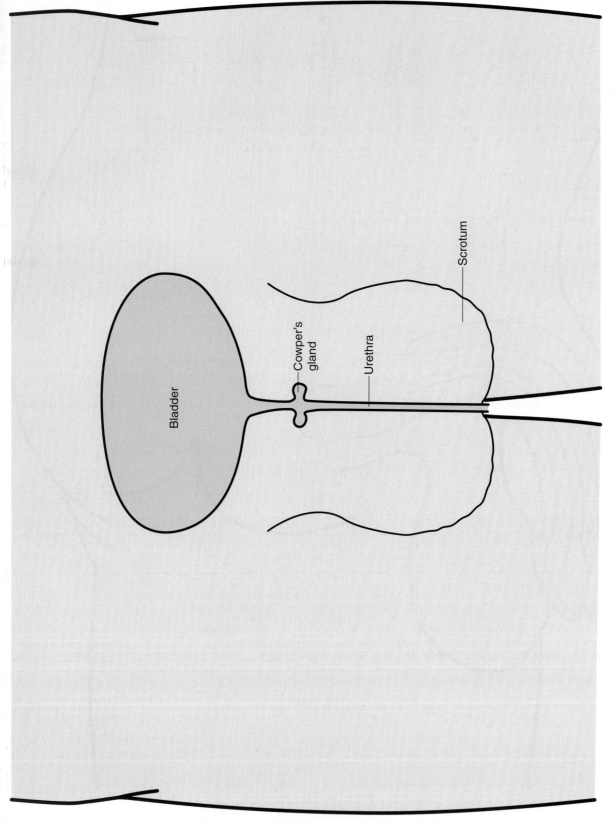

Bladder

Cowper's gland

Urethra

Scrotum

Male front

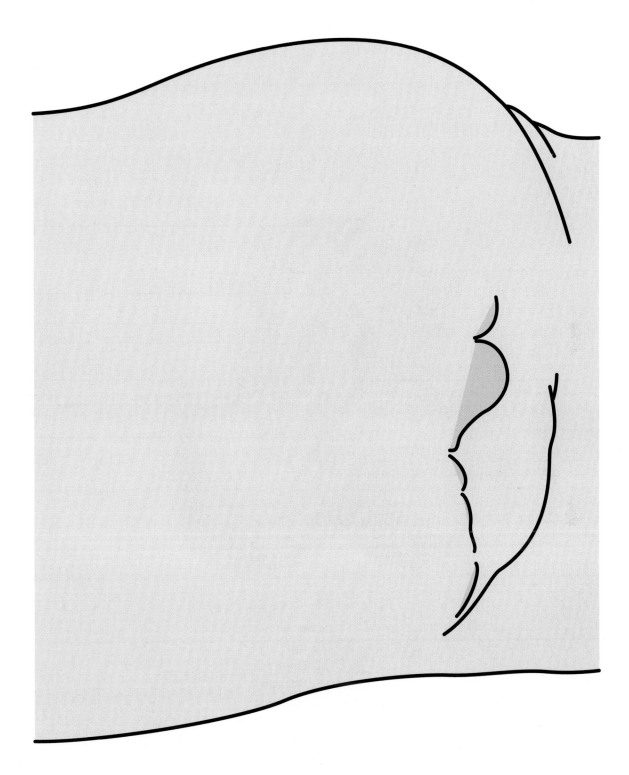

Female side

Study Guide and Self-Assessment

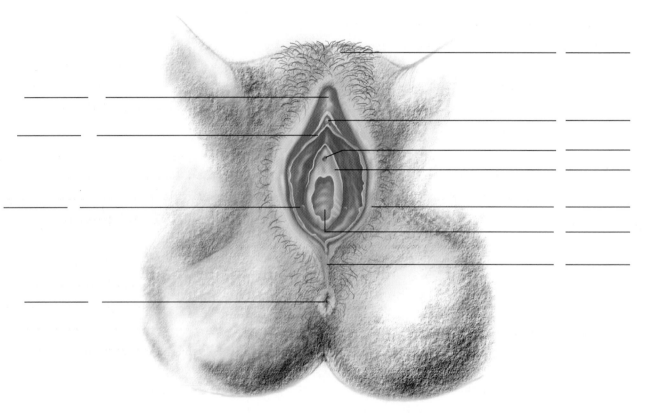

Label

1. Anus
2. Clitoris
3. Labia majora
4. Labia minora
5. Mons veneris
6. Perineum
7. Prepuce (hood)
8. Urinary meatus
9. Vaginal orifice

8.2 My Sexual Attitudes

Steer clear of the front of a billygoat, the back of a horse, and all sides of a fool.
—Yiddish proverb

Write a one-paragraph response to the following questions. Your responses will be read only by the instructor and will be kept strictly confidential.

1. Describe how your current sexual attitudes and beliefs compare to those of your parents (give examples).

2. Describe the ways religious/spiritual values affect your sexuality and sexual behavior.

3. What is the importance of sex in human relationships?

4. By what criteria, if any, is sexual intercourse before marriage permissible? How would you advise your own child on having premarital sex?

5. Describe two social expectations of you as a member of your sex.

Complete the following statements based upon your experiences and thoughts.

6. When I was growing up, talking about sexual matters with my parents . . .

7. As a child and teenager I learned the most about sex from . . .

8. The way I reacted to how my body changed at puberty was . . . especially . . .

9. My first significant sexual experience (not necessarily intercourse) taught me that . . .

10. From my parents' marriage I learned . . .

8.3 My Sexual Values

We do not see things as they are. We see things as we are.
—Talmud

For each statement, indicate the response that most closely identifies your beliefs and attitudes. Use the following code:

A = I strongly agree   B = I slightly agree

C = I slightly disagree   D = I strongly disagree

_____ 1. Men are by nature more sexually aggressive than women are and enjoy sex more than women do.

_____ 2. Sex-role definitions and stereotypes get in the way of mutually satisfying sexual relations.

_____ 3. Concern over sexual performance is quite common.

_____ 4. Psychologically healthy people don't experience any guilt over their sexual activities.

_____ 5. If a woman doesn't experience orgasm, it is generally because the man has not been sensitive enough to her needs.

_____ 6. If a man experiences erection problems, it is generally because of the woman's lack of appreciation of his manhood.

_____ 7. In a sexual relationship, it is the job of each partner to make the other feel like a woman or a man.

_____ 8. Getting in touch with our sexual attractions and feelings toward others generally leads to overt sexual behavior.

_____ 9. The quality of a sexual relationship is usually parallel to the quality of the partners' relationship in general.

_____ 10. Sexual freedom implies doing whatever consenting adults agree to.

_____ 11. If we want to, we can reeducate ourselves so that we can experience sexual relationships with numerous partners without feeling guilty.

_____ 12. Sexual freedom ought to be counterbalanced by sexual responsibility.

_____ 13. We will probably be no more sexually attractive to others than we are to ourselves.

_____ 14. Discussing sexual wants and needs generally leads to mechanical and unspontaneous sex.

_____ 15. Extramarital sex inevitably causes dissatisfaction in the marital relationships.

_____ 16. Today's generation is really unconcerned about being sexually inadequate.

_____ 17. Most people who are intimate with each other find it relatively easy to talk openly and honestly about the intimate details of sexuality.

_____ 18. The key to improving sexual satisfaction is to master sexual techniques and skills.

_____ 19. Sex without love is unsatisfying.

Study Guide and Self-Assessment

8.4 Sexual Communication

If the person you are talking to doesn't appear to be listening, be patient. It may simply be that he has a piece of fluff in his ears.
—A. A. Milne, Winnie-the-Pooh

Communication skills contribute to rewarding relationships in many ways. Many of the problems couples experience could be avoided or easily resolved with more effective communication skills. How are your communication skills?

For each statement, circle the appropriate number of points.

	Usually	Sometimes	Seldom
1. I find it easy to express my nonsexual needs and feelings to others.	2	1	0
2. I find it easy to express my sexual needs and feelings to others.	2	1	0
3. I am sensitive to the needs and feelings expressed by others, and especially their nonverbal expressions.	2	1	0
4. My relationships with other people are pleasant and rewarding.	2	1	0
5. When a conflict arises in one of my relationships, it is resolved with ease.	2	1	0
6. I find it easy to communicate with people of both genders.	2	1	0
7. I can communicate effectively with people of various ethnic groups.	2	1	0
8. I can find the right words to express the ideas I want to convey.	2	1	0
9. I am good at interpreting nonverbal messages from other people.	2	1	0
10. I try very hard not to interrupt someone who is speaking to me.	2	1	0
11. I try very hard to be nonjudgmental in my responses when people share their ideas and feelings with me.	2	1	0
12. When a discussion is causing me to feel uncomfortable, I try hard not to withdraw from the discussion or change the subject.	2	1	0
13. I try to help people open up by asking open-ended, rather than yes-or-no questions.	2	1	0
14. When I want to express my feelings, I try to phrase them as "I" statements, rather than "you" statements.	2	1	0
15. I feel that I am adequately assertive.	2	1	0
16. I let someone know when they are not respecting my rights or feelings.	2	1	0
17. I find it easy to say no to pressure for unwanted sexual activity.	2	1	0
18. I find it easy to talk to a potential sexual partner about prevention of sexually transmitted diseases.	2	1	0
19. When conflicts arise in my relationships, I am, if necessary, willing and able to make a compromise to resolve the conflict.	2	1	0
20. When conflicts arise in my relationships, I try to find a resolution that satisfies the needs of both persons involved.	2	1	0

TOTAL POINTS: _____

Interpretation:

36 to 40 points: You have developed highly effective patterns of communication and assertiveness.

32 to 35 points: You have above-average communication and assertiveness skills.

28 to 31 points: You have about-average communication and assertiveness skills. Sharpening these skills will improve your relationships and need fulfillment.

27 points or less: It would be very rewarding for you to improve your communication skills. Your relationships would function much better, and you would experience much greater need fulfillment.

Source: Byer, C. O., Shainberg, L. W., & Galliano, G. (1999). *Dimensions of human sexuality,* 5th ed. Boston, MA: McGraw-Hill College, p. 68. Reprinted with permission from The McGraw-Hill Companies, Inc.

Study Guide and Self-Assessment

8.5 My Attitudes About Love

We must always follow somebody looking for truth, and we must always run away from anyone who finds it.
—Andre Gide

Directions

For each of the following statements, circle the number that most closely approximates your response.

	Strongly agree	Somewhat agree	Strongly disagree
1. I don't believe that research should be done on love, because love should remain mysterious.	3	2	1
2. Love is the most important thing in my life.	3	2	1
3. My life is very unhappy when I am not in love.	3	2	1
4. I am able to function very well without someone to love.	1	2	3
5. Love is a fantasy that is popular with 13-year-old girls.	1	2	3
6. Each of us has our "one and only" somewhere out there, if only we can find that person.	3	2	1
7. Once you find your "one and only," you will never feel attracted to anyone else.	3	2	1
8. If you love too much, you will only get hurt.	1	2	3
9. I am able to function very well without someone loving me.	1	2	3
10. The smartest people don't get hung up on someone.	1	2	3
11. You can tell when you first see someone if you are going to love that person.	3	2	1
12. The best relationships have some basis more important than love.	1	2	3
13. If you love someone enough, any kind of problem in the relationship can be overcome.	3	2	1
14. If I had to choose between living in poverty or living without love, I would choose to love in poverty.	3	2	1
15. As soon as someone thinks you love them, that person will start to take advantage of you.	1	2	3
16. You're a sucker if you fall in love with someone who has no money.	1	2	3

TOTAL POINTS: _____

Interpretation:

40 to 48 points: You have very romantic ideas about love. You might put too much emphasis on love as a basis for a partnership, while ignoring other important considerations.

24 to 39 points: You have more realistic ideas about love. Love is important to you, but you also are aware of the many other bases of a smoothly functioning partnership.

16 to 23 points: You appear to be pretty cynical about love. Maybe you previously have been hurt or come from a family where romance was not emphasized. Your attitudes might insulate you from getting hurt again but could also be preventing you from enjoying the benefits of a loving relationship.

Source: Byer, C. O., Shainberg, L. W., & Galliano, G. (1999). *Dimensions of human sexuality,* 5th ed. Boston, MA: McGraw-Hill College, p. 86. Reprinted with permission from The McGraw-Hill Companies, Inc.

Study Guide and Self-Assessment

8.6 My Relationship Wants and Needs

A second touching a hot stove seems like an hour. An hour touching a pretty girl seems like a second. Now that's relativity.

　　　　　　　　　　　　　　　　　—Albert Einstein

Directions

1. What are your wants and needs in a love relationship? Choose the three most important items from the list below.

　　_____

　　_____

　　_____

2. Consider the list again and choose the singlemost important item.

　　_____

3. Write your choices and the reasons for choosing them.

　　_____

　　_____

　　_____

4. Optional: Which items does your partner choose?

　_____

I want someone to . . .

Love me
Confide in me
Show me affection
Respect my needs
Appreciate what I wish to achieve
Understand my moods
Help me make important decisions
Stimulate my ambition
Look up to
Give me self-confidence
Stand by me in difficulty
Appreciate me as I am
Admire my ability
Make me feel that I count for something
Relieve my loneliness
Support me and our children
Accept my need to be self-sufficient and independent

8.7 My Relationship Values

Love is many things, but more than anything it is a disturbance of the digestive system.
—Gabriel Garcia Marquez, February 14, 1995

What are your priorities in a love relationship? Rate the items in the list below with a number from 1 to 10, using 1 to indicate least importance to you and 10 most importance to you.

Write a one-page essay in which you describe the three items you feel most strongly about and why.

_____ Being able to talk comfortably to my partner about my innermost feelings

_____ Having my partner share with me his/her innermost feelings

_____ Sharing with my partner nearly all of my leisure time

_____ Both of us having similar political beliefs

_____ Each of us having our own careers

_____ Being able to express anger to my partner

_____ Having my partner express his/her anger to me

_____ Being able to have sexual relations with other people

_____ Having good relations with my parents and family

_____ Enjoying what we have now without concern for a lifelong relationship

_____ Having mutual close friends

_____ Having similar religious beliefs

_____ Having major interests and friendships of my own outside the relationship

_____ Wanting the same material possessions (house, car, etc.)

_____ Being able to tell my partner when I feel jealous

_____ Having the most influence over how we as a couple spend money

_____ Trying with my partner new sexual experiences and techniques

_____ Working together on tasks rather than dividing them between us

_____ Having children

8.8 Listening Exercise

One of the lessons of history is that nothing is sometimes a good thing to do,
and often a clever thing to say.
—Will Durant

Directions

Ask someone to be the speaker for this exercise. Carry out steps 1–4 below. So that you can observe body language (very important for discerning the speaker's emotions), do the assignment in person, not on the phone or via e-mail or IM, or text messaging.

Step 1. Topic 1: Ask the speaker to tell you something that's important to her or him. The first time you do this it's better that the topic *not* involve you personally or your relationship with the speaker. Let the speaker talk for up to five minutes.

Step 2. While the speaker is talking, *just listen,* and notice any urges you have to stop paying attention or to interrupt with suggestions or comments. Notice where your attention goes, for example, if your mind drifts to other topics or you daydream. Notice if you feel critical or if you have the urge to comment or advise.

Step 3. When the speaker has finished, tell her or him what you experienced. Share with the speaker if you were able to pay full attention to what was being said or if your mind was busy with something else. If you're new at this, you'll probably notice that it's difficult simply to listen.

Step 4. Topic 2: Do the exercise a second time. Ask the speaker to address a topic different from that addressed in step 1. Also, instead of telling the speaker your experience with listening, tell the speaker a paraphrase of what she or he said using

- an *emotion word* that describes the speaker's feelings (not yours!)
- a *because statement* that describes the reason for that emotion from the speaker's point of view (not yours!)

As a noun, the word *paraphrase* means a condensed rewording of a statement, given in simple language for clarity. As a verb, *paraphrase* means to render a paraphrase.

Example: The speaker talks about being worried that she has not found an occupation that seems interesting. The listener responds:

"You seem nervous because you haven't found a job you want to do in the future."

nervous = emotion word that describes the speaker's feelings
because you haven't found a job you want to do in the future = reason for the feelings

Do not offer the speaker

- your advice ("You should . . . ")
- your opinion ("I think . . . ")
- your judgments ("That's crazy/stupid/weird")
- your life history ("Here's what happened to me . . . ")
- your predictions ("It/he/she will . . . ")

At first, listening and paraphrasing may feel uncomfortable because it is not how we usually converse. But with a little practice you'll get good at it, and those with whom you communicate—family, friends, lovers, and coworkers—will appreciate you greatly for it.

Reaction Essay

Respond in writing to the following questions.

1. With whom did you carry out the Listening Exercise?

2. In step 1, what topic did the speaker address?

3. In step 1, what did you notice your mind doing while the speaker was talking?

4. In step 4, what was the topic of the speaker's remarks?

5. In step 4, write the paraphrase you offered the speaker, using the speaker's emotion word (not yours!) and the speaker's because statement (not yours!).

   Correct: "You're nervous because you cannot find a job you want to do."
   Incorrect: "The speaker was nervous about not finding a job."
   Incorrect: "I was bored because I've heard this complaint a million times."

6. What effect did this exercise have on your usual listening style?

As a noun, the word *paraphrase* means a condensed rewording of a statement, given in simple language for clarity. As a verb, *paraphrase* means to render a paraphrase.

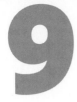

CHAPTER 9

9.1 Parenthood and Me

It's better to know some of the questions than all of the answers.
—James Thurber

Directions

In the list below, indicate how strongly you agree with each motivation for becoming a parent. Can you add any motivations to the list?

Motivation	Strongly agree	Agree	Disagree
To have a child who looks like me			
To have child who will carry on the family name			
To have a child who will be successful			
To have someone to inherit my money or property			
To have someone who will regard me highly			
To have someone who will return my love			
To do something I know I can do well			
To feel pride in creating another human being			
To keep me young at heart			
To help me feel fulfilled			
To make my marriage happier			
To make me feel masculine/feminine			
To please my family and society			
To teach someone about the beauty of life			
To help someone grow and develop			
Other			
Other			

10.1 Contraception

I believe in looking reality straight in the eye and denying it.
—Garrison Keillor

Directions
Respond to the questions below for any contraceptive method you are considering using.

Check **Yes** or **No** for each of the following questions:	Yes	No
1. Have I had problems using this method before?	_____	_____
2. Have I or my partner ever become pregnant while using this method?	_____	_____
3. Am I afraid of using this method?	_____	_____
4. Would I really rather not use this method?	_____	_____
5. Will I or my partner have trouble remembering to use this method?	_____	_____
6. Will I or my partner have trouble using this method correctly?	_____	_____
7. Do I still have unanswered questions about this method?	_____	_____
8. Does this method make menstrual periods longer or more painful?	_____	_____
9. Does this method cost more than I can afford?	_____	_____
10. Could this method cause me or my partner to have serious complications?	_____	_____
11. Am I opposed to this method because of my religious or moral beliefs?	_____	_____
12. Is my partner opposed to this method?	_____	_____
13. Am I using this method without my partner's knowledge?	_____	_____
14. Will using this method embarrass my partner?	_____	_____
15. Will using this method embarrass me?	_____	_____
16. Will I or my partner enjoy intercourse less because of this method?	_____	_____
17. If this method interrupts lovemaking, will I avoid it?	_____	_____
18. Has a nurse or physician ever told me or my partner *not* to use this method?	_____	_____
19. Is there anything about my or my partner's personality that could lead me or my partner to use this method incorrectly?	_____	_____
20. Am I or is my partner at risk of being exposed to HIV or another STD if I use or my partner uses this method?	_____	_____

Most persons will have a few "yes" answers. "Yes" answers mean that problems might arise. If you have more than a few "yes" responses, you may want to talk with a physician, counselor, partner, or friend to help you decide whether to use this method or how to use it so that it will really be effective for you. In general, the more "yes" answers you have, the less likely you are to use this method consistently and correctly at every act of intercourse.

Source: Byer, C. O., Shainberg, L. W., & Galliano, G. (1999). *Dimensions of human sexuality,* 5th ed. Boston, MA: McGraw-Hill College, p. 455. Reprinted with permission from The McGraw-Hill Companies, Inc.

10.2 Choosing a Contraceptive

Love is giving someone the space to be the way they are—and the way they are not.
—Edmund Burke

Directions
Rate the contraceptives in the list below and give reasons for your choices.

Method	Very suitable	Suitable	Not suitable	Reasons
Abstinence	_____	_____	_____	_____
Condom (female)	_____	_____	_____	_____
Condom (male)	_____	_____	_____	_____
Diaphragm	_____	_____	_____	_____
Fertility awareness	_____	_____	_____	_____
Hormonal pill	_____	_____	_____	_____
Hormonal patch	_____	_____	_____	_____
Hormonal ring	_____	_____	_____	_____
Intrauterine device (IUD)	_____	_____	_____	_____
Progestin-only method	_____	_____	_____	_____
Spermicidal foam/gel	_____	_____	_____	_____
Tubal ligation	_____	_____	_____	_____
Vasectomy	_____	_____	_____	_____

Study Guide and Self-Assessment

11.1 AIDS and Me

> *A loving heart is the beginning of all knowledge.*
> —Thomas Carlyle

How has HIV/AIDS touched your life? Write a response to this question considering the following aspects:

1. Personal experience with someone with HIV/AIDS

2. Whether HIV/AIDS has affected your personal behaviors

3. The ways HIV/AIDS has affected your community and society

4. The ways the worldwide HIV/AIDS epidemic affects your life

11.2 AIDS in Film

Hope is a waking dream.
—Aristotle

1. Watch the HBO film "And the Band Played On," a dramatization of the beginnings of the AIDS epidemic in the 1980s.

2. After viewing the film, write a reaction paper in which you respond to these questions:

   - What was your overall impression of the film?

   - What were the two most interesting things about HIV/AIDS that you learned?

   - What is your opinion of the scientists who do HIV/AIDS research?

   - What effect did the video have on your attitudes about HIV/AIDS?

   - Would you recommend that others watch this film? Why or why not?

Note: The 2008 Nobel Prize in Medicine was awarded to two of the scientists portrayed in the film, Luc Montagnier and Françoise Barre-Sinoussi (see the Nobel Foundation Web site: http://nobelprize.org/nobel_prizes/).

Study Guide and Self-Assessment

©Jones and Bartlett Publishers 2004

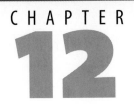

C H A P T E R

12

12.1 My Vaccination Record

There is an alchemy in sorrow. It can be transmuted into wisdom,
which, if it does not bring joy, can yet bring happiness.
—Pearl Buck

Directions
Make a record of your vaccinations using the chart below.

Vaccine	Year initial series completed	Years revaccinated					
Diphtheria							
Hepatitis A							
Hepatitis B							
Influenza							
Measles							
Mumps							
Pertussis (whooping cough)							
Polio							
German measles (rubella)							
Tetanus							
Tuberculosis							
Other							

13.1 My Cancer Risks

Judge thyself with the judgment of sincerity, and thou will judge others with the judgment of charity.
—John Mitchell Mason

Directions

1. Go to the online assessment tool Your Disease Risk (http://www.yourdiseaserisk.wustl.edu/).

2. Click on "What Is Your Cancer Risk?"

3. Assess your risks for any three of the cancers listed here:

   Bladder
   Breast
   Cervix
   Colon
   Kidney
   Lung
   Skin
   Ovary
   Pancreas
   Prostate
   Stomach
   Uterus

13.2 My Environmental Cancer Risks

Never confuse movement with action.
—Ernest Hemingway

Many environmental factors are linked to cancer, including those in the list below.

Directions

1. Estimate your exposure to each potential carcinogen listed in the chart below.

2. Write down some ideas about how you could reduce your exposure to some of them.

Potential Carcinogen	Exposure			
	High	Moderate	Low	None
Personal cigarette smoking	_____	_____	_____	_____
Secondhand smoke	_____	_____	_____	_____
Smokeless tobacco	_____	_____	_____	_____
Asbestos (in old buildings, including schools)	_____	_____	_____	_____
Radon (a radioactive gas in soil)	_____	_____	_____	_____
Indoor solid fuel (wood, coal) burning	_____	_____	_____	_____
Photochemical smog (from cars)	_____	_____	_____	_____
Human papillomavirus	_____	_____	_____	_____
Human immunodeficiency virus	_____	_____	_____	_____
Hepatitis B virus	_____	_____	_____	_____
Epstein-Barr virus	_____	_____	_____	_____
Helicobacter pylori infection	_____	_____	_____	_____
Sun exposure (or artificial tanning)	_____	_____	_____	_____
Well-done cooked meats	_____	_____	_____	_____
Postmenopausal estrogen therapy	_____	_____	_____	_____
Diethylstilbestrol (DES)	_____	_____	_____	_____
Benzene	_____	_____	_____	_____
Formaldehyde	_____	_____	_____	_____
Nickle-containing materials	_____	_____	_____	_____
Gamma irradiation	_____	_____	_____	_____
X-rays	_____	_____	_____	_____
Radioactive chemicals	_____	_____	_____	_____
Dioxin	_____	_____	_____	_____
Vinyl chloride	_____	_____	_____	_____
Coal tars	_____	_____	_____	_____
Soot	_____	_____	_____	_____
Wood dust	_____	_____	_____	_____

CHAPTER

14

14.1 My Risk for Heart Disease

Do not protect yourself by a fence, but rather by your friends.
—Czech Proverb

Directions

1. Go to the online assessment tool Your Disease Risk (http://www.yourdiseaserisk.wustl.edu/).

2. Click on "What Is Your Heart Disease Risk?"

3. Complete the Questionnaire.

4. List any risk factors that you could/should lower, and for each, identify one health behavior you could change that would help reduce that risk.

CHAPTER

15

15.1 My Family Medical History

Get your facts first, and then you can distort them as much as you please.
—Mark Twain

Directions

1. In the chart below, mark an "X" in a column to indicate the occurrence of a particular disease in a family member.

	Disease						If deceased, age at death	Cause of death
	Cancer	Diabetes	Heart disease	Hypertension	Stroke	Other		
Father								
Mother								
Brother								
Brother								
Sister								
Sister								
Father's father								
Father's mother								
Father's brother or sister								
Mother's father								
Mother's mother								
Mother's brother or sister								

2. For any "X" in your chart, research any possibility that the disease has some degree of inherited component.

16

16.1 Being Knowledgeable About Drugs

When you win, say nothing. When you lose, say less.
—Paul Brown

What do you know about the drugs and medicines that you consume?

Directions

1. Go to one of the Web sites listed on this page (or an authoritative alternative) to learn about any medications or dietary supplements you are taking or have taken or a particular "recreational" or social drug you currently use or once used.

2. Describe something of interest that you learned.

_____

_____

_____

_____

Medicines

MedlinePlus Drug Information, http://www.nlm.nih.gov/medlineplus/druginformation.html

Dietary Supplements

U.S. National Center for Complementary and Alternative Medicine, http://nccam.nih.gov/health/supplements.htm

Nonmedical Drug Use

U.S. National Institute on Drug Abuse, http://www.nida.nih.gov/

Alcohol Use and Abuse

U.S. National Institute on Alcohol Abuse and Alcoholism, http://www.niaaa.nih.gov/

16.2 Medicines I Take

Do not throw the arrow which will return against you.
—Kurdish proverb

Directions

1. In the chart below, list any medicines you are taking. Consult the product packaging, your doctor, the pharmacist, authoritative books (e.g., *Physician's Desk Reference*), or the Internet for information about side effects and reasons not to take the medicine (*contraindications*).

2. Assess the risks of taking a medicine in relation to its therapeutic benefits.

   _____

   _____

3. Search for nondrug alternatives to the drugs on your list.

   _____

   _____

Drug	Side effects	Contraindications

16.3 Nonessential Drugs I Consume

Of all forms of caution, caution in love is perhaps the most fatal to true happiness.
—Bertrand Russell

Americans consume too many drugs, in part because of the belief (promoted by drug manufacturers) that health and well-being are enhanced by chemicals. Whereas many drugs, when used appropriately, can promote wellness and relieve illness, too often people consume drugs unnecessarily.

Directions

1. For 1 week, make a list of the nonessential drugs you ingest. Be sure to include coffee, tea, and cola and "energy" drinks, all of which contain caffeine; alcohol, nicotine, and pain relievers.

2. After recording your nonessential drug consumption during Week 1, for another week try to eliminate one of the nonessential drugs you ingest and make notes about how you feel.

Week 1	Sun	Mon	Tues	Wed	Thurs	Fri	Sat
Caffeine (How many cups of coffee or 12-oz. servings of cola drinks per day?)							
Alcohol (How many 12-oz. beers, glasses of wine, or mixed drinks per day?)							
Nicotine (How many cigarettes, cigars, pipes, or dips of snuff or chewing tobacco per day?)							
Pain relievers (How many tablets per day?)							
Other:							
Other:							

Week 2	Sun	Mon	Tues	Wed	Thurs	Fri	Sat
Caffeine (How many cups of coffee or 12-oz. servings of cola drinks per day?)							
Alcohol (How many 12-oz. beers, glasses of wine, or mixed drinks per day?)							
Nicotine (How many cigarettes, cigars, pipes, or dips of snuff or chewing tobacco per day?)							
Pain relievers (How many tablets per day?)							
Other:							
Other:							

Study Guide and Self-Assessment

16.4 Drugs in Media and Advertising

Make the most of yourself, for that is all there is of you.
—Ralph Waldo Emerson

Directions

Find two examples of advertising in magazines, newspapers, radio, film, TV, or the Web that promote or facilitate the use of alcohol, tobacco, or prescription and nonprescription drugs. For each example, write an analysis in which you do the following:

1. Describe the images in the advertisement (e.g., the ages, appearance, and activities of the models; if a story is being depicted).

    _____

    _____

2. Identify the means by which the advertiser links the images in the ad to the product being sold.

    _____

    _____

3. Identify the audience to which the ad is directed and how the imagery is used to "grab" that audience.

    _____

    _____

4. Offer your opinion of the commercial effectiveness of the ad (i.e., does it sell?).

    _____

    _____

    _____

    _____

5. Offer your opinion of the effect of the ad on society.

    _____

    _____

    _____

    _____

Study Guide and Self-Assessment

17

17.1 Why Do I Smoke?

To be conscious that you are ignorant is a great step to knowledge.
—Benjamin Disraeli

Smoking can provide a variety of rewards. Knowing the reasons you smoke can help you quit and stay smoke-free.

Directions

1. Answer the 18 questions below.

2. Use the scoring section to calculate your score for each of the smoking categories.

3. Consult the scoring interpretation page to find out what your scores mean.

	Always	Frequently	Occasionally	Seldom	Never
A. I smoke cigarettes to keep myself from slowing down.	5	4	3	2	1
B. Handling a cigarette is part of the enjoyment of smoking it.	5	4	3	2	1
C. Smoking cigarettes is pleasant and relaxing.	5	4	3	2	1
D. I light up a cigarette when I feel angry about something.	5	4	3	2	1
E. When I have run out of cigarettes I find it almost unbearable until I can get them.	5	4	3	2	1
F. I smoke cigarettes automatically without even being aware of it.	5	4	3	2	1
G. I smoke cigarettes to stimulate me, to perk myself up.	5	4	3	2	1
H. Part of the enjoyment of smoking a cigarette comes from the steps I take to light up.	5	4	3	2	1
I. I find cigarettes pleasurable.	5	4	3	2	1
J. When I feel uncomfortable or upset about something, I light up a cigarette.	5	4	3	2	1
K. I am very much aware of the fact when I am not smoking a cigarette.	5	4	3	2	1
L. I light up a cigarette without realizing I still have one burning in the ashtray.	5	4	3	2	1
M. I smoke cigarettes to give me a "lift."	5	4	3	2	1
N. When I smoke a cigarette, part of the enjoyment is watching the smoke as I exhale it.	5	4	3	2	1
O. I want a cigarette most when I am comfortable and relaxed.	5	4	3	2	1
P. When I feel "blue" or want to take my mind off cares and worries, I smoke cigarettes.	5	4	3	2	1
Q. I get a real gnawing hunger for a cigarette when I haven't smoked for a while.	5	4	3	2	1
R. I've found a cigarette in my mouth and didn't remember putting it there.	5	4	3	2	1

Source: Smoker's Self-Testing Kit developed by Daniel Horn, Ph.D. Originally published by National Clearinghouse for Smoking and Health. Department of Health, Education, and Welfare.

How to Score

1. Enter the numbers you have circled in the spaces below, putting the number you have circled to question A over line A, to question B over line B, etc.

2. Add the three scores on each line to get your totals. For example, the sum of your scores over lines A, G, and M gives you your score on *Stimulation,* lines B, H, and N give the score on *Handling,* and so on.

Totals

_____	+	_____	+	_____	=	_____
A		G		M		Stimulation
_____	+	_____	+	_____	=	_____
B		H		N		Handling
_____	+	_____	+	_____	=	_____
C		I		O		Pleasurable relaxation
_____	+	_____	+	_____	=	_____
D		J		P		Crutch: tension reduction
_____	+	_____	+	_____	=	_____
E		K		Q		Craving: psychological addiction
_____	+	_____	+	_____	=	_____
F		L		R		Habit

Scores of 11 or above indicate that this factor is an important source of satisfaction for the smoker. Scores of 7 or less are low and probably indicate that this factor does not apply to you. Scores in between are marginal. A description of what your scores mean can be found on the next page.

What My Scores Mean

Scores can vary from 3 to 15 in each category. A score of 11 or above is high; a score of 7 or less is low.

Stimulation

Smoking stimulates/energizes you. You believe smoking helps you wake up, concentrate, organize your energies, and keep going. If you scored more than 11 in this category, you need to find other ways to feel energized, such as the following:

- Avoid fatigue: get sufficient sleep so you won't feel tired.

- Take a walk (or do other exercise) to get yourself moving.

- Meditate to clear your mind and prepare yourself for a day's activities.

- Do some yoga or stretching exercises to balance your energy.

- Use a journal to plan your day's activities.

- Talk to someone or log on to a chat room.

- Chew cinnamon gum (or another strong flavor) to stimulate your sense of taste.

Handling

You like to handle cigarettes, a lighter, or matches. If you scored more than 11 in this category, you need to find other ways to satisfy your desire to handle things, such as the following:

- Hold a special object that has healing significance for you (a stone, beads, etc.).

- Hold a pen or pencil (or plastic cigarette).

- Doodle.

- Play with a coin, a piece of jewelry, or some other harmless object.

- Clean and polish your nails.

Pleasure

Smoking gives you pleasure (or reduces unpleasant feelings). If you scored more than 11 in this category, you need to find alternative ways to feel pleasure, such as the following:

- Meditate.

- Do a pleasurable activity.

- Remind yourself of the harmful effects of smoking.

- Chew a flavored gum that you like.

- Talk to someone or log on to a chat room.

Reduction of negative feelings or crutch

Smoking helps you cope with uncomfortable feelings and stress. If you scored more than 11 in this category, you need to find alternative ways to deal with unpleasant feelings, such as the following:

- Meditate.

- Write your thoughts and feelings in a journal.

- Talk to someone about your feelings.

- Take a walk or exercise.

- Listen to music.

- Identify common stressful situations in your life and experiment with nonsmoking coping methods to find ones that work best.

Craving

You experience cravings for cigarettes. If you scored more than 11 in this category, you need to find other ways to cope with cravings, such as the following:

- Become mindful of—and avoid—situations and circumstances that "trigger" smoking.

- Use deep breathing or meditation to help you let cravings pass.

- Use nicotine replacement products (patch or gum).

- Use craving-reducing medications (e.g., buproprion).

- Take soothing baths or showers.

Habit

For you, smoking is virtually automatic. You do it without thinking. If you scored more than 11 in this category, you need to replace smoking-related habits with nonsmoking ones, such as the following:

- Remove ash trays, cigarettes, and other smoking-related paraphernalia from your house, office, and car so they won't trigger automatic/mindless smoking.

- Designate smoke-free places in your home and office; make your car smoke-free.

- Sit in nonsmoking sections of restaurants.

- Don't go to bars and other locales that permit (and encourage) smoking.

- Make a pact with friends and coworkers who smoke not to smoke around you.

Study Guide and Self-Assessment

17.2 Am I Addicted to Nicotine?

*I have come to believe that the whole world is an enigma, a harmless enigma
that is made terrible by our own mad attempt to interpret it as though it had
an underlying truth.*

—Umberto Eco

Nicotine addiction (also called physical dependence) is a major reason for tobacco addiction. Without nicotine, a tobacco-addicted person experiences
withdrawal syndrome consisting of being grouchy and irritable, having
headaches, having trouble sleeping, feeling depressed, and having intense
cravings for cigarettes.

Directions

- For questions 1–6, circle the answer that best represents you.

- Add your points in column 3.

- Refer to the scoring section below to determine your level of nicotine
  addiction.

Questions	Answers	Points
1. How soon after you wake do you smoke your first cigarette?	Within 5 minutes	3
	6 to 30 minutes	2
2. Do you find it difficult to refrain from smoking in places where it is forbidden (e.g., in church, at the library, at the movies)?	Yes	1
	No	0
3. Which cigarette would you most hate to give up?	The first one in the morning	1
	All others	0
4. How many cigarettes per day do you smoke?	10 or less	0
	11 to 20	1
	21 to 30	2
	31 or more	3
5. Do you smoke more frequently during the first hours after waking than during the rest of the day?	Yes	1
	No	0
6. Do you smoke if you are so ill that you are in bed most of the day?	Yes	1
	No	0

Scoring

0 to 2—very low dependence

3 to 4—low dependence

5—medium dependence

6 to 7—high dependence

8 to 10—very high dependence

Source: Fagerström, K. O., Heatherton, T. F., & Kozlowski, L. T. (1991). Nicotine addiction and its assessment. *Ear, Nose, and Throat Journal, 1990, 69,* 763–765.

Study Guide and Self-Assessment

Am I Addicted to Nicotine?

17.3 If You Want to Quit

Every patient carries her or his own doctor inside.
—Albert Schweitzer

Cigarette smoking is the worst thing one can do to one's health, worse than all other unhealthy behaviors (not exercising, eating too much fat, etc.) combined.

- Cigarette smoke contains over 4000 chemicals, about 40 of which cause cancer.

- Cigarette smoking increases the risk of heart disease, emphysema (a fatal lung disease), and all types of cancer.

- About 1000 people die each day as a long-term consequence of their smoking habit.

- 40 million Americans have quit smoking, and most of them are glad they did, so you know it can be done.

- Quitting can be difficult, so the quitters motto should be "If at first you don't succeed, try, try again."

Why People Start Smoking

- Smoking almost always begins in late childhood or adolescence because of peer pressure, modeling after family members and media personalities, and the influence of advertising.

Why People Continue to Smoke

- Nicotine is highly addicting.

- Cigarettes are easy to get.

- Smoking becomes linked to a wide variety of emotional states, social situations, and activities.

- Nicotine is used to change one's mental state
  - to arouse ('a wake me up")
  - to sedate ("a calm me down")
  - to change a mood (dampen unpleasant emotions)

- Smokers often deny that their health is at risk.

How to Quit

Step 1: Understand the Quitting Process

- The smoker must be ready to stop. When the mind is ready to stop smoking, steps can be taken to bring the body along.

- There is no single method for quitting successfully.

- Many people try several times before achieving permanent success. Relapse can be seen as a step to a final goal rather than a defeat.

Step 2: Precontemplation

- Understanding why you smoke cigarettes (see Exercise 17.1)

- Accepting that smoking is harmful to one's own health and the health of others

- Believing that one can quit successfully

- Having social support during the quitting and maintenance phases of quitting

Step 3: Understanding Withdrawal and Urges

- The first few days are the toughest; withdrawal symptoms peak in 2–4 days.

- After withdrawal, ex-smokers may continue to experience the urge to smoke in situations in which they smoked in the past (e.g., stress, anger, after a meal, talking on the phone, etc.).

- An urge to smoke rarely lasts for more than a few seconds . . . so have a way to chill while it passes.

- During the quitting process, consider using nicotine-containing gum, the nicotine patch, and any of a variety of medications that lessen the urge to smoke. Be aware of the *denial trap, which is believing* that by choosing pharmacological help you are substituting one habituating drug for another. Stop-smoking medications are used only during the few weeks of the quitting process. And they work!

Step 4: Set a quit date—the Day You Will Stop Smoking Forever

- Put it on your calendar.

- Announce it to your family and friends.

Step 5: Prepare for the Quit Date

- Cut back on the number of cigarettes smoked (see Exercise 17.4).

- Find alternatives to smoking in the usual smoking situations.

- Come up with strategies for dealing with the urge to smoke after you've quit.

- Stop smoking in your car; clean your car and clothes of cigarette smell.

Step 6: On the Quit Date and for the Next 14 Days

- Discard all cigarettes and smoking paraphernalia (lighters, ashtrays).

- Limit time spent with smokers and in smoking situations.

- Employ alternative behaviors to smoking.

- Employ your strategies for dealing with urges to smoke.

Step 7: Preparing for Possible Relapse

- Be aware that nearly all ex-smokers are tempted to smoke again during the first few months after quitting.

- Never delude yourself into thinking "I'll have only this one."

- Relapse tends to occur during negative emotional states, so quitters should develop alternatives to smoking (e.g., meditating, walking, journal-writing, etc.) for the times of difficult emotions.

- Relapse should be seen as a normal step in the quitting process and not a sign of failure (which can trigger negative, punishing inner self-talk, the soothing of which can be to smoke).

Online Resources for help with quitting:

- QuitNet

- SmokeFree.gov . . . Quitting info from the U.S. National Cancer Institute

- You Can Quit Smoking Now . . . a guide from the U.S. National Institutes of Health

- Quit Smoking Program . . . from the Canadian Lung Association

- The Quit Smoking Company . . . information and products to help smokers quit including learning how to set a quit date, quit and avoid weight gain, and making quitting easier . . . lots of resources

©Jones and Bartlett Publishers 2004

17.4 The Cut-Back Method for Quitting Smoking

You gain strength, courage, and confidence by every experience in which you really stop to look fear in the face. You must do the thing you think you cannot do.

—Eleanor Roosevelt

Prepare for Quit Day (see Exercise 17.3) by cutting back on the number of cigarettes smoked.

- Buy only ONE pack of cigarettes at a time (no more cartons!).
- Change to a less desirable brand of cigarettes.
- Cut cigarettes in half before smoking them.
- Don't carry cigarettes with you so you will have to "bum" them from others.
- Don't smoke on breaks at work, prior to a class, at clubs, or in your car.

Keep a smoking diary to help cutting back on smoking.

Step 1: For two days that are *representative* of your usual smoking pattern, keep a list of all the cigarettes you smoke. For each cigarette record:

- the time of day it was smoked
- how much you wanted/needed the cigarette—1 = not much, 2 = medium, 3 = a lot
- your feelings at the time it was smoked (happy, sad, neutral, depressed, angry, bored, etc.)
- what you were doing when it was smoked (eating, watching TV, driving, etc.)
- whom you were with when it was smoked it (alone, with friends or family, etc.).

Step 2: Refer to your smoking diary and identify the cigarettes that you need the least (score of "1" or "2") and cut back on one cigarette a day for as many cigarettes as you can. When you are ready, come up with a plan for eliminating them from your life.

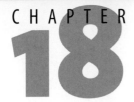

CHAPTER
18

18.1 My Alcohol Use

Every man is guilty of all the good he didn't do.
—Voltaire

The CRAFFT and AUDIT (Alcohol Use Disorders Identification Test) questionnaires were developed to identify persons whose alcohol consumption may be hazardous to their health.

Directions:

- Visit the Web sites listed below and do the online questionnaires.

- If your scores indicate a drinking problem, talk with your doctor or a counselor.

CRAFFT:

http://www.drugfree.org/Intervention/Quiz/CRAFFT_Quiz

AUDIT:

http://www.counseling.caltech.edu/drug/selftest/test1.html

18.2 Cutting Down on Drinking

If you do not wish to be prone to anger, do not feed the habit; give it nothing which may tend to its increase.

—Epictetus (A.D. 55–135)

Directions

1. Respond to these questions:

   - Do you drink alone when you feel angry or sad?

     _____

     _____

   - Does your drinking ever make you late for work?

     _____

     _____

   - Does your drinking worry your family?

     _____

     _____

   - Do you ever drink after telling yourself you won't?

     _____

     _____

   - Do you ever forget what you did while you were drinking?

     _____

     _____

   - Do you get headaches or have a hangover after you have been drinking?

     _____

     _____

If you answered yes to any of the questions, you may have a drinking problem. If you want to cut down on your drinking, follow these steps:

1. Write your reasons for cutting down or stopping.

   _____

   _____

2. Set a drinking goal.

   Choose a limit for how much you will drink. You may choose to cut down or not to drink at all. If you are cutting down, keep below these limits:

   - Women: No more than one drink a day
   - Men: No more than two drinks a day

Now write your drinking goal on a piece of paper. Put it where you can see it, such as on your refrigerator or bathroom mirror. Your paper might look like this:

My drinking goal

   I will start on this day _____.
   I will not drink more than _____ drinks in 1 day.
   I will not drink more than _____ drinks in 1 week.
   or
   I will stop drinking alcohol.

3. Keep a diary of your drinking. Write down every time you have a drink for three to four weeks.

Week:			
	No. of Drinks	Type of Drinks	Place Consumed
Mon			
Tues			
Wed			
Thurs			
Fri			
Sat			
Sun			

Now you know why you want to drink less and you have a goal. There are many ways you can help yourself to cut down. Try the tips.

4. Watch it at home.

Keep a small amount or no alcohol at home. Don't keep temptations around.

5. Drink slowly.

When you drink, sip your drink slowly. Take a break of 1 hour between drinks. Drink soda, water, or juice after a drink with alcohol. Do not drink on an empty stomach! Eat food when you are drinking.

6. Take a break from alcohol.

Pick a day or two each week when you will not drink at all. Then, try to stop drinking for one week. Think about how you feel physically and emotionally on these days. When you succeed and feel better, you may find it easier to cut down for good.

7. Learn how to say *NO*.

You do not have to drink when other people drink. You do not have to take a drink that is given to you. Practice ways to say *no* politely. For example, you can tell people you feel better when you drink less. Stay away from people who give you a hard time about not drinking.

8. Stay active.

9. Get support.

Cutting down on your drinking may be difficult at times. Ask your family and friends for support to help you reach your goal. Talk to your doctor if you are having trouble cutting down. Get the help you need to reach your goal.

10. Watch out for temptations.

Watch out for people, places, or times that make you drink when you do not want to. Stay away from people who drink a lot or bars where you used to go. Plan ahead of time what you will do to avoid drinking when you are tempted.

Do not drink when you are angry or upset or have a bad day. These are habits you need to break if you want to drink less.

11. Do not give up!

Most people do not cut down or give up drinking all at once. Just like a diet, it is not easy to change. That is okay. If you do not reach your goal the first time, try again. Remember, get support from people who care about you and want to help.

Source: National Institute on Alcohol Abuse and Alcoholism, National Institutes of Health, March 1996, NIH Publication No. 96-3770.

Study Guide and Self-Assessment

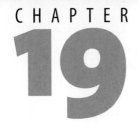

CHAPTER

19

19.1 My Medical History

If you can find a path with no obstacles, it probably doesn't lead anywhere.
—Frank A. Clark

As you are likely to have more than one health care provider in your life (thus increasing the risk of record-keeping errors), use the charts below to keep (and update regularly) your own medical records.

Illness History

Illness	No	Yes	When	Treatment	Special problems
German measles					
Mumps					
Chicken pox					
Scarlet fever					
Diphtheria					
Pneumonia, bronchitis, asthma					
Arthritis					
Rheumatic fever					
Heart disease or heart murmur					
Anemia					
Bleeding problem					
Ulcer, colitis					
Epilepsy					
Severe headaches					
Mononucleosis					
Jaundice or hepatitis					
Eye injury					
Ear disease or injury					
Skin disease					
Varicose veins					
Kidney or bladder problem					

Surgical History

What	When	Where	Physician

19.2 Am I an Intelligent Health Consumer?

Every increased possession loads us with new weariness.
—John Ruskin

This exercise can help you determine the extent to which you act intelligently when exposed to misleading and inaccurate health information, health fraud, and health quackery.

Directions

Place an X in the column that best represents your answer.

	VM	M	S	L	N
Are you sufficiently informed to be able to make sound decisions?					
Where do you go for information when needed?					
Professional health organizations or individuals					
Health books, magazines, newsletters					
Government health agencies					
Advertisements					
Newspapers or magazines					
Radio or television					
People you know					
To what extent do you accept statements appearing in news reports or advertisements at face value?					
To what extent can you identify quacks, quackery, fraudulent schemes, and hucksters?					
When selecting health practitioners to what extent do you:					
Talk with or visit before first appointment					
Check or inquire regarding qualifications or credentials					
Ask friend or neighbor about reputation					
Inquire about fees and payment procedures					
When you have been exposed to a fraudulent practice, quack, quackery, or a poor product or service, to what extent do you report your experience?					

Key: VM = very much; *M* = much; *S* = some; *L* = little; *N* = none.

Source: Comacchia, H. J., & Barrett, S. (1993). *Consumer health: A guide in intelligent decisions* (5th ed.). St. Louis, MO: Mosby, p. 11.

19.3 Using the Internet for Health Research

Words that come from the heart enter the heart.
—The Sages

Your tax dollars are definitely at work at the U.S. National Library of Medicine (part of the U.S. Department of Health and Human Services), the most comprehensive medical library in the world. One of the library's services is providing consumers with accurate, up-to-date, authoritative health and medical information through its MedlinePlus Web site: http://www.medlineplus.gov.

Directions

1. Visit the MedlinePlus Web site and click any links that interest you.

2. Describe your experience.

_____

_____

_____

_____

_____

_____

Study Guide and Self-Assessment

19.4 Web Field Trips

People grow through experience if they meet life honestly and courageously.
This is how character is built.

—Eleanor Roosevelt

There are more than 10,000 health-related Web sites. The purpose of most of them is to sell you something. A few health-related Web sites are not commercial; they are dedicated to providing authoritative health information to help people. The purpose of the Web Field Trips exercise is to help you assess health-related Web sites to determine those that are most authoritative, reliable, and helpful.

Directions

Visit, evaluate, and write a review of three health-related Web sites. The review should evaluate each Web site by addressing these questions:

1. What is the purpose of the Web site?

2. What does the site contain?

3. Who is responsible for the Web site's content?

4. How is the Web site funded and does the sponsorship influence the site's content?

5. How well is the Web site constructed?

6. How well does the Web site fulfill its purpose?

A list (with links) of authoritative health Web sites is on the *Health and Wellness* Web site. The list includes Web sites in the following categories:

Comprehensive Health Web sites	Nutrition
Mental Health	Alcohol and Drug Use and Abuse
Cancer	Human Genetics
Sexuality and Reproductive Health	Ear and Eye
Respiratory System and Allergy	Digestive System and Liver
Brain and Nervous System	Bones and Joints

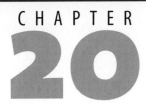
20.1 Exploring Complementary and Alternative Medicine

I've missed more than 9,000 shots in my career. I've lost almost 300 games. Twenty-six times, I've been trusted to take the game winning shot and missed.
I've failed over and over and over again in my life. And that is why I succeed.

—Michael Jordan

Directions

1. Visit the Web site of the National Center for Complementary and Alternative Medicine (http://nccam.nih.gov/), a division of the U.S. National Institutes of Health (NIH).

2. On the home page, click the link Making Decisions About Using CAM, and write a paragraph summary on what you find.

3. Browse the Web site and write a paragraph describing something of interest that you discover.

21

21.1 Preventing Intentional Injury

When I do good, I feel good; when I do bad, I feel bad, and that is my religion.
—Abraham Lincoln

Directions

Answer the questions in number 1 below and then respond to 2 and 3.

1. Answer *yes* or *no* to the following questions.

1. I have guns in my home.	Y	N
If yes, are they stored safely?	Y	N
When used, are they always used safely?	Y	N
2. I am involved in an abusive relationship.	Y	N
3. I live in a heavy-crime area.	Y	N
4. I abuse alcohol or other drugs.	Y	N
5. I work in a high-risk job.	Y	N
6. I clearly communicate my intentions and boundaries in a dating situation.	Y	N
7. I know, and have immediate access to, emergency phone numbers.	Y	N
8. I have sources of personal support.	Y	N
9. I know the warning signs of suicide.	Y	N
10. I know resources for mental health counseling in my community.	Y	N

2. Based on your responses to the questions in question 1, are there behaviors or situations in your life that need to be addressed? If so, what are they?

   _____

   _____

   _____

   _____

   _____

3. What concerns do you have, both as an individual and a member of your community, related to intentional injury and death?

   _____

   _____

   _____

   _____

   _____

Source: D. Birch and M. Creary. *Managing your health: Assessment and action.* © 1996 by Jones and Bartlett Publishers, Inc.

21.2 Preventing Unintentional Injury

Hate no one; hate their vices, not themselves.
—J. G. C. Brainard

Directions
Answer the questions in number 1 below and then respond to 2 and 3.

1. Answer *yes* or *no* to the following questions.

   1. I abuse alcohol or other drugs.   Y   N
   2. I wear seat belts when driving or riding in a car.   Y   N
   3. I have a car with front air bags.   Y   N
   4. I drive defensively rather than competitively.   Y   N
   5. I drive appropriately for weather conditions.   Y   N
   6. I maintain my car's tires, wipers, brakes, and lights.   Y   N
   7. I wear a helmet when riding on a bicycle, motorcycle, or roller blades.   Y   N
   8. I follow safety rules when riding a bicycle.   Y   N
   9. I keep gasoline, paint, oily rags, newspapers, plastics, and other flammable materials away from sources of heat.   Y   N
   10. I avoid overloading electrical circuits.   Y   N
   11. I use only safe sources of heat in my living quarters.   Y   N
   12. I avoid smoking in bed.   Y   N
   13. I have a smoke detector on each floor of my house.   Y   N
   14. I have a fire extinguisher in my house.   Y   N
   15. I keep a first-aid kit at home and in my car.   Y   N
   16. I post local emergency numbers and the poison control center number.   Y   N
   17. I follow safety procedures when involved in recreational activities.   Y   N

2. Based on your responses to the questions in question 1, are there behaviors or situations in your life that need to be addressed?

   _____

   _____

   _____

3. What concerns do you have, both as an individual and a member of the community, related to unintentional injury and death?

   _____

   _____

   _____

Study Guide and Self-Assessment

22.1 Healthy Aging

A great many people think they are thinking when they are really rearranging their prejudices.
—Edward R. Murrow

The health habits you observe as a young and middle-aged adult will greatly determine your health as an older person.

Directions

1. Indicate how frequently you practice each of the health behaviors listed below.

2. Among the health behaviors you do you not practice regularly, choose one that you could work on this year to make it a regular part of your life.

Health behavior	Frequency		
	Regularly	Once in a while	Rarely
Do not smoke	_____	_____	_____
Consume recommended amount of fiber	_____	_____	_____
Consume recommended amount of calcium	_____	_____	_____
Consume five servings of fruits and vegetables per day	_____	_____	_____
Limit consumption of well-done meat	_____	_____	_____
Maintain normal body weight	_____	_____	_____
Practice physical activity 3–4 times a week	_____	_____	_____
Have social relationships and ties	_____	_____	_____
Have daily quiet time	_____	_____	_____
Consume minimal or no alcohol	_____	_____	_____
Consume minimal or no fast food	_____	_____	_____
Brush teeth twice a day	_____	_____	_____
Floss teeth once a day	_____	_____	_____
Obtain flu shots	_____	_____	_____
Obtain mammograms (if over age 40)	_____	_____	_____
Obtain Pap smear	_____	_____	_____
Practice human papillomavirus prevention	_____	_____	_____
Practice AIDS prevention	_____	_____	_____
Obtain colorectal screening (if over age 50)	_____	_____	_____
Obtain blood pressure screening	_____	_____	_____
Obtain cholesterol check screening	_____	_____	_____

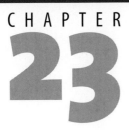

23.1 Do I Protect Myself from Crime?

Whatever you do will be insignificant, but it is very important that you do it.
—Mahatma Gandhi

Crime Protection

Rate yourself on a scale of 1 to 5 to show how often you follow these crime prevention methods.

1 = always
2 = frequently
3 = sometimes
4 = rarely
5 = never

_____ 1. I walk in well-lit areas.
_____ 2. I watch where I am going and what is happening to me.
_____ 3. I try to avoid walking alone at night.
_____ 4. I carry a whistle in my hand when walking alone.
_____ 5. I lock my car doors and do not leave valuables in sight.
_____ 6. I get out my car keys before I reach my car.
_____ 7. I park in well-lit and well-traveled areas of the parking lot.
_____ 8. I know the location of campus pay phones and call boxes.
_____ 9. I always carry cash in case of an emergency.
_____ 10. I avoid working or studying in buildings alone.
_____ 11. I take the safest, not the fastest, route when walking on campus.
_____ 12. I use shuttle buses or a campus escort service after dark.
_____ 13. I have memorized the phone number of the campus police.
_____ 14. When jogging or biking, I go with a friend and exercise on well-traveled routes.
_____ 15. If strangers harassed me, I would leave the scene and go to an open store, gas station, or anywhere people are present.
_____ 16. If I were held up, I would give the perpetrator my possessions and not fight.
_____ 17. If I were assaulted, I would try not to panic and look at the attacker carefully in order to give a good description to police.

Adapted from Ball State University's Campus Safety Tips (www.bsu.edu), Las Positas College's Campus Crime Prevention Web site (www.laspositascollege.edu), and information from the Columbus, Ohio, Police Department (www.columbuspolice.org).

24.1 Environmental Awareness Questionnaire

Success usually comes to those who are too busy to be looking for it.
—Henry David Thoreau

Directions

Circle the number that is your most appropriate response to each question.

Do you use pesticides in the house to kill insects, such as ants, roaches, or flies?

1. Frequently
2. Occasionally
3. Almost never

Do you use pesticides or herbicides around the garden and yard to kill insects and weeds?

1. Frequently
2. Occasionally
3. Almost never

Do you recycle newspapers or other kinds of paper?

1. Almost never
2. Sometimes
3. Regularly

Do you recycle bottles, cans, or plastics?

1. Hardly ever recycle these items
2. Some of these items sometimes
3. Most of the items regularly

When you go on a picnic or hike do you pack up and dispose of all trash in proper trash receptacles?

1. Very infrequently
2. Sometimes
3. All the time

If you need to run an errand that is less than a half mile away, do you walk or bike instead of drive?

1. Almost never
2. Occasionally
3. Most of the time

Do you conserve electricity by turning off unneeded lights and by not running appliances when you don't really need to (like the air conditioner)?

1. Hardly ever
2. Some of the time
3. Almost always

Do you make an effort to conserve water when showering, flushing, washing the car, etc.?

1. Almost never
2. Sometimes
3. Almost always

Do you pour dangerous chemicals such as gasoline or paint solvents down the drain or into sewer systems instead of arranging for proper disposal?

1. Often
2. Sometimes
3. Almost never

Have you thrown an empty can or bottle into the environment?

1. Within the past week
2. Within the past month
3. Not within the past year that you can remember

If you smoke, do you throw your butts into the environment when smoking outside?

1. Usually
2. Occasionally
3. Never

What kind of mileage does your automobile average?

1. Less than 20 miles per gallon
2. 20 to 30 miles per gallon
3. More than 30 miles per gallon

If you play a radio outdoors, how loud do you play it?

1. About as loud as it will go
2. Just loud enough for me to hear
3. Never play a radio outdoors where it might disturb others

When shopping for needed products, do you look for environmentally safe ones?

1. Never, just look for the cheapest and best product

2. Sometimes, depends on what is needed

3. Almost always, if I can find one

How many motor vehicles do you own, including cars, motorcycles, motorboats, jet skis, and others?

1. More than four

2. Two to four

3. Only one

A perfect score on these specific environmental questions is 45, but remember that no one is perfect. Perhaps by reviewing your answers you can find ways to improve your environmental awareness—and also contribute to your own health.

24.2 How Environmentally Friendly Is My Car?

Do not condemn the judgment of another because it differs from your own. You may both be wrong.
—Dandemis

Directions

1. Go to the U.S. Department of Energy's air pollution Web site (http://www.fueleconomy.gov).

2. Click the link at the upper left called Find and Compare Cars and report the annual greenhouse gas emissions in tons per year and the air pollution score (if given) of your current car. (If you don't drive a car, acquire the data for the car of someone you know.)

3. Compare the greenhouse gas emissions and air pollution scores of your present car with your prior car. Any improvements?

24.3 How Healthy Is My Drinking Water?

Arithmetic is being able to count up to twenty without taking off your shoes.
—Mickey Mouse

The Environmental Protection Agency sets health standards for drinking water. Obtain a report from your local water supplier's most recent report on the quality of the water distributed to you. The easiest way to do this is to contact your local water system (phone or e-mail) and ask. An alternative is to use the EPA Web site: http://www.epa.gov/safewater/dwinfo/index.html.

PHOTO CREDITS

Part Opener 1 © JohnnyZ/ShutterStock, Inc.

Chapter 1

Opener © Photos.com; **page 6** © aricvyhmeister/ShutterStock, Inc.; **page 9** © Photos.com; **page 11** © Cora Reed/ShutterStock, Inc.; **page 12 (left)** © Photos.com; **page 12 (right)** © John Wollerth/ShutterStock, Inc.; **page 15 (left)** © Skip Nall/Photodisc/Getty Images; **page 15 (right)** © Karl Weatherly/Photodisc/Getty Images

Chapter 2

Opener © Photodisc; **page 28** © Muriel Lasure/ShutterStock, Inc.; **page 34** © Photos.com; **page 38** © ThinkStock LLC/Index Stock Imagery

Chapter 3

Opener © paulaphoto/ShutterStock, Inc.; **page 50** © AbleStock; **page 51** © Florea Marius Catalin/ShutterStock, Inc.; **page 53** © UPI Photo/Monika Graff/Landov; **page 54** © Photos.com; **page 56** © Photos.com

Chapter 4

Opener © LiquidLibrary; **page 73** © Phototake, Inc./Alamy Images; **page 77** © LiquidLibrary; **page 80** © Don Hammond/Design Pics, Inc./age fotostock; **page 83 (top)** © Rob MeInychuk/Photodisc/Getty Images; **page 83 (bottom)** © Photos.com

Part Opener 2 © Creatas Image/Jupiterimages

Chapter 5

Opener © bilderlounge/Alamy Images; **page 98** © Photodisc; **page 103** © Photodisc; **page 106** © Photos.com; **page 110 (top)** © Photodisc; **page 110 (bottom)** © Radu Razvan/ShutterStock, Inc.; **page 121** © MIXA/age fotostock

Chapter 6

Opener © Galina Barskay/ShutterStock, Inc.; **page 136** © Dennis MacDonald/age fotostock; **page 141** © Anton Albert/ShutterStock, Inc.; **page 143** © Daniel Acker/Bloomberg News/Landov; **page 144** Courtesy of Mayo Clinic; **page 149 (left)** © Photodisc

Chapter 7

Opener © AMA/ShutterStock, Inc.; **page 160** © Dynamic Graphics Group/Creatas/Alamy Images; **page 164** © Photodisc; **page 165** © Peter Mumford/Alamy Images; **page 170** © Phil Date/ShutterStock, Inc.; **page 172 (left)** © Photos.com; **page 172 (middle)** © SW Productions/Photodisc/Getty Images; **page 172 (right)** © AbleStock

Part Opener 3 © Photos.com

Chapter 8

Opener **(top left)** © AbleStock, **(top right)** © Photos.com, **(bottom)** © Doug Menuez/Photodisc/Getty Images; **page 197** © Photodisc; **page 198** © AbleStock; **page 199** © Philip Date/ShutterStock, Inc.

Chapter 9

Opener © LiquidLibrary; **page 211** © Andrew Taylor/ShutterStock, Inc.; **page 213** © Bill Crump/Brand X Pictures/Alamy Images; **page 217** © Karl Weatherly/Photodisc/Getty Images

Chapter 10

Opener © Rubberball Productions; **page 233** © Jeff Greenberg/PhotoEdit, Inc.; **page 239** © Creatas; **page 242 (left)** © Reuters/Joshua Roberts/Landov; **page 242 (right)** © UPI Photo/Yuri Gripas /Landov

Chapter 11

Opener © Corbis; **page 252** Courtesy of Dr. Hermann/CDC; **page 253** Courtesy of Susan Lindsley/CDC

Part Opener 4 © Orange Line Media/Dreamstime.com

Chapter 12

Opener © Ron Chapple/Thinkstock/Creatas; **page 267 (top)** Courtesy of Dr. Fred Murphy/Cynthia Goldsmith/CDC; **page 267 (bottom)** Courtesy of Elizabeth H. White, M.S., and Peggy S. Hayes/CDC; **page 272** © David M. Phillips/Photo Researchers, Inc.; **page 293** Courtesy of CDC

Chapter 13

Opener Courtesy of the National Cancer Institute; **page 301** © Photodisc; **page 309** © Photodisc; **page 313** © Zsolt, Biczó/ShutterStock, Inc.

Chapter 14

Opener © Galina Barskaya/ShutterStock, Inc.; **page 331** © BananaStock/age fotostock; **page 337** © AbleStock

Chapter 15

Opener © Billy Lobo/ShutterStock, Inc.; **page 348** © Phototake, Inc./Alamy Images; **page 351** © Photodisc; **page 353** © Simon Pederson/ShutterStock, Inc.; **page 358** © Reuters/HO/Landov

Part Opener 5 © Pixtal/age fotostock

Chapter 16

Opener © Photodisc/Creatas; **page 380** © Photos.com; **page 382** © Vladimir Pomortzeff/ShutterStock, Inc.

Chapter 17

Opener © Kenneth William Caleno/ShutterStock, Inc.; **page 396** © Mary Evans Picture Library/Alamy Images; **page 399** © Photos.com; **page 403** © AP Photos

Chapter 18

Opener © iofoto/ShutterStock, Inc.; **page 413 (left)** © Ximagination/ShutterStock, Inc.; **page 413 (middle)** © Photodisc; **page 413 (right)** © Photo-

disc; **page 416** © www.imagesource.com/Jupiter images; **page 418** © Bill Aron/PhotoEdit, Inc.

Part Opener 6 © ImageDJ/age fotostock

Chapter 19

Opener © Ryan McVay/Photodisc/Getty Images; **page 434** © AbleStock; **page 437** © AbleStock; **page 438** © Reuters/Rebecca Cook/Landov

Chapter 20

Opener © Karin Lau/ShutterStock, Inc.; **page 452** © Terry Walsh/ShutterStock, Inc.; **page 456** © Paul Biddle/Science Source/Photo Researchers, Inc.

Chapter 21

Opener © LiquidLibrary; **page 471** © Jean Schweitzer/ShutterStock, Inc.; **page 473** © Creatas/Jupiterimages; **page 475** Courtesy of U.S. Coast Guard; **page 478** Courtesy of Photographer's Mate Airman Paul H. Laverty, Jr./U.S. Navy; **page 479** © BananaStock/age fotostock

Part Opener 7 © Image100/Jupiterimages

Chapter 22

Opener © Photodisc; **page 488** © Comstock/Jupiterimages; **page 489** © Monkey Business Images/ShutterStock, Inc.; **page 494** © Photodisc; **page 496** © LiquidLibrary; **page 500** © Big Cheese Photo/Jupiterimages

Chapter 23

Opener © James Dawson/Image Farm Inc./Jupiterimages; **page 510** © Sean O'Brien/Custom Medical Stock Photo

Chapter 24

Opener © Photodisc; **page 528** © Photodisc; **page 539** © Photodisc; **page 541** © Pixtal/age fotostock; **page 544** © Jason Stitt/ShutterStock, Inc.

Study Guide

Page 599 © Photos.com

Unless otherwise indicated, all photographs and illustrations are under copyright of Jones and Bartlett Publishers, LLC, or have been provided by the author(s).